Clinical Psychiatry
for Medical Students

Clinical Psychiatry for Medical Students

Third Edition

Edited by

Alan Stoudemire, M.D.

Professor of Psychiatry
Department of Psychiatry and Behavioral Sciences
Emory University School of Medicine
Atlanta, Georgia

52 Contributors

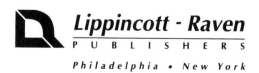

Lippincott - Raven
P U B L I S H E R S
Philadelphia • New York

Acquisitions Editor: Richard Winters
Developmental Editor: Erin O'Connor
Manufacturing Manager: Dennis Teston
Production Manager: Robert Pancotti
Production Editor: Loretta Cummings
Cover Designer: Karen Quigley
Indexer: Katherine Pitcoff
Compositor: Circle Graphics
Printer: R. R. Donnelley

Printed in the United States of America

9 8 7 6 5 4 3 2 1

Library of Congress Cataloging-in-Publication Data
Clinical psychiatry for medical students / edited by Alan Stoudemire.
　　— 3rd ed.
　　　　p.　　cm.
　　Companion v. to: Human behavior / edited by Alan Stoudemire. 3rd
ed. c1998.
　　Includes bibliographical references and index.
　　ISBN 0-397-58460-1
　　1. Psychiatry.　I. Stoudemire, Alan.　II. Human behavior.
　　[DNLM:　1. Mental Disorders.　2. Psychophysiologic Disorders.　WM
140 C641 1998]
　　RC454.C539　1998
　　616.89—dc21
　　DNLM/DLC
　　for Library of Congress　　　　　　　　　　　　　　　　　98-12186
　　　　　　　　　　　　　　　　　　　　　　　　　　　　　　CIP

Care has been taken to confirm the accuracy of the information presented and to
describe generally accepted practices. However, the authors, editor, and publisher
are not responsible for errors or omissions or for any consequences from application of the information in this book and make no warranty, express or implied, with
respect to the contents of the publication.
　　The authors, editor, and publisher have exerted every effort to ensure that drug
selection and dosage set forth in this text are in accordance with current recommendations and practice at the time of publication. However, in view of ongoing
research, changes in government regulations, and the constant flow of information
relating to drug therapy and drug reactions, the reader is urged to check the package insert for each drug for any change in indications and dosage and for added
warnings and precautions. This is particularly important when the recommended
agent is a new or infrequently employed drug.
　　Some drugs and medical devices presented in this publication have Food and
Drug Administration (FDA) clearance for limited use in restricted research settings. It is the responsibility of the health care provider to ascertain the FDA status
of each drug or device planned for use in their clinical practice.

Dedicated to the memory of Boyce Blake and to his family

Contents

Contributing Authors

David B. Abrams, Ph.D.

Professor
Department of Psychiatry and Human Behavior
Brown University School of Medicine
97 Waterman Street
Providence, Rhode Island 02912

David Bienenfeld, M.D.

Professor and Vice Chair
Department of Psychiatry
Wright State University School of Medicine
P.O. Box 927
Dayton, Ohio 45401

Robert J. Boland, M.D.

Assistant Professor
Department of Psychiatry and Human Behavior
Brown University School of Medicine
97 Waterman Street
Providence, Rhode Island 02912

Thomas M. Brown, M.D.

Associate Clinical Faculty
Department of Psychiatry and Neurology
Tulane University School of Medicine
900 Powell's Point
Gautier, Mississippi 39553

Jerry L. Carter, M.D.

Assistant Professor of Psychiatry and Internal Medicine
Medical College of Pennsylvania and
Allegheny University of the Health Sciences
320 East North Avenue
Pittsburgh, Pennsylvania 15212

Dennis S. Charney, M.D.

Deputy Chair of Academic and Scientific Affairs
Department of Psychiatry
Yale University School of Medicine
P.O. Box 208055
333 Cedar Street
New Haven, Connecticut 06520

Matthew M. Clark, Ph.D.

Assistant Professor
Department of Psychiatry and Human Behavior
Brown University School of Medicine
97 Waterman Street
Providence, Rhode Island 02912

Alberto Diaz, Jr., M.C., U.S.N.

RADM, Fleet Surgeon
CINCPAC FLT
250 Makalapa Drive
Attn: N01M
Pearl Harbor, Hawaii 96860

Arden D. Dingle, M.D.

Assistant Professor
Department of Psychiatry and Behavioral Sciences
Emory University School of Medicine
1440 Clifton Road, Northeast
Atlanta, Georgia 30322

Karl Doghramji, M.D.

Associate Professor of Psychiatry
Department of Psychiatry and Human Behavior
Jefferson Medical College
1025 Walnut Street
Philadelphia, Pennsylvania 19107

William R. Dubin, M.D.

AmeriChoice Behavioral Health
100 Penn Square East
Philadelphia, Pennsylvania 19107

Mina K. Dulcan, M.D.

Professor of Psychiatry and Behavioral Sciences
Northwestern University Medical School
303 East Chicago Avenue
Chicago, Illinois 60611

Peter J. Fagan, Ph.D.

Associate Professor
Department of Psychiatry
Johns Hopkins University School of Medicine
720 Rutland Avenue
Baltimore, Maryland 21205

Eugene W. Farber, Ph.D.

Assistant Professor
Department of Psychiatry and Behavioral Sciences
Emory University School of Medicine
1440 Clifton Road, Northeast
Atlanta, Georgia 30322

David G. Folks, M.D.

Professor and Chair
Department of Psychiatry
University of Nebraska College of Medicine
600 South 42nd Street
Omaha, Nebraska 68198

Charles V. Ford, M.D.

Professor of Psychiatry
University of Alabama School of Medicine, Birmingham
1813 Sixth Avenue, South
Birmingham, Alabama 35294

George K. Ganaway, M.D.

Clinical Assistant Professor of Psychiatry
Emory University School of Medicine
1440 Clifton Road, Northeast
Atlanta, Georgia 30322

Richard J. Goldberg, M.D.

Professor
Department of Psychiatry and Human Behavior
Brown University School of Medicine
97 Waterman Street
Providence, Rhode Island 02912

Michael G. Goldstein, M.D.

Associate Professor of Psychiatry and Human Behavior
Brown University School of Medicine
97 Waterman Street
Providence, Rhode Island 02912

Gregg E. Gorton, M.D.

Assistant Professor
Department of Psychiatry and Human Behavior
Jefferson Medical College
1201 Chestnut Street
Philadelphia, Pennsylvania 19107

Barrie J. Guise, Ph.D.

Clinical Psychologist
Lenox Hill Hospital
100 East 77th Street
New York, New York 10021

Carl A. Houck, M.D.

Associate Professor
Department of Psychiatry
University of Alabama School of Medicine, Birmingham
1813 6th Avenue, South
Birmingham, Alabama 35294

Gerald Hurowitz, M.D.

Assistant Professor
Department of Psychiatry
Columbia College of Physicians and Surgeons
630 West 168th Street
New York, New York 10032

Mark E. James, M.D.

Clinical Assistant Professor of Psychiatry and Behavioral Sciences
Emory University School of Medicine
1440 Clifton Road, Northeast
Atlanta, Georgia 30322

Nadine J. Kaslow, Ph.D.

Associate Professor of Psychiatry
Emory University School of Medicine
1440 Clifton Road, Northeast
Atlanta, Georgia 30322

Roger G. Kathol, M.D.

Professor of Internal Medicine and Psychiatry
University of Iowa College of Medicine
200 Medicine Administration Building
Iowa City, Iowa 52242

John H. Krystal, M.D.

Associate Professor of Psychiatry
Yale University School of Medicine
P.O. Box 208055
333 Cedar Street
New Haven, Connecticut 06520

James L. Levenson, M.D.

Professor of Psychiatry, Medicine, and Surgery and
Vice Chair of the Department of Psychiatry
Virginia Commonwealth University
Medical College of Virginia
Campus Box 980268
Richmond, Virginia 23298

Steven T. Levy, M.D.

Bernard C. Holland Professor of Psychiatry and
Vice Chair of Academic Affairs
Department of Psychiatry
Emory University School of Medicine
1440 Clifton Road, Northeast
Atlanta, Georgia 30322

Richard R. J. Lewine, Ph.D.

Professor
Department of Psychiatry and Behavioral Sciences
Emory University School of Medicine
1440 Clifton Road, Northeast
Atlanta, Georgia 30322

Rosalind M. Mance, M.D.

Associate Professor
Department of Psychiatry and Behavioral Sciences
Emory University School of Medicine
1440 Clifton Road, Northeast
Atlanta, Georgia 30322

Constance J. McKee, M.D.

Clinical Assistant Professor
Department of Psychiatry and Behavioral Sciences
Emory University School of Medicine
1440 Clifton Road, Northeast
Atlanta, Georgia 30322

Michael G. Moran, M.D.

Associate Professor
Department of Psychiatry
University of Colorado School of Medicine
4200 East Ninth Avenue
Denver, Colorado 80262

William D. Murphy, Ph.D.

Professor of Clinical Psychology
Department of Psychiatry
University of Tennessee College of Medicine, Memphis
800 Madison Avenue
Memphis, Tennessee 38163

Linda M. Nagy, M.D.

Department of Psychiatry
Dartmouth Medical School
Hanover, New Hampshire 03755

Philip T. Ninan, M.D.

Associate Professor of Psychiatry
Emory University School of Medicine
1440 Clifton Road, Northeast
Atlanta, Georgia 30322

Julie A. Rand, M.D.

Assistant Clinical Professor of Psychiatry
Emory University School of Medicine
1440 Clifton Road, Northeast
Atlanta, Georgia 30322

Mickey R. Riggs, M.D.

Staff Psychiatrist
Veterans Affairs Medical Center
950 Campbell Avenue
West Haven, Connecticut 06516

Emile D. Risby, M.D.

Associate Professor
Department of Psychiatry and Behavioral Sciences
Emory University School of Medicine
1440 Clifton Road, Northeast
Atlanta, Georgia 30322

Laurie Ruggiero, Ph.D.

Associate Professor
Department of Psychology
University of Rhode Island
2 Chafee Road
Kingston, Rhode Island 02881

Chester W. Schmidt, Jr., M.D.

Professor of Psychiatry
Johns Hopkins University School of Medicine
4940 Eastern Avenue
Baltimore, Maryland 21224

Elizabeth D. Schwarz, M.D.

Department of Psychiatry
University of Tennessee College of Medicine, Memphis
800 Madison Avenue
Memphis, Tennessee 38163

Edward K. Silberman, M.D.

Clinical Professor
Department of Psychiatry and Human Behavior
Jefferson Medical College
1025 Walnut Street
Philadelphia, Pennsylvania 19107

Jonathan M. Silver, M.D.

Associate Professor
Department of Psychiatry
Columbia University College of Physicians and Surgeons
630 West 168th Street
New York, New York 10032

Alan Stoudemire, M.D.

Professor of Psychiatry
Department of Psychiatry and Behavioral Sciences
Emory University School of Medicine
2302 Dellwood Drive, Northwest
Atlanta, Georgia 30305

Robert M. Swift, M.D., Ph.D.

Associate Professor
Department of Psychiatry and Human Behavior
Brown University
Veterans Administration Medical Center
830 Chalkstone Avenue
Providence, Rhode Island 02908

Robert J. Ursano, M.D.

Professor of Psychiatry and Neuroscience and
Chair of Department of Psychiatry
Uniformed Services University of the Health Sciences
4301 Jones Bridge Road
Bethesda, Maryland 20814

Scott VanSant, M.D.

Assistant Clinical Professor
Department of Psychiatry and Behavioral Sciences
Emory University School of Medicine
1440 Clifton Road, Northeast
Atlanta, Georgia 30322

Joel Yager, M.D.

Professor and Vice Chair for Education
Department of Psychiatry
University of New Mexico School of Medicine
2400 Tucker, Northeast
Albuquerque, New Mexico 87131

William R. Yates, M.D.

Professor and Chair
Department of Psychiatry
University of Oklahoma College of Medicine, Tulsa
2808 South Sheridan Road
Tulsa, Oklahoma 74129

Stuart C. Yudofsky, M.D.

D.C. and Irene Ellwood Professor and Chair
Department of Psychiatry and Behavioral Sciences
Baylor College of Medicine
One Baylor Plaza
Houston, Texas 77030

Foreword

We marvel at the clinical, technological, and research advances which have the potential to significantly impact the delivery of health care in America, and we imagine that there may be no limits to scientific progress. However, no technology, no discovery, no pharmacological intervention has transported us beyond the reality that at the essence of health care remains the relationship between a doctor and a patient, and this is most fundamentally true in understanding the emotional and psychological needs of every patient.

Despite our efforts to reduce the stigma of mental illness and emotional problems, millions of Americans are still very fearful about the difficulties that affect their mental, emotional, and social well-being. Patients and their families are afraid to identify these problems, in many instances frightened about what others will think, and often need the help of a physician to understand the nature of their illness and validate the need for help. While we may not be able to overcome this fear and stigma overnight, it is the relationship between doctor and patient which offers an opportunity to be fully responsive to each patient's needs.

The high prevalence of mental and emotional disturbances in the community creates a responsibility for doctors to be sensitive to and cognizant of the mental and emotional needs of their patients and also to develop the readiness to refer them to appropriate specialists when necessary. This requires the study and understanding of human behavior and psychiatry as part of medical education as well as familiarity with mental disorders that are prevalent in medical settings, such as anxiety disorders, depression, alcoholism, and substance abuse. More than just education, this requires a willingness to clearly hear the mental and emotional concerns of a patient and to make accurate psychiatric diagnoses. The model presented in this text underscores the importance of a carefully cultivated doctor-patient relationship and points to the possibilities for improved quality of care when this framework is conscientiously and consistently applied.

Mrs. Rosalynn Carter

Foreword

There are many reasons why physicians should be knowledgeable about clinical psychiatry. First, individuals who are experiencing emotional distress usually seek help initially not from mental health professionals but from their primary care physicians. Since psychological distress is often accompanied by stress-related symptoms such as headaches, tinnitus, indigestion, loss of appetite, fatigue, and insomnia, it is often the task of the physician to ascertain when such physical complaints actually represent "masked" psychiatric illness. Conservative estimates have established that approximately 20–25% of office visits to primary care physicians are primarily for psychiatrically-related reasons.

It is well-known, however, that primary care physicians, as well as other medical and surgical subspecialists, frequently overlook or minimize the psychiatric problems of their patients. Misdiagnosis of psychiatric illness can lead to prolonged and unnecessary suffering, disability, and excessive health care expenditures. Early recognition and prompt treatment of psychiatric conditions that initially present in the general medical setting would result not only in better medical and psychological care for patients but would also result in the elimination of misdirected medical expenses in the form of unnecessary laboratory testing and surgical procedures.

The first task for medical students in gaining the knowledge and skills necessary to care for the psychiatric and emotional needs of their patients is to develop the ability to properly recognize psychiatric illness in the medical setting. A major goal of this text is to assist future physicians in that task. In this spirit, special emphasis has also been placed on practical treatment strategies suitable for the medical setting as well as the indications for psychiatric referral.

While this text emphasizes practical aspects of diagnosis and treatment, recent research that has yielded many exciting discoveries in detecting the neurochemical basis of the major psychiatric disorders is also discussed. State-of-the-art scientific information is provided on advances in areas such as genetics, neuroimaging, psychopharmacology, and other neurobiological aspects of psychiatric disorders. The text, however, strives toward an integrated biopsychosocial model in understanding the etiology of psychiatric disorders and considers biological, psychological, and social factors in the development of treatment strategies.

Dr. Stoudemire has organized a superb third volume of this text and is very well qualified to do so based on his experience as both an educator and clinician. He served as Director of Medical Student Education in Psychiatry at Emory University School of Medicine for a number of years and developed first hand knowledge of medical students' interests and needs regarding clinical psychiatry. Dr. Stoudemire also founded and served as Director of the Medical–Psychiatry Unit at Emory University Hospital, a nationally recognized program designed to treat patients with combined medical and psychiatric illness. These experiences have enabled him to interact on a daily basis with physicians in many other specialties and, thereby, to see what they most want and need to learn about psychiatry to be better able to care for their patients. From these experiences, Dr. Stoudemire distilled the framework of this textbook, which specifically focuses on the basic clinical psychiatric knowledge and skills needed by medical students for their future careers regardless of their clinical specialty.

Dr. Stoudemire then assembled a group of chapter authors from across the country who meet two criteria. First, they are skilled psychiatric educators with a great deal of personal experience teaching medical students. Second, they have up-to-date scientific knowledge of their topic and have refined their ideas on their topic by teaching and receiving feedback from medical students. The result is a rare combination of new and exciting psychiatric knowledge that is clearly, concisely, and practically discussed at the level of medical students in their clinical years. This also makes this text a superb overview for first or second year psychiatry residents and residents in primary care disciplines. A number of psychiatrists preparing for the written and oral specialty Board examinations also have told me this text served as a well-organized and -edited, crisply reasoned, and up-to-date review of major psychiatric topics.

I hope the physicians who care for me and my family and friends in future years are well-grounded in the basic biopsychosocial and psychiatric knowledge, skills, and physicianly attitudes embodied in this excellent text.

Troy L. Thompson II, M.D.
The Daniel Lieberman Professor
Department of Psychiatry and Human
* Behavior*
Jefferson Medical College and Hospital
Philadelphia, Pennsylvania

Preface

It is the fundamental premise of this text that psychiatric illness must be understood, evaluated, and treated in a multidimensional manner. Hence, biological, psychological, and sociological factors are all considered to be potentially important in evaluating and treating psychiatric illness. While it will be noted in the introductory chapter on assessment that the amount of attention given to any particular area will vary depending on the clinical situation, the complexity of psychiatric illness requires that a comprehensive assessment of the patient be performed to facilitate accurate diagnosis and effective treatment.

Recent developments in descriptive and biological psychiatry have provided physicians with more exact methods of diagnosis as well as psychopharmacologic treatments that are often dramatically effective. Some psychiatrists, while acknowledging the importance of recent developments in the classification of psychiatric disorders and biologic treatments, have been concerned that the importance of understanding developmental and experiential aspects of the patient's life and the role of psychotherapy in treatment are being neglected in the process. A fundamental premise that has guided the development of this text is that multiple perspectives (biological, psychological, sociological) must be simultaneously integrated in research and clinical practice to fully understand and effectively treat psychiatric disorders. While controversy still reigns as to which *forms* of treatment are most effective for certain disorders and to what the relative contribution of psychological and biological factors is in determining disease vulnerability, clinicians should always strive to understand patients and their illnesses in the context of their developmental life experiences and their current interpersonal relationships. Those who still argue the "nature vs. nurture" issue are fundamentally missing the point: Elements of both almost always influence vulnerability to emotional illness and need to be considered in treatment.

A new generation of psychiatrists is gradually emerging who will be able to fully integrate both the perspectives of developmental psychology and biological understanding of the etiology and treatment of psychiatric disorders. It is this integrated psychobiologic paradigm in research and clinical practice that forms the future for psychiatry. While the complete scientific integration of psychoanalytic, behavioral, sociological and biological theories is not yet possible, the inability to do so is primarily the result of our insufficient understanding of the etiology of psychiatric illness.

As will be noted in the first chapter, this text will advocate a structured approach to psychiatric diagnosis within the matrix of the biopsychosocial model. In addition, as will be discussed in Chapter 2, the importance of understanding the patient's developmental life experiences and quality of their interpersonal relationships is considered to be of crucial importance in personality formation, vulnerability or resistance to stress, as well as susceptibility and adaptability to both medical and psychiatric illness. Comprehensive patient care must be based on assessing and treating each patient from the biological, psychological, and social perspectives.

This text is unique in that it deals with the major clinical psychopathological syndromes from this perspective as well as specifically addressing, in the second half of the text, the practical management of the common psychiatric disorders encountered in medical and surgical practice. These latter chapters are all written by clinicians who have extensive experience in working with physicians in medical settings, so readers should find them both precise and practical. In addition, Chapter 16 addresses the major childhood psychiatric disorders that are likely to be encountered in family and pediatric practice and emphasizes their diagnosis and treatment.

Finally, it should be noted that this text provides only an overview and covers the essential aspects of clinical psychiatry that are most pertinent for medical students. Each chapter is followed by an annotated bibliography of recommended references that students are referred to for more extensive reading, and a general reading list if provided. It should also be noted that this text is best used when it is preceded by reading the companion volume to this series, *Human Behavior: An Introduction for Medical Students*, which covers the fundamental principles of human behavior in health and illness using the biopsychosocial model and a psychobiological perspective.

It is hoped that in using and studying this text students will gain some appreciation the exciting developments that have evolved in psychiatry and will be able to use this knowledge in providing excellent integrated medical and psychiatric care to their patients.

Alan Stoudemire, M.D.

The Calling of a Physician

The thought that I had been granted such a specially happy youth was ever in my mind; I felt it even as something oppressive, and ever more clearly there presented itself to me the question whether this happiness was a thing that I might accept as a matter of course. Here, then, was the second great experience of my life, viz., this question about the right to happiness. As an experience it joined itself to that other one which had accompanied me from my childhood up; I mean my deep sympathy with the pain which prevails in the world around us. These two experiences slowly melted into one another, and thence came definiteness to my interpretation of life as a whole, and a decision as to the future of my own life in particular.

It became steadily clearer to me that I had not the inward right to take as a matter of course my happy youth, my good health, and my power of work. Out of the depths of my feeling of happiness there grew up gradually within me an understanding of the saying of Jesus that we must not treat our lives as being for ourselves alone. Whoever is spared personal pain must feel himself called to help in diminishing the pain of others. We must all carry our share of the misery which lies upon the world. Darkly and confusedly this thought worked in me, and sometimes it left me, so that I breathed freely and fancied once more that I was to become completely the lord of my own life. But the little cloud had risen above the horizon. I could, indeed, sometimes look away and lose sight of it, but it was growing nevertheless; slowly but unceasingly it grew, and at last it hid the whole sky!

"The Right to Happiness" from *Memoirs of Childhood and Youth* by Dr. Albert Schweitzer, translated by C. T. Campion. Used with permission of The Macmillan Company, publishers.

Acknowledgments

The contributors to this textbook are all dedicated clinicians and researchers who represent the very best in academic psychiatry. It has been a pleasure and a privilege to work with them over the years. Their dedication to patient care and medical education will be evident in the quality of the chapters contained herein.

This text could not have been completed without the tireless dedication, loyalty, and effort of my administrative assistant, Ms. Lynda Matthews. Her contribution to this book is greatly appreciated.

Thanks is extended to Dr. Jim Andrews, Clinical Assistant Professor of Psychiatry at Emory University School of Medicine, for his careful and thoughtful review of this text.

Thanks are also extended to the students and faculty of Emory University School of Medicine, as well as to those of other medical schools. Their suggestions regarding the first two editions of this text have, I hope, resulted in a more complete and refined third edition.

Special appreciation is extended to Dr. Steve Rosenberg and his dedicated staff at the National Cancer Institute, National Institutes of Health, who represent the highest ideals of medical science and practice.

Shannon and Dan Amos of Columbus, Georgia provided support, enthusiastic encouragement, and faith in my work that was essential to bringing this third edition to a reality.

Finally, special thanks to Mrs. Rosalynn Carter, Mr. Sam Donaldson, and Senator Max Cleland for their help and advice during difficult times.

Recommended Reference Textbooks

Diagnostic and Statistical Manual of Mental Disorders, 4th ed. Washington, DC. American Psychiatric Association, 1994

> This is the "bible" of descriptive psychiatry. It contains epidemiological and descriptive data of the major psychiatric disorders.

Hales RE, Yudofsky S, Talbott J (eds): Textbook of Psychiatry, 2nd ed. Washington, DC, American Psychiatric Press, 1994

> This is an excellent textbook of clinical psychiatry that is eminently readable and practical. The chapters will provide a more expanded discussion of the psychopathological syndromes contained in this text.

Kaplan HI, Sadock BJ (eds): Comprehensive Textbook of Psychiatry, 6th ed, Vols 1 and 2. Baltimore, Williams & Wilkins, 1994

> This is an encyclopedic textbook that covers all areas of psychiatry. Detailed and comprehensive, it should be primarily used as a reference source.

Michels R (ed): Psychiatry, Vols I–III. Philadelphia, Lippincott–Raven Publishers, 1996

> This is an excellent, up-to-date, comprehensive textbook of clinical psychiatry. Published in three volumes, the chapters are lucid, well edited, and are kept fresh by a subscription process that periodically updates the material.

Stoudemire A, Fogel BS (eds): Psychiatric Care of the Medical Patient. New York, Oxford University Press, 1993

> This comprehensive textbook is a detailed reference on the psychiatric disorders as encountered in medically ill patients. It contains detailed information regarding diagnosis, psychotherapy, and psychopharmacologic modifications that are required in treating psychiatric disorders in the medically ill.

Clinical Psychiatry
for Medical Students

1 Psychiatric Assessment, DSM-IV, and Differential Diagnosis

William R. Yates,
Roger G. Kathol, and
Jerry L. Carter

During the past 25 years, advances in psychiatric research have led to a better understanding of mental and emotional disorders. This improved knowledge has modified the approach to evaluating and treating patients with psychiatric conditions. This chapter focuses on how to perform a basic and practical evaluation of psychiatric problems. It provides a method of psychiatric evaluation, useful in both the psychiatric and medical setting, that increases the likelihood that the most effective treatment will be given.

The *biopsychosocial* approach currently is advocated as the best paradigm of psychiatric assessment (Fink, 1988). Using a model of assessment based on general systems theory, this approach suggests that equal emphasis be given to the evaluation of the psychological, social, and biological factors impacting on the patient's clinical presentation. In the clinical setting, however, the importance of each of these areas of assessment varies at any given moment in time, depending on the emotional or behavioral difficulty with which the patient presents. For example, in a patient experiencing marital problems and when neither spouse has interfering medical difficulties, the psychological assessment (the patient's view of his or her role in the relationship, the patient's expectations of the marriage, the patient's ultimate life goals) and the social assessment (the relationship with the spouse, the causes of conflicts, family member influences, economic constraints) would receive greater attention than the biological assessment. Thus, therapeutic intervention directed toward the psychological and social realms would receive the most emphasis, unless a concurrent medical illness in one of the family members was a primary cause of the crisis. Alternatively, if a patient is delirious, biological factors (underlying medical differential diagnosis, likelihood of improvement, or complications with various interventions) become paramount.

As in all areas of medicine, students learn to balance their evaluations to best explore the complaints and needs of the patient. The astute clinician develops skills in each area of assessment and incorporates them as the clinical situation dictates.

In this introductory chapter, a biopsychosocial approach to patient assessment using a structured system of psychiatric diagnosis will be presented. In addition, the importance of understanding patients in light of both their present and past experiences will be emphasized. Students are referred to the companion volume, on human behavior, for background information and substantiated evidence for the biopsychosocial model of human disease and illness (Stoudemire, 1998). Chapter 2 of this text will discuss the practical aspects of the biopsychosocial model as it relates to psychodynamic and psychosocial assessment of patients.

VALUE OF A DIAGNOSIS

Although many psychiatrists spend a good deal of their time assisting *normal* patients in their adjustment to *normal* life experiences, the main reason for psychiatric evaluation is the identification of mental and emotional disorders. To do this effectively, clinicians must develop a basic understanding of what constitutes "abnormal" behavior.

During medical training, students and residents learn to differentiate the normal human condition from the abnormal. When is the liver enlarged? When is a cardiac murmur clinically significant? How high does the alkaline phosphatase level have to go before further diagnostic testing is needed? Implicit in the answers to these questions is an understanding of what is "normal." In most medical disciplines, the distinction between normal and abnormal has been quantified. Laboratory tests list a "normal range," which indicates an acceptable deviation from the mean for a control population. Alternatively, the presence of certain findings indicates abnormality. Examples would include fungating skin lesions or rales in the chest, which are uniformly absent in normal individuals.

One of the most perplexing but seldom asked questions in psychiatry is, "What constitutes normal emotion and behavior?" Without an answer to this question, is it possible to define the "abnormal?" In a somewhat contrived study, Rosenhan (1979) reported that nonpsychiatrically ill "pseudopatients" who faked having heard the words "hollow," "thud," and "empty" for several days presented themselves for psychiatric evaluation. The pseudopatients were diagnosed as having schizophrenia, in remission, during 11 of 12 inpatient encounters at independent hospitals. One must question if so few symptoms, which cause no incapacity and resolve spontaneously and immediately after the initial evaluation, are sufficient to label a person schizophrenic, with its attendant personal, social, legal, and economic repercussions.

Although there are diverse opinions on what constitutes "normalcy," most consider it to be defined by behavior that falls within a commonly recognized "standard" within a given culture. Aberrant behavior can be identified by this method, although the reliability of such an approach, especially in mild conditions, is limited by the cultural diversity of the United States (ethnic—white, black, Asian; religious—Hari Krishna, Jehovah's Witness, fundamentalist; organizational—Ku Klux Klan, motorcycle gangs) and by the cultural background, personal biases, and norms of the person performing the examination. Essentially, what is deemed "normal" ends up being that which is not too different from the accepted cultural and behavioral norms of the evaluator!

Mere recognition of those with "abnormal" behavior is insufficient for diagnosing a psychiatric disorder. That would be equivalent to calling a jockey who races horses and a person who plays center on a basketball team medically ill because they fall at the extremes of the bell-shaped curve for height. However, doctors often consider those who do not conform to their concept of appropriate behavior psychologically unstable.

Despite the difficulty in specifying abnormal emotions and behavior, there are clearly individuals who are *functionally impaired* as a result of emotion, thought, or behavior. Few would argue that a delirious or profoundly depressed patient represents a variant of normal behavior. *It is, in fact, impairment of function that distinguishes "eccentric behavior" from psychiatric illness.* As with all other medical disorders, psychiatric *disease* includes conditions associated with pain, disability, death, or an increased liability to these states (Robins and Guze, 1970).

A disease is more than just a *descriptor* of conditions causing human suffering. Perhaps more importantly, it is a *predictor.* Consistent and reliable identification of syndromes with specific symptoms and signs allows documentation of the condition's cause, the mode of transmission, family involvement, the age of onset, the natural course of the symptoms, and the treatments that might alter the ultimate outcome. One of the primary objectives of the rapidly changing editions of the *Diagnostic and Statistical Manual of Mental Disorders-IV* (DSM-IV; American Psychiatric Association, 1994) is categorization of incapacitating aberrant behavior (see Appendix to this chapter). Reliable identification using this "cookbook" approach can improve our ability to study these predictive factors. This nomenclature system has been a major advance in psychiatric diagnosis during the past 25 years.

The following case study will be presented and then used throughout the chapter as a teaching example of the correct way to perform a medical/neurological assessment (which includes the mental status examination) in a patient with psychiatric symptoms and as an example of use of the DSM-IV classification scheme. Readers should study it carefully because reference to this case will be made throughout the first part of this chapter. Reasons for the therapeutic intervention will be provided at the conclusion of the chapter.

A CASE STUDY

Patient Identification
Admitted to the emergency room, RH is a 57-year-old alcoholic man who is drowsy and somewhat combative after being brought from a boarding house by the police.

Chief Complaint
"Bugs crawling on my skin, and the mob is after me."

History of Present Illness
The patient was marginally responsive and was unable to say why he was brought to the hospital. He had been drinking his usual fifth of whiskey until 2 days before admission when "the mob stole" his social security check, and he had no money for liquor. Since then he had "holed up" in his room and "nearly starved to death." He refused to give more history for fear that it might have "repercussions."

After the patient gave reluctant permission, the family was contacted. They stated that the patient had been drinking since the age of 13 and had been hospitalized on numerous occasions for alcohol-related problems. Volumes of hospital charts on the patient confirmed this information. He had binged since age 16 and had been drunk nearly every day, except when in treatment, since his mid-30s. His first blackout occurred at age 22, "the shakes" had predictably come on with abstinence of greater than 18 hours for many years, and he had had several episodes of "the DTs." There was no history of withdrawal seizures, however. Short periods of enforced sobriety occurred when the patient was hospitalized for hemorrhaging gastric ulcers. Numerous alcohol rehabilitation programs failed to change his drinking habits.

The family kept track of the patient because "he was a good man when he wasn't drinking," but they didn't want him home because he was abusive during periods of inebriation and was arrested frequently for public intoxication. He had not had a job for many years and had a strong family history for alcoholism. When he was feeling remorseful about his effect on his family, he became despondent and talked of killing himself, but he had never attempted suicide. His suicidal tendencies did not occur during periods of abstinence.

Medical and Psychiatric History
The patient had a 120-pack-a-year smoking history and had been treated for hypertension unsuccessfully, due to noncompliance. He had been given benzodiazepines in an apparent attempt to help

curb his drinking, but he denied nervousness or panic attacks in the absence of alcohol intoxication or during withdrawal. He had numerous alcohol-related injuries and sequelae. His history did not include abuse of controlled substances or over-the-counter medication. He was prone to fighting while under the influence but had no difficulty with the law when sober.

Developmental/Social History

The patient was the only son in a family of four. There were no known problems with gestation, delivery, or reaching developmental milestones. His childhood was disturbed by frequent fights between his parents, mainly over his father's drinking. He was raised largely by his mother, who was nurturing and attentive to his needs until he was in high school, when he began getting into trouble with authorities. He was suspended and eventually expelled for drinking on school premises, when he had "run-ins" with his teachers. While in school he had a close group of friends, was reasonably successful in organized sports, and participated in extracurricular activities. After holding numerous small jobs, he spent 3 years in military service and received a general discharge. He was married at age 23, when he was working as a laborer in a steel mill, and had two daughters. After 14 years of marriage, the patient's wife divorced him because "it was apparent that nothing was going to change." Since then, the patient had lived in numerous places on social security and provided little in the way of child support.

Family History

The patient's father, paternal uncle, and paternal and maternal grandfathers were alcoholics. One paternal aunt saw doctors nearly all the time for health problems. Deaths in the family were mainly due to liver and heart problems. There were no other known family illnesses.

Review of Systems

Could not be obtained from the patient.

Physical Examination

The patient was disheveled and cachectic and had poor hygiene. Blood pressure was 160/94 mm Hg. Pulse was 98 and regular. Respirations were 20 and unlabored. Temperature was 36.2°C. The skin revealed profuse sweating, several ecchymoses, palmar erythema, and numerous spider angiomata, but no jaundice. There was a recent bruise on the patient's forehead. Poor compliance prevented observation of the patient's fundi. The heart examination revealed no murmurs or rubs, and there were diffuse pulmonary rhonchi. The liver was enlarged and tender. No ascites could be *demonstrated. Stool was brown and positive for occult blood. Cranial nerves were "grossly intact," and the patient could move all extremities. There was no strabismus. The patient was tremulous and responsive to pinching in all extremities. Deep tendon reflexes were 1+ and symmetrical, and the plantar response was downgoing bilaterally. Gait was unsteady, and the patient refused to tandem walk.*

Mental Status Examination

The mental status examination revealed the patient to be drowsy, uncooperative, and intermittently agitated. His speech was slurred and coherent, but his responses to questions were appropriate only occasionally. He remained silent and lying flat with eyes closed when not pressed to respond, but lashed out when shaken. His mood was angry and distrustful. Affect was exaggerated but appropriate to the stimulus. He denied thoughts of harming himself or others but stated that he sure would protect himself if anyone "came at" him. The patient's statements were understandable but laced with concerns about being imprisoned and tortured (by the mob). He had difficulty maintaining a coherent train of thought. Complaints of the floor crawling with snakes or other repulsive animals and feeling bugs under his skin were frequent. The patient could not maintain attention long enough for full assessment of cognitive function with the Mini-Mental State Examination.

Screening Laboratory

The patient's sodium, magnesium, and calcium levels were low, and his liver enzymes and amylase levels were elevated. B_{12} was normal, but folate was low. There was a macrocytic anemia and thrombocytopenia; however, bleeding parameters were normal. Blood alcohol level was 2 mg/dl (intoxicated 50 to 100 mg/dl). Urine screen for other drug abuse was negative. Chest X-ray and electrocardiogram were normal.

Hospital Course

The patient initially required large doses of chlordiazepoxide for alcohol withdrawal. This was tapered during the first 9 days of his hospital stay with gradual resolution of the changes in mental state. Sodium, magnesium, and calcium levels returned to normal with replacement and adequate nutrition. Thiamine and multivitamins were given. When the patient became less paranoid and confused, he scored 29/30 on the Mini-Mental State Examination. Elevated amylase levels spontaneously returned toward normal, and blood in the stool disappeared after treatment of alcoholic gastritis documented by endoscopy.

The patient expressed remorse for his drinking behavior and promised to attend Alcoholics Anonymous (AA) meetings when released from the hospital. Contact was made with AA during his hospitalization. He demonstrated no evidence of depression when his withdrawal symptoms had resolved. After 3.5 weeks of treatment, he was preparing for discharge when he had a grand mal seizure. Electroencephalogram demonstrated diffuse slowing with increased prominence on the right. Computed tomography of the head revealed a large right frontoparietal subdural hematoma. The hematoma was surgically evacuated, and the patient was discharged to his boarding house 6 weeks later with the intent to initiate alcohol outpatient treatment. An AA sponsor was contacted to ensure the patient's participation in outpatient treatment.

HISTORY, PHYSICAL EXAMINATION, AND LABORATORY ASSESSMENT IN THE PSYCHIATRIC EVALUATION

Psychiatric evaluations can be conveniently divided into those that take place in the *psychiatric* setting (inpatient psychiatric hospital, outpatient psychiatry clinic, psychiatry consultation service, or other situations in which the patient expects to see a psychiatrist for possible psychiatric problems) and those that take place in the *medical* (nonpsychiatric) setting. In the first situation, patients are referred or are being treated specifically for psychiatric problems. In the second instance, the patient's principal problem is probably nonpsychiatric in nature, but psychiatric factors could be involved. Because misconceptions exist about what constitutes an appropriate psychiatric evaluation in these two situations, they will be addressed separately.

Psychiatric Evaluation in a Psychiatric Setting

The principal features of the psychiatric evaluation are the *psychiatric history* and the *mental status examination.* These establish the presence of a psychiatric syndrome. A medical history, physical examination, and laboratory assessment also are included in psychiatric evaluations, although little emphasis is placed on their role during medical training when patients are assumed to have "primarily psychiatric problems." *Because 30 to 50% of psychiatric inpatients and outpatients have medical disease concurrent with their psychiatric symptoms (LaBruzza, 1981), 5 to 30% of which either actually cause or exacerbate the psychiatric problem, it is inappropriate for psychiatrists or medical students to neglect the medical part of the evaluation in patients with psychiatric symptoms.*

It may not be reasonable to expect psychiatrists to complete a full medical history and a physical examination every time they see a patient, just as it is not logical for primary care physicians to perform complete psychiatric examinations on all the patients they see. In two studies, however, medical findings in 45% of psychiatric patients led to reconsideration of the psychiatric diagnosis, and in 6 to 9% they led to a *major* alteration in the approach to treatment (Hoffman, 1982; Chandler and Gerndt, 1988). *It is therefore essential to include the physical examination as an integral part of the psychiatric evaluation in all first-time inpatients and outpatients being appraised for a psychiatric disease.* This point is particularly true when the risk of a metabolic or neurologic component is high, such as in patients over 50 years old, in those with atypical psychiatric presentations or adverse (or no) responses to treatment for disorders in which improvement should be expected, or in patients with known or suspected underlying medical conditions that could contribute to their symptoms.

Psychiatric Evaluation in the Medical Setting

Medical students are usually taught psychiatric evaluation in *psychiatric* settings. In most medical centers, little or no instruction is given for initiating psychiatric questions in patients seen in primarily medical settings, even though 80% of patients with psychiatric conditions are seen by primary care physicians (Regier et al., 1978). Medical students frequently are indoctrinated with the idea that "nonpsychiatric patients shouldn't be asked embarrassing psychiatric questions." The end result of this advice is that, in their future practices, psychiatric problems in many if not most of their primary care patients are overlooked.

Psychiatrists have little difficulty asking patients referred for psychiatric evaluation personal and confidential questions. That, after all, is what psychiatrists are trained to do. Medical patients, however, come to see nonpsychiatric physicians for "physical" problems. To embark on a series of psychological questions usually is unexpected and may be viewed initially by the patient as an invasion of privacy unless the reasons for the questions are explained or the patient can be led to see a possible connection to the presenting complaint or general condition. The patient also may be both relieved and reassured that the physician is interested in him or her "as a person" and may use the opportunity to express worries and emotional and psychological distress.

Because psychiatric questions are not asked routinely in the medical setting, psychiatric illness frequently remains undetected, or, alternatively, a psychiatric illness may be diagnosed presumptively without just cause. The prevalence of mental illness, the availability of effective treatments for many psychiatric disorders, and the harm of inappropriate diagnosis make it imperative that all physicians develop the skills for initiating psychiatric evaluations. Nothing can replace specific psychiatric questions in documenting the presence or absence of a psychiatric disorder.

Psychiatric Interviewing

The psychiatric interview is an interaction between patient and physician designed to assess psychiatric status or to provide treatment of an emotional or behavioral problem. During the first interview, patients typically describe their perception of the difficulty. The physician clarifies the chief complaint and enhances the patient's history by observing the patient's behavior during the interaction (*infra vide*) and by listening to the patient's responses to open-ended questions. During this encounter, the physician should establish a rapport, if possible, by being honest and straightforward during the interview, by showing empathy for the patient's condition or situation, and by demonstrating his or her willingness and ability to improve the patient's problem.

Ideally, when the patient is coherent, the patient and physician arrive at a general understanding of the nature of the problem and agree on the form and duration of treatment. This approach clearly and unambiguously defines the limits of the relationship, the goals, and the expectations of each party. Such an approach is particularly important when working with patients with certain psychiatric disorders. For instance, patients with psychotic disorders or borderline/antisocial personality disorders often distort, misinterpret, or manipulate what is said; thus, initial clarification and guidelines are necessary.

Certain critical ingredients are important during the initial interview. First, *adequate time* should be set aside for the interview. This entails not only time to obtain the necessary information to make a diagnosis, but also time to initiate the interview on a personal note. Patients can then feel that you are seeing and treating them as individuals. Second, if possible, steps should be taken to ensure that there are no interruptions. Third, the patient should be put at ease. Such details as providing adequate space for patient movement, equal eye level of the examiner and patient, the presence or absence of other support personnel or the patient's acquaintances, and limiting noise can make significant differences in the patient's willingness to share pertinent information about problems. Fourth, note-taking should be limited, especially if it makes the patient feel uncomfortable. These simple, seemingly inconsequential details can affect not only the type of behavior demonstrated and information obtained during the initial interview, but also the course of treatment. Finally, if the situation permits, the physician should usually *sit down* when speaking to the patient and avoid standing over and shifting around him or her when standing at the bedside.

There are some who consider the psychiatric interview to be different and distinct from the interview performed in primary care. In fact, considerable importance is given to observing behavior and obtaining data related to psychiatric issues during the general medical history-taking process (Bates and Hoekelman, 1983). The primary care physician, however, is usually dealing with signs and symptoms of medical conditions in the absence of psychiatric involvement. Therefore, observations such as the color of the patient's skin, the rapidity of his or her breathing, and the coarseness of a tremor take on greater clinical importance. When complaints in the primary care setting point to a psychiatric problem, nonpsychiatric physicians, like psychiatrists, merely need to extend their observations to include mood, behavior, and thought processes. Additional questions to confirm or deny the presence of a psychiatric syndrome complete the history. There is no magic in this as long as the basics about psychiatric syndromes and symptoms are known.

A good deal of emphasis in psychiatry is placed on the interpretation of answers to questions or manifest behaviors. When a patient who obviously looks depressed because of poor eye contact, tearfulness, apparent fatigue, latency of response, or stooped posture says he or she does not feel sad (essentially denying being depressed), how should this be handled? It is best to take what the patient says at face value initially and try to make sense of it in relation to the remainder of the clinical picture before suggesting that the patient is unable to identify emotions, is unable to report accurately, is lying, or is massively denying. It is just as possible that the patient with the symptoms described above is suffering from anemia or cancer.

Psychiatric interviews are designed to be predominantly diagnostic or therapeutic, but elements of both often are contained in initial evaluations. Primarily diagnostic interviews detect and characterize psychiatric illness. Interviews arranged to follow the course of psychiatric illness or response to therapy might also be considered partly diagnostic because they provide a steady flow of information that allows for ongoing assessment of the patient's condition. Therapeutic interviews involve the use of psychotherapeutic techniques. These are primarily intended to provide treatment in the form of support, reassurance, and exploration of the patient's past history and current stresses to facilitate expression of painful feelings and to provide insight.

The form of psychotherapy employed may influence the nature of patient questioning beyond that required to make a DSM-IV diagnosis. For example, the cognitive therapist might pursue details regarding the manner in which one deals with current life problems, whereas the psychoanalyst or psychodynamically oriented psychiatrist might be interested in details regarding one's perceptions of, and emotional reactions to, historical life events. These forms of therapy and special interview techniques will be covered elsewhere in this text (see Chapter 17).

In addition to gathering historical data narrated by the patient, the physician derives diagnostic data by observing and assessing the patient's appearance, behavior, and various aspects of mental functioning during the interview process. Thus, in addition to assessing the *content* of the patient's history, the psychiatrist routinely looks beyond the narrative to assess the patient's mental apparatus that perceives, formulates, and elaborates the history and the behavior that emanates from it. This will provide objective data in a manner analogous to the physical examination of the internist. For example, patients with major depression frequently demonstrate poor eye contact, stooped posture, latency of response, and psychomotor retardation. When a patient presents with a history that corresponds to the clinical picture, an initial diagnosis can be made with more confidence.

The importance of documenting information from both the history (including history provided by the patient's family) and direct observation of the patient is essential because signs and symptoms during the interview may be limited. For instance, there are medical conditions that show no evidence of disease on physical examination (e.g., migraine headache), just as there are patients with certain psychiatric conditions who may demonstrate completely normal mental function and behavior during the examination (e.g., alcohol dependence, eating disorders, sexual disorders, and so forth). The reverse is also true for patients with dementia, who may have no idea that problems exist, although their behavior may demonstrate the opposite.

One means of acquiring more accurate information, as well as a better understanding of the mental and emotional state, is to perform the interview using open-ended, unstructured questions. Many medical and psychiatric interviews resemble interrogations, with rapid-fire questions that require yes or no answers and leave almost no chance for the patient to elaborate on his or her own perception of the problem, much less express painful emotions or experiences. Avoiding leading questions allows patients to provide an unbiased account of their perception of the problem. Contextually accurate information is obtained by following the patient's lead with questions directed at clarifying or enlarging on historical items. As the interview progresses, it may become increasingly structured and specific to fill in details and to complete the history, as detailed in following sections.

Many physicians are afraid of open-ended, unstructured questions because time constraints do not allow the luxury that questioning during numerous hour-long psychotherapy sessions provides. For this reason, psychiatric questions are often avoided altogether. Nonetheless, a limited amount of time devoted to this type of questioning is essential for a more accurate diagnostic impression, regardless of time constraints. The accomplished physician develops skill in providing a balance between the open-ended, person-to-person questions and the single-answer questions that are required to make a diagnosis. In this way, critical information from and about the patient can be obtained while controlling interviewing time and maintaining a more predictable schedule.

Factors Affecting the Interview

Patients present to psychiatrists in a variety of situations that greatly influence the form of the interview, the nature of patient–physician interaction, and the overall goals. These situations range from the highly functioning patient presenting for an outpatient evaluation of a moderate depression to the emergency evaluation of a hostile, psychotic patient taken to the emergency room in restraints by police officers, as in the case presented at the beginning of this chapter. In the first situation (moderate depression in an outpatient), one might obtain a meticulous psychiatric and medical history, physical and mental status examination, and screening laboratory evaluation. Such interviews facilitate therapeutic decision making. In the situation of an agitated, medically ill alcoholic, the evaluation initially would include documenting the presence of delirium, performing the physical examination, and admitting the patient for inpatient care. Only later, when information can be obtained from charts, relatives, and the patient, when he or she becomes better controlled, will a comprehensive, accurate understanding of the case become possible.

Other factors also may influence the ability to conduct a thorough psychiatric interview. For instance, some patients may be so fatigued from medical illness that they require a concise interview. Alternatively, some patients refuse to cooperate. Often, this can be a clue to their diagnosis, as in the case of a patient with borderline personality or paranoid disorder. In such cases, additional information from the patient's doctor, nursing personnel, or descriptions in the chart can provide valuable insight into the nature and cause of the patient's difficulties and perhaps lead to more effective management. Thus, the skilled interviewer must be flexible and ever mindful of not only the details of a patient's psychiatric condition, but also the interwoven social, legal, and medical factors that complicate psychiatric assessment and intervention.

Specific Interview Situations

Although each patient is unique, necessitating a flexible and individualized interview style, many psychiatric disorders influence aspects of the interview in a manner that is predictable and characteristic of that disorder. Thus, the following comments are not intended to offer a "cookbook" approach to these patients, but rather offer suggestions in the interpretation and planning of specific interview situations.

The Depressed Patient

A prominent feature of severe depression is the tendency for all perceptions to be colored by bleakness, pessimism, sadness, and hopelessness. When the history is taken, therefore, it is essential to keep in mind that many descriptions presented by the patient in a negative light by way of a depressed state may actually be more positive or at least neutral. For example, it is common for depressed patients to think that they are going bankrupt or doing terrible things for which they feel guilty to family and friends. Information from other sources may reveal that the situation is not nearly so dismal.

Depressed patients often are in desperate need of hope and reassurance. They may repeatedly ask whether they are bad persons or if they can be helped. Nonetheless, when reassurance is provided, it may be received with quiet skepticism and generally results in only temporary relief.

Depressed persons often have their own ways of accounting for suffering. For example, they may be convinced that they are being justly punished by

God for transgressions. Such beliefs may become delusional in psychotic depressions, such as when patients think they have committed the "unforgivable" sin; think they, or the world, no longer exists (nihilistic); or think they are riddled with cancer (somatic). Explaining that such ideas are the result of depression and will go away with treatment offers momentary hope, but the patient is unlikely to alter such opinions until improvement occurs.

The Psychotic Patient

The term *psychosis* includes a broad range of clinical presentations unified by loss of contact with reality and the presence of delusions or hallucinations. Such presentations range from the patient who appears to function normally (with the exception of a well-circumscribed paranoid delusional system) to the acutely disorganized, agitated, vividly hallucinating patient. The severity of the patient's thought disorder and degree of departure from reality will determine the structure of the interview. The former patient may be able to provide a history that is complete and reliable, with the exception of issues relating to the delusional system. When the patient discusses these beliefs, details should be sought regarding the nature and extent of the delusions and how the patient makes sense of them. These details, as well as the degree of conviction in the delusional beliefs, can be followed to assess the course of and response to treatment. When delusions are persecutory in nature, the patient may be reluctant or unwilling to provide information or even consent to be interviewed for fear that the interviewer is an agent of the persecutory process. Such was the situation in the case presented earlier.

When a patient is floridly psychotic, the interview may involve little more than observing the patient as findings are noted. Interacting with such patients often provides stimulation that may make evidence of psychosis more apparent. In addition to grossly distorting reality, acutely psychotic patients are often very frightened. Both of these factors can result in unpredictable and, rarely, even violent behavior. Although such patients should be treated with kindness and understanding, necessary precautions must be taken. *Florid psychosis should not deter the physician from performing the physical examination or laboratory assessment, although special care and techniques may be required. These are essential to rule out a neurologic, metabolic, or toxic cause for the psychosis* (see also Chapters 4, 5, and 19).

The Hostile Patient

When assessing a hostile patient, interviewers must take whatever precautions are necessary to ensure their safety. The initial step is identification of the potentially violent patient. Clues include a previous history of violent behavior, such as that often seen in patients with antisocial personality disorder, alcoholism, and substance abuse; a paranoid psychosis; and a person who is angry and threatening violence, even in the absence of a psychiatric disorder.

One sensitive indicator of whether the situation is becoming dangerous is your emotional response to the patient's behavior, that is, your "gut level" reaction. If the interviewer feels uncomfortable or fearful of the patient, precautions should be taken *immediately* to ensure safety. If concern is minimal, precaution may involve nothing more than sitting between the patient and an open door or making sure other personnel are nearby. When the index of concern is higher, one or several security officers—without guns—may be stationed in the interview area or be used to restrain the patient if needed during the interview. Such precautions are often a relief to confused, psychotic, or agitated patients because they provide the situation with structure and absolve patients of the necessity of making decisions at a time when they may not be in control of their actions. Chapter 19 on emergency psychiatry also discusses special considerations in interviewing violent and hostile patients.

The Somatic Patient

Many psychiatric disorders manifest somatic symptoms in which a medical disorder is not readily found. These include conversion disorder, hypochondriasis, somatization disorder, and nonspecific complaints associated with anxiety or depression. Such complaints, however, may just as likely be the result of medical disease too early in onset to diagnose, due to insensitivity of the physical examination and laboratory tests; a medical problem more benign than the evaluation needed to diagnose it; or merely the patient's attempt to receive attention. Care must be taken, therefore, in diagnosing somatoform disorders (see Chapter 9).

A convenient way to categorize patients with unexplained somatic complaints is to determine whether the complaints are *single or multiple.* If the somatic complaint is single, the evaluation should proceed until a physical cause has been reasonably excluded *and* a psychiatric cause is deemed possible. This evaluation may entail no more than a careful history with a brief physical examination; occasionally, it requires more extensive testing.

If the complaints are multiple and somatization disorder is a possibility, then symptoms must be *seriously listened to,* but only objective evidence of disease on basic evaluation should lead to further workup. At the first evaluation, time should be taken to obtain a directed history about the main complaint and each complaint with a potentially dangerous cause. A complete physical examination and basic laboratory evaluation (if not already done) are required. Records from prior physicians and hospitals are particularly helpful and should be obtained before further workup unless eminent problems are evident. Any objective finding on the physical examination or laboratory evaluation should prompt further investigation or treatment after the nature and extent of previous evaluations have been delineated. It also should be noted that some patients have a very limited "psychological vocabulary," and when in emotional distress, communicate their feelings predominantly in physical or somatic terms. This trait has been called *somatothymic* and is a very common form of "emotional language" in many cultures worldwide and in certain types of patients in the United States (Stoudemire, 1991a & b). This concept is discussed further in Chapter 9.

In patients with multiple somatic complaints, the physician should place particular emphasis on the terms of agreement regarding specific responsibilities of physician and patient. The physician should agree to evaluate symptoms when deemed appropriate and to follow the patient at regular intervals to assess change. The patient should allow the physician adequate time to complete the evaluation and should seek no other medical evaluations unless consent is first obtained from the physician. This approach will not guarantee ease in caring for such patients, but may result in the development of rapport and trust, which are essential if the patient's suffering is to be eased and the pursuit of evaluations slowed. The diagnosis and management of patients with chronic somatic complaints are further discussed in Chapter 9.

The Psychiatric History

Many psychiatric patients make the process of obtaining an accurate history a challenge for a variety of reasons. First, they may have illnesses, such as dementia or delirium, that prevent them from revealing details related to the onset and type of symptoms that brought them to the physician's attention. Second, they may wish to hide salient facts related to their difficulties because of embarrassment, mistrust, or outright deception. Third, they may present with symptoms that follow a variable pattern or are difficult to describe. It is for these reasons that *obtaining additional information from a second or, preferably, a third and fourth source, such as family members, friends, or police,* as well as scrutinizing available information in the patient's records, is *critical* to ensure that the correct diagnosis is made and appropriate treatment is given. Table 1–1 outlines the main sections of the psychiatric history. Important factors related to each part of the psychiatric history are enumerated below.

Identifying Information

Chief Complaint
Often the patient's chief complaint differs from the examining physician's perception of the problem. In this situation, the primary problem that the patient perceives should be addressed first while the "real" problem waits. In this way, the patient is indirectly told that his or her complaint is important, thus creating an alliance in trying to clarify and relieve both the perceived and the "real" problem.

History of Present Illness
As with any medical evaluation, clarification of the chief psychiatric complaint lies at the heart of the psychiatric history. Pertinent information includes an accurate description of the difficulty, the mode of onset

Table 1–1 **The Psychiatric History**

Identifying Information
    Sociodemographic Summary
Chief Complaint
History of Present Illness
    Extended information About Chief Complaint
    Onset
    Duration/Course
    Precipitants
    Exaggerating and Alleviating Factors
Psychiatric Review of Systems
    Psychological Symptom Inventory
    Review of Major DSM-IV Psychiatric Diagnostic Symptoms
Medical History
Personal/Family History of Psychiatric Disorders and Treatment
Personal History
    Prenatal/Birth History
    Childhood
    Adolescence
    Adulthood
        Educational
        Occupational
        Interpersonal/Social
        Sexual (Table 1–2)
        Habits—Alcohol, other Drugs

and duration, the course of the symptoms (steady, intermittent, progres-sively worse), exacerbating and alleviating factors (medication, position, time of day), and factors such as recent deaths or illnesses in the family, marital or family relationship problems, financial or legal problems, med-ical illness, problems at work, or intractable social problems with which the patient feels unable to cope, possibly associated with the onset and con-tinuation of the symptoms. These details relevant to the chief complaint are supplemented with pertinent features from the past medical and psychiatric history, past personal history, family history, sexual history, and review of sys-tems. The objective in obtaining this information is to typify the difficulty that the patient is experiencing, to establish whether it warrants psychiatric diagno-sis, and to consider ways in which the problem might be alleviated, whether or not a psychiatric disease is present.

Information obtained in this data-gathering section of the interview is coupled with observations made during the interaction with the patient that con-stitutes part of the mental status examination. It is important that the patient's history and clinical presentation be consistent with the psychiatric condition under consideration; otherwise, alternative explanations should be explored. As might be recalled in the study by Rosenhan alluded to earlier, which used "fake" patients presenting with artificial complaints of hearing the words "hollow," "thud," and "empty" (auditory hallucinations?), there was neither a syndrome picture (early age of onset, chronic deteriorating clinical course, and so forth) nor other past or present clinical signs (thought disorder, blunted affect, ambivalence, anhedonia) that suggested schizophrenia as a primary diagnostic entity.

Review of Systems

One of the principal ways in which unexplained somatic complaints are identified is through a review of the symptoms the patient has experienced. The review of systems also serves as a means of reviewing potential medical causes for the principal complaint of the patient. Frequently, it will uncover a problem that has a direct and pertinent relation to the chief complaint. Each positive finding on the review of systems should be understood well enough to know whether further investigation is needed. Such investigation may include anything from a spot physical examination to an invasive X-ray procedure.

In medical settings, most patients with psychiatric problems initially present with *physical* symptoms (such as in depression). Physical symptoms of anxiety and depression may be mixed with symptoms of concurrent underlying medical illness as well, thus further complicating the clinical assessment. For example, somatic symptoms associated with depression include sleep fragmentation (usually early morning awakening with an inability to get back to sleep), headaches, constipation, physical fatigue, decreased appetite, weight loss, and gastrointestinal distress.

Psychophysiological symptoms of anxiety include palpitations, tachycardia, diaphoresis, hyperventilation, diarrhea, urinary urgency and frequency, restlessness, chronic fatigue, insomnia, dry mouth, blurred vision, nausea, vomiting, chest pain, dizziness, choking, difficulty swallowing, headaches, muscle aches, and pain. Patients with schizophrenia occasionally will have bizarre physical sensations, such as their brain dissolving or body parts feeling disconnected. Patients with somatoform disorders such as hypochondriasis are preoccupied with physical complaints to an excessive, unrealistic degree. Hence, while somatic complaints are nonspecific, they often constitute a predominant component of the signs and symptoms of psychiatric disorders. Care must be taken, however, since it is all too easy to ascribe a physical complaint to a psychiatric condition when, in fact, it is caused by an underlying medical illness.

Medical History

Any medical history pertinent to the chief complaint is included in the history of the present illness. Such information usually becomes evident during the careful questioning used in delineating the chief complaint. Thus, current medical illnesses, which might be contributing to the symptoms and medications, and familial medical illnesses that are known to be associated with the development of psychiatric symptoms would be enumerated in the history of present illness and their possible association with the current psychiatric condition suggested.

In addition to the review of pertinent physical factors in the history of present illness, other seemingly less relevant medical or surgical difficulties, allergies, and medications also should be recorded. Even though they may not be helpful in understanding the patient's reason for seeking psychiatric assistance, they frequently become important when assessing the need for additional information concerning the patient's case when deciding on the type of treatment to be given. For instance, in the case of RH, if it had been known that he had a bleeding disorder, then the bruise on his head might have precipitated a more extensive neurologic investigation before the development of the seizure.

Personal and Family History of Psychiatric Disorders and Treatment

As with the past medical history, pertinent past psychiatric history related to the chief complaint should be included in the history of present illness. *The longitudinal course of psychiatric symptoms and responses to treatment is one of the most important ingredients in making a psychiatric diagnosis.* It is known, for instance, that alcoholism often begins in the teenage years to the 20s, has a fluctuating but progressive course unless the individual maintains prolonged abstinence, and often leads to chronic disability. Had patient RH had a good premorbid history and only started drinking weeks to months before his admission, then the primary diagnosis of alcoholism with alcohol withdrawal delirium (delirium tremens) would have become suspect. Alternative explanations for the drinking behavior and delirium would have been required.

Other factors related to the psychiatric history should be reported under a separate heading. Even though no apparent relation to the current presentation can be shown, they sometimes can provide additional insight into the patient's problem and may alter the course of treatment or investigation. Past suicide attempts should be carefully documented.

Specific questions that delineate the past psychiatric history include the following: First, patients can be asked, using colloquial terms, if they have ever had difficulties with nerves or emotions or whether or not they have ever had a "nervous breakdown." Often, patients will not remember or do not think they should reply in the affirmative unless they were hospitalized for the problem. Therefore, patients should be asked whether they have been given medication by a primary physician for "nerves" or emotional problems or whether they have seen a counselor, pastor, psychologist, social worker, or physician for counseling.

Second, patients should be asked if there has ever been a time when they felt they needed help but did not get it. Hence, the history should involve both untreated and formally treated bouts of psychiatric illness. If the patient did get treatment, where did they get it and for how long were they treated? Were they ever hospitalized for a psychiatric problem? If they did get treatment, including medications, what drugs were given and what was their response? Were there any side effects that caused problems?

Third, and perhaps most important, the same questions should be asked of someone who knows the patient well enough to confirm or deny the patient's answers.

A family history of psychiatric illness is crucial because certain psychiatric disorders have a genetic component (schizophrenia, mood disorders, alcoholism, Alzheimer's disease; Baron, 1994). In fact, a strong family history of affective disorder can be used to reinforce a diagnostic impression in a patient with an otherwise confusing presentation. It is important to ask about the nature of symptoms, type of treatment (medication or electroconvulsive treatment), response to treatment, complications, and hospitalizations for involved family members. A family history of suicide and violence also should be elicited.

Personal History

The personal history includes information about the patient's relationships, schooling, employment, personal achievements and failings, and goals. As might be expected, each of these areas can impact in a major way on the course and duration of psychiatric symptoms.

A person's prenatal history and development through the various stages of infancy, childhood, and adolescence are the principal areas of interest in the personal development section of the examination. Items such as birth trauma, developmental physical and emotional milestones, illnesses, parental and sibling relationships, important memories, rewards and punishments, exposure to abuse, and the establishment of independence are addressed. Major milestones, frustrations, and problems in childhood and adolescence should be identified, when appropriate, along with the quality of family and peer relationships during each phase of development.

One frequently *unasked* question is whether or not sexual molestation occurred as a child. Patients should be asked about sexual molestation in a frank and straightforward manner, although some tact may be required. For example, one might ask, "Were you ever sexually molested or attacked as a child by anyone, including members of your family?" Most patients harbor severe shame and guilt about incest in particular, requiring special sensitivity to this issue in the session.

When pursuing a psychodynamic understanding of the patient's problems, a chronological picture of the patient's developmental history, including their adult history, should be reconstructed, and events or experiences that may have been psychologically or emotionally traumatic should be noted. Past life experiences that appear to correlate with current life events or stresses should be noted by the examiner and explored with the patient.

Social History

This part of the psychiatric history recounts the patient's educational background and functioning in the school system; encounters with the law; lawsuits or criminal connections; premarital, marital, postmarital, and extramarital relationships; relationships and problems with children; employment (types, frequency of change, reasons for job changes, compensation issues) and fiscal responsibility; military history (assignment and nature of discharge, history of combat experience); and personal goals and expectations. Criminal charges, arrests, convictions, or time served in prison should be carefully addressed, as should the circumstances leading up to the encounter with the law. During the process of gathering this information, the physician can identify areas in the patient's life that might serve as precipitating stresses or recurrent patterns of problematic social relationships. *All social factors of importance to the presenting complaint should be included in the history of present illness, while the remainder are recorded under the personal or social history section of the examination.*

When considering those areas of the social history that may be stresses involved in precipitating the patient's presenting complaint, it should be remembered that life is literally a "series of crises." It is always possible to point to a flat tire, fight with a relative or friend, failed test, or unpaid bill as a potential stressor for the development of symptoms. A means of placing social factors in proper perspective is to establish whether current stressors in relation to other stressors the patient has previously experienced are of sufficient magnitude to influence the patient's ability to cope.

Interpersonal Relationships. Of major importance in the patient's social history is the nature, pattern, and stability of his or her interpersonal relationships, whether they relate to romantic involvements, friendships, occupational relationships, or relationships with authorities. For example, is the patient capable of forming stable relationships based on trust? Is the patient capable of forming close friendships? What is the pattern of the patient's romantic and sexual involvements? How successful have they been in working with peers, within teams, and for those in authority? Problematic patterns in interpersonal and social relationships often indicate the presence of a personality disorder. One of the cardinal symptoms of a personality disorder is the tendency of the individual to "repeat mistakes" in their interpersonal and social relationships, to fail to learn from experience, and to assign fault to others rather than to accept responsibility for their life difficulties.

The Sexual History. There are occasional situations in which the sexual history is of significant importance in understanding the patient's problem. Certainly, basic questions concerning sexual function, such as whether the patient is sexually active, what the sexual preference is, and whether there is concern about a venereal disease, should always be asked because most persons cannot be expected to volunteer such information. When the problem involves potential difficulty within relationships, sexual deviancy, or other problems that may influence sexual function, then more detailed information may be necessary. Because this area of questioning is highly personal, the physician may encounter more resistance than in other areas of the examination. As the doctor–patient relationship becomes better established, however, patients will often become more willing to talk about such matters. Details of a comprehensive sexual history are listed in Table 1–2 and also are discussed in Chapter 14. Physicians should focus on various parts of the history as the clinical situation dictates.

The basic sexual history is best customized to the individual patient. Reducing the level of anxiety surrounding discussion of sexual issues is particularly important for adolescents. Female adolescents may be more comfortable discussing sexual interests with female health professionals. For adolescents, issues of first sexual experiences become more important. Since sexual behavior can be affected by alcohol and drugs, the relationship between substance use and sexual behavior should be explored. Sexual histories in adolescents may need to be obtained over several interviews to allow for the development of trust and confidence in the relationship with the physician. Among geriatric

Table 1–2 Basic Sexual History (Modified to Age of Patient and Clinical Circumstances)

Introductory comments about why the interview is being conducted and its routine or special nature given the clinical situation at hand; reassurance about confidentiality
Open-ended question to give the patient an opportunity to voice any areas of special worry or concern regarding the part of the interview or sexual concerns in general
Source of information about sex in growing up
Attitudes of the parents toward sex
Age of onset of puberty
Age of menarche and menstrual history in women
Age of first intense romantic or sexually oriented relationship
History of childhood molestation or incest
History of venereal diseases
Attitudes about masturbation and frequency of masturbation
Age of first intercourse; number of partners
General pattern of attraction to person of the opposite or same sex; general patterns of heterosexuality or homosexuality
Abortions, miscarriages, pregnancies
Method(s) of birth control
Frequency of current sexual activity and its nature
Physical discomfort with sexual activity:
  Men: Problem with arousal or achieving/maintaining erection, ejaculation control
  Women: Problems with arousal, lubrication, achieving orgasm, physical comfort with intercourse
Conflicts in relationship or marriage over sexual matters: frequency, methods of birth control, sexual dysfunction
Medications or illness that seem to negatively affect sexual desire or functioning
Issues regarding decision to avoid or achieve conception and have children
Risk factors for AIDS or other concerns regarding this disease

(From Becker JV, Johnson BR, Hunter JA: Human sexual development and physiology. In Stoudemire A (ed): Human Behavior: An Introduction for Medical Students. 3rd Ed. Philadelphia, Lippincott–Raven Publishers, 1998)

patients, the decline of sexual functioning can be a significant stress and a source of worry and concern. Potential reversible medical factors that impair sexual functioning should be reviewed. The physician should understand how changes in sexual functioning affect the geriatric patients' self-esteem and relationship with their partners.

Alcohol and Substance Dependency/Abuse. Obtaining a substance-abuse history should be of paramount importance in the history, given the prevalence of alcoholism and drug abuse in our society. Use of alcohol, cocaine, marijuana, stimulants, sedative-hypnotics, analgesic opiates, and sleeping pills should be rigorously investigated, including age at first use, frequency of use, amount, and complications in the interpersonal, occupational, medical, and legal spheres that may have resulted. A history of the results of intoxication, withdrawal, and "bad trips" should be explored. The use of caffeine (coffee, tea, soft drinks, chocolate) almost always is overlooked by examiners, even though caffeine may be addicting and is associated with a withdrawal syndrome. The use of tobacco products, perhaps the most lethal substance abused in our society, should also be documented. Pertinent aspects of the substance use history are also discussed in Chapter 10.

Assimilation of the Psychiatric History

When a psychiatric syndrome is suggested by the information gathered during the psychiatric history, only the beginning of the diagnostic process has been completed. Depressive symptoms, anxiety symptoms, psychosis, and symptoms from most other psychiatric syndromes can, after all, be caused by a spectrum of psychiatric and medical diseases and can even be seen in some normal individuals. For instance, some clinicians automatically think that patients who meet criteria for major depression develop their symptoms in response to a primary psychiatric illness. Medical conditions such as hypothyroidism and cancer are frequently responsible for the production or exacerbation of depression or symptoms that mimic depression. Even patients with other psychiatric conditions, such as somatization disorder or alcoholism, can have a depressive symptom complicating their primary psychiatric condition. It is for these reasons that the psychiatric history should not be limited to the identification of symptom complexes themselves, but should incorporate pertinent medical, personal, and social information to complete the assessment. This additional information can have a substantial impact on the approach taken in the patient's treatment.

Preparing Medical Patients
for Psychiatric Evaluation

How can a physician lead into psychiatric screening questions without antagonizing or threatening the patient? First, it cannot be avoided in every case. Regardless of how tactful you are, some may be offended at first. Table 1–3 outlines a way to decrease the likelihood of offending medical patients. This approach will often "break the ice" and allow the patients to describe areas in their lives that have been troubling, but that they find difficult to discuss. Occasionally these questions will lead to the most dreaded reactions of all: "What! Do you think I'm putting this on?" or "Do you think this is all in my head?" or "Do you think I'm crazy?" In response to this, the patient might be told, "Emotional factors and stress can influence physical symptoms (some people get headaches, some ulcers from stress). The medical problem is real, but can be triggered by stress. I routinely ask these and other questions of all my patients so that I can give the best and most appropriate treatment and don't miss anything important." Thereafter, additional psychiatric screening questions (Table 1–4) can be asked if circumstances warrant. If screening questions are positive, a more detailed psychiatric history can be obtained.

When Is It Appropriate to Ask Medical Patients Psychiatric Questions?

In many patients, psychiatric illness with or without concurrent medical illness is readily apparent. Presence of a persistent and pervasive depressed mood, frank psychosis, or an agitated confusional state are clear indications to pursue further psychiatric evaluation. Unfortunately, psychiatric illness often is not so apparent. The following indicators are helpful in detecting patients with psychiatric disorders presenting in a subtle or ambiguous manner: (1) nonresponse to treatment in situations in which it is usually effective, particularly when litigation is pending; (2) multiple somatic complaints not accounted for by known medical conditions or symptoms not conforming to the bounds of anatomy or physiology; (3) a chaotic lifestyle (e.g., unstable relationships, frequent job changes, substance abuse, frequent legal problems, and so forth); (4) a history of "hopping" from one physician to another (doctor shopping); (5) symptoms related to stress, anxiety, or depression; (6) a personal or family history of psychiatric illness; (7) a degree of disability or resultant lifestyle changes out of proportion to symptoms; and (8) suspected or known alcohol

---

Table 1–3 **Initiating Psychiatric Questions in Patients with Nonpsychiatric Complaints**

Discuss and define the nonpsychiatric problem with the patient first (it may be related to the emotional problem).

If there is some question about whether the nonpsychiatric complaint is "real," do not challenge the patient with this possibility. You don't have to state that you feel the complaint is or isn't real, but you can acknowledge the patient's perception of its presence.

Ask, "Do you think your symptom(s) is (are) affected by nerves or emotions?" "Do you think that your symptom(s) is (are) related to stress?"

Table 1–4 **Psychiatric Screening Questions for Patients in the Primary Care Setting**

Depression

"Have you been feeling sad or depressed? Is this accompanied by trouble with sleep or appetite, low energy, or decreased interest in doing things? Do you have feelings of guilt or thoughts of harming yourself?"

Mania

"Do you feel on top of the world? Is this out of proportion to your usual self such that you talk more, don't need as much sleep, your thoughts race, or your enthusiasm gets you into trouble?"

Psychosis

"Have you heard or seen things that others didn't? Do you feel that you have special powers?

Have you felt that others were watching or following you? Have you received peculiar or special messages or felt that others knew or controlled your thoughts?"

Alcoholism

"Have others thought you had a drinking problem? Has drinking alcohol caused problems with friends or relatives, caused you to miss work or lose a job, resulted in arrest, or caused health problems? Do you use recreational drugs?"

Anxiety Disorder

"Have you had trouble with nervousness, anxiety, or feeling like you are going to panic?"

Anorexia Nervosa

"Do you take special measures to keep your weight at its current level?"

and substance abuse. Although none of these indicators is pathognomonic, they suggest the possibility of psychiatric illness.

Perhaps of equal importance are factors indicating that psychiatric illness should be viewed with a relatively *lower* index of suspicion than other possible causes of the patient's symptoms. This determination is particularly important because inappropriately labeling a patient's symptoms as "psychiatric" can lead to delay in identifying the correct primary diagnosis. Items in this category include (1) any *objective* finding on physical examination or laboratory evaluation that appears directly related to the symptom; (2) previous emotional *stability,* as reflected by work responsibilities, family relationships, and personal endeavors, in a person with questionable "psychiatric" symptoms; (3) an unusual psychiatric presentation of the characteristics of the possible psychiatric syndrome under consideration; and (4) the lack of any acute or chronic stressors in the patient's life. It is in these patients that there is a high risk of labeling the symptoms "psychiatric" when there actually is an underlying medical disease. This brings us to the importance of the physical assessment as part of the evaluation process.

Physical Examination

The physical examination currently is included in 0 to 11% of outpatient psychiatric evaluations and in 4 to 40% of inpatient evaluations (Krummel and Kathol, 1987). Ideally, all psychiatric patients should receive a physical examination. Unfortunately, many psychiatrists, like other medical specialists, logically focus their examination on areas related to their specialty. Few "primary" psychiatric diagnoses can be confirmed by positive findings on the physical examination; thus, it is often bypassed altogether.

Of what importance, then, is the physical examination in the evaluation of psychiatric patients? Unlike many subspecialties in medicine, psychiatry deals with clinical presentations that frequently have as their origin a primary medical disorder that causes the patient's symptoms. The list for major depression alone includes diseases from most organ systems (Hall et al, 1980). To exclude an underlying medical disorder as a cause of the patient's symptoms, a systematic evaluation that traditionally has included a physical examination is required.

The next obvious question is whether clinical tradition is correct in requiring the performance of a physical examination as a part of the assessment because most medical diagnoses are made from historical information alone. Hampton et al (1975) answered this question when they found that the physical examination confirmed, denied, or narrowed the differential diagnosis arrived at from historical information in 30% of patients in a primary medical setting. In 7.5%, it uncovered unexpected yet important findings that led to the diagnosis of a disease that was not necessarily related to the chief complaint. Considering that Chandler and Gerndt (1988) showed similar findings in 224 consecutively examined psychiatric inpatients, the need for a physical examination to confirm or deny medical factors is evident. It is for these reasons that psychiatrists should include a physical examination in psychiatric patients at risk of medical illness co-morbidity. This would include (1) any new patient with a psychiatric disorder, (2) patients older than 50 years of age, (3) patients with an unusual psychiatric presentation or response to treatment, (4) patients with medical conditions known to cause or exacerbate psychiatric symptoms, and (5) patients with significant complaints from the review of systems.

There are some clinicians who think that adding a neurological examination to the psychiatric interview is sufficient to exclude most underlying medical causes of psychiatric symptoms. Although there are certainly a number of neurologic conditions that can cause behavioral or emotional problems (Taylor et al, 1987), medical illness frequently mimics psychiatric disorders (Chandler and Gerndt, 1988). For this reason, it is important to perform a complete physical examination. Hall et al (1980) showed that a cursory physical examination was unreliable in identifying physical changes when they were present; thus, a complete physical is required. When findings are identified, they should be explained and treated along with the psychiatric manifestations accompanying them.

The scope of this chapter does not allow individual treatment of the different sections of the physical examination. These can be reviewed in Bates' (1995) *A Guide to Physical Examination and History Taking.* A word can be said, however, about the difficulties encountered in performing the physical examination in the psychiatric setting. This portion of the psychiatric evaluation is often neglected, only partially because it is not patently pertinent to the presenting complaint. Other factors also are involved. These include (1) worry about missing abnormalities due to lack of experience, (2) no examination facilities, (3) no assistant (or chaperone) for the examination, (4) no reimbursement for the "extra effort," (5) concern that the examination might influence the therapeutic relationship, and (6) dislike for doing physical examinations.

The student should know that, with a little effort in setting up an office or hospital practice, examination facilities and support personnel can be made available. This will permit more frequent physical examinations and thus reduce concern about the quality of the examination. Payment schedules often can be set up to provide fair reimbursement for time used in adding this essential aspect to the remainder of the psychiatric assessment.

Koranyi (1980) showed that physical examination did not adversely affect the therapeutic relationship in over 2,000 psychiatric outpatient evaluations although it was not clear if breast and genital examinations were completed on all patients, or if there was any effect caused by the gender of the examiner and the gender of the patient. Those who claim transference and countertransference problems due to the physical examination may be creating imaginary dragons because the psychoanalytic/psychodynamic process involves working through these and other psychological conflicts. More likely, those who suggest this reason for avoiding the physical examination are merely rationalizing their dislike of or lack of skill in doing them. In many outpatient settings, however, it may be more realistic for the psychiatrist to insist that a physical examination be performed by a family physician or internist as part of the overall evaluation before formal psychiatric treatment proceeds. In any case, breast and genital exmainations by a psychiatrist should receive special consideration and, if performed, should always be chaperoned.

Laboratory Assessment

Laboratory assessment, like the physical examination, should be performed in patients at risk of medical co-morbidity (*supra vide*). Screening tests included in an initial evaluation are a complete blood count, electrolytes, blood chemistry screen, and urinalysis. Medication blood levels and urine screen for drug abuse should be included when indicated. In patients over 50 years old, an electrocardiogram and chest X-ray may be added. Depressed and anxious patients should have a thyroid-stimulating hormone level drawn, even in the absence of clinical symptoms or signs.

Although there is a great deal of interest in the measurement of other hormones and neurotransmitters in patients with psychiatric disorders, none of these have been found to be useful in diagnostic or therapeutic decision making. Even the dexamethasone suspension test, once widely investigated in patients with mood disorders, has some potential value only in predicting who is likely to relapse when it remains positive after successful treatment.

The basic evaluation listed above provides a screen for metabolic or neurologic factors that might be contributing to the psychiatric presentation. This evaluation does not replace the need to perform specific laboratory tests when the clinical history dictates. For instance, a chronic schizophrenic patient from a state hospital who presents with a documented 2-month history of weight loss and low-grade fevers even in the absence of "basic" laboratory abnormalities requires further workup to explain the presenting complaints. Just such a case was diagnosed as having tuberculous meningitis on a recent admission to our institution.

Although all diagnostic testing procedures, regardless of complexity and invasiveness, should be considered when the clinical assessment dictates, computed tomography (CT) of the head, magnetic resonance imaging (MRI) of the head, and electroencephalography (EEG) deserve special attention because they are frequently considered in the evaluation of patients presenting with psychiatric symptomatology. Head CT is a specialized, noninvasive X-ray technique that allows visualization of the anatomy of the head in slices of various thickness. MRI, using an entirely different imaging technique, provides similar slices; however, it has an advantage in that radiation is not involved, the images are not interfered with by bony structures, the images can be obtained in multiple planes, and the differentiation between gray and white matter is better delineated. EEG is the measurement of electrical activity on the surface of the brain. (Use of these techniques in neuropsychiatric assessment also is discussed in Chapter 4.)

There is no simple formula to cover all the indications for these procedures. Simply stated, MRI is the most expensive, but the most sensitive, test to pick up anatomic pathology. Because the images obtained using this technique are not altered by bony structures and can be seen in multiple projections, posterior fossa and brain stem abnormalities are better seen with MRI. For these reasons, some authorities consider it the noninvasive test of choice. Some types of pathology can be seen on MRI that cannot be seen on CT. Examples would include strokes within the first 3 to 7 days of occurrence and multiple sclerosis lesions. Basically, all that can be seen on head CT can be seen on MRI, but the cost, accessibility, limits in interpretation, and problems with patient cooperation in lying still during a relatively lengthy period make it unlikely that it will replace head CT completely.

EEG complements MRI and CT, but does not replace them. EEG is not a tool that separates normal from abnormal anatomy; rather, it separates normal and abnormal electrical physiology. In some situations, the two can correspond, as is seen with some brain tumors. In others, the EEG may identify changes (epilepsy) while the imaging procedures remain normal or vice versa.

MRI, CT, and EEG all should be used to detect structural, metabolic, and seizure-related causes of psychiatric syndromes. One study found increased use of MRI, CT, and EEG studies in patients with a mental disorder compared with patients without a mental disorder (Olfson, 1992). Clinical clues about when the EEG, CT, and MRI are more likely to be abnormal are: (1) if there are focal neurological deficits; (2) if there has been a recent and marked change in mental status; (3) if there is a history of substance abuse/alcoholism, head trauma, or other central nervous system (CNS) pathology; (4) if the patient is elderly; and (5) if the patient presents in an atypical fashion and has a history that does not suggest psychiatric involvement. It should be remembered that medicine is based on probability. A certain number of normal tests are necessary to ensure that abnormal tests aren't missed.

The Mental Status Examination

The term *mental status examination* is somewhat misleading because it suggests a circumscribed period of assessment that takes its turn, as would auscultation of the heart or inspection of the fundi. To the contrary, the skilled interviewer gathers data regarding the multiple facets of mental functioning as they are observed and elicited during the psychiatric interview. For example, performing tests of recent memory imparts little information not already apparent in a patient who provides an accurate, detailed history. In fact, such exercises may convey a sense of rote mechanical detachment, rather than empathy and positive regard for the patient. Furthermore, some aspects of the mental status examination, such as judgment, can be better assessed by what brought the patient to your attention than by asking the patient artificial questions.

Not all areas of the mental status examination are adequately covered during the psychiatric interview. These must be addressed more directly with questions specifically formulated to assess mental function or emotional state. In developing a technique that is both thorough and personalized, it is essential to have a clear understanding of each of the mental status parameters.

A rational method of organizing the mental status examination is to follow the order in which findings are apparent during the interview. Appearance, level of consciousness, psychomotor activity, behavior, and general mood state are observed before and also throughout the interview. Speech, thought content and form, orientation, and memory are appraised throughout the interview. Insight and judgment are usually determined at the conclusion of the interview.

This overview of the basic aspects of the mental status examination is intended to provide a guide to the many areas of inquiry that should be evaluated and recorded in the process of patient assessment. Assignment of a formal psychiatric diagnosis requires complete integration of the patient's psychiatric and medical history and laboratory assessment with the findings on mental status examination. Knowledge of how certain signs and symptoms "fit" into certain categories in the current psychiatric nomenclature system determines the diagnosis.

The mental status examination is a systematic method to gather behavioral and psychological data with the understanding that such data is then processed, analyzed, and integrated to determine whether or not a diagnosis of a formal psychiatric disease should be made. The principal features can be found in Table 1–5. Even if the degree and severity of the patient's symptoms do not warrant formal DSM-IV diagnosis, one may nevertheless assess the possible relationship between the symptoms and current stresses to identify a point of therapeutic intervention.

Appearance, Attitude, and Behavior

Any clues regarding the patient's mental functioning and emotional state should be noted. A slovenly appearance, tattered and dirty clothes, pungent body odor, unkempt hair, and dirty hands are often seen in patients with undifferentiated schizophrenia, alcoholism, or dementia. Stooped posture, poor eye contact, tearing, and slow response to questions in a person with an otherwise normal appearance, on the other hand, are more likely to be seen in patients with depression. Other facets of a patient's appearance and behavior include the patient's apparent health (well developed, bedridden), nutritional state (well nourished, emaciated), posture (catatonic, vigilant), mannerisms (tics, hand-wringing), and actions (compulsions, apparent response to hallucina-

Table 1–5 **Basic Mental Status Examination Outline**

Appearance, attitude and behavior
   Description of appearance, hygiene
   Attitude toward examiner
   Psychomotor activity
Speech
Mood and affect
   Subjective and objective mood
   Affect variability and appropriateness
   Presence of anxiety
   Assessment of suicidality
Thought and language
   Production
   Form
   Content (obsessions/delusions)
Perceptions
   Hallucinations/illusions
   Depersonalization
   Derealization
Cognitive function
   Level of consciousness
   Orientation
   Concentration
   Memory
   Intelligence
Insight and judgment

tions, random acts). Behavioral and neurological signs and symptoms of intoxication or medication side effects should be noted here, as well.

Another aspect of observing behavior is noting the attitude toward the interviewer. For instance, patients who are unusually guarded and suspicious suggest paranoia. Patients who are flattering and ingratiating, but then demand special privileges or request disability compensation, suggest the manipulative behavior of antisocial, histrionic, or borderline personality disorders. Other descriptors of attitudes toward the interviewer include friendly, cooperative, hostile, threatening, seductive, challenging, and competitive. Each provides a clue to normal and abnormal function when coupled with other aspects of the patient's presentation.

Speech

Tone, rate, and volume of speech should be noted. Depressed patients may speak slowly and quietly with effort, whereas the speech of the manic patient is often rapid, pressured, and resists interruption. The speech of an anxious patient may be both rapid and frantically expressive. Intoxicated patients often speak with loud, slurred speech and are disinhibited in *what* they say.

Mood and Affect

Mood describes the *prevailing* subjective emotional state of the patient, whereas "affect" generally refers to how the patient's mood is expressed or exuded. The mood may be euthymic (normal mood state), happy, sad, euphoric, suicidal, guilty, bored, anxious, irritable, agitated, panicky, terrified, angry, enraged, or sensual. If affect (the way the patient outwardly expresses or exhibits mood state) varies appropriately with the content of the patient's thoughts (becomes bright and warm when discussing close relatives or sad when discussing the death of a friend), the patient is demonstrating a *full* and *appropriate* affect. When the patient is depressed or in a manic euphoria, the affect is characteristically *confined* to that particular range of mood. In some patients with depression or schizophrenia, the affect may be described as *blunted* or *flat* when it is static, regardless of the environmental stimuli. Patients with schizophrenia, and occasionally other conditions, may also demonstrate *inappropriate* affect by laughing or grinning while describing an unfortunate or tragic event. Other descriptors of affect are *superficial, shallow,* or *labile.*

Depressed mood is characterized by general hopelessness, passivity, lifelessness, dysphoria, demoralization, and pessimism. Patients often are irritable, labile, and querulous. Some patients may be profoundly agitated and anxious, whereas others may be quietly apathetic and vegetative. Crying spells may be frequent and uncontrollable. Anhedonia, the inability to experience pleasure and interest in life, is a cardinal symptom of depression. Physical symptoms also may be prominent in depression. In psychotic depression, paranoia and somatic delusions of parasitic infestation or venereal infection may be present. Other symptoms of depression include low self-esteem, feelings of inadequacy, helplessness, guilt, unlovability, worthlessness, excessive self-criticism, and suicidal thoughts. Many, if not most, patients will initially present with physical or somatic complaints as the primary manifestation of their depression (insomnia, headache, G.I. distress, fatigue, loss of appetite and weight, etc.). If the complaints are persistent and patients display little ability to verbalize their feelings, or are unable to make a connection between somatic complaints and their depression, they may be somatothymic, a condition discussed earlier in this chapter, in which patients use physical symptoms to express emotional distress.

In mania, the mood is inappropriately euphoric, giddy, silly, disinhibited, or extremely irritable. Grandiose ideas and schemes, as well as an inflated self-image, may be observed. Emotional expansiveness and excessive and intrusive gregariousness may be observed with the patient's manic mood.

Anxiety. Components of acute or chronic anxiety are often reported by way of the expression of psychophysiologic symptoms. Subjectively, patients may complain of being tense, nervous, fearful, frightened, anxious, worried, fretful, or unable to relax or sleep. Phobic symptoms may be present, such as circumscribed simple phobias (of snakes or spiders, for example), social phobia, or agoraphobia (fear of being alone or being in open or crowded spaces). Anxiety, as part of an obsessive–compulsive disorder, can lead to severe crippling anxiety usually centered on intrusive thoughts or fears. Patients with posttraumatic stress disorders are often chronically anxious and plagued by nightmares and startle responses and are hypervigilant. Symptoms of anxiety often are mixed with those of depression.

Assessment of suicide potential is a key feature of the psychiatric evaluation and mental status evaluation. The clinician should be able to answer three questions to estimate the suicide potential (Table 1–6). First, what is the current extent of the patient's thinking and behavior regarding suicide? Both thoughts and plans about suicide should be examined. Second, does the patient demonstrate historical and sociodemographic risk factors for completed suicide? The more risk factors present, the higher the risk of completed suicide. However, one should note that if no risk factors are present, this does not mean the risk of completed suicide is zero. Third, does the patient meet criteria for a psychiatric disorder that has been associated with completed suicide? The clinician develops an estimate of suicide risk based on the comprehensive evaluation of these three areas for an individual patient.

The patient also should be asked if he or she has had thoughts of hurting others, and if so, what the thoughts have been and how far the planning has progressed. Has he or she been violent before? Toward whom? What were the circumstances and consequences? Does he or she have weapons in his/her possession or access to them? Where are the weapons stored? Has she/he ever been arrested or incarcerated for violence? Were drugs or alcohol involved? Does he/she feel in control of their impulses at the current time?

Thought and Language

An impairment in the ability to translate thoughts into symbols or to use symbols in communication (*language disorder*) differs from a *thought disorder* in that the latter implies a compromised ability to organize, coherently associate, and effectively use information and ideas. Both problems are identi-

Table 1–6 **Assessment of Suicidality**

1. What is the extent of the patient's thinking and behavior related to suicide?
   Passive death wish versus a desire to kill self
   Hopelessness about situation and future
   Specific plan to commit suicide
   Means to commit suicide by the plan
   Lethality of suicide plan
   Arrangements made to accomodate completed suicide
   Suicide note
2. Does the patient have historical and sociodemographic risk factors for completed suicide?
   History of aggressive and violent behavior
   Family history of suicide
   History of prior suicide attempts
   Male gender
   White race
   Single, divorced, widowed, or recently separated
3. Does the patient have a severe psychiatric disorder associated with completed suicide?
   Major depressive disorder
   Schizophrenia
   Bipolar mood disorder
   Panic disorder
   Active alcohol or drug dependence
   Personality disorder with Axis I comorbidity

fied during the process of human interaction and usually require the production of speech. Examples of language disorders include aphasias, alexias, and agraphias and are by definition the result of focal brain dysfunction. A screening examination for language disorders includes the evaluation of spontaneous speech, repetition of words and sentences, comprehension of spoken and written language, the ability to produce names of objects on confrontation, and the ability to write. These areas of assessment are found on the Mini-Mental State Examination (MMSE), discussed at some length in Chapter 4.

Thought is subdivided into *production of thought, form of thought* (thought process), and *content of thought* and can be disordered in several ways.

Disorders of the Production of Thought. The production of thought refers to the abundance of thought, as evidenced by a persons interactional capabilities. In most situations, thought production is assessed by observation of the patient's verbal communication; however, those with speech impediments or congenital mutism also can demonstrate difficulties in this area through other modalities of communication. *Poverty of thought* is characterized by a decrease in the apparent ability or interest in interacting with the environment and other people. This is seen most frequently in schizophrenia and major depression. In some situations, one's thoughts race ahead of one's ability to communicate them (*flight of ideas*); this phenomenon is usually seen in mania. *Thought blocking* is characterized by an abrupt cessation of communication before the topic of discussion can be completed. The delay that follows may be prolonged, following which patients are often unable to recall the topic. Patients sometimes explain this occurrence by stating that their "mind went blank."

Disorders of the Form of Thought. *Form of thought or thought process* refers to the manner in which thoughts are connected or associated. Normal thinking is goal directed, with sequential thoughts having logical connections. The "train of thought" can be easily followed, and the communicant reaches the intended goal. Conditions characterized by abnormalities in thought processing, such as psychotic disorders, may be manifested in several ways (Table 1–7).

Disorders of Thought Content. Disorders of thought content are often divided into two broad categories—preoccupations and delusions. Preoccupations include phobias, obsessions, and compulsions. A *phobia* is an irrational, pathologic dread of a specific type of stimulus or situation that results in marked anxiety and avoidance of the situation. An *obsession* is a disturbing, persistent, and usually intrusive thought, feeling, or impulse that cannot be eliminated from consciousness. Common obsessions include fear of contamination or of losing control and harming others. Obsessions may involve fear of self-harm or suicide, even though the patient may deny feeling depressed or wishing to die. Such suicidal thoughts would be properly included in this portion of the mental status examination. *Compulsions* are irresistible urges to perform meaningless, often ritualistic motor acts, such as handwashing.

Delusions are fixed, false beliefs that have no basis in reality, are not generally held by one's culture, and from which the patient will not be dissuaded, despite evidence to the contrary. Delusions can be mood congruent

---

Table 1–7 **Disorders of Thought Processing**

Circumstantiality
Marked by tedious and unnecessary details but eventually reaches the point

Tangentiality
Marked by skirting the question rather than directly answering it. Connections between subsequent thoughts are apparent, but a goal is never reached

Loosening of Associations
A jumping from subject to subject without apparent logical or sequential connections

Verbigeration
Conveys little information despite adequate volume of speech due to vagueness, empty repetitions, or obscure phrases

"Word Salad"
An incoherent collection of words and phrases

Neologisms
Made-up words that have meaning only for the patient

Clang Associations
Words or phrases connected due to characteristics of the words themselves (rhyming, punning) rather than the meaning they convey

Echolalia
Repetitive, often playful repetition of the words of others

with the psychiatric state, such as those of *nihilism* (life or world is ending), *poverty* (all life possessions have been lost), *somatic* distress [a serious illness (cancer) has invaded the body], or *sin* (heinous sins have been committed for which punishment is necessary), as is sometimes seen in depression. Delusions of *grandeur,* in which special powers are claimed, are characteristically found in mania. Delusions also can be incongruent with the prevailing mood, such as delusions of reference (unrelated events apply to oneself) or control (outside force controlling actions). These usually are more characteristic of schizophrenia. Karl Schneider described a group of delusions characterized by externally imposed influences concerning thought, feelings, and somatic function. These are referred to as the "first-rank symptoms of schizophrenia," although they are known to occur in affective psychoses and delirium, as well (Table 1–8). These symptoms also are reviewed in the chapter on schizophrenia (Chapter 5).

Perception

Perceptual disturbance involves disordered processing of sensory information. Hallucinations are perceptions that occur in the absence of actual stimuli. Illusions are misinterpretations of existing stimuli. Auditory hallucinations occur most frequently in the psychoses of schizophrenia, mania, or other "functional" disorders. Visual hallucinations occur more frequently than auditory hallucinations in psychotic episodes due to medical, neurologic and toxin-induced

Table 1–8 **Schneider's First-Rank Symptoms of Schizophrenia***

	BELIEF
Thought insertion	An external agency is inserting thoughts into the passive mind.
Thought withdrawal	An external agency is removing thoughts from the passive mind.
Thought broadcasting	Thoughts are audible to others.
Made feelings (passivity feelings)	Feelings being experienced are imposed by an external source.
Made drives (passivity feelings)	Powerful drives (to which the patient usually responds) are being imposed by an external agency.
Made volitional acts (passivity feelings)	Actions are completely under the control of an external influence.
Somatic passivity (passivity feelings)	Bodily sensations are being imposed by an external agency against the will.
Delusional perception	A two-stage phenomenon in which a normally perceived stimulus is followed by a delusional belief regarding the meaning of the stimulus.

* Other first-rank symptoms involve specific types of auditory hallucinations.

disorders (i.e., substance abuse, toxins, and intrinsic brain disease), although visual hallucinations are often associated with primary psychiatric disease. Olfactory and gustatory hallucinations often occur as prodromal symptoms of complex partial seizures. Haptic hallucinations, especially the sensation of bugs crawling on one's skin (formication), frequently occur in delirium induced by sedative withdrawal. There is considerable overlap in these symptoms, however, and none is specific to, or pathognomonic of, the disorders noted.

Paranoid delusions may be highly systematized (such as elaborate systems of observations by the FBI, or CIA plots) or bizarre (Martians peering at one from outer space). Paranoia as an isolated symptom is not specifically diagnostic. It is the nature, duration, *and* severity of the paranoia in the context of the patient's history that relates it to one particular diagnosis or the other. For example, the isolated delusion that one's wife is having an affair in the absence of other signs or symptoms would be diagnosed as delusional disorder. A severely depressed patient who had paranoid delusions of being persecuted would most likely have a major depression with psychotic features; a woman with paranoid delusions of being watched and followed by the CIA, with a deteriorating longtitudinal course and other more pervasive symptoms of a thought disorder, might be diagnosed as having paranoid schizophrenia; a man with paranoid ideation in the context of amphetamines might be considered to have a substance-induced delusional disorder. Somatic delusions such as feelings of rotting inside, being infected with a venereal disease, or having AIDS may be seen in psychotic depression. Alternatively, general suspiciousness, mistrust, cynicism, and querulousness of others that does not reach overtly delusional proportions may be seen as a trait of a paranoid personality disorder.

Depersonalization refers to feelings that one is falling apart, fragmenting, "not the same," not one's self, becoming unreal, or detached and may be seen in a number of psychiatric disorders—principally anxiety disorders, but also delirious states, including those that are substance induced. Symptoms of *derealization* include the feeling that the world is not real, people are not real, or things are becoming distant, alien, or strange. Both types of symptoms are variations on the same theme and may be seen in CNS disease, such as complex partial epilepsy.

Cognitive Functioning

Level of Consciousness. It is best to describe patients' levels of consciousness by their ability to respond to the environmental stimuli. Extremes include hyperalertness and coma. *Hyperalertness* is characterized by hypervigilance, often with agitation or tremulousness, and is seen most often in mania or delirium. *Alert* describes normal wakefulness and awareness of the environment. *Lethargic* indicates that the patient has a tendency to drift into unresponsiveness if left alone, but is easily roused to verbal stimulus. *Stupor* reflects the need for continual stimulation to maintain consciousness, and *coma* is characterized by unconsciousness and the absence of response to any stimuli.

Orientation. Orientation assesses awareness of identity, time (day of week, month, exact day of month, year, time of day), place, and situation. Awareness of person usually indicates that a person can remember his or her name. Awareness of time and place involves the ability to provide the correct date and current location, while awareness of situation suggests a grasp of the circumstances surrounding the patient's current plight. In confusional states, the first manifestation of disorientation normally involves time and situation, and these are usually the last to normalize with recovery.

Concentration (Attention). Concentration refers to the ability to direct and sustain attention. Patients with impaired attention require repetition of questions and may be distracted by seemingly inconsequential stimuli. Concentration is formally tested by performance of serial 7s or 3s (counting backward from 100 by 7s or 3s). Alternatively, the patient can be asked to repeat strings of random numbers forward (average normal—seven digits) or in reverse (average normal—five digits). Failure is identified by two unsuccessful attempts at the same number. Gross impairment of concentration (attention) is characteristic of delirium and is usually recognized by the patient's inability to respond to your requests consistently and coherently.

Memory. Tests of memory assess the ability to retrieve and recite information previously stored (retrograde memory) and to form new memories (anterograde memory). Remote memory (usually retrograde) involves remembering events that occurred many years ago, such as the name of a school attended, the nature of previous jobs, and so forth. With disorders of declining intellectual function, remote memory is usually one of the last to be affected. Recent past memory (retrograde and/or anterograde) involves remembering events occurring months ago and may be assessed as the patient provides believable and/or confirmed details of the present illness or events leading up to the assessment.

Inability to form new memories (anterograde) is clinically identified when patients are unable to recall events that have just occurred or people they have just met. Less obvious forms of anterograde memory dysfunction can be assessed by providing the names of three unrelated objects that the patient immediately repeats (immediate recall) and then recalls after 5 minutes (short-term memory). Impairment of immediate recall, especially with repeated attempts, suggests an attention deficit that precludes further anterograde memory testing. Intact immediate recall with impaired recall after 5 minutes suggests impairment of short-term memory.

Isolated deficits in cognitive function are diagnostically nonspecific because they can occur with intellectual decline of varied cause. If identified by the screening tests performed on the mental status examination, they should be further characterized by more formal neuropsychological testing (*infra vide*). The MMSE is a convenient brief physician-administered mental status examination (Folstein et al, 1975). The MMSE assesses orientation, attention, memory, verbal fluency, ability to follow complex commands, and visuographic skills. Using it routinely in psychiatric evaluations allows for screening for many of the cognitive components of the mental status examination. Scores of 24 or less out of a possible 30 are suggestive of cognitive difficulties and may be confirmed with more extensive neuropsychological testing. The use of the MMSE is addressed in more detail in Chapter 4.

Intelligence. Some observations may be made about the patient's general education level and the ability to learn, integrate, and process new information and to solve problems. Formal education level does not necessarily indicate intelligence, because intelligence, most basically, is an assessment of the individual's ability to learn new information, process that information, and solve problems. Individuals with relatively little or no formal education can be quite intelligent. On the other hand, a person who has completed his or her doctorate would not be expected to function in the range of those with borderline intellectual function. Formal psychological testing may be needed, especially in children or when mental retardation is expected, to assess the patient's intelligence level accurately (see also Chapter 3 on psychological testing).

Insight and Judgment

Insight refers to awareness of factors influencing one's situation. When a patient has a psychiatric illness, insight refers to the appreciation that an illness or psychiatric difficulty is occurring, recognition of its impact on the ability to function, and awareness of the need to take steps to correct it. The most meaningful method of assessing insight is to gather data about these factors throughout the history. The presence or absence of insight has profound impact on adjustment to illness, compliance with treatment, and consequent level of function. Thus, an estimation of a patient's insight is helpful in planning an effective treatment strategy.

The patient's capacity for self-observation and demonstration of empathy are also measures of insight that are helpful in assessing the presence of a personality disorder. Patients with a personality disorder are often egocentric, tend to blame others for their problems, resist self-examination to determine their personal contribution to their difficulties in life, and lack insight into their behavior.

Empathy refers to the ability to identify with the feelings of others and to "feel with them." It is also a measure of consideration for the feelings, welfare, and rights of others. Patients with some personality disorders (antisocial, paranoid, narcissistic, and borderline personality disorders) often show a lack of empathy for others and exploit other people for their own gratification. Traits found in personality disorder and details about their diagnosis are discussed in Chapter 6.

Judgment refers to a person's ability to handle finances; manage day-to-day activities; and avoid danger, including exposure to heat, cold, malnutrition, and crime. Insight into factors influencing a person's well-being must be present before options and priorities can be weighed and judgment exercised.

Standardized methods of assessment, such as asking what a person would do if he or she found a stamped, addressed envelope on the sidewalk, are inadequate for most purposes. It is more helpful to rely on an understanding of the circumstances that led to the patient's seeking psychiatric attention in assessing judgment. For instance, a person walking in the snow with shorts and no shoes would, in the absence of extenuating circumstances, be exhibiting poor judgment. Despite the subjective nature of the assessment, impaired judgment resulting from mental illness or substance dependence that directly or indirectly places the patient or others in danger is a prerequisite for involuntary commitment in many states.

PSYCHOLOGICAL AND NEUROPSYCHOLOGICAL TESTING

The clinical indications and usefulness of psychological and neuropsychological testing are discussed in Chapter 3, but a brief overview of the place of such testing in the general psychiatric assessment will be mentioned here.

Tests of psychological and neuropsychological function complement, but do not replace, the psychiatric history and mental status examination, just as laboratory and radiologic procedures complement, but do not replace, the medical history and physical examination. This is a particularly important point, because no standardized test used in clinical practice provides an assessment that allows a psychiatric diagnosis to be made, with the possible exception of dementia. There is a tendency among nonpsychiatrists to use psychological tests, such as the Minnesota Multiphasic Personality Inventory (MMPI) or the General Health Questionnaire (GHQ), to establish whether a psychiatric disorder may be involved in a patient's symptom picture. As will be discussed later, use of these instruments can lead to inappropriate labeling and ineffective treatment. When correctly used, however, psychological and neuropsychological tests provide an important adjunct to the psychiatric evaluation and treatment plan.

Neuropsychological tests assess cognitive abilities and require the expertise of a psychologist who has received specialized training in their administration and interpretation (a neuropsychologist). *Psychological tests* were developed to identify the presence and frequency of psychological symptoms in various populations. Some psychological tests are easily administered or self-administered and can be readily scored merely by reading a short description of the test. Others are more complex and require skills in the interpretation and quantification of the behaviors being tested. Those with master's degrees or doctorates in psychology usually possess the skills necessary to perform these tests if they choose to emphasize this area in their work. Not all psychologists, however, specialize in giving and interpreting psychological tests, so care should be taken to ensure that the person doing the testing has an adequate background and interest.

As is discussed in Chapter 3, psychological and neuropsychological tests are best used to clarify specific important questions during patient assessment and management. Although the multitude of standardized tests cannot be covered in this chapter, four common clinical questions in which psychological and neuropsychological tests can help with clinical decision making will be addressed here: (1) Are psychiatric factors involved in the patient's clinical presentation? (2) Can the severity of the patient's psychiatric symptoms be reproducibly assessed and used to monitor improvement? (3) Does the patient's personality assessment give a clue about psychiatric involvement? and (4) Does the patient have impaired brain function? Because it is impossible to review all the tests that could potentially assist in answering these questions, only a few widely used and well-standardized tests will be discussed. More extensive discussion of these and other tests can be found in the book by van Riezen and Segal (1988). Psychological tests are used to address the first three questions, whereas neuropsychological tests are used in the last.

Screening Tests for Psychiatric Involvement

Are there screening tests that detect the presence of specific psychiatric disorders? *No!* There are, however, self-administered screening questionnaires (which can be used before a psychiatric assessment) that identify those at risk of psychiatric difficulties and measure psychiatric symptoms. These instruments are best used in primary care outpatient and inpatient settings. Because these tests often are exquisitely sensitive, but have limited specificity, it is necessary to be aware of the need for more formalized psychiatric assessment before a diagnosis is considered and treatment for a "psychiatric" condition is instituted.

The General Health Questionnaire (GHQ) is a widely studied self-report instrument validated primarily in nonpsychiatric outpatient populations. A low score on this test predicts that a psychiatric disorder is unlikely and that psychiatric factors are probably not involved in the symptom presentation. High scores suggest the need for further questioning if the presentation of the patient suggests that psychiatric factors may be playing a role. The GHQ can save valuable time in screening new outpatients attending a primary care clinic by alerting the clinician to patients who might require more careful psychiatric evaluation in addition to the medical workup.

Depression is one of the most common psychiatric disorders seen in primary care medical populations. The Center for Epidemiologic Studies-Depression Scale (CES-D) is a self-report questionnaire that has been standardized to identify those at risk of depression in the general population. It lists the presence of a number of depressive symptoms but does not, even when the score is elevated, suggest that a pathological, clinical depression is present or that treatment should be administered. In clinical samples, the CES-D is a sensitive screen for depression. A clinical diagnostic interview is necessary to confirm the presence of a mood disorder

Screening for Severity of Illness

One of the most important tasks of the clinician is to establish a baseline level of symptoms and to confirm that the treatment being given results in their reduction. Although the patient interview is the principal means of accomplishing this purpose, several tests that reliably document psychiatric symptoms can improve consistency. Depression severity and change can be monitored with the Beck Depression Inventory (self-report) or the Hamilton Rating Scale for Depression (interviewer-rated). However, these scales should not be used for diagnosis, as they can frequently misclassify medically ill patients (Kathol et al, 1990). The Hamilton Rating Scale for Anxiety (interviewer-rated) is available to quantitate symptoms of anxiety. General psychiatric severity can be assessed with the Hopkins Symptoms Checklist 90 (HCL-90) (self-report), whereas psychotic symptoms can be enumerated with the Brief Psychiatric Rating Scale (interviewer-rated). Because the HCL-90 is divided into subscales pertaining to specific areas of psychiatric symptoms, the questions pertinent only to that area can be repeatedly administered during treatment.

Screening with Personality Questionnaires

Although personality disorders have received relatively little rigorous, systematic research attention, there is growing evidence that the presence of personality disorder in patients with other major psychiatric disorders is associated with increased severity and poorer outcome. Additionally, personality disorder may increase the likelihood of contact with health professionals for medical conditions (Reich, 1987).

The MMPI is perhaps the most commonly used personality assessment instrument. It has nine clinical scales from which profiles of behavioral patterns are derived and, when originally formulated (1939), was well standardized in a large control population. Two problems arise with the use of the MMPI in current practice. First, the MMPI was standardized when cultural mores were considerably different from today and well before the psychiatric diagnostic system in current use. The importance of this problem is emphasized by the fact that restandardization of the MMPI in a contemporary population showed that there was a 20 to 30% difference in the identification of dysfunction between the old and new standards (Colligan et al, 1983). Despite these findings, which suggest that many patients are being misclassified, few testing centers have switched to the new standards, and the revised MMPI is just beginning to be implemented at the level of the general community practice setting.

Not only are there problems with the use of a dated population standard, but there are also difficulties in the interpretations made based on test results. In the 1940s, interpretation was based on a conceptualization of psychiatric disease very different from that espoused today. The relevance of "standard" (often computer-generated) personality profiles from the MMPI to current psychiatric disorders is uncertain because they are based on different theoretical constructs. Significant differences can therefore occur between the MMPI results and a diagnosis revealed through clinical interview.

The second major problem with the MMPI is that it is commonly used to assess patients with medical illness. Because the test was standardized in a nonmedically ill control group, using this instrument to determine whether psychiatric factors may be involved in the complaints of patients with real or potential medical illness is inappropriate (Osborne, 1987). Such patients will routinely rate high on the hypochondriacal and depressive scales because a number of the questions in these scales reflect the presence of physical symptoms (real or imagined). Unfortunately, those evaluating patients in whom a functional cause is in the differential are frequently enamored of the fact that the MMPI gives real and reproducible numbers to quantitate psychiatric disturbances while forgetting that the results are of questionable validity. *For this and the reasons listed above, the MMPI is not recommended as a routine adjunct to the clinical interview,* and its use should be limited to special situations.

Screening for Impaired Brain Function

The principal aims of neuropsychological testing are to provide an estimate of the severity of cognitive deficit, to localize the areas of the brain that are impaired, and to assess the degree and estimated duration of functional limitations. The Halstead–Reitan Battery and the Luria–Nebraska Inventory are two extensive test batteries that help answer questions related to the areas above. Unfortunately, the length of testing makes these tests unsuitable in severely ill psychiatric patients. The Wechsler Adult Intelligence Scale–Revised and other briefer screens (Berg et al, 1987) of cognitive function now frequently replace the more comprehensive batteries (Table 1–9). When mental retardation in children is the focus of assessment, specialized age-specific measurements of intelligence can be used. These tests include the Wechsler Intelligence Scale Children–Revised and the Wechsler Preschool and Primary Scale of Intelligence. These tests require the assistance of a neuropsychologist for administration and interpretation. Additionally, the comprehensive neuropsychological batteries can be expensive. Nevertheless, complete neuropsychological batteries may be helpful in defining subtle cognitive deficits and are indicated in some clinical situations, such as in evaluating patients who have sustained severe head injuries or occupational exposure to potential neurologic toxins, patients who may have temporal lobe seizures, or patients with cerebrovascular disease. Comprehensive neuropsychological inventories also can be helpful when legal compensation issues are important or for planning rehabilitation programs. The use of neuropsychological testing is discussed further in Chapter 3.

Table 1–9 **Comprehensive Neuropsychologic Batteries and Specific Function Tests**

NEUROPSYCHOLOGIC BATTERIES	NUMBER OF SECTIONS	COMMENTS
Halstead-Reitan Battery (HRB)	10	Includes MMPI and WAIS. Full test may take several days
Luria-Nebraska Inventory	11	Provides score on 14 measures of cognitive function with *t* scores
Tests of Specific Function	**Function Tested**	
Wechsler Adult Intelligence Screen-R (WAIS)	Verbal and nonverbal skills	Provides verbal and performance intelligence scores as well as a full-scale IQ
Token Test	Speech	Can be used as a screening test for aphasia
Wechsler Memory Scale	Memory	Seven subtests; provides memory quotient similar to IQ
Wisconsin Card Sort	Abstraction—conceptual shifting	Considered a test of frontal lobe function
Trail-Making Test	Visuomotor tracking	Contains parts A and B; performance decreases with age
Seashore Rhythm Test	Nonverbal auditory	Part of HRB; tests ability to discriminate between two tone groups
Finger-Tapping Test	Motor	Cortical damage slows tapping speed

CLASSIFICATION OF PSYCHIATRIC DISEASE: DSM-IV

As in all medical disciplines, the nature of the information obtained during the diagnostic interview conforms to the classification of illness used. The classification, in turn, should be derived from the ability to identify consistently complexes of signs and symptoms that predict etiology, natural course, family involvement, outcome, and response to treatment of a condition that causes or leads to impairment. DSM-IV reflects the state of the art in classifying psychiatric disease in the United States and, at least in part, stems from three previous classification systems used since the mid-1970s in psychiatric research [the "Feighner criteria" (Feighner et al, 1972) and Research Diagnostic Criteria (Spitzer et al, 1978)].

DSM-IV uses a signs-and-symptoms, criterion-based approach to psychiatric diagnosis. If certain symptoms are present in sufficient degree and for sufficient duration, then the diagnosis can be made. Those meeting "criteria" are thus more likely to conform to the predictive factors known about the disease being diagnosed. As might be expected, some conditions have greater validity than others. For instance, depression, mania, schizophrenia, panic disorder, alcohol and substance dependency/abuse, and somatization disorder can be reproducibly identified. As a result, definite statements can be made regarding the likely age of onset, sex distribution, familial involvement, course if untreated, and probability of response to certain interventions in those carrying these diagnoses. Other diagnoses, however, such as personality disorder (with the exception of antisocial personality disorder), adjustment disorders, and psychosexual disorders, currently have less predictive value. As more research is performed, these will be further refined or deleted, depending on the findings.

Those who do not meet criteria for diagnosis according to DSM-IV can be diagnosed with "no psychiatric disorder" or the possible/probable distinction for a certain condition. This occurrence results when DSM-IV is correctly used and does not preclude that such patients be treated. What such diagnoses say is that these patients do not warrant a label with its positive and negative connotations, although a clinical trial may be attempted to see whether symptoms improve.

In an attempt to ensure that information of value in planning treatment and predicting outcome is recorded, DSM-IV uses a multiaxial system of evaluation. Axes I and II comprise mental disorders; Axis III, general medical conditions; Axis IV, psychosocial and environmental problems; and Axis V, global assessment of functioning (GAF).

Axis I diagnoses include clinical syndromes that represent a deterioration from a previous level of functioning, such as schizophrenia, major depression, and substance-abuse disorders. Axis II includes personality disorders. Patients with Axis II diagnoses, in contrast to Axis I, usually have symptoms extending back into their early developmental years. Axis I and II disorders frequently coexist, requiring careful evaluation for Axis I disorders in patients with personality disorder. Physical disorders (Axis III) either exacerbate or cause Axis I and II disorders in up to 50% of patients with psychiatric conditions (LaBruzza, 1981). It is therefore very important to document the medical conditions present and assess whether they may be impacting on the psychiatric symptoms. Axis II is also used for mental retardation diagnoses.

Although DSM-IV does not identify stress as a major cause of psychiatric disorders, the importance of psychosocial and environmental stressors is noted in Axis IV. Axis V rates the current GAF in terms of social, occupational, or academic activity. Ratings of impairment are made on a 0 (most) to 90 (least) scale. An example of the multiaxial patient assessment as it relates to RH is listed in Table 1–10.

V (the letter) codes ("vee" codes) constitute emotional situations not attributable to a mental disorder. Examples include marital problems, uncomplicated bereavement, and so forth, and were described previously as "problems in living." V codes allow description of the presenting problem without assigning the patient a formal psychiatric diagnosis.

Table 1–10 **DSM-IV Multiaxial Evaluation for Patient RH**

Axis I:	Alcohol Dependence
	Alcohol-Induced Psychotic Disorder
	Delirium due to multiple etiologies
	Delirium Due to General Medical Conditions
	Alcohol Withdrawal Delirium
Axis II:	Diagnosis deferred on Axis II
Axis III:	Status post-head trauma
	Subdural hematoma
	Alcoholic cirrhosis
	Alcoholic gastritis
	Pancreatitis
	Hyponatremia
	Hypomagnesemia
	Hypocalcemia
	Macrocytic anemia
	Thrombocytopenia
	Essential hypertension
Axis IV:	Psychosocial and Environmental Problems
	Primary support group
	Social environment
	Occupational
Axis V:	GAF*: 10

* GAF, global assessment of function.

Important Diagnostic Issues

Two medical problem-solving principles are important in identifying psychiatric illness (Elstein et al, 1978). First, common diseases are the most likely to be seen and should not be overlooked. Table 1–11 shows that mood disorders, anxiety disorders, alcohol and substance abuse, and adjustment dis-

Table 1–11 **Rank Order of Psychiatric Diagnoses by Site of Encounter**

SURVEY OF OUTPATIENT PHYSICIANS	GENERAL HOSPITAL PSYCHIATRIC CONSULTATION	INPATIENT PSYCHIATRIC SERVICE	COMMUNITY SURVEY
Anxiety disorders	Mood disorders	Mood disorders	Substance abuse
Mood disorders	Adjustment disorders	Schizophrenia	Anxiety disorders
Substance abuse	No psychiatric diagnosis	Substance abuse	Mood disorders
Psychophysiologic disorders	Substance abuse	Delirium, dementia	Antisocial personality
Adjustment disorders	Delirium	Adjustment disorders	Schizophrenia

orders are seen often in several clinical settings. They therefore deserve special attention and consideration. Second, uncommon problems have increased importance when effective treatment is available. Missing an uncommon problem in this situation can be catastrophic and frequently happens in patients with reversible organic causes of psychiatric syndromes.

Finally, diagnosis of psychiatric disorders that may be complicated by suicidal or homicidal ideation should not be overlooked. Depression, schizophrenia, substance abuse, and antisocial personality deserve serious attention because all may endanger the patient or others.

Differential Diagnosis

Identifying the underlying psychiatric problem(s) and the variables that might be impacting on it (them) involves a stepwise process. Initially, the chief complaint and associated symptoms related to the history of present illness will suggest the major DSM-IV diagnostic category (see also Fig. 1–1). Once the principal symptoms or problems are identified, refinements (first differential) are made during the history-taking process to help establish which diagnostic

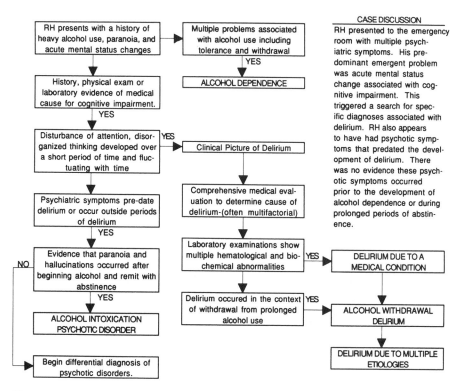

Figure 1–1. *Diagnostic issues in the case of RH.*

category best describes the clinical situation. Because the end product of this process will influence the treatment or assistance given to the patient, thoroughness is very important.

In the differential diagnosis of primary psychiatric disease, medical factors should be identified at the onset of the evaluation. If they are, then the clinician should aggressively pursue medical, neurologic, or toxic factors before planning a specific psychiatric treatment modality. In some cases, this is possible, since such conditions as steroid psychosis or systemic lupus cerebritis (both examples of delirium) are often readily identifiable at the onset, thus facilitating the recognition of the medical nature of the mental symptoms.

Much more often, the patient will present with no evidence or limited evidence of medical conditions that might be related to the psychiatric symptoms. In these circumstances, decisions about the psychiatric syndromes in question are made based on the assumption that symptoms are unrelated to medical illness. For instance, a patient with undiagnosed hypothyroidism who has many symptoms in common with depression (Table 1–12) presents to a primary physician or psychiatrist with complaints of weakness, constipation, crying spells, difficulty sleeping, and weight gain. Because the patient appears depressed and, in fact, has many symptoms of depression, the differential for mood disturbance is entertained. Sure enough, the patient meets all the criteria for a severe single major depressive episode, and yet the underlying problem is hypothyroidism.

This suggests that even after a presumed psychiatric condition is diagnosed, it is often necessary to run through another differential (the second) of conditions that may be causally or casually related to the syndrome. In the case of major depression, for instance, symptoms could be the result of underlying medical conditions, such as endocrine disease, cancer, anemia, hypoxemia, medication reaction, epilepsy, and so forth. It could be the result of stress, such as the death of a loved one. It could be secondary to a preexisting psychiatric condition, such as antisocial personality disorder, alcoholism, and so forth, or it could be feigned by someone who wants compensation, attention, and so forth.

Table 1–12 **Comparison of Psychological Symptoms in Hypothyroidism and Depression**

HYPOTHYROIDISM (%)	DEPRESSION
Loss of energy (25–98)	Loss of energy
Weakness (25–95)	Weakness
Poor concentration	Poor concentration
Memory loss (48–66)	Memory loss
Slowed actions (48–91)	Motor retardation
Decreased sex drive	Decreased libido
Constipation (38–61)	Constipation
Insomnia (25–98)	Insomnia
Nervousness (13–58)	Agitation

The reason that this second differential is important in the care of patients is that, depending on the complicating circumstances, major differences may occur in the way the patient is handled. This is illustrated in Table 1–13. DSM-IV lists secondary categories for most symptom groups. For example, depression due to hypothyroidism would be designated "Mood Disorder Due to Hypothyroidism, With Depressive Features."

The psychiatric evaluation, as outlined in this chapter, helps to perform this function in a time-efficient, yet thorough manner. The chief complaint and history of present illness are used to identify the principal difficulty of the patient. The history of present illness helps determine whether a syndrome of behavior is present and how typical it is. It also documents the presence of variables that may directly influence the production or continuation of symptoms.

The past medical and psychiatric history, personal and social history, and review of systems uncover information and discrepancies that could have a bearing on the presenting complaints but do not, at first glance, appear to have a relationship. The physical examination and laboratory assessment confirm or deny suspicions derived from the history about possible medical/neurologic involvement and check for signs of diseases not entertained.

One help in differentiating primary psychiatric disorders from those related to the secondary conditions noted is to have a good understanding of the primary psychiatric disorders. Such knowledge includes symptom presentation, age of onset, sex ratio, natural course, family involvement, and likelihood

Table 1–13 **Sample Treatment Strategies In the Treatment of Patients with Depression**

CLINICAL SITUATION	TREATMENT
Primary major depression	Antidepressant medication Psychotherapy Social support mobilization
Depression secondary to hypothyroidism	No antidepressant medication Supportive psychotherapy Reassurance and social support Thyroid replacement Education about when symptoms will resolve
Adjustment disorder with depression in histrionic personality disorder and somatization	No antidepressant medication Supportive psychotherapy Social support mobilization
Depression in a patient caught faking the symptoms	Empathic confrontation No antidepressant medication Supportive psychotherapy
Depression 2 weeks after mother's death	Supportive psychotherapy Social support reinforcement

of response to treatment. For example, major depression is more frequent in women, has its onset during the 20s to 40s, runs a recurrent course, has a higher incidence in other members of the family, has few or no residual symptoms between episodes, and has a good likelihood of response to cyclic antidepressants or other antidepressant therapies. Therefore, if a patient presents for the first time in his or her 70s, has no history of emotional problems, other family members have had no difficulty with affective problems, and the symptoms are cluttered with unusual complaints, then causes for the psychiatric presentation other than primary depression should be given greater consideration.

DSM-IV Case Formulation

Refer to, or reread, the case of RH presented at the beginning of this chapter. This case presentation describes a middle-aged man with a lifelong history of alcohol abuse that progressed to the point that he abstained only when sleep, unconsciousness, illness, or the inability to procure more intervened. He was admitted agitated and incoherent with paranoid thoughts and physical signs and symptoms suggesting alcohol withdrawal. Other causes of delirium were possible because the patient had liver enzyme and electrolyte disturbances, pancreatitis, a gastrointestinal bleed, and cerebral trauma. Nonetheless, because the clinical history from the patient, the police, and the family was most compatible with alcohol withdrawal delirium (delirium tremens), it was considered the most likely Axis I diagnosis (Table 1–10). Despite this working diagnosis, other possible causes of the patient's mental state were being considered or corrected while the patient was treated for alcohol withdrawal.

During the years before admission, he demonstrated dependence and tolerance to alcohol. His education was shortened, marriage broken, job lost, and health impaired because of alcohol consumption. Despite attempts at in- and outpatient treatment, he persisted in nearly continuous intoxication. He showed drinking behavior consistent with that of other first- and second-degree family members. This tight history of mental and emotional problems related to alcohol ingestion supports the Axis I diagnosis of alcohol dependence (see DSM-IV for criteria). Figure 1–1 outlines additional diagnostic issues for RH. RH displayed evidence of delirium, which should trigger a search for specific causes. It is common for multiple causes of delirium to be identified.

Other psychiatric syndromes are seen frequently in patients with alcohol dependence. These include depression, other forms of substance abuse, antisocial personality disorder, anxiety, and dementia. RH had a history of antisocial traits, but these were insufficient to make the diagnosis of antisocial personality disorder. Furthermore, the antisocial traits that were present (school expulsion, difficulties with teachers, frequent fights, arrests) always occurred under the influence of alcohol. RH denied abuse of other substances, and his denial was confirmed, at least at the time of admission, by the absence of other substances of abuse in his urine. The family also confirmed that he didn't use "pills."

RH had a history of depressed affect during intoxication or withdrawal, accompanied by suicidal ideation on several occasions. During periods of abstinence, depression had never been a problem. Both during and after treatment of the patient's withdrawal delirium, there was no evidence of depression, despite an apparently dismal life situation. Despite treatment with antianxiety medications, he showed no evidence for current or past anxiety disorder. RH reported significant paranoid delusions. Although these may have occurred as part of a recurrent withdrawal pattern, it appears that paranoid symptoms also occurred independent of withdrawal. DSM-IV would classify this alcoholic paranoia as an alcohol psychotic disorder, with delusions.

It was impossible to assess cognitive function of the patient during the delirious state. After adequate treatment, however, he was able to score 29 of 30 on the MMSE (see screening tests section and Chapter 4). Although his performance does not exclude the possibility that more subtle evidence for cognitive impairment is present in this high-risk patient, it does suggest that dementia is not a major problem. More specialized cognitive testing was not performed in RH for reasons that will be discussed later. As in many patients with alcohol dependence, the patient exhibits some traits of avoidant, dependent, and schizoid personality disorders. There is insufficient evidence to make the diagnosis of any one of these or to make a diagnosis of mixed personality disorder because the influence that alcohol has on these traits cannot be parceled out, even when the chart is reviewed thoroughly. The Axis II diagnosis is therefore deferred. As previously mentioned, antisocial personality disorder, which has greater validity and reliability than other personality disorders, has been excluded.

The Axis III diagnoses for RH are listed in Table 1–10 and are primarily related to complications of alcohol abuse. The patient, however, had a seizure 3 weeks into his hospital stay. Although alcohol withdrawal seizure is a logical choice in the differential, it occurred outside the expected period (3 to 14 days) for this complication to happen. The EEG and CT, documenting a subdural hematoma, were done not only because the presentation was atypical (although this would have been enough), but also because RH was at high risk for an alternative cause of new seizure onset because of his history of alcohol abuse and thrombocytopenia. In addition, it may be recalled that the patient had a head bruise on physical examination, and the fundoscopic examination had not been performed because of poor patient compliance.

The subdural hematoma could have been identified earlier had a more aggressive CNS workup for delirium been done at the outset. This is the point at which systematic and thorough examination and informed clinical judgment become so important. The patient is at a high risk of other causes of CNS pathology because of the unreliable alcoholic state, and a fundoscopic examination was not initially possible during the delirium. Delirium alone should be sufficient to warrant further evaluation in such a case. Decisions such as these have important implications regarding patient care.

Before the onset of this admission, the patient experienced no acute stressors (Axis IV) that would have predisposed him to admission. Although not receiving his disability check could have been considered an acute stressor, it is more likely that the lack of alcohol was a major factor in his presentation. However, he was unemployed, had no social support system, and suffered from intermittent medical problems related to his alcohol abuse, which qualify as severe, enduring stressful circumstances. The patient's global assessment of function during the delirious state suggests that he wouldn't have been able to maintain his personal care on his own (Axis V).

RH responded well to high-dose benzodiazepines for withdrawal within a few days of initial hospitalization. Other medical factors were evaluated and treated during the initial hospital stay. As the patient's delirium resolved, further information was obtained from the patient. His behavior was observed to confirm the initial impression and determine whether other psychiatric conditions might be present, especially those with a high frequency in alcohol dependence. Particular emphasis was placed on observing the patient's ability to identify familiar personnel, locate his room, and perform activities of daily living. He accomplished these tasks without trouble after the delirium cleared, suggesting that he would be able to function satisfactorily outside a structured environment. Furthermore, documenting these behaviors obviated the need to perform more formalized and expensive neuropsychological testing.

RH had participated in several alcohol treatment programs without lasting benefit. For this reason, legal commitment to an inpatient treatment center was deemed unlikely to benefit him. This particular admission was occasioned by a serious threat to the patient's life. It is at times like these that some alcoholics become sufficiently frightened that they enter and follow through on their resolve to stay sober. During his hospital stay, he expressed an interest and was encouraged to reinitiate contact with Alcoholics Anonymous. Such a program, if adhered to, effectively uses group support, confrontation, religious motivation, and behavior modification to modify the long-term behavior of alcoholics. Because it is run by former alcoholics, rationalizations and evasive ploys are much more difficult to get away with than when mental health professionals administer treatment.

Social factors also often play a role in when and how much alcoholics drink. One thing that has not been done is to have the patient live in a more structured environment such as a nursing home in the hope that opportunities to imbibe would not be as frequent. The patient would have to agree to this arrangement and be willing to cooperate with the personnel in abiding by rules at the facility.

When the clinical situation warrants, a systematic psychiatric assessment is important for appropriate patient care, regardless of the setting. It requires an understanding of current psychiatric nomenclature (DSM-IV) and predictive value of the disorders being diagnosed. Because psychiatric conditions are no longer diagnosed merely by excluding other illnesses that can cause similar complaints, it is important to know what questions to ask and how to ask them, as well as to observe accurately the behaviors that lead to making a psychiatric diagnosis. The skilled use of the mental status examination, psychological and neuropsychological tests, and laboratory evaluations will help to differentiate medical from psychiatric problems or to identify the relationship between the two. DSM-IV provides a framework, albeit not perfect, for considering psychiatric diagnosis in the differential diagnosis of many patient problems. Chapter 2 discusses basic aspects of the psychosocial and psychodynamic assessment. Other chapters will discuss the major psychiatric diagnostic categories in more detail, including specific issues relevant to clinical diagnosis and treatment.

CLINICAL PEARLS

- The principles of psychiatric assessment are identical to those of physical disorder assessment. Symptoms are elicited and signs are reviewed. Differential diagnosis is carried out using all available evidence including laboratory and X-ray findings.
- Medical patients will usually accept psychiatric assessment when it is explained as part of a comprehensive assessment of the role of physical and stress factors influencing their symptoms.
- Because psychiatric symptoms are many times colored by subjective factors, the extra effort to interview the patient's family and friends often pays off in more accurate assessment.
- Thyroid function abnormalities are a common medical cause of psychiatric symptoms.
- The setting of a patient encounter will influence the types of common psychopathology. However, mood disorders, anxiety disorders, and alcohol/drug disorders are commonly found in all settings.
- All mental status examination reports should indicate whether homicidal or suicidal ideation present.
- When a patient is unable to relate an understandable history, consider cognitive impairment disorder and psychiatric disorders associated with thought disorder such as schizophrenia or bipolar disorder.
- An EEG may be helpful when there is a question of whether a patient's symptoms are due to brain dysfunction or a functional psychiatric disorder.
- Presenting an extensive five-axis formulation will provide the major aspects of a biopsychosocial assessment.
- New psychiatric symptoms in a geriatric patient should trigger a vigorous search for mental disorders due to medical, neurologic, toxic, or medication-related factors.

ANNOTATED BIBLIOGRAPHY

American Psychiatric Association: Diagnostic and Statistical Manual of Mental Disorders, 4th ed. Washington, DC, American Psychiatric Association, 1994

> Contains diagnostic criteria for over 200 defined psychiatric diagnoses. Also includes information about age of onset, predisposing factors, prevalence, sex ratios, and differential diagnosis for each disorder.

Berg R, Franzen M, Wedding D: Screening for Brain Impairment. New York, Springer-Verlag, 1987

> Excellent summary of neuropsychological tests that have relevance for evaluation of psychiatric patients. Gives historical information about individual tests and reviews briefer neuropsychological screening batteries.

Frances AJ, First MB, Widiger TA, et al: An A to Z guide to DSM-IV conundrums. J Abnormal Psychol 100:407–412, 1991

> This article outlines the changes in DSM-IV.

Goodwin DW, Guze SB: Psychiatric Diagnosis, 5th ed., New York, Oxford University Press, 1996.

> Reviews essentials of diagnosis for major psychiatric disorders and provides summary of clinical validation for each disorder, including epidemiology, natural history, and family studies.

Kaufman D: Clinical Neurology for Psychiatrists. New York, Grune & Stratton, 1987

> For students interested in details of the neurological exam as applied to psychiatric patients, this is a practical and lucid guide.

MacKinnon RA, Yudofsky SC (eds): The Psychiatric Evaluation in Clinical Practice. Philadelphia, JB Lippincott, 1986

> This book provides an authoritative and well-written discussion of the psychiatric interview and history from a psychodynamic perspective. It also provides excellent discussions of the mental status examination and other aspects of the neuropsychiatric evaluation.

Mesulam M (ed): Principles of Behavioral Neurology. Philadelphia, FA Davis, 1985

> This is a splendid presentation of the basic science and clinical application of behavioral neurology with a strong emphasis on neuropsychiatric assessment.

van Riezan H, Segal M: Comparative Evaluation of Rating Scales for Clinical Psychopharmacology. Amsterdam, Elsevier, 1988

> Extensive review of psychiatric rating scales used for research and clinical purposes. Includes information on how to obtain scales and copyright considerations.

REFERENCES

American Psychiatric Association: Diagnostic and Statistical Manual of Mental Disorders, 4th ed. Washington, DC, American Psychiatric Association, 1994

Baron M: Behavioral genetics. In Stoudemire A. (ed): Human Behavior: An Introduction for Medical Students, 2nd ed. Philadelphia, J. B. Lippincott Company, 1994

Bates B, Bickley LS, Hoekelman RA. A Guide to Physical Examination and History Taking, 6th ed., New York, Lippincott–Raven Publishers, 1995

Berg R, Franzen M, Wedding D: Screening for Brain Impairment. New York, Springer-Verlag, 1987

Chandler JD, Gerndt JE: The role of medical evaluation in psychiatric inpatients. Psychosomatics 29:410–416, 1988

Colligan RC, Osborne D, Swenson WM, Offord KP: The MMPI: A Contemporary Normative Study. New York, Praeger, 1983

Elstein AS, Shulman LS, Sprafka SA: Medical Problem Solving: An Analysis of Clinical Reasoning. Cambridge, MA, Harvard University Press, 1978

Feighner JP, Robins E, Guze SB, et al: Diagnostic criteria for use in psychiatric research. Arch Gen Psychiatry 26:57–63, 1972

Fink PJ: Response to the presidential address: Is "biopsychosocial" the psychiatric shibboleth? Arch Gen Psychiatry 145:1061–1067, 1988

Folstein MF, Folstein SE, McHugh PR: "Mini-Mental State": A practical method for grading the cognitive state of patients for the clinician. J Psychiatr Res 12:189–198, 1975

Hall RCW, Gardiner ER, Stickney SK, et al: Physical illness manifesting as psychiatric disease: II. Analysis of a state hospital inpatient population. Arch Gen Psychiatry 35:989–995, 1980

Hampton JR, Harrison MJG, Mitchell JRA, et al: Relative contributions of history-taking, physical examination, and laboratory investigation to diagnosis and management of medical outpatients. Br Med J 2:486–489, 1975

Hoffman RS: Diagnostic errors in the evaluation of behavioral disorders. JAMA 248:964–967, 1982

Kathol RG, Mutgi A, Williams J, Clamon G, Noyes R: Diagnosis of major depression in cancer patients according to four sets of criteria. Am J Psychiatry 147:1021–1024, 1990

Koranyi EK: Somatic illness in psychiatric patients. Psychosomatics 21:887–891, 1980

Krummel S, Kathol RG: What you should know about physical evaluations in psychiatric patients: Results of a survey. Gen Hosp Psychiatry 9:275–279, 1987

LaBruzza AL: Physical illness presenting as psychiatric disorder: Guidelines for differential diagnosis. J Operational Psychiatry 12:24–31, 1981

Osborne D: The MMPI in medical practice. Psychiatr Ann 15:534–541, 1985

Olfson M: Utilization of neuropsychotic diagnostic tests for general hospital psychiatry patients with mental disorders. Am J Psychiatry 149:1711–1717, 1992

Regier DA, Goldberg ID, Taube CA: The de facto U.S. mental health system. Arch Gen Psychiatry 35:685–693, 1978

Reich J: Personality disorders in primary care. In Yates WR (ed): Primary Care Clinics—Psychiatry Issue, Vol 14. Philadelphia, WB Saunders, 1987

Robins E, Guze SB: Establishment of diagnostic validity in psychiatric illness: Its application to schizophrenia. Am J Psychiatry 126:983–987, 1970

Rosenhan DL: On being sane in insane places. Science 179:250–258, 1979

Spitzer RL, Endicott J, Robins E: Research diagnostic criteria. Rationale and reliability. Arch Gen Psychiatry 35:773–782, 1978

Stoudemire A: Somatothymia: Part I. Psychosomatics 32:365–370, 1991a

Stoudemire A: Somatothymia: Part II. Psychosomatics 32:371–381, 1991b

Stoudemire A (ed): Human Behavior: An Introduction for Medical Students, 2nd ed. Philadelphia, JB Lippincott, 1994

Taylor MA, Sierles FS, Abrams R: The neuropsychiatric evaluation. In Hales RE, Yudofsky SC: Textbook of Neuropsychiatry. Washington, DC, American Psychiatric Press, 1987

van Riezen H, Segal M: Comparative Evaluation of Rating Scales for Clinical Psychopharmacology. Amsterdam, Elsevier, 1988

Appendix to Chapter One

DSM-IV Classification *

NOS = Not Otherwise Specified.

An *x* appearing in a diagnostic code indicates that a specific code number is required.

An ellipsis (. . .) is used in the names of certain disorders to indicate that the name of a specific mental disorder or general medical condition should be inserted when recording the name (e.g., 293.0 Delirium Due to Hypothyroidism).

Numbers in parentheses are page numbers.

If criteria are currently met, one of the following severity specifiers may be noted after the diagnosis:
  Mild
  Moderate
  Severe

If criteria are no longer met, one of the following specifiers may be noted:
  In Partial Remission
  In Full Remission
  Prior History

Disorders Usually First Diagnosed in Infancy, Childhood, or Adolescence

MENTAL RETARDATION
Note: *These are coded on Axis II.*
317   Mild Mental Retardation
318.0   Moderate Mental Retardation
318.1   Severe Mental Retardation
318.2   Profound Mental Retardation
319   Mental Retardation. Severity Unspecified

LEARNING DISORDERS
315.00   Reading Disorder
315.1   Mathematics Disorder

*Reprinted with permission from ASM-IV American Psychiatric Association. Washington, DC, 1994, 13–24, 32(GAF).

315.2 Disorder of Written Expression
315.9 Learning Disorder NOS

MOTOR SKILLS DISORDER
315.4 Developmental Coordination Disorder

COMMUNICATION DISORDERS
315.31 Expressive Language Disorder
315.31 Mixed Receptive-Expressive Language Disorder
315.39 Phonological Disorder
307.0 Stuttering
307.9 Communication Disorder NOS

PERVASIVE DEVELOPMENTAL DISORDERS
299.00 Autistic Disorder
299.80 Rett's Disorder
299.10 Childhood Disintegrative Disorder
299.80 Asperger's Disorder
299.80 Pervasive Developmental Disorder NOS

ATTENTION–DEFICIT AND DISRUPTIVE BEHAVIOR DISORDERS
314.xx Attention-Deficit/ Hyperactivity Disorder
.01 Combined Type
.00 Predominantly Inattentive Type
.01 Predominantly Hyperactive-Impulsive Type
314.9 Attention-Deficit/ Hyperactivity Disorder NOS
312.8 Conduct Disorder
Specify type: Childhood-Onset Type/Adolescent-Onset Type
313.81 Oppositional Defiant Disorder
312.9 Disruptive Behavior Disorder NOS

FEEDING AND EATING DISORDERS OF INFANCY OR EARLY CHILDHOOD
307.52 Pica
307.53 Rumination Disorder
307.59 Feeding Disorder of Infancy or Early Childhood

TIC DISORDERS
307.23 Tourette's Disorder
307.22 Chronic Motor or Vocal Tic Disorder
307.21 Transient Tic Disorder
Specify if: Single Episode/ Recurrent
307.20 Tic Disorder NOS

ELIMINATION DISORDERS
——.– Encopresis
787.6 With Constipation and Overflow Incontinence
307.7 Without Constipation and Overflow Incontinence
307.6 Enuresis (Not Due to a General Medical Condition)
Specify type: Nocturnal Only/Diurnal Only/Nocturnal and Diurnal

OTHER DISORDERS OF INFANCY, CHILDHOOD, OR ADOLESCENCE
309.21 Separation Anxiety Disorder
Specify if: Early Onset
313.23 Selective Mutism
313.89 Reactive Attachment Disorder of Infancy or Early Childhood
Specify type: Inhibited Type/ Disinhibited Type
307.3 Stereotypic Movement Disorder
Specify if: With Self-Injurious Behavior
313.9 Disorder of Infancy, Childhood, or Adolescence NOS

Delirium, Dementia, and Amnestic and Other Cognitive Disorders

DELIRIUM

293.0   Delirium Due to . . . *[Indicate the General Medical Condition]*

——.–   Substance Intoxication Delirium *(refer to Substance-Related Disorders for substance-specific codes)*

——.–   Substance Withdrawal Delirium *(refer to Substance-Related Disorders for substance-specific codes)*

——.–   Delirium Due to Multiple Etiologies *(code each of the specific etiologies)*

780.09   Delirium NOS

DEMENTIA

290.xx   Dementia of the Alzheimer's Type, With Early Onset *(also code 331.0 Alzheimer's disease on Axis III)*

.10   Uncomplicated
.11   With Delirium
.12   With Delusions
.13   With Depressed Mood
Specify if: With Behavioral Disturbance

290.xx   Dementia of the Alzheimer's Type, With Late Onset *(also code 331.0 Alzheimer's disease on Axis III)*

.0   Uncomplicated
.3   With Delirium
.20   With Delusions
.21   With Depressed Mood
Specify if: With Behavioral Disturbance

290.xx   Vascular Dementia
.40   Uncomplicated
.41   With Delirium
.42   With Delusions
.43   With Depressed Mood
Specify if: With Behavioral Disturbance

294.9   Dementia Due to HIV Disease *(also code 043.1 HIV infection affecting central nervous system on Axis III)*

294.1   Dementia Due to Head Trauma *(also code 854.00 head injury on Axis III)*

294.1   Dementia Due to Parkinson's Disease *(also code 332.0 Parkinson's disease on Axis III)*

294.1   Dementia Due to Huntington's Disease *(also code 333.4 Huntington's disease on Axis III)*

290.10   Dementia Due to Pick's Disease *(also code 331.1 Pick's disease on Axis III)*

290.10   Dementia Due to Creutzfeldt-Jakob Disease *(also code 046.1 Creutzfeldt-Jakob disease on Axis III)*

294.1   Dementia Due to . . . *[Indicate the General Medical Condition not listed above] (also code the general medical condition on Axis III)*

——.–   Substance-Induced Persisting Dementia *(refer to Substance-Related Disorders for substance-specific codes)*

——.–   Dementia Due to Multiple Etiologies *(code each of the specific etiologies)*

294.8   Dementia NOS

AMNESTIC DISORDERS

294.0   Amnestic Disorder Due to. . .
        *[Indicate the General Med-
        ical Condition]*
        Specify if: Transient/Chronic

——.—   Substance-Induced Persist-
        ing Amnestic Disorder *(refer
        to Substance-Related Disor-
        ders for substance-specific
        codes)*

294.8   Amnestic Disorder NOS

OTHER COGNITIVE DISORDERS

294.9   Cognitive Disorder NOS

Mental Disorders Due to a General Medical Condition Not Elsewhere Classified

293.89 Catatonic Disorder Due to . . .
        *[Indicate the General Med-
        ical Condition]*

310.1   Personality Change Due
        to . . . *[Indicate the General
        Medical Condition]*
        Specify type: Labile Type/
        Disinhibited Type/Aggressive Type/
        Apathetic Type/Paranoid Type/
        Other Type/Combined Type/
        Unspecified Type

293.9   Mental Disorder NOS Due
        to. . . *[Indicate the General
        Medical Condition]*

Substance-Related Disorders

[a] *The following specifiers may be
applied to Substance Dependence:*
   With Physiological Dependence/Without
     Physiological Dependence
   Early Full Remission/Early Partial Remis-
     sion
   Sustained Full Remission/Sustained Partial
     Remission
   On Agonist Therapy/In a Controlled Envi-
     ronment

*The following specifiers apply to
Substance-Induced Disorders as noted:*
[I]With Onset During Intoxication/[W]With
   Onset During Withdrawal

ALCOHOL-RELATED DISORDERS

Alcohol Use Disorders

303.90 Alcohol Dependence[a]
305.00 Alcohol Abuse

Alcohol-Induced Disorders

303.00 Alcohol Intoxication
291.8   Alcohol Withdrawal
        Specify if: With Perceptual Distur-
        bances
291.0   Alcohol Intoxication Delir-
        ium
291.0   Alcohol Withdrawal Delir-
        ium
291.2   Alcohol-Induced Persisting
        Dementia
291.1   Alcohol-Induced Persisting
        Amnestic Disorder
291.x   Alcohol-Induced Psychotic
        Disorder
   .5   With Delusions[I,W]
   .3   With Hallucinations[I,W]
291.8   Alcohol-Induced Mood Dis-
        order[I,W]
291.8   Alcohol-Induced Anxiety
        Disorder[I,W]
291.8   Alcohol-Induced Sexual Dys-
        function[I]
291.8   Alcohol-Induced Sleep Dis-
        order[I,W]
291.9   Alcohol-Related Disorder
        NOS

AMPHETAMINE (OR AMPHETAMINE-LIKE)– RELATED DISORDERS

Amphetamine Use Disorders

304.40 Amphetamine Dependence[a]
305.70 Amphetamine Abuse

Amphetamine-Induced Disorders

292.89 Amphetamine Intoxication
Specify if: With Perceptual Disturbances

292.0 Amphetamine Withdrawal

292.81 Amphetamine Intoxication Delirium

292.xx Amphetamine-Induced Psychotic Disorder

.11 With Delusions[I]

.12 With Hallucinations[I]

292.84 Amphetamine-Induced Mood Disorder[I,W]

292.89 Amphetamine-Induced Anxiety Disorder[I]

292.89 Amphetamine-Induced Sexual Dysfunction[I]

292.89 Amphetamine-Induced Sleep Disorder[I,W]

292.9 Amphetamine-Related Disorder NOS

CAFFEINE-RELATED DISORDERS

Caffeine-Induced Disorders

305.90 Caffeine Intoxication

292.89 Caffeine-Induced Anxiety Disorder[I]

292.89 Caffeine-Induced Sleep Disorder[I]

292.9 Caffeine-Related Disorder NOS

CANNABIS-RELATED DISORDERS

Cannabis Use Disorders

304.30 Cannabis Dependence[a]

305.20 Cannabis Abuse

Cannabis-Induced Disorders

292.89 Cannabis Intoxication
Specify if: With Perceptual Disturbances

292.81 Cannabis Intoxication Delirium

292.xx Cannabis-Induced Psychotic Disorder

.11 With Delusions[I]

.12 With Hallucinations[I]

292.89 Cannabis-Induced Anxiety Disorder[I]

292.9 Cannabis-Related Disorder NOS

COCAINE-RELATED DISORDERS

Cocaine Use Disorders

304.20 Cocaine Dependence[a]

305.60 Cocaine Abuse

Cocaine-Induced Disorders

292.89 Cocaine Intoxication
Specify if: With Perceptual Disturbances

292.0 Cocaine Withdrawal

292.81 Cocaine Intoxication Delirium

292.xx Cocaine-Induced Psychotic Disorder

.11 With Delusions[I]

.12 With Hallucinations[I]

292.84 Cocaine-Induced Mood Disorder[I,W]

292.89 Cocaine-Induced Anxiety Disorder[I,W]

292.89 Cocaine-Induced Sexual Dysfunction[I]

292.89 Cocaine-Induced Sleep Disorder[I,W]

292.9 Cocaine-Related Disorder NOS

HALLUCINOGEN-RELATED DISORDERS

Hallucinogen Use Disorders

304.50 Hallucinogen Dependence[a]

305.30 Hallucinogen Abuse

Hallucinogen-Induced Disorders

292.89 Hallucinogen Intoxication

292.89 Hallucinogen Persisting Perception Disorder (Flashbacks)

292.81   Hallucinogen Intoxication
Delirium

292.xx   Hallucinogen-Induced Psychotic Disorder

.11   With Delusions[I]

.12   With Hallucinations[I]

292.84   Hallucinogen-Induced Mood
Disorder[I]

292.89   Hallucinogen-Induced Anxiety Disorder[I]

292.9   Hallucinogen-Related Disorder NOS

INHALANT-RELATED DISORDERS

Inhalant Use Disorders

304.60   Inhalant Dependence[a]

305.90   Inhalant Abuse

Inhalant-Induced Disorders

292.89   Inhalant Intoxication

292.81   Inhalant Intoxication Delirium

292.82   Inhalant-Induced Persisting
Dementia

292.xx   Inhalant-Induced Psychotic
Disorder

.11   With Delusions[I]

.12   With Hallucinations[I]

292.84   Inhalant-Induced Mood Disorder[I]

292.89   Inhalant-Induced Anxiety
Disorder[I]

292.9   Inhalant-Related Disorder
NOS

NICOTINE-RELATED DISORDERS

Nicotine Use Disorder

305.10   Nicotine Dependence[a]

Nicotine-Induced Disorder

292.0   Nicotine Withdrawal

292.9   Nicotine-Related Disorder
NOS

OPIOID-RELATED DISORDERS

Opioid Use Disorders

304.00   Opioid Dependence[a]

305.50   Opioid Abuse

Opioid-Induced Disorders

292.89   Opioid Intoxication
Specify if: With Perceptual Disturbances

292.0   Opioid Withdrawal

292.81   Opioid Intoxication
Delirium

292.xx   Opioid-Induced Psychotic
Disorder

.11   With Delusions[I]

.12   With Hallucinations[I]

292.84   Opioid-Induced Mood Disorder[I]

292.89   Opioid-Induced Sexual Dysfunction[I]

292.89   Opioid-Induced Sleep Disorder[I,W]

292.9   Opioid-Related Disorder
NOS

PHENCYCLIDINE (OR PHENCYCLIDINE-LIKE)–RELATED DISORDERS

Phencyclidine Use Disorders

304.90   Phencyclidine Dependence[a]

305.90   Phencyclidine Abuse

Phencyclidine-Induced Disorders

292.89   Phencyclidine Intoxication
Specify if: With Perceptual Disturbances

292.81   Phencyclidine Intoxication
Delirium

292.xx   Phencyclidine-Induced Psychotic Disorder

.11   With Delusions[I]

.12   With Hallucinations[I]

292.84   Phencyclidine-Induced Mood
Disorder[I]

292.89 Phencyclidine-Induced Anxiety Disorder[I]

292.9 Phencyclidine-Related Disorder NOS

SEDATIVE-, HYPNOTIC-, OR ANXIOLYTIC-RELATED DISORDERS

Sedative, Hypnotic, or Anxiolytic Use Disorders

304.10 Sedative, Hypnotic, or Anxiolytic Dependence[a]

305.40 Sedative, Hypnotic, or Anxiolytic Abuse

Sedative-, Hypnotic-, or Anxiolytic-Induced Disorders

292.89 Sedative, Hypnotic, or Anxiolytic Intoxication

292.0 Sedative, Hypnotic, or Anxiolytic Withdrawal
Specify if: With Perceptual Disturbances

292.81 Sedative, Hypnotic, or Anxiolytic Intoxication Delirium

292.81 Sedative, Hypnotic, or Anxiolytic Withdrawal Delirium

292.82 Sedative-, Hypnotic-, or Anxiolytic-Induced Persisting Dementia

292.83 Sedative-, Hypnotic-, or Anxiolytic-Induced Persisting Amnestic Disorder

292.xx Sedative-, Hypnotic-, or Anxiolytic-Induced Psychotic Disorder
  .11   With Delusions[I,W]
  .12   With Hallucinations[I,W]

292.84 Sedative-, Hypnotic-, or Anxiolytic-Induced Mood Disorder[I,W]

292.89 Sedative-, Hypnotic-, or Anxiolytic-Induced Anxiety Disorder[W]

292.89 Sedative, Hypnotic, or Anxiolytic-Induced Sexual Dysfunction[I]

292.89 Sedative-, Hypnotic-, or Anxiolytic-Induced Sleep Disorder[I,W]

292.9 Sedative-, Hypnotic-, or Anxiolytic-Related Disorder NOS

POLYSUBSTANCE-RELATED DISORDER

304.80 Polysubstance Dependence[a]

OTHER (OR UNKNOWN) SUBSTANCE-RELATED DISORDERS

Other (or Unknown) Substance Use Disorders

304.90 Other (or Unknown) Substance Dependence[a]

305.90 Other (or Unknown) Substance Abuse

Other (or Unknown) Substance-Induced Disorders

292.89 Other (or Unknown) Substance Intoxication
Specify if: With Perceptual Disturbances

292.0 Other (or Unknown) Substance Withdrawal
Specify if: With Perceptual Disturbances

292.81 Other (or Unknown) Substance-Induced Delirium

292.82 Other (or Unknown) Substance-Induced Persisting Dementia

292.83 Other (or Unknown) Substance-Induced Persisting Amnestic Disorder

292.xx   Other (or Unknown) Substance-Induced Psychotic Disorder
.11   With Delusions[I,W]
.12   With Hallucinations[I,W]
292.84   Other (or Unknown) Substance-Induced Mood Disorder[I,W]
292.89   Other (or Unknown) Substance-Induced Anxiety Disorder[I,W]
292.89   Other (or Unknown) Substance-Induced Sexual Dysfunction[I]
292.89   Other (or Unknown) Substance-Induced Sleep Disorder[I,W]
292.9   Other (or Unknown) Substance-Related Disorder NOS

Schizophrenia and Other Psychotic Disorders

295.xx   Schizophrenia

The following Classification of Longitudinal Course applies to all subtypes of Schizophrenia:

Episodic With Interepisode Residual Symptoms (*specify if:* With Prominent Negative Symptoms)/Episodic With No Interepisode Residual Symptoms
Continuous (*specify if:* With Prominent Negative Symptoms)
Single Episode in Partial Remission (*specify if:* With Prominent Negative Symptoms)/Single Episode In Full Remission
Other or Unspecified Pattern

.30   Paranoid Type
.10   Disorganized Type
.20   Catatonic Type
.90   Undifferentiated Type
.60   Residual Type

295.40   Schizophreniform Disorder
         Specify if: Without Good Prognostic Features/With Good Prognostic Features
295.70   Schizoaffective Disorder
         Specify type: Bipolar Type/Depressive Type
297.1   Delusional Disorder
         Specify type: Erotomanic Type/Grandiose Type/Jealous Type/Persecutory Type/Somatic Type/Mixed Type/Unspecified Type
298.8   Brief Psychotic Disorder
         Specify if: With Marked Stressor(s)/Without Marked Stressor(s)/With Postpartum Onset
297.3   Shared Psychotic Disorder
293.xx   Psychotic Disorder Due to ... *[Indicate the General Medical Condition]*
.81   With Delusions
.82   With Hallucinations
——.–   Substance-Induced Psychotic Disorder (*refer to Substance-Related Disorders for substance-specific codes*)
         Specify if: With Onset During Intoxication/ With Onset During Withdrawal
298.9   Psychotic Disorder NOS

Mood Disorders

Code current state of Major Depressive Disorder or Bipolar I Disorder in fifth digit:
1 = Mild
2 = Moderate
3 = Severe, Without Psychotic Features
4 = Severe, With Psychotic Features
   Specify: Mood-Congruent Psychotic Features/Mood-Incongruent Psychotic Features
5 = In Partial Remission
6 = In Full Remission
0 = Unspecified

The following specifiers apply (for current or most recent episode) to Mood Disorders as noted:

[a]Severity/Psychotic/Remission Specifiers/[b]Chronic/[c]With Catatonic Feature/[d]With Melancholic Features/[e]With Atypical Features/[f]With Postpartum Onset

The following specifiers apply to Mood Disorders as noted:

[g]With or Without Full Interepisode Recovery/ [h]With Seasonal Pattern/ [i]With Rapid Cycling

DEPRESSIVE DISORDERS

296.xx   Major Depressive Disorder
  .2x   Single Episode[a,b,c,d,e,f]
  .3x   Recurrent[a,b,c,d,e,f,g,h]
300.4   Dysthymic Disorder
          Specify if: Early Onset/Late Onset
          Specify: With Atypical Features
311   Depressive Disorder NOS

BIPOLAR DISORDERS

296.xx   Bipolar I Disorder
  .0x   Single Manic Episode[a,c,f]
          Specify if: Mixed
  .40   Most Recent Episode
            Hypomanic[g,h,i]
  .4x   Most Recent Episode
            Manic[a,c,f,g,h,i]
  .6x   Most Recent Episode
            Mixed[a,c,f,g,h,i]
  .5x   Most Recent Episode
            Depressed[a,b,c,d,e,f,g,h,i]
  .7   Most Recent Episode
            Unspecified[g,h,i]
296.89   Bipolar II Disorder[a,b,c,d,e,f,g,h,i]
          Specify (current or most recent episode): Hypomanic/Depressed
301.13   Cyclothymic Disorder
296.80   Bipolar Disorder NOS
293.83   Mood Disorder Due to. . .
          [Indicate the General Medical Condition]

Specify type: With Depressive Features/With Major Depressive-Like Episode/With Manic Features/With Mixed Features

——.—   Substance-Induced Mood Disorder *(refer to Substance-Related Disorders for substance-specific codes)*
          Specify type: With Depressive Features/With Manic Features/ With Mixed Features
          Specify if: With Onset During Intoxication/With Onset During Withdrawal
296.90   Mood Disorder NOS

Anxiety Disorders

300.01   Panic Disorder Without Agoraphobia
300.21   Panic Disorder With Agoraphobia
300.22   Agoraphobia Without History of Panic Disorder
300.29   Specific Phobia
          Specify type: Animal Type/Natural Environment Type/Blood-Injection-Injury Type/Situational Type/ Other Type
300.23   Social Phobia
          Specify if: Generalized
300.3   Obsessive-Compulsive Disorder
          Specify if: With Poor Insight
309.81   Posttraumatic Stress Disorder
          Specify if: Acute/Chronic
          Specify if: With Delayed Onset
308.3   Acute Stress Disorder
300.02   Generalized Anxiety Disorder
293.89   Anxiety Disorder Due to. . . *[Indicate the General Medical Condition]*

Specify if: With Generalized Anxiety/With Panic Attacks/With Obsessive-Compulsive Symptoms

——.– Substance-Induced Anxiety Disorder *(refer to Substance-Related Disorders for substance-specific codes)*
Specify if: With Generalized Anxiety/With Panic Attacks/With Obsessive-Compulsive Symptoms/With Phobic Symptoms
Specify if: With Onset During Intoxication/ With Onset During Withdrawal

300.00 Anxiety Disorder NOS

Somatoform Disorders

300.81 Somatization Disorder
300.81 Undifferentiated Somatoform Disorder
300.11 Conversion Disorder
Specify type: With Motor Symptom or Deficit/With Sensory Symptom or Deficit/With Seizures or Convulsions/ With Mixed Presentation
307.xx Pain Disorder
    .80 Associated With Psychological Factors
    .89 Associated With Both Psychological Factors and a General Medical Condition
Specify if: Acute/Chronic
300.7 Hypochondriasis
Specify if: With Poor Insight
300.7 Body Dysmorphic Disorder
300.81 Somatoform Disorder NOS

Factitious Disorders

300.xx Factitious Disorder
    .16 With Predominantly Psychological Signs and Symptoms

.19 With Predominantly Physical Signs and Symptoms
.19 With Combined Psychological and Physical Signs and Symptoms
300.19 Factitious Disorder NOS

Dissociative Disorders

300.12 Dissociative Amnesia
300.13 Dissociative Fugue
300.14 Dissociative Identity Disorder
300.6 Depersonalization Disorder
300.15 Dissociative Disorder NOS

Sexual and Gender Identity Disorders

SEXUAL DYSFUNCTIONS
The following specifiers apply to all primary Sexual Dysfunctions:
Lifelong Type/Acquired Type
Generalized Type/Situational Type
Due to Psychological Factors/Due to Combined Factors

Sexual Desire Disorders
302.71 Hypoactive Sexual Desire Disorder
302.79 Sexual Aversion Disorder

Sexual Arousal Disorders
302.72 Female Sexual Arousal Disorder
302.72 Male Erectile Disorder

Orgasmic Disorders
302.73 Female Orgasmic Disorder
302.74 Male Orgasmic Disorder
302.75 Premature Ejaculation

Sexual Pain Disorders

302.76　Dyspareunia (Not Due to a General Medical Condition)

306.51　Vaginismus (Not Due to a General Medical Condition)

Sexual Dysfunction Due to a General Medical Condition

625.8　Female Hypoactive Sexual Desire Disorder Due to. . . *[Indicate the General Medical Condition]*

608.89　Male Hypoactive Sexual Desire Disorder Due to. . . *[Indicate the General Medical Condition]*

607.84　Male Erectile Disorder Due to. . . *[Indicate the General Medical Condition]*

625.0　Female Dyspareunia Due to. . . *[Indicate the General Medical Condition]*

608.89　Male Dyspareunia Due to. . . *[Indicate the General Medical Condition]*

625.8　Other Female Sexual Dysfunction Due to. . . *[Indicate the General Medical Condition]*

608.89　Other Male Sexual Dysfunction Due to. . . *[Indicate the General Medical Condition]*

——.–　Substance-Induced Sexual Dysfunction *(refer to Substance-Related Disorders for substance-specific codes)*
Specify if: With Impaired Desire/ With Impaired Arousal/With Impaired Orgasm/With Sexual Pain
Specify if: With Onset During Intoxication

302.70　Sexual Dysfunction NOS

PARAPHILIAS

302.4　Exhibitionism

302.81　Fetishism

302.89　Frotteurism

302.2　Pedophilia
Specify if: Sexually Attracted to Males/Sexually Attracted to Females/Sexually Attracted to Both
Specify if: Limited to Incest
Specify if: Exclusive Type/ Nonexclusive Type

302.83　Sexual Masochism

302.84　Sexual Sadism

302.3　Transvestic Fetishism
Specfiy if: With Gender Dysphoria

302.82　Voyeurism

302.9　Paraphilia NOS

GENDER IDENTITY DISORDERS

302.xx　Gender Identity Disorder

　.6　　　in Children

　.85　　in Adolescents and Adults
Specify if: Sexually Attracted to Males/ Sexually Attracted to Females/Sexually Attracted to Both/Sexually Attracted to Neither

302.6　Gender Identity Disorder NOS

302.9　Sexual Disorder NOS

Eating Disorders

307.1　Anorexia Nervosa
Specify type: Restricting Type; Binge-Eating/Purging Type

307.51　Bulimia Nervosa
Specify type: Purying type/Nonpurging Type

307.50　Eating Disorder NOS

Sleep Disorders

PRIMARY SLEEP DISORDERS

Dyssomnias

307.42　Primary Insomnia

307.44　Primary Hypersomnia
Specify if: Recurrent

347   Narcolepsy
780.59   Breathing-Related Sleep Disorder
307.45   Circadian Rhythm Sleep Disorder
   Specify type: Delayed Sleep Phase Type/Jet Lag Type/Shift Work Type/Unspecified Type
307.47   Dyssomnia NOS

Parasomnias
307.47   Nightmare Disorder
307.46   Sleep Terror Disorder
307.46   Sleepwalking Disorder
307.47   Parasomnia NOS

SLEEP DISORDERS RELATED TO ANOTHER MENTAL DISORDER
307.42   Insomnia Related to . . . *[Indicate the Axis I or Axis II Disorder]*
307.44   Hypersomnia Related to. . . *[Indicate the Axis I or Axis II Disorder]*

OTHER SLEEP DISORDERS
780.xx   Sleep Disorder Due to. . . *[Indicate the General Medical Condition]*
   .52   Insomnia Type
   .54   Hypersomnia Type
   .59   Parasomnia Type
   .59   Mixed Type
——.–   Substance-Induced Sleep Disorder *(refer to Substance-Related Disorders for substance-specific codes)*
   Specify type: Insomnia Type/ Hypersomnia Type/Parasomnia Type/ Mixed Type
   Specify if: With Onset During Intoxication/With Onset During Withdrawal

Impulse-Control Disorders Not Elsewhere Classified

312.34   Intermittent Explosive Disorder
312.32   Kleptomania
312.33   Pyromania
312.31   Pathological Gambling
312.39   Trichotillomania
312.30   Impulse-Control Disorder NOS

Adjustment Disorders

309.xx   Adjustment Disorder
   .0   With Depressed Mood
   .24   With Anxiety
   .28   With Mixed Anxiety and Depressed Mood
   .3   With Disturbance of Conduct
   .4   With Mixed Disturbance of Emotions and Conduct
   .9   Unspecified
   Specify if: Acute Chronic

Personality Disorders

Note: *These are coded on Axis II.*
301.0   Paranoid Personality Disorder
301.20   Schizoid Personality Disorder
301.22   Schizotypal Personality Disorder
301.7   Antisocial Personality Disorder
301.83   Borderline Personality Disorder
301.50   Histrionic Personality Disorder
301.81   Narcissistic Personality Disorder

301.82 Avoidant Personality
Disorder

301.6 Dependent Personality
Disorder

301.4 Obsessive–Compulsive
Personality Disorder

301.9 Personality Disorder NOS

Other Conditions That May Be a Focus of Clinical Attention

PSYCHOLOGICAL FACTORS AFFECTING MEDICAL CONDITION

316 . . .*[Specified Psychological Factor]*
Affecting. . .*[Indicate the General Medical Condition]*
Choose name based on nature of factors:
Mental Disorder Affecting Medical Condition
Psychological Symptoms Affecting Medical Condition
Personality Traits or Coping Style Affecting Medical Condition
Maladaptive Health Behaviors Affecting Medical Condition
Stress-Related Physiological Response Affecting Medical Condition
Other or Unspecified Psychological Factors Affecting Medical Condition

MEDICATION-INDUCED MOVEMENT DISORDERS

332.1 Neuroleptic-Induced Parkinsonism

333.92 Neuroleptic Malignant Syndrome

333.7 Neuroleptic-Induced Acute Dystonia

333.99 Neuroleptic-Induced Acute Akathisia

333.82 Neuroleptic-Induced Tardive Dyskinesia

333.1 Medication-Induced Postural Tremor

333.90 Medication-Induced Movement Disorder NOS

OTHER MEDICATION-INDUCED DISORDER

995.2 Adverse Effects of Medication NOS

RELATIONAL PROBLEMS

V61.9 Relational Problem Related to a Mental Disorder or General Medical Condition

V61.20 Parent–Child Relational Problem

V61.1 Partner Relational Problem

V61.8 Sibling Relational Problem

V62.81 Relational Problem NOS

PROBLEMS RELATED TO ABUSE OR NEGLECT

V61.21 Physical Abuse of Child *(code 995.5 if focus of attention is on victim)*

V61.21 Sexual Abuse of Child *(code 995.5 if focus of attention is on victim)*

V61.21 Neglect of a Child *(code 995.5 if focus of attention is on victim)*

V61.1 Physical Abuse of Adult *(code 995.81 if focus of attention is on victim)*

V61.1   Sexual Abuse of Adult
         (code 995.81 if focus of
         attention is on victim)

**ADDITIONAL CONDITIONS
THAT MAY BE A FOCUS
OF CLINICAL ATTENTION**
V15.81 Noncompliance With Treatment
V65.2   Malingering
V71.01 Adult Antisocial Behavior
V71.02 Child or Adolescent Antisocial Behavior
V62.89 Borderline Intellectual Functioning
         Note: This is coded on Axis II.
780.9   Age-Related Cognitive Decline
V62.82 Bereavement
V62.3   Academic Problem
V62.2   Occupational Problem
313.82 Identity Problem
V62.89 Religious or Spiritual Problem
V62.4   Acculturation Problem
V62.89 Phase of Life Problem

Additional Codes

300.9   Unspecified Mental Disorder
         (nonpsychotic)
V71.09 No Diagnosis or Condition on
         Axis I
799.9   Diagnosis or Condition
         Deferred on Axis I
V71.09 No Diagnosis on Axis II
799.9   Diagnosis Deferred on Axis II

Multiaxial System

Axis I   Clinical Disorders
          Other Conditions That May
          Be a Focus of Clinical Attention
Axis II   Personality Disorders
          Mental Retardation
Axis III General Medical Conditions
Axis IV   Psychosocial and Environmental Problems
Axis V   Global Assessment of Functioning

Axis IV:
Psychosocial and Environmental Problems

Check:
_____ Problems with primary support group
_____ Problems related to the social environment
_____ Educational problems
_____ Occupational problems
_____ Housing problems
_____ Economic problems
_____ Problems with access to health care services
_____ Problems related to interaction with the legal system/crime
_____ Other psychosocial and environmental problems

Global Assessment of Functioning (GAF) Scale[1]

Consider psychological, social, and occupational functioning on a hypothetical continuum of mental health–illness. Do not include impairment in functioning due to physical (or environmental) limitations.

Code (**Note:** Use intermediate codes when appropriate, e.g., 45, 68, 72.)

100 | **Superior functioning in a wide range of activities, life's problems never seem to get out of hand, is sought out by others**
|
91 | **because of his or her many positive qualities. No symptoms.**

90 | **Absent or minimal symptoms** (e.g., mild anxiety before an exam),
| **good functioning in all areas, interested and involved in a wide**
| **range of activities, socially effective, generally satisfied with**
| **life, no more than everyday problems or concerns** (e.g., an occa-
81 | sional argument with family members).

80 | **If symptoms are present, they are transient and expectable**
| **reactions to psychosocial stressors** (e.g., difficulty concentrating
| after family argument); **no more than slight impairment in social,**
| **occupational, or school functioning** (e.g., temporarily falling
71 | behind in school work).

70 | **Some mild symptoms** (e.g., depressed mood and mild insomnia) **OR**
| **some difficulty in social, occupational, or school functioning**
| (e.g., occasional truancy, or theft within the household), **but gener-**
| **ally functioning pretty well, has some meaningful interpersonal**
61 | **relationships.**

60 | **Moderate symptoms** (e.g., flat affect and circumstantial speech,
| occasional panic attacks) **OR moderate difficulty in social, occu-**
| **pational, or school functioning** (e.g., friends, conflicts with peers
51 | or co-workers).

50 | **Serious symptoms** (e.g., suicidal ideation, severe obsessional rituals,
| frequent shoplifting) **OR any serious impairment in social, occu-**
| **pational, or school functioning** (e.g., no friends, unable to keep
41 | a job).

[1] The GAF Scale is a revision of the GAS (Endicott J, Spitzer RL, Fleiss, et al: The Global Assessment Scale: A procedure for measuring overall severity of psychiatric disturbance. *Archives of General Psychiatry* 33:766–771, 1976) and the CGAS [Shaffer D, Gould MS, Brasic J, et al: Children's Global Assessment Scale (CGAS). *Archives of General Psychiatry* 40:1228–1231, 1983]. These are revisions of the Global Scale of the Health-Sickness Rating Scale (Luborsky L: Clinicians' judgments of mental health. *Archives of General Psychiatry* 7:407–417, 1962).

40
     Some impairment in reality testing or communication (e.g., speech is at times illogical, obscure, or irrelevant) **OR major impairment in several areas, such as work or school, family relations, judgment, thinking, or mood** (e.g., depressed man avoids friends, neglects family, and is unable to work; child frequently beats up
31
     younger children, is defiant at home, and is failing at school).

30
     Behavior is considerably influenced by delusions or hallucinations OR serious impairment in communication or judgment (e.g., sometimes incoherent, acts grossly inappropriately, suicidal preoccupation) **OR inability to function in almost all areas** (e.g.,
21
     stays in bed all day; no job, home, or friends).

20
     Some danger of hurting self or others (e.g., suicide attempts without clear expectation of death, frequently violent, manic excitement) **OR occasionally fails to maintain minimal personal hygiene** (e.g., smears feces) **OR gross impairment in communication** (e.g.,
11
     largely incoherent or mute).

10
     Persistent danger of severely hurting self or others (e.g., recurrent violence) **OR persistent inability to maintain minimal personal hygiene OR serious suicidal act with clear expectation of**
1
     death.

0
     Inadequate information.

2 Biopsychosocial Assessment and Case Formulation

Alan Stoudemire and James L. Levenson

The preceding chapter focused on the basics of the psychiatric history, mental status examination, physical and laboratory assessment, and the *Diagnostic and Statistical Manual of Mental Disorders* (DSM-IV) as a descriptive psychiatric classification system. Based on the information gathered in this type of initial assessment, a preliminary diagnosis and treatment plan can be made. A more in-depth psychological evaluation, however, is then required. Examples of patients in whom an in-depth psychosocial assessment is called for include the following:

1. Patients who appear to have complex or problematic family, marital, or interpersonal problems.
2. Patients who appear to have *repetitive* patterns of conflicts or difficulties in their interpersonal relationships.
3. Individuals who appear to have psychiatric disorders and symptoms that are apparently precipitated or exacerbated by social, occupational, family, or interpersonal factors.
4. Patients who have unexplained somatic symptoms that cannot be explained on the basis of physical or laboratory findings.
5. Children and adolescents with psychiatric symptoms.

By emphasizing the importance of psychosocial assessment, one should not necessarily assume that such factors are the direct *cause* of the patient's psychiatric disorder. This may or may not be the case. The relative contribution of psychosocial factors in precipitating the onset or exacerbation of psychiatric disorders and symptoms varies, depending on the disorder being evaluated.

Moreover, the relative contribution of psychosocial factors to the cause of many psychiatric disorders remains highly controversial in the psychiatric literature. To take the position that psychosocial factors are important in the assessment of a patient who has a psychiatric disorder such as schizophrenia, however, is not the same as saying that schizophrenia is *caused by* psychosocial factors, because schizophrenia is now considered to derive primarily from predisposing genetic and biological factors. Nevertheless, few psychiatrists would argue against the position that psychosocial and environmental factors may be involved in relapses of schizophrenia or that schizophrenia has profound effects on the patient's social and interpersonal functioning. Likewise, vulnerability to panic disorder and the major mood disorders appears to be strongly determined by biological factors, yet for certain patients the symptoms may be precipitated or exacerbated under certain types of emotionally stressful conditions. *Hence, even though certain disorders may have a primarily genetic and biological basis in respect to their underlying pathophysiology, the disorder's onset and relapse may be affected by social or environmental factors in the biologically predisposed individual.* Even in physical disorders, acute and chronic medical illness always poses a form of stress for the individual that may potentially affect every aspect of their family, social, and occupational life. For example, cancer and chronic renal disease may have devastating effects on the patient's emotional and social functioning (Green, 1994). Psychological reactions to physical illness are discussed further in Chapters 9 and 20.

GOALS OF PSYCHOSOCIAL ASSESSMENT

The primary goals of a comprehensive psychosocial evaluation are to (1) assess whether psychological or social factors are important in contributing to the patient's vulnerability to psychiatric illness, (2) assess whether psychosocial factors are significant in causing relapse or exacerbation of symptoms, and (3) identify areas in the psychological or social realm where treatment efforts might be focused. In addition, such an assessment also will identify areas in the patient's support system that may be a resource. In patients who suffer primarily from repetitive problems in their interpersonal relationships or who have dysfunction within the family system, the psychosocial assessment may be the only means of fully understanding their condition and of planning an effective course of treatment.

PSYCHODYNAMIC ASSESSMENT

A *psychodynamic* assessment is a more specialized form of psychological evaluation that is usually performed by a psychiatrist who endorses and is trained in this method of evaluation. An in-depth psychodynamic assessment may be needed as part of the psychosocial assessment in some situations and involves examining the key developmental life experiences that may have affected the patient's personality formation, the nature of the patient's past and current family relationships, the patient's strengths and vulnerabilities, and the patient's characteristic psychological defense mechanisms. A psychodynamic assessment also evaluates current interpersonal stresses that may be affecting the patient and, therefore, overlap with the general psychosocial evaluation. Individuals and important environmental and family events that have influenced the patient in either a positive or negative manner are identified, and the effect they currently have or have had on the patient is evaluated. Psychodynamic assessment is often critical not only in developing a comprehensive understanding of the patient's personality and current difficulties, but also in determining whether or not psychotherapy is required, and, if so, what type of psychotherapy would be most appropriate.

Psychodynamic assessment is a form of evaluation somewhat more specialized than a general psychosocial assessment and is largely based on a psychoanalytic frame of reference. Psychodynamic assessment imparts major significance to developmental influences on the patient within the family system and potential unconscious factors that may be affecting the patient's behavior, motivations, and interpersonal relationships. Psychodynamic assessment thus focuses on the influence of early relationships on the patient's personality formation, the patient's ego defense mechanisms, and the effects that these early relationships have on their interpersonal relationships.

Some psychoanalytic and psychodynamic theorists have attempted to explain all psychiatric illness—including major disorders such as schizophrenia, major depression, and anxiety disorders—in their most doctrinaire form as deriving from intrapsychic and unconscious mental processes. Personality disorders and other disturbances in behavior also are explained primarily on a psychodynamic basis as deriving from abnormal or otherwise conflicted childhood developmental experiences and dysfunction within the family system.

Recent advances in biological psychiatry and psychopharmacology in some instances have almost completely usurped primarily psychoanalytic and psychodynamic viewpoints with respect to *etiological* explanations for the major mental disorders such as schizophrenia, major depression, and bipolar disorder. In addition, psychoanalytically oriented therapies for these disorders based on these types of purist etiological explanations have been under serious criticism. Although considerable polarization and strain exist within the field of psychiatry regarding the relative contribution of psychodynamic factors in the causation of the major psychiatric disorders, there has been a recent trend to attempt to integrate biological and psychological viewpoints regarding the etiology and treatment of psychiatric illness (Cooper, 1985; Kandel, 1979, 1983; Reiser, 1984; van der Kolk, 1998). In addition, it is recognized that the relative contribution of psychological and biological factors varies with the psychiatric disorder being studied and that even within a given disorder (such as major depression), considerable heterogeneity exists among patients who may carry the same primary diagnosis.

Further discussion of this area is beyond the scope of this text. It is the philosophy of this text that, given our limited knowledge of the precise cause of most psychiatric disorders, a balanced approach should be taken in patient evaluation: the possible contributions of biological, psychological, and sociological factors relevant to the patient's condition are always considered. In every case, however, a psychosocial assessment should be part of the patient's evaluation. If a detailed assessment of the patient's personality structure is indicated, this is often best performed by a psychoanalyst or psychodynamically oriented psychotherapist. The theoretical bases for such assessments are primarily based on psychoanalytic theory that is discussed in depth in the companion text (on human behavior) to this volume (Inderbitzen and James, 1998).

THE PRIMARY PHYSICIAN'S ROLE IN PSYCHOSOCIAL ASSESSMENT

It should be emphasized that a complete psychosocial assessment may be a complex and time-consuming process. In many cases, performing such an evaluation will exceed the skills and time of even the most psychologically minded physician. In such situations, it may be necessary to refer the patient to a psychiatrist for a more indepth assessment. Nevertheless, it is still the responsibility of the primary physician to gather certain basic information and to assess and identify patients who may need referral.

The responsibility of the primary physician to elicit basic psychosocial data in this situation has analogies in general medical practice. For example, a general internist will assess the signs and symptoms of a patient with chest pain and, after this initial assessment, might then refer the patient to a cardiologist for possible cardiac catheterization and definitive cardiologic diagnosis and treatment. The internist would hardly consider initiating such a referral without gathering the basic medical history and performing a physical examination. Similarly, gathering basic psychosocial information about the patient will ensure that patients in need of more specialized evaluation will be identified appropriately.

PSYCHOSOCIAL ASSESSMENT: BASIC APPROACHES

When the psychosocial assessment is conducted, several fundamental questions should be posed to the patient, and if adequate time is allowed for exploration of the patient's responses, an excellent initial data base can be assimilated by the primary physician (regarding the patient's general developmental history and current psychosocial status.) For example, the physician may ask questions directed toward determining the key events and important people in the patient's childhood, adolescence, and adulthood that appear to have had or continue to have an effect on the patient. Were there past traumas, losses, or problems within the family system, or difficulties in other childhood and adult relationships that had a major impact on the patient? Are there conflicted or unresolved relationships with family, friends, or significant other individuals that are a source of distress for the patient? Have there been particularly difficult times in the patient's life? What have been the patient's sources of happiness and satisfaction or unhappiness and frustration? Answers to open-ended questions of this sort will usually yield information that will form the rubric of a preliminary psychosocial and psychodynamic understanding of the patient. Patients who are guarded or who deny the significance or importance of psychological matters will require more extended psychiatric evaluations, or the physician will need to gather information from other sources such as family members.

PSYCHOSOCIAL STRESSES AND SOMATIC SYMPTOMS

Many patients under psychosocial stress in the general medical setting will present to their primary care physicians with somatic symptoms (insomnia, headaches, gastrointestinal distress). Somatic symptoms are also extremely common and may develop as a response to even minor stresses (e.g., tension headaches). Patients will also seek help in the medical sector for somatic symptoms that are part of a major depressive disorder long before the symptoms are recognized or considered as part of a primary psychiatric syndrome.

Somatothymia

Some patients have a limited capacity to describe their feelings verbally. This limitation in the ability to articulate and communicate feeling states in verbal language has been termed *somatothymia,* a term derived from the Greek meaning "a bodily state of feeling." Research in child development has shown that the fundamental "language" children use to communicate physical or emotional distress is in somatic or physical terms. It is only later in development that children begin to learn "feeling" words to label and verbally communicate internal emotional distress, fear, or alternatively, their affectionate feelings. In some individuals, because of cultural, educational, intellectual, familial, and psychological factors, the ability to articulate and communicate emotional states is never developed or is developed to a very limited degree. The multiple determinants of the capacity for emotional language have been discussed in detail elsewhere (Stoudemire, 1991a, b).

In some cultures, the *primary* means of communicating emotional distress remains based on the use of somatic language. The tendency to describe strong emotional reactions persists in our own culture ("the news just made me *sick*"; "he died of a *broken heart*"; "the news gave me great *pain*"; etc.). Hence, the capacity for directly communicating emotional distress in abstract "psychological" language varies from individual to individual and is subject to strong cultural and subcultural influences. The task of the physician is to learn the "emotional language" of the patient and to interpret it appropriately. For many patients, the language of emotion will continue to be predominantly based on somatic or physical words. The concept of somatothymia will also be mentioned in respect to the somatoform disorders in Chapter 9, as well as in the somatic presentations of depression in Chapter 7. Particularly in respect to depression, it should be noted that somatic symptoms are the principle way that disturbances in mood present in the medical setting.

Two Caveats

It should not, however, be assumed that all physical symptoms with a negative medical workup are "psychosomatic" or "stress related" in nature. Two caveats should always be kept in mind: first, symptoms of medical illness and stress/psychiatrically related symptoms may coexist and be enmeshed; hence, even if stress-related symptoms are identified as such, this does not rule out the possibility of concurrent medical illness. Second, stress and the presence of a concurrent psychiatric illness, such as depression, may greatly magnify the symptoms of clearly documented underlying physical illnesses.

BIOPSYCHOSOCIAL ASSESSMENT

The DSM-IV system discussed in Chapter 1 (see Chapter 1 Appendix) is used primarily for purposes of description and classification and is based on data that can be documented objectively. Integrating the descriptive approach of DSM-IV with a psychosocial and psychodynamic understanding of the patient, however, is useful in determining what types of psychiatric treatment would be most helpful for the patient, especially in determining the need for psychotherapy.

As mentioned in Chapter 1, the biopsychosocial model uses a systems approach in attempting to integrate biological, psychological, and social aspects of the patient's condition (Alexander, 1950; Bertalanffy, 1968; Cole and Levinson 1998; Engel, 1977; Fink, 1988; Meyer, 1957; Reiser, 1988). This approach inherently validates the potential importance of biogenetic, psychological, social, and environmental factors in the diagnosis and treatment of the patient.

The basic clinical principles of the type of biopsychosocially oriented case assessment of patients in medical *or* psychiatric settings presented in this text would take the following into consideration:

1. Genetic and biological factors are deemed to be of major importance in the pathogenesis and treatment of certain psychiatric disorders (such as schizophrenia and mood disorders) and also may play a part in determining the patient's resilience or vulnerability to stress.
2. Certain problematic developmental experiences and conflicted relationships within the family and social system may confer vulnerabilities to certain types of psychiatric illness; alternatively, positive developmental experiences and relationships and good social support may provide a buffering effect.
3. Current life stresses may precipitate the onset of certain psychiatric disorders and symptoms or contribute to relapses of preexisting conditions.

This chapter focuses on the practical clinical applications of these principles, and space does not permit a critical review of the overwhelming scientific evidence to support the biopsychosocial model. In the companion volume on human behavior for medical students, the scientific basis for the biopsychosocial model is discussed in depth, particularly by Cole and Levinson (1998). Students are referred to selected articles in the annotated bibliography and reference list and other chapters in the companion text on human behavior for substantiating information (Aneshensel and Stone, 1982; Bifulco et al, 1987; Birley and Brown, 1970; Bolton and Oatley, 1987; Breier et al, 1988; Bryer et al, 1987; Cadoret et al, 1985; Coyne, 1991; Dew et al, 1992; Doane et al, 1981; Galanter, 1988; Goldberg et al, 1990; Greenblatt et al, 1982; Harris et al, 1986, 1987; Kendler 1988; MacMillan, Gold, Crow et al, 1986; Miklowitz Goldstein, Neuchterlein et al, 1988; Miller et al, 1976; Parry and Shapiro, 1986; Pellegrini, 1990; Penkower et al, 1988; Romans et al, 1992; Roy, 1980; Rutter, 1985; Schwartz and Myers, 1977a, b; Stansfeld et al, 1991; Tennant, 1983, 1988; Tennant et al 1982; Tennant et al, 1982a, b; Tennant et al, 1981; Uhlenhuth and Paykel, 1973; van der Kolk, 1986, 1998; Weissman et al, 1987).

CLINICAL APPLICATIONS

Diagnosis and treatment using the biopsychosocial model are multimodal and are directed toward stabilizing each sphere of the patient's life that appears to be under stress—biological, psychological, and/or social. To reiterate, in this conceptual framework it is essential to (1) assess accurately the pertinent biological and physical factors associated with the patient's condition; (2) evaluate the effects of past and present environmental, social, and family stressors; and (3) appraise the psychological significance of the illness for the patient (e.g., how the patient experiences the illness in light of significant current and past life experiences).

The following prototypical case describes how the biopsychosocial model, the DSM-IV descriptive approach, and a psychosocial/psychodynamic formulation can be integrated into patient evaluation and comprehensive treatment planning.

CASE STUDY: MR. A

Mr. A, a 50-year-old married attorney, presented to his internist 4 weeks after successful coronary artery bypass surgery. He appeared to have deteriorated after his successful surgery, was chronically fatigued, had severe insomnia, had lost his appetite, and had lost interest in doing almost everything, including returning to work. Because of his inability to return to work, he was sinking into financial debt, and his position in his law firm was in jeopardy. Although he had little interest in sex, he did attempt intercourse with his wife several times, but was impotent.

The internist performed a complete medical evaluation and checked his laboratory profile. He was slightly hypokalemic because of the use of a thiazide diuretic. He was also taking high doses of the agent alpha-methyldopa (Aldomet) for hypertension. Other than being overweight and continuing to smoke two packs of cigarettes a day, his examination, including a screening thyroid profile, was unremarkable.

The internist assessed that the patient was primarily depressed, so he tapered and discontinued his propranolol (the physician knew the drug has been associated with inducing depression). He "reassured" the patient and prescribed a low dose of a cyclic antidepressant and a benzodiazepine sleeping medication and scheduled a follow-up appointment for 4 weeks.

Despite these measures, the patient continued to deteriorate. He began to have crying spells, guilty ruminations, and suicidal thoughts. He took his antidepressant inconsistently. He returned to the internist after a week, at his wife's insistence. The internist felt a psychiatric consultation was then necessary.

The psychiatrist evaluated the patient and, because the patient had recently had an extensive physical and laboratory evaluation, he decided to begin treatment with a cyclic antidepressant with incremental increases, no more than a week's supply at a time, because of the possibility of a suicidal overdose. Because the patient's wife could stay with him during the day and the patient denied any suicidal plans, the decision was made to treat him initially as an outpatient with twice-weekly visits.

Before deciding on this treatment plan, however, the psychiatrist first performed a full psychiatric history and mental status examination. The patient was found to be cognitively intact, and his symptoms were all consistent with the diagnosis of major depression. The patient's personality assessment revealed marked obsessive–compulsive traits in that he was a "workaholic," a perfectionist, driven to achieve, and rarely ever "relaxed." He was generally rigid and strict with his children and emotionally aloof. Although he loved and was devoted to his family, he had severe difficulty in directly expressing any affection or personal feelings toward them or other people. Although things had gone well for him professionally, he believed he was never totally happy and had a tendency to be chronically mildly depressed, dysphoric, and dissatisfied with himself and life in general. He never believed he had "done enough" professionally and always thought he had to prove himself to others, and he had doubts about his basic self-worth. He had marked difficulties in expressing not only affectionate feelings, but anger, as well. When angry, he would generally "bottle it up," become preoccupied with the person or situation he was angry with, and "stew" for days.

Exploration of his developmental history revealed that his mother was generally available to him, but she had periods of apparent depressive episodes that were disabling, and she would emotionally withdraw from the family. She had never sought or received professional treatment for these apparent depressive episodes. His father was emotionally remote, cold, critical, and "pushed" him to do well in school. Because of the pressure and criticism from his father (and the fact that he felt he had to "earn" his father's love and approval), he gradually became more distant from him, silently resenting him, and sometimes "wished he were dead."

His father died suddenly of a myocardial infarction at age 49 when the patient was 15. The patient described his father's death as traumatic, not only because of the loss of his father, but because he felt as if the anger and hostility he felt toward his father "had something to do with his death." Although he realized that this was not rationally possible, he nevertheless felt guilty about having been angry at his father and felt that he had to make it up to him "in some way." In addition, he felt that when his father died, he had forever lost the chance to be close to him.

The patient ultimately went on to finish high school and college and decided to become an attorney, similar to his father. The patient always had a fear of dying at an early age—of a heart attack, similar to his father—but nevertheless smoked, was over-weight, and did not exercise.

Based on the patient's chronic history of depression, the psychiatrist believed that, in addition to his antidepressant treatment, the patient could benefit from psychotherapy. The psychiatrist, who had a psychodynamic orientation, initially formulated the patient's case as follows: Part of the patient's problems with depression and low self-esteem were associated with problematic relationships with his parents. His mother's periodic depressions would, at times, make her unavailable to him when the patient needed support as a child, and he often interpreted her lack of interest and responsiveness as a sign of rejection. Moreover, his father was hypercritical and demanding, leaving the patient with feelings of worthlessness and guilt when he did not perfectly please his father, and he was frustrated by his inability to be emotionally close to him. In addition to this frustration, he was also resentful and angry and hated his father at times, although he also loved him and craved his attention and approval. When his father died, the patient was stricken with not only a sense of loss, but also remorse and guilt. His guilt centered on his hostility toward his father in that he may have unconsciously related his father's death to his hostile feelings and blamed himself for it.

Because both parents often were unavailable to him emotionally and because communication of feelings in the family was poor, he felt trapped with his loneliness and did not know to whom or how he could express his inner feelings. Because of his guilt and pattern of having to "achieve" and produce to maintain his self-esteem, he gradually became more engrossed in school and work. His compulsive work habits also served to help him avoid his inner feelings of mild depression and contributed to his compulsive personality traits. The patient nevertheless channeled his compulsive style and need for achievement into his work and did well academically and professionally. His marriage was generally stable, although his wife felt that he was always emotionally remote from her, neglected the family for his work, and could not express his feelings, repeating the pattern of his own father. He tended to be distant, hypercritical, and demanding of his own children. He had drifted further and further from both his wife and children.

The psychiatrist believed that the patient's own heart attack could have reactivated the memories and feelings associated with the grief surrounding his father's death. The patient may have identified with the father, and his own heart attack fulfilled his lifelong fear that he too would die at an early age. The psychiatrist also believed that the patient was genetically at high risk for depression because of his mother's probable history of depression and the patient's use of the antihypertensive agent alpha-methyldopa. Both of these factors may have contributed to his biological vulnerability to depression, as may have the acute stress of his coronary artery bypass surgery.

In the course of the patient's subsequent psychotherapy, the memories and feelings related to his childhood experiences were explored. The patient gained a new understanding of the impact that his father's death had on him and came to realize fully that his angry feelings toward his father were largely justified and had nothing to do with his father's death; thus, his sense of guilt, which had been largely unconscious, was relieved. He began to realize more fully how he was still trying to "earn" approval by way of work and achievement, a central conflict related to his need to be close to his father and earn his love.

Concurrent with his psychotherapy and antidepressant medication, the patient was referred to a cardiac rehabilitation program, where he was placed on a diet, an exercise regimen, and a smoking cessation program. Brief office counseling with the patient's wife reassured them both about the safety of gradually resuming normal sexual activity.

The patient complied with this multimodal approach and responded well to his antidepressant, psychotherapy, and cardiac rehabilitation program and returned to work. Formal psychotherapy was terminated after 6 months, although he continued on his antidepressant for 1 year, after which it was gradually tapered and discontinued. The patient did well subsequently.

DIAGNOSIS AND BIOPSYCHOSOCIAL ASSESSMENT

In the DSM-IV schemata, the patient initially would have been diagnosed as follows:

Axis I: Major depression, single episode, severe, without psychotic features
Dysthymic disorder, early onset (provisional diagnosis)
Nicotine dependence
Axis II: Obsessive–compulsive personality traits (premorbid)
Axis III: Coronary artery disease, status post-coronary artery bypass surgery. Status post-hypokalemia, essential hypertension, overweight
Axis IV: Psychosocial and environmental problems: threat of job loss
Axis V: Global assessment of functioning (GAF): 45

The biopsychosocial assessment applied to this case provided a structured and systematic way of understanding the patient's condition by attributing significance to each sphere of his life—psychological, biological, and social—as well as understanding key developmental influences that affected the patient's personality development and vulnerability to depression (Fig. 2–1). In this manner, the treatment interventions that were devised (medical/biological, psychotherapeutic, and rehabilitative/social) addressed *each aspect* of the patient's life and sources of stress. Hence, the descriptive approach of DSM-IV, which is based clearly on the biopsychosocial model with its multiaxial system, combined with a basic psychodynamic assessment that attempts to analyze the meaning of an illness for patients from the standpoint of both past and current life experiences, provides a comprehensive method to formulate an integrated plan of treatment. Table 2–1 summarizes a structured treatment approach to psychiatric assessment and treatment planning based on this approach.

Although the relative *weight* attached to biological, psychological, and social aspects of each individual patient varies, it is essential that each area at least be considered to be potentially important. This philosophy and approach to patient care is the essential theme that runs throughout the course of this text.

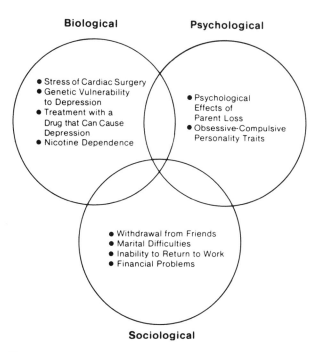

Figure 2–1. *The interaction of biological, psychological, and social factors in the case of Mr. A.*

Table 2–1 **Outline of Psychiatric Assessment and Treatment Planning**

Psychiatric history
Mental status examination
Medical evaluation
Differential diagnosis: psychiatric and medical
DSM-IV diagnoses (definitive or provisional)
   Psychiatric disorders (Axis I)
   Personality diagnoses (Axis II)
   Medical diagnoses (Axis III)
   Psychosocial and environmental problems (Axis IV)
   Assessment of psychosocial functioning (Axis V)
Psychosocial assessment and case formulation
Treatment plan
   Psychological—need for and choice of psychotherapy; inpatient or outpatient
   treatment
   Biological—need for further medical/neurological evaluation or treatment;
   psychopharmacological treatment; rehabilitation programs
   Social—need for intervention in environmental conditions and social conditions; re-
   ferral to support agencies, occupational counseling, financial or legal assistance

---

CLINICAL PEARLS

The following ten questions, which should be modified by the interviewer to be asked in an open-ended manner, will facilitate uncovering the source of psychosocial stress connected with the onset or relapse of psychiatric symptoms, assuming the patient is open and cooperative with the interviewer.

- Has there been any recent serious illness or death in your family?
- Have you been having any problems with money or with your job? Are you seriously in debt?
- Have you had any serious problems with your children, your marriage, or other close relationships?
- Have you had any recent illness or surgery, and are you on any medications?
- Have you ever thought you might have a problem with drinking too much alcohol or taking drugs?
- Have you been under any stress or pressure recently that has been difficult for you to manage?

Regarding the patient's past history, the following questions will help to identify any significant psychodynamic problems or major stresses in the patient's developmental years. These are "lead" questions that will identify any major developmental traumas, but the development history should not be limited solely to these four questions.

- Tell me about growing up with your family and your relationship with your parents. Did you have any special problems with your parents or within your family when you were growing up? Was there frequent fighting between your parents when you were a child or teenager?
- Did either one of your parents have a problem with alcohol or drugs?
- Did your parents divorce or separate when you were a child, or did one of your parents die when you were young?
- Were you ever physically or sexually molested when you were a child or teenager?

In the remaining chapters of this text, students will become familiar with major psychopathological syndromes in clinical psychiatry and the management of behavioral and psychiatric disorders that are encountered in medical, surgical, and pediatric settings. As the student studies these conditions and encounters them in his or her future medical practice, it is hoped that they will take an integrated approach to patient assessment and treatment based on the biopsychosocial model presented in these introductory chapters.

ANNOTATED BIBLIOGRAPHY

Nemiah JC: Foundations of Clinical Psychopathology. New York, Oxford University Press, 1961
> This is an intriguing and beautifully written text that remains a classic as an introduction to psychodynamic theory.

Balint M: The Doctor, His Patient and the Illness. New York, International University Press, 1957
> Balint was a psychoanalyst who worked extensively with primary care doctors in evaluating and treating the common psychiatric conditions of general medical patients. This text remains a classic for exploring and understanding the psychological aspects of medical practice.

For students interested in excellent resources on psychiatric interviewing, the following books are recommended:

Shea SC: Psychiatric Interviewing. The Art of Understanding. Philadelphia, WB Saunders, 1988

Cohen-Cole SA: The Medical Interview: The Three-Function Approach. Washington DC, CV Mosby Company, 1991

REFERENCES

Alexander F: Psychosomatic Medicine. Its Principles and Applications. New York, Norton, 1950
American Psychiatric Association: Diagnostic and Statistical Manual of Mental Disorders, 4th ed. Washington, DC: American Psychiatric Association, 1994
Aneshensel CS, Stone JD: Stress and depression: A test of the buffering model of social support. Arch Gen Psychiatry 39:1392–1396, 1982
Bertalanffy L von: General system theory: A critical review. In Buckley W (ed): Modern Systems Research for the Behavioral Scientist, pp 11–30. Chicago, Aldine, 1968
Bifulco AT, Brown GW, Harris TO: Childhood loss of parent, lack of adequate parental care and adult depression: A replication. J Affective Disord 12:115–128, 1987
Birley JLT, Brown GW: Crises and life changes preceding the onset or relapse of acute schizophrenia: Clinical aspects. Br J Psychiatry 116:327–333, 1970
Bolton W, Oatley K: A longitudinal study of social support and depression in unemployed men. Psychol Med 17:453–460, 1987
Breier A, Kelsoe JR, Kirwin PD, et al: Early parental loss and development of adult psychopathology. Arch Gen Psychiatry 45:987–993, 1988
Bryer JB, Nelson BA, Miller JB, et al: Childhood sexual and physical abuse as factors in adult psychiatric illness. Am J Psychiatry 144:1426–1430, 1987
Cadoret RJ, O'Gorman TW, Troughton E, et al: Alcoholism and antisocial personality: Interrelationships, genetic and environmental factors. Arch Gen Psychiatry 42:161–167, 1985
Cobb S: Social support as a moderator of life stress. Psychosom Med 38:300–314, 1976
Cole SA, Levinson R: The biopsychosocial model in medical practice. In Stoudemire A (ed): Human Behavior: An Introduction for Medical Students, 3rd ed. Philadelphia, Lippincott–Raven Publishers, 1998

Cooper AM: Will neurobiology influence psychoanalysis? Am J Psychiatry 142:1395–1402, 1985

Coyne JC: Social factors and psychopathology: stress, social support, and coping processes. Annu Rev Psychol 42:401–425, 1991

Dew MA, Bromet EJ, Penkower L: Mental health effects of job loss in women. Psycho Med 22:751–764, 1992

Doane JA, West KL, Goldstein MJ, et al: Parental communication deviance and affective style: Predictors of subsequent schizophrenia spectrum disorders in vulnerable adolescents. Arch Gen Psychiatry 38:679–685, 1981

Engel GL: The need for a new medical model: A challenge for biomedicine. Science 196:129–136, 1977

Fink PJ: Response to the presidential address: Is "Biopsychosocial" the psychiatric shibboleth? Am J Psychiatry 145:1061–1067, 1988

Galanter M: Research on social supports and mental illness. Am J Psychiatry 145:1270–1272, 1988 (editorial)

Goldberg D, Bridges K, Cook D, et al: The influence of social factors on common mental disorders. Br J Psychiatry 156:704–713, 1990

Green SA: Supportive psychological care of the medically ill: A Synthesis of the Biopsychosocial Approach in Medical Care. In Stoudemire A (ed): Human Behavior: An Introduction for Medical Students 2nd ed. Philadelphia, JB Lippincott, 1994

Greenblatt M, Becerra R, Serafetinides EA: Social networks and mental health: An overview. Am J Psychiatry 8:977–984, 1982

Harris T, Brown GW, Bifulco A: Loss of parent in childhood and adult psychiatric disorder: The role of lack of adequate parental care. Psychol Med 16:641–659, 1986

Harris T, Brown GW, Bifulco A: Loss of parent in childhood and adult psychiatric disorder. The role of social class position and premarital pregnancy. Psychol Med 17:163–183, 1987

Inderbitzin LB, James ME: Psychoanalytic Psychology. In Stoudemire A (ed): Human Behavior: An Introduction for Medical Students, 3rd ed. Philadelphia, Lippincott–Raven Publishers, 1998

Kandel ER: Psychotherapy and the single synapse. The impact of psychiatric thought on neurobiologic research. N Engl J Med 301:1028–1037, 1979

Kandel ER: From metapsychology to molecular biology: Explorations into the nature of anxiety. Am J Psychiatry 140:1277–1293, 1983

Kendler KS: Indirect vertical cultural transmission: A model for nongenetic parental influences on the liability to psychiatric illness. Am J Psychiatry 145:657–665, 1988

Leavy RL: Social support and psychological disorder: A review. Community Psychol 11:3–21, 1983

Lindberg F, Distad L: Post-traumatic stress disorders in women who experienced childhood incest. Child Abuse Negl 9:329–334, 1985

MacMillan JF, Gold A, Crow TJ, et al: The Northwick Park study of first episodes of schizophrenia: IV. Expressed emotion and relapse. Br J Psychiatry 148:133–143, 1986

Meyer A: Psychobiology, A Science of Man. Springfield, IL, Charles C Thomas, 1957

Miklowitz DJ, Goldstein MJ, Neuchterlein KH, et al: The family and the course of recent-onset mania. In Hahlweg K, Goldstein MJ (eds): Understanding Major Mental Disorder: The Contribution of Family Interaction Research, pp 195–211. New York, Family Process Press, 1987

Miklowitz DJ, Goldstein MJ, Neuchterlein KH, et al: Family factors and the course of bipolar affective disorder. Arch Gen Psychiatry 45:225–231, 1988

Miller PM, Ingham JG, Davidson S: Life events, symptoms and social support. J Psychosom Res 20:515–522, 1976

Parry G, Shapiro DA: Social support and life events in working class women. Arch Gen Psychiatry 43:315–323, 1986

Pellegrini DS: Psychosocial risk and protective factors in childhood. Dev Behav Pediat 11:201–209, 1990

Penkower L, Bromet EJ, Dew MA: Husbands' layoff and wives' mental health. Arch Gen Psychiatry 45:994–1000, 1988

Reiser MF: Mind, Brain, Body. New York, Basic Books, 1984

Romans SE, Walton VA, Herbison GP, et al: Social networks and psychiatric morbidity in New Zealand women. Aust N Z J Psychiatry 26:485–492, 1992

Roy A: Parental loss in childhood and onset of manic-depressive illness. Br J Psychiatry 136:86–88, 1980

Rutter M: Psychopathology and development: Links between childhood and adult life. In Rutter M, Hersov L (eds): Child and Adolescent Psychiatry. London, Blackwell Scientific Publications, 1985

Schwartz CC, Myers JK: Life events and schizophrenia. I: Comparison of schizophrenics with a community sample. Arch Gen Psychiatry 34:1238–1241, 1977a

Schwartz CC, Myers JK: Life events and schizophrenia. II: Impact of life events on symptom configuration. Arch Gen Psychiatry 34:1242–1245, 1977b

Stansfeld SA, Gallacher JEJ, Sharp DS, et al: Social factors and minor psychiatric disorder in middle-aged men: A validation study and a population survey. Psychol Med 21:157–167, 1991

Stoudemire A: Somatothymia: Part I. Psychosomatics 32:365–370, 1991a

Stoudemire A: Somatothymia: Part II. Psychosomatics 32:371–381, 1991b

Tennant C: Life events and psychological morbidity: The evidence from prospective studies. Psychol Med 13:483–486, 1983

Tennant C: Parental loss in childhood: Its effect in adult life. Arch Gen Psychiatry 45:1045–1050, 1988

Tennant C, Bebbington P, Hurry J: Social experiences in childhood and adult psychiatric morbidity: A multiple regression analysis. Psychol Med 12:321–327, 1982

Tennant C, Hurry J, Bebbington P: The relation of childhood separation experiences to adult depressive and anxiety states. Br J Psychiatry 141:475–482, 1982a

Tennant C, Hurry J, Bebbington P: The relationship of different types of childhood separation experiences to adult psychiatric disorders. Br J Psychiatry 141:475–482, 1982b

Tennant C, Smith A, Bebbington P, et al: Parental loss in childhood: Relationship to adult psychiatric impairment and contact with psychiatric services. Arch Gen Psychiatry 38:309–314, 1981

Uhlenhuth EG, Paykel ES: Symptom intensity and life events. Arch Gen Psychiatry 28:473–477, 1973

van der Kolk B: The psychological consequences of overwhelming life experiences. In van der Kolk B (ed): Psychological Trauma. Washington, DC, American Psychiatric Press, 1986

van der Kolk B: Behavioral and psychobiological effects of developmental trauma. In Stoudemire A (ed): Human Behavior: An Introduction for Medical Students, 3rd ed. Philadelphia, Lippincott–Raven Publishers, 1998

Vaughn CE, Snyder KS, Jones S, et al: Family factors in schizophrenic relapse: Replication in California of British research on expressed emotion. Arch Gen Psychiatry 41:1169–1177, 1984

Warr P, Jackson P: Factors influencing the psychological impact of prolonged unemployment and of re-employment. Psychol Med 15:795–807, 1985

Weissman MM, Gammon GD, John K, et al: Children of depressed parents: Increased psychopathology and early onset of major depression. Arch Gen Psychiatry 44:847–853, 1987

3 Psychological Testing in Medical Practice

Nadine J. Kaslow and
Eugene W. Farber

A cornerstone of good clinical care is that the physician gather as much information as possible when working up or evaluating a diagnostically complex patient or when trying to ascertain the efficacy of a therapeutic intervention. Psychological testing data provide an important source of information about an individual's cognitive, neuropsychological, psychiatric, and personality functioning. Psychological test findings can aid the physician in diagnosis, case formulation, treatment planning, prediction of behavior, and assessment of treatment progress and outcome. This chapter focuses on the nature and uses of psychological testing. Specific attention is given to referral questions and how the information gleaned from testing can be used in formulating and implementing a treatment plan. Case vignettes illustrate several major assessment instruments and how findings obtained are used to assist with clinical care.

NATURE OF PSYCHOLOGICAL TESTING

The process of psychological assessment encompasses the collection, organization, and interpretation of information about a person's psychological functioning and the contexts of behavioral difficulties. Psychological tests provide a standardized empirical means of measuring, describing, evaluating, and predicting some types of human behavior.

Psychometric Properties

A determination of the usefulness of the findings from a given test is based on three psychometric properties: standardization, reliability, and validity. A test is considered *standardized* when consistent stimuli are used to elicit information, when the test is administered in a uniform manner, and when norms are available using data from demographically and clinically representative samples (Anastasi, 1988). *Reliability* refers to the consistency, accuracy, and reproducibility of the test results. If a measure is reliable, scores obtained are relatively consistent within the given test (internal consistency reliability), across administrations (test–retest reliability), and across examiners (interrater reliability) (Anastasi, 1988). A test is said to have *validity* to the extent that it measures what it is purported to assess. Valid tests include items that accurately represent the psychological domain being assessed (content validity), that are effective in predicting a person's performance in a specific area of functioning (predictive validity), and that adequately measure the theoretical construct or trait for which the test was developed (construct validity) (Anastasi, 1988).

Format of Administration

Tests may be administered in individual or group format. *Individually administered* tests allow for careful observation and evaluation of psychological functioning in a given person. Psychological tests administered individually often include those used to gather diagnostic information (e.g., Structured Clinical Interview for Diagnosis), detailed information about personality functioning (e.g., Rorschach Inkblot Test), and in-depth evaluation of cognitive functioning (e.g., Wechsler Intelligence Scale for Children, Wechsler Adult Intelligence Scale). *Group tests* offer the advantage of easy administration and scoring and thus are time and cost efficient. Achievement and aptitude tests (e.g., Scholastic Aptitude Test, Medical College Admission Test) often are administered in a group format.

Structure of Tests

Psychological tests vary in their structure, depending on the nature of the task, the stimuli involved, and the degree to which interpretation on the part of the examiner is required to evaluate test findings. In general, three classes of tests can be distinguished: objective, projective, and semistructured. *Objective tests* typically are self-report pencil and paper measures using specific questions and a standardized response format that can be mechanically scored and statistically analyzed. Although the format of such tests is objective, the meaning of the results and scores requires interpretation by a skilled clinician. Common examples of objective tests include the Beck

Depression Inventory, Symptom Checklist-90-Revised, Family Environment Scale, Minnesota Multiphasic Personality Inventory II, and Millon Clinical Multiaxial Inventory.

In contrast to objective measures, *projective tests* are less structured with regard to response format and scoring and require the testee to provide responses based on his/her perception and interpretation of relatively ambiguous stimuli for which a range of responses is possible. It is posited that such perceptions and interpretations are influenced by core aspects of psychological functioning, as the individual projects his/her characteristic modes of organizing experience, needs, motivations, feelings, meanings, and salient intrapsychic and interpersonal conflicts and psychodynamics. This has been referred to as the *projective hypothesis* (Frank, 1939). Proponents of projective techniques, who often use a psychodynamic approach to test interpretation, assert that this method of assessment is particularly effective in revealing unconscious aspects of personality functioning. The most frequently cited examples of projective tools include the Rorschach Inkblot Test, Thematic Apperception Test, and Sentence Completion Test.

Semistructured tasks require the patient to respond to specific questions in an open-ended manner. Typically these are interview evaluations in which the examiner follows a structured line of questioning but has the flexibility to ask individualized follow-up questions that explore specific responses of the examinee. Common semistructured measures include the Structured Clinical Interview for Diagnosis, Diagnostic Interview Schedule for Children, Brief Psychiatric Rating Scale, Hamilton Rating Scale for Depression, and Structured Clinical Interview for the Positive and Negative Syndrome Scale.

Functional Domains

Psychological tests differ according to format of administration and structure of the task and also vary in terms of the areas of mental functioning assessed. Tests with medical and psychiatric patients often are used to assess intelligence, educational achievement, aptitude, adaptive behavior functioning (e.g., effective use of skills to accomplish activities of daily living and engage in interpersonal interactions), vocational skills and interests, neuropsychological functioning, psychiatric symptomatology and diagnosis, and personality.

Intelligence tests assess an individual's present level of cognitive functioning and capacity to understand and cope with the world (Wechsler, 1991). These tests assess a broad range of intellectual functions: verbal and nonverbal reasoning, capacity for abstraction, fund of knowledge, attention and concentration, visual-spatial skills, and facility with simultaneous (concurrent processing of many stimuli) and sequential (arrangement of stimuli in sequential or serial order) processing. Based on an individual's performance on verbal and performance tasks, an overall Intelligence Quotient (IQ) can be determined. IQ scores, a quantitative interpretation of a total test score in relation to appropriate group norms, are derived using the following formula: IQ = MA/CA × 100. Mental age (MA) is the average intellectual level of a particular age, and chronological age (CA) is the individual's chronological age. People with average IQs have equivalent mental and chronological ages; thus, their IQ scores approximate 100. An IQ of 100 is the mean score, with a standard deviation of 15 points on the major intelligence tests. When a psychologist provides feedback regarding the intellectual functioning of a particular individual, the psychologist offers an IQ score and describes the individual's level of functioning according to the classification listed in Table 3–1. Recently, the meaningfulness of IQ scores interpreted in isolation has been questioned. For example, some authors assert that the IQ classification schema are arbitrary, varying according to test authors, diagnostic and classification manuals, and government criteria (Kaufman, 1990). In this regard, two individuals with comparable IQ scores will not necessarily demonstrate similar intellectual capabilities. Concurrent with the concern about the usefulness of IQ scores is an increased emphasis on qualitative evaluation of the individual's intellectual strengths and weaknesses relative to overall IQ. In addition, the past decade has witnessed increased attention to an individual's IQ score in the context of sociocultural factors and adaptive behavior functioning.

Educational achievement tests measure the effects of a specific educational program of study on academic achievement (Anastasi, 1988). These tests identify academic difficulties and are used to develop interventions addressing achievement concerns (Sattler, 1992). In combination with intelligence test results, achievement test findings identify specific learning disabilities or DSM-IV academic skills disorders (i.e., developmental arithmetic, expressive writing, or reading disorders).

Table 3–1 **IQ Score Classification of Intellectual Functioning Level**

CLASSIFICATION	CORRESPONDING IQ RANGE
Very superior	130 and above*
Superior	120–129*
High average	110–119*
Average	90–109*
Low average	80–89*
Borderline	70–79*
Mild mental retardation	50–55 to approximately 70[†]
Moderate mental retardation	35–40 to 50–55[†]
Severe mental retardation	20–25 to 35–40[†]
Profound mental retardation	Below 20 or 25[†]

* Criteria correspond to those described in the WAIS-R Manual
[†] Criteria correspond to those described in the DSM-IV

Aptitude tests measure abilities in specified skill domains and are employed to predict subsequent performance. For example, the Medical College Admission Test, which measures competencies important for medical practice, is an aptitude test presumed to have predictive validity for medical school performance.

Tests of adaptive behavior measure the capacity to meet the natural and social demands of one's environment effectively in accord with cultural and age expectations. The areas of personal and social sufficiency addressed include independent functioning, social and communication skills, physical skill capacities, language development, and academic competencies. In the *Diagnostic and Statistical Manual of Mental Disorders,* 4th ed. (DSM-IV), a diagnosis of mental retardation includes documentation of an IQ less than 70 and adaptive functioning impairments.

Vocational skills and interest tests assess job and career preferences. These tests are used most often by career counselors, industrial/organizational psychologists, school psychologists, and guidance counselors. Information obtained from these tests can provide a useful guide for career planning.

Neuropsychological tests measure brain–behavior relationships in the following domains: orientation, language, memory, perception, perceptual-motor, attention and concentration, concept formation, and executive functions (planning and problem-solving abilities). Neuropsychological tests help detect the presence of organic brain pathology and evaluate the nature of associated cognitive or behavioral deficits (Lezak, 1995). The data from these tests can be helpful for the development and implementation of cognitive rehabilitation programs.

Semistructured diagnostic interviews permit more precise and standardized psychiatric diagnoses than unstructured clinical interviews (Widiger and Frances, 1987). These measures assess symptom and personality patterns consistent with DSM-IV Axis I and Axis II diagnoses. Semistructured interview data can be used in conjunction with information obtained from self-report measures and clinical interviews in assessing symptom severity and refining diagnostic impressions.

Personality tests measure emotional, motivational, interpersonal, and attitudinal characteristics of the individual (Anastasi, 1988). Information gathered from personality measures provide a description of stylistic and phenomenological aspects of personality functioning. These data can be of use in formulating clinical diagnoses and can aid in the identification of salient psychological and interpersonal issues that may be relevant to psychotherapy.

See Table 3–2 for examples of test instruments according to the classification scheme outlined above. Table 3–3 presents a synopsis of clinical questions, types of psychological tests indicated, and pertinent information derived.

Table 3–2 **Classification of Commonly Used Psychological Testing Instruments**

TEST TYPE	EXAMPLES
Intelligence	Wechsler Scales (WAIS-III, WISC-III, WPPSI); Stanford Binet, 4th ed.; Kaufman Assessment Battery for Children (K-ABC)
Achievement	Wide Range Achievement Test-Revised (WRAT-R); Woodcock-Johnson Psychoeducational Battery; Kaufman Test of Educational Achievement (K-TEA)
Aptitude	Scholastic Aptitude Test (SAT); Medical College Admission Test (MCAT); Graduate Record Examination (GRE)
Adaptive behavior	Vineland Adaptive Behavior Scales; Scales of Independent Behavior
Vocational	Strong Vocational Interest Blank (SVIB)
Neuropsychological	Halstead-Reitan Test Battery (HRB); Luria-Nebraska Neuropsychological Battery (LNNB); Bender Visual Motor Gestalt Test; Wechsler Memory Scales-Revised (WMS-R); Wisconsin Card Sort
Symptoms and Diagnosis	Symptom Checklist-90-Revised (SCL-90-R); Structured Clinical Interview for Diagnosis Revised (SCIDR); Diagnostic Interview Schedule for Children (DISC)
Personality Objective	Minnesota Multiphasic Personality Inventory (MMPI-2); MMPI-Adolescent; Millon Clinical Multiaxial Inventory (MCMI); Myers-Briggs Type Indicator (MBTI)
Projective	Rorschach Inkblot Test; Thematic Apperception Test (TAT); Sentence Completion Test (SCT); House-Tree-Person Test (HTP)
Individual	WAIS-III; Rorschach
Group	MCAT, SAT, GRE

USES OF PSYCHOLOGICAL TESTING

Physicians may request psychological testing when further information is needed regarding a patient's intellectual and neuropsychological functioning, presence of underlying psychotic processes and affective disturbances, quality of ego functioning, intrapsychic and interpersonal dynamics and personality style, and veracity of patient's complaints. Findings from testing can then be integrated with other forms of pertinent clinical data, including behavioral observation, clinical presentation, and psychiatric and medical history, to provide the most comprehensive portrait of the individual's psychological functioning. Additionally, psychological testing data is useful in systematically and empirically evaluating and documenting treatment progress and outcome.

Psychological testing is most helpful to the physician who clearly delineates the reasons for referral. When referring a patient for psychological testing, the physician should specify what information is needed, how the findings

Table 3–3 **Examples of the Clinical Uses of Common Psychological Tests**

CLINICAL QUESTION	TEST(S) INDICATED*	DATA DERIVED
Intellectual functioning	WAIS-III; WISC-III; Stanford Binet	IQ estimate, cognitive strengths and weaknesses
Academic achievement	WRAT-R; K-TEA	Academic skills and deficits
Skill/aptitude	SAT, MCAT, GRE	Skill level and prediction of performance
Adaptive behavior	Vineland	Capacity to meet environmental demands effectively
Vocational skills	SVIB, MBTI	Job and career suitability and interest
Organic brain impairment	HRB; LNNB	Presence and effects of brain lesions
Psychiatric diagnosis	SCID-R; DISC	DSM-IV diagnostic considerations
Psychosis	SCID-R; Rorschach; MMPI-2; SCI-PANSS	Disordered thinking, impaired reality testing
Mood disorder	Beck Depression Inventory, SCL-90-R; SCID; Rorschach; MMPI-2	Depression, mania, affect regulation
Global personality functioning	MMPI-2; MMPI-A; MCMI; TAT; Rorschach	Self-esteem, interpersonal style, dynamic conflicts

* For definitions, See Table 3–2.

will be helpful in assessment and treatment planning, and for what it will be used. Once the physician makes the referral for testing, it is the psychologist's responsibility to select the appropriate test or battery of tests (i.e., a combination of tests that measure different psychological domains) that can best address the specific referral questions.

Formulating Referral Questions

Psychological testing can be useful in addressing a range of issues. Brief vignettes will be used to illustrate circumstances in which the physician may request psychological testing.

Cognitive Abilities

Mr. and Mrs. Jones, Adam's parents, spoke with their pediatrician about Adam's school performance. Although Adam was well behaved and popular, he was not learning as quickly as his classmates and was feeling frustrated that "the other kids were smarter." The pediatrician made a referral to a child psychologist for psychological testing to receive information regarding Adam's intellectual abilities.

In cases like Adam's, psychologists typically will focus their evaluation in the area of abilities testing. Abilities testing provides an estimation of intellectual ability (e.g., IQ score) and gives information about the person's cognitive and intellectual strengths and weaknesses (e.g., learning disabilities). Test findings can aid in the formulation of appropriate modes of clinical intervention (i.e., how to communicate information in a manner consistent with the person's level of cognitive functioning and intellectual strengths and weaknesses). These data also may be used to help the individual obtain necessary remedial services for intellectual handicaps or learning disabilities. If questions about mental retardation arise, measures of adaptive functioning can also be administered.

In making a referral for abilities testing for a child or adolescent, the physician should specifically ask about (1) the child's developmental progress in cognitive, emotional, and interpersonal functioning, adaptive behavior, and skill acquisition; (2) comparison of the child's intellectual functioning and achievement, to diagnose learning disabilities; and (3) differential diagnosis of psychopathological conditions (Racusin and Moss, 1991). This information can facilitate treatment planning, predict the course of therapy, and provide the necessary documentation for the child or adolescent to receive special services (e.g., classes for the intellectually gifted, behaviorally or emotionally disordered, or learning disabled, services for the mentally retarded, residential placement).

For adults, abilities testing can provide information with regard to the following types of referral questions: (1) What is the overall level of this person's intellectual functioning, including areas of relative strength and weakness? (2) Is this person able to understand the nature of his/her physical condition and follow instructions for self-care? and (3) For this individual, who is currently receiving Workmen's Compensation or disability payments for a physical disability, which cognitive strengths can be used in pursuing occupational alternatives?

Neuropsychological Functioning

Dr. Stuart, a neurologist, was consulted by a colleague, a hematologist, who was treating a sickle cell patient who had recently suffered a cerebral vascular accident (CVA). This sickle cell patient had functioned effectively prior to his CVA and was now reporting difficulties with language comprehension and distractibility. As part of the workup, the neurologist requested a neuropsychological evaluation.

For patients such as the one referred by Dr. Stuart, neuropsychological testing can be useful in ascertaining the organic contributions to the symptom picture or in assessing the impact of brain impairments/lesions on cognitive functioning. In conjunction with neurological data, neuropsychological test findings can answer questions regarding the nature, extent, and impact of the brain impairment and provide directions for cognitive rehabilitation. Common types of questions that the physician may pose when referring for neuropsychological testing may include: (1) What impact does this CVA have on this person's cognitive functioning? (2) What is the impact of this temporal lobe lesion on this individual's memory? (3) What type of cognitive rehabilitation programming would be most efficacious for this patient? and (4) Is there evidence of an organic component to this person's impulse control problems?

Thought Disorder and Reality Testing

Dr. Costner, a psychiatric resident, was treating an intelligent 26-year-old man in outpatient psychotherapy. As the patient became more self-revealing, Dr. Costner found it difficult to follow his line of thinking, which appeared odd. The physician also noticed that the patient misinterpreted events and displayed magical thinking. The patient, however, denied hallucinations and delusions. Dr. Costner requested psychological testing to assess for the presence of an underlying thought disorder and difficulties with reality testing.

For referrals such as the one made by Dr. Costner, the testing is geared toward assessing the nature and severity of the patient's thought disorder and the degree of impaired reality testing. The information obtained from the testing process may aid the psychiatry resident in making the differential diagnosis among a schizophrenia spectrum disorder, a personality disorder with transient psychotic symptoms, a drug-induced psychosis, or a mood disorder with psychotic features. Specific questions that Dr. Costner might ask include: (1) Does this person have difficulties with accurate perception of events and stimuli, and how pervasive and serious are these impairments? (2) Is there evidence of disorganized thinking? (3) What are the specific conditions under which thought disturbance or reality testing problems might emerge and/or be exacerbated? and (4) What clinical strategies might the treatment team use to help improve this person's thinking and reality testing?

Mood Disorder

Dr. Newman, an internist, was following Suzanne, a 31-year-old woman with a diagnosis of chronic fatigue syndrome. For the past year, Suzanne had complained of fatigue, low energy, and anhedonia. Her symptoms recently had worsened, and she reported such extreme bouts of tiredness and low energy that she was no longer able to maintain her full-time job. Dr. Newman requested psychological testing to ascertain whether or not Suzanne was experiencing a depressive disorder in addition to chronic fatigue syndrome.

Data regarding an affective component to Suzanne's difficulties may be gleaned from multiple tests of psychiatric symptoms and more subtle indications of a mood disturbance. Information regarding the nature and severity of the person's affective distress may assist in differential diagnosis when the following diagnoses are being considered: major depression with or without psychotic features, dysthymia, bipolar disorder with or without psychotic features, schizoaffective disorder, or affective instability secondary to the presence of a personality disorder. Examples of specific referral questions regarding the presence and nature of a mood disorder may include: (1) Is this woman with chronic fatigue syndrome also experiencing a major depressive episode or dysthymia? (2) Is this mother's difficulty caring for her newborn consistent with a diagnosis of a major depressive episode in the postpartum period or reflective of an underlying personality disorder? and (3) This patient evidences both psychotic and depressive symptoms. Which symptom complex is primary, and what are appropriate treatment recommendations?

Ego Functioning

Dr. Jennings, a forensic psychiatrist, was asked to evaluate the violence potential of Ms. Terry, a prison inmate. Ms. Terry was incarcerated for her involvement in a cocaine distribution ring. She had provided key evidence enabling law enforcement personnel to make arrests of the leaders of the drug ring. As the trial date approached, in which she would be asked to testify against her former bosses, she became increasingly emotionally labile, and at one point was overheard making suicide threats. In an effort to gather a more complete picture of Ms. Terry's impulse control, frustration tolerance, and affect regulation, Dr. Jennings requested a psychological evaluation.

To evaluate someone like Ms. Terry, the psychologist will administer a testing battery that can assess impulse control, frustration tolerance, and affect regulation. These data provide information about the quality of ego functioning and defenses used to cope with stress. Questions may include: (1) What is this individual's potential for losing control, and under what circumstances may his/her impulse control be most problematic? (2) Under what conditions is this person likely to become suicidal or violent? (3) What is this person's capacity for delaying gratification? (4) How does this person manage affective stimulation and his or her own emotional responses? and (5) What are the prominent defenses or adaptive mechanisms this person employs to cope with stressful circumstances?

Psychodynamics and Personality Functioning

George, a successful stockbroker, was significantly disfigured by burns suffered in an automobile accident. Upon discharge from the burn unit, he returned home to his family and soon thereafter resumed his work. His physician, Dr. Hawthorne, was concerned that George did not appear to be adjusting to his disfigurement and recommended psychotherapy. During psychotherapy sessions, George was guarded and often silent. While his distress about his disfigurement was understandable, his inability to articulate his thoughts and feelings left his therapist uncertain about how to be most helpful. Thus, psychological testing was requested to assist in more fully understanding the psychodynamic issues contributing to George's adjustment difficulties.

Psychological testing with someone like George can be useful in providing information regarding his self-esteem, identity formation, major areas of conflict, and typical interpersonal modes of relating and interacting. Pertinent questions may include: (1) How has this patient's physical condition affected his self-concept? (2) What types of interpersonal difficulties is this person most likely to encounter? and (3) How will this individual's personality style influence his interactions in the doctor–patient relationship and treatment compliance?

Validity of Complaints

Pete Donaldson, a 23-year old first-year law student, fractured his pelvic bone in a rock climbing accident. Although X-rays and computed tomography (CT) scans revealed no additional complications, Pete complained that he was unable to walk because his legs did not "feel right." His orthopedist, Dr. Wilkins, found no physical reason to explain Pete's complaints. The physical therapy team also could find no underlying physical reason that Pete could not walk once his pelvic bone had healed. Dr. Wilkins and members of Pete's medical team began to question the validity of his complaints. He was thus referred for psychological testing to ascertain whether or not there was a significant psychogenic basis for his alleged inability to walk.

To aid Pete's medical team in making a differential diagnosis of malingering, a factitious or somatoform disorder, and other DSM-IV Axis I and Axis II disorders, the psychologist would administer tests that could yield information about the presence of a primarily psychological etiology of his medical complaints (Schretlen, 1988). Examples of questions Dr. Wilkins may ask are as follows: (1) Is there a significant discrepancy between symptom claims and psychological test findings suggestive of malingering? and (2) Are the test results consistent with a conversion or dissociative disorder?

PROCESS OF TESTING

Once a patient is referred for testing, the psychologist meets with the patient to explain the testing process and the rationale for testing. Background information pertinent to the reasons for evaluation is obtained. Then the psychologist selects and administers the appropriate tests. Depending on the breadth of the psychological functions being evaluated and the severity of the patient's impairments, the duration of the testing process may vary from a relatively brief amount of time (e.g., 1 to 2 hours) to lengthy and/or numerous testing sessions (e.g., 10 to 15 hours).

To illustrate the testing process in some detail, the following vignettes introduce commonly used psychological tests, information gleaned from the assessment process, and treatment implications of test results. After presenting the vignettes, a brief discussion of the communication of test findings is offered, as this is the final stage in the testing process.

Vignette I

Mr. Jordan, a 32-year-old single advertising executive, presented to his primary care physician complaining of chest pain. He jogged 4 miles three times a week and played tennis on the weekend. He denied smoking cigarettes, and his weight was within the normal range. He denied prior history of cardiac difficulties, although his family history was positive for heart disease. Specifically, his paternal and maternal grandfathers died secondary to myocardial infarctions in their sixties. While he reported that work typically was fast paced, he did not report subjective feelings of anxiety or stress. Additionally, he stated that his personal life was satisfactory. A thorough physical examination was conducted, including an electrocardiogram, and all findings were negative. His primary care physician recommended that Mr. Jordan recontact her should his symptoms continue or worsen. A few weeks later, the patient was seen for a follow-up appointment with complaints of continued intermittent chest pains. He was then referred for a full cardiology workup, which was negative. At this point, his primary care physician and cardiologist referred him for psychological evaluation because his pain symptoms defied etiological diagnosis, and they were interested in information regarding a functional component to his physical distress.

Having received a referral with the question, "Does this individual evidence personality characteristics consistent with persons who experience chronic pain with no apparent organic etiology?," the psychologist elected to administer the Minnesota Multiphasic Personality Inventory-2 (MMPI-2; Hathaway and McKinley, 1989).

Minnesota Multiphasic Personality Inventory-2

The MMPI-2, a 567-item personality inventory, is the most commonly used and thoroughly researched objective self-report personality inventory. It is a psychometrically valid and reliable test that has been well standardized across representative demographic groups (Graham, 1993). The MMPI-2 requires the respondent to answer true or false to statements describing psychological symptoms, preferences, interpersonal relationships, and emotional responses to commonly encountered situations. The MMPI-2 provides indices addressing response style, including measures of guardedness, underreporting or overreporting of psychological difficulties, and random responding. The measure also provides information on ten clinical scales: Hypochondriasis,

Depression, Hysteria, Psychopathic Deviate, Masculinity-Femininity, Paranoia, Psychasthenia, Schizophrenia, Hypomania, and Social Introversion. A brief description of the three validity scales and the ten clinical scales can be found in Table 3–4.

The MMPI-2 also includes supplementary and content scales measuring a variety of personality characteristics that aid in the interpretation of the results obtained on the main clinical scales. A high score on a given scale does not necessarily indicate that the respondent has that psychiatric disorder. For example, a high score on the hypomania scale does not necessarily imply a

Table 3–4 **MMPI-2 Validity (L, F, K) and Clinical (Hs, D, Hy, Pd, Mf, Pa, Pt, Sc, Ma, Si) Scales**

SCALE	CONTENT
L: Lie	Measures frankness in responding to test items, including willingness to admit minor shortcomings; detects deliberate and unsophisticated efforts to present oneself in a positive light
F: Infrequency	Detects atypical response sets; serves as an index of overall degree of psychopathology
K: Suppressor	Measures subtle forms of defensive responding and conversely, responding that suggests an unusually frank or self-critical approach; adjusts clinical scale elevations according to degree of response defensiveness
1. Hypochondriasis (Hs)	Measures somatic focus and preoccupations with bodily functioning
2. Depression (D)	Measures symptomatic depression, including low morale, lack of hope, and general dissatisfaction with one's life situation
3. Hysteria (Hy)	Measures tendency to rely on "hysteroid" defenses including denial, repression, and inhibition, and proneness to conversion of somatoform symptoms in response to stress
4. Psychopathic deviate (PD)	Measures general social maladjustment, family conflict, authority problems, rebelliousness, and antisocial patterns
5. Masculinity-femininity (Mf)	Measures a range of personality and interest areas, including aesthetic interests, sensitivity, and passivity, as well as sex-role stereotyped behavior patterns
6. Paranoia (Pa)	Identifies paranoid symptoms and assesses interpersonal sensitivity, suspiciousness, vigilance, and distrust
7. Psychasthenia (Pt)	Measures anxiety, fear, tension, and obsessive–compulsive tendencies
8. Schizophrenia (Sc)	Measures bizarre thinking, unusual perceptions, social alienation, identity confusion, and feelings of general inadequacy
9. Hypomania (Ma)	Measures degree of hypomanic personality features, including elated but unstable mood, psychomotor excitement, flight of ideas, and overactivity
10. Social introversion (Si)	Assesses level of comfort in social situations, degree of withdrawal or gregariousness, and extent of social anxiety and social inhibition

diagnosis of bipolar disorder; this elevation may be seen in active, accomplished, and extroverted individuals with no history of a mood disorder.

The MMPI-2 and its predecessor, the MMPI, often are used in medical practice (e.g., Osborne, 1985), as in the psychological evaluation of chronic pain patients (Keller and Butcher, 1991). The MMPI/MMPI-2 have been used with medical patients to screen for serious psychopathology and substance abuse, to ascertain the patient's likely responses to medical interventions and psychosocial adjustment to their medical condition, and to distinguish between functional and organic illness (Graham, 1993; Osborne, 1985). It is important to underscore, however, that the MMPI/MMPI-2 cannot and should not be used in isolation to diagnose or rule out the presence of an organic condition; rather, MMPI/MMPI-2 data regarding personality functioning can be used along with other available medical and psychological information to make inferences regarding the compatibility of personality characteristics expressed on the MMPI/MMPI-2 and a functional etiology for physical symptoms (Graham, 1993).

Interpretation of Test Findings. Mr. Jordan provided a valid MMPI-2 protocol according to the validity scales. He showed a mild elevation on scale 7, the Psychasthenia scale, and scale 9, the Hypomania scale. These elevations typically are indicative of tension, anxiety, obsessive–compulsive traits, and the use of hypomanic defenses (i.e., high activity level as defense against an underlying depression) that make it difficult for him to relax (Greene, 1991). There were no additional elevations on the main clinical scales.

Mr. Jordan's profile was not consistent with protocols typically obtained from chronic pain sufferers. Such patients most frequently exhibit one of the following profiles: (1) clinically significant elevations on scale 1 (Hypochondriasis), scale 2 (Depression), and scale 3 (Hysteria); (2) clinical scale scores within the normal range, with scales 1, 2, and 3 being the most elevated, although not significantly so; and (3) clinically significant elevations on several clinical scales, in addition to scales 1, 2, and 3, namely, scale 6 (Paranoia), scale 7 (Psychasthenia), and scale 8 (Schizophrenia) (Strassberg et al, 1992).

While Mr. Jordan's profile is not consistent with that of chronic pain sufferers, his elevation on scale 7 may suggest that he is frightened and worried about the possibility of having cardiac difficulties. Alternatively, his profile might reflect a type A behavior pattern characterized by high levels of competitiveness and achievement strivings, hard-driving behavior, and high levels of hostility. The type A behavior pattern has been found by some researchers to be a risk factor for cardiac disease (Friedman and Rosenman, 1974; Williams, 1986; see Thoresen and Powell, 1992 for recent critical review of this literature). An examination of his MMPI-2 content and supplementary scale scores revealed a significant elevation on the type A subscale.

Based on these MMPI-2 findings, the psychologist informed the referring physician that the patient's self-reported personality style was not consistent with that of individuals who somatize; rather, while the results from psychological testing cannot be used as documentation of cardiac difficulties, they are indicative of an individual whose behavior and personality style may put them at risk for cardiovascular symptoms. Thus, the psychologist and cardiologist spoke together with the patient and recommended psychotherapy to help Mr. Jordan address the dynamics associated with his anxious, obsessive and hard-driving style, combined with cognitive–behavioral interventions, including relaxation training.

Vignette 2

Ms. Foster, a 21-year-old cashier, was brought into the psychiatric emergency room by her coworker because she had been acting "strange" the past few days. Her coworker reported that Ms. Foster was "suspicious and became angry a lot." Upon evaluation, she appeared disorganized, her affect was labile and often inappropriate to content, and she reported hearing her dead grandmother's voice calling her name. She acknowledged suicidal ideation and had contemplated using a knife to stab herself. A complete mental status examination revealed that she was alert and fully oriented and that her cognitive functions were intact. She acknowledged occasional alcohol use, denied past or current drug abuse, and her toxicology findings were negative. Her family history was significant for maternal depression and a paternal uncle who was hospitalized for "nerve problems." A breakup with her boyfriend of 2 years precipitated her recent deterioration. According to reports obtained from family members, Ms. Foster had no previous psychiatric history. She was hospitalized, and a complete psychiatric and medical evaluation was conducted. Laboratory findings were within normal limits, and head CT and electroencephalogram were normal. Within 3 days of being on the inpatient unit, she denied psychotic symptoms and showed evidence of increasing personality reorganization without antipsychotic medication treatment. She acknowledged mild depressive symptoms, but demanded discharge as soon as possible. The psychiatric resident requested a testing consultation to aid in differential diagnosis. The resident queried whether or not the patient's psychological functioning was consistent with that of an individual with a personality disorder manifesting a transient psychotic episode, an underlying thought disorder consistent with a schizophrenia spectrum diagnosis, or a mood disorder with psychotic features.

Due to the complexity and variability of the patient's symptom picture and the importance of a thorough psychological assessment given that this patient presented with her first psychotic episode, the psychologist conducted a relatively standard battery of psychological tests, including the Wechsler Adult Intelligence Scale-Third Edition (WAIS-III; Wechsler, 1997), the Rorschach Inkblot Test (Rorschach, 1921/1949), the Thematic Apperception Test (TAT; Murray, 1943), and the MMPI-2.

Wechsler Adult Intelligence Scale-Third Edition (WAIS-III)

The WAIS-III, the most widely used and psychometrically sound intelligence test for adults, is comprised of 11 subtests, including 6 subtests measuring verbal IQ (information, digit span, vocabulary, arithmetic, comprehension, similarities) and 5 subtests measuring predominantly nonverbal perceptual and motor capacities, termed performance IQ (picture completion, picture arrangement, block design, object assembly, digit symbol). The range of functions measured allows the psychologist to determine areas of strength and weakness relative to the individual's overall intellectual functioning and to make comparisons with an age-matched national sample. Additionally, for purposes of interpretation, Kaufman (1990) has suggested three major domains of intellectual functioning assessed by the WAIS-III, namely, verbal comprehension (information, vocabulary, comprehension, similarities subtests), perceptual organization (picture completion, block design, object assembly subtests), and freedom from distractibility (arithmetic, digit span subtests). Furthermore, subtest score patterns can be used as a screening device for neuropsychological deficits (Lezak, 1995). Table 3–5 presents descriptions of the WAIS-III subtests.

Rorschach Inkblot Test

The Rorschach, a projective instrument, consists of ten symmetrical inkblot designs of varying complexity and color, administered in a standardized order. The examiner records verbatim responses to each card. Although a number of systems have been devised to score the patient's responses, psychologists rely increasingly on the scoring guidelines delineated by Exner (1991, 1993), a highly structured and psychometrically reliable scoring system. Based on certain combinations of scores, indices related to key diagnostic questions are computed, assessing schizophrenia, depression, coping deficits, suicide potential, hypervigilance, and obsessive style. Systematic analysis of Rorschach content material is used to obtain information regarding intrapsychic conflicts, predominant defenses, and patterns of interpersonal relationships.

Thematic Apperception Test

The TAT, a projective device, consists of 30 pictures representing a particular scene or interpersonal situation and one blank card. Examiners administer approximately ten cards selected based on common interpersonal situations depicted in the cards and information about interpersonal dynamics relevant to the given patient. In response to each card, the patient is asked to make up a story about what is being depicted in the card, and the examiner records these responses verbatim.

The TAT investigates personality dynamics manifested in interpersonal relationships via the patient's meaningful interpretations (apperceptions) of the environment as depicted on the cards. The TAT differs from the Rorschach

Table 3–5 **Description of WAIS-III Subtests**

	SUBTEST	DESCRIPTION
Verbal Scales	Information	Measures range of general factual knowledge
	Digit Span	Measures immediate rote recall/reversibility skills and involves short-term auditory memory, sequential and attentional processes
	Vocabulary	Measures word knowledge and provides index of language development
	Arithmetic	Measures computational skill and taps attentional, sequential, and numerical reasoning processes
	Comprehension	Measures social judgment, practical knowledge, and ability to apply past experience in formulating solutions to specific problems
	Similarities	Measures verbal concept formation and verbal reasoning skills
Performance Scales	Picture Completion	Measures ability to differentiate essential from nonessential details and taps long-term visual memory skills
	Picture Arrangement	Measures planning ability, the capacity to anticipate consequences, and temporal sequencing and time concepts
	Block Design	Measures nonverbal concept formation, spatial visualization skills, and the capacity for analysis and synthesis of abstract visual stimuli
	Object Assembly	Measures anticipation of relations among parts to form familiar objects, and ability to benefit from sensory-motor feedback
	Digit Symbol	Measures speed and accuracy of visual-motor coordination, psychomotor speed, and visual short-term memory

by providing less ambiguous stimuli, a more clearly specified task structure, and a greater focus on interpersonal dynamics than on perceptual functioning and reality testing. The absence of accepted formal scoring procedures has resulted in a standard practice of qualitative analysis of test data requiring clinical acumen and experience. Typical categories that provide a systematic focus for TAT interpretation include interpersonal relationships, significant intrapsychic and interpersonal conflicts, and adequacy of ego and superego functioning (Bellak and Abrams, 1993).

Interpretation of Test Findings. Ms. Foster's WAIS-R results placed her in the superior range of overall intellectual functioning, as she obtained a Full Scale IQ of 127. Her Verbal IQ was 119 and her Performance IQ was 127. There was no statistically significant difference between her verbal and performance scores. Her verbal comprehension and perceptual organization scores were comparable, suggesting that these abilities were fairly evenly developed; however, her performance on the Digit Span subtest, which loads on the freedom from distractibility factor, was significantly lower than all other subtest scores, suggesting that psychological factors impaired her attention and concentration. These results were not indicative of any neuropsychiatric condition or learning disability. Additionally, the comparability in verbal and performance subscale scores was not consistent with what might be expected from a depressed person whose depressive symptoms would probably interfere with performance on nonverbal timed tasks. Qualitative and quantitative analyses of the data revealed no evidence of a thought disorder, as might be expected from an individual with a schizophrenia spectrum disorder.

Despite the lack of evidence for a thought disorder on the WAIS-R, Ms. Foster showed signs of a mild thought disorder on the Rorschach, a test sensitive in detecting subtle underlying disturbances in thinking. Although she did not offer responses reflective of a severe thought disorder, on occasion, she provided realistically implausible and odd responses, including "two pigs fighting over a baseball bat" and responses reflecting boundary disturbance, such as "two women joined at the hip." Ms. Foster's overall Rorschach protocol also revealed reality testing difficulties; however, no gross perceptual distortions were noted.

Her Rorschach responses suggested difficulties with impulse control and a tendency to become overwhelmed by her feelings. On the first card in which there is some color present (red blot areas), she commented, "Oh boy, this makes me nervous! Wait a minute. I'm confused. Okay. That looks like blood, like menstrual blood, like when I have my period." The manner in which color is incorporated into percepts indicates the degree of emotional control, with more emphasis on color than form suggesting that affect is likely to be expressed more intensely. Ms. Foster provided a significant number of Rorschach responses depicting aggressive activity and interaction, including "an angel and a devil in a fist fight." This response also suggests the use of splitting as a defense, as she offers a "good" object (angel) fighting with a "bad" object (devil).

Finally, her Rorschach Coping Deficit Index and Suicide Constellation were positive. These findings are indicative of chronic susceptibility to difficulties coping with everyday stressors and interpersonal conflicts and increased risk for suicidal ideation and/or behavior.

Her TAT responses were consistent with her Rorschach results. Her responses reflected aggressive themes and tumultuous interpersonal relationships, marked by impulsivity, difficulty with affect regulation, and a propensity to consider suicidal behavior to cope with stress. For example, on a card in which a woman is touching the shoulders of a man who is turned away from her as if he were trying to pull away, Ms. Foster produced the following story: "They are having an argument over whether he's having an affair. She yells that she has always been faithful and he constantly betrays her. She demands that he stay with her because if he leaves, she will overdose. The fight started because he came home a half hour late from work and wasn't very sociable when he arrived. She was furious and he didn't seem to care. As always, they will probably make up, but fight about the same problem later, or he may leave and she may take an overdose."

Her MMPI-2 was valid and interpretively useful. It yielded a 3-point code (three highest clinical scale elevations) of 8-4-2 (Schizophrenia, Psychopathic Deviate, and Depression Scales). Individuals with this profile typically present with social alienation and social adjustment difficulties, proneness to frequent relationship conflicts, angry and impulsive behavior, and underlying dysphoria. Additionally, such persons often present with identity confusion and distortions in thinking.

Taken together, Ms. Foster's test findings are consistent with a diagnosis of borderline personality disorder with a propensity to experience transient psychotic episodes under stress and chronic depression. At her best, which occurs in relatively structured and affectively neutral circumstances, she is an intelligent woman with a capacity for positive interpersonal interactions. Given the extent of her coping deficits, however, her equilibrium becomes easily disrupted under stressful conditions, particularly those marked by interpersonal conflict. At these times, she may become affectively labile, impulsive, and hostile. Under conditions that she experiences as extremely stressful, namely, when confronted with threats of abandonment and actual loss, she may become actively suicidal, and the quality of her thinking and reality testing are likely to deteriorate, giving way to psychotic distortions of reality. However, her thinking and reality testing impairments are not so severe as to be consistent with a diagnosis of schizophrenia or major depression with psychotic features. Based on these results, long-term psychodynamic psychotherapy was recommended to help the patient develop more effective coping strategies for dealing with interpersonal conflicts and painful affects. Additionally, group therapy was deemed advisable, as this is a particularly effective modality for addressing interpersonal difficulties (Yalom, 1995).

Vignette 3

Mr. Lee, a 40-year-old computer software specialist, was diagnosed positive for the human immunodeficiency virus (HIV) 4 years prior to being referred by his internist for psychiatric evaluation of his complaints of unmanagable anxiety and insomnia. These difficulties began 4 months earlier, concurrent with his first HIV/acquired immunodeficiency syndrome-related hospitalization for pneumocystis pneumonia. He had no previous psychiatric history, although he reported a tendency to worry and to be "high strung." During the evaluation, the psychiatrist conducted a Mini-Mental Status Examination (Folstein et al, 1975), which suggested possible difficulties with short-term memory. Upon questioning, Mr. Lee acknowledged that he had "not been as sharp as usual at work." As it was unclear whether or not his memory difficulties were secondary to his anxiety problems or indicative of deteriorated cognitive functioning associated with HIV-related neurocognitive impairments, head CT and magnetic resonance imaging were ordered. The results were negative. Thus, the psychiatrist referred Mr. Lee for neuropsychological evaluation to ascertain whether or not there was an organic basis to his short-term memory difficulties not detected on neurological work-up.

The psychologist conducted a brief screening evaluation for specific memory deficits, which included the WAIS-III, Trail-Making Test (a subtest of the Halstead-Reitan Battery), Bender Visual-Motor Gestalt Test (Bender-Gestalt), and California Verbal Learning Test (CVLT). The MMPI-2 was administered to assess personality functioning.

Trail Making Test

The Trail Making Test, assessing motor speed, visuomotor tracking, and attention, is sensitive to the effects of brain injury (Lezak, 1995). Part A asks the patient to draw lines to connect consecutively numbered circles on a worksheet. For Part B, the patient is asked to connect consecutively numbered and lettered circles by alternating between the two sequences (i.e., 1-A-2-B-3-C, etc.). For both Parts A and B, the respondent is asked to complete the task as quickly as possible without lifting the pencil from the paper.

Bender Visual Motor Gestalt Test

The Bender-Gestalt, a visual motor task widely used as a screen for physical brain impairment, consists of nine simple designs displayed on separate cards presented to the patient one at a time. The patient is instructed to copy each design exactly as it appears on the card in front of them (Direct Copy Trial). Objective scoring systems provide a means to evaluate whether or not there is likely to be organic impairment. The Bender-Gestalt can also be used to assess visual memory deficits. For these purposes, after the direct copy trial, the patient is asked to recall the nine designs from memory by drawing them (Immediate Recall Trial). Then, after working for 20 minutes on an interference task, the respondent is again asked to draw the nine designs from memory (Delayed Recall Trial).

California Verbal Learning Test

The CVLT assesses retention, recognition, and recall in the verbal memory system. Results enable the examiner to distinguish deficits in these three areas. The CVLT assesses the capacity to learn new orally presented material, retain this information in short- and long-term memory, and recall this information in the context of semantic cues. Additionally, it assesses long-term recognition memory.

Interpretation of Test Findings. Results of the brief neuropsychological evaluation suggested that Mr. Lee's memory difficulties may reflect both high levels of anxiety and organic difficulties. On the WAIS-R, Mr. Lee obtained a Full Scale IQ of 110, Verbal IQ of 115, and Performance IQ of 104, placing him in the average range of intellectual functioning. The 11-point Verbal-Performance IQ difference is statistically significant, but not an abnormally large discrepancy, suggesting that his verbal skills are better developed than his nonverbal skills. Intra- and inter-subtest scatter on the Performance sub-tests was minimal, revealing relatively consistent intellectual functioning in the nonverbal area. Although five of the six Verbal subtest scores were above average, on the Digit Span subtest, he evidenced moderate impairments on the digits forward portion and considerable difficulty repeating digits backward. This suggests that his anxiety interfered with his capacity to attend (digits forward) and raised the possibility of short-term auditory memory difficulties (significant discrepancy between digits forward and digits backward).

On the Trail Making Test, Mr. Lee's time in completing Parts A and B were not significantly different; however, his time to completion on both sections was slower than expected for an individual achieving an average Full Scale IQ and fell below the average time to completion for persons without brain impairment.

Mr. Lee's direct copy of the Bender-Gestalt yielded an overall score in the borderline range for the task, raising questions about possible organic impairment. His immediate and delayed recall trials were slightly below average, suggesting mild impairment of short- and long-term visual memory.

On the CVLT, he evidenced considerably more difficulty in learning newly presented material than would be expected for an individual with an average IQ. Furthermore, he demonstrated impaired short- and long-term retention, with minimal improvement noted when semantic cues were provided. In addition, he demonstrated only slightly improved performance on the delayed recognition portion of the CVLT. This overall pattern of results on the CVLT and Bender-Gestalt suggests the presence of verbal and visual memory deficits. Specifically, the results are indicative of encoding, retention, and recall difficulties inhibiting his capacity to learn and retain new information.

The patient provided a valid MMPI-2, albeit with some indication of guardedness (mild elevation on the K validity scale). All his clinical scale scores were in the normal range, except for scales 2 (Depression) and 7 (Psychasthenia), which were mildly elevated. This profile typically is seen in individuals who feel nervous, tense, guilty, and dysphoric. Such persons are also prone to excessive worry and obsessional thinking.

Overall, results from this screening battery led the psychologist to conclude that Mr. Lee's overall intellectual functioning is in the average range. The findings showed evidence for mild attentional difficulties and specific memory deficits. Mr. Lee appears to experience significant levels of anxiety that may exacerbate his encoding and retention difficulties, although his anxiety is unlikely to account for the extent of his apparent memory deficits; however, his pattern of results does not suggest impairments significant enough to interfere profoundly with his capacity to function effectively at work. Finally, there were some data suggesting possible diffuse organic brain impairment (e.g., borderline performance on the Bender-Gestalt and Trail Making tests, Verbal-Performance IQ difference on the WAIS-III).

Based on these findings, the psychologist recommended further and more complete neuropsychological evaluation to ascertain the presence and extent of diffuse organic brain impairment and its impact on cognitive functioning. The psychologist also recommended that the internist provide written instructions regarding medical management to enhance proper compliance. Furthermore, a combination of stress management, cognitive-behavioral interventions, and evaluation for anxiolytic medications was suggested as a means to address the patient's anxiety. Finally, the importance of helping him develop strategies for coping with his memory deficit was underscored.

Communication of Findings

Once the testing has been completed and interpreted and the evaluator is prepared with answers to the referral questions and other pertinent information, it is essential that the information gleaned from the testing be provided to the relevant parties. Providing feedback regarding test results is an interactive process in which all concerned parties discuss the findings, their meanings, and the limitations of the results (Pope, 1992). The format and content of the communication of test findings vary, depending on the referral source, the questions being addressed, and the person(s) to whom the results are being presented. In addition to receiving verbal feedback, test results will be communicated to the physician via a testing report. The testing report involves analysis, synthesis, and integration of the material gathered during the testing (Tallent, 1993). Testing reports typically include the following sections: identifying information, reason for referral, pertinent background information, behavioral observations, intellectual and neuropsychological functioning, achievement and aptitude, personality and/or emotional functioning, summary and recommendations.

SUMMARY AND CONCLUDING COMMENTS

Psychological assessment is a process that entails collecting, organizing, and interpreting information about a person's cognitive and emotional functioning and situational influences. Psychological tests permit the measurement, description, evaluation, and prediction of some human behaviors. The reliability and validity of the results are influenced by the patient's attitudes toward testing and degree of compliance, the psychometric properties of the assessment devices used, the manner in which the testing is conducted (i.e., degree of standardization of test administration), and the ways in which the examiner interprets the findings. Choices of assessment devices and interpretation of findings often are guided by the referral questions, theoretical biases of the examiner, and context in which the testing is conducted. Physicians may request psychological testing when further information is needed regarding a patient's intellectual and neuropsychological functioning, presence of underlying psychotic processes and affective disturbances, quality of ego functioning, intrapsychic and interpersonal dynamics and personality style, and veracity of patient's complaints. Psychological testing results, if communicated clearly and in a manner relevant to the referral questions, can be used by the referring physician to aid in diagnosis, case formulation, and treatment planning.

Mental health professionals may request a psychological testing consultation during any phase of psychotherapy. In the evaluation phase, test results may be useful in matching patients to treatment modality, theoretical orientation, and clinician. In the early stages of psychotherapy, testing may provide a comprehensive understanding of the patient's psychological functioning across functional domains. This helps the therapist anticipate potential difficulties that may complicate the therapeutic alliance, sensitize the therapist to central areas of conflict, suggest areas of focus in treatment, elucidate potentially useful intervention strategies, and assist the therapist in more effectively managing resistances. In the later stages of psychotherapy, testing can be of value when therapeutic impasses emerge, and testing may be useful as a barometer of therapeutic progress and future areas of work.

Like all assessment tools, psychological tests are not without their limitations. Interpretation of test findings often varies between psychologists, who may differentially emphasize various pieces of test data. Interpretation is influenced by the interpersonal dynamics of the testing situation (Schafer, 1954), the theoretical orientation of the psychologist, the types and format of the tests utilized, and the interpretive systems employed. These factors influence which psychological themes become the focus of the assessment and treatment process.

Another potential limitation of psychological assessment is the questionable applicability of tests for individuals from various cultural and ethnic groups. Psychological tests vary with regard to the degree of cross-cultural standardization used in their psychometric construction. As such, psychologists must use care in test selection, to determine the psychometric appropriateness of a given test for use with persons from a specific cultural group. Furthermore, knowledge of normative differences in performance among different ethnic and cultural groups is essential to the interpretive process.

Some have argued that a potential limitation of the psychological testing process is an excessive emphasis on deficits and pathology to the relative exclusion of the person's strengths and health. They advocate a more balanced approach in test design and the interpretation of test findings. They stress the importance of identifying the individual's adaptive modes of functioning. Finally, research regarding the psychometric soundness (e.g., adequacy of reliability and validity) of various assessment instruments has yielded equivocal results, which, in turn, lead to questions regarding the usefulness and meaningfulness of test findings. Some researchers and clinicians assert that many of the psychological tests described in this chapter, particularly personality inventories and projective tests, are of minimal value. For example, behavioral psychologists avoid subjective interpretation of the person, as they eschew the notion of internal psychological dynamics or traits in favor of an emphasis on functional analysis of observable behavior patterns and associated environmental events (Skinner, 1974).

These potential limitations underscore the importance of interpreting psychological test findings in the context of a person's medical status, psychiatric presentation, and sociocultural milieu. Thus, the integration of interdisciplinary sources of assessment data allows for comprehensive patient evaluation and well-informed treatment planning sensitive to the uniqueness of each person and his or her situation.

CLINICAL PEARLS

- Referral for psychological testing is appropriate when there is a need to assess intellectual, neuropsychological, and personality functioning, as well as questions pertaining to diagnostic clarification.
- Psychological testing results should be integrated with other pertinent clinical data when tests are used to aid in diagnosis, case formulation, treatment planning, and prediction of behavior.
- To maximize the usefulness of testing results, it is important that the physician clearly articulate specific referral questions to be addressed in the psychological evaluation.
- The utility of a given psychological test instrument should be evaluated on the basis of the psychometric properties of standardization, reliability, and validity.
- Although psychological tests are standardized instruments, individual differences, as well as the person's developmental and sociocultural context, must be taken into account in test interpretation.

ANNOTATED BIBLIOGRAPHY

Anastasi A: Psychological Testing, 6th ed. New York, Macmillan, 1988

This classic text provides an introduction to the nature and uses of psychological testing. It includes a review of the history of psychological testing, a discussion of ethical considerations in testing, an overview of basic psychometric issues pertaining to psychological tests, and a description of a wide range of commonly used tests.

Exner, JE: The Rorschach: A Comprehensive System. Vol 1: Basic Foundations, 3rd ed. New York, John Wiley and Sons, 1993

> This is an excellent introduction to the Comprehensive System of Rorschach administration, scoring, and basic interpretation. It also includes a brief history of the Rorschach as a clinical assessment tool, as well as a discussion of research findings relevant to Rorschach interpretation.

Exner JE: The Rorschach: A Comprehensive System. Vol 2. Interpretation, 2nd ed. New York, John Wiley and Sons, 1991

> A companion to Exner's first volume, this text offers a detailed focus on methods of Rorschach interpretation, including discussion of issues in diagnosis and treatment planning. It also outlines changes and revisions in scoring and interpretation made subsequent to publication of the first volume.

Greene RL: The MMPI-2/MMPI: An Interpretive Manual. Needham Heights, MA, Allyn and Bacon, 1991

> An excellent introduction to the MMPI-2 is presented in this book. In addition to an overview of basic psychometric properties of the MMPI-2, a comprehensive step-by-step discussion of test interpretation is also provided.

Kaufman AS: Assessing Adolescent and Adult Intelligence. Boston, Allyn and Bacon, 1990

> This book offers a detailed discussion of intellectual testing with an emphasis on the WAIS-R, providing an excellent detailed account of the breadth and depth of interpretive usefulness of intellectual test results. An overview of important issues and debates relevant to intellectual testing is also included.

Lezak MD: Neuropsychological Assessment, 3rd ed. Oxford, Oxford University Press, 1995

> This classic reference offers an overview of the nature and uses of neuropsychological testing. It provides descriptions of a wide range of available test instruments and includes discussion of their interpretive usefulness.

Sattler JM: Assessment of Children, 3rd ed. San Diego, Jerome M. Sattler, 1992

> This standard reference text offers an overview and introduction to psychological assessment with children. The emphasis is on assessment of abilities (e.g., intellectual functioning, achievement). Such specialized topics as mental retardation, learning disabilities, developmental disorders, attention-deficit hyperactivity disorder, and adaptive behavior are also discussed.

Tallent N: Psychological Report Writing, 4th ed. Englewood Cliffs, NJ, Prentice Hall, 1993

> An introduction to considerations in communication of test findings in a report is provided in this text. Even for those who are not likely to need knowledge of how to write a report, this book may offer insights into the types of information that might be derived from psychological testing.

REFERENCES

Anastasi A: Psychological Testing, 6th ed. New York, Macmillan, 1988

Bellak L, Abrams DM: The T.A.T, C.A.T, and S.A.T in Clinical Use, 5th ed. Boston, Allyn and Bacon, 1993

Exner JE: The Rorschach: A Comprehensive System. Vol 1: Basic Foundations, 3rd ed. New York, John Wiley and Sons, 1993

Exner JE: The Rorschach: A Comprehensive System. Vol 2. Interpretation, 2nd ed. New York, John Wiley and Sons, 1991

Folstein MF, Folstein SE, McHugh PR: Mini-mental state. J Psychiatr Res 12:189–198, 1975

Frank LK: Projective methods for the study of personality. J Psychol 8:389–413, 1939

Friedman M, Rosenman RH: Type A Behavior and Your Heart. New York, Knopf, 1974

Graham JR: MMPI-2: Assessing Personality and Psychopathology, 2nd ed. New York, Oxford University Press, 1993

Greene RL: The MMPI-2/MMPI: An interpretive Manual. Needham Heights, MA, Allyn and Bacon, 1991

Hathaway SR, McKinley JC: The Minnesota Multiphasic Personality Inventory, rev. ed. Minneapolis, University of Minnesota Press, 1943

Hathaway SR, McKinley JC: The Minnesota Multiphasic Personality Inventory–2. Minneapolis, University of Minnesota Press, 1989

Kaufman AS: Assessing Adolescent and Adult Intelligence. Boston, Allyn and Bacon, 1990

Keller LS, Butcher JN: Assessment of Chronic Pain Patients with the MMPI-2. Minneapolis, University of Minnesota Press, 1991

Lezak MD: Neuropsychological Assessment, 3rd ed. Oxford, Oxford University Press, 1995

Murray HA: Thematic Apperception Test Manual. Cambridge, Harvard University Press, 1943

Osborne D: The MMPI in medical practice. Psychiatr Ann 15:534–541, 1985

Pope KS: Responsibilities in providing psychological test feedback to clients. Psychol Assessment 4:268–271, 1992

Racusin GR, Moss NE: Psychological assessment of children and adolescents. In Lewis M (ed): Child and Adolescent Psychiatry: A Comprehensive Textbook. Baltimore, Williams & Wilkins, 1991:472–485

Rorschach H: Psychodiagnostics. New York, Grune & Stratton, 1921/1949

Sattler JM: Assessment of Children, 3rd ed. San Diego, Jerome M. Sattler, 1992

Schafer R: Psychoanalytic Interpretation in Rorschach Testing. New York, Grune & Stratton, 1954

Schretlen DJ: The use of psychological tests to identify malingered symptoms of mental disorder. Clin Psychol Rev 8:451–476, 1988

Skinner BF: About Behaviorism. New York, Vintage Books, 1974

Strassberg DS, Tilley D, Bristone S, Oei TPS: The MMPI and chronic pain: A cross-cultural view. Psychol Assessment 4:493–497, 1992

Tallent N: Psychological Report Writing, 4th ed. Englewood Cliffs, NJ, Prentice Hall, 1993

Thoresen CE, Powell LH: Type a behavior pattern: New perspectives on theory, assessment, and intervention. J Consult Clin Psychol 60:595–604, 1992

Wechsler D: Manual for the Wechsler Adult Intelligence Scale, 3rd ed. New York, Psychological Corporation, 1997

Wechsler D: Manual for the Wechsler Intelligence Scale for Children, 3rd ed. New York, Psychological Corporation, 1991

Widiger TA, Frances A: Interviews and inventories for the measurement of personality disorders. Clin Psychol Rev 7:49–75, 1987

Williams RB: Biobehavioral factors in cardiovascular disease. In Houpt JL, Brodie HKH (eds): Psychiatry, Vol 3: Consultation—Liaison Psychiatry and Behavioral Medicine. New York, Basic Books, 1986:391–399

Yalom IB: The Theory and Practice of Group Psychotherapy, 4th ed. New York, Basic Books, 1995

4

Delirium, Dementia, and Other Disorders Associated with Cognitive Impairment

Alan Stoudemire, James L. Levenson, and Thomas M. Brown

This chapter will discuss diagnosis and treatment of delirium, dementia, and other psychiatric conditions associated with cognitive impairment. The term *cognitive impairment* has replaced the anachronistic term "organic" in DSM-IV because it is now recognized that *many* of the *major* psychiatric disorders involve some degree of neuropsychological dysfunction and that all behavior has a neurochemical (organic) substrate. Taken as a whole, dementia, delirium, and other cognitive impairment disorders are among the most common psychiatric disorders encountered by general medical and surgical physicians in clinical practice.

Before proceeding in this area, a few basic terms will be defined to guide the discussion (Tucker et al, 1992; Popkin and Tucker, 1992).

1. *Delirium.* Delirium is a disorder, usually acute and fluctuating, characterized by an altered state of consciousness (that is, reduced awareness of and ability to respond to one's environment) (Table 4–1). Cognitive deficits in attention, concentration, thinking, memory, and goal-directed behavior are almost always present. Delirium may be accompanied by hallucinations, misperceptions of sensory stimuli (illusions), emotional lability, alterations in the sleep–wake cycle, psychomotor slowing, or hyperactivity. The onset of delirium is often abrupt, but

The editor gratefully acknowledges the help of Drs. Marshall Folstein and Paul McHugh who supplied textual material for the original version of the chapter in the first edition of this textbook.

Table 4–1 **Major Signs and Symptoms of Delirium**

Altered state of alertness, awareness, and consciousness (hyper-alert or obtunded; patient's level of consciousness may vary from time to time; lucid intervals may occur)

Fluctuating course—as above

Onset may be dramatic but may be subtle and evolve over days or weeks

Disorientation and confusion

Decreased attention, concentration, and memory

Psychotic symptoms—paranoia, hallucinations (often visual), delusions

Behavioral disinhibition, emotional lability, irritability

Psychomotor retardation or agitation—may vary in a 24-hour period

Fragmented sleep/wake cycle; increased agitation at night

Usually reversible with correction of underlying etiology

Apraxia, dysgraphia, dysnomia and tremors, abnormal reflexes (myoclonus or asterixis)

---

may be insidious in nature. The cause is usually traced to a medication side effect, metabolic abnormalities, toxic agents, acute central nervous system (CNS) abnormalities, or medication/drug intoxication or withdrawal. If the cause of the delirium can be identified and corrected, the condition usually remits relatively promptly. In DSM-IV the subtypes "substance-induced delirium" and "delirium due to multiple etiologies" are listed.

2. *Substance-induced delirium.* Substance-induced delirium is associated with psychoactive agents due to either intoxication or withdrawal. This category of mental disorders is used to designate behavioral abnormalities caused by direct effects of psychoactive agents on the brain. DSM-IV addresses the following drugs associated with intoxication syndromes: alcohol, amphetamines (and similar sympathomimetics), caffeine, cannabis, opioids, cocaine, hallucinogens, inhalants, phencyclidine (and similarly acting arylcyclohexylamines), sedative-hypnotics, and anxiolytics. *Withdrawal* deliria are possible with alcohol, sedative-hypnotics, and anxiolytics. Many medical drugs (including narcotics) can cause delirium, e.g. histamine (H-2) blocking agents, digitalis, and anticholinergics. In many cases, it is difficult to ascertain a precise etiology of the patient's delirium (such as a patient who has fever, electrolyte abnormalities, and renal failure being treated with multiple medications including narcotic), in which case the delirium is noted to be caused by

"multiple etiologies." Table 4–2 is a *partial* listing of drugs that have been reported to cause delirium. They are discussed further in Chapter 10 by Dr. Swift.

3. Dementia is a disorder of cognitive impairment (Table 4–3). *In addition* to impairments in short- and long-term memory, prob-

Table 4–2 **Drugs That May Cause Psychiatric Symptoms***

Depression

*Antihypertensives (especially reserpine, methyldopa, beta-blockers, clonidine)	Indomethacin (and other nonsteroidal antiinflammatory drugs)
Amphotericin B	Antineoplastic drugs
*Corticosteroids	Procarbazine
Anticonvulsants	Tamoxifen
*Sedative-hypnotics	Vinblastine
Oral contraceptives	Asparaginase
Antipsychotics	Ethionamide
Metoclopramide	Acetazolamide

Mania

*Corticosteroids	Dopamine agonists
Sympathomimetics (esp. nonprescription decongestants and bronchodilators)	Antidepressants
	Zidovudine (AZT)
Isoniazid	Stimulants

Anxiety

*Sympathomimetics	Stimulants
*Theophylline	Antidepressants
*Caffeine	*Sedative-hypnotics (withdrawal)

Psychosis (Hallucinations or Delusions)

*Anticholinergics	Antiviral drugs
Antihistamines (cimetidine, ranitidine, diphenhydramine, etc)	Acyclovir
	Vidarabine
Antiarrhythmics (esp. lidocaine, tocainide, mexiletine, quinidine)	Interferon
	Zidovudine (AZT)
*Dopamine agonists	Podophyllin
L-dopa	Antineoplastic drugs
Bromocriptine	Asparaginase
Amantadine	Methotrexate
*Corticosteroids	Vincristine
Digitalis	Cytarabine
Antidepressants	Fluorouracil
Opiates	Disulfiram
Meperidine	Sympathomimetics
Pentazocine	Metrizamide
Antimalarials	Methysergide
Anticonvulsants	Baclofen
Beta-blockers	Cycloserine
	Cyclosporine

*   Denotes especially "high-risk" drugs for causing symptoms in question.

Table 4–3 **Summary of the Major Signs and Symptoms of Dementia**

Alzheimer's type
Multiple cognitive deficits characterized by:
  Memory impairment
  At least one of the following disturbances:
    Aphasia
    Apraxia
    Agnosia
    Executive functioning (planning, organizing, sequencing, abstraction) impaired
Gradual onset and continued decline
Cognitive deficits lead to significant impairment in social and/or occupational function-
  ing and represent decline from previous level of functioning
Cognitive deficits are *not* due to another identifiable metabolic, or neurologic disorder,
  or due to another psychiatric disorder (such as depressive pseudodementia or schizo-
  phrenia)
Cognitive deficits are not primarily caused by delirium

Vascular Dementia
Multiple cognitive, deficits characterized by:
  Memory impairment
  At least one of the following disturbances:
    Aphasia
    Apraxia
    Agnosia
    Executive functioning (planning, organizing, sequencing, abstraction) impaired
Focal neurologic signs (see text) or radiographic evidence of cerebral vascular disease
Cognitive deficits lead to significant impairment in social and/or occupational function-
  ing and represent decline from previous level of functioning
Cognitive deficits are not due to a delirium

Dementia Due to Other Conditions
Multiple cognitive deficits characterized by:
  Memory impairment
  At least one of the following disturbances:
    Aphasia
    Apraxia
    Agnosia
    Executive functioning (planning, organizing, sequencing, abstraction) impaired
Cognitive deficits lead to significant impairment in social and/or occupational function-
  ing and represent decline from previous level of functioning
Cognitive deficits not primarily caused by delirium
Evidence exists from physical exam or laboratory or radiographic evidence that the cog-
  nitive dysfunction is caused by one or more of the following:
    HIV
    Head trauma
    Parkinson's disease
    Huntington's disease
    Pick's disease
    Creutzfeldt-Jakob disease
    Other causes (hypothyroidism, B_{12} deficiency, normal pressure hydrocephalus,
      brain tumors, etc.; see Table 4–4)

(Adapted from American Psychiatric Association: Diagnostic and Statistical Manual of Mental Disorders, 4th
ed. Washington, DC, American Psychiatric Association, 1994)

lems exist in abstract thinking, logical judgment, personality changes, orientation, interpersonal relationships, and higher cortical functions, such as language and calculations. The onset is usually insidious and slowly progressive. As noted above, unlike in delirium, the patient's *level of awareness and alertness is usually intact* in the early and middle stages of the illness and usually becomes impaired only in the *latter stages* of the illness; the retention and stability of *alertness* is a primary symptom that distinguishes *dementia* from *delirium.* Examples of dementia include Alzheimer's disease, Pick's disease, AIDS-related dementia, vascular (multi-infarct) dementia, dementia of Parkinson's disease, and normal pressure hydrocephalus (Table 4–4). Table 4–5 contrasts the clinical differences between delirium and dementia. Alzheimer's-type dementia *must* also be accompanied by one more of the following signs or symptoms (indicating dementia is more than just a memory disorder): aphasia (language dysfunction), apraxia (difficulty or inability to carry out most activities), agnosia (difficulty or failure to recognize or identify objects), and disturbances in executive functioning (DSM-IV; American Psychiatric Association, 1994).The course is usually chronic and deteriorating unless an identifiable, treatable cause of the brain dysfunction is identified (such as B_{12} deficiency or hypothyroidism).

The most common form of dementia is Alzheimer's disease and can be associated with superimposed delirium, delu-

Table 4–4 **Causes of Dementia (Partial Listing)**

Alcohol-related dementia
Alzheimer's disease
Chronic granulomatous meningitis (tuberculous, fungal)
Folic acid deficiency
Head trauma
Human immunodeficiency virus
Huntington's chorea
Hypothyroidism
Multiinfarct dementia
Multiple sclerosis
Neoplasms
Normal-pressure hydrocephalus
Parkinson-dementia complex
Postanoxic states
Progressive supranuclear palsy
Tertiary neurosyphilis
Transmissible virus dementia (Jakob-Creutzfeldt disease)
Vitamin B_{12} deficiency

Table 4–5 **Differential Diagnosis of Delirium and Dementia**

FEATURE	DELIRIUM	DEMENTIA
Onset	Acute, often at night	Insidious
Course	Fluctuating, with lucid intervals, during day; worse at night	Stable over course of day
Duration	Hours to weeks	Months or years
Awareness	Reduced	Clear
Alertness	Abnormally low or high	Usually normal
Attention	Lacks direction and selectivity, distractibility, fluctuates over course of day	Relatively unaffected
Orientation	Usually impaired for time, tendency to mistake unfamiliar for familiar place and persons	Often impaired
Memory	Immediate and recent impaired	Recent and remote impaired
Thinking	Disorganized	Impoverished
Perception	Illusions and hallucinations, usually visual and common	Often absent
Speech	Incoherent, hesitant, slow or rapid	Difficulty in finding words
Sleep–wake cycle	Always disrupted	Fragmented sleep
Physical illness or drug toxicity	Either or both present	Often absent, especially in Alzheimer's disease

(Used with permission from Lipowski ZJ: Delirium (acute confusional states). JAMA 258:1789–1792, 1987)

sions, and symptoms of depressed mood. If the patient's depressive symptoms are of such severe proportion to meet diagnostic criteria for major depression, then major depression should be listed as a separate concurrent diagnosis.

The other major cause of dementia in the elderly is *vascular dementia* (also referred to as multi-infarct dementia or cerebrovascular dementia). In DSM-IV, its criteria differ little from those of Alzheimer's disease, except that evidence of focal neurologic signs and symptoms should be present [e.g., hyperactive deep tendon reflexes, extensor plantar (Babinski) response, pseudobulbar palsy, gait abnormalities, weakness, etc.] *or* radiographic evidence of cerebral vascular disease, such as multiple infarction of the cerebral cortex or white matter. Vascular dementia can be "subtyped" based on the presence or absence of concurrent deliria, delusions, or depressive symptoms (American Psychiatric Association, 1994).

4. *Substance-induced dementia.* Dementia syndromes induced by substances are also characterized by multiple cognitive deficits and by memory impairment (usually the inability to learn new information or to recall previously learned information) along with one or more of the following symptoms: aphasia, apraxia, agnosia, or disturbances in executive functioning (planning, organization, and abstract thought). The symptoms should represent a change in the patient's usual level of functioning. The primary substance associated with this form of dementia is *alcohol,* but it may occur with certain types of inhalants, as well.

5. *Amnestic disorders.* These are disorders characterized by a relatively focal disorder of short-term memory, characterized by the inability to learn new information or the inability to recall previously learned information; other cognitive functions are intact. The memory disturbance must be accompanied by impaired social or occupational functions. The memory problem should not occur as part of a primary delirium or dementia syndrome. The most common cause of substance-induced amnestic disorders is alcoholism. The most common neuroanatomic abnormality that has been described with the amnestic syndrome is bilateral sclerosis of the mamillary bodies, probably due to hemorrhage. Degenerative changes also have been described in the dorsal medial nucleus of the thalamus, which serves as a relay point between memory centers and the frontal cortex.

    Transient global amnesia (TGA) is a form of amnestic disorder that usually occurs in middle-aged or elderly individuals and is characterized by the sudden loss of memory of recent events and the inability to recall new information. In DSM-IV, TGA would be coded as an *amnestic disorder with transient features.* The essential feature of this condition is the transitory inability to learn new information (encoding memory problems) with a variable retrograde amnesia that "shrinks" following recovery such that the amnestic gap is confined to that time period predominantly between the acute onset of the disorder and its resolution (Caine, 1993). The level of consciousness usually is normal during the course of TGA, and personal identity remains intact. Patients are aware of their deficits and may ask questions about their circumstances. Such episodes may last from minutes to hours, and attacks usually are episodic. The "spells" often remit within 24 hours. Most experts consider the episodes to be caused by transient vascular insufficiency of the mesial temporal lobe, but other disorders such as tumors, use of short-acting benzodiazepines (such as triazolam), cardiac arrhythmias, cerebral embolism, migraine, polycythemia vera, and mitral valvular disease have been reported to cause episodes of TGA. Most patients with TGA also have associated risk factors for cerebrovascular stroke. Amnestic disorders may be classified based upon whether they are due to medical causes or due to psychoactive substances (Caine, 1993). Amnestic disorders are characterized as being either *transient or chronic,* based on the time course and persistence of the amnesia.

6. *Anxiety, mood, and psychotic disorders due to general medical conditions and substances.* These diagnoses are made when evidence of brain dysfunction affecting behavior (anxiety, mood, psychosis) exists but a *primary* dementia or delirium has been ruled out; the symptoms should occur in the presence of a relatively clear mental status. These conditions involve abnormalities in *mood, anxiety,* or *the presence of psychotic symptoms, delusions,* and *hallucinations* that can usually be attributed directly to some specific cause or agent. *As noted above, these diagnoses should not be made if the patient primarily meets diagnostic criteria for delirium or a dementia.*

   A patient with a clear mental status who becomes depressed because of *hypothyroidism* would be considered to have a depressive disorder due to a general medical condition. A complete review of these syndromes is beyond the scope of this text, but the most common causes of these mood and psychotic disorders are summarized in Tables 4–6, 4–7, and 4–8.

7. *Personality change due to a general medical condition.* This disorder applies to situations where patients develop personality changes from the usual pattern due to a specific medical or neurological condition (such as temporal lobe epilepsy). The disorder is subtyped into the following categories: *labile, disinhibited, aggressive, apathetic,* and *paranoid,* although mixtures of symptoms are perhaps most common clinically (combined type) (Table 4–9).

8. *Catatonic disorder due to a general medical condition.* Catatonic behavior is characterized by negativism, profound withdrawal, mutism, motor rigidity, and catalepsy ("waxy" flexibility that may alternate with severe agitation). The disorder is most commonly associated with mood disorders, but may also occur as a presenting symptom of a variety of medical and neurological disorders such as herpes encephalitis, vascular insults, or as a profound parkinsonian-like reaction to neuroleptics (neuroleptic-induced catatonia) (Popkin and Tucker, 1992; Stoudemire, 1982). In DSM-IV, the category is deemed

Table 4–6 **Major Reported Causes of Depressive Syndromes Due to General Medical Conditions, Medications, and Other Substances**

Medications and Substances

Antihypertensives (reserpine, methyldopa, propranolol)
Barbiturates
Corticosteroids
Ethanol
Indomethacin
Levodopa
Psychostimulants (amphetamine and cocaine in the postwithdrawal phase)

Medical Illnesses

Carcinoid syndrome
Carcinomas (pancreatic)
Cerebrovascular disease (stroke)
Collagen-vascular disease (systemic lupus erythematosus)
Endocrinopathies (Cushing's syndrome, Addison's disease, hypoglycemia, hyper- and hypocalcemia, hyper- and hypothyroidism)
Lymphomas
Parkinson's disease
Pernicious anemia (B_{12} deficiency)
Viral illnesses (hepatitis, mononucleosis, influenza)

(Adapted from Stoudemire A: Selected organic mental disorders. In Hales RE, Yudofsky SC (eds): Textbook of Neuropsychiatry. Washington, DC, American Psychiatric Press, 1987)

"catatonic disorder due to a general medical condition" where medical and neurologic disorders are the causative factor.

9. *Postconcussional syndrome* (included in DSM-IV as a diagnosis for further study). This syndrome follows a history of head trauma resulting in significant cerebral concussion, manifested in loss of consciousness, posttraumatic amnesia, and, less commonly, post-traumatic seizures. Evidence should exist from neuropsychological testing of impairments in attention, concentration, performing simultaneous cognitive tasks, and impairments in learning new information or recalling information that occurs shortly after the traumatic injury. Other symptoms associated with the postconcussive syndrome include easy fatiguability, vertigo, dizziness, irritability, emotional lability, impulsivity (sometimes involving aggression), anxiety, depression, personality changes, inappropriate sexual or social behaviors, and apathy. Patients should not meet criteria for dementia, including dementia due to head trauma. Hence, the

Table 4–7 **Major Reported Causes of Manic Syndromes Due to General Medical Conditions, Medications, and Other Substances**

Medications

Antidepressants
Corticosteroids/ACTH
Decongestants (containing phenylephrine)
Levodopa
Monoamine oxidase inhibitors
Sympathomimetics/bronchodilators (containing theophylline and/or ephedrine/isophedrine)

Metabolic Abnormalities

Hyperthyroidism

Seizure/Neurologic Disorders

Multiple sclerosis
Right hemispheric damage
Temporal lobe seizures

Neoplasms

Human Immunodeficiency Virus Infection

(Adapted from Stoudemire A: Selected organic mental disorders. In Hales RE, Yudofsky SC (eds): Textbook of Neuropsychiatry. Washington, DC, American Psychiatric Press, 1987)

postconcussive syndrome is *not* a form of dementia. This disorder is listed in the Appendix to DSM-IV and will undergo further study before becoming an "official" disorder in this diagnostic manual (American Psychiatric Association, 1994).

Arriving at the diagnosis of delirium, dementia, and other cognitive impairment disorders requires a carefully structured cognitive and behavioral assessment of the patient. The following section discusses the clinical assessment of the patient's condition.

CLINICAL EXAMINATION OF THE PATIENT WITH COGNITIVE DYSFUNCTION: USE OF THE MINI-MENTAL STATE EXAMINATION

Perhaps the most serious clinical error made in medicine is underdiagnosis of cognitive disorders in medical and surgical settings. It is common for physicians to label erroneously a patient's abnormal behavior caused by a cognitive disorder as "functional" (that is, due to a "psychiatric" or emotional problem). Although the reasons for underdiagnosis or misdiagnosis of cognitive

Table 4–8 **Major Reported Causes of Psychotic Disorders Due to General Medical Conditions, Medications, and Other Substances (Partial Listing)**

CNS Disorders	**Endocrinopathies**
Cerebrovascular disease	Adrenal insufficiency
Idiopathic basal ganglia calcification	Cushing's disease
Multiple sclerosis	Hyperthyroidism
Neoplasms	Hypothyroidism
Parkinson's disease	Hypo- and hypercalcemia
Spinocerebellar degeneration	Panhypopituitarism
Temporal lobe epilepsy	**Miscellaneous**
Connective Tissue Disease	Amphetamines
Systemic lupus erythematosus	Bromide
Temporal arteritis	Corticosteroids
Deficiency States	Heavy metal toxicity
B$_{12}$	Huntington's chorea
Folate	Pentazocine
Niacin	Porphyria
Drug/Medications	
Antidepressants	
Antihypertensives	
Antimalarials, anticonvulsants	
Antiparkinsonian agents	
Antituberculosis agents	
Hallucinogens	

(Adapted from Stoudemire A: Selected organic mental disorders. In Hales RE, Yudofsky SC (eds): Textbook of Neuropsychiatry. Washington, DC, American Psychiatric Press, 1987)

impairment disorders are multiple, the most common explanation is the failure to perform a mental status examination. Because of this pervasive problem in clinical medicine, a significant portion of this chapter is devoted to presenting in some detail a structured cognitive mental status examination using the Mini-Mental State Examination (MMSE) (Folstein et al, 1975). The MMSE is a prac-

Table 4–9 **Major Reported Causes of Personality Changes Due to Medical and Neurological Conditions**

Adrenocortical disease
Head trauma
Heavy metal poisoning
Hypothyroidism
Multiple sclerosis
Neoplasms
Systemic lupus erythematosus
Temporal lobe, seizure disorders
Vascular disease

tical and efficient instrument for assessing, documenting, and tracking a patient's cognitive functioning over time. This cognitive screening instrument has been extensively validated in both clinical and research settings. Its brevity, accuracy, and efficiency make it immensely practical for routine clinical use (see Appendix at end of chapter).

There are, however, several disadvantages to this approach. Symptoms such as delusions and hallucinations, which could not be quantitated as easily, are not included. A total score does not specifically characterize the patient's cognitive capacity in terms such as amnesia, aphasia, or apraxia. A stereotyped exam like the MMSE will be less sensitive in the highly intelligent and less specific in those below average intelligence. Hence, the MMSE is *not* to be considered a comprehensive behavioral or cognitive mental status examination, but a reliable means of screening and monitoring gross changes in cognitive functioning.

More extensive mental status examinations are described elsewhere (Trzepacz and Baker, 1993).

Mini-Mental State Examination

The MMSE briefly surveys important cognitive functions, including language function, that are omitted from most other brief psychiatric screening tests (Chapter 4 Appendix). It is useful in screening patients and also is useful in teaching aspects of the cognitive examination. It can be embellished by the examiner's asking for such things as the interpretation of proverbs, a listing of the presidents in reverse order, or a drawing of a cube or a clock. It also can be amplified by the addition of more formal neuropsychological testing, including symbol digit and trails tests, to delineate in more detail preserved and impaired functions.

The MMSE begins with a set of questions about orientation in time and place. The patient is asked, "Where are you?" and the patient is expected to be able to tell us the place they are in space and time, specific to the day of the week and the month of the year. Thus, orientation to time and place can be graded, and a patient is *more or less* oriented, rather than *absolutely* disoriented or oriented. Patients can acquire 10 points out of 30 on the examination for giving a complete answer to the questions concerning *orientation.* Orientation is the first and easiest capacity to assess because it is so frequently disturbed among patients. Although disorientation can be as subtle as a mild sense of bewilderment over the date, it can be so severe that patients may not know whether they are indoors or outdoors, standing or lying, in the hospital or at home.

Because one cause of disorientation might be the inability of patients to learn from an assessment of their surroundings, the disorientation could be the outcome of a memory disorder. The next set of probes tests the ability of the patient to learn and remember.

Questions in this segment of the exam begin with the test of the patient's capacity to register and repeat three simple words that are presented orally. The patient is asked to repeat three words given approximately 1 second apart, such as pony, quarter, and orange, and is given one point *for* each of the three correctly repeated. This task is also an assessment of the patient's capacity to hear, attend, and repeat words, as well as the capacity to remember three objects mentioned in a very short period of time. To determine their capacity to recall for a longer period of time, the patient is asked to recall the three objects a short while later, after which he or she performs another task that is presented to prevent constant rehearsal of the three objects.

During this interval, another capacity is tested; the patient is asked to attend to a task and carry it through to completion. The best tasks testing attention and concentration are those that demand a continuing focus on and performance of a serial problem. Thus, a subtraction of 7 from 100 for five consecutive subtractions requires patients to be able to attend and at the same time perform an arithmetic function without losing track of the task that they are performing. Another similar, but less difficult, task is the spelling of the word "world" backward. This task is offered to patients only when they refuse to perform the serial 7s, because the serial 7s task is more difficult.

After the assessment of attention and calculation by the serial 7s task, it is determined whether patients can recall three words presented to them previously in the registration task; thus, they are able to tap a longer-term aspect of memory.

This completes the *first section* of the MMSE. Many aspects of the tests of orientation, registration, attention and calculation, and recall depend to some extent on the patient's capacity to comprehend and use language. The second part of the examination is designed explicitly to test the patient's language capacity. It is then determined whether the patient can name a visually presented object; repeat the phrase "No ifs, ands, or buts"; follow a three-stage verbal command—"Take this piece of paper in your right hand, fold it in half, and put it on the floor"; read a simple sentence—"Close your eyes"; write a sentence spontaneously; and copy a design. This aspect of the MMSE can be supplemented with evaluation by the physician of the patient's speech, whether it is fluent, dysarthric, or of normal rate, rhythm, and prosody. Thus, one then makes a judgment as to whether the patient speaks clearly with normal intonation or whether the speech is monotonic or slurred. In addition, it is noted whether the patient uses appropriate vocabulary or whether mistakes are made in the meaning of particular words, such as when new words are constructed or old words are pronounced incorrectly. It is also noted whether patients use appropriate syntax with complex or simple sentences in their response to questions, and finally, whether the patient in the course of the examination addresses the examiner in the expected fashion, with appropriate eye contact and demeanor. In this way, in addition to being able to score the patient's performance on a series of simple tasks, it is possible to appraise the patient's phonology; semantics, syntax, and pragmatics of language function. These last aspects are not scored, but should be entered as commentary on the patient's performance on the examination. The language section of the MMSE can be affected by disease processes of several types, including focal brain diseases of the left hemisphere, such as a stroke, as well as by diffuse brain disease, such as Alzheimer's disease.

The examination is concluded by an assessment of the patient's level of consciousness, which is rated on an analog scale from comatose to fully alert. This rating can be performed reliably and is a measure of the patient's alertness, responsiveness, and accessibility to the examiner (Anthony et al, 1985). Although this aspect of the examination is not taken into the total score, it serves to distinguish those patients who are cognitively impaired in a clear state of consciousness, as in dementia, from those who are cognitively impaired with an altered state of alertness and consciousness, as in delirium.

In a medical setting, the usual procedure is to try to determine whether the impairments as assessed by the MMSE in fact cluster into groups of symptoms, such as the syndromes of dementia and delirium. After that assessment, one then attempts to determine whether an *identifiable* pathological process is present, such as a stroke, Alzheimer's disease, or drug intoxication. In a final step of the overall evaluation, it is determined whether a recognizable risk factor or causal agent is present, such as hypertension or a genetic abnormality. Thus, one reasons from symptoms and signs to syndromes to pathology to etiology.

THE SYNDROMES

One conceptual approach to syndromes of cognitive impairment is to divide them into two main groups, the *developmental syndromes* and the *deteriorations*. The *developmental syndromes* include those aspects of *mental retardation, developmental dyslexia, and attention-deficit hyperactivity disorders,* which are present from *birth or early childhood.* These syndromes are contrasted with the *deteriorations* of cognition, which represent a decline from a previous level of functioning. Examples of deteriorations of cognition include dementia, delirium, aphasic syndromes, and amnestic syndromes. In this chapter, we consider only the *deteriorations* that are called dementia and delirium. Several of the developmental syndromes are discussed in Chapter 16 on child psychiatry by Dr. Dulcan.

DEMENTIA

Dementia is a deterioration of multiple cognitive functions occurring in clear consciousness and alertness and may have multiple causes (Tables 4–3 and 4–4). Dementia should be distinguished from cognitive impairments that are not deteriorating in nature and from more focal deteriorations of the brain, which may affect single functions such as language.

The determination of brain deterioration requires confirming evidence other than what is observed directly or elicited from the patient (e.g., family members or employers who can give examples of functions that the patient could once perform but in which there has been a change). Useful functions that can be evaluated and that may indicate cognitive decline include the ability to manage finances and a checkbook, the capacity to travel without becoming lost, the ability to use the telephone and take messages, and the ability to recall the place of objects, such as the patient's wallet, keys, and eyeglasses. Observations such as these from the patient's family are correlated with impairments in orientation, recall, attention, and sometimes language function, which can be documented with the MMSE. When a decline has been reported and found to be accompanied by multiple cognitive impairments on formal examination, the syndrome of dementia can be diagnosed if the patient is otherwise generally alert.

Contrary to some expectations, the syndrome of dementia can occur *suddenly,* as seen after stroke or hypoxic insults, but it more commonly develops *insidiously and progresses gradually,* as seen in Alzheimer's disease. The syndrome may at times be totally or partially reversible, such as in hypothyroidism, although the patient may be left with permanent impairments. Most dementia is irreversible, such as that associated with Alzheimer's disease. From an epidemiological point of view, most cases of dementia seen in the community are insidious, gradually progress, and are, at the present time, not reversible (Folstein et al, 1985). These facts clearly are subject to revision, however, if adequate treatments are discovered. The epidemiology of dementia in elderly patients is discussed in Chapter 11 on geriatric psychiatry.

Some authorities have found it useful to divide dementia into two types, the *cortical* type and the *subcortical* type. The former is associated with lesions in the cerebral cortex (gray matter) and the latter with lesions in the deeper, white matter. Clinically, this distinction is based on the symptomatic impression or "gestalt" of the presentation of patients. For example, dementias of the *cortical* type, as in Alzheimer's disease, tend to be characterized by a profound memory deficit and often a semantic aphasia, but the patient is fluent, moderately attentive, normally responsive to questions, and normally active in his environment at home or in the office (Brandt et al, 1987).

In contrast, patients with the *subcortical* dementing illness, such as Huntington's disease and normal pressure hydrocephalus, are relatively alert, but slowly responsive and inactive and usually are not fluent in their language. They are often dysarthric and have difficulty with forming complex sentences. These patients have little difficulty with semantic processing, however, and usually comprehend language fully, even when severely affected. They may have relatively mild disorders of memory or have marked attentional problems and show difficulty with "executive" functions, such as changing from one cognitive "set" to another, as demonstrated by the Wisconsin Card Sort Task or the Trail-Making Test (Brandt and Butters, 1986). In addition to their cognitive features, patients with subcortical dementia frequently suffer from motor disorders such as involuntary movements, as seen in Parkinson's disease and Huntington's disease. They often are found to have a depressive syndrome in addition to their cognitive syndrome. Thus, the patient with subcortical dementia is slow in response, apathetic, behaviorally inactive, and has a cognitive disorder associated with disorders of movement and mood. The distinction between cortical and subcortical dementias is not universally accepted by clinicians, and a significant amount of overlap exists between symptoms and pathology in the two categories.

Noncognitive Symptoms Accompanying Dementia

Disorders of mood, perception, belief, and behavior are often associated with dementia. Disorders of mood of several types are seen. A sustained depressive syndrome occurs in 30 to 60% of patients with subcortical dementia and 10 to 20% of cortical dementia patients (Rovner et al, 1986). Hence, dementia and depressive states can coexist, and the mood disorder component of the patient's condition can be responsive to antidepressants or electroconvulsive therapy.

Pathological laughter or crying occurs when the dementia syndrome is caused by bilateral corticobulbar lesions, such as in multiple strokes and multiple sclerosis. The disruption in mood may be transient, lasting seconds or minutes, and is often prompted by a meaningful psychological stimulus, such as a conversation, music, or a sentimental memory. The laughter or crying observed is often abnormal because it is expressed against the will of the patient, who does not always actually feel sad or happy and in fact is often embarrassed by it. It tends to be exaggerated, a caricature of normal crying or laughing.

Irritability and explosiveness is another type of emotional disorder seen with dementia, especially with the dementia of Huntington's disease. Excessive emotional outbursts that occur after task failure have been called "catastrophic reactions" and may occur in any dementia. Catastrophic reactions can be avoided or modulated by educating family members to avoid confrontations of memory deficits.

Delusions and hallucinations occur about 10 to 20% of the time at some phase of the dementia process. Paranoid delusions may arise out of the cognitive impairment, as when misplaced objects are reported by the patient to be stolen; hence, the patient attempts to make "sense" out of the fact that an object is gone by arriving at what he or she believes must be a logical explanation. It is not "there" because someone has apparently stolen it.

Hallucinations of all types occur, but visual hallucinations tend to be the most common. In Parkinson's disease or diencephalic vascular disease, peduncular hallucinosis is seen. In this condition, pleasant or relatively benign simple visions, such as falling handkerchiefs, usually occur. Lilliputian hallucinations of small people often dressed in colorful costumes also occur. In addition to these primary hallucinatory experiences, patients with dementia also experience a variety of misinterpretations of environmental stimuli (illusions). Patients with agnosia often misinterpret their environment and become fearful or aggressive (Cummings et al, 1987). A wide variety of abnormal behaviors is encountered, including suicide, aggression, agitation, emotional lability, wandering, and insomnia.

The relationship of dementia to other psychiatric disorders, such as depressive disorders, schizophrenia, and hysterical disorders, requires some clarification. Cognitive dysfunction also may occur in severe depression to the extent that it has been reported to "mimic" dementia in some respects. When cognitive dysfunction occurs in depression or in another psychiatric disorder, it may be referred to as "pseudodementia," the "dementia syndrome of depression," or "dementia of schizophrenia" (Folstein and McHugh, 1978). Perhaps more accurately, one may refer to it as *depression-related cognitive dysfunction*. Clinically, cognitive dysfunction due to depression *rarely*, if ever, resembles the global progressive deficits seen in dementia unless the patient already has a preexisting dementia on which the depressive disorder becomes superimposed. Primary dementia and depression may be superimposed on each other, although depression is frequently overlooked, dismissed, or otherwise not aggressively treated in patients with dementia (Stoudemire et al, 1988).

Causes of Dementia

Among the 6% of elderly individuals in the general population who are suffering from a dementia syndrome of some sort, approximately one-third to one-half are suffering from Alzheimer's disease, and approximately one-fifth to one-third are suffering from dementia related to stroke, with the remaining 20 to 30% suffering from other causes, including head trauma, alcoholism, Parkinson's disease, human immunodeficiency virus (HIV), and miscellaneous causes (Table 4–4).

In the general community, dementia related to *reversible* disorders is extremely low. In hospital settings, however, individuals with dementia syndromes often are suffering from reversible cognitive dysfunction that requires treatment (Rocca et al, 1986). It is also extremely common for delirium to occur concurrently with dementia in the hospitalized elderly because of unstable metabolic problems and medications (see following section on delirium).

The full evaluation of dementia [which consists of history, physical examination, laboratory tests for drug levels and toxins, electrolytes, liver function tests, calcium, phosphorus, thyroid, fluorescent treponemal antibody (FTA) test, serum B_{12} and folate levels sedimentation rate, chest X-ray, electrocardiogram (ECG), magnetic resonance imaging (MRI), computed tomography (CT), and electroencephalogram (EEG)] is usually unrevealing of reversible causes of cognitive dysfunction, although about 5 to 15% of patients may have a reversible or partially reversible condition affecting their cognitive dysfunction (Table 4–10).

Cortical Dementia

Alzheimer's Disease

The leading example of a cortical dementia syndrome is Alzheimer's disease (AD; Alzheimer, 1907). Approximate estimates of the prevalence of

Table 4–10 **Comprehensive Workup of Dementia and Delirium**

Physical exam, including thorough neurologic exam
Vital signs
Mental status examination
Mini-Mental State Exam (MMSE)
Review of medications and drug levels
Blood and urine screens for alcohol, drugs, and heavy metals*
Physiologic workup
    Serum electrolytes/glucose/Ca^{2+}, Mg^+
    Liver, renal function tests
    Urinalysis
    Complete blood cell count with differential
    Thyroid function tests (including TSH level)
    RPR or FTA
    Serum B_{12}, folate levels
    Ceruloplasmin*
    Erythrocyte sedimentation rate (Westergren)
    Antinuclear antibody*, C_3C_4, anti-DS DNA*
    Arterial blood gases*
    HIV screen*[†]
Chest X-ray
Electrocardiogram
Neurologic workup
    CT or MRI scan of head*[‡]
    Lumbar puncture*
    EEG*
Neuropsychological testing[§]

* If indicated by history and physical examination.
[†] Requires special consent and counseling.
[‡] See Table 4–11 for relative discriminating power.
[§] May be useful in differentiating dementia from other neuropsychiatric syndromes if this cannot be done clinically.
(Adapted with permission from Stoudemire A, Thompson TL: Recognizing and treating dementia. Geriatrics 36:112–120, 1981)

Alzheimer's disease in the community vary from 2 to 10% of the population over age 65 and from 15 to 20% of the population over age 85 (Rocca et al, 1986). Patients with Alzheimer's disease constitute more than half of all patients in nursing homes. These patients in the community or in nursing homes seldom have access to adequate psychiatric care and thus present a major public health problem in terms of the prevention of complications that result from the secondary symptoms of the disease.

AD is a dementia syndrome consisting of prominent memory deficits that usually begin with short-term memory and then progress to more pervasive memory deficits and global cognitive deficits such as aphasia, apraxia, and agnosia. Alzheimer's disease has an insidious onset and a gradual progression to death on average 7 years after onset, although great variability exists in the course of the illness (Katzman, 1986). The MMSE score in AD is approximately 14 (of 30) after 4 years of illness.

A firm diagnosis of AD requires pathological verification. On postmortem examination, the brain is found to be small and atrophic with a remarkable accumulation of neurofibrillary tangles and neuritic plaques with amyloid core and a deposition of amyloid in blood vessels in most cases. The composition of the neuritic tangle is under active investigation; however, there is some evidence that it consists of an amyloid fibril decorated with a variety of proteins, including ubiquitin and tau. The neuritic plaque consists of a beta pleated sheet of amyloid, probably derived from a transmembrane protein. Embedded in the amyloid mass are bits of neurons derived primarily from *cholinergic* and *adrenergic* systems.

Two systems of neurons appear to be primarily involved in AD. One of them is the cholinergic system originating in the basal forebrain, the so-called *nucleus basalis of Meynert*. Reductions in brain acetylcholine and its rate-limiting enzyme choline acetyltransferase *are* the most consistent neurotransmitter abnormalities observed in the brains of AD patients. The other neurotransmitter system also consistently observed to be abnormal is the *adrenergic* system originating in the *locus ceruleus* (Resser and Iverson, 1986). There is some evidence that these two systems are affected independently in the disease because some patients can be found with more or less adrenergic involvement. Involvement of the adrenergic system may be at least partially responsible for the high degree of disruptions in mood and anxiety regulation seen in AD.

Genetics. The cause of the neuronal death and subsequent deposition of neurofibrillary plaques and tangles is currently unknown; however, some cases have been found to be linked to a restriction fragment length polymorphism marker on chromosome 21, and others have been found to be associated with trisomy 21. Furthermore, the gene for the regulation of the protein that is precipitated in amyloid is also found on chromosome 21. In addition, Down's syndrome appears more likely to occur in families with AD than in families without histories of AD (Heston et al, 1981). DNA markers on chromosome 21 have been linked to the genetic defect causing familial AD in three of four large pedigrees (St George-Hyslop et al, 1987). The gene that encodes amyloid, which is a major component in neuritic plaques, is located nearby on chromosome 21.

Several family lines have been identified in which the early onset of AD appears to segregate in an autosomal dominant pattern and in a subset of early-onset familial AD kindreds, mutations of the amyloid precursor protein (APP) gene appear to be responsible for the disease (Schellenberg, 1995). At least 95% of early-onset familial AD families, however, do not show linkage or have mutations on the APP gene. The most severe form of AD in terms of age of onset and rate of decline is associated with a familial AD locus on chromosome 14 (Schellenberg, 1995). The most current data suggests that AD is a genetically heterogeneous disease caused by two or more genes located on two or more chromosomes (14, 19, and 21 have been most consistently implicated to date). Identifying the gene loci involved is a much more complex process, but one that will eventually unravel the core biochemical defect of the disease, as well as resolve the issue as to whether or not abnormalities in beta amyloid metabolism are a primary or secondary element of the disease.

Other theories of causation of AD included the excess deposition of aluminum in the brain and the possibility of a slow viral infection. A review of current theories of Alzheimer's disease is beyond the scope of this discussion, but students should be aware that research is moving so rapidly in this area that "dated" information may be only a few months old.

For many years, AD was thought to be a disorder with an early age of onset (before age 65) that was distinct from so-called senile dementia, which occurred much later and was common in the elderly. Because the neuropathology and the clinical presentation of Alzheimer's disease, or "presenile dementia," and "senile dementia," are the same, the early-onset and later onset types are considered to have the same pathophysiology. In recent years, however, evidence has been emerging that the disorder might very well be heterogeneous, with one form having an early age of onset that is associated with more severe neuropathological changes, more rapid progression, dermatoglyphic changes similar to those found in Down's syndrome, and platelet membrane abnormalities (such as increased platelet membrane fluidity).

In the families in which there appears to be a genetic component in the development of AD, several investigators have attempted to estimate the morbid risk among first-degree relatives of patients with AD. One method involves the life-table method, which estimates the age-specific cumulative incidence of a disease in a manner that adjusts for the fact that individuals die of other causes before the disease's onset (Breitner and Folstein, 1984; Mohs et al, 1987; Zubenko et al, 1988). Using this technique, the morbid risk among first-degree relatives of patients has been estimated to be as high as 50% by age 90 (Mohs et al, 1987). These calculations have been used to suggest that there is a dominant mode of inheritance for the AD gene, although it appears that the genetic predisposition to the illness shows variable penetrance.

During the next several years, the genetic basis of AD may be defined, along with the factors that may influence its expression. AD is probably not a single disease entity, but rather a heterogeneous disorder with varying degrees of behavioral, neurochemical, and neuropathological differences (Small and Greenberg, 1988).

Brain Imaging. Abnormalities have also been noted on CT, MRI, single-photon emission computed tomography (SPECT), and positron emission tomography (PET) scanning (Jobst et al, 1994), though PET and Spect are not used as part of standard clinical care. Cerebral atrophy, cortical sulci widening, deep white matter lesions with periventricular distribution, and ventricular enlargement changes have been observed on CT/MRI scanning, but these changes also can be seen in elderly patients without AD; alternatively, many patients *with* AD will have normal CT/MRI scans. The primary purpose of CT/MRI scanning is to *exclude* any potentially treatable causes of cognitive dysfunction, such as a brain tumor or chronic subdural hematoma.

The most consistent observations made to date with PET scanning have been decreases in the regional cerebral metabolic rate of glucose using the marker F-18-deoxyglucose. These findings also appear to correlate with decreased cerebral blood flow, as measured by SPECT techniques (Bonte et al, 1990). The deficits that have been observed are predominantly in the *temporoparietal area,* but are also in *frontal* regions in more severe cases. Decreased glucose use observed by PET scanning, however, is not always uniform or symmetric in the hemispheres. In addition, there is a significant amount of interpatient variability (Salmon et al, 1994). Metabolic dysfunction revealed by PET is an indication of the first cortical degeneration, while the anatomic changes with CT and MRI reflect later manifestations of the disease (Faulstich, 1991; Albert and Lafleche, 1991).

Pick's Disease and Jakob-Creutzfeldt Disease
Two other disorders that are differentiated from AD and are primarily cortical in their expression are *Pick's disease* and *Jakob-Creutzfeldt disease.* Pick's disease typically occurs in patients in their 60s and 70s and presents with an insidious and progressive change in behavior and cognition. Usually the patients show marked unpredictable and unexplainable behavioral abnormalities in association with relatively mild cognitive problems early in the illness. Although the patient subsequently develops a clear dementia syndrome, the disease is characterized by a lobar or focal atrophy that often affects the *frontal and temporal lobes* and is clearly detectable with CT or MRI scans.

Jakob-Creutzfeldt disease is a subacute dementia syndrome that affects the same age groups as AD and Pick's disease and presents with a cortical syndrome that is both insidious and rapidly progressive, usually over a period of weeks to months, rather than months to years. The patient becomes moderately to severely demented 6 months to a year after the initial symptom. Patients have a typical cortical dementia syndrome with amnesia, aphasia, apraxia, and agnosia, but in addition, often have tremor, ataxia of gait, and a *typical burst pattern on the EEG.* It is the rapid course of the illness that suggests the diagnosis. This condition is associated with a spongiform degeneration of the brain that is transmissible to animals and has been found to be caused by a slow virus (prion) of the scrapie type. The disease is remarkable in that it has a long latent period between exposure to the virus and subsequent expression of its effects. Although it is caused by an infectious agent, the typical inflammatory changes in the brain, which are usually associated with infection, are absent. This observation has led to the speculation that perhaps other psychiatric disorders, including Alzheimer's disease and even schizophrenia, could be caused by a similar virus; however, there has been no evidence of transmissibility in any of the other disorders, with the exception of the so-called Gerstmann syndrome.

Pick's disease and Jakob-Creutzfeldt disease are rare disorders. There are other cerebral degenerations, even more rare, that are occasionally seen presenting as a dementia syndrome. These include Kufs' disease or a late-onset form of Tay-Sachs disorder, cortical striatal degenerations, and a variety of dementia syndromes associated with atypical neuropathological findings, and occasionally, a case of dementia syndrome of the cortical type with an apparently normal brain. Although all these disorders are extremely rare, they are exceptions that might reveal important mechanisms of disease.

Subcortical Dementia

The subcortical dementias are distinguished from the cortical dementias by symptoms and pathology. An important clinical distinction is that patients with disease entities causing a subcortical dementia often have a gait disorder in the presence of a moderate dementia, whereas with AD and other cortical dementias, a gait disorder occurs late in the illness.

The discussion of subcortical disorders will begin with multi-infarct dementia. Although this is clearly a disorder that could have either cortical or subcortical signs, depending on the location of the lesions, small lacunar infarctions associated with hypertension are most often found in the basal ganglia and in the subcortical white matter.

Multi-infarct dementia is a term used for a dementia syndrome associated with prominent infarctions of the brain, which can be due to a variety of causes, but is most commonly associated with either hypertension or atrial fibrillation with multiple cerebral emboli. The clinical diagnosis is based on the sudden and episodic appearance of worsening of the patient's mental state, usually associated with asymmetrical motor signs and CT or MRI signs of cerebral infarction. Claims have been made that its course may be altered by vigorous treatment of hypertension (Hachinski et al, 1974).

Occult hydrocephalus or "normal pressure" hydrocephalus is a more typical subcortical disorder, characterized by a triad of *dementia, ataxia,* and *urinary incontinence* and associated with a large dilatation of the cerebral ventricles with relatively mild cerebral atrophy. The disorder is caused by the defective drainage of cerebrospinal fluid. (CSF), which is usually due to a blockage of reabsorption sites secondary to head trauma, previous hemorrhage, or infection. Some of these cases respond to surgical drainage of the CSF, but the technique remains controversial, and response to shunting procedures is not always predictable; thus, diagnosis is important (McHugh, 1964; Vanneste, 1994)

Huntington's disease is a hereditary disease with autosomal dominant transmission. Chorea is the most common clinical manifestation; however, behavioral abnormalities, psychosis, and a subcortical dementia syndrome are more disabling. The caudate nucleus and eventually other striatal centers atrophy. Cortical atrophy is sometimes seen. The cause of the disease is an abnormal gene on the long arm of chromosome 4 whose specific mutation is now known. A marked loss of N-methyl-D-aspartate receptors in the striatum is noted. The abnormality in this receptor could lead to excessive cellular excitation by incoming glutaminergic fibers and then to cell death through calcium influx, kinase activation, and eventually, free radical oxygen accumulation (Folstein et al, 1986). Genetic testing (including prenatal) is available, raising difficult ethical and psychological issues.

Another subcortical dementia disorder is associated with *Parkinson's disease,* which is characterized by the triad of akinesia, rigidity, and tremor, associated with degeneration of the dopamine-containing neurons of the substantia nigra. In recent years, Parkinson's disease has been divided into two types, that associated with the neuritic plaques and tangles of AD and that with a pure nigral degeneration. At this point, the clinical distinction between these types is uncertain.

While Parkinson's disease is associated with a clear dementia syndrome, a high proportion of patients with Parkinson's disease also develop depressive disorders. Treatment of the depressed parkinsonian patient often includes L-dopa and an antidepressant or electroconvulsive therapy, which is effective in the motoric, cognitive, and mood features of the disorder. Delusions and hallucinations also are commonly seen in Parkinson's disease and may at times be caused by L-dopa itself.

HIV (AIDS)-Related Dementia

AIDS-related cognitive disorders are not fully addressed in this chapter and are dealt with in depth by Moran in Chapter 21. One should note, however, that AIDS involvement in the central nervous system has been well documented to occur as a *primary symptom of the illness with clinical signs and symptoms that may appear well before any systemic signs of immunosuppression.* In the later, more advanced stages of AIDS, behavioral observations of both delirium and dementia may be seen as a direct result of HIV infection or secondary fungal, parasitic, viral, or neoplastic disease (Grant et al, 1987; Ostrow et al, 1988).

CNS involvement with HIV pervades the course of the illness from beginning to end. The initial infection of HIV likely involves the brain in almost all cases, and this initial vital infection may be neurologically asymptomatic or be accompanied by aseptic meningitis or meningoencephalitis. The most common symptom of acute infection involves flulike symptoms and headache (Robertson and Hall, 1992). Bell's palsy and other cranial nerve abnormalities may occur soon after acute exposure, as well as peripheral neuropathy. Seizures may occur at any time during the course of infection and demand a search for the cause (infections, tumors), but in about 50% of cases, no specific etiology is identified (Wong et al, 1990).

Some reports demonstrate signs of neuropsychologic dysfunction early in the course of HIV infection, but others do not. Cognitive dysfunction parallels signs of neuroanatomic changes (Masde et al, 1991; Hall et al, 1996). As has been emphasized by others (Robertson and Hall, 1992), despite evidence that the CNS is affected early in the course of HIV, general intellectual functioning remains relatively intact until the later stages of AIDS.

In latter phases of the illness, patients with HIV dementia show a variety of intellectual and motor impairments. Delays in response time and shortening of the attention span are common. Functional areas of impairment include not only attention, concentration, and speed of processing but also memory, visuospatial skills, and mental flexibility (Robertson and Hall, 1992).

Motor decline tends to parallel intellectual decline and may include impairments in fine motor skills, gait difficulties, incoordination, a fine or coarse tremor, and general "clumsiness." Bradykinesia, apraxia, and abnormalities of saccadic and pursuit eye movements are common. Muscle stretch (deep tendon) reflexes may be hyperactive, or possibly decreased, indicating a concomitant peripheral neuropathy. Plantar (Babinski) responses may be extensor. Primitive reflexes may be observed, including grasp, suck, snout, and palmomental responses. Diffuse muscle weakness is also typical. (Price, 1996) More details regarding neuropsychiatric aspects of HIV/AIDS are found in Chapter 21.

Other Types of Dementia

Multiple Sclerosis

Multiple sclerosis (MS) is characterized by multifocal lesions in the white matter of the central nervous system. Neuropsychiatric symptoms in patients with MS are, therefore, relatively common, particularly as the disease progresses. Because of the shifting and transient nature of both the neurological and neuropsychiatric symptoms associated with MS, many of these patients may be diagnosed as "hysterical," or as having conversion disorder, early in the course of their illness. In the advanced stages, global dysfunction may occur in cognitive and behavioral functioning and a dementia syndrome results. In addition, depression is relatively common in MS. Mood disorders such as depression or mania in MS may be caused by treatment with exogenous steroids or adrenocorticotropic hormone treatment.

Vitamin B$_{12}$ Deficiency

Failure of the gastric mucosa to secrete intrinsic factor results in abnormal absorption of vitamin B$_{12}$ from the ileum. B$_{12}$ deficiency can result in peripheral neuropathy and a variety of neuropsychiatric disturbances. Megaloblastic anemia (pernicious anemia) is the most obvious hematologic manifestation of the illness. Nevertheless, *neurological changes, including CNS degeneration, may appear before megaloblastic changes.* Behavioral changes associated with vitamin B$_{12}$ deficiency include depression, emotional lability, irritability, and the spectrum of signs and symptoms associated with dementia. Similar symptoms may result from deficiencies in folate or other B vitamins. Screening for serum B$_{12}$ and folate levels is a standard component of a dementia evaluation.

Hypothyroidism (Myxedema)

Hypothyroidism may cause a form of dementia, in addition to a depressive disorder. The onset may be insidious and may be overlooked for months or years. The psychiatric picture is usually characterized by lethargy, mental sluggishness, and slowing of cognition. These symptoms occur in concert with the typical physical signs of the illness, which include dry skin, slow reflexes, bradycardia, nonpitting edema over the face and limbs, hair loss, menstrual changes, and a "froglike" voice due to laryngeal edema. A variety of metabolic findings may be seen, including hyponatremia and hypokalemia. With progression of disease, there is increased cognitive dysfunction. Gross psychosis (myxedema madness), in addition to the cognitive and depressive features, rarely may be seen. In screening patients for possible hypothyroidism, it is essential to obtain a serum thyroid-stimulating hormone level to detect subclinical levels of the illness.

Wilson's Disease

A dementia is also caused by Wilson's disease, which is an inherited defect in copper metabolism that affects the putamen of the lenticular nucleus and the liver (hepatolenticular degeneration). Neuropsychiatric symptoms often precede overt manifestations of the dementia syndrome. This is a disorder that usually presents in the second decade of life and is associated with cirrhosis, golden brown pigmentation on the posterior corneal surface (Kayser-Fleischer rings), tremor, and rigidity. The diagnosis can be made by the presence of decreased serum ceruloplasmin in association with aminoaciduria.

Diagnostic Evaluation of Dementia

The screening diagnostic evaluation for dementia is relatively straight-forward and parallels the evaluation for a delirium, although usually without the same dramatic urgency that accompanies a patient with delirium. The basic diagnostic workup is listed in Table 4–10, but a few special points might be considered:

1. If AIDS-related dementia is suspected, special consent and counseling will be required for HIV antibody testing.
2. As noted above, the serum B_{12} and folate levels should be ascertained.
3. The serum VDRL may be negative in older patients with tertiary syphilis, and a serum FTA is usually recommended for a definitive answer. If the serum FTA is positive, the same test should be performed on the CSF to confirm tertiary CNS syphilis.
4. CT and MRI scanning have differential powers in assessing for dementia and other CNS lesions. While Table 4–11 (AMA Council Report, 1988) offers a guide to their relative sensitivities, consultation with a neuroradiologist may save both money and patient duress (the isolation involved in MRI scanning may be stressful for older patients with cognitive impairment) (see also Chapter 1 by Drs. Yates, Kathol, and Carter).
5. The EEG is not sensitive for detecting dementia (high rate of false negatives) and is often normal in both the early and middle phases of AD; however, the EEG is quite sensitive for detecting delirium.

Physician's Role in the Management of Dementia

Beyond the diagnostic evaluation, the role of the general medical physician in the care of dementia patients is as follows:

1. Provide long-term supportive medical care for the patient.
2. Provide emotional support for the patient and family as a triage point for medical and community resources.
3. Provide assistance with management of disruptive behavior.

In respect to the latter items, major behavioral difficulties often arise in patients with dementia, most commonly dementia of the Alzheimer's type. The

Table 4–11 **CT Versus MRI as a Neurodiagnostic Probe***

DISEASE	MRI	CT	METRIZAMIDE-ENHANCED CT
Cerebrovascular Disease			
TIA-RIND	+ +	±	—
Emboli	+ + +	+	—
Ischemic infarction	+ + + +	+ + +	—
Vasculitis	+++	±	—
Intracerebral hemorrhage	+ + +	+ + + +	—
Trauma			
Craniocerebral	+ +	+ + +	—
Spinal	+ + +!	+ + +	+ + +
Tumors			
Glioma			
Low-grade (1–2)			
Supratentorial	+ + +	+ +	—
Infratentorial	+ + + +	+ +	—
High-grade (3–4)			
Supretentorial	+ + + +	+ + + +	—
Infratentorial	+ + + +	+ +	—
Metastases			
Supretentorial	+ + +	+ +	—
Infratentorial	+ + +	+	—
Meningioma			
Supratentorial	+ +	+ + + +	—
Infratentorial	+ +	+ +	—
Pituitary	+ +	+ + + +	—
Sinuses and orbits	+ + + +	+ + +	—
Demyelinating disease	+ + + +	+ +	—
Dementia			
SAE	+ + + +	+ +	—
Alzheimer's, Huntington's, and PSP	±	±	—
NPH	+	+	+ + +
Cervicomedullary Junction and Cervical Spinal Cord			
Syrinx (and congenital anomalies)	+ + + +	+	+ +
Tumors (intraaxial)			
Brain stem	+ + + +	+	+ +
Cerebellopontine angle	+ + +	+ +	+ + +
Cervical spine	+ + + +	±	+ +
Tumors (extraaxial)			
Brain stem	+ + + +	+	+ +
Cervical spine	+ + + +	±	+ + +
Cervical disk disease	+ + +	+ + +	+ + + +
Lumbar disk disease	+ + +	+ + +	+ + + +
Regional Cerebral Blood Flow	***	+ + + #	—

*MRI, magnetic resonance imaging; CT, computed tomography; TIA-RIND transient ischemic attacks and reversible ischemic neurological deficits; SAE, subcortical arteriosclerotic encephalopathy; PSP, progressive supranuclear palsy; NPH, normal-pressure hydrocephalus.

most problematic are agitation, insomnia, emotional lability, personality changes, and psychotic symptoms (most often paranoia). There are, however, a surprisingly small number of systematic studies of the psychopharmacologic treatment of the behavioral disorders of dementia. Low doses of neuroleptic agents, such as haloperidol or risperidone, will help control agitation, emotional lability, and paranoia, but often symptoms are only suppressed rather than eliminated. Disturbed sleep is an extremely common component of dementia and is the symptom that most exhausts caregivers. Again, low-dose neuroleptic agents near bedtime may help, but sedative-hypnotics may be needed. Low doses of shorter acting benzodiazepines such as temazepam, which has a short half-life (13 to 16 hours) and whose metabolism is not affected by aging, can help on an "as needed" basis. Benzodiazepines however, sometimes aggravate confusion. More recently, some clinicians have reported the efficacy of trazodone (50 to 200 mg), a sedating antidepressant also effective for nocturnal agitation. The anxiolytic agent buspirone may also have some efficacy in the control of agitation in dementia. This drug has no habit-forming or sedating properties and takes 2 to 4 weeks to reach its full therapeutic effect.

If possible, psychotropic drugs should be used on an "as needed" basis, rather than given automatically for long periods of time, until the necessity of their ongoing use becomes absolutely necessary. Caution should be used, especially with the high-potency neuroleptic agents (e.g., haloperidol), because elderly patients are quite prone to extrapyramidal reactions (see Chapter 18). Psychotropic agents are often used excessively and inappropriately in nursing home patients because they are frequently used as "chemical restraints" by overextended staffs (Beers et al, 1988). Physicians should carefully reassess the need for psychotropic agents in this population on a regular basis.

Perhaps one of the most valuable things a physician can do for a patient's family is to refer them to a community social worker or other geriatric specialist who has an interest in geriatrics to assist in resource planning. In addition, a referral to a support organization, such as the Alzheimer's Association, will assist the family in receiving help through support groups and education as to

---

±, of questionable value;

+, of some value, but other technologies are definitely superior;

+ +, of moderate value at present and frequently competitive with other technologies, but should not be considered as the initial diagnostic approach;

+ + +, of definite value;

+ + + +, of definite value and the preferred initial approach;

*** research phase—of great potential importance for the future as a first-line diagnostic tool;

!, roentgenographic CT is superior in visualizing bone abnormalities, whereas MRI may be superior in demonstrating blood and spinal cord injury;

#, roentgenographic CT combined with inhalation of stable xenon or intravenous administration of contrast medium. (Used with permission from American Medical Association Council on Scientific Affairs, Report of the panel on Magnetic Resonance Imaging: Magnetic resonance imaging of the central nervous system. JAMA 259:1211–1222, 1988)

the patient's care and management. Referral to an attorney for legal planning, in addition to getting a durable power of attorney for the family to be made when the diagnosis becomes evident, will save the family enormous amounts of time, trouble, and money (Overman and Stoudemire, 1988).

Finally, physicians should be careful to follow the patient periodically for concurrent medical problems and to continue as a source of support and information for the family. Many families often feel abandoned by their physicians if no regular plans for follow-up appointments are made. Dementia is a *chronic* illness, continuing until death, during which the family will often be under enormous emotional stress. The primary physician's role in the ongoing support of the patient and family is crucial. (Students are referred to Chapter 11 for more information regarding the overall management of psychiatric illness in the elderly.)

DELIRIA

As noted in the introductory comments, delirium (previously known as acute organic brain syndrome) is characterized by an alteration in the level of consciousness that often fluctuates. Patients may have either a clouding or fogging of consciousness, or they may be hyperalert and agitated at times, as in alcohol withdrawal delirium. Multiple signs and symptoms may accompany delirium and include gross psychotic symptoms such as paranoia, delusions, and hallucinations (tactile, auditory, visual, and olfactory). Patients also may exhibit evidence of thought disorganization and incoherent language that may resemble a schizophrenic psychosis.

The sleep–wake cycle may be grossly disrupted, with agitation often exacerbated during the evening hours (the same observation may be seen in relatively stable dementias)—the "sundowning" syndrome. Cognitive signs usually receive the most attention, but they may be subtle and undetected in patients who are "quietly delirious" and are not exhibiting any overt behavioral disturbances or who are overmedicated with sedatives and tranquilizers. Cognitive dysfunction may be exhibited in defects in memory, attention, concentration, and orientation. Behaviorally, the patients may be agitated, combative, and hostile. Many times, the uncooperative, irritable, and aggressive nature of the delirious patient, combined with his paranoia, is assumed to be a "functional psychosis," and the underlying metabolic component driving the patient's abnormal behavior overlooked.

As noted earlier, the primary feature of a delirium is a diminution in the level of consciousness that fluctuates over time. Consistent with this pattern, patients may actually experience *periods of relative lucidity.* As noted above, "clouding" of consciousness and decreased alertness are the most common symptoms. Some patients can also show hyperalert activity. Sleep is usually fragmented and poor, with the patients being anxious, irritable, and restless.

Disturbances in psychomotor functioning vary from hyperactivity to lethargy, stupor, obtundation, and catatonia. Neurological signs and symptoms may be seen, such as tremor, asterixis (particularly in deliria caused by metabolic and hepatic encephalopathies), or drug intoxications or withdrawal.

Deliria by definition are usually "acute" in onset, but some, particularly those due to subtle or insidious metabolic deficits, may develop and persist over days, weeks, or months with fluctuating cognitive dysfunction. Most cases of delirium should improve or resolve quickly if the underlying cause can be identify and corrected.

Delirium is an extremely common disorder within the general hospital population with an average prevalence of about 20% in general hospital populations, higher in the elderly (Trzepacz, 1996). Delirium is common after major surgery, and in patients with preexisting cognitive dysfunction, especially dementia. Delirium is associated with adverse outcomes, including increased hospital length of stay, more likely discharge to nursing home, and increased mortality (Francis et al, 1990; Marcantonio et al, 1994; Schor et al, 1992). Delirium is often missed by physicians, especially when the patient is "quietly confused" rather than agitated and disrupted. Delirious patients frequently jeopardize their own care through removing tubes (ventilator hose, IV, etc.) and assaulting care-givers.

Diagnosis

The diagnosis of delirium is made by a combination of clinical observations and formal changes in the patient's mental status. Of paramount importance is checking on the observations of the nursing staff either verbally or by reviewing the chart. This is especially helpful in assessing for fluctuations in the patient's mental status over a 24-hour period. Documenting the patient's baseline mental status before the hospitalization or onset of the cognitive dysfunction from information provided by the family is essential. The family will also be helpful in documenting the use of drugs or alcohol.

Factors Associated with Delirium and High-Risk Groups

Lipowski (1983) has documented the most common physical illnesses associated with delirium (in the elderly). These include congestive heart failure, pneumonia, urinary tract infections, cancer, uremia, malnutrition, hypokalemia, dehydration, hyponatremia, and cerebrovascular accidents (Trzepacz, 1996). Systemic illnesses that result in brain dysfunction are more common causes of delirium than are primary CNS disorders. Intoxication with medical drugs and psychotropic agents is probably the most common cause of delirium in the elderly patient, particularly iatrogenic drugs that have sedative and anticholinergic side effects, such as amitriptyline (Lipowski, 1983, Tune et al,

1993). Delirium is frequent after cardiac surgery and other major operations, particularly in patients with other risk factors (older age, prior cognitive dysfunction, history of alcohol abuse, etc.) (Marcantonio et al, 1994).

Alcoholics, particularly those with a history of recent heavy drinking where there is a possibility of a withdrawal syndrome, should be watched very closely. Patients with a history of other drugs that involve significant potential withdrawal, such as barbiturates, sedative-hypnotics, and benzodiazepines, should also be monitored carefully and treated with the appropriate detoxification regimen (see Chapters 10 and 19).

Patients with a history of trauma, especially head trauma, are at extremely high risk medically for complications. Patients with sensory impairment (blindness, deafness, history of cataract surgery, or those facing extensive bandaging or casting) are prone to become delirious because of sensory deprivation and may need special care to promote orientation to the environment. Patients with preexisting cognitive dysfunction, mental retardation, or dementia have less ability to organize and adjust to the strangeness of the hospital and also are prone to delirium.

The differentiation between dementia and delirium is important. Table 4–5 lists key differentiating factors (Lipowski, 1987). It is essential to note, however, that dementia and delirium may coexist and be superimposed on one another.

Etiology

Delirium can derive from failure or dysfunction in any organ system (e.g., pulmonary, cardiac, hepatic, renal, endocrine, gastrointestinal) because of either direct or secondary metabolic abnormalities of the central nervous system (e.g., electrolyte imbalances, hypoglycemia, adrenal insufficiency, hyperosmolarity or hypoosmolarity, uremia, hypoxemia, hypercarbia, hypercalcemia or hypocalcemia, or severe hypertension). Decreases in cardiac output from congestive heart failure can lead to decreased perfusion of the CNS and to confusion. Peripheral as well as central nervous infections can cause fever and sepsis, leading to altered mental status. Infiltration of the meninges from certain forms of leukemia can also cause delirium.

Direct insults to the CNS from bacterial meningitis, viral encephalitis, cerebrovascular hemorrhage, subdural hematoma, strokes, and vasculitis from connective tissue diseases, such as systemic lupus erythematosus, may cause delirium with or without psychotic symptoms. Gliomas and meningiomas may cause delirium or resemble dementia, and their onset may be insidious if the tumor is growing slowly and may not be associated with focal neurological findings in their early stages.

Patients who suffer from intermittent delirium (often with psychotic features), in addition to having a history of chronic abdominal pain and a peripheral neuropathy, should be suspected of having acute intermittent porphyria.

The family history, if it can be reconstructed, is usually positive. Although the diagnosis is confirmed by special urine tests (porphobilinogen levels), the diagnosis occasionally has been made by exposing the patient's urine to sunlight, in which it turns beet red.

Medication side effects, particularly in the elderly and even in "therapeutic" doses, may cause delirium, especially when there are coexisting medical problems that may alter the pharmacokinetics of the drug. Common offenders include narcotic analgesics, barbiturates, benzodiazepines, and other sedative-hypnotics. Antidepressant drugs, particularly cyclic antidepressants with strong anticholinergic and sedating side effects, such as amitriptyline, are notorious for causing delirium in the elderly (anticholinergic delirium).

A variety of nonpsychiatric medications cause symptoms of delirium. These include antihistamines (some of which also have relatively potent anticholinergic effects), atropine-like drugs, H-2 (histamine receptor) blockers (cimetidine, ranitidine), phenytoin, phenobarbital, digitalis (even at "therapeutic levels"), procainamide, lidocaine, L-dopa, and antihypertensive agents, if they are sedating (such as clonidine). Steroids, particularly when administered rapidly in high doses, can cause a delirium usually known as "steroid psychosis." Table 4–2 presents a partial listing of drugs reported to potentially cause delirium.

Delirium and Intensive Care Unit Syndromes

Special note should be made of the so-called intensive care unit (ICU) syndrome, ICU psychosis, and postcardiotomy syndrome. Although the abnormalities that have been described in intensive care unit patients often have been called *postoperative psychosis,* most of these patients suffer from what is best characterized as a delirium with psychotic components. Delirious states in the ICU are usually multifactorially determined and may be aggrevated (but not caused) by the inherent stresses of the ICU itself, particularly its sleep-depriving effects. The environmental stresses of the ICU may include being placed in a strange, technologically oriented environment; incapacitation; noisy monitors; restriction in movement by intravenous lines and catheters; and the lack of privacy. Most patients in the intensive care unit are gravely ill and compromised medically and receive multiple medications. In addition, sleep deprivation and loss of the normal diurnal light–dark rhythm in units without windows may be biologically disrupting.

Delirium after cardiothoracic surgery also has been described and has been termed *postcardiotomy delirium* (Smith and Dimsdale, 1989). This condition classically occurs 3 or 4 days after surgery. The patient may be lucid, but then suffers from progressive deterioration, confusion, and other features of delirium such as psychosis. Factors that may contribute to the development of postcardiotomy delirium include increasing age, total time spent on cardiopulmonary bypass, intraoperative hypotension, severity of illness, sleep deprivation, and sensory monotony. Postcardiotomy delirium may be related to decreased postoperative cardiac index, leading to a greater likelihood of impaired cerebral perfusion and oxygenation. (Heller et al, 1979).

Diagnosis

The cardinal rule in evaluating patients with delirium is to detect and correct the underlying disorder contributing to the patient's cerebral dysfunction. Appropriate treatment must be preceded by an extensive and thorough search for the cause of the patient's cognitive dysfunction. Although the differential diagnosis of potential causes of delirium is extensive, the actual diagnostic workup is straightforward.

First, a review of all factors leading up to the patient's hospitalization is essential. If the patient is postsurgical, the operative record is reviewed for potential causes like severe hypotension. Premorbid factors include the presence of alcoholism, medication use, or coexisting dementia. Because medications are almost always high on the list in the hospitalized elderly, the cumulative dose of medications received over the past week should be reviewed, along with serum levels for drugs when possible (anticonvulsants, digoxin, theophylline, and so forth). Any psychotropics that the patient has been taking should be scrutinized, particularly the relationship between the onset of cognitive dysfunction and any new drugs or changes in doses. Anticholinergic agents are especially troublesome in the elderly.

Once the patient has been examined medically and neurologically, the history has been reviewed, and the events leading up to the hospitalization or surgery have been documented, the patient should undergo a physical and mental status examination. Following review of vital signs, the assessment is based on an organ system-by-organ system search for evidence of metabolic dysfunction, such as cardiovascular and pulmonary (arterial blood gasses, chest X-ray), renal (electrolyte imbalance, uremia), endocrine (thyroid panel, glucose, calcium), and liver (hepatic function tests). A search for infection (sepsis, occult abscess, meningitis, urinary tract infection, pneumonia) is crucial. *The fundamental clinical principle remains that of detecting and correcting to whatever extent possible the underlying abnormality causing the patient's altered mental status.*

Special note should be made regarding the use of the EEG in the evaluation of delirium. Although the EEG may be normal in dementia, it is almost always abnormal in delirium, making it a very sensitive test in this clinical situation. Typically, the EEG shows diffuse slowing in delirium, but the EEG is not very helpful in pinpointing a specific cause of delirium. The EEG abnormalities, are not always characterized by slowing, and the patterns can be low amplitude–fast activity, as may be found in alcohol withdrawal and sedative-hypnotic withdrawal. EEG abnormalities, which almost always accompany delirium, may persist after the clinical manifestations of the brain syndrome remit.

Treatment

The treatment of patients with delirium primarily involves treating the underlying cause of the cerebral dysfunction, as noted above. Until that can be identified and corrected, however, some environmental and psychopharmacologic strategies can facilitate keeping patients safe and stabilizing their behavior. Environmental strategies include having a window from which the patient can observe normal light–dark cycles to help correct the diurnal rhythm (windows should be secured to prevent jumping). A familiar family member should be allowed at the bedside if at all possible to facilitate orientation. Large calendars on which days can be marked off, clocks, familiar photographs, and having a radio or television playing during waking hours can also help the patient stay connected to the outside world and provide sensory stimulation. Providing night-lights and other types of additional sensory input for heavily bandaged or casted patients can be helpful. Elderly patients with cataracts are at risk for delirium, leading to the practice of performing such procedures "one eye at a time" to prevent "black patch delirium." Making sure eyeglasses or hearing aids are in place for those who use them is a simple but often overlooked step. Patients who are on ventilators or are unable to speak because of tube placement or mechanical problems should nevertheless be communicated with by handwriting, hand signals, or lap-computer keyboards.

Pharmacologic Strategies

The psychopharmacologic management of agitated and psychotic behavior will be described in other sections of this text, particularly Chapters 10, 18, and 19. In general, however, the "higher potency" antipsychotic agents such as haloperidol are the drugs of choice in this setting because they have minimal effects on blood pressure. These drugs tend to be less sedating and also have very few cardiac or anticholinergic side effects. "Lower potency" antipsychotic agents such as chlorpromazine and thioridazine tend to cause hypotension.

The prototypical drug used for stabilization of delirium is haloperidol, which can be given in tablet or liquid form orally or through the intramuscular and intravenous routes (see Chapter 18). A typical starting dose of haloperidol would be 1 to 2 mg p.o. or i.m. q1h or until the patient is sedated. Some clinicians advocate the use of parenteral benzodiazepines such as lorazepam for this purpose, as well. For example, lorazepam may be used by giving the patient 1 to 2 mg orally, sublingually, or intramuscularly every hour until the patient is calm and slightly drowsy. Lorazepam, however, can cause anterograde amnesia when given in this manner, and benzodiazepines may exacerbate disinhibited behavior.

If a patient is suffering from a severe anticholinergic delirium, physostigmine salicylate 1 to 2 mg can be given slowly intravenously or intramuscularly and repeated after 15 minutes. Contraindications to using this potent cholinergic agonist include a history of heart disease, asthma, diabetes, peptic ulcer disease, or the possibility of bladder or bowel obstruction (Lipowski, 1987).

After the patient is stabilized, haloperidol may then be given in supplemental doses every 3 to 4 hours as needed. The need for continuous medication should then be reevaluated every 24 hours and the doses decreased and discontinued as rapidly as possible commensurate with stabilization of the patient medically and the patient's overall mental status. In most instances, resolution of the delirium should be accompanied by discontinuation of the antipsychotic agent as soon as possible.

Patients also should be carefully monitored for the presence of extrapyramidal side effects, neuroleptic-induced catatonia, and neuroleptic malignant syndrome. Diagnosis and management of these side effects of neuroleptics are discussed in Chapters 5 and 18. Chapter 11 on geriatric psychiatry discusses special considerations in using psychotropic drugs in the elderly.

CLINICAL PEARLS

- Several of the most frequently underdiagnosed disorders in medicine are delirium and early dementia.
- The most common causes of delirium in hospitalized patients are medication side effects.
- Delirious patients are not always either obtunded or agitated; some may be hyperaroused and excitable or quietly delirious.
- The EEG is very sensitive for delirium, but relatively insensitive in dementia.
- A mild dementia may be one of the earliest signs of HIV infection occurring before signs of systemic immunosuppression.
- Intravenous haloperidol may be give for rapid control of severely agitated delirious patients, but the necessity of its use should be carefully documented.
- Neurological signs and symptoms of B_{12} deficiency have been reported before hematologic changes and in the presence of a normal serum B_{12} level.
- Depression and dementia may coexist, and the mood disturbance may exacerbate the cognitive and psychosocial dysfunction of the demented patient. Major depression rarely mimics the pervasive and progressive picture of dementia unless the patient already has some degree of underlying dementing illness.

ANNOTATED BIBLIOGRAPHY

Lishman WA: Organic Psychiatry, 2nd ed. Oxford, Blackwell Scientific Publication, 1987

  This is a classic textbook that reviews neuropsychiatric disorders in detail.

Trzepacz PT: Delirium: Advances in diagnosis, pathophysiology, and treatment. Psychiatr Clin North Am 19:429–448, 1996

Slaby AE, Erie SR: Dementia and Delirium. In Stoudemire A, Fogel BS (eds): Psychiatric Care of the Medical Patient, pp 415–453. New York, Oxford University Press, 1993

> This is an excellent and in-depth overview of the diagnosis and management of delirium and dementia.

Yudofsky SC, Hales RD (eds): Textbook of Neuropsychiatry, 2nd ed. Washington, DC, American Psychiatric Press, 1992

> This is an eminently readable textbook that provides practical reviews of the major disorders in clinical neuropsychiatry.

REFERENCES

Albert MS, Lafleche G: Neuroimaging in Alzheimer's disease. Psychiatr Clinics N Am 14:443–459, 1991

Alzheimer A: About a peculiar disease of the cerebral cortex. Alzheimer Dise Associated Disorders 1:7–8, 1987. Jarvik L, Greenson H, translators

Alzheimer A: Uber eine eigenartige Erkrankund der Hirnrinde. Allg Z Psychiatric Psychisch-Gerichtlich Med 64:146–148, 1907

American Medical Association Council on Scientific Affairs, Report of the Panel on Magnetic Resonance Imaging: Magnetic resonance imaging of the central nervous system. JAMA 259:1211–1222, 1988

American Psychiatric Association: Diagnostic and Statistical Manual of Mental Disorders, 4th ed. Washington DC, American Psychiatric Association, 1994

Anthony JC, LeResche LA, Von Korff MR, et al: Screening for delirium on a general medical ward: The tachistoscope and a global accessibility rating. Gen Hosp Psychiatry 7:36–42, 1985

Beers M, Avorn J, Soumerai SB, et al: Psychoactive medication use in intermediate-care facility residents. JAMA 260:3016–3020, 1988

Bonte FJ, Hom J, Tintner R, et al: Single photon tomography in Alzheimer's disease and the dementias. Semin Nucl Med 20:342–352, 1990

Brandt J, Butters N: The neuropsychology of Huntington's disease. Trends Neurosci 93:118–120, 1986

Brandt J, Folstein S, Folstein M: Differential cognitive impairment in Alzheimer's disease and Huntington's disease. Ann Neurol 9:21, 1987

Breitner JCS, Folstein MF: Familial Alzheimer's dementia: A prevalent disorder with specific clinical features. Psychol Med 14:63–80, 1984

Caine ED: Amnesic disorders. J Neuropsychiatry Clin Neurosci 5:6–8, 1993

Cummings JL, Miller B, Hill MA, et al: Neuropsychiatric aspects of multiinfarct dementia and dementia of the Alzheimer type. Arch Neurol 44:389–393, 1987

Engel GL, Romano J: Delirium, a syndrome of cerebral insufficiency. J Chronic Dis 9:260, 1959

Faulstich ME: Brain imaging in the dementia of the Alzheimer type. Int J Neurosci 57:39–49, 1991

Folstein MF, Anthony JC, Parhad I, et al: The meaning of cognitive impairment in the elderly. J Am Geriatr Soc 33:228–235, 1985.

Folstein MF, Folstein SE, McHugh PR: Mini-Mental State. A practical method for grading the cognitive state of patients for the clinician. J Psychiatr Res 12:189–198, 1975

Folstein S, Leigh RJ, Parhad I, et al: Diagnosis of Huntington's disease. Neurology 36:1279–1283, 1986

Folstein MF, McHugh PR: Dementia syndrome of depression. In Katzman R, Terry RD, Rick KL (eds): Alzheimer's Disease: Senile Dementia and Related Disorders, Vol 7. New York; Raven Press, 1978:87–96

Francis J, Martin D, Kapoor WN: A prospective study of delirium in hospitalized elderly. JAMA 263:1097–1101, 1990

Grant I, Atkinson JH, Hesselink JR, et al: Evidence for early nervous system involvement in the acquired immunodeficiency syndrome (AIDS) and other human immunodeficiency virus (HIV) infections. Ann Intern Med 107:828–836, 1987

Hachinski VC, Lassen NA, Marshall J: Multi-infarct dementia: A cause of mental deterioration in the elderly. Lancet 2:207–210, 1974

Hall M, Whaley R, Robertson K, et al: The correlation between neuropsychological and neuro-anatomic changes over time in asymptomatic and symptomatic HIV-I-infected individuals Neurology 46:1697–1702, 1996

Heller SS, Kornfeld DS, Frank KA, et al: Postcardiotomy delirium and cardiac output. Am J Psychiatry 136:337–339, 1979

Heston LL, Mastri AR, Anderson E, et al: Dementia of the Alzheimer type: Clinical genetics, natural history, and associated conditions. Arch Gen Psychiatry 38:1085–1090, 1981

Jobst KA, Hindley NJ, King E, et al: The diagnosis of Alzheimer's disease: A question of image? J Clin Psychiatry 55[Suppl]:22–31, 1994

Katzman R: Alzheimer's disease. Trends Neurosci 9:522–525, 1986

Lindenbaum J, Healton EB, Savage DG, et al: Neuropsychiatric disorders caused by cobalamin deficiency in the absence of anemia or macrocytosis. N Engl J Med 318:1720–1728, 1988

Lipowski ZJ: Transient cognitive disorders (delirium, acute confusional states) in the elderly. Am J Psychiatry 140:1426–1436, 1983

Lipowski ZJ: Delirium (acute confusional state). JAMA 258:1789–1792, 1987

McHugh PR: Occult hydrocephalus. Q J Med 33:297–308, 1964

Marcantonio ER, Goldman L, Mangione CM, et al: A clinical prediction rule for delirium after elective non-cardiac surgery. JAMA 271:134–139, 1994

Masde JC, Yudd A, Van Heertum RI, et al: Single-photon emission computed tomography in human immunodeficiency virus encephalopathy: A preliminary report. J Nucl Med 32:1471–1475, 1991

Mohs RC, Breitner JCS, Silverman JM, et al: Alzheimer's disease: Morbid risk among first-degree relatives approximates 50% by 90 years of age. Arch Gen Psychiatry 44:405–408, 1987

Ostrow D, Grant I, Atkinson H: Assessment and management of the AIDS patient with neuropsychiatric disturbances. J Clin Psychiatry 49:14–22, 1988

Overman W, Stoudemire A: Guidelines for legal and financial counseling of Alzheimer's disease patients and their families. Am J Psychiatry 145:1495–1500, 1988

Popkin MK, Tucker GJ: "Secondary" and drug-induced mood, anxiety, psychotic, catatonic, and personality disorders: A review of the literature. J Neuropsychiatr Clin Neurosci 4:369–385, 1992

Price RW: Neurological complications of HIV infection. Lancet 348:445–452, 1996

Robertson KR, Hall CD: Human immunodeficiency virus-related cognitive impairment and the acquired immunodeficiency syndrome dementia complex. Semin Neurol, 12:18–27, 1992

Rocca WA, Amaducci LA, Schoenberg BS: Epidemiology of clinically diagnosed AD. Ann Neurol 19:415–424, 1986

Rosser M, Iverson LL: Non-cholinergic neurotransmitter abnormalities in Alzheimer's disease. Br Med Bull 42:70–74, 1986

Rovner BW, Kafonek S, Flipp L, et al: The prevalence of mental illness in a community nursing home. Am J Psychiatry 143:1446–1449, 1986

Salmon E, Sadzot B, Maquet P, et al: Differential diagnosis of Alzheimer's disease with PET. J Nucl Med 35:391–398, 1994

Schellenberg GD: genetic dissection of Alzheimer disease, a heterogeneous disorder. Proc Natl Acad Sci USA 92:8552–8559, 1995

Schor JD, Levkoff MD, Lipsitz LA, et al: Risk factors for delirium in hospitalized elderly. JAMA 267:827–831, 1992

Small GW, Greenberg DA: Biologic markers, genetics, and Alzheimer's disease. Arch Gen Psychiatry 45:945–947, 1988

Smith LW, Dimsdale JE: Postcardiotomy delirium: Conclusions after 25 years? Am J Psychiatry 146:452–458, 1989.

St George-Hyslop PH, Tanzi RE, Polinsky RJ, et al: The genetic defect causing familial Alzheimer's disease maps on chromosome 21. Science 235:885–890, 1987

Stoudemire A: Selected organic mental disorders. In Hales R, Yudofsky S (eds): Textbook of Neuropsychiatry. Washington, DC, American Psychiatric Press, 1987

Stoudemire A: The differential diagnosis of catatonic states. Psychosomatics 23:245–252, 1982

Stoudemire A, Hill C, Kaplan W, et al: Clinical issues in the assessment of dementia and depression in the elderly. Psychiatr Med 6:40–52, 1988

Stoudemire A, Thompson TL: Recognizing and treating dementia. Geriatrics 36:112–120, 1981

Strub KL, Black FW: The mental status connection in neurology. 2nd ed. Philadelphia: FA Davis, 1985

Trzepacz PT: Delirium: Advances in diagnosis, pathophysiology, and treatment. Psychiatr Clin North Am 19: 429–448, 1996

Trzepacz PT, Baker RW: The Psychiatric Mental Status Examination. New York, Oxford University Press, 1993

Tucker GJ, Caine ED, Folstein MF, et al: Introduction to background papers for the suggested changes to DSM-IV: Cognitive disorders. J Neuropsychiatr Clin Neurosci 4:360–368, 1992

Tune L, Carr S, Cooper T, Klug B, Golinger RC: Association of anticholinergic activity of prescribed medications with post-operative delirium. J Neuropsychiatr Clin Neurosci, 5:208–210, 1993

Vanneste JA: Three decades of normal pressure hydrocephalus: Are we wiser now? J Neurol Neurosurg Psychiatry 57:1021–1025, 1994

Wong MC, Suite ND, Labar DR: Seizures in human immunodeficiency virus infection. Arch Neurol 47:640–642, 1990

Zubenko GS, Huff FJ, Beyer J, et al. Familial risk of dementia associated with a biologic subtype of Alzheimer's disease. Arch Gen Psychiatry 45:889–893, 1988

Appendix to Chapter 4: Mini-Mental State Examination and Instructions

Patient _____

Examiner _____

Date _____

MINI-MENTAL STATE EXAMINATION

Maximum

Score	Score	
		Orientation
5	( )	What is the (year) (season) (date) (day) (month)?
5	( )	Where are we: (state) (county) (town) (hospital) (floor)

		Registration
3	( )	Name three objects: 1 second to say each. Then ask the patient all three after you have said them. Give 1 point for each correct answer. Then repeat them until he learns all three. Count trials and record.

Trials _____

(Used with permission from Folstein MF, Folstein SE, McHugh PR: Mini-Mental State: A practical method for grading the cognitive state of patients for the clinician. J Psychiatr Res 12:189–198, 1975)

Attention and Calculation

5 ( ) Serial 7s. 1 point for each correct. Stop after five answers. Alternatively, spell "world" backwards

Recall

3 ( ) Ask for the three objects repeated above. Give 1 point for each correct.

Language

9 ( ) Name a pencil, and watch. (2 points).
Repeat the following: "No ifs, ands, or buts." (1 point)
Follow a three-stage command:
    "Take a paper in your right hand, fold it in half, and put it on the floor." (3 points)
Read and obey the following:
    Close your eyes. (1 point)
    Write a sentence. (1 point)
    Copy design. (1 point)

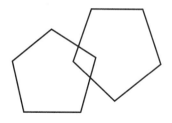

Total Score

Perfect score = 30
Any score below 25 indicates the presence of significant cognitive dysfunction.

Assess the level of consciousness along a continuum:
    Alert   Drowsy   Stupor   Coma

INSTRUCTIONS FOR ADMINISTRATION OF MINI-MENTAL STATE EXAMINATION

Orientation

(1) Ask for the date. Then ask specifically for parts omitted, e.g., "Can you also tell me what season it is?" One point for each correct.

(2) Ask in turn "Can you tell me the name of this hospital?" (town, county, etc.). One point for each correct.

Registration

Ask the patient if you may test his or her memory. Then say the names of three unrelated objects, clearly and slowly, about 1 second for each. After you have said all three, ask him or her to repeat them. This first repetition determines the score (0–3) but keep saying them until he or she can repeat all three, up to six trials. If he or she does not eventually learn all three, recall cannot be meaningfully tested.

Attention and Calculation

Ask the patient to begin with 100 and subtract backwards by 7. Stop after 5 subtractions (93, 86, 79, 72, 65). Score the total number of correct answers.

If the patient cannot or will not perform this task, ask him or her to spell the word "world" backwards. The score is the number of letters in correct order, e.g., dlrow = 5, dlorw = 3.

Recall

Ask the patient if he or she can recall the three words you previously asked him or her to remember. Score 0–3.

Language

Naming: Show the patient a wrist watch and ask him or her what it is. Repeat for pencil. Score 0–2.

Repetition: Ask the patient to repeat the sentence after you. Allow only one trial. Score 0 or 1.

Three-stage command: Give the patient a piece of plain blank paper and repeat the command. Score 1 point for each part correctly executed.

Reading: On a blank piece of paper print the sentence "Close your eyes," in letters large enough for the patient to see clearly. Ask him or her to read it and do what it says. Score 1 point only if he or she actually closes his eyes.

Writing: Give the patient a blank piece of paper and ask him or her to write a sentence for you. Do not dictate a sentence; it is to be written spontaneously. It must contain a subject and verb and be sensible. Correct grammar and punctuation are not necessary.

Copying: On a clean piece of paper, draw intersecting pentagons, each side about 1 in., and ask him or her to copy it exactly as is. All ten angles must be present, and two must intersect to score 1 point. Tremor and rotation are ignored.

Estimate the patient's level of sensorium along a continuum, from alert on the left to coma on the right.

5 Schizophrenia and Other Psychotic Disorders

Philip T. Ninan,
Rosalind M. Mance,
and Richard R. J. Lewine

Traditionally, psychoses have been termed either "organic" (caused by underlying neurological or metabolic abnormalities) or "functional." This differentiation is now obsolete because even "functional" psychotic disorders have an underlying anatomic and biochemical substrate in the brain. This chapter will discuss schizophrenia, schizophreniform disorder, brief psychotic disorder, schizoaffective disorder, and delusional disorder. DSM-IV labels psychotic disorders resulting from neurologic and metabolic conditions as "Psychotic Disorder Due to a General Medical Condition." Mood disorders with psychotic features (psychotic depression) will be dealt with in Chapter 7.

Psychosis is a generic descriptive term applied to behavior marked by a *break from reality*. This often presents as disorganization of mental processes, emotional aberrations, difficulty in interpersonal relationships, and a decrease in functional capacity. Mundane daily responsibilities can become burdensome or impossible to manage. Schizophrenia is the prototypical psychotic disorder and hence will be the primary focus of this chapter.

It should be emphasized that psychotic symptoms may occur in multiple medical, neurological, and substance-abuse disorders, and a vigorous search should be made for a medical or neurologic cause of the patient's psychiatric symptoms before a primary psychiatric diagnosis is made (Table 5–1). In addition, psychotic symptoms may occur in a *variety* of psychiatric disorders and are *not* by any means specific for schizophrenia (Table 5–2). For example, psychotic symptoms may be seen in mood disorders (psychotic depression and mania), in personality disorders

Table 5–1 **Brief Differential Diagnosis of Psychosis**

Medical, Neurologic, and Substance-Induced Disorders
Psychotic disorders due to general medical conditions
Dementia
Delirium (includes side effects of medications)
Substance-induced (e.g., amphetamine, phencyclidine, etc.)
  psychotic disorder

Mood Disorders
Bipolar disorder (mania)
Major depression with psychotic features

Psychotic Disorders
Brief psychotic disorder
Schizophreniform disorder
Schizophrenia
Schizoaffective disorder
Delusional disorder

Personality Disorders*
Schizotypal
Schizoid
Paranoid
Borderline

* Usually have brief psychotic disorders. See Chapter 6

Table 5–2 **Schizophrenia and Other Psychotic Disorders***

Schizophrenia
  Catatonic
  Disorganized
  Paranoid
  Undifferentiated
  Residual
Schizophreniform Disorder
Schizoaffective Disorder
Delusional Disorder
Brief Psychotic Disorder
Shared Psychotic Disorder
Psychotic Disorder Due to a General Medical Condition
Substance-Induced Psychotic Disorder
Psychotic Disorder Not Otherwise Specified

* Derived from DSM-IV (American Psychiatric Association, 1994).

(often during brief psychotic breaks), and in "encapsulated" form as part of a delusional disorder. Psychotic symptoms found in psychotic depression and mania are discussed in chapters elsewhere in this text (Chapter 7). The differential diagnosis for psychosis in dementia, delirium, and neurologic disorders may be found in Chapters 4 and 19.

SCHIZOPHRENIA

Schizophrenia is an illness that is present in all cultures. Early writings indicating the presence of schizophrenia go back to the twelfth century B.C. Contemporary epidemiological studies suggest that there is a 1 to 2% chance that an individual will develop an episode of schizophrenia during his or her lifetime (Robins et al, 1984). The cost to society is substantial—over 100,000 psychiatric beds are occupied by patients suffering from schizophrenia in the United States, and their treatment costs are estimated at $7 billion annually. What cannot be quantified is the enormous emotional cost to the patient, family, and society at large.

Phenomenology and Diagnosis

Schizophrenia is a *brain disorder* characterized by abnormalities in thinking, emotions, and behavior. Because we have no laboratory test yet that can confirm the diagnosis of schizophrenia, we are dependent on a descriptive or phenomenological definition of the disorder. Unfortunately, *there is no symptom that is pathognomonic of the illness or a symptom that is present in every patient with the illness.* Thus, no one symptom is necessary or sufficient for the diagnosis. The criterion diagnosis is a particular *constellation of symptoms* rather than a single symptom.

Such a diagnostic system does not define a homogenous group of patients with a single etiology, pathophysiology, treatment response, and outcome but a *heterogenous* group of disorders. This *heterogeneity* of schizophrenia has been a significant hurdle to the advancement of our understanding of schizophrenia because findings relevant to one subgroup of schizophrenic patients are obscured by the heterogeneity of the population studied.

Various attempts have been made to describe the constellation of symptoms that would best make the diagnosis of schizophrenia. Different diagnostic criteria can either define the illness broadly, which results in a large number of patients meeting the criteria for the illness, or provide a narrow definition of the illness, which would result in just a small (presumably core) group of patients being diagnosed. If the illness lies along a spectrum of severity, then casting a wide net would include those patients with milder, nonpsychotic versions of the illness (schizophrenia spectrum disorders), but would also risk some nonschizophrenics being given the label (i.e., a false–positive diagnosis).

The most reliably recognized symptoms of the illness are its more dramatic ones, such as hallucinations, delusions, and bizarre behavior. These are called "positive" symptoms because they are symptoms that are added to the premorbid state. By contrast, "negative" symptoms, such as *emotional blunting, apathy,* and *avolition,* are symptoms marked by the absence of functions. These negative symptoms, although less dramatic in presentation, are postulated by some to be the core elements of schizophrenia. In practice, there is considerable variability among individuals in the schizophrenic symptoms they exhibit when ill.

Historical Development

Emil Kraepelin (1907) coined the term *dementia praecox,* which he differentiated from manic-depressive (bipolar) illness. Dementia praecox, or the precocious development of intellectual impairment, was based on acute symptomatology marked by hallucinations, delusions, withdrawal, loss of interest, and poor attention associated with a dissociation of thought content and affect. Kraepelin believed that the illness usually began early in life and tended to result in an end state of dementia. The cause was postulated to be a disease process that affected cortical neurons. Inherent in Kraepelin's definition of dementia praecox was a constellation of psychotic symptoms that included both positive and negative symptoms, an early onset, and a deteriorating course over time.

Eugen Bleuler (1911) coined the term *schizophrenia* and described it as a group of illnesses. *He shifted the focus from the course of illness to a purely cross-sectional approach* in making the diagnosis of schizophrenia. He described schizophrenia as being marked by problems with thought association, affect, autistic thinking, and intense, pervasive ambivalence, referring to these as the fundamental symptoms of the illness. He did *not* consider that a deteriorating course was necessarily characteristic of the illness. Bleuler believed that the delusions and hallucinations often associated with schizophrenia were really secondary and derived from the fundamental symptoms. Bleuler also postulated a basic neurologic or metabolic defect as the cause of schizophrenia. He believed that the illness of schizophrenia could present with the fundamental symptoms without the secondary manifestations of delusions and hallucinations and called it "simple schizophrenia." Bleuler also thought that the basic defect causing schizophrenia could exist without expressing itself in either the fundamental symptoms or the secondary manifestations, and called this condition "latent schizophrenia."

A significant problem with the approach taken by Bleuler in diagnosing schizophrenia was the lack of a well-defined threshold of how prominent a symptom (e.g., autistic thinking) had to be before the diagnosis of schizophrenia should be made. Thus, nonpsychotic individuals with personality aberrations (for example, the current concept of schizotypal personality disorder) were diagnosed as having schizophrenia. The concepts of latent and simple schizophrenia blurred the distinction between patients who had schizophrenia and those who had nonpsychotic pathology.

Subsequent authors tried various methods to address the basic conflict of diagnosing an illness that required *both* cross-sectional symptomatology *and* longitudinal course of illness in its diagnostic criteria. For example, Langfeldt (1956) developed the term *schizophreniform* to define a group of patients who had psychotic symptoms, but did not have a deteriorating course.

Current Nomenclature

The DSM-IV has a relatively stringent approach to the diagnosis of schizophrenia that requires specific psychotic symptoms to be present for at least a month (Table 5–3). A *deteriorating course* is one of the diagnostic criteria. This combination of a cross-sectional and longitudinal approach provides for improved reliability in the diagnosis. Patients who might have an illness that is related to schizophrenia in some ways but is atypical in others are given other diagnostic labels. For example, patients who have the symptoms of schizophrenia but recover without residual symptoms within a 6-month period of time are classified as having *schizophreniform disorder.* Patients with schizophreniform disorder also may be subclassified into those with or without good prognostic features. Good prognostic features include an acute onset, good premorbid functioning, and absence of flat affect. The diagnosis is provisional in patients who meet the criteria for schizophreniform disorder but have not yet recovered.

If a patient has symptoms of depression or mania with psychotic symptoms, then the diagnoses of either *schizoaffective disorder* or a primary *mood disorder* with psychotic features should be considered. *Schizoaffective disorder* is usually diagnosed when depressive or manic symptoms are a promi-

Table 5–3 **Key Features of Schizophrenia***

Psychotic symptoms, *at least two*, present for at least a month
  Hallucinations
  Delusions
  Disorganized speech (incoherence, evidence of a thought disorder)
  Disorganized or catatonic behavior
  Negative symptoms (affective flattening, lack of motivation)
Impairment in social or occupational functioning
Duration of the illness for at least 6 months
Symptoms not primarily due to a mood disorder or schizoaffective disorder
Symptoms not due to a medical, neurological or substance-induced disorder

* Summarized from DSM-IV. See DSM-IV (American Psychiatric Association, 1994) for specific diagnostic criteria.

nent and consistent feature of a patient's long-term psychotic illness. The diagnosis of schizoaffective disorder is supported if the longitudinal course of the patient's condition is consistent with schizophrenia and if residual schizophrenic-like symptoms persist when the patient is not depressed or manic. If the psychotic symptoms are present *only* when the patient is depressed or manic, and the patient has relatively good interim functioning between episodes, then the patient should be considered to have a primary *mood disorder* (major depression or bipolar disorder) with psychotic features.

Schizophrenia has been subclassified into *catatonic* (dominated by motoric abnormalities such as rigidity and posturing), *disorganized* (marked by flat affect and disorganized speech and behavior), *paranoid* (paranoid symptoms in the absence of catatonic and disorganized features), and *undifferentiated* types. The *prodromal phase* of the illness refers to the period when the patient's functioning changes before the onset of frank psychotic symptoms. Because it is difficult to "predict" prospectively when a schizophrenic break will occur, the prodromal phase is most safely labeled retrospectively. Residual symptoms exist when the frank psychotic features, such as prominent delusions, hallucinations, incoherence, and bizarre behavior, are controlled but other symptoms (e.g., negative symptoms) remain. The course of the illness is classified into continuous or episodic with complete or incomplete remissions.

DELUSIONAL DISORDER AND BRIEF PSYCHOTIC DISORDER

Delusional disorder is a condition in which the patient has a delusion lasting for at least 1 month in the absence of prominent hallucinations or bizarre behavior. The delusion is usually confined to a single area or person (i.e., it is encapsulated or relatively confined to a specific idea). Other gross psychotic symptoms evident in schizophrenia are absent in delusional disorder. Patients with delusional disorder are subclassified into erotomania, grandiose, jealous, persecutory, somatic, and mixed types based on their symptomatic presentation.

Brief psychotic disorder is characterized by a relatively sudden onset of psychosis that lasts for a few hours to a month with a return to premorbid functioning afterwards. The psychotic symptoms could be, though not necessarily, in response to a significant stressor or occur during 4 weeks postpartum. The patient should recover and return to premorbid levels of functioning within approximately a month to receive this diagnosis.

DIFFERENTIAL DIAGNOSIS

The psychotic disorders described above should be differentiated from psychotic disorders due to substances such as hallucinogens, as well as those caused by primary medical and neurologic conditions. This can be done by gathering historical information that would provide clues as to the presence of a specific diagnosis that could be etiologically related to the psychosis. Principal among these would be a history of alcohol or substance abuse, especially of the stimulant (e.g., amphetamine) type. Amphetamine-induced psychosis is clinically indistinguishable in acute presentation from paranoid schizophrenia. Any person developing a psychotic illness for the first time should have a comprehensive evaluation. A complete physical examination, with particular emphasis on the neurological examination, is essential. In the mental status examination, clouding of consciousness or fluctuating levels of consciousness, memory difficulties, disorientation, and confusion should raise the possibility of a neurologic or metabolic process underlying the psychotic presentation (see Chapter 4).

The diagnostic criteria for *psychotic disorders implies that medical, including neurological and toxic, causes have been ruled out as part of the diagnostic evaluation.*

CASE STUDY
Clinical Case Vignette of Schizophrenia

Jim was 20 years old when his family and friends started to see a change in his behavior. During the previous months, he had begun to withdraw from those around him, preferring to spend more and more time by himself. He lost interest in his scholastic work and his extracurricular activities. He seemed less interested in his personal appearance. He developed a sudden interest in philosophy and spent hours reading philosophical texts.

He had difficulty sleeping for a few nights, and his mother discovered him mumbling to himself. She noticed that he would talk to himself and pause as though he were listening, and then start talking again. When questioned about his behavior, he would stop, turn, and walk away. He began getting suspicious, telling his mother that his friends had turned against him and were plotting to kill him. He subsequently began to read special meanings into the everyday events in his life. Thus, a blue car parked on the road meant that somebody was trying to contact him.

When taken for an evaluation, he told the psychiatrist that a voice was suggesting to him that he jump in front of traffic. He was hospitalized. After a full medical and neurological workup, he was started on medication. Within a few days his sleep pattern seemed to improve considerably, and he became more interested in his hygiene. Within a week, he was able to follow the routine on the ward and take part in the structured activities. He seemed much less focused on the internal concerns that had preoccupied him before admission and was able to talk about current affairs without interjecting his pathological symptoms into the conversation. Although he did not think there was anything seriously wrong with him, he was willing to take medications and was discharged to out-patient treatment.

Within a few months of his hospitalization, he was doing relatively well, and he attempted to return to college. He became more paranoid, however, and refused to take his medication. Over a period of a week, he became more symptomatic and developed gross psychotic symptoms, resulting in a repeat hospitalization.

The next 5 years were marked by periodic hospitalizations, lasting a few days to a week at a time, and outpatient treatment, which included medications and individual and family sessions. The family sessions were aimed at educating the family about the illness and helping them accept Jim's limitations. Interpersonal problems in the family were dealt with by improving communication skills. Stress-management and problem-solving skills were also addressed.

Jim finally began to accept the fact that he had an illness and that he needed long-term treatment. He attended day treatment for a while and then was able to use vocational rehabilitation to begin to look for a job within his limitations. He moved out of his parents' home into a semistructured group home. He was compliant with his medication and was able to tell his therapist when he felt an impending relapse.

Symptoms of Schizophrenia

Psychotic symptoms are marked by abnormalities in the form of thought (called *formal thought disorder*), content of thought, perceptual disturbances, and alterations in emotions and behavior (Andreasen, 1987).

Formal thought disorder is an abnormality in the form of thought. It is differentiated from lack of speech, which is called poverty of speech. The extreme form of poverty of speech can present itself as muteness. Examples of formal thought disorders are as follows:

1. *Derailment or loose associations* is a condition in which the sequential connection between ideas is difficult or impossible to follow because the patient wanders to unrelated subjects. This can be present in a single sentence or in a series of sentences.

2. *Tangentiality* is the tendency to wander to ideas that are distantly connected, but be unable to return spontaneously to the original point. Returning to the original line of thought through a circuitous, detailed, and overly elaborate route is called *circumstantiality*.

3. *Incoherence* is a condition in which even sentences are impossible to follow. It is different from derailment and loose

associations, in which the connections between clauses or sentences are problematic. Lack of understanding because of incomprehensible verbalization of speech is excluded from this description.

Delusions are the result of an abnormality in the *content* of thought. Delusions are false beliefs that are often fixed and cannot be explained based on the cultural background of the individual. If the intensity of the delusions is minor, patients may have some insight into their nonsensical nature and therefore may doubt them. An individual's belief in his or her delusion will often vary as the severity of the illness varies. Beliefs that can be possibly explained within the realm of reality (e.g., the patient has paranoid delusions that someone is trying to kill him) are differentiated from bizarre delusions that can have no basis in reality (e.g., the television is controlling the patient's behavior against his or her will). A systematized delusion (compared with an encapsulated one) is one that is complex, with elaborate connections and multiple implications.

The concept of *mood congruence and incongruence* refers to the extent to which the delusions are consistent with the overall affective state of the patient. Thus, delusions of grandeur are often associated with manic states, and nihilistic delusions can be seen in major depression with psychotic features. Mood-*incongruent* delusions are more likely to be associated with schizophrenic states.

The intensity of a delusion is based on how firmly the belief is held, lack of insight, whether the delusion preoccupies the individual to the exclusion of other concerns, and whether the individual bases his or her actions on the delusion. The different types of delusions are as follows:

1. *Paranoid* delusions are convincing feelings that one is being persecuted, in the absence of such a reality. Paranoid patients may believe that they are being followed, their personal belongings are being tampered with, their telephone is tapped, and they are being harassed. The persecution can come from individuals or organizations (such as the FBI or CIA). The delusion can be a simple, isolated one or an intricate one that pervades all aspects of the individual's life such that all experiences are explained by the delusion.

2. *Ideas and delusions of reference* occur when the patient believes that some event, often of no consequence, is uniquely related to them (i.e., a baby in a stroller signifies that the patient should cross the street). Often the delusions can have a paranoid theme, whereby someone talking in the distance is misinterpreted as talking about and having designs on the patient; or a statement made on the radio or television has special reference to the patient. The questioning of these

beliefs by the patient would make them ideas of reference, while their acceptance as reality would make them delusions. These experiences should be differentiated from anxiety, in which one feels the focus of attention with a fear of social embarrassment.

3. *Delusion of being controlled* is the belief that one's actions are under the control of someone or some external force with malicious intent. The patient feels powerless in the face of such a force and will often relinquish responsibility for their actions or thoughts. The voluntary release of control over one's beliefs and actions, which is seen in cult situations, is not delusional because control is real and given voluntarily.

4. *Thought broadcasting* is the delusion that one's thoughts are broadcast so that they can be heard by others or transmitted to others, even in the absence of vocalizations. Some patients might feel that their thoughts are heard audibly by themselves, or that their mind can be read by someone, even in the absence of speaking.

5. *Thought insertion and withdrawal* are delusions that the patient's mind is having alien thoughts inserted or thoughts withdrawn outside of their control. These thoughts are experienced by the patient as "ego alien," that is, not belonging to the patient.

6. Delusions of *jealousy* are ones in which the individual believes that a loved one is being unfaithful, in the absence of such a reality. The love might be real or imagined (where the recipient of the love does not know that he or she is the object of such admiration by the patient).

7. Delusions of *guilt* are ones in which patients feel that, by acts of omission or commission, they are guilty of some deed for which they blame themselves excessively. Often the delusion is based on an insignificant detail in the patient's past that he or she is unable to forget. At times, the patient will confess to being the cause of major catastrophes or confess to a deed that is obviously not of their doing. Delusions of guilt are often in the context of overzealous religious beliefs. Delusions of guilt are not specific for schizophrenia and are also common in psychotic depressions. Care should be taken to differentiate delusions of guilt from ruminations seen in nonpsychotic depression and obsessions seen in obsessive–compulsive disorder.

8. *Grandiose* delusions are delusions in which the patient believes he or she has special powers that are beyond those of the normal individual. The patient may think that he or she is

someone special, such as Jesus or the president, or believe that he or she has a special mission or significance to society and the world (e.g., developing a theory that would finally explain all of nature). A paranoid theme is at times associated with grandiose delusions. Grandiose delusions are often associated with manic states and frequently are accompanied by excess irritability. Because paranoid delusions can be present in mania, they provide little help in differentiating schizophrenia from manic psychosis.

9. *Religious* delusions also are a frequent phenomenon and include exaggerations of conventional religious beliefs. The beliefs have to be taken within a sociocultural context before they are labeled as delusional. These can be seen in schizophrenic and affective psychoses.

10. *Somatic* delusions are false beliefs related to the body. These frequently take the form that the body or a part of it is rotting or does not exist. Similar delusions may occur in major depression with psychotic features. Somatic concerns of less than delusional degree are seen in hypochondriasis, various anxiety disorders, and body dysmorphic disorder.

Hallucinations are the experiencing of stimuli in any of the senses in the absence of external stimulation. Based on the particular sense involved, the hallucination is called auditory, visual, tactile, olfactory, or gustatory. In functional psychotic conditions, auditory hallucinations are frequent, visual hallucinations are relatively uncommon, and hallucinations in the other senses are rare. The presence of visual hallucinations raises the possibility of primary neurologic disorders or the presence of metabolic or toxin/drug/medication-induced delirium, whereas the presence of olfactory hallucinations raises the likelihood of seizure disorders, especially complex partial seizures.

Auditory hallucinations are the most frequently reported hallucinations in schizophrenic patients. These include one or more voices talking to or about the patient. Infrequent calling of the patient by name is not by itself evidence that the patient is schizophrenic, but continuous hallucinations lasting all day or on and off for a couple of weeks are indicative of a schizophrenic psychosis. Typically, the patient experiences them as unpleasant, although he or she can get used to them and miss them in their absence. The voices can keep a running commentary of the patient's actions as they happen or can predict actions. The auditory hallucinations can be heard either inside the patient's head or coming from outside. At times, patients responding to treatment will report the progression of voices from outside to inside the head, to audible thoughts that may initially be alien, but may later be their own before they go away. Auditory hallucinations of a self-critical or damning nature also may appear in major depression with psychotic features.

Visual hallucinations that occur with the use of hallucinogenic drugs or transiently just as the patient is about to fall asleep (hypnagogic) or wake up (hypnopompic) should not be considered schizophrenic in nature.

Bizarre behaviors include socially inappropriate behaviors, such as dressing totally out of context (e.g., wearing a heavy woolen coat in the middle of summer), or disinhibition of behavior that would not be socially accepted, such as masturbating in public. The sociocultural contexts of the behavior should be taken into consideration before they are labeled as bizarre. Stereotyped behaviors are repetitive actions, often symbolic, that have some contextual meaning to the patient.

Catatonic behavior is the presence of a marked reduction of psychomotor activity. This may present as rigidity, causing passive resistance to movement, or waxy flexibility, in which the patient maintains postures induced by the examiner. Lesser forms of catatonic behavior include mutism and negativism (passive resistance to any attempt to move).

Psychotic depression also may present with catatonic states, and catatonia is more frequently associated with depressive states than schizophrenia. Catatonia also may be caused by a variety of medical and neurological disorders or may be a side effect of neuroleptic treatment.

Affect is the outward expression of emotion and is observed in facial features that routinely accompany the experience of emotions during communication. In schizophrenic patients, there is a paucity of emotional expression or affect, and terms such as emotional blunting or flat affect are used to describe this situation. A dissociation between affect and behavior or cognition is described as incongruent affect.

Positive–Negative Symptoms Dichotomy

The symptoms of schizophrenia can be categorized as positive or negative. Positive symptoms are subjective experiences or behaviors that are added on to the premorbid mental state and include delusions, hallucinations, and bizarre behaviors. Negative symptoms are marked by the loss or reduction in areas of functioning that are normally present in the premorbid state. Andreasen (1982) created a rating scale based on the following broad areas of negative symptoms: *affective flattening, alogia, avolition, anhedonia,* and *attentional impairment.* There is some difficulty in differentiating negative symptoms from the "defect state" (which is the end state of chronic schizophrenia), from depressive symptoms, and (neuroleptic) medication-induced side effects such as bradykinesia.

On the basis of the positive–negative symptom dichotomy, Crow (1985) postulated a two-syndrome concept of schizophrenia in which *type I schizophrenia* was marked by a predominance of *positive symptoms,* reversible outcome, good response to neuroleptic medications, and lack of intellectual impairment, and *type II schizophrenia* was characterized by *negative symptoms,* possible irreversible outcome, poor responsiveness to neuroleptics, and intellectual impairment.

Although such a division is potentially useful, it is difficult to divide schizophrenia into such syndromes because the vast majority of patients seem to have a clinically mixed picture symptomatically and to be partially responsive to treatment. However, a theory that attempts to explain the clinical manifestations of the illness, and correlate psychopathological findings, cognitive changes, and response to treatment is a significant advance because it allows the proposal of testable hypotheses.

Factors in the Expression of Schizophrenia

Environmental Factors

Historical Overview. At the turn of the century, late contemporary European researchers in schizophrenia such as Kraepelin focused on the phenomenology and definition of psychotic disorders. Adolf Meyer (1866–1950) introduced the first empirical approach to investigating the role of environmental factors in the development of psychiatric disorders. Meyer's "psychobiologic" approach advocated the use of a life chart to map life events so that the relationship of life events to the development of psychotic behavior and symptomatology could be examined. Meyer's techniques formed the basis for the biopsychosocial model, although he is rarely given credit for his original contribution to this conceptual model.

The subsequent development of psychoanalytic theory led to interest in the childhood experiences that might be responsible for the development of schizophrenia. The focus was on the child's interpersonal experience within the family, which might lead to faulty ego development and intrapsychic conflict, which in turn put the child at risk for psychotic regression in adult life. The role of the mother was the first to be cited in the search for a cause. Freida Fromm-Reichmann coined the term *schizophrenogenic mother* to describe the emotionally withholding, domineering, and rejecting attitudes she believed to be present in an excessive number of mothers whose children developed schizophrenia. The mother's attitudes, she theorized, led to the child growing up feeling in conflict with, distrustful of, and angry toward others, which later is expressed as a psychotic illness. Other theorists noted evidence of overprotection or rejection in the mothers of schizophrenic individuals.

In the 1950s, interest shifted toward patterns of family or parental interaction that could be responsible for the development of schizophrenia in a child. Three major groups of theorists emerged with different hypotheses. Bateson et al (1956) described the concept of the *double-bind* type of communication, which, they argued, could cause schizophrenia in a child who was repeatedly exposed to it. In a double-bind message, meaning is conveyed by communication on different levels or in different modes—for example, literal or metaphorical meaning, verbal expression, and body language. Conflicting messages may thus be given simultaneously, and Bateson suggested that this type of communication could lead to deficits in interpreting meaning, which progress to a disorder of cognition and metacommunication that is seen in schizophrenia

Theodore Lidz (1958) looked more specifically at two types of dysfunctional parental interaction that, he hypothesized, interfere with personality maturation in the offspring and lead to the development of schizophrenia. In the *schismatic* marriage, parental conflict and lack of trust and communication are seen, whereas in *skewed* marriages, the serious psychopathology of one parent is supported by the masochistic and submissive attitude of the other.

Lyman Wynne and Margaret Singer (1963) at the National Institute of Mental Health (NIMH) developed the concept of *communication deviance.* They argued that parents of schizophrenics show idiosyncratic, disconnected, and confused patterns of speech analogous to the thought disorder seen in schizophrenic patients.

In spite of significant methodologic problems associated with these studies, these theorists postulated that serious disturbances are found in a majority of families with a schizophrenic offspring. Later studies have revealed that the original studies on which these psychological theories were based had seriously flawed methodologies and did not confirm their findings. Dysfunction in families in which a member had already developed schizophrenia *may be due to the effects of living with a disturbed person.* Retrospective reports of early life experience are unreliable, especially in someone who has become ill; the reported abnormal interaction patterns also are found in families of alcoholic and mood disordered patients, making the findings nonspecific.

The etiological significance of communication deviance is continuing to be explored. It could be a subclinical manifestation of schizophrenia present in family members, a reflection of the social isolation resulting from the stigma of mental illness, or an environmental inducer of schizophrenia (a vulnerability or a causative factor) (Doane et al, 1981). A recent study using childhood home videotapes suggests that siblings who later develop schizophrenia can be distinguished from their control siblings on subtle motor and interpersonal behaviors early in childhood (Walker and Lewine, 1990).

Expressed Emotion

Once established, schizophrenia and the major psychoses have considerable variability in their course and outcome. Only part of this variance is related to response to medication. Thus, environmental influences on the course of illness have become a fertile area of investigation.

The course of the illness may be measured by the frequency and severity of relapse and the level of functioning between acute episodes. Follow-up studies of schizophrenic patients returning home have identified certain styles of communication in families that are positively correlated with earlier relapse (Leff and Vaughn, 1981). The critical factors as measured during a standardized family interview are criticism, hostility, and overinvolvement, known as *expressed emotion* (EE). Based on specific criteria when families were divided into "high and low" degrees of EE, there were large differences in relapse rates. Patients from high EE families relapsed at a higher rate than those from low EE families. These relapse rates were not correlated with severity of illness in the patient. Similar results were found for families of depressed patients. In high EE families, fewer hours of face-to-face contact between patients and adult relatives significantly reduced the relapse rate in the schizophrenic, but not the depressed group of patients. Use of prophylactic medications reduced the relapse rate in schizophrenics returning to high EE homes.

Life Events

Stressful life events seem to relate to the onset of relapse in major psychotic illnesses. Stressors can be divided into those that are acute and independent of the person's behavior and influence (such as an acute illness or death of a relative) and those that are chronic (such as poverty or difficulties at work or in the family environment), which also may be dependent on illness factors in the patient. In the 3 weeks before a psychotic relapse (in both schizophrenia and depression), it has been shown that there is a high frequency of independent social stressors (Brown and Birley, 1968). Moreover, the use of prophylactic medication in schizophrenic patients may protect against relapse under circumstances of acute stress though this is less likely when imposed on a situation of chronic life stress.

When discussing the role of stress in the precipitation or maintenance of psychotic symptoms, one must also take into account each individual's variable response to that stress, his or her resources for dealing with it, and the degree to which he or she had control over its occurrence (Dohrenwend and Dohrenwend, 1978).

Social Class

Schizophrenia clusters in the lower socioeconomic classes (especially in urban environments), which is different from other psychotic conditions such as bipolar disorder. A contributing factor to this clustering is the phenomenon of *social drift.* The higher representation of schizophrenia in lower socioeconomic classes has been shown to relate in part to the downward mobility experienced by schizophrenic individuals secondary to their disability. Studies of the occupations of both biological and adopted fathers of schizophrenics show that patients frequently fail to reach the occupational level of their parents, thus confirming that social drift occurs.

Social Network

The interaction between the effects of the environment on schizophrenia and the effects of schizophrenia on social experience is illustrated again in studies of social network. Social network refers to the circle of family members, friends, and associates with whom support and social activity is shared. Schizophrenics tend to have networks that are smaller, more family oriented, and less intimate than those of controls. This tendency becomes more prominent after repeated hospitalizations, and in many cases, family members will eventually disengage and be replaced by more formal professional contacts, such as mental health staff. This finding can be explained by the difficulties schizophrenic patients have in initiating and sustaining social relationships. Because an individual's social network serves as a major buffer against the stresses of life, the patient's shrinking social network also tends to influence the progression of the illness.

Genetic Factors

There is considerable evidence that schizophrenia is an illness that runs in some families, although most of the patients evaluated do not have a first-degree relative (i.e., sibling, parent, or child, each of whom probably shares half of the patient's genes) with schizophrenia. The overall morbid risk of a schizophrenic patient's first-degree relative developing schizophrenia is between 4 and 9%, based on different studies. Family members more distantly related to a schizophrenic patient have a lesser risk for the development of schizophrenia. What exactly is transmitted is not clear. Twin studies report that monozygotic twins are more likely to be concordant for schizophrenia (range in different studies 31 to 78%) than dizygotic twins (range in different studies 0 to 28%). However, the concordance for monozygotic twins is not absolute, suggesting that the illness is transmitted only in a subset of the twins or that environmental influences can have either a triggering or protective influence in individuals.

Various studies have shown that the likelihood of monozygotic twins being concordant for schizophrenia is over *four times* greater than that for dizygotic twins. It is important to note that approximately 50% of monozygotic twin pairs are discordant for schizophrenia, suggesting that what is transmitted is not the illness per se, but the *vulnerability* for the development of it. Adoption studies of offspring of schizophrenic patients show that they have a greater likelihood of developing schizophrenia than do the adopted offspring of healthy individuals. The estimated heritability of a diathesis for schizophrenia based on such studies is between 60 and 90%.

Advances in molecular biology allow chromosomal analysis in which a search for linkage with known genetic markers can be done in families in which schizophrenia is prevalent. The gene that transmits schizophrenia was reported to be situated in close proximity to a known DNA marker on the *fifth chromosome* in one study of a large extended family, although a number of attempts to replicate this finding have failed. Questions about the statistical assumptions used in studies like this have been raised. Failure to replicate the original report could also be the result of the heterogeneity of schizophrenia. Another approach is to explore candidate genes, i.e., the D_2 receptor gene, as possibly involved in the transmission of schizophrenia. Attempts to link candidate genes to schizophrenia have failed so far.

Schizophrenic mothers are more likely to have pregnancy problems and perinatal problems with their children; thus, their offspring might have not only the genetic diathesis, but also both intrauterine and perinatal insults. Furthermore, children of schizophrenic mothers are more likely to have disruptive early life experiences that contribute to developmental aberrations, including psychological ones.

There is a complex interaction between the genetic influences and environmental variables leading to the phenotypic expression of schizophrenia. These variables are interactive, not just additive. This complex interaction of nature and nurture affects not only the development of schizophrenia, but also its course. In different individuals, differing genetic and environmental factors may thus play lesser or greater roles in cause and pathogenesis, thus contributing to the heterogeneity of the disorder. The most widely accepted view of the pathogenesis of schizophrenia is the *stress diathesis* model, in which constitutional factors determined by heredity (the diathesis) interact with environmental influences (stress) that precipitate overt expression of the clinical symptoms.

Anatomical Factors

Neuropathological studies of postmortem schizophrenic brains have attempted to find lesions that would explain the symptoms of schizophrenia. The search for pathological lesions in schizophrenia has focused on the frontal and medial temporal lobes, particularly the hippocampus and adjacent entorhinal cortex. The pathological findings include nonspecific gliosis and cellular loss and disordered orientation of the pyramidal cells in the hippocampus, suggesting a developmental rather than a degenerative disturbance. However, there is still insufficient evidence to indicate clearly a specific site for a pathological lesion in most schizophrenic patients.

Although a resurgence of interest exists in postmortem neuropathological studies of schizophrenic brains, there are a number of potential pitfalls in this methodology. These include the difficulty in dissociating the etiological factors from effects that might be the result of long-term chronic illness and effects of treatment. Other difficulties include changing ideas about diagnosis, the question of appropriate controls, the cause of death, delays in obtaining and fixing the brain after death, and so forth.

Neurochemistry also has been used in postmortem studies to unravel the mysteries of schizophrenia. A number of studies have documented increases in the number of type 2 dopamine (D_2) receptors in areas such as the basal ganglia, caudate nucleus, and nucleus accumbens, although such an increase appears to be the result of neuroleptic treatment in some cases.

Imaging techniques, as they have become available, have been used to understand better the morphology and pathophysiology of schizophrenia. Computed tomography (CT) allows a noninvasive technique to be used to obtain X-rays of the brain in transverse slices. Numerous studies have documented *enlargement of the lateral ventricles, increased width of the third ventricle, and sulcal enlargement suggestive of cortical atrophy.*

Lateral ventricular enlargement is reported in schizophrenic patients in the majority of controlled studies (Fig. 5–1). Enlargement of the lateral ventricles is not necessarily sufficient to be read as clinically abnormal in these

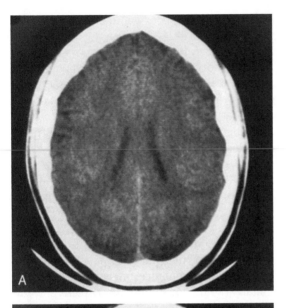

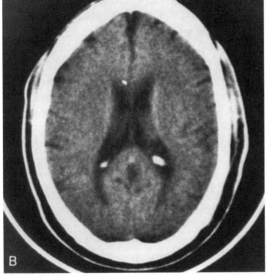

Figure 5–1. *(A)* CT scan of patient with schizophrenia with normal lateral ventricles. *(B)* CT scan of patient with schizophrenia taken at level of bodies of lateral ventricles with enlarged lateral ventricles.

cases. However, planimetric and automated measurements clearly show that statistically significant enlargement of the lateral ventricle exists in many schizophrenic patients. Lateral ventricular enlargement is *not specific* to schizophrenia. It is found in a number of neurological conditions and also in nonschizophrenic psychiatric conditions such as bipolar disorder.

The lateral ventricular enlargement is seen very early in the onset of the illness, suggesting that it precedes the psychosis and is probably not progressive. Lateral ventricular enlargement has been correlated with cognitive disturbances, negative symptoms, poor premorbid psychosocial functioning, poor response to treatment, and poor outcome.

The third ventricle is situated close to anatomical areas of particular interest in schizophrenia. It has been measured in a number of studies, and the majority report its enlargement. Sulcal enlargement also has been reported in a significant number of schizophrenic patients, suggesting diffuse cortical atrophy.

Magnetic resonance imaging (MRI) techniques provide significant advantages over CT scan studies, including better resolution; lack of exposure to radiation; the capacity for transverse, sagittal, and coronal cuts; and the capacity for three-dimensional reconstruction of the brain. MRI studies generally confirm the CT findings of enlarged lateral ventricles (Fig. 5–2). In addition, some (but not all) studies report a 3 to 5% reduction in total brain area and/or volume in schizophrenia. MRI studies focusing on the temporal lobe and limbic structures report a reduction in temporal lobe, hippocampal, and amygdala volumes in schizophrenia. The abnormalities are found more often on the left side.

Morphological studies can provide only a limited understanding of an illness that has some functional basis to it. Hence, static measures of structure are one step removed from physiological processes that need to be studied.

Physiological Factors

Physiological studies connect mental function to underlying physiological processes that are measurable and thus provide insights into normal and pathological psychological functioning. Physiological studies of cerebral blood flow in schizophrenia have been done with xenon 133 inhalation, positron emission tomography (PET), and single-photon emission computed tomography. Xenon is an inert gas that does not affect physiological or biochemical processes. Thus, measurement of radioactivity using gamma detectors, after inhalation of radiolabeled xenon, is a measure of regional blood flow in the brain. As neuronal activity is directly correlated with blood flow, regional cerebral blood flow is a measure of local neuronal activity. Physiological studies with xenon have the advantage of allowing repeat measures in individuals because of the limited radioactivity involved, but they give us only information about surface activity. To get an idea about deeper parts of the brain, we turn to techniques such as PET studies. PET allows three-dimensional quantification of physiological activity of the brain, either of blood flow or of receptor activity.

There does not seem to be a difference in the total cerebral blood flow between schizophrenic patients and normal controls. Attempts to study differences in the resting state have resulted in inconsistent results. A number of studies have suggested a *hypofrontal pattern* to the regional distribution of cerebral blood flow with a *decrease* of blood flow to *the frontal lobes* relative to other brain areas.

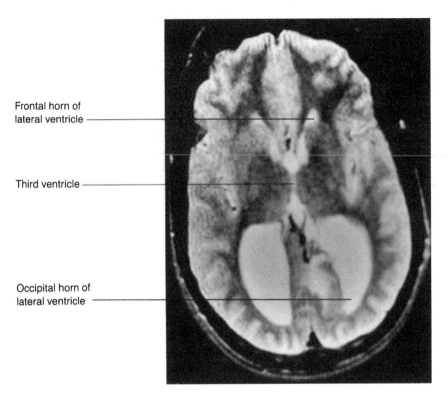

Frontal horn of
lateral ventricle

Third ventricle

Occipital horn of
lateral ventricle

Figure 5–2. *Axial MRI scan (T_2 = weighted image) of a patient with schizophrenia showing enlarged lateral ventricles.*

Under behavioral activation paradigms, the functional responsivity of the various cerebral areas can be assessed. A series of studies using this methodology has involved the use of a cognitive task (the Wisconsin Card Sort [WCS]) that activates the dorsolateral prefrontal cortex (DLPFC) in comparison with the use of a nonspecific cognitive task. Schizophrenic patients failed to activate the DLPFC, and the lack of activation was associated with the number of errors made on the WCS. Similar results have been obtained using a paradigm that activates the left medial frontal cortex with schizophrenic patients failing to activate, compared with controls. The interpretation of this series of studies is that some schizophrenic patients have a specific abnormality in activating the prefrontal cortex, part of the brain that is physiologically important in planning, altering strategies in problem solving, and coping with change.

Biochemical Factors

The search for a biochemical understanding of schizophrenia has been plagued by numerous discoveries that have failed to be replicated. The dopamine system has been a primary focus as a mediator of pathology that could explain the illness of schizophrenia. There is mostly indirect evidence to support a causal role of dopamine in schizophrenia. Thus, all typical antipsychotic medications (that is, the "older" ones) have the common capacity to block D_2 (non-adenylate cyclase) dopamine receptors. Furthermore, indirect dopamine agonists have the capacity to induce a condition that is clinically indistinguishable from schizophrenia (as in amphetamine psychosis) or exacerbate a psychotic condition, although neither of these effects is consistent in all patients. The affinity that various typical neuroleptic agents have for the D_2 receptor correlates highly with the average therapeutic dose used for the control of psychotic symptoms. Such data strongly suggest that the neuroleptic action at the D_2 receptor is pharmacologically relevant for the clinical benefits (Table 5–4).

With the cloning of several dopamine receptors, multiple types that could not be delineated using previous methodologies are now recognized (Table 5–5). Of particular interest, the D_4 receptor has a higher affinity for the atypical neuroleptic clozapine and could mediate its greater antipsychotic potency. A number of dopamine systems exist in the mammalian brain. The ones of particular relevance to schizophrenia include the mesolimbic and mesocortical systems, which are thought to be integrally related to schizophrenia, and the nigrostriatal and tuberoinfundibular, which are thought to be related more to the side effects of neuroleptics (Table 5–6).

Crow's typology of schizophrenia suggests two different pathological processes in the development of schizophrenia. The first involves the negative symptoms of schizophrenia, which could be reflections of pathological processes in the prefrontal cortex. Damage to the prefrontal cortex results in an amotivated withdrawn state with lack of initiative, thought, and emotion (Fuster, 1980). The positive symptoms, such as hallucinations and delusions, seem to be the result of pathology in the limbic system (Schmajuk, 1987).

Because both the limbic and prefrontal cortex have dopamine projections from the midbrain, it is interesting to look at these systems and their relation to pathology in schizophrenia. There are some differences between the mesocortical and mesolimbic dopamine pathways. The mesocortical dopamine pathway, like the tuberoinfundibular one, does not seem to have autoreceptors on the cell bodies and nerve terminals (Bannon and Roth, 1983). It is believed that as a result of this lack of autoreceptors, the mesocortical dopamine neurons have a higher rate of physiological activity, are less responsive to dopamine agonists and antagonists, and do not develop tolerance to chronic neuroleptic treatment. Thus, it is possible that neuroleptics are used at therapeutic doses that have their predominant effect on the nigrostriatal and the mesolimbic dopamine systems, which result in control of the positive psychotic symptoms and the development of extrapyramidal side effects. At higher doses, neuroleptics may also have an effect on the mesocortical system, whereby they can exacerbate negative symptoms.

Lesion studies of the mesocortical dopamine system (Pycock et al, 1980) in rats result in disinhibition of the mesolimbic dopamine system with the

Table 5-4 Side-Effect Profiles and Dose Equivalents of Commonly Used Neuroleptics*

DRUG	EQUIVALENT DOSE (MG)	DOSAGE FORMS	SIDE EFFECTS			
			SEDATIVE	Extra-pyramidal	Hypo-tensive	ANTI-CHOLINERGIC
Phenothiazines						
Chlorpromazine	100	t,i,c,s,r	+++	++	i.m. +++ Oral ++	+++
Thioridazine	95	t,c,s	+++	+	+	++++
Mesoridazine	50	t,i,c	+++	+	++	+++
Fluphenazine	2	t,i,d,s,c	+	+++	+	+
Perphenazine	10	t,i,c	++	++	+	++
Trifluoperazine	5	t,i,c	+	+++	+	+
Butyrophenones						
Haloperidol	2	t,i,c,d	+	+++	+	+
Thioxanthenes						
Thiothixene	5	t,i,c	+ to ++	++	+	+
Dihydroindolone						
Molindone	10	t,c	++	+	0	+
Dibenzoxazepine						
Loxapine	15	t,i,c	+	++	+	++
Diphenylbutylpiperidine						
Pimozide†	2	t	+	+	+	+
Atypical Neuroleptics						
Clozapine	50	t	+++	+	+++	++++
Quetiapine	50	t	++	+	++	—
Neuroleptics						
Risperidone	2	t	+	+	+	—
Olanzapine	2	t	++	+/–	+	+/–

* 0, none; +, slight; ++, moderate; +++, marked; ++++, pronounced; +/–, ; t, tablet or capsule; i, injectable; c, concentrate; s, suspension; r, rectal suppository; d, depot injection.
† Pimozide may have a greater propensity for prolonging the QT interval than other neuroleptics. Information in table extracted in part from: Mason A, Granacher RP: *Clinical Handbook of Antipsychotic Drug Therapy*, pp 19–108. New York, Brunner/Mazel, 1980 and Baldessarini RJ: Chemotherapy. In Nicholi AM (ed): *The Harvard Guide to Modern Psychiatry*, p. 390. Cambridge, Harvard University Press, 1978. (Used with permission from Stoudemire A, Fogel BS: Psychopharmacology in the medically ill. In Stoudemire A, Fogel BS (eds): Principles of Medical Psychiatry, p. 89. Orlando, Grune & Stratton, 1987)

Table 5–5 **Cloned Dopamine Receptors**

TYPE	EFFECT ON ADENYLATE CYCLASE	ANATOMIC LOCALIZATION
D$_1$	Stimulates	Cerebral cortex
D$_2$	Inhibits	Striatum and limbic cortex
D$_3$	? Inhibits	Limbic areas
D$_4$	? Inhibits	Frontal cortex, midbrain, amygdala, medulla
D$_5$	? Stimulates	Limbic system (including hippocampus and amygdala)

resulting functional overactivity and upregulation of the dopamine receptors. Such a finding is congruent with postmortem studies of schizophrenic brains (Weinberger and Kleinman, 1986). These data can suggest a model for explaining the symptomatology in schizophrenia whereby underactivity of the mesocortical dopamine system results in an overactivity of the mesolimbic system, which results in the positive symptoms of schizophrenia (Davis, 1991).

Weinberger (1987) has suggested that insult to the prefrontal cortex early in life would be silent through prepubertal development. However, when the prefrontal cortical functions come on-line with normal brain development associated with sexual maturity and the attainment of early adulthood, such a "lesion" could express itself (possibly triggered by stress) in the form of a psychotic episode. The pathophysiology of this abnormality would be in the form of decreased inhibition of subcortical dopamine systems, which are expressed as psychotic symptoms. Such a model would potentially explain the age of onset of schizophrenia.

There is a growing body of evidence suggesting that in schizophrenia, the cell migration, synapse formations, and programmed cell death might be abnormal in the frontal and temporal cortex and the hippocampus and surrounding areas. Cell migration is most intense in the early and middle second trimester. Such a period of development might be particularly vulnerable to specific viral infections, failure of gene expression, or other etiological mechanisms that can leave the individual vulnerable to the development of schizophrenic symptoms during adulthood. The influenza epidemic in 1957 has been

Table 5–6 **Dopamine Systems Relevant to Schizophrenia**

SYSTEM	CELL BODIES	PROJECTIONS
Nigrostriatal	Substantia nigra (A9)	Neostriatum (putamen + caudate)
Mesolimbic	Ventral tegmental area (A10) Substantia nigra (A9)	Accumbens, olfactory tubercle, amygdala
Mesocortical	Ventral tegmental area (A10)	Prefrontal cortex

associated with an increased incidence of schizophrenia in children whose mothers were in the second trimester of pregnancy.

Acute treatment with typical neuroleptic agents results in an increase in the firing rate of the dopamine cells and an increasing turnover of dopamine at the synaptic sites. However, chronic treatment results in a decrease in the firing rate related to depolarization block of the dopamine cells and the down-regulation of the receptor sensitivity. The decrease is reflected in the reduction of both plasma and cerebrospinal fluid (CSF) homovanillic acid (HVA), a metabolite of dopamine. This reduction in HVA is temporally associated with clinical improvement.

Thus, a number of different lines of information from the clinical, anatomical, physiological, biochemical, and pharmacological areas are coming together to aid in understanding the complex enigma of schizophrenia.

Treatment of Schizophrenia

Pharmacological Management

The pharmacology of neuroleptic (antipsychotic) medications is covered in Chapter 18. This section will focus on clinical issues in the use of neuroleptics in the treatment of schizophrenia.

Neuroleptic agents are significantly more powerful in controlling the symptoms of psychosis than are antianxiety, antidepressant, and antimanic agents, none of which is any better than placebo. There are two indications for neuroleptic agents in the treatment of schizophrenia. The first is to control the active symptoms of the illness, and the second is to provide a prophylactic effect in preventing relapse. The first is aimed at controlling the acute episode, whereas the second is aimed at maintenance management. In a significant number of patients, however, the control of symptoms is only partial, and therefore, the palliative and prophylactic indications for the neuroleptics are often combined.

The typical predominately D_2 receptor-blocking neuroleptic agents in use today are all equally effective in the treatment of psychosis (Table 5–4). Thus, in choosing a particular neuroleptic for the treatment of a patient, therapeutic effectiveness is not a factor that guides the physician in the choice of a particular neuroleptic. Even neuroleptics that have a greater sedating effect (e.g., chlorpromazine, thioridazine) seem to improve psychomotor retardation associated with psychosis, whereas less sedating neuroleptic agents (e.g., haloperidol) have a calming effect in agitated patients.

Side effects should be considered when choosing which neuroleptic should be used in a particular individual. Major side effects include anticholinergic ones, postural hypertension, and extrapyramidal ones (acute dystonic reactions, pseudoparkinsonism, akathisia, and tardive dyskinesia). Less common, but with considerable morbidity and mortality, is neuroleptic malignant syndrome (see Chapter 18).

For the acute episode of schizophrenia, doses in the range of 400 to 600 mg of chlorpromazine or its equivalent are necessary for successful treatment (Kane, 1987). Megadoses of neuroleptics (over 2,000 mg of chlorpromazine or its equivalent) do not seem to result in any greater or faster improvement of schizophrenia. Combining benzodiazepines with neuroleptic agents in the early part of the treatment of an acute schizophrenic episode can be an appropriate strategy to induce sedation and control agitated behavior while using lower doses of neuroleptic agents. Use of benzodiazepines for such an indication should not be for more than a few days at a time because of the potential development of physiological dependence.

The maintenance strategy is to find the lowest useful dose of neuroleptic that will continue to provide protection against psychotic relapse while not interfering with the psychosocial functioning of the individual and reducing the risk for tardive dyskinesia. If high doses of neuroleptics are required for control of an acute episode of schizophrenia, one should consider a slow and gradual reduction in dose once the patient has stabilized and is relatively free of stressful situations. One approach would be to reduce the dosage of chlorpromazine or its equivalent at the rate of 100 mg a month. Such a decrease in dosage should be coupled with education of the patient and significant others and attempts to monitor the development of early warning signs indicative of impending relapse. An unstable environment around the patient and emotional hostility and intrusiveness (high EE) that the patient might have to endure from close relationships are much more likely to be associated with a psychotic relapse. Hence, patients with these situations should have their medications reduced in a more conservative manner.

Neuroleptic Side Effects

Neuroleptics have numerous side effects; this chapter focuses exclusively on the extrapyramidal side effects. These are important because they have a major impact on the patient's compliance with neuroleptic medications.

The extrapyramidal systems are involved in the nonconscious control of all voluntary musculature. Neuroleptics have complex effects on the extrapyramidal systems that are exacerbated by anxiety, disappear during sleep, and can be consciously controlled for a limited time with effort. Extrapyramidal side effects can be classified into those that happen early or late in treatment.

Among the early extrapyramidal side effects are *acute dystonic reactions.* These are involuntary spasms of voluntary muscle groups that are often painful and frightening to patients. Frequently, they involve the orofacial and head and neck areas, although any part of the body may be involved. Young men on high-potency neuroleptics (e.g., haloperidol) are at the greatest risk for the development of acute dystonic reactions. Low-potency neuroleptics, especially ones that have significant anticholinergic effects (e.g., thioridazine), have less likelihood of inducing acute dystonic reactions. Acute dystonic reactions tend to happen relatively early in treatment, and there is some tolerance that develops to them. The presumed mechanism of action is an imbalance induced by neuroleptic agents blocking dopamine receptors that are in balance with the cholinergic system. The use of neuroleptics with anticholinergic agents or dopamine agonists results in reestablishment of this dopamine–cholinergic balance and the control of the acute dystonic reaction. Considering the impact of such reactions on compliance of the patient, it is worthwhile to consider using antiparkinsonian agents in a prophylactic manner in patients who are started on neuroleptics, especially the high-potency ones such as haloperidol.

Parkinsonian side effects also associated with the use of neuroleptics include tremor, rigidity, and bradykinesia. These symptoms are indistinguishable from the symptoms of Parkinson's disease, which is caused by degeneration of the dopamine cells in the substantia nigra. Neuroleptic-induced parkinsonian side effects are responsive to anticholinergic and dopamine agonist agents.

Bradykinesia is a state associated with diminished spontaneous motor movements associated with a reduction in spontaneous speech, general apathy, and difficulty initiating activities. Bradykinesia can be difficult to differentiate from depression and negative symptoms. Because anticholinergic agents are effective in treating bradykinesia, such symptoms should be aggressively treated with these agents.

Akathisia is a subjective sense of motor restlessness and is often mistaken for agitation. It is not as responsive as other extrapyramidal side effects to anticholinergic agents. Some patients with akathisia respond to the use of beta-blockers such as propranolol. The most effective treatment for akathisia is a reduction in neuroleptic dose.

Tardive dyskinesia (TD) is a late complication of neuroleptic treatment and has been described as "a syndrome consisting of abnormal stereotyped involuntary movements, usually of choreoathetoid type principally affecting the mouth, face, limbs and trunk, which occurs relatively late in the course of drug treatment and the etiology of which the drug treatment is a necessary factor" (Jeste, 1982). There is roughly a 3% annual risk for the development of TD, which is cumulative annually. About one-third of patients treated with neuroleptics seem to be at risk for the development of TD. If detected early, and the neuroleptic is discontinued, the TD is often reversible. Continued treatment with neuroleptics results in potential worsening of the symptoms of TD and makes them more likely to be irreversible. Risk factors for the development of TD include total lifetime exposure to the dose of neuroleptic medications, older age, female sex, a history of extrapyramidal side effects, and mood disorders.

The presumed pathogenesis of TD is the development of supersensitive dopamine receptors in response to chronic blockade by neuroleptics. However, such supersensitivity probably develops in all patients treated chronically with neuroleptics, but only some go on to develop TD. Hence, supersensitive dopamine receptors might be necessary but not sufficient for the development of TD. Currently, there is no clinically successful strategy for the treatment of TD. Thus, the best approach for avoiding the risk of TD is the use of neuroleptics at the lowest possible dose necessary, regular evaluation for development of the symptoms of TD, and periodic voluntary informed consent for the continued use of neuroleptics.

The "Atypical" Antipsychotic Medications. Clozapine, risperidone, olanzapine, and quetiapine are antipsychotic agents recently available in the United States, that have a significantly greater effect on the serotonergic system than the "typical" antipsychotics. As a consequence, these medications, especially clozapine, are more effective than older medications in the treatment of negative symptoms (Fleisch-hacker and Hummer, 1997). The efficacy of these newer antipsychotic medications, via both serotonergic and dopaminergic effects, suggest that positive and negative schizophrenial symptoms may be mediated by different biochemical pathways (Meltzer, 1991). Clinical studies, furthermore, have shown superior efficacy of clozapine over typical neuroleptics in the treatment of refractory schizophrenic patients. Clozapine is not associated with significant extrapyramidal side effects, including the development of TD. However, there is a 1 to 2% risk for the development of agranulocytosis requiring the weekly monitoring of white cell count (Lieberman, 1989). Other common side effects include sedation, sialorrhea (excessive salivation), hyperthermia, hypotension, grand mal seizures, sexual dysfunction, and enuresis (see also Chapter 18).

Psychosocial Treatment

Psychosocial treatment of the major psychoses is best conceptualized as an essential part of an integrated plan involving a range of therapies matched to the phase of illness and the individual characteristics of each patient. Underlying goals are the treatment of symptoms, reduction of stress, mobilization of social supports, assistance with deficits in daily living skills caused by the illness, and gradual rehabilitation to the most autonomous level of functioning possible for the individual patient. Psychosocial treatment modalities include the use of hospitalization, partial hospitalization or day treatment programs, crisis intervention, individual therapy, and family treatment, including psychoeducational approaches, social skills and behavioral training, and case management.

Individuals with all major psychotic disorders are likely to need long-term, often lifetime treatment. A consistent relationship with a primary clinician is of key importance to provide support and guidance through different phases of the illness and to coordinate the different treatment modalities that may be needed. Careful attention to maintaining continuity of care between hospital and outpatient clinic, day treatment, vocational rehabilitation, and family treatment programs is of particular importance for patients whose illness may make it difficult for them to make transitions and new relationships, or to negotiate complex institutional barriers. Integration of medication and psychosocial programs is essential. Psychosocial treatments are used to target problems not responsive to medications, such as negative symptoms and social and occupational deficits, to support medication strategies that have maximal therapeutic efficacy with the least possible side effects, and to assist patients in gaining knowledge and confidence in how best to manage their illness. Studies indicate that the combination of medication and psychosocial programs is significantly more effective than either used alone (Falloon and Lieberman, 1983).

Acute Phase. In the acute phase of a psychotic illness, hospitalization is often necessary to contain disruptive and dangerous behavior and to remove the individual from everyday stresses and responsibilities. Patients should always be medically reevaluated for the presence of medical, neurological, or substance abuse disorders that may be etiologically related to the psychotic break or may have precipitated a relapse.

The push toward deinstitutionalization and community care (founded on the advent of neuroleptics), concern over the iatrogenic effects of long-term institutionalization, and the shifting of public money from state hospitals to community mental health centers have dramatically reduced the length of stay for most psychotic patients. Studies show short-term hospitalization to be at least as effective as longer stays. Interest in partial hospitalization, in which the patient lives at home but attends a structured daily program, has grown. Several studies show that this is feasible and works as well as inpatient treatment for patients who do not present a risk of violence or suicide (Weiss and Dubin, 1982).

The goals of psychosocial intervention in the acute phase of a psychotic experience are to reduce stimulation and to provide a safe and structured environment in which clear communication, little demand for performance, and firm limit setting by tolerant and supportive staff can complement the use of medication in achieving a rapid resolution of symptomatic behavior. Immediate contact with the family is important in developing an alliance, providing crisis intervention to resolve stress that may have caused or been caused by the patient's relapse, and planning for future treatment. Connecting the patient with appropriate aftercare treatment is an essential part of the treatment of the acute phase of illness. This coordination requires careful attention because in many public care systems, inpatient and outpatient staff are segregated into different institutions and agencies under different funding and administration, resulting in a high failure rate in keeping first outpatient appointments.

Follow-up Treatment. After an acute psychotic episode, only limited resumption of normal roles and activities should be expected of the patient for several months. The principal goals of treatment at this stage are to prevent relapse while adjusting medication to a maintenance level, and to help the patient reintegrate into the community. The home environment is now often the major treatment milieu, and it is important for the clinician to attend to the major impact that an acute psychotic episode has on the family system. Emotional turmoil, disruption of family routine and coping strategies, stigma, and restriction of social network are all dimensions that need to be addressed while the family is helped to provide the most therapeutic milieu. Attempts to change specific aspects of family interaction that correlate with higher relapse rates, such as high EE or communication deviance, may be warranted. Family treatment programs involving crisis intervention, education about the illness, stress reduction, and communication skills training have been shown to reduce the risk of relapse in the first year after hospitalization. Day hospital programs can play a useful role in assisting the patient's gradual readjustment to community living and also have been shown to reduce the risk of relapse. They may be particularly helpful for many chronic patients who have little family support and return to boarding homes, halfway houses, or cooperative living arrangements, which provide little in the way of treatment. Psychosocial programs that are too demanding or stimulating are not appropriate for this phase of treatment. Major role therapy, an intensive problem-solving approach used with schizophrenic outpatients, has been shown to improve social functioning after 18 months of treatment, but if it is offered without the use of prophylactic medication, it is associated with a lower level of adjustment, indicating that too much pressure can be detrimental to patients in the recovery process.

Individual psychoanalytic psychotherapy has not been shown to improve the outcome for schizophrenic patients over the use of medication alone. This does not preclude its use for a few high-functioning schizophrenic patients. Supportive psychotherapy to help patients develop a language to discuss and integrate the traumatic experience of psychosis is important. This is best provided by a consistent primary clinician who is both flexible in his/her approach and knowledgable about schizophrenia. For many patients recovering from an acute psychotic episode, help with living accommodations, food, clothing, income, child care, and medical care is needed immediately. Case management is the term used to describe the social work function of helping the patient access the services that will meet these needs. This model of care is now part of many aftercare systems for psychotic patients. Case management functions may be provided by the primary clinician or may be allocated to separate case managers who work with a specific target population.

For the many patients who do not return to a premorbid level of adjustment following reentry into the community, other psychosocial interventions may be indicated. Social skills training programs using behavioral techniques focus on teaching patients verbal and nonverbal behaviors necessary for independent living and everyday social interaction. Assessment of strengths and weaknesses is followed by instruction, modeling, rehearsal (often in role play), and positive reinforcement of behavior that is correctly carried out. This approach has been shown to be helpful for chronic patients left with marked negative symptoms.

Group psychotherapy is useful in developing social skills, as well as in encouraging supportive interpersonal relationships, reality testing, giving and receiving advice with practical problems of living, and exploring fears and feelings in a safe environment. With patients who have been psychotic, the group should have a structured, task-oriented focus rather than an exploratory focus. Many mental health centers use a biweekly or monthly medication group to provide an opportunity for patient evaluation, education, and socialization, as well as an extension of each patient's social network.

Patients who recover sufficiently from the acute psychotic episode may need assistance in returning to work. Vocational rehabilitation programs such as workshops, job training programs, and transitional employment are offered by state and private agencies, which usually provide a structured and sheltered work environment in which patients may rehearse general job-related skills, such as being on time, completing tasks, and responding to supervision, as well as acquire new skills in preparation for a specific job. Little research has been done to measure the effectiveness of such programs, but they nevertheless address an area of recovery that is sorely in need of help, considering that less than 30% of schizophrenic patients return to work postdischarge. Vocational programs need to be open ended with the expectation that many patients will need ongoing support such as that provided by supported employment programs.

CONCLUSIONS

Schizophrenia is an illness that is heterogenous in its cause, pathophysiology, response to treatment, and long-term outcome. Thus, generalizations about the illness and predictability in treatment response and outcome are important factors to consider. Their predictive capacity, however, is small.

CLINICAL PEARLS

- Pyschotic symptoms are nonspecific and occur in a variety of medical, psychiatric, neurological, and substance-induced disorders.
- Always rule out a medical, neurological or substance-induced disorder first before assuming that any patient with psychotic symptoms has a "functional" psychiatric disorder.
- First-onset psychosis after age 45 generally indicates a neurological, medical or substance-induced disorder or a psychotic depression; the onset of schizophrenia after age 45 is relatively rare.
- It is now believed that schizophrenia is primarily a brain disorder with a strong genetic component; it is possible, however, that certain types of environmental or developmental stresses in individuals who are genetically vulnerable may contribute to the onset of the illness.
- It has been well demonstrated that the most effective treatment for schizophrenia involves a combination of neuroleptic medication and psychosocial treatment modalities.
- After years of research, abnormalities in the dopaminergic system of the brain remain the most consistent theory for the biological basis of schizophrenia. This theory has been elaborated to consider dysfunctional serotonergic neurotransmission as well.
- In treating schizophrenia, neuroleptics should be used at the lowest possible dose, and the patient should be monitored closely for tardive dyskinesia. Informed consent regarding tardive dyskinesia should be given at least every 6 months.

ANNOTATED BIBLIOGRAPHY

Andreasen NC: The diagnosis of schizophrenia. Schizophr Bull 13:9–22, 1987

>An overview of the development of the criteria for diagnosing schizophrenia. Assesses both the strengths and limitations of nomenclature in psychiatry.

Arieti S: The Interpretation of Schizophrenia, 2nd ed. New York, Basic Books, 1974

>For students interested in an eloquent, psychoanalytically oriented view of the inner world of the schizophrenic, this text is a classic. Its fundamental flaw is that it considers psychological factors as being primary in the etiology of the illness, but it nevertheless enables one to understand the evolution of schizophrenia from the internal world of the patient.

Bloom FE: Advancing a neurodevelopmental origin for schizophrenia. Arch Gen Psychiatry 50:224–227, 1993

>Detailed discussion of neurodevelopment theories on schizophrenia.

Kendler KS: The genetics of schizophrenia: A current perspective. In Meltzer HY (ed): Psychopharmacology: The Third Generation of Progress, pp 705–713. New York, Raven Press, 1987

>A brilliant review of a confusing area. Frames the right questions and reviews the literature to delineate the answers that are known, and discusses the areas in which knowledge is lacking.

Kane JM: Treatment of schizophrenia. Schizophr Bull 13:133–156, 1987

>A detailed overview of the state-of-the-art knowledge on pharmacological treatment of schizophrenia. Includes strategies on how to address patients who are nonresponders.

Lieberman JA, Kane JM, Johns CA: Clozapine: Guidelines for clinical management. J Clin Psychiatry 50:329–338, 1989

>Everything you wanted to know about clozapine clinically.

Meltzer HY: The mechanism of action of novel antipsychotic drugs. Schizophrenia Bulletin, 17:263–288, 1991

>In reviewing the pharmacologic action of newer antipsychotic medications, old theories about a simple relationship between dopamine and schizophrenia are challenged.

Weinberger DR: Implications of normal brain development for the pathogens of schizophrenia. Arch Gen Psychiatry 44:660–669, 1987

>An interesting hypothesis that potentially explains the disparate aspects of schizophrenia, including its symptomatology, age of onset, biochemistry, and pharmacological response. The hypothesis connects morphological abnormality, brain development, and pathogenesis of schizophrenia.

Woods BT, Yurglun-Todd D, Goldstein JM et al: MRI brain abnormalities in chronic schizophrenia: One process or more? Biological Psychiatry 40:585–596, 1996

>Addresses the issue of heterogeneity in schizophrenia.

REFERENCES

Akbarian S, Bunney WE, Potkin SG, et al: Altered distribution of nicotinamide-adenine dinucleotide phosphate-diaphorase cells in frontal lobe of schizophrenics implies disturbances of cortical development. Arch Gen Psychiatry 50:169–177, 1993

American Psychiatric Association: Diagnostic and Statistical Manual of Mental Disorders, 4th ed., Washington, DC, American Psychiatric Association, 1994

Anderson CM: Family intervention with severely disturbed patients. Arch Gen Psychiatry 34:697–702, 1977

Andreasen NC: Negative symptoms in schizophrenia: Definition and reliability. Arch Gen Psychiatry 39:784–788, 1982

Andreason NC: Comprehensive Assessment of Symptoms and History. Department of Psychiatry, University of Iowa College of Medicine, 1987

Andreason NC, Rezai K, Alliger R, et al: Hypofrontality in neuroleptic-naive patients and in patients with chronic schizophrenia. Arch Gen Psychiatry 49:943–958, 1992

Baldessarini RJ, Cohen BM, Teicher MM: Significance of neuroleptic dose and plasma level in the pharmacological treatment of psychosis. Arch Gen Psychiatry 45:79–91, 1988

Bannon MJ, Roth RH: Pharmacology of mesocortical dopamine neurons. Pharmacol Rev 35:53–68, 1983

Bateson G, Jackson DD, Haley J, et al: Toward a theory of schizophrenia. Behav Sci 1:251–264, 1956

Bleuler E: Dementia Praecox or the Group of Schizophrenias. Zinkin J (trans): New York, Int University Press, 1960 (German ed, 1911)

Brier A, Buchanan RW, Elkashef A, et al: Brain morphology and schizophrenia: A magnetic resonance imaging study of limbic prefrontal cortex and caudate structures. Arch Gen Psychiatry 49:921–926, 1992

Brown GW, Birley JLT: Crises and life changes and the onset of schizophrenia. J Health Soc Behav 9:203–214, 1968

Crow TJ: The two-syndrome concept: Origins and current status. Schizophr Bull 11:471–485, 1985

Crowe RR, Black DW, Wisner R, et al: Lack of linkage to chromosome 5q11–q13 markers in six schizophrenia pedigrees. Arch Gen Psychiatry 48:357–361, 1991

Davis KL, Kahn RS, Ko G, et al: Dopamine and schizophrenia: Review and reconceptualization. Am J Psychiatry 148:1474–1486, 1991

Doane J, West KL, Goldstein MJ, et al: Parental communication deviance and affective style. Arch Gen Psychiatry 38:679–685, 1981

Dohrenwend BS, Dohrenwend BP: Some issues in research on stressful life events. J Nerv Ment Dis 166:7–15, 1978

Falloon IRH, Lieberman RP: Interactions between drug and psychosocial therapy in schizophrenia Schizophr Bull 9:543–544, 1983

Farde L, Weisel FA, Stone-Elander S, et al: D2 dopamine receptor in neuroleptic-naive schizophrenic patients; a position emission tomography study with [^{11}C] raclopride. Arch Gen Psychiatry 47:213–219, 1990

Fromm-Reichmann F: Notes on the development of treatment of schizophrenics by psychoanalytic psychotherapy. Psychiatry 11:263–273, 1948

Fuster J: The Prefrontal Cortex. New York, Raven Press, 1980

Garmezy N, Neuchterlein K: Invulnerable children: Fact and fiction of competence and disadvantage. Presented at the annual meeting of the American Orthopsychiatric Association, Detroit, Michigan, 1972

Gibbons R, Lewine R, Davis J, et al: An empirical test of a Kraepelinian vs a Bleulerian view of negative symptoms. Schizophr Bull 11:390–396, 1985

Gottesman II, Shields J: Schizophrenia: The Epigenetic Puzzle. New York, Cambridge University Press, 1982

Herz M: Prodromal symptoms and prevention of relapse in schizophrenia J Clin Psychiatry 46:22–25, 1985

Hogarty GE, Anderson CM, Reiss DJ, et al: Family psychoeducation, social skills training and maintenance chemotherapy in the aftercare treatment of schizophrenia. Arch Gen Psychiatry 43:633–642, 1986

Hollingshead AB, Redlich FC: Social Class and Mental Illness: A Community Study. New York, John Wiley & Sons, 1958

Holzman PS: Eye movement dysfunction and psychosis. Int Rev Neurobiol 27:179–205, 1985

Jeste DV, Wyatt RJ: Understanding and Treating Tardive Dyskinesia, p 84. New York, Guilford Press, 1982

Kendler KS: The genetics of schizophrenia: a current perspective. In Mettzer HY (ed): Psychopharmacology: The Third Generation of Progress, pp 705–713. New York, Rowen Press, 1987

Kraepelin E: Textbook of Psychiatry (abstr). Diefendorf AR (trans): London, Macmillan, 1907

Langfeldt G: The prognosis in schizophrenia. Acta Psychiatr Neurol Scand 110:7–66, 1956

Left JP: Schizophrenia and sensitivity to the family environment. Schizophr Bull 2:566–574, 1976

Leff J, Vaughn C: The role of maintenance therapy and relatives' expressed emotion in relapse of schizophrenia: A two-year follow-up. Br J Psychiatry 139:102–104, 1981

Lidz T: Schizophrenia and the family. Psychiatry 21:21–27, 1958

Maser JD, Keith SJ: CT scans and schizophrenia—report on a workshop. Schizophr Bull 9:265–283, 1983

Meyer A: The dynamic interpretation of dementia praecox. Am J Psychol 21:385–403, 1910

Moises HW, Gelernter J, Giuffra LA, et al: No linkage between D_2 dopamine receptor gene region and schizophrenia. Arch Gen Psychiatry 47:643–647, 1990

O'Callaghan E, Shaw P, Takei N, et al: Schizophrenia after prenatal exposure to 1957 AZ influenza epidemic. Lancet 337:1248–1250, 1991.

Pycock CJ, Kerwin RW, Carter CJ: Effect of lesion of cortical dopamine terminals on subcortical dopamine receptors in rats. Nature 286:74–76, 1980

Robins LN, Helzer JE, Weissman MM, et al: Lifetime prevalence of specific psychiatric disorders in three sites. Arch Gen Psychiatry 41:949–958, 1984

Scheibel AB, Conrad AS: Hippocampal dysgenesis in mutant mouse and schizophrenic man: Is there a relationship? Schizophr Bull 19:21–33, 1993

Schmajuk NA: Animal models for schizophrenia. The hippocampally lesioned animal. Schizophr Bull 13:317–327, 1987

Schneider K: Clinical Psychopathology. Hamilton MW (trans): New York, Grune & Stratton, 1959

Sherrington R, Brynjolfsson J, Petursson H, et al: Localization of a susceptibility locus for schizophrenia on chromosome 5, Nature, 336:164–167, 1988

Tienari P, Sorri A, Lahti I, et al: The Finnish adoptive family study of schizophrenia. Yale J Biol Med 58:227–237, 1985

Vaughn CE, Leff JP: The influence of family and social factors on the course of psychiatric illness. Br J Psychiatry 129:125–137, 1976

Walker E, Lewine RJ: Prediction of adult-onset schizophrenia from childhood home movies of the patients. Am J Psychiatry 147:1052–1056, 1990

Weinberger DR: Implication of normal brain development for the pathogens of schizophrenia. Arch Gen Psychiatry 44:660–669, 1987

Weinberger DR, Berman KF, Zec RF: Physiological dysfunction of the dorsolateral prefrontal cortex in schizophrenia. Arch Gen Psychiatry 43:114–124, 1986

Weinberger DR, Kleinman JE: Observations on the brain in schizophrenia. In Hales RE, Frances JA (eds): Psychiatry Update, American Psychiatric Association Annual Review, Vol 5, pp 42–67. Washington, DC, American Psychiatric Press, 1986

Weiss KJ, Dubin WR: Partial hospitalization: State of the art. Hosp Community Psychiatry 33:923–928, 1982

Wong DF, Wagner HN, Tune LE, et al: Positron emission tomography reveals elevated D2 dopamine receptors in drug-naive schizophrenics. Science 234:1558–1563, 1986

Wynne L, Singer M: Thought disorder and family relations of schizophrenia I: Research strategies. Arch Gen Psychiatry 9:191–198, 1963

6 *Personality Disorders*

Gregg E. Gorton

The success or failure of any doctor–patient encounter, and indeed, of any long-term relationship between doctor and patient, is to a great extent determined by the capacity of each party not only to tolerate, but to adapt to and collaborate with the other. Many factors are involved in determining whether both doctor and patient can muster the required degree of psychological and social flexibility that will allow them to collaborate most effectively in the service of the patient's best interests and, ideally, the doctor's professional gratification. Not least among these determinant factors are the personalities of each party in this complex and potentially profound human relationship. Francis Peabody, in his classic essay "The Care of the Patient" (1928), part of which was quoted in Dr. Stoudemire's preface to this text, says that "The good physician knows his patients through and through, and his knowledge is bought dearly, but the reward is to be found in that personal bond which forms the greatest satisfaction of the practice of medicine." If, indeed, doctor and patient are able to form such a bond, the relationship can serve both parties well; however, if the pathway leading to that ideal collaborative relationship is strewn with enough obstacles, the journey will be less than satisfying, or even downright frustrating, with dissatisfaction and premature termination likely outcomes.

For the patient, failure to form a workable attachment compounds his or her suffering, thereby adding insult to the original malady for which help had been sought in the first place. For the doctor, a dysfunctional or failed relationship with a patient deprives him or her of the usual professional gratification earned through helpful physicianly work and, if chronic or recurrent, may create a source of nagging stress. Physicians can barely treat if they cannot relate, and, when they cannot meaningfully relate (whether or not their medical bag of tricks is exhausted), then they cannot provide even that simplest of remedies, human comfort, which is the last resource they have to offer when all else fails (Tumulty, 1970).

Behavioral disturbance in the patient must be accorded a high rank on the list of obstacles most likely to obstruct formation of a good, working collaboration between doctor and patient. *Since the focus of this chapter is personality disorders, it is crucial to appreciate that maladaptive personality traits are only one of the many causes of behavioral disturbance, whether in the doctor or the patient.* Also, as we shall see, personality disorder represents one end of the continuum of behavioral disturbance whose dimensions include temporality (transitory, episodic, or chronic), severity (mild, moderate, extreme), and pervasiveness (partial, global), with only the truly chronic, extreme, and global conditions being properly labeled as personality disorder.

Other causes of behavioral problems in medically ill patients must always be carefully sought. These include medical problems (e.g., brain tumor, hyperthyroidism, medication side effect, etc.), major *psychiatric disorders* (e.g., the many Axis I disorders described elsewhere in this book), extreme *reactions to the stress of the illness experience, or to reality-based conflicts with the social environment (e.g., racism, homophobia, etc.), or to the healthcare system (e.g., lack of insurance coverage, limitations to access to services, etc.).*

Within the crucible of physical (or psychiatric) illness, concomitant emotional crisis and behavioral regression (i.e., a revival of more child-like behaviors and coping strategies that are more characteristic of earlier life stage) are so common that they should routinely be expected. For most patients, however, such emotional upset will be transitory (or, in chronic illness, episodic), mild-to-moderate in severity, and less than global in its manifestations. *Most patients possess a reasonable capacity for psychosocial coping with the stress of illness,* which means that they are able to use psychological defenses (see Inderbitzin, Furman, and James, 1998), coping strategies, and social supports successfully to overcome whatever is most frightening and overwhelming to them.

Because patients with preexisting Axis I disorders are, as a group, more prone to behavioral difficulties in the healthcare setting than are patients without such problems, their course of medical treatment and recovery is often more complicated and costly when psychiatric problems are not addressed in a timely and effective manner. What information about Axis II disturbances will be most useful to the physician—whether this disturbance takes the form of full-blown personality disorder or a more circumscribed constellation of maladaptive traits that we will call "personality style"? How is an Axis II disorder best defined? How common is it? What causes it? How is it best treated? And how can it be most efficiently recognized and managed in the medical setting?

DIFFICULT-TO-HELP PATIENTS

For most physicians, *the first clue to the possible presence of personality disorder in a patient will consist of some notable difficulty the patient is having in emotionally traversing the psychological tasks that accompany any significant illness.* Perry and Viederman (1981) have outlined these tasks nicely: first, the task of acknowledging to oneself and others that one has an illness; second, the task of permitting oneself to depend on others for care; and, third, the task of resuming normal functioning as the illness improves. *At any point in this process, one or more of the following difficulties may be seen: problematic behavior,* such as extreme denial, anger, manipulativeness, or inordinate attention seeking; *trouble collaborating with providers and poor adherence to treatment recommendations; symptoms of common Axis I psychiatric disturbances,* such as depression, anxiety, somatoform disorders, or substance-related disorders (since patients with personality disorder have a higher prevalence of many Axis I conditions); *an unusually intense and uncharacteristic emotional reaction by the doctor* to the patient, such as anger or dread or intense attraction; or *uncharacteristic behavior on the doctor's part,* such as marked impatience, avoidance of the patient, inappropriate attempts to rescue the patient, or even unprofessional conduct of some sort, such as yelling at a patient or becoming sexually involved. It cannot be overemphasized that *the patient should never be blamed for the doctor's inappropriate, uncharacteristic, or unprofessional responses, although these can often be understood as having been in part elicited by some aspect of that particular patient.*

Patients who elicit unusually intense reactions in the physician most often appear not so much psychiatrically disturbed—with one or another clear-cut psychopathologic syndrome—as exhibiting what feels to the doctor as sheer "obnoxiousness" of some sort. They "get under the skin" of the doctor by behaving in a way that is so striking or distressing as to feel like a personal assault or burden. Often, while doctors believe that these patients simply *won't* collaborate, these patients act as if—or even tell us—that they *"can't"* change their behavior (Anscombe, 1986). *One of the classic hallmarks of personality disorder is, in fact, a marked tendency to blame others for one's interpersonal difficulties and therefore to expect others to change.*

Perhaps as many as 20% of medical patients are perceived by physicians as frustrating or difficult, and among high users of medical care the percentage may be as high as 40% (Mayou and Sharpe, 1995). These patients do not conform to physicians' expectations of prototypical "good" patients. These are the apparently "bad" patients a physician is most likely to find himself or herself silently dreading, cursing, avoiding—even wishing dead!—or at least wishing they would quickly leave the physician's office or hospital service.

Besides the terms "frustrating" and "difficult," such patients have variously been referred to as "crocks," "thick-chart," "heartsink," "hateful," "hated," "angry," "annoying," "overly dependent," "hysterical," "manipulative," "overdemanding," "undesirable," "attention-seeking," "hypochondriacal," "somatic," "masochistic," "impossible," "difficult-to-help," and a host of other often disrespectful and pejorative, if colorful, terms, *most of which have no proper place in actual discourse with patients.*

In my experience, *the most clinically useful among these labels is "difficult-to-help"* (Mayou and Sharpe, 1995), *since it locates the "difficulty" not solely within the patient, but within the doctor–patient relationship, thereby mitigating against blaming and stigmatizing the patient.* The descriptive label "difficult-to-help" also reminds us that the doctor must also play some role in the perceived difficulty! In this sense, students would do best to move away from the ideal of "managing the patient" (Tumulty, 1970) toward that of *managing the doctor–patient relationship.* In fact, evidence suggests that *"it is the perceived mismatch between the care the doctor feels able to offer and the patient's expressed hopes that gives rise to the doctor's experience of difficulty"* (Mayou and Sharpe, 1995).

Thus, *the doctor's expectations of the patient are a crucial variable in the interactive process that, in fact, produces the difficult-to-help patient,* although it may appear as if the patient is imbued with "difficulty" as one of his or her innate traits. Put another way, *not all physicians find the same patients "difficult,"* since physicians naturally vary in their own personalities, life experience, coping skills, psychosocial vulnerabilities and biases, and degree of willingness to change their own behavior according to the *patient's* needs.

Likely, only a significant *minority* of difficult-to-help patients have a full-blown personality disorder, but even in its absence, these patients may have maladaptive personality traits (or a "personality style") comprising subthreshhold personality disorder that puts them at higher than average risk for emotional and behavioral difficulty under stress. *However, medical students must always bear in mind that the stress of illness, with its attendant anxiety, loneliness, fear, and helplessness, may elicit situation-dependent maladaptive responses in any of us.* Such states of distress should not be taken as prima facie evidence of true personality disturbance!

This chapter will discuss disturbances of personality from a number of perspectives, including the descriptive perspective embodied by the Diagnostic and Statistical Manual of Mental Disorders, 4th edition (DSM-IV; American Psychiatric Association, 1994), the psychoanalytic perspective embodied in psychodynamic theory and technique, and the behavioral perspective— embodied for our purposes in a variety of behavioral techniques that are useful in working effectively with many of these patients, as we shall see below.

Different personality styles may predict differential responses to illness, to healthcare providers, and to the healthcare system itself. This is one reason that since at least the time of Hippocrates physicians have been interested in discerning, categorizing, and understanding different personality types.

For much of medical history, interest in patients' personalities took the form of a search for particular behavioral traits that might correlate with—or even cause—particular medical diseases. The great physician William Osler, for example, knew 100 years ago that high-strung, physiologically reactive patients (today called Type A or obsessive–compulsive personalities) were at risk for heart disease. However, with the possible exception of coronary artery disease, there has been no convincing evidence that any specific type of personality trait alone can account for the development of a particular physical illness (Stoudemire, 1995).

Instead, focus has shifted toward patients' reactions to being sick as a function of their personality and psychological defenses; the effects of their maladaptive responses to illness on themselves, their families, and their healthcare providers (Gorlin and Zucker, 1983); the impact of personality factors on the course of medical and psychiatric illnesses; and techniques for managing the doctor–patient relationship so as to foster optimal collaboration with the physician and the healthcare system.

Today, it is clear that medical students who aspire to practice medicine humanely, cost effectively, and with the greatest degree of professional satisfaction must learn, whatever their future specialty will be, to appreciate not only the nature of "personality disorder" per se, but also the way in which different personality styles and reactions to illness can be discerned and usefully responded to by the doctor in routine fashion in every doctor–patient encounter (Kahana and Bibring, 1965; Tumulty, 1970; Geringer and Stern, 1986; Lipp, 1986; Cohen-Cole, 1991; Fogel, 1993; Widiger and Sanderson, 1997). Physicians can develop a practical approach to recognition of and collaboration with patients whose behaviors and ways of relating demand much more of doctors than they would often wish, but who can be immensely gratifying to treat if only doctors can successfully adapt to each of these unique human beings yet also consistently expect such patients to take responsibility for their own health.

DEFINITIONS

Personality or personality "style" consists of enduring, habitual patterns of thinking, feeling, behaving, and relating that determine a person's adaptation and reaction to the two worlds he or she inhabits—that is, both the inner psychological world and the outer environment. Taken collectively, these patterns—or "personality traits"—constitute the distinctive and predictable qualities that make a person unique. For example, we typically draw on our perception of a person's personality when we are asked to describe him or her so that another person can imagine what this particular individual must be like.

A personality disorder exists when a sufficient number of a person's personality traits are sufficiently inflexible and maladaptive that significant impairment in relating, loving, working, and enjoying life is produced.

DIAGNOSIS

Personality disorders, or maladaptive personality traits that do not constitute a full-blown personality disorder, are listed on Axis II of the five-axis diagnostic system that is used in psychiatry today. The creation of a separate diagnostic axis for personality disturbance was designed to highlight the clinical importance of these conditions both in their own right and in terms of their interaction with the disorders coded on Axis I and Axis III. Many studies have indicated that *the comorbid presence of both Axis I and Axis II disorders tends to predict a worse prognosis,* whether the issue is recovery from major depression or substance dependence, response to electroconvulsive therapy (ECT), outcome of anorexia nervosa or obsessive–compulsive disorder, predisposition to cardiovascular disease, response to treatment of anxiety disorders, or course of human immunodeficiency virus (HIV) infection, to name only a few such situations.

In order for a patient's personality to be diagnosed in a scientifically valid way as a personality disorder, the "General Diagnostic Criteria for a Personality Disorder" listed in DSM-IV must first be scrupulously applied. These criteria are crucial because they embody the fundamental nosologic principles that make true personality disorder—by definition, a long-term *trait* condition—different from a change in personality *state,* which is a time-limited alteration in adaptation or coping. For example, behavioral regression due to illness or injury is extremely common, yet regressed patients may or may not have displayed a chronic pattern of maladaptive behaviors prior to their current medical illnesses. Had they done so, they may, indeed, meet criteria for personality disorder; had they not, however, personality disorder is a very unlikely diagnosis.

CLINICAL VIGNETTE

Mr. A, a 64-year-old, happily married, successful real estate manager, entered the hospital for evaluation of bladder dysfunction. While somewhat anxious about the realistic possibility of having cancer, he readily accepted the need to be in the hospital, since he was in a great deal of discomfort. He cooperated pleasantly with a series of at times prolonged and uncomfortable urologic tests.

On the second hospital day, however, he became increasingly frustrated at the lack of communication from Dr. B, his newly assigned urologist, about what the test battery had thus far revealed. He "raised some hell," as he later described it, but was not able to see his doctor that day. Since it wasn't clear to him why he needed to stay longer in the hospital, and since "I wasn't getting any results," he stormed out abruptly, against the advice of the nursing staff, who tried to convince him to wait to talk to Dr. B. He shot back that he would have none of "this charade" any longer. After he left, one of the nurses commented, "I had no idea he was such a time bomb—he seemed really polite and pleasant!"

When Mr. A saw Dr. B the following week in the doctor's office, he was still angry, and he blurted out, "Maybe I'm a lousy patient, and maybe you're a good doctor, but you weren't so good to me last week!" Dr. B, despite feeling personally attacked and wanting to lash out in return, tried his best to listen attentively and empathically. He wanted to say, "You have no idea what a terrible day I had last week when you were trying to get ahold of me!" Instead, he found himself responding "I can understand how angry and upset you were, and obviously you still are, and I want to apologize for leaving you in that terrible position of not knowing whether or not you had cancer, or what else was going on. I should have been able to do better for you, and I certainly want to work out this problem so that your care is not interrupted."

Mr. A's anger subsided somewhat, as he listened to Dr. B's explanation of why he had been unable to meet with Mr. A on the second day of his recent hospitalization. Dr. B reminded him that prior to the admission, they had discussed the need for a 2 or 3-day stay, as well as the fact that test results might not all be available even by the time Mr. A left the hospital. Mr. A acknowledged that he had "forgotten" these things in his anxious state and said, "It's not like me to blow my stack and walk out like that! I'm just so used to being in control of what's happening around me—that's the way I run my business, and that's the way I like my life to be. My wife can tell you—she knows I'm a real control freak! I've been that way as long as I can remember. No question I get a little hot under the collar if things don't go the way I want, that's for sure! But to really lose it like that— I'm real sorry. You probably thought I was some kind of genuine jerk!" Dr. B replied, "Well, I realized that there was some misunderstanding, and that you had a pretty good reason to be upset."

This vignette illustrates a patient's maladaptive reaction to the stress of illness. Not only was Mr. A in physical discomfort, he also had no idea what was causing his problem, and he feared that it was something life-threatening. This patient was a man with some obsessive–compulsive personality traits, and when he felt abandoned he regressed from his polite, cooperative, and pleasant—if anxious, but tightly controlled—demeanor and behaved like a naughty child who could only act out his feelings angrily rather than tolerate the intense frustration of waiting for his doctor.

If a naive diagnostician had happened to see only Mr. A's demanding, entitled, and raging behavior, followed by his impulsive flight to avoid feeling abandoned by his doctor when his needs were not immediately gratified, the observer might have inappropriately concluded that this apparently petulant man had a personality disorder with narcissistic, borderline, and obsessive–compulsive traits. In fact, he is a well-adjusted, somewhat obsessive–compulsive man with a good deal of pride who regressed in the medical setting. His lack of significant prior maladaptation and his rapid return to a more appropriate level of adaptive coping when the stress was reduced both confirm this formulation.

The *General Diagnostic Criteria for a Personality Disorder* are as follows:

1. An enduring pattern of inner experience and behavior that deviates markedly from the expectations of the individual's culture. This pattern is manifested in two (or more) of the following areas:
   a. Cognition (i.e., ways of perceiving and interpreting self, other people, and events)
   b. Affectivity (i.e., the range, intensity, lability, and appropriateness of emotional response)
   c. Interpersonal functioning
   d. Impulse control
2. The enduring pattern is inflexible and pervasive across a broad range of personal and social situations.
3. The enduring pattern leads to clinically significant distress or impairment in social, occupational, or other important areas of functioning.
4. The pattern is stable and of long duration, and its onset can be traced back to adolescence or early adulthood.
5. The enduring pattern is not better accounted for as a manifestation or consequence of another mental disorder.
6. The enduring pattern is not due to the direct physiological effects of a substance (e.g., a drug of abuse, a medication) or a general medical condition (e.g., head trauma) (American Psychiatric Association, 1994, p 633).

If, and only if, all these General Criteria are met, then consideration of the various traits of specific personality disorder diagnoses can begin. One must always keep in mind that *lack of sufficient information in the clinical setting should invariably militate against any overly eager assumption that the General Criteria have truly been met.*

Note that *patients who undergo a personality change in middle or late adulthood would not meet these criteria.* Should this not uncommon situation confront the physician, he or she must always consider the high likelihood that the personality change is due to a general medical condition or some unidentified Axis I condition.

Classic examples of medical conditions causing personality change include hyperparathyroidism and other endocrinopathies, HIV infection, neurosyphilis, sleep apnea, brain tumor, head injury, multiple sclerosis, Huntington's disease, and covert substance dependence. *The relevant DSM-IV diagnosis in these situations is "Personality Change Due to . . . [Indicate the General Medical Condition],"* with the specific type of Personality Change indicated as either labile, disinhibited, aggressive, apathetic, paranoid, other, combined, or unspecified (American Psychiatric Association, 1994, pp. 171–174). If chronic substance use is associated with the personality change, the diagnosis should be [Name of substance]-Related Disorder Not Otherwise Specified.

CLASSIFICATION

The system of disease classification used in DSM-IV is an example of a *categorical,* compared with a *dimensional,* diagnostic system. From this perspective, each of the ten personality disorders in DSM-IV is taken as a qualitatively distinct clinical syndrome. Even if a patient has a mixture of traits from more than one personality disorder—but not enough of any single personality disorder to qualify for that particular diagnosis—and taken together these traits meet the General Diagnostic Criteria for a personality disorder, then the patient is placed into an 11th diagnostic category called Personality Disorder Not Otherwise Specified (NOS). By this way of thinking, clear boundaries are seen to exist between the different disorders, although in reality human nature cannot so easily be carved up, as if it had obvious, naturally occurring joints.

Under a dimensional taxonomy, personality traits are considered to exist on a broad continuum of qualitative personality shadings that merge imperceptibly into normality, into one another, and even into various of the Axis I disorders. Many different dimensional models have been proposed in an effort to define this broad palette of possible personality components that blend in a myriad of constellations to produce the normative range of adaptive and maladaptive personalities in a given population and perhaps across the species (McCrae and Costa, 1997). A good deal of research is under way to assess the validity and utility of these dimensional models, but since they are rarely routinely applied in clinical work, nothing further about them will be said here (interested readers should consult Millon and Davis, 1996).

Cluster Classification

The DSM-IV personality disorders are grouped into three clusters, according to basic similarities in their features (Table 6–1). *This tripartite division of the ten disorders provides the easiest way to recall them quickly in the clinical setting, since each cluster is associated with*

Table 6–1 **The Three Clusters of Personality Disorders**

CLUSTER A (ODD, ECCENTRIC)	CLUSTER B (DRAMATIC, EMOTIONAL)	CLUSTER C (ANXIOUS, FEARFUL)
Schizotypal	Histrionic	Avoidant
Schizoid	Narcissistic	Dependent
Paranoid	Antisocial	Obsessive–compulsive
	Borderline	

specific descriptive adjectives that conjure up the fundamental qualities of the associated disorders. Once these adjectives are learned, the behaviors they describe may jog the doctor's memory about different personality types when he or she is confronted with a patient manifesting any of those qualities.

   Cluster A includes the odd, eccentric (historically called "pre-psychotic") personality disorders: paranoid, schizoid, and schizotypal. *Cluster B includes the dramatic, emotional (also called labile and impulsive) personality disorders:* antisocial, borderline, histrionic, and narcissistic. *Cluster C includes the anxious, fearful (or "neurotic") personality disorders:* avoidant, dependent, and obsessive–compulsive.

   Finally, patients with mixtures of the above traits, or with personality disorders that are not included here, such as self-defeating and depressive, both of which are included in an appendix to DSM-IV, as well as hypomanic personality, sadistic, passive–aggressive, and others, can be diagnosed as "Personality Disorder NOS," with the specific type of disorder indicated (e.g., "with self-defeating and passive–aggressive traits").

   Some personality disorders co-occur in the same patient more frequently than would be expected based on chance association alone. For example, borderline personality is often found in association with partial or full expressions of antisocial personality, schizotypal personality, and histrionic personality. Antisocial personality often overlaps with histrionic or narcissistic personality. Avoidant personality often coexists with dependent personality, and it can be difficult to distinguish from schizoid personality, which some feel is just another variant of the same disorder. Many patients who meet criteria for histrionic personality also have dependent traits, and dependent personality disorder often coexists with passive–aggressive personality traits or full-blown passive–aggressive personality disorder, which would be documented as personality disorder not otherwise specified, passive–aggressive type. Paranoid and narcissistic personalities frequently coexist, in a particularly malignant combination. Finally, and especially important in the medical setting, passive–aggressive traits often coexist with self-defeating (historically, "masochistic") traits to produce a form of personality disorder not otherwise specified that is particularly frustrating to caring, well-intentioned physicians.

   The interface between personality disorders and Axis I disorders is important both conceptually and clinically and can be outlined as follows: certain personality traits may (1) predispose toward, (2) modify, (3) represent a complication of, (4) represent an attenuated form, or (5) coexist independently with specific Axis I disorders (Marin et al, 1994). We will look only at the latter two possibilities. Certain personality disorders can be understood as being nosologic and perhaps etiologic "cousins," or attenuated forms, of specific major mental illnesses, and at times the personality disorder may be difficult to distinguish from the Axis I condition. For example, schizotypal, paranoid, and possibly schizoid personality disorder may represent partial, perhaps genetically based expressions of schizophrenia, or conditions that are prodromal to full-blown schizophrenic illness. Borderline personality may in some patients represent a variant of a mood disorder or an impulse control disorder. Avoidant personality may be related to social phobia, and depressive personality may lie on the mood disorder spectrum.

On the other hand, in terms of the independent coexistence of Axis I and Axis II disorders, or true comorbidity, some of the most frequent epidemiologic associations between independently coexisting Axis II and Axis I diagnoses include borderline personality with mood disorders; mood disorders, including bipolar disorder, with any personality disorder; antisocial, borderline, narcissistic, and histrionic personalities with substance-related disorders; substance-related disorders with any personality disorder; cluster C disorders with anxiety disorders; avoidant personality with social phobia; bulimia with cluster B and C disorders; obsessive–compulsive disorder with histrionic, dependent, obsessive–compulsive and schizotypal personality disorders; and somatoform disorders with cluster C or other personality disorders (Gorton and Akhtar, 1990, 1994; Marin et al, 1994).

METHODS OF DIAGNOSTIC ASSESSMENT

The clinical interview is the most commonly used diagnostic method in the clinical setting for assessing a patient's mental status, personality, interactive style, degree of denial or acceptance of illness, capacity to cope with illness, capacity for collaboration with healthcare, degree of likability, and amount of professional energy that will likely be required to provide the necessary care. Information from collateral informants such as family or other providers is extremely useful and can substantially enhance the reliability of such assessments. In nonpsychiatric settings, the standard doctor–patient interaction appropriate for that medical specialty and that service arena serves as the vehicle for this data gathering.

In other words, the early phase of a doctor–patient relationship should include evaluation of how easy or difficult it will likely be to develop an optimally collaborative treatment relationship with that particular patient. Patients who behave in ways that are difficult, and especially those who are also inordinately rigid, and therefore unresponsive to feedback about their problematic behaviors, should cause the doctor to take note. Inexperienced clinicians too often learn this the hard way, that is, only when they encounter difficulty with a patient do they begin to wonder how they might collaborate more effectively. On the other hand, seasoned clinicians often evaluate the quality of the relationship subconsciously. They are able to deploy seamlessly this or that interpersonal approach or communicative style as needed for the interaction to proceed most smoothly. As Tumulty noted, "What the scalpel is to the surgeon, words are to the clinician. . . . A first-rate clinician trains himself to do two things exceedingly well: to talk to his patients and to listen to them" (1970). In other words, not only are the technical knowledge and medical skills of the physician vital to an ability to help the patient, but the physician's "emotional intelligence" in knowing how best to relate to the patient is equally vital (Goleman, 1995).

Often, difficult-to-help patients will have their first visible impact on the larger treatment system, causing extraordinary chaos and turbulence among and between health professionals involved in their care. McDaniel et al (1992) describe a striking example of the complexities that can arise in such a situation, when a patient with cardiomyopathy presented extreme behavioral difficulties for the medical team.

Finally, in the psychiatric setting, diagnostic instruments may at times be deployed for personality assessment, including self-report inventories such as the Minnesota Multiphasic Personality Inventory (MMPI) and the Millon Clinical Multiaxial Inventory (MCMI). These are easily administered and machine scored, yet they may not correlate particularly well with results obtained through the variety of semistructured interviews that may also be used, including the Structured Clinical Interview for DSM-III-R (SCID), the Diagnostic Interview for Borderlines, Revised (DIB-R), and the Structured Interview for the Diagnosis of Personality Disorders (SIDP). These instruments are time consuming but have the advantage of being systematic; however, reliability of personality disorder diagnosis is no better than fair when these instruments are compared with one another.

EPIDEMIOLOGY

Unfortunately, there are as yet no systematic data on the prevalence of all DSM personality disorders in the general population. Most pre-DSM-IV studies of personality disorder epidemiology either used clinical populations, or screened for only one type of personality disorder, or, if they were pre-DSM-II, did not use standardized diagnostic criteria. The average prevalence of personality disorders in a series of pre-DSM-III studies was between 6 and 10%, but many of these studies counted alcoholism and drug abuse as types of personality disorder (Merikangas and Weissman, 1986), a diagnostic approach that did not change until DSM-III in 1980.

The Epidemiological Catchment Area Study of the National Institute of Mental Health, the largest psychiatric epidemiology study ever done on the general population in the United States, did not screen for any personality disorders except antisocial personality, for which the lifetime prevalence was 2.6% (Robins and Regier, 1991). A number of more recent studies have used family members of control and patient populations as subjects and have revealed lifetime rates for any personality disorder ranging from 10 to 13% (Oldham, 1994). In these studies, among personality disorders within cluster A, schizotypal was most common; within cluster B, borderline was most common; and within cluster C, dependent and obsessive–compulsive were most common.

Overall, personality disorders as a whole affect each gender about equally, although some, such as antisocial and narcissistic, are diagnosed more often in men, and another, borderline personality, more often in women. Personality disorders appear to be more common in lower socioeconomic groups. In many studies, especially those that use semistructured interviews as the diagnostic method, *the percentage of subjects with a single, pure personality disorder diagnosis is less than that of subjects with either more than one such diagnosis or a mixture of traits (i.e., personality disorder not otherwise specified) but no single personality disorder.* This is important in the clinical setting, in which patients should not necessarily be expected to fit neatly into one or another of the Axis II categories.

On average, *as many as half of individuals carefully screened for personality disorder in psychiatric inpatient or outpatient treatment settings may manifest the disorder.* Few data are available that speak to the prevalence of personality disorder in *medical* inpatient or outpatient settings, yet based on clinical experience, personality disorder appears to be quite common (Oldham, 1994). *It is a well-established clinical tenet that medical/surgical patients with comorbid personality disorders tend to have a more difficult clinical courses, and they also tend to utilize a higher than expected amount of healthcare resources.*

ETIOLOGY

Each of our personalities is the product of a complex maturational-developmental process that begins with our genetic endowment and encompasses our intrauterine experience, our earliest physiologic responses and behavioral expressions (or temperament), and our life experiences. Thus, *an individual's personality is the sum total of a mixture of inherited tendencies, inborn temperamental traits, and learned responses that have familial and other sociocultural sources.* Although debate goes on about the degree of influence that each of these factors should be assigned in the final multifactorial equation that describes personality, it is clear that the biopsychosocial etiologic model provides the best perspective on personality disorder. Let us briefly examine each of these factors—biological, psychological, and social—more closely.

Many recent studies have focused on *biological correlates* of various personality traits, dimensions, and disorders. I will not review these data in detail, since their clinical applications are as yet few, but some examples will illustrate some of the research frontiers, and interested readers can explore relevant references.

The heritability of normal personality traits is generally believed to range from 40 to 60%, and it appears that this holds also for traits involved in personality disorder (Livesley et al, 1993), which leaves unanswered the tantalizing question of whether nature or nurture plays the final determinate role in our personality makeup. How exactly genes operate to produce particular personality traits is still not clear, although variation in neurotransmitter systems and in receptor sensitivity has been advanced as a possible partial explanation for why a person tends to react to the environment in certain stereotyped ways (Cloninger et al, 1993). Further studies must examine not only how genetically based vulnerabilities influence responses to adverse environmental circumstances, but how environmental effects may modulate the expression of genetically based tendencies.

The personality dimensions with the most current evidence in favor of a neurobiological substrate are mood regulation, impulse control, and cognitive/perceptual functioning (Kavoussi and Coccaro, 1995). Some evidence for each of these has come from genetic/family studies, central nervous system neurochemical studies (e.g., cerebrospinal fluid analysis), neuroendocrine challenge studies (e.g., the responses of specific neurotransmitter systems stimulated by a specific psychopharmacologic agent), and psychophysiologic studies (e.g., brain evoked potentials, electroencephalography, smooth pursuit eye movements, etc.). Specific examples include the finding of apparent differences in serotonin metabolite levels in the cerebrospinal fluid of highly aggressive and impulsive antisocial personality disorder subjects, blunted prolactin response to stimulation with fenfluramine in impulsive, aggressive personality disorder subjects (Kavoussi and Coccaro, 1995), and significant differences in smooth pursuit eye movements in schizotypal patients compared with controls.

Preliminary evidence also suggests that at least some subsets of specific personality disorder populations have subtle neuropsychological impairment (Gorton et al, in press). Certainly, abnormalities in central nervous system structure and function can be hypothesized to impinge on normal personality development. The all-too-prevalent history of physical abuse among patients with certain personality disorders may, for example, be a marker for subtle brain injury that manifests not as overt "brain damage," but as apparent personality disorder.

Regarding *psychological etiologic factors,* significant difficulties in the child–parent interaction during particular phases of development are believed to produce particular lasting personality deformations, including personality disorder. Early causal theories of personality disorder emphasized either the primary presence in the developing infant of excessively strong "instinctual drives," such as sexuality (libido) or aggression, or, the presence of instinctual drives that, while not themselves overly strong, were either too greatly frustrated or excessively indulged by the parents. The resultant mismatch between the infant's needs and his or her environmental nurturance was believed to produce traumatic experiences that distorted the developing personality.

Such primary or secondary disturbances in the relationship between the young person and his or her social environment were seen to produce either the relatively circumscribed symptoms of "neurosis" (e.g., such problems as difficulty completing important projects, or undue guilt, or a pattern of repeated failures in intimate relationships), or the more pervasive symptoms of true personality disorder.

In fact, neurotic symptoms closely resemble the maladaptive personality traits that, when clustered in sufficient quantity, comprise personality disorder. Traditionally, neurotic symptoms are hypothesized to be more bothersome, conflictual, and alien to the individual (that is, "ego-dystonic") compared with the maladaptive traits of personality disorder, which feel to the individual simply like a way of life, an appropriate preference, or even an ideal way of "doing business" in the world (that is, "ego-syntonic"). Another traditional distinction between personality disorder and neurosis has to do with whether the bearer of symptoms tends to adapt to the social context ("autoplastic"), as is true of neurosis, or whether he or she expects other people to adapt ("alloplastic"), as is true of personality disorder. This conceptual distinction, while not always completely predictive of patients' behavior, is also very useful in the clinical setting. *When a physician feels that certain difficult-to-help patients rigidly and consistently expect the physician to change his or her behavior in order for the physician–patient relationship to succeed in its goals, such patients should be considered among those who may perhaps have personality disturbance or even full-blown personality disorder.*

In general, personality disorder *involves use of developmentally early or "lower level" cognitive–behavioral strategies that are known as psychological defenses* (introduced by Inderbitzin, Furman, and James, 1998, in Chapter 5 of the companion volume to the present text). Vaillant (1977) and others have put forward schematic hierarchies of psychological defense mechanisms that range across the most developmentally primitive or "immature" defenses, the midlevel or "neurotic" defenses, and the most adaptive, high-level, or late-developing defenses, called "mature." *As a general rule, personality disorder patients are less able to sustain use of mature defenses than are neurotic or more healthy individuals; they tend to be "stuck" with using neurotic and immature defenses.* They are also more prone than neurotic or psychologically mature individuals to slip transiently into states of Axis I disturbance, such as psychosis, in which immature defenses are dominant.

As discussed by Inderbitzin, Furman, and James (1998), *immature defenses* include psychotic denial, delusional projection, projection, distortion, and schizoid fantasy. *Neurotic defenses,* which are seen most consistently among people with neurosis and personality disorder, include acting-out, hypochondriasis, passive–aggressive behavior, splitting, projective identification, dissociation, repression, reaction formation, displacement, and intellectualization. While at times such individuals may manifest *mature defenses* such as altruism, humor, suppression, anticipation, or sublimation, they are unable to sustain use of these higher level defenses.

The reader should keep in mind that this conceptual hierarchy of defenses is a schematic model that is not to be taken as a literal reflection of all human psychological structure and function. Under certain conditions of stress, illness, confusion, social turmoil, and so forth, any of us may deteriorate in our psychosocial functioning, as did Mr. A, above; conversely, the sickest among us may rise to remarkable heights in a time of crisis. An example would be a patient with catatonic schizophrenia who had not spoken in more than 20 years, yet who rounded up his fellow patients and told them coherently and succinctly how to proceed in an orderly fashion out of doors during a fire on a state hospital ward; afterward he lapsed into his former state of profound impairment.

Examples of how specific defenses operate in personality disorder would include a taxicab driver with paranoid personality who is prone to projection and schizoid fantasy in his imagining that others always seem to harbor malevolent motives toward him, and who therefore retreats into his fantasies of retaliation, meanwhile failing to earn a living because he doesn't feel safe with passengers in his back seat; the college student with borderline personality who is prone to splitting, projective identification, and acting-out in her experience of herself as a disgusting person whom others seem often to mistreat, and who has no choice but to react impulsively through aggression or flight; the obsessive–compulsive executive with narcissistic traits who manages his intense emotions by intellectualizing endlessly, but becomes overwhelmed by his own need for perfection and ends up acting out his helplessness and frustration by distorting his monthly statistical reports to his superior so he can hide his self-perceived defectiveness.

Personality disorders *differ in terms of the severity of disturbance in psychological structure that underlies the overt symptoms of the personality disturbance.* In general, schizotypal, paranoid, borderline, and antisocial personality disorders are the most disturbed. Borderline individuals may, however, present with less severity, as is also true of schizoid and avoidant patients. Narcissistic, histrionic, dependent, and other personalities such as passive–aggressive, self-defeating, and hypomanic have variable levels of severity. Typically, obsessive–compulsive and subsyndromal "near-personality-disorders" are the least severe. *However, the degree of severity of personality pathology does not necessarily correlate with the degree of subjective distress, actual social or occupational dysfunction, or difficulties in the medical setting.* As a rule of thumb for medical practitioners, *the degree of dysfunction in the medical setting should be the most important consideration in the initial assessment and intervention process.*

Within the confines of this text, it is not possible to explicate thoroughly psychoanalytic and other theories of the etiology of personality disorders, although the impact of early life experiences, as well as of the family, social, and cultural milieux, including both positive and negative experiences, cannot be overemphasized. At the same time, it is becoming increasingly clear that genetic influences, and perhaps intrauterine conditions, also play an important role and that the term "maturation," referring to the shaping of the person by innate biological predispositions and tendencies, should be used in conjunction with "development," which carries a largely psychosocial connotation, when discussing the origin of personality and personality disorder.

Readers should consult comprehensive textbooks of psychiatry (e.g., Meissner, 1985), the companion volume to this text (Stoudemire, 1998), Millon and Davis (1996), Neubauer and Neubauer (1990), Kegan (1982), Ratey (1995), Stone (1993), and Zuckerman (1991) for more in-depth discussions and alternative perspectives on normal personality development and on the genesis of personality disorders.

The particular etiology of a given patient's Axis II disorder(s) may be of little immediate consequence in the clinical setting. Physicians can serve patients best by careful biopsychosocial assessment followed by consistent focusing on crucial and achievable clinical tasks such as developing a working treatment relationship and a common set of treatment goals.

COURSE OF ILLNESS, MORBIDITY, MORTALITY, AND SOCIAL IMPACT

Although, by definition, personality disorder begins in the teens or early twenties, it is also generally assumed that the course extends across the life span, even if some attenuation of symptoms may occur in late life. In fact, despite recent findings of more personality disorders than had been expected in certain populations of elderly psychiatric patients, little research has been conducted on the course of personality disorder across the life span. What studies do exist have mostly focused on borderline subjects, and they show that roughly half of individuals with borderline personality disorder retain that diagnosis at follow-up some years after the initial diagnosis. The same is true for antisocial personality disorder (McDavid and Pilkonis, 1996). Nevertheless, *whether or not personality disorder persists over the lifespan in the average patient with such a disorder, its impact as measured by a number of key psychosocial indicators can be severe.*

Personality disorders *are associated with high rates of marital problems such as divorce or separation, unemployment, work inefficiency, lack of work satisfaction, and disability.* Functional impairment has been found in a recent study to be greater in patients with personality disorder than in patients with other psychiatric disorders without personality disorder (Nakao et al, 1992). Antisocial personality in men, for example, may be associated with greater loss of income than even schizophrenia. Both antisocial and borderline personalities, in particular, are associated with increased lifetime risk for suicide (as high as 10 to 15% in some series), and antisocial personality is associated with increased risk of homicide and accidental death.

TREATMENT

In general, personality change in those with personality disorder occurs quite slowly, although, as suggested above, there is some evidence that the course of personality disorder includes a developmental "maturing out" process that may lead eventually to apparent remission of some or all symptoms, whether treated or not (McDavid and Pilkonis, 1996). *The central treatment principle in personality disorder is to try in whatever ways are most effective to facilitate the patient's highest level and most flexible degree of adaptive interpersonal functioning.*

Perhaps the most critical aspect of treatment is to avail the patient of a person (or institution, such as a clinic or group practice) to whom he or she can learn to attach and in whom he or she can trust. In the medical setting, this may, of necessity, involve a relationship with a primary provider or clinic. Less frequently, some form of psychotherapeutic relationship may be available and desirable, and here the patient may learn gradually to modify his or her maladaptive ways of "doing business" in the spheres of self-protection, self-care, relationships, intimacy, work, and leisure (McLemore and Brokaw, 1987).

Among the treatment modalities for personality disorders are psychoanalytic, supportive, interpersonal, cognitive, behavioral, and psychopharmacologic therapies, all of which may draw in one degree or another from psychodynamic theory (see Chapter 17 of this text for detailed discussion of these treatment modalities). Experienced *medical* providers can and often do draw from one or a combination of these techniques in fashioning a collaboration with difficult-to-help patients. I will illustrate some such approaches below when discussing particular personality disorders and associated maladaptive behaviors.

In the mental health setting, psychoanalytic psychotherapy or psychoanalysis are the treatments that specifically target personality structure, rather than just the individual's symptoms and functional capacity. Typically, personality disorder requires relatively lengthy treatment—often, years—if definitive change in personality is the goal. The requisite vehicles upon which this form of treatment depends are *the patient's motivation to change,* his or her *capacity for insight,* and his or her *capacity to engage in a therapeutic relationship* that can serve as an interpersonal "laboratory" for psychosocial learning.

By drawing connections between the patient's symptoms, developmental history, current life situation, and the treatment relationship, the patient becomes more aware of habitual maladaptive responses and therefore may be better able to self-direct alternative ways of thinking, feeling, behaving, and relating. Principal sources of the enhanced interpersonal flexibility than can emerge from treatment are enhanced capacities for recognition, understanding, and self-modulation of internal states.

Personality disorders that may most benefit from psychodynamic or psychoanalytic treatment include the cluster C disorders (avoidant, dependent, and obsessive–compulsive), and most of the cluster B disorders (histrionic, borderline, and narcissistic). Personality disorders that are most resistant include the cluster A disorders (paranoid, schizoid, and schizotypal) and antisocial personality disorder.

Supportive psychotherapy, in contrast, attempts to aid patients without challenging their basic defenses or attempting to change their fundamental personality structure. Supportive treatment can help the patient through periods of medical, social, occupational, or other stress by minimizing regression to even more maladaptive behaviors and by maximizing collaboration with the doctor and the treatment system (Marin et al, 1994). Personality disorder patients frequently benefit most from a combination of supportive and psychoanalytic approaches and, depending on the severity of the personality disorder, adjunctive use of behavioral, interpersonal, and psychopharmacologic strategies.

Interpersonal psychotherapies, including individual, marital or couple, family, and group approaches, rely on the observation that personality traits often elicit complementary responses in others, including the therapist. Thus, he or she may deploy an interpersonal style that best facilitates more flexible and adaptive coping on the part of the patients. Through generalization of learning from the therapeutic context to various life situations, the overall impact of personality disorder may be mitigated (Marin et al, 1994; McLemore and Brokaw, 1987).

Behavioral therapy can be used to reduce specific problematic behaviors in selected patients. Particular techniques include behavioral contracting, contingency contracting, limit-setting, assertiveness training, relaxation training, token economy (a system that rewards desirable behaviors), and exposure therapy, to name only a few.

Cognitive therapy, an approach that grew out of psychoanalytic theory, relies on the observation that many individuals remain "stuck in a rut" of certain habitual responses due in part to their underlying belief system or schematic set of rules for living, which generates certain stereotyped ways of thinking, feeling, and behaving. These stereotyped responses, in turn, serve to reinforce the subconscious beliefs, and people then repetitively experience the very things that they expect to experience, even though, in reality, they themselves have "constructed" this way of being, and it bears no necessary correspondence to what may actually be possible. The classical example is of depressed persons who, because they cannot experience pleasure, come to believe that there is no more pleasure available anymore to them; conversely, because they are convinced that no pleasure can be had, then no pleasure can be experienced. Most importantly, this self-reinforcing system of belief, feeling, and thought creates and is created by increasingly ineffectual attempts to change, often with resultant helplessness.

By pointing out these various forms of self-entrapment in certain maladaptive strategies for living, the therapist who has a good collaborative relationship with the patient may be able very gradually to nudge him or her toward trying slightly modified strategies, but the work is often arduous (Beck and Freeman, 1989). Cognitive strategies are often combined with behavioral approaches, with the proper admixture titrated for a given patient. For example, a flexible, cognitive–behavioral approach has been developed and found to be quite effective for selected borderline patients (Linehan, 1993).

Psychopharmacologic treatment is essential for ameliorating the frequent comorbid Axis I conditions that have overwhelmed the maladaptive defenses of the patient with Axis II pathology. In addition, many studies have indicated that specific target symptoms and behaviors of some personality disorder patients (especially borderline and schizotypal) are at least partly responsive to certain medications.

Potentially useful drugs and their associated target symptoms include the following: for cognitive distortions, paranoia, or psychotic symptoms: low-dose antipsychotics; for the spectrum of irritability, impulsivity, dyscontrol, rage, and violence against self or others: lithium, anticonvulsants, serotonin-reuptake-inhibiting antidepressants, or antipsychotics; for affective lability: lithium or anticonvulsants; for persistent anxiety: buspirone, benzodiazepines, beta-blockers, or antidepressants; for dysphoria and depression: antidepressants, including monoamine oxidase inhibitors, or lithium; for acute insomnia: low-dose trazodone, a sedating tricyclic antidepressant, or short-term use of a hypnotic drug such as zolpidem; for persistent and pervasive attentional difficulties: stimulants, bupropion, or desipramine; for severe obsessive–compulsive symptoms: clomipramine or serotonin-reuptake-inhibiting antidepressants; for depersonalization or derealization: antipsychotics or benzodiazepines; and, for acute conversion symptoms: benzodiazepines (Gorton and Akhtar, 1990).

As always when prescribing medications, care should be taken to be scrupulous in providing an on-going informed consent process, to limit the dose and duration of medication, to specify target symptoms and mitigate against unrealistic expectations, to avoid nonrational polypharmacy, to ensure adherence to the recommended regimen (e.g., through contingency contracting), to monitor for concurrent use or abuse of intoxicants, to monitor for drug interactions (especially with the serotonin-reuptake-inhibiting antidepressants), and to safeguard against potentially fatal suicide attempts by careful drug selection and provision of small supplies.

Although, in general, medical practitioners are unlikely to become involved in the complexities of definitive psychiatric treatment of patients with personality disorder, they should be aware of what treatments are available, and they may become comfortable deploying some of these strategies to mitigate both distress and poor collaboration in the medical setting. Examples might include: a low dose of risperidone or haloperidol in an irritable patient with borderline traits who is awaiting a surgical procedure; or a small amount of a benzodiazepine for a non-substance-abusing woman with avoidant and dependent traits who feels overwhelmed by the burden of acute illness in her mother, who is her sole social support.

With the growing recognition of the importance played by maladaptive personality traits and personality disorders in shaping the course of both Axis I mental disorders and Axis III medical/surgical conditions, medical and psychiatric practitioners are now better equipped to design specific interventions and treatment strategies and to coordinate the care provided by a healthcare team or system so as to give the patient optimal care and conserve increasingly scarce healthcare resources.

RELATIONSHIP BETWEEN MALADAPTIVE REACTIONS TO ILLNESS AND DIFFERENT TYPES OF PERSONALITY DISORDER

Keeping in mind that not all medical patients with personality disorder are difficult-to-help, and certainly that not all difficult-to-help patients have personality disorder, we can outline for heuristic purposes (as shown in Table 6–2) the possible relationships between four aspects of the psychosocial illness experience: first, a variety of personality styles; second, the prototypical meaning that patients with each style often ascribe more or less unconsciously to the illness experience; third, typical associated maladaptive responses to illness; and, finally, the particular corresponding type(s) of personality disorder found in DSM-IV. Many authors have advanced their own approach to the relationship between two or more of these four variables, all of them originating with Kahana and Bibring's seminal work (1965), and some of these have been incorporated into Table 6–2. (See also Adler, 1981 on the hypochondriacal patient, and Ness and Ende, 1994 on the patient in denial.)

Of course, none of these stylistic responses to illness are mutually exclusive or necessarily as clear-cut as they appear in this schematic. However, such a chart can at least provide a starting point for clinicians who wish to troubleshoot a problematic relationship with a patient in order to formulate the best responses in that particular situation. At first, the mass of possible personality styles and personality disorders may seem complex and overwhelming! Through regular use of such a schematic, however, students will be better equipped to bring themselves most effectively to each patient. More patients will then feel helped, and more will probably collaborate with the healthcare system for their own benefit. Likewise, more physicians will feel competent and effective, and more will be able to avail patients of their medical–technical expertise. Both parties to this noble project will be more likely to reap the rewards to which they are entitled as patient and healer.

Consistent with their different personality styles, patients will frequently present typical help-seeking themes or demands to the physician, as presented in a schematic series of narrative statements in Table 6–3, arranged according to personality disorder.

Although we cannot expect patients to make such statements in literal fashion, these can be thought of as summary entreaties that more or less embody the general themes running through the relationship with that particular sort of person. These statements comprise the larger message or underlying demand that is encoded within that patient's way of relating to the doctor, if only the doctor can listen for it and recognize it. (Note that "denial" can be a highly adaptive way of coping, and is by no means necessarily pathologic, as discussed by Ness and Ende, 1994.)

For example, take a look at how the statement that correlates with obsessive–compulsive personality disorder in Table 6–3 can be utilized to make sense out of what Mr. A was indirectly saying in the case vignette above. Recall also that although Mr. A did not have a personality disorder per se, he did manifest an obsessive–compulsive personality style. Thus, Tables 6–2 and 6–3 can be useful whenever we are confronted with a particular maladaptive reaction or personality style, or what appears to be personality disorder, in our patients.

DSM-IV PERSONALITY DISORDERS

Included in each of the descriptions of the disorders discussed below are the key diagnostic criteria, typical presentation in the medical setting, management strategies for the nonpsychiatric physician, and possible psychiatric treatment approaches. The key personality traits for each DSM-IV and one DSM-III (revised) personality disorder are also summarized in Table 6–4. Whenever personality disorder is being considered, the doctor must first determine whether the apparent personality disturbance is, indeed, a symptom of a long-lasting disorder, or only a relatively recent change. In either case, medical causes of the interpersonal problem must first be considered. Next, substance-related disorders must be entertained and carefully investigated for their role in causing the problem. Finally, other comorbid or look-alike Axis I conditions must be thoughtfully ruled out, such as bipolar disorder, schizophrenia, major

(text continues on page 210)

Table 6–2 Schematic Relationship of Maladaptive Behaviors and Personality Styles to DSM-IV Personality Disorders and the Meanings of Illness

MALADAPTIVE BEHAVIORS	PERSONALITY STYLES							DSM-IV PDs*	MEANINGS OF ILLNESS
	KAHANA AND BIBRING (1965)	GROVES (1978)	LURIE (1982)	LIPP (1986)	SCHWENK AND ROMANO (1992)	FOGEL (1993)	GOLDBERG (1995)		
1 Angry, Hostile, Threatening, Demanding	1 Oral, Narcissistic	1 Entitled demander	1 Hostile	1 Borderline, Complaining, Demanding, Angry, Manipulative	1 Angry, Demanding, Complaining	1 Least Mature	1 Borderline, Narcissistic, Antisocial	1 BPD NPD ASPD	1 BPD: Threat to self-cohesion; abandonment NPD: Threat to self-image of omnipotence and perfection ASPD: Opportunity for advantage/revenge
2 Mistrustful, Suspicious, Guarded, Querulous	2 Paranoid	2 Self-destructive denier	2	2 Paranoid	2	2 Least Mature	2 Paranoid	2 PPD STPD	2 Threat of external control and/or attack
3 Helpless, Self-defeating, Martyrlike,	3 Masochistic	3 Manipulative help-rejecter	3	3 Manipulative (passive)	3 Long-suffering, Masochistic	3	3 Long-suffering, Self-sacrificing, Masochistic	3 SDPD, PAPD, DPD, HPD	3 Deserved punishment
4 Emotional, Dramatic	4 Hysterical, Oral	4 Dependent clinger	4 Seductive	4 Overly Affectionate, Borderline	4 Dramatic, Emotionally Involved, Seductive, Affectionate	4 Variably Mature	4 Histrionic	4 HPD, BPD	4 Threat of rejection and/or of damage to masculinity/femininity

5 Passive-Aggressive, Resistant	5	5 Manipulative (covert) help-rejecter	5	5 Dependent, Passive	5 Passive, Dependent, Over-demanding	5 Variably Mature	5 Passive-Aggressive	5 PAPD, SDPD, DPD	5 Opportunity for resistance to and punishment of helpers
6 Controlling, Rigid	6 Compulsive	6 Entitled demander	6 Rigid, Competitive, Perfectionistic	6	6	6 More Mature	6 Obsessive-Compulsive	6 OCPD	6 Threat of loss of self-control/helplessness
7 Hypochondriacal	7	7 Manipulative (somatic) help-rejecter	7 Somatization, Hypochondriasis, Chronic Pain	7	7 Somatizing	7	7	7 DPD, SDPD, HPD, Other PD	7 Threat of endless suffering/pain
8 Pathologic denial of Illness	8	8 Self-destructive denier	8	8 In Denial	8	8	8	8 Any PD	8 Altogether too threatening/overwhelming
9 Overly Dependent	9 Oral, Masochistic	9 Dependent clinger	9 Dependent	9 Dependent, Passive	9 Passive, Dependent, Over-demanding	9 Variably Mature	9 Dependent	9 DPD, SDPD, BPD	9 Threat of abandonment/helplessness
10 Distant, Aloof, Uninvolved	10 Schizoid	10 Self-destructive denier	10	10	10	10 Less Mature	10 Schizoid	10 SPD, STPD, PPD, APD	10 Threat of intrusion/inner turmoil

* PD, Personality Disorder; ASPD, Antisocial PD; APD, Avoidant PD; BPD, Borderline PD; DPD, Dependent PD; HPD, Histrionic PD; NPD, Narcissistic PD; OCPD, Obsessive-compulsive PD; PPD, Paranoid PD; PAPD, Passive-aggressive PD; SPD, Schizoid PD; STPD, Schizotypal PD; SDPD, Self-defeating PD.

Table 6–3 **Typical Help-Seeking Themes or Demands in Various Personality Types***

TYPE	DEMAND
1 BPD:	"Help me!—Take care of me!—Don't ever leave me or I'll totally freak out!—and there will be HELL to pay!"
NPD:	"Help me, and do precisely what I demand! Never forget that I don't really need you and that I expect obedience at all times! Don't cross me, or I'll chop you down to size, have you removed from my case, or throw a tantrum!"
ASPD:	"Help me, because I'm so charming and I hurt so much, but you'd better do it just the way I want, and let me take advantage of you! Otherwise, WATCH OUT!"
2 PPD:	"I need your help, but I certainly can't trust that you're really trying to help me! In fact, maybe you're trying to harm me—it's people like you who probably caused my problem in the first place!"
3 SDPD:	"Help me, but it won't do any good, so forget I ever asked!—But why don't you ever want to help me?—You don't like me, do you?"
4 HPD:	"Help me, because I can't cope!—and don't reject me, or I'll fall apart and be a total mess!"
5 PAPD:	"Help? I don't need help! Why would I need help? Oh, I see you're busy—can you help me NOW?"
6 OCPD:	"Help me, right now, in just the way I want, or I'll feel like I've lost control!—That's when I get angry!"
7 Any PD:	"Help me! I hurt all over! I have diseases you can't even find—nothing in my body works—it's hopeless!"
8 Any PD:	"Help? For what? I'm sorry, doctor, I'm just fine, and I'm sure it's nothing, anyway!"
9 DPD:	"Help me! Don't leave me—I'll do whatever you say! Talk to me, take care of me. . . ."
10 SPD:	"Help me, but don't intrude too much, because I want to believe that I'm really okay and that I don't need anyone."
STPD:	"Help me, but I don't really need any help because nothing is really the matter, or, if it is, I already understand it and it doesn't really trouble me, so don't make a big deal out of it, or I'll get really nervous. . . ."
APD:	"Help me, but I feel like an idiot because things can't really be that bad—I'm so ashamed, don't look at me!"

* Note that the sequence of personality disorders in this table corresponds to the numbered sequence of maladaptive behaviors used in Table 6–2. See footnote to Table 6–2 for abbreviations.

depression, posttraumatic stress disorder, obsessive–compulsive disorder, attention deficit disorder, dissociative disorder, sleep apnea, subtle dementia, intermittent explosive disorder, chronic adjustment disorder, and so forth. Psychiatric consultation will be extremely useful here.

I have proposed a mnemonic tool for all 17 categories of psychopathology in DSM-IV, which can aid in rapid and comprehensive recall of the differential diagnostic possibilities: "DSM-F-SCOPE: SAM IS SAD." In other words,

Table 6–4 **Summary of the Key Personality Traits for DSM-IV and Other Personality Disorders***

CLUSTER	TRAITS
A	*Paranoid:* pervasive distrust and suspiciousness, such that, without sufficient basis, others' motives are interpreted as malevolent, exploitative, harmful, or deceptive; therefore is reluctant to confide, holds grudges, overreacts with anger, and suspects disloyalty or infidelity *Schizoid:* detachment from and lack of enjoyment in social relationships; therefore socially isolated, celibate, lacking pleasure in activities, apparently aloof from praise or criticism, and emotionally restricted *Schizotypal:* paranoid, with ideas of reference, odd beliefs and thought patterns, unusual perceptions and speech, constricted or peculiar affect, eccentric behavior, lack of close friends, and excessive social anxiety
B	*Antisocial:* prior to age 15—aggression against people or animals, destruction of property, deceitfulness, theft, and serious violations of rules; after age 15—unlawful behavior, lying or conning, impulsivity, irritability or fights, disregard of safety, failure to take responsibility in work or financial affairs, and lack of remorse about harming others *Borderline:* unstable and intense relationships, frantic efforts not to be abandoned, marked identity disturbance, harmful impulsivity, recurrent self-harm or suicidality, affective lability, chronic emptiness, intense and poorly controlled anger, and transient paranoia or dissociation *Histrionic:* demanding of attention, inappropriately seductive or provocative; shallow, but labile and dramatic emotionality; vague and impressionistic speech; easy suggestibility; and a false sense of intimacy with acquaintances *Narcissistic:* grandiosity and a sense of social specialness, fantasies of ideal personal qualities or unlimited power, excessive entitlement and need for admiration, a tendency to exploit others, lack of empathy, arrogance and enviousness
C	*Avoidant:* fears criticism, embarrassment, shame or rejection in work, social activities, or other new activities; therefore, unwilling to become involved or intimate unless certain of being liked; feels socially inept, inferior, and unappealing *Dependent:* difficulty making everyday decisions, needing others to assume responsibility; nonassertive due to fear of disapproval or loss of support; lacking confidence, with trouble functioning autonomously; obsequiously seeking of nurturance, and desperate to find substitute caretakers when unsupported; helpless, anxious and fearful of being overwhelmed when alone *Obsessive–compulsive:* excessively preoccupied with details and orderliness; perfectionistic; driven to work very hard and exclude leisure activities; scrupulous and inflexible regarding morality, ethics, or values; compulsively hoards worthless objects; too scrupulous about money; rigid and stubborn, with difficulty in teamwork

(continued)

Table 6–4 *(continued)*

CLUSTER	TRAITS
Other (Personality Disorder Not Otherwise Specified)	*Passive–aggressive:* negativistic and passively resistant to authority; given to procrastination and "forgetting" so as to avoid responsibility; given to protesting the unreasonableness of others' expectations; sulking, scornful, critical, or deliberately obstructive and inefficient in performance, yet resentful of helpful feedback
	Self-defeating: self-sacrificing and self-sabotaging to maintain relationships and self-esteem; may feel exploited; tends to defeat others' efforts to help, yet complains about suffering; humiliated and angry, with grudges against others; intolerant of success and positive experiences, with paradoxically negative reactions to any situational improvement; rejects pleasure and won't admit to enjoyment

* Adapted from DSM-IV, with the exception of self-defeating personality disorder (from DSM-III, revised). Note that only some *subsets* of the listed traits are required to diagnose that personality disorder.

doctors should look through their "DSM-F(our)-SCOPE" and consider what is ailing "SAM(uel)" or "SAM(antha)," i.e., the male or female patient who is difficult to help. Each letter in the mnemonic corresponds to a major diagnostic category in DSM-IV: D, Delirium, Dementia, and Amnestic and Cognitive Disorders; S, Substance-Related Disorders; M, Mood Disorders; F, Factitious Disorders; S, Schizophrenia and Other Psychoses; C, Child, Infant, and Adolescent Disorders; O, Other Disorders That May Be a Focus of Clinical Attention; P, Personality Disorders; E, Eating Disorders; S, Somatoform Disorders; A, Anxiety Disorders; M, Mental Disorders Due to a General Medical Condition; I, Impulse Control Disorders; S, Sexual and Gender Identity Disorders; S, Sleep Disorders; A, Adjustment Disorders; and D, Dissociative Disorders (Gorton, in press). As already noted, the presence of any personality disorder predicts a greater likelihood that an Axis I disorder will also be found, so both may certainly exist concurrently.

Cluster A: The Odd, Eccentric Disorders

Paranoid Personality Disorder

CASE VIGNETTE

Mr. C., a 46-year-old man, presented to the medical clinic with the chief complaint of feeling weak and tired. He said, "I need a checkup to find out what's wrong so I don't have to feel this way anymore." He tended to dominate the interview with the resident, raising his voice and talking more rapidly whenever the doctor would attempt to redirect him toward some aspect of the relevant medical history or review of systems.

During the interaction, Mr. C was intensely vigilant of the doctor's every movement. After the verbal control struggle had gone on for about 10 minutes, the doctor said: "I can't help you if you won't cooperate with me." The patient leaned forward, glowered threateningly, and said: "I figured when I came in here that you'd try to screw me over. You're just like all the rest—all you do is want to mess with me, ask stupid questions, and then tell me what to do!"

The hallmark of paranoid personality is a pervasive suspiciousness, mistrust, and expectation of harm, with great sensitivity to any perceived slight or criticism, since this is automatically taken as a manifestation of some malevolent intention toward the paranoid person. The lack of clear-cut delusions, hallucinations, or any evidence of frank psychosis, differentiates this personality disorder from schizophrenia and from the delusional disorders. (Naturally, medical and other psychiatric causes of paranoia must be ruled out; see Block and Pristach, 1992.).

Paranoid beliefs are associated with anxiety that is often masked by arrogance, defensiveness, secretiveness, hostility, anger, jealousy, or an anti-authoritarian attitude laced with sarcasm, cynicism, bitterness, and sometimes litigiousness. These patients fear being controlled, invaded, exploited, and damaged, and they typically resist intimacy with all except perhaps one other person whom they observe vigilantly for any sign of disloyalty or betrayal. Prevalence of paranoid personality in the general population is roughly between 0.5 and 1.5%.

The etiology of this personality disorder is unclear, although a significant genetic contribution may be present. Traumatic and shame-inducing experiences in the very earliest developmental phases may play a role, but so might the effects of parental modeling of mistrust, scapegoating, and perceived or actual experiences of mistreatment or discrimination. Sometimes entry into a foreign environment, such as occurs during immigration to a new country or culture, correlates with onset of a paranoid tendency.

Paranoid personality is one among a number of personality disorders that are theorized to have their psychological foundation in the cognitive strategy called "splitting" (Akhtar, 1992). This is a psychological defense mechanism by which perceptions and feelings about oneself, others, and the world are divided rigidly between "bad" and "good" categories. This way of organizing experience originates with the infantile ego's sorting of its pleasurable and unpleasurable moments into "all" or "nothing"—idealized or hated—compartments in emotional life and in memory. Paranoid thoughts are symptoms of the way the mind defends against inwardly directed feelings of badness and hatred by misattributing these perceptions to other people via the defense mechanism of projection.

Thus, although this process is automatic, such patients might, in effect, explain their situation as follows: "I am not bad—I feel this way because *they* hate me! In fact, *they* are bad, and I must protect myself by being ever on the alert and fighting back if necessary. I can never be too careful!"

In the medical setting, *it is as if such patients are saying, "I need your help, but I certainly can't trust that you're really trying to help me! In fact, maybe you're trying to harm me—it's people like you that probably caused my problem in the first place!"* In this situation, the physician should err far on the side of carefully explaining all treatment plans, procedures, medications, lab results, and above all, his or her intent not to harm the patient. For example, the doctor might say, "Even though this test may cause some discomfort, I certainly hope that it is tolerable, because I do not mean to cause you more pain than you already have!" An attitude of seriousness, respect, and consistent concern; acknowledgement of the patient's feelings of being put upon; and nonjudgmental conveying of information, will all go a long way toward fostering a workable doctor–patient relationship.

Psychiatric treatment, if a paranoid patient is willing to accept referral, should ideally consist of supportive psychotherapy and low-dose antipsychotic medication, with group therapy and partial hospitalization as possible adjuncts to this regimen. Naturally, paranoid patients will initially be suspicious of medication, but if a somewhat trusted doctor can identify a target symptom that such patients can agree with, they may be willing to try a tiny trial dose. The doctor might introduce it by saying, "I know you're highly stressed by this feeling of being mistreated—it's enough to upset anyone! The medicine I am recommending will, hopefully, take the edge off of the stress so you won't feel quite so miserable. Please be sure to tell me right away if it doesn't agree with you, since I certainly don't want to make things worse!"

If only the physician can "hang in there" with these patients, enough trust may develop such that they can become quite attached, and a mutually satisfying collaboration can result.

Schizoid Personality Disorder

CASE VIGNETTE

Mr. B, a lanky 49-year-old man with long hair, a thin face, and a sallow complexion, complained to his family doctor of difficulty concentrating on his reading. He described a routine of spending all day in the public library, where he would request a stack of obscure philosophy books whose contents he felt he needed to absorb in order to be able to write his comprehensive treatise on the nature of reality and the human condition. He told the doctor, "I wonder if there's something wrong with my brain function—or maybe I'm developing some kind of viral condition."

Mr. B lived alone in a cheap rooming house, having quit his job in a bookstore 3 years previously because "They were making me work with a new employee all the time—you know, like an appren-

tice—it was too much!—I'd rather live on welfare 'til I can get my book done. I'm just not cut out for working around other people!" He described infrequent visits home to see his aging parents, who still hadn't given up on trying to "fix him up" with various single younger women in the old neighborhood where he had grown up as an only child.

When Mr. B's doctor explored whether he might be depressed, as a possible explanation for his difficulty concentrating, Mr. B adamantly denied this: *"I'm fine, I really am!—After all, it's the human condition to feel alienated—it's not about what you feel or don't feel—I'm dealing with it the best way I know how! Just run a few tests, please—maybe it's all the dust I'm inhaling in the library stacks. . . ."*

The central feature of this disorder is a pattern of pervasive social detachment, with a narrowed range of emotional expression in social settings. Schizoid persons seem to be more or less content with their lack of emotional intimacy, their lack of close friends (other than a relative or two) and sexual experiences, their solitary activities, and their lack of much pleasure. However, they are often lonely and easily perturbed by what they feel to be the hassles and complexity of ordinary relationships. Thus, they may display an apparently sturdy self-sufficiency, are often indifferent to others' praise or criticism, and, in general, have difficulty expressing much anger or any other intense feeling. They lack the perceptual distortions and bizarreness of schizotypal patients and the frank psychotic symptoms of schizophrenia and delusional disorders. Prevalence in the general population appears to be between 0.5 and 1%.

Schizoid individuals as patients may react with a stoic acceptance that masks a defensive withdrawal in the face of what they perceive as threatened intrusion. Their need for a protective "shell" of privacy and emotional distance is best not confronted, yet clinicians should not neglect to offer empathic support and reassurance, since these patients yearn, in fact, for some degree of soothing and comfort from medical authority figures. *They seem to be saying, "Help me, but don't intrude too much, because I want to believe that I'm really okay and that I don't need anyone."*

Psychiatric treatment of schizoid personality disorder usually occurs in the context either of overwhelming depression or anxiety, or of transitory paranoia or frank psychotic decompensation. Maintenance use of antipsychotic medication is rarely necessary after resolution of the acute episode. Supportive psychotherapy that focuses on everyday issues and obstacles and is not too uncovering or intrusive usually suffices to facilitate relatively stable coping, albeit at a functional level that may be suboptimal when one considers the individual's innate capacities (e.g., high intelligence).

Schizotypal Personality Disorder

CASE VIGNETTE

A 38-year-old man who appeared somewhat haphazardly attired and poorly groomed spoke to his doctor in long, involved sentences that lacked a consistent focus and blended overly concrete statements with highly abstract generalities: "I'm just about all the way down the road to being able to exist now that I figured out the flow of energy I need every day—particularly food such as vegetables, sunflower seeds, and all that organic stuff that doesn't poison your system! As a doctor, you know about that, but I'm doctoring myself—as part of this Big Tribe, you've gotta heal yourself before you can heal everybody else, yes, oh yes. So that's where I am in my life—what can I do for you, doc?"

The patient appeared not to have any particular complaint to present; he seemed to want to engage in a peculiar reversal of roles. But when the doctor said, "Well, I don't know whether I'm going to be of much use to you today—you seem to be doing fine," the patient allowed as how he was concerned that maybe something he had eaten was making his "energy flow too slowly." The doctor determined that he seemed to have developed generalized fatigue over the past several weeks. He reassured the man that he would do his best to "get to the bottom of this," and, in fact, was able to detect a mild anemia due, it turned out, to inadequate iron intake.

At no point did the doctor challenge or try to "correct" the patient's odd way of understanding himself and his body, except to recommend several iron-rich foods that the patient was willing to integrate into his idiosyncratic diet. At no time did this man manifest frank symptoms of psychosis, and he had no interest in mental health care, since he did not perceive any problem within himself, yet appropriate medical care was delivered once it was couched in terms the patient could accept.

Schizotypal individuals manifest oddness or eccentricity that may include peculiar behaviors, thoughts, and perceptions, as well as speech that is idiosyncratic. They are often socially awkward and isolated, with a number of eccentric beliefs, unusual perceptual experiences, a paranoid tendency, unusual dress and/or grooming, and inappropriate or constricted affect. At the same time, they lack the frank psychotic symptoms of schizophrenia or other psychotic illnesses. They are apt to interpret their physical ailments in light of their unusual beliefs and superstitions.

This personality disorder is present at a higher than expected rate in families of patients with schizophrenia, with an overall prevalence in the population of roughly 1 to 3%, and is believed to be a partial expression of that more severe disorder. It differs from schizoid and paranoid personality disorders in the greater preponderance of cognitive distortions and the greater degree of overt oddness. Episodes of florid psychosis may occur under stress, but these remit once the situation stabilizes. If psychotic symptoms do not remit after an acute episode, the diagnosis of a Cluster A disorder must be reconsidered, since schizotypal personality is often indistinguishable from the symptomatic prodrome that heralds onset of schizophrenia.

Whether schizotypal cognitive–perceptual disturbance can develop in the absence of a genetic predisposition is not known. A plausible model for this disorder is that defects in attentional, perceptual, and information-processing areas of the brain cause difficulty in evaluating and appropriately interacting with the social environment. This in turn may lead to mistrust, suspiciousness, and maladaptive coping through elaboration of odd explanatory hypotheses about self and others, and social isolation.

The social anxiety present with schizotypal personality tends to remain fairly constant for these patients, even when they achieve some familiarity, say, with their physician. *These patients seem to be saying. "Help me—but I don't really need any help because nothing is really the matter, or, if it is, I already understand it and it doesn't really trouble me—so don't make a big deal out of it or I'll get really nervous. . . ."* Physicians who deploy a consistently educative, reality-clarifying strategy, while at the same time suggesting that maybe the patient has "just a *little* bit of concern or worry" about their medical status, will find the interaction going most smoothly.

These individuals use psychological defenses of denial, distortion, projection, schizoid fantasy, and acting-out through interpersonal distancing; by these means they manage to keep most of their anxiety out of conscious awareness. Therefore, supportive, empathic statements by the doctor should never take an overly emotional form, such as "I can see how terribly frightened and overwhelmed you are!" This will only make matters worse, since the patient will have to deny and project all the more, with resultant increase in paranoia and withdrawal.

Physicians often underestimate the degree of trust and attachment these patients actually have to them, partly out of physicians' own anxiety about interaction with "weird" people. In fact, if schizotypal patients' perspectives can be appreciated as "the particular pair of glasses through which they see their world," providers can make allowance for their peculiarities and allot them the dignity, privacy, aloofness, but also support, that they need to make their way through the healthcare environment.

As with the paranoid personality patient, if the schizotypal patient is willing to accept a referral, psychiatric treatment consists of supportive, reality-based therapy and perhaps a low dose of an antipsychotic medication and/or a touch of a benzodiazepine such as clonazepam, which will ameliorate anxiety.

Even if the condition evolves into overt psychosis under severe stress, long-term use of an antipsychotic agent should not be necessary.

Cluster B: The Dramatic, Impulsive, Emotional Disorders

Antisocial Personality Disorder

CASE VIGNETTE

Mr. C, a 31-year-old roofer with a history of multiple episodes of trauma from fights, motorcycle accidents, and falls, presented to the orthopedic clinic with a chief complaint of back pain. He was a pleasant, charming fellow who was now living with his second (common-law) wife. He had grown up with his mother and two younger sisters, his father's having abandoned the family when he was 11, after a tumultuous decade with the patient's mother. The boy had witnessed frequent beatings of the mother by the father and had himself been struck several times when the father was in drunken rages.

After the father left, the mother went through a period of depression, and the patient was left to wander the neighborhood with a ragtag group of older youths who smoked, drank, and played hooky from school. He became increasingly defiant of authority, lied about his activities, began to get into fights (often while high on alcohol and marijuana), and engaged in shoplifting and petty theft. On one occasion he killed a stray cat by stomping on it, which greatly impressed his older pals.

At age 14 he was arrested during a crackdown on neighborhood crime, but charges were dropped when an uncle, who had recently taken an interest in the lad, agreed to supervise his activities. He settled down significantly and was able to finish high school. He became an apprentice roofer, but after an argument with a supervisor during which Mr. C threatened to "beat the shit out of him," he was fired. After a period of unemployment, he got married and lived off his wife's income from waitressing, supplemented by his small-time marijuana dealing. He began to strike his wife when he felt she disrespected him, so she retreated to her parents' home and filed for divorce.

Within 3 months, he had secured a part-time, non-union roofing job and found a girlfriend who enjoyed motorcycles. It was the third crash of his second-hand bike that brought him into the clinic with persistent back pain. Mr. C was clear with the surgeon that what he needed was "something to kill the pain" so that he could get back to work, since he had no disability benefits or health insurance. The doctor advised him that he needed further tests and provided him with just enough of a weak opiate analgesic to last until the man returned following the magnetic resonance imaging scan that had been ordered. Mr. C thanked the doctor, but failed to return for the follow-up appointment 2 weeks later.

Antisocial personality is characterized by a pervasive pattern of disregard for, and violation of, the rights of others that begins by middle adolescence (at 14 years old) and continues into adulthood. What begins as "conduct disorder" (see Chapter 16 for childhood and adolescent disorders) becomes, in time, a personality marked by superficial—but seductive—charm, deceit, manipulation, and aggressive behaviors in the service of the individual's own needs, as the principal means of negotiating social life. Impulsive behaviors are common, with frequent disregard for the safety of self or others, along with irresponsibility and often a lack of remorse or empathic appreciation regarding the impact of the person's antisocial behaviors on others. Acting-out, rationalization, bland denial and minimization, splitting, and hypochondriasis are commonly used defenses.

The most common comorbid condition found in antisocial patients is substance-related disorder, although mood and anxiety disorders are also common. A watershed change in the General Diagnostic Criteria for all personality disorders occurred in DSM-IV which distinguishes antisocial personality disorder from antisocial behaviors that occur as a consequence of substance-related disorders such as alcohol or drug dependence. Clinicians should also be mindful that many individuals develop both antisociality and substance abuse more or less simultaneously during adolescence. In this case, although one can legitimately diagnose both disorders, a growing body of research has revealed that many of these individuals' antisocial behaviors will disappear once their addictive disorders are in remission (Gorton and Akhtar, 1994).

Thus, it is crucial in differential diagnosis not to reduce a substance-related disorder to "sociopathy," "psychopathy," or some other version of erstwhile "addictive personality" that today might be called—with the best of intentions!—"antisocial personality disorder." In fact, there is no evidence that some monolithic "addictive" profile of personality disturbance of any type either exists or can be said to cause addiction (Gorton and Akhtar, 1994).

Whereas severe antisocial personality disorder attracts a disproportionate amount of society's attention and resources, it is important to keep in mind that, on the one hand, adult criminal behavior by itself does not constitute a personality disorder, and, on the other hand, that less severe forms of this personality, marked by relative lack of guilt and of willingness to accept responsibility, as well as a tendency to lie and cheat when convenient to do so, are relatively common. In fact, some people with traits of antisocial personality disorder are quite successful in their chosen career! Overall, perhaps 2 or 3% of the population has this personality disorder, which is less than had previously been believed.

More men than women have antisocial personality. A genetic predisposition may be at work, which may establish the biological substrate for the apparent failure of many of these people to develop conditioned responses to stimuli related to fear. Neuropsychological dysfunction may also play a role (Gorton et al, in press), as may attentional problems and impulsivity. Failure to develop appropriate self-restraint and a socially suitable conscience may certainly reflect the high degree of family dysfunction found in most of these individuals, although parental criminality, even though it clearly runs in families, does not always correlate with onset of antisocial personality disorder. Factors related to family dysfunction that may mediate likelihood of developing antisocial personality disorder include inconsistency in or lack of discipline and limit-setting; this may at times be a function of parental loss or separation, which is more common in this disorder. Low family income, large family size, and low intelligence are other social factors that appear to play a role in etiology in some cases.

Management of the relationship with the antisocial patient may be extremely challenging because of the often intense reactions that many doctors have in response to the interpersonal maneuvers of these demanding patients. Many doctors have a highly attuned sense of when they are feeling disrespected, manipulated, or controlled, and this tends to clash with their own need to take pride in, be in control of, and feel competent in the medical encounter. *Often physicians feel as if these patients are saying, "Help me, but you'd better do it just the way that I want, and let me take advantage of you! Otherwise, watch out!"* The implied threat can result in the doctor's feeling fearful of what may happen if the patient's demands are not gratified. In such situations, it is imperative that the doctor create an atmosphere of safety for all parties, which at times may require the presence of multiple staff members or even a security officer.

Other *guidelines for intervention include:* (1) once aware of a power struggle, avoid participating in it and point out that it will not be productive; (2) use respectful, but firm, confrontation to clarify roles, boundaries, and the consequences of noncollaborative behavior; (3) rather than getting pulled into formulating treatment based on the emotional currents in the encounter, and rather than being maneuvered either into taking "special" care of the patient, or reacting according to your harsh judgment of the patient and depriving him or her of deserved professional assistance, thereby step back and think about the medical issues as clearly as possible, and do your best to provide the "routine" care that every patient deserves; (4) remember that no matter how noxious these patients' attitudes or behaviors, very likely they learned their particular approach to authority figures through difficult life experiences in which they themselves felt controlled, manipulated, attacked, or exploited; (5) try not to react in kind, but tell the patient, "It's clear that you need and deserve help, and I will do my best to provide it, but I will ask you to pay me the same respect that I hope to give to you, so that we can work together on your behalf"; (6) be clear with the patient that the two of you may not always agree—in fact, you may have to agree to disagree!—and that he or she doesn't have to like everything that you recommend, yet for you to be their doctor, the patient must at least *try* to do what you think is best; and (7) advise the patient that if the two of you cannot work things out then you will do your best with a referral to someone else, but that you'd really rather try to make the present treatment relationship work.

If the doctor can find a way to "hang in there" with these off-putting patients, a mutually grudging respect may develop, and a meaningful and rewarding relationship may emerge.

Definitive psychiatric treatment of antisocial personality disorder is elusive, although these patients adapt to highly structured settings such as prisons (Vaillant, 1975). Generally, if any headway is to be made in a less structured context, a combination of individual and group therapy is best, with firm limit-setting a crucial component.

Borderline Personality Disorder

CASE VIGNETTE

A 28-year-old woman came to an internist's office with intermittent low-grade pelvic pain of long standing. She appeared rather depressed and vulnerable, with a soft voice and a tendency to lapse into a sullen silence. The routine history took much longer than usual to elicit. After the physical examination, which revealed an incidental finding of extensive, healed lacerations on her left wrist, she became irritable after being told that no cause for her discomfort could thus far be identified. She was advised to return for repeat assessment in 1 month, or to call if the pain worsened. Upon hearing this plan, she burst into tears, but then abruptly yelled, "I can't deal with this!—It's too much!—Two weeks is forever! I'll probably be dead by then, but you wouldn't give a damn! This is the story of my life!"

Borderline personality disorder appears to be the most common personality disorder in inpatient and outpatient psychiatric settings; it is also one of the most common personality disorders in the general population, with a prevalence of about 2%. It carries with it a high lifetime risk of suicide, and a high degree of psychosocial morbidity. The essential feature is a pervasive pattern of instability in interpersonal relationships, identity, self-image, mood states, and behavior. These individuals desire intensely to be taken care of, yet they are terrified of closeness. Their attachments to others have a desperate and frenetic quality, with wide swings between loving idealization and hateful devaluation.

The features of this personality disorder have been captured in a mnemonic device for the nine DSM-IV criteria: "BP: AAIILRS" (Gorton, 1996), which is designed to remind clinicians that these patients truly are "ailing" and that they are not simply trying to hassle or harrass us or manipulate the system for no good reason. Here are the criteria, with a capitalized initial letter of each word that corresponds to the mnemonic: profound emptiness or Boredom; brief stress-related Paranoia or dissociative symptoms; inappropriate, intense Anger; frantic efforts to avoid real or imagined Abandonment; Impulsive behavior in at least two areas that are self-damaging (sex, spending, gambling, binge eating, substance abuse, etc.); lack of cohesive Identity, with markedly unstable sense of self; marked Lability of mood; markedly unstable social Relationships; and recurrent Suicidal or Self-mutilating behavior (American Psychiatric Association, 1994).

The etiology of borderline personality disorder remains controversial. Many of these patients have a history of physical, sexual, and/or psychological trauma in early life, or even throughout childhood, yet many—particularly males with this disorder—also show evidence of subtle brain dysfunction of uncertain origin (Gorton et al, in press). Additionally, most have mood disturbance that may have partial genetic loading, and many suffer anxiety disorders (including posttraumatic stress disorder), substance-related disorders, or even dissociative disorders, some of which likely have genetic underpinnings. Borderline personality probably represents a final common pathway disorder, since in fact it seems to be comprised of a variety of different subtypes, including populations that overlap with antisocial, schizotypal, and histrionic personality disorders, and others that have comorbidity with many Axis I conditions, such as anxiety and depression, psychosis NOS, cyclothymic (atypical bipolar) disorder, attention deficit disorder, eating disorders, substance-related disorders, and dissociative disorders.

The fundamental psychological defenses typically used by borderline individuals include splitting of self-image and image of others into "all good" (idealized) and "all bad" (devalued) categories, projective identification (unconsciously attributing to and identifying with aspects of others that are, in fact, projected images of aspects of oneself), and acting out (often aggressively) toward self and others. During crises, transitory paranoid or dissociative states may emerge that last for hours to days. These patients frequently reenact unconsciously many of the dysfunctional features of past relationships, such as abuse, power struggles, deprivation, boundarylessness, and pathologic dependency. They often have undue entitlement and grandiose expectations of being cared for that, if frustrated, may lead to intense anger, behavioral regression, and suicidal emptiness and dysphoria. For some of these patients, self-mutilation, such as by self-cutting, becomes a means of reestablishing a sense of self through the experience of pain or the sight of blood—in effect becoming an eerie kind of soothing mechanism.

In the medical setting, these patients often appear attractive, vulnerable, and hopeful. *They seem to say to the doctor. "Help me—take care of me— don't ever leave me!—"* Inevitably, however, they experience disappointment at the doctor's hands, when the idealized treatment does not eventuate or the doctor's perfect availability is tarnished, and they often up the ante by revealing in no uncertain terms the second half of their initial plea: *"—or there will be hell to pay!"* They are intense and unstable and extremely rejection sensitive. When their needs are frustrated, anger, hostility, and aggression are quick to emerge, and behavioral regression, often with manipulative attacking/self-defeating (sado-masochistic) overtones, may become the order of the day.

Some guidelines for working with these patients include (1) maintain a realistic perspective—and be clear with the patient—about treatment options, as these patients will pull very strongly for a dramatic rescue; (2) communicate in a simple, straightforward way that is least likely to be distorted or misinterpreted; (3) when what you have said is, indeed, distorted or misconstrued, clarify what was intended, but also point out that the patient may have a tendency to distort in ways that are not productive, and that the two of you will have to watch for this; (4) establish and explain the reasons for clear, consistent boundaries and realistic, nonpunitive limits, as well as role expectations and ground rules—and try not to make exceptions to these!; (5) tell the patient what her responsibilities are if she (or he) wishes you to be their doctor (e.g., to arrive on time for appointments, to avoid calling you in nonemergency situations, not to yell at your staff, to cooperate with lab tests, etc.); (6) point out if you feel blackmailed or manipulated, and reassess with the patient ways that the treatment relationship can function more collaboratively—if none can be agreed upon, then treatment may have to be terminated in a clinically and ethically appropriate manner; on the other hand, written agreements and "contracts" can be very usefully drawn up when problematic issues recur; (7) try always to avoid responding to hostility with hostility, but rather with calm acknowledgment that the patient is angry; then allow for further ventilation before finally inquiring as to what may be making the patient so upset; (8) watch for a wide range of reactions to the patient among the team of providers, and beware of "splits" that may develop in response to the patient's own unintegrated emotions toward herself and others (McDaniel et al, 1992); (9) be alert to the potential impact on the patient of any breaks in the treatment, such as illness or vacation, or rotation to another site, and prepare the patient in advance; (10) be mindful of your own limits and monitor your emotional reactions for clues as to how you are doing with managing the doctor–patient relationship; and (11) seek and use consultation, both informal ("blowing off steam" with a colleague) and formal ("please assist in the care of this patient. . ."), so as not to devolve into therapeutic martyrdom or nihilism, both of which will likely be reflections of what these patients themselves often feel—and often manage to make others feel! (See also Stoudemire and Thompson, 1982; Groves, 1991; and Searight, 1992 for additional tips on management.)

The mainstay of psychiatric treatment of borderline personality disorder is the establishment of a psychotherapeutic relationship that can flexibly draw from a combination of modalities (including behavioral, cognitive, psychoanalytic, interpersonal, and psychopharmacologic therapies), with treatment tailored according to the case formulation for that particular patient. Typically, definitive treatment takes several years, or longer, and the therapist must carefully walk a line between too much gratification and too much deprivation with regard to the patient's need to be taken care of. Details of such treatment are available elsewhere (Horwitz et al, 1996).

Medications that may be useful for selected borderline patients include selective use of low doses of antipsychotic agents (for irritability, hostility and paranoia, especially), serotonin-reuptake-inhibiting antidepressants (which should be considered for all borderline patients), and mood stabilizers or anticonvulsants (for irritability, aggression, mood lability, or impulsivity), all of which have been shown in controlled studies to be of benefit in selected cases.

Medical practitioners should be aware that their own consistent, supportive presence with such patients can be enormously important in patients' being able to maintain some degree of stable, adaptive coping with both ill health and other life stressors. For borderline patients to have reliable access to a concerned, caring professional who is also consistent, firm, and nonpunitive—but not afraid to confront the patient in an empathic manner about his or her unwillingness or apparent incapacity to engage in appropriate self-care—can be enormously stabilizing in the short run and developmentally growth promoting over the longer term. These oft-hated and maligned patients are fully capable of metamorphizing in surprising ways, if only we can find a way of respecting, tolerating, and getting along with them without unduly compromising ourselves in the process!

Histrionic Personality Disorder

CASE VIGNETTE

Ms. E, a 34-year-old divorced, childless woman with few friends and a host of bodily complaints for which little cause could be found, regularly arrived for her monthly medical appointment in a state of visible emotional distress. Dr. K, who had been in a group practice with a number of other primary care physicians for 3 years, dreaded these visits, since he rarely felt that there was anything he could do to alleviate his patient's apparent misery. A variety of tranquilizers, painkillers, sleeping pills, and even an antidepressant agent had done little to help her; they had only caused side effects, of which she had complained bitterly. "I just don't know what to do to help you," he would say over and over again to Ms. E, yet he would offer various sorts of advice about all of her many problems, both medical and social, and inevitably each visit would be long and drawn-out, leaving other of Dr. K's patients to wait with mounting frustration in the crowded waiting room.

Often he would take "urgent" calls from her during the week, only to find that she wanted help with some relatively minor problem that could have waited for a regular appointment. She seemed to need constant attention, and Dr. K began to have thoughts of making home visits to see her on his way home in the evening. Somehow he imagined that this might be less stressful for him and more palliative for her. He was confused by his tremendous sense of ambivalence toward his patient, something he had never before experienced so starkly.

Finally, Dr. K happened to attend a Continuing Education Lecture at the local medical school on the treatment of anxiety disorders in primary care. He approached the lecturer, a prominent Professor of Psychiatry, as she gathered her slides together afterward. Without identifying his patient, he briefly outlined his dilemma as to how to best help Ms. E. The psychiatrist noted that he seemed to feel he had to take care of Ms. E's every need in one way or another and that she probably had regressed to a rather childlike state in which she felt helpless and alone unless Dr. K were ministering to her. The consultant suggested that he begin to talk with her about the importance of her taking responsibility for the things she could do something about and that he also gently begin to set limits on the phone calls and the length of her appointments. She suggested further that he give her homework assignments such as keeping a log of all her symptoms, but also finding time to go out with a friend once a week and perhaps learn some relaxation techniques. Indeed, when Dr. K applied these techniques over a period of weeks, she responded favorably, especially when he made it clear that he very much wanted to continue to be her doctor and had no intention of abandoning her.

The essential feature of histrionic personality is a pervasive pattern of excessive emotionality and attention-seeking behavior. These individuals are uncomfortable in situations in which they are not the center of attention, and they will consistently use physical appearance to garner such attention, including using inappropriately seductive or sexually provocative behavior. They are given to histrionic displays of self-dramatization, theatricality, and rapidly shifting emotionality that is actually quite shallow, although by its being exaggerated it may appear deeply felt. The content of their speech is also often shallow, lacking in substance and appropriate detail, and replete with overgeneralizations and vague impressions. Finally, such individuals are vulnerable to social influence, suggestion, and romantic fantasy. They often feel themselves to be more deeply connected and intimate with others than is truly the case, their whole list of acquaintances consisting putatively of "dear friends."

Approximately 2% of the general population probably has histrionic personality disorder. One etiology is thought to reside in developmental disturbance between ages 3 and 6 or 7 that involves an overly heated relationship ("sexualization") with the parent of the opposite sex, although this is believed to represent a defensive adaptation to significant deprivation by the maternal (or other primary) caretaker in earlier childhood. Hence, in females, the need for nurturing and attention that is not forthcoming from their mothers is sought by attempting to attract the attention of their fathers. The use of theatrical and seductive behavior is really pseudosexual; as adults, sexuality is used to attract, control, and manipulate men. Histrionic behavior is by no means limited to females; male "hysterics" are often recognized in the form of excessive "machoism."

There is a tendency toward depression, substance abuse, sexual promiscuity, and suicidal threats during times of crisis, such as after an acute rejection. Regression to childlike behaviors, such as clinging, temper tantrums, and impulsivity, is an ever-present possibility that not infrequently occurs under the stress of medical illness. High anxiety, helplessness, and demandingness may occur. *It is as if the patient is saying, "Help me—because I can't cope!—and don't reject me, or I'll fall apart and be a total mess!"*

Management of the relationship with such a patient should include maximal support, reassurance, and structured availability by members of the treatment team. Attentiveness and expressed admiration of the patient's adaptive capabilities, as well as firm limit-setting and reality-based education about the medical situation will usually mitigate regressive and maladaptive behavior. Antianxiety medication may be indicated, in the absence of a substance-abuse/dependence history.

Definitive psychiatric treatment usually requires long-term psychotherapy or psychoanalysis, and these patients generally have a good prognosis.

Narcissistic Personality Disorder

CASE VIGNETTE

Mr. D, a 60-year-old business executive, presented to his new cardiologist with a chief complaint of "I want a tune-up, because I'm going on a golf vacation and this damn chest pressure is going to ruin my plans! I know that you don't know me, but if Dr. Z hadn't worked himself to death, I wouldn't have to break in a new cardiologist! Don't worry, I'll tell you exactly what I need. I might as well have an honorary medical degree, with everything I know about my heart!" He then proceeded to dictate to the doctor exactly what medicines he needed. When the doctor began to ask Mr. D some questions about his medical history, Mr. D said, "That's not necesssary, believe me—I'll fill you in some other time. Right now, I just need prescriptions, so I can catch my plane. I've got a helluva golf game when this damned old ticker is cooperating!"

Essential features of narcissistic personality are a grandiose sense of self-importance, need for excessive admiration, undue entitlement, and lack of empathy for others. These individuals possess an unquestioned belief that they are very special and that they deserve only the best of everything. They are preoccupied with fantasies of success, power, brilliance, attractiveness, or perfect love, and in one way or another they take advantage of others to achieve these ends. If necessary, they will inflate their image in others' eyes, creating falsehoods when expedient, and rationalizing if caught in their lies: "Well, I might as *well* have gotten into Harvard—I'm smarter than most of the *professors* there!" Thus, typical defenses against their covert envy of others are haughty omnipotence and devaluation.

Narcissistic personality appears to be one of the less common personality disorders, though narcissistic traits often coexist with other Cluster B disorders, or paranoid personality, as well as obsessive–compulsive personality. Narcissistic personality appears to develop as a result of disturbed parenting between the ages of 6 months and 2$^1/_2$ years. This may take the form either of unempathic overintrusiveness and overcontrol of the child, or unempathic neglect. In both cases the child's own separateness, individuality, and potential for successful development are undermined and devalued by the parent(s). Thus, there is a failure to provide that "good enough" empathic attunement and responsiveness that appears to be necessary for optimal emergence of the child's self-esteem and self-care functions. The result is an individual who in fact has an unconscious sense of profound inadequacy, hidden low self esteem, and for whom any need to depend on others is profoundly humiliating. This must be masked, even from the individual's own awareness, by an armorlike exterior that requires constant polishing by the admiring gaze of others. Self-worth is therefore achieved only through external reward, even as the individual with narcissistic personality believes all the while that, in fact, "I don't need ANYONE—you can all go to hell, as far as I'm concerned!" But this provides only temporary surcease from inner doubt and self-hatred.

As patients, these people may be quite difficult-to-help, especially when their demands are thwarted, even if only through the routines of the healthcare system, which do not necessarily recognize them as more "special" than anyone else. When they truly *are* VIPs—say, if Mr. D had donated a lot of money to the hospital for which Dr. Z worked—the combination of extreme narcissism and high social status can present some of the most problematic situations any doctor will encounter. *In effect, these patients say to the doctor, "Help me, and do precisely what I demand! Never forget that I don't really need you and that I expect obedience at all times! Don't cross me or I'll chop you down to size, get rid of you, or get really hacked off!"*

The best way to deal with this sort of "entitled demander" (see Table 6–3) is to try not to get rattled and to resist becoming defensive or getting into a power struggle. A polite firmness regarding your expectations, your limits, and the fact that your capacity to help the patient depends on his or her acceptance of these "realities" will go a long way toward settling him or her down a bit, even if grudgingly at first. Consistent maintenance of this stance, which respects *both* the doctor and her patient, actually reassures him or her that you *are* available, that you *are* willing to help, and that his or her power and importance will not drive you away.

In the best case scenario, the patient begins to admire and idealize the doctor! This may also be problematic, but gentle reminders that you are not perfect and that you *do* make mistakes usually help to mitigate this: "Well, thank you for your compliment, but I'm sure at times I *do* let you down in some way—though you may be too polite to complain—and I certainly want you to let me know so we can get back in synch with each other!" By giving "permission to complain," the doctor paradoxically hedges against the patient's need to "turn up the heat" when he or she is frustrated.

Psychiatric treatment, of course, requires acceptance by these patients that there is something about themselves that they want to change, a notion that is especially threatening to these individuals. Psychoanalytic and supportive psychotherapy, in the proper admixture, are the best approach should patients wish to embark on treatment. Since they are especially prone to depression, anxiety, and substance abuse, crises brought about by these comorbid conditions are often what leads them to give treatment a try, although they may flee as soon as they can convince themselves that they are once again impervious to distress.

Cluster C: The Anxious, Fearful, "Neurotic" Personality Disorders

Avoidant Personality Disorder

CASE VIGNETTE

Ms. E, a 39-year-old office worker, and the only child of aging, possessive parents, presented to her internist with a chief complaint of chronic insomnia. She was soft-spoken and hesitant and tended to avert her eyes while speaking. She was dressed according to a fashion that had faded from popularity many years before. No obvious cause for her sleep disturbance could be identified, although the doctor wondered whether she wasn't a tad depressed.

After two different sedating antidepressant agents were tried at bedtime, both having caused side effects that the patient resented,

she accepted psychiatric referral reluctantly. Apparently, prior psy-
chotherapy had not been very helpful, so she had dropped out. While
she knew that the sleep disturbance was by no means her only prob-
lem, she held out virtually no hope that she would be able to meet
someone with whom she might have a meaningful, intimate rela-
tionship, although her deepest fear was of being left alone in the
world after her parents died. She simply found it impossible to initi-
ate social contact with anyone new to her. It was unthinkable that
she should have anything meaningful to offer anyone, so she was
convinced that she would be discovered to be a "fraud and a freak,"
as she put it, if she allowed anyone to get to know her at all.

This personality disorder is characterized by a pervasive pattern of social inhibition, feelings of inadequacy, and hypersensitivity to criticism. Individuals with avoidant personality are riddled with self-doubt or even a stubborn certainty that they are inferior, stupid, unattractive, socially inept, uninteresting, or worthless. Observers perceive them as shy, timid wallflowers who are reluctant to enter into new social situations unless they have a virtual guarantee of approval and acceptance. In general, despite an intense desire for contact that, at least theoretically, differentiates them from people with schizoid personality disorder, they avoid work or social situations that involve an intense interaction, fearing they will be judged negatively and rejected. Shame and self-blame are ever-present bugaboos. So, too, is an undue vulnerability to embarrassment, blushing, or crying that adds the disturbing possibility of additional injury to their fragile sense of self.

The general prevalence of avoidant personality is thought to be 0.5 to 1%, and this disorder is frequently associated with anxiety disorders such as social phobia or panic disorder with agoraphobia, as well as with depression. The etiology is thought to involve a combination of a problematic inborn temperamental tendency and a suboptimal parental response. The temperament is toward shyness, social anxiety, and harm avoidance, manifest as undue early-life fear of strange situations and anxious attachment to caregivers. While some individuals "grow out" of these tendencies, those who develop full-blown avoidant personality seem to become increasingly shy, avoidant, and awkward during adolescence and early adulthood. Perhaps this happens most often when one or both parents are unable to foster gradually increasing exploratory movements toward greater independence on the part of the avoidant child. Parents who are needy, dependent, anxious, and relatively socially isolated themselves may get immense gratification out of having a child they can always depend on for the parents' own needs, but although the child may in the short run be comforted by this "holding," in the long run it will feel more and more like an imprisonment. Depression may ensue, and sometimes this is when doctors encounter these sufferers.

These patients are often quite embarrassed and anxious in the medical setting. A consistent thematic refrain goes something like this: "Help me, but I feel like an idiot because things can't really be that bad!—After all, I brought this all on myself!—I'm so ashamed—don't look at me!" Management of the helping relationship with them should include diligent empathy, consistent support, reassurance, and encouragement, as well as gentle admiration ("You know, I don't know how you do it—feeling so bad and alone all the time!"). Subtly letting these individuals know that you perceive them as having some positive qualities may enhance the rapport, as will your letting them know that they often seem to be much too hard on themselves. When irritable, they are much more often mad at themselves than at you, and if treated well they can usually collaborate responsibly.

Psychiatric treatment involves long-term psychotherapy with adjunctive use of anxiolytic and antidepressant medications. Social phobia must be carefully sought and aggressively treated with medication and cognitive–behavioral therapy. Group therapy may be feasible and very useful in the middle or later stages of treatment.

Dependent Personality Disorder

CASE VIGNETTE

Ms. F, a 47-year-old unemployed woman with insulin-dependent diabetes, was admitted in a hyperosmolar state 2 weeks after her husband of 28 years had had surgery for two ruptured disks. He was now convalescing at home. She was tearful and whiney in a childlike sort of way, and persistently demanded of the doctor "What should I do?—Just tell me what to do!—I can't take it!—Everything's hopeless!" Within minutes after the end of the interview, a nurse summoned the doctor to the phone at the nurse's station. Ms. F's husband was calling from home to be sure the doctor was aware that Ms. F will need "round the clock" assistance—even in choosing her menu selections from the hospital dining service, for example. "She's always been this way doctor—I'm sorry I can't be there to take care of her myself—if it weren't for my surgery. . . ."

Dependent personality is characterized by a pervasive and excessive need to be taken care of that is manifest as a clinging submissiveness with tremendous separation anxiety. Passivity is a striking and ever-present feature, and assertiveness is notably lacking. Initiative and independent action seem nearly impossible much of the time. Routine, everyday decisions such as clothing selection typically require guidance from a caretaking person who has also been allowed to assume responsibility for major areas of the person's life. In the absence of this nurturant figure, dependent people feel helpless, overwhelmed, and fearful that they cannot cope on their own. If abandoned in one way or another (e.g., illness in the caretaker, as in the above vignette), frantic efforts at finding a replacement will ensue. Self-esteem is very low and self-denigration very high.

This personality is associated with a high incidence of anxiety and depression. The general prevalence of extreme dependency may be as high as 3%, with perhaps more women than men. Etiology may include an anxious-inhibited temperament and/or a clinging, overly protective parent who infantilizes the child and prevents separation and individuation. Such individuals may then seek out a parental caretaker from whom they garner support, reassurance, and guidance since they cannot independently generate the self-sustenance and self-governance requisite for everyday life.

In the medical setting, these individuals present as "dependent clingers" (see Table 6–3) who are unable to make decisions or take responsibility and are eager to do "whatever you [the doctor] say!" This attitude may at first appear as a willingness to adhere perfectly to recommended treatment; however, it is soon revealed as the pathologic dependency that it actually is, when the patient seems incapable of returning to some reasonable level of self-care as illness subsides. In reality, extremely dependent persons are bottomless pits of neediness and helplessness, and they want the doctor to take control of their lives. Offering consistently empathic, but appropriately limited, availability, with reassurance, clarification, and clear expectations, will help them to collaborate. Giving "homework" assignments focused on particular problems that need solving, with the clear expectation that they must participate in order to receive optimal care, may foster a higher level of function.

Psychiatric treatment consists of a psychotherapeutic approach that avoids the taking of control and any ill-advised collusion in pathologic dependency. Cognitive–behavioral techniques can help address the poor self-esteem and sense of incompetence. Assertiveness and social skills training, as well as problem-solving exercises, perhaps in conjunction with group therapy, may be very helpful. Treatment of associated Axis I disorders, such as depression and anxiety, is critical.

Obsessive–Compulsive Personality Disorder

CASE VIGNETTE

Mr. J, a 50-year-old lawyer with no prior medical history, presented to the emergency room with crushing substernal chest pain, shortness of breath, and nausea. He had reluctantly cancelled a business meeting to come for an evaluation under extreme pressure from his partner. Laboratory studies and an electrocardiogram confirmed an acute myocardial infarction. The patient adamantly refused admission, stating that his work could not go unattended. His wife described him as a perfectionist "workaholic" who worked 7 days a week without vacations and saved virtually all his earnings "just in case." He adhered to this rigid and demanding schedule and faulted those who did not subscribe to his standards and morals. He was extremely proud of how he was in command of his professional practice and personal affairs, and he could not imagine letting his health interfere with his many important obligations, since he thought of himself as irreplaceable.

After some discussion about the clinical, ethical, and legal issues involved, the treatment team elected to have the patient and his wife sign a carefully worded statement that they were accepting full responsibility for any consequences that would befall Mr. J as a result of his leaving the hospital against medical advice. His wife's parting words to the doctor were, "I'm just really sorry about all of this! I can never get through to him either—thanks for trying so hard to convince him to stay, but I think he's just one of those people who will have to drop dead before he ever changes!" (adapted from Marin et al, 1994)

Obsessive–compulsive personality is characterized by a pervasive need for orderliness, perfection, and mental and interpersonal control, even if achieving these means sacrificing efficiency. Preoccupation with rules, lists, details, schedules, and organization leads to obliviousness to the overall goal. Completion of tasks is impeded by a tenacious perfectionism, which often leads to sacrifice of other activities, including socializing and relaxation, especially since the individual can rarely delegate something so important to someone else's control without a guarantee of adherence to exacting standards. Rigidity in moral concerns and general inflexibility in values, along with stubbornness and lack of openness, are common. Pointless retention of worn-out or useless items "just in case" they may prove useful leads to peculiar collections of things without particular sentimental value. Money is also withheld and hoarded "just in case" disaster should strike.

All in all, this personality disorder causes the person to appear neurotically rigid and finicky, and although possessing only *some* of these traits may be quite adaptive, in the extreme this disorder deprives the person of most of life's pleasures. Anger, resentment, power struggles, lack of emotional sensitivity, competitiveness, time urgency, and general world-weariness are the inevitable consequences. Burn-out, depression, and exhaustion, and even higher risk of cardiovascular disease may occur in these close cousins to the Type A (or "workaholic") personality associated with risk for heart attack.

Prevalence is roughly 1%. Etiology may be at least partly due to inherited tendencies toward obsessionality, constraint, and the temperament of attentional self-regulation. Relative developmental fixation in the anal phase (approximately age 3) probably also contributes in many cases. Unconscious shame and guilt, with associated need to control rigidly one's impulses, feelings, and desires, may underlie this personality disorder.

Doctors who encounter these individuals as patients tend to react with frustration and anger unless they can recognize these patients' excessive need for control as a coping style and not take it as a personal affront. Doctors should rather provide these patients with as much control as is reasonable, as well as all appropriate and up-to-date information about the medical situation. Sometimes, pointing out that "a stitch in time saves nine"—that is, taking the time for treatment in the short run—may well save them a much longer interruption in their schedule over the long run. Engaging them in planning for recovery can help keep these patients focused usefully rather than fretting unproductively. If the patient's anger should boil over, a calm, firm, reassuring tone, with polite clarification of any undue expectations on the patient's part that the medical system should function perfectly, will usually smooth ruffled feathers. Clear limit-setting may also be necessary at times, especially if narcissistic traits are prominent.

Psychiatric treatment depends not only on the patient's willingness to admit to some problem with their approach to life, but also on their willingness to cede some degree of control to the doctor. When this can occur, these patients are often notably dutiful, except that their tendency to intellectualize can make progress dauntingly slow.

However, in general the prognosis is fairly good when psychotherapy or psychoanalysis is used.

Personality Disorders (and Traits) Not Otherwise Specified

I will briefly mention only two additional personality disorders since they can offer particular challenges, and some of their traits often intermix with those of the ten official Axis II disorders to produce particularly thorny interpersonal dilemmas.

Passive–Aggressive Personality Disorder

Passive–aggressive personality is listed in an appendix to DSM-IV. It is characterized by a pervasive pattern of negativistic attitudes and passive resistance to authority, demands, responsibilities, or obligations. These individuals tend to complain, grumble, whine, argue, and be generally discontented and resentful. They have an angry, bitter, hostile perspective on the world, and generally scorn that which appears constructive and productive. Their stubborn sullenness can be extraordinarily difficult to tolerate by physicians, who not uncommonly become enraged at these patients. Acknowledging patients' frustration and encouraging them to be assertive and to complain freely, while also noting their tendency to be their own worst enemy, can ease things somewhat. The wise clinician avoids power struggles and does not expect great joy from them when their health improves!

Self-Defeating Personality Disorder

Self-defeating personality was listed in an appendix to DSM-III (revised), but has not been retained in DSM-IV. It remains a somewhat controversial diagnosis, due to its former name of masochistic personality, which was too often associated with "blaming the victim" (usually female) of domestic violence, as if she were the *cause* of her victimization! However, in the medical setting this disorder is characterized by a pervasive tendency to create (unconsciously) situations that frustrate the patient's own needs and desires, with an associated incapacity on the part of the patient to free himself or herself from such entrapments. These individuals feel angry and resentful, and, not appreciating their own role in creating the problem, collect grudges against those whom they feel have wronged and harmed them. These are individuals who can snatch defeat from the joys of victory and then make a show of their suffering.

In the doctor–patient relationship, they inevitably feel worse. Even when they have actually improved they cannot admit it, and when it is pointed out, they regress and feel worse again. They feel undeserving and are ridden with shame and guilt; pleasure is typically unthinkable. If the doctor can acknowledge their suffering and their "courage to go on," and frame recovery as "some of the hardest work any person can ever do," slow progress and decreased need for attention to their helplessness may ensue. Inviting the patient to be curious about how it is that they consistently work against themselves is the most useful form of gentle confrontation that should be deployed. Finally, if the self-defeating process is stopping progress altogether, and assuming that the patient is competent to refuse treatment, the doctor may have to acknowledge that he or she can no longer be useful to the patient—this in itself may be the very thing that engenders some collaborative response from the patient (see also Levy et al, 1988).

GENERAL PRINCIPLES OF MANAGEMENT OF MALADAPTIVE BEHAVIORS AND PERSONALITY DISORDERS IN THE MEDICAL SETTING

The first step in the process of optimal intervention is the recognition that a problematic interpersonal dilemma is obstructing the delivery of routine care. Naturally, *intervention should focus on facilitating the patient's collaboration with the doctor and the healthcare system.* Determining how this can best be accomplished will depend on *identifying the specific behaviors that are making the patient difficult-to-help.* This can lead to *selection of management techniques appropriate for the interactive difficulty at hand.* Although this may not necessarily include psychiatric referral of the patient, *consultation with a psychiatrist can be enormously helpful in managing the situation,* whether or not the psychiatrist actually interviews the patient.

Following are some *guiding tenets* that may be helpful in effective intervention with difficult-to-help and personality disorder patients (some are drawn from Vaillant, 1975, and Lipp, 1986):

Maintain a respectful, nonjudgmental attitude toward the person as a whole; avoid pejorative and critical comments and reserve judgmental and confrontational remarks for the maladaptive behaviors you are targeting for change. This requires self-awareness and constant monitoring and self-vigilance. Become aware of your typical, average, or routine attitudes and feelings toward your patients and your work. Only if you have such a sense of your emotional and attitudinal "background" will you become adept at noticing potentially problematic reactions and attitudes (Longhurst, 1988; Stern et al, 1993). Keep in mind that you don't necessarily have to like every patient (and you won't!) in order to help them!

To arm yourself consistently with the optimal empathic, nonjudgmental approach to patient care, you will need good stress management strategies. You will need to take care of yourself in both your personal and professional life. You will need to be able to notice when you're tired, less than sharp, frustrated, having a "bad day," and so forth. To work with our routine easy-to-help patients, much less the difficult-to-help ones, we need to avoid developing habits that will set us up for professional burnout, when we have no tolerance or patience, and little more of ourselves to give.

Be as honest as possible at all times. The burden of proof is on you if you choose some degree of dishonesty as a therapeutic maneuver. Don't get defensive. Don't take things personally. Assume the patient is reacting the way he or she is *for some good reason,* such as a lifetime spent trying to survive in his or her own hellish world. Take time to listen and get to know people: "My goodness, you must have been through a lot to react with such [fill in the blank with a problematic behavior]!" Showing respect for people's travail and suffering goes a long way toward garnering at least a grudging respect!

Once you notice some unusually strong reaction in yourself, consider as one possibility that what you are feeling mirrors the patient's feeling, e.g., helplessness, frustration, apathy, etc. In an effort to enhance collaboration, it's okay to say things like "I wonder if you're feeling as helpless as I am!"

Try to do *with,* not *to* the patient: foster *collaboration, not submission and unquestioning obedience.* Compliment patients for asking questions, or even for complaining: "I'm glad to see that you're willing to speak up for yourself—you've gotta be able to do that in order to get along in this world!" Not only will the patient feel understood; they will also complain less, or at least more usefully.

Expect the unexpected. Don't try to outwit, but to understand. Don't be afraid to feel confused, and don't try to save face if criticized or fooled by the patient. *The doctor–patient relationship should not be a competition.*

Don't punish the patient or blame inappropriately—but *expect and require them to take responsibility.* Don't try to insist on a behavioral contract that doesn't allow room for the pathology, because you can't legislate personality change. Patients will rightly be convinced that you'd just as soon get rid of them as give them a chance to learn a different way of doing things.

Set limits and provide consistent structure. Limits are best set on your own capabilities and behaviors: "No matter how much I want to help, there is a limit to how much I can do for someone who so consistently displays [name maladaptive behavior]!" "I will be unable to see you anymore if you continue to [name problematic behavior]." This approach puts the responsibility to change squarely on the patient, but it also demonstrates your willingness to work with them, within certain limits and under certain conditions: "I wish I were the kind of doctor who wasn't bothered by [name the difficulty in the doctor–patient relationship], but unfortunately I'm not, so you'll have to decide whether you want to try a different approach." And so forth.

Help patients think through the consequences of their behaviors and arrive at their own conclusions. *Your job is not to tell them what to do, to run their life, or to take over. You are a consultant they have hired to consult about their health. Make your best recommendations, but be clear whose job it is to accept or reject them, and to reap the consequences, whether good or bad.* Use Socratic dialogue to facilitate their insight into how their maladaptive traits end up defeating certain of their goals. Try to be matter-of-fact, avoiding sarcasm or teasing, such as "Well, if you want to kill yourself by [name maladaptive habit or behavior], go right ahead. . . ."

When you find yourself reacting strongly with one of those "Gee, that's not my typical reaction!—what's going on?!" feelings, listen to yourself, and *delay responding.* Give yourself time to reflect and analyze the situation. If you're not sure why you're about to say something, or whether you really mean it to be a *constructive* comment, then shut up! Tincture of time is an excellent solution to many difficult situations—you can always take a "time out" or ask the patient to do so: "Would you mind waiting in the Waiting Area while I think about this situation for a moment?"

Acknowledge the emotional content of the patient's communication (Goleman, 1995). This is a way of indicating that you understand, but it also buys some time for you to think how best to respond: "I don't blame you for feeling angry—please tell me more about how you feel about our work together."

Always consider whether an apology is the better part of valor when the doctor–patient relationship has gone awry: "I'm sorry that I didn't realize how sensitive a person you are. . . ." Since patients with personality disorder tend to externalize blame, don't be above apologizing for whatever it may have been in *your* behavior that, to their way of thinking, caused *their* transgressions of social rules or boundaries, even if you don't really think that what they did was justified: "I'm sorry that you thought I said that I don't care about you—that's certainly not what I intended at all! I can understand why you started to threaten me; however, you must understand that threats cannot be tolerated because I'll be scared and I won't be able to give you the help you need!"

CLINICAL PEARLS

- A personality disorder is evident by early adulthood and presents as a severe disturbance in a person's capacity for flexible adaptation and coping with the social environment due to a sufficient number of symptoms in at least two of the psychosocial spheres of thinking, feeling, behaving, and relating.
- Maladaptive personality symptoms, or traits, are enduring and pervasive, cause significant distress or impairment in terms of biopsychosocial functioning, and deviate markedly from the typical expectations of the individual's culture.
- Personality disorders or subsyndromal forms called personality styles are fairly common and are associated with specific kinds of maladaptive behaviors in the medical/surgical setting; such patients are especially prone to behavioral regression under the stress of illness or injury.
- Due to maladaptive and problematic responses in the healthcare environment, these patients often present as especially difficult-to-help, and evoke uncharacteristic and often intense emotional responses in healthcare providers; thus, when a physician dreads seeing a patient, or feels angry, frustrated, helpless, fearful, manipulated, seduced, overly charmed, or some other extreme or unusual response, this should be understood as providing critically useful data about the patient's personality, coping style, and response to illness.
- Physicians who routinely take note of their reactions to all patients will be in the best position to understand and most effectively relate to them so as to facilitate acceptance of illness, need for help, the necessary degree of dependency on the doctor, optimal collaboration, reasonable coping, and return to routine functioning.
- Assessment of what makes patients difficult-to-help can best be achieved by the doctor's stepping back and reflecting on why the interaction is not proceeding smoothly. The next step is consultation with a medical/surgical or psychiatric colleague and formulation of a specific way of managing the situation respectfully so as to preserve both the doctor's and the patient's dignity and to create a better match between each person's expectations of the other.
- Contributing medical/surgical or Axis I psychiatric conditions must always be considered in understanding the patient's interactive difficulties, and symptomatic reaction to the illness experience itself may by itself account for the turbulence between patient and health provider(s).
- General rules of thumb for coping with difficult-to-help patients, whether they have personality disorder or not, include the following: be scrupulously respectful, but request the same in return; listen attentively to what is being said, what is being implied, and what is not being said; communicate clearly; be clear about your own limits as far as what you can tolerate and what you expect; avoid meeting hostility with hostility or getting into power struggles; try to judge particular problem behaviors—but not the whole person—as needing to be changed; try to find something positive about the person, so as to remind yourself that they are, after all, fundamentally human; admit your mistakes, apologize for your errors, and be prepared to apologize even for the patient's transgressions if the better part of valor demands it; avoid burnout through proper caring for yourself in both your personal and professional life—otherwise, you will improperly burden your patients and confuse your needs with theirs.
- Although referral to a psychiatrist will be required for definitive treatment of personality disorder, which assumes that the patient is motivated to change, medical doctors can play a critical role as sustaining figures in the patient's life, and, in consultation with a psychiatrist may, in many cases, provide the mainstay of treatment, which may include appropriate psychopharmacologic treatment of both Axis I disorders and Axis II traits.

Never hesitate to get help from a colleague. The process of stepping back and getting a different perspective is often the single most important intervention in helping yourself help your difficult-to-help patients:

> The refusal to acknowledge that we have reached an impasse, and a martyr-like and obstinate determination to persevere in the face of manifest failure and to avoid seeking help from colleagues, are bad for the patient and for the [doctor]. One should get credit for courage and for thoughtful application to one's tasks. No credit can be claimed for the symbolic self-flagellation which includes the patient in its lacerating blows, and which denies the healing potential of fellow-workers (Grant, 1980).

SUMMARY

Physicians must pay careful attention to patients' capacity to collaborate in their treatment; when patients are having difficulty doing so, a methodical search for the causes of this problem must be initiated. Once major psychiatric illness, behavioral disturbance due to the direct effects of medical illness, problems within the treatment system, and the physician's own personality and demeanor are all excluded, then the possibility of personality disturbance in the patient should be entertained. Maladaptive reactions to the many stresses of the illness experience may mimic personality disorders, so patients should never be prematurely labeled with an Axis II diagnosis. Until the diagnosis is sorted out, however, the type of maladaptive reaction and the apparent personality style of the patient can be extremely useful pieces of data in planning how best to facilitate optimal collaboration with the patient. Thus, careful attention should be paid to managing the doctor–patient relationship by taking into account the idiosyncrasies of the unique individual the doctor is attempting to help. Self-awareness, informal and formal consultation with medical and psychiatric colleagues, and frank and respectful discussion with the patient and family can all be enormously useful in ironing out wrinkles in the fabric of what, at its best, can be a profoundly meaningful relationship through which healing of body, mind, and spirit can occur.

ANNOTATED BIBLIOGRAPHY

Akhtar S: Broken Structures. Northfield, NJ, Jason Aronson, 1992

   A clear, encyclopedic synthesis of the psychoanalytic and descriptive psychiatric
   literatures on severe personality disorders, with a succinct discussion of treatment.

American Psychiatric Association: Diagnostic and Statistical Manual of Mental Disorders, 4th ed:
Primary Care Version. Washington, DC, American Psychiatric Association, 1994

An indispensable, user-friendly distillation for medical practitioners of the nuts and bolts diagnostic methodology of DSM-IV. Extremely helpful for recognition and differential diagnosis of psychiatric disorders by means of very clear and useful algorithms.

Fogel BS: Personality disorders in the medical setting. In Stoudemire A, Fogel BS (eds): Psychiatric Care of the Medical Patient, pp 289–305. New York, Oxford University Press, 1993

A useful review of specific strategies for assessment and management of patients with personality disorders in the medical setting.

Geringer ES, Stern TA: Coping with medical illness: The impact of personality types. Psychosomatics 27:251–261, 1986

Usefully discusses the relationship between specific personality types and reactions to medical illness, as well as the corresponding DSM-III PD diagnoses and some intervention techniques.

Gorlin R, Zucker HD: Physicians' reactions to patients: A key to teaching humanistic medicine. N Engl J Med 308:1059–1063, 1983

A unique and lovely explication and typology of why and how physicians react in particular ways to particular patients and particular clinical situations; bears repeated reading at different stages of professional development.

Groves J: Taking care of the hateful patient. N Engl J Med 298:883–887, 1978

A classic article on managing the treatment relationship with four types of difficult-to-help patients.

Kahana RJ, Bibring GL: Personality types in medical management. In Zinberg NE (ed): Psychiatry and Medical Practice in a General Hospital, pp 108–123. New York, International Universities Press, 1964

The article that laid the foundation for modern approaches to difficult-to-help patients in the medical/surgical setting.

Lipp M: Respectful Treatment: A Practical Handbook of Patient Care, 2nd ed. New York, Elsevier, 1986

A wonderful, highly readable and truly practical handbook that addresses all aspects of the doctor–patient relationship, including how best to communicate and how to work with difficult-to-help patients.

Oldham J: Personality disorders: Current perspectives. JAMA 272:1770–1776, 1994

An up-to-date review for the medical practitioner, with many useful references.

Tumulty PA: What is a clinician and what does he do? N Engl J Med 283:20–24, 1970

A beautifully written classic that exhorts young physicians to develop fully and use their human qualities in order to establish the best kind of healing relationship with their patients.

REFERENCES

Adler G: The hypochondriacal patient. N Engl J Med 304:1394–1396, 1981

Akhtar S: Quest for Answers: A Primer of Understanding and Treating Severe Personality Disorders. Northvale, NJ, Jason Aronson, 1995

American Psychiatric Association: Diagnostic and Statistical Manual of Mental Disorders, 4th ed. Washington, DC, American Psychiatric Association, 1994

Anscombe R: Treating the patient who "can't" versus treating the patient who "won't." Am J Psychotherapy 40:26–35, 1986

Beck AT, Freeman A: Cognitive Therapy of Personality Disorders. New York, Guilford, 1989

Block B, Pristach CA: Diagnosis and management of the paranoid patient. Am Fam Physician 45:2634–2640, 1992

Cohen-Cole SA: The Medical Interview: The Three-Function Approach. St. Louis, Mosby Year Book, 108–145, 1991

Cloninger CR, Svrakic DM, Przybeck TR: A psychobiological model of temperament and character. Arch Gen Psychiatry 50:975–990, 1993

Goldberg RJ: Practical Guide to the Care of the Psychiatric Patient, pp 199–208. St. Louis, Mosby, 1995

Goleman D: Emotional Intelligence. New York, Bantam, 1995, pp 164–185

Gorton GE: A mnemonic device for borderline personality disorder. Am J Psychiatry 153:582, 1996

Gorton GE, Akhtar S: The literature on personality disorders, 1985–88: Trends, issues, and controversies. Hosp Community Psychiatry 41:39–51, 1990

Gorton GE, Akhtar S: The relationship between addiction and personality disorder: Reappraisal and reflections. Integrative Psychiatry 10:185–198, 1994

Gorton GE, Swirsky-Sacchetti T, Sobel R, et al: Neuropsychological dysfunction in personality disorder. In Calev A (ed): Neuropsychological Functions in Psychiatric Disorders. Washington, DC, American Psychiatric Press, in press

Grant WB: The hated patient and his hating attendants. Med J Aust 2:727–729, 1980

Groves JE: Patients with borderline personality disorder. In Cassem NH (ed): Massachusetts General Hospital Handbook of General Hospital Psychiatry, 3rd ed, pp 191–215. St. Louis, Mosby, 1991

Horwitz L, Gabbard GO, Allen JG, et al: Borderline Personality Disorder: Tailoring the Psychotherapy to the Patient. Washington, DC, American Psychiatric Press, 1996

Inderbitzin LB, Furman A, James ME: Psychoanalytic psychology. In Stoudemire A (ed): Human Behavior: An Introduction for Medical Students. Philadelphia, JB Lippincott, 1998

Kavoussi RJ, Coccaro EF: Neurobiological approaches to disorders of personality. In Ratey J (ed): Neuropsychiatry of Personality Disorders, pp 17–34. Cambridge, Blackwell Scientific, 1995

Kegan R: The Evolving Self. Cambridge, Harvard, 1982

Levy ST, Lyle C, Cohen-Cole SA: Masochistic character pathology in medical settings. In Ross JM, Myers WA (eds): New Concepts in Psychoanalytic Psychotherapy, pp 80–93. Washington, DC, American Psychiatric Press, 1988

Linehan MM: Cognitive-Behavioral Treatment of Borderline Personality Disorder. New York, Guilford, 1993

Livesley WJ, Lang KL, Jackson DN, Vernon PA: Genetic and environmental contributions to dimensions of personality disorder. Am J Psychiatry 150:1826–1831, 1993

Longhurst M: Physician self-awareness: The neglected insight. Can Med Assoc J 139:121–124, 1988

Lurie HJ: Practical Management of Emotional Problems in Medicine. New York, Raven Press, 28–42, 1982

McCrae RR, Costa PT: Personality trait structure as a human universal. Am Psychol 52: 509–516, 1997

McDaniel JS, Stoudemire A, Riether AM, et al, Terminal cardiomyopathy, splitting, and borderline personality organization. Gen Hosp Psychiatry 14:277–284, 1992

McDavid JD, Pilkonis PA: The stability of personality disorder diagnoses. J Pers Disord 10:1–15, 1996

McLemore CW, Brokaw DW: Personality disorders as dysfunctional interpersonal behavior. J Pers Disord 1:270–285, 1987

Marin DB, Frances AJ, Widiger T: Personality disorders. In Stoudemire A (ed): Clinical Psychiatry for Medical Students, 2nd ed. Philadelphia, JB Lippincott, 172–195, 1994

Mayou R, Sharpe M: Patients whom doctors find difficult to help. Psychosomatics 36:323–325, 1995

Meissner WW: Theories of personality and psychopathology: Classical psychoanalysis. In Kaplan HI, Sadock BJ (eds): Comprehensive Textbook of Psychiatry, 4th ed, vol 1. Baltimore, Williams & Wilkins, 1985

Merikangas KR, Weissman MM: Epidemiology of DSM-III Axis II personality disorders. In Frances AJ, Hales RE (eds): American Psychiatric Association Annual Review, vol 5, pp 258–278. Washington, DC, American Psychiatric Press, 1986

Millon T, Davis R: Disorders of Personality: DSM-IV and Beyond, 2nd ed. New York, John Wiley, 1996

Nakao K, Gunderson JG, Phillips KA: Functional impairment in personality disorders. J Pers Disord 6:24–33, 1992

Ness DE, Ende J: Denial in the medical interview: Recognition and management. J Am Med Assoc 272: 1771–1781

Neubauer PB, Neubauer A: Nature's Thumbprint: The New Genetics of Personality. New York, Addison-Wesley, 1990

Peabody F: The care of the patient. J Am Med Assoc 88: 882, 1927

Perry S, Viederman M: Management of emotional reactions to acute medical illness. Med Clin North Am 65:3–14, 1981

Ratey J (ed): Neuropsychiatry of Personality Disorders. Cambridge, Blackwell Scientific, 1995

Robins L, Regier D: Psychiatric Disorders in America: The Epidemiologic Catchment Area Study. New York, Free Press, 1991

Schwenk TL, Romano SE: Managing the difficult physician-patient relationship. Am Fam Physician 46:1503–1509, 1992

Searight HR: Borderline personality disorder: Diagnosis and management in primary care. J Fam Pract 34: 605–612, 1992

Stern TA, Prager LM, Cremens MC: Autognosis rounds for medical house staff. Psychosomatics 34:1–7, 1993

Stone MM: Abnormalities of Personality. New York, WW Norton, 1993

Stoudemire A: Human Behavior: An Introduction for Medical Students, 3rd ed. Philadelphia, Lippincott–Raven Publishers, 1998

Stoudemire A (ed): Psychological Factors Affecting Medical Conditions. Washington, DC, American Psychiatric Press, 1995

Stoudemire A, Thompson TL II: The borderline personality in the medical setting. Ann Int Med 96:76–79, 1982

Vaillant G: Sociopathy as a human process. Arch Gen Psychiatry 32:178–183, 1975

Vaillant G: Adaptation to Life. Boston, Little Brown, 1977

Widiger T, Sanderson CJ: Personality Disorders. In Tasman A, Kay J, Lieberman JA (eds): Psychiatry, vol 2, pp 1291–1317. Philadelphia, WB Saunders, 1997

Zuckerman M: Psychobiology of Personality. New York, Cambridge University, 1991

7 *Mood Disorders*

Emile D. Risby, Scott VanSant, and Alan Stoudemire

The *mood disorders* are a heterogeneous group of clinical syndromes with a disturbance in mood as their predominant feature. Although a mood disorder generally involves varying degrees of depression, elation, or irritability, the presence of an altered mood state by itself is usually not sufficient to warrant a diagnosis of a mood disorder. A formal diagnosis of a mood disorder can only be made if the individual develops significant *functional impairment* as a result of the mood disturbance and/or its associated symptoms. Currently, the *Diagnostic and Statistical Manual of Mental Disorders-IV* (DSM-IV; American Psychiatric Association, 1994) provides the most widely used criteria for diagnosing psychiatric illnesses in the United States (see Chapter 1).

The mood disorders themselves are divided into the depressive disorders (which include Major Depressive Disorder, Dysthymic Disorder, and Depressive Disorder Not Otherwise Specified) and the bipolar disorders (which include Bipolar I Disorder, Bipolar II Disorder, Cyclothymic Disorder, and Bipolar Disorder Not Otherwise Specified). If a clinically significant primary mood disturbance occurs that does not meet the diagnostic criteria for a depressive disorder or a bipolar disorder, then the diagnosis of Mood Disorder Not Otherwise Specified can be applied. For clinically significant mood disturbances secondary to the *physiological* effects of a medical condition, or secondary to an ingested substance (i.e., medication or illegal drug), the diagnosis of Mood Disorder Due to a General Medical Condition or Substance-Induced Mood Disorder should be applied (Table 7–1). In addition to subtyping the various mood disorders, the DSM-IV also provides for the designation of a number of "specifiers" that further describes the mood disorder's clinical characteristics and longitudinal course.

A recent study estimates that the annual cost of mood disorders in the United States is about $43 billion. Direct costs are estimated to be $12 billion a year. Indirect costs are estimated to be $31 billion a year, of which $8 billion is due to premature death and $23 billion to absenteeism and lost productivity in the workplace. These estimates are felt to be conservative and include the costs for Major Depression, Bipolar Disorder, and Dysthymia, with Major Depression accounting for over 85% of the total cost (Finkelstein et al, 1996; Greenburg et al, 1993; Hall and Wise, 1995).

MOOD EPISODES

Major Depressive Episode

The word *depression* is often used to describe an array of conditions, such as feelings of demoralization, disappointment, or transient psychological reactions to an injury or loss. In addition, the complaint of "depression" can be seen in almost every psychiatric disorder. A major depressive episode however, is a *syndrome* that *usually* includes the presence of a depressed mood plus other associated symptoms such as an appetite disturbance, sleep disturbance, psychomotor disturbance, decreased energy, decreased libido, feelings of worthlessness or guilt, difficulty with concentration and memory, and thoughts of death or suicide (Weissman and Klerman 1992; Preskorn and Burke, 1992). The diagnostic criteria for a Major Depressive Episode are listed in Table 7–2.

The hallmarks of a Major Depressive Episode are a subjective sense of dysphoria (sadness) and a loss of interest or pleasure in all activities and pastimes that were previously enjoyed (anhedonia). Depressed individuals

---

Table 7–1 **Mood Disorders**

Depressive Disorders
Major Depressive Disorder
Dysthymic Disorder
Depressive Disorder NOS

Bipolar Disorders
Bipolar I Disorder
Bipolar II Disorder
Cyclothymic Disorder
Bipolar Disorder NOS

Secondary Mood Disorders
Mood Disorder Due to a General Medical Condition
Substance-Induced Mood Disorder

Table 7–2 **Key Features of Major Depressive Episodes***

At least a 2-week period of maladaptive functioning that is a clear change from previous levels of functioning. At least five of the following symptoms must be present during that 2-week period, one of which must be a or b:

   a. depressed mood
   b. inability to experience pleasure or markedly diminished interest in pleasurable activities
   c. appetite disturbance with weight change (change >5% of body weight within 1 month)
   d. sleep disturbance
   e. psychomotor disturbance
   f. fatigue or loss of energy
   g. feelings of worthlessness or excessive or inappropriate guilt
   h. diminished ability to concentrate or indecisiveness
   i. recurrent thoughts of death or suicidal ideations

The mood disturbance causes marked distress and or significant impairment in social or occupational functioning.

There is no evidence of a physical or substance-included etiology for the patient's symptoms or presence of another major mental disorder that accounts for the patient's depressive symptoms.

* Summarized from DSM-IV. See DSM-IV (American Psychiatric Association, 1994) for specific diagnostic criteria.

often feel discouraged, defeated, helpless, hopeless, and unable to cope with the stresses of everyday life. Severely depressed individuals may find it impossible to motivate themselves to carry out even the most common day-to-day tasks. Physical activity may be either decreased (psychomotor retardation) or purposelessly increased (psychomotor agitation). Depressed patients may begin to think of themselves in negative terms, feel like failures, or feel that their families would be better off without them. The thought processes of some severely depressed people may become so distorted that their thinking becomes delusional and psychotic. Clearly, major depression is a serious and often disabling psychiatric disorder.

Although a depressed mood is frequently the most common complaint in depressed patients, a subjective sense of depression may not be present in every patient who has a major depressive episode. Elderly patients in particular may complain of anxiety, irritability, weakness, or multiple somatic complaints, rather than verbalize complaints of depression per se. Somatic symptoms of depression include pain syndromes (headaches, backaches), gastrointestinal complaints, neurological complaints (dizziness, numbness), and general fatigue and lethargy. It is important to remember that major depression may present with somatic symptoms as the predominant complaint (see below: Diagnosis and Treatment of Mood Disorders in Medical Settings).

After a diagnosis of depression has been made, the clinician should further characterize the syndrome using the specifiers of the DSM-IV. Specify if this is the first or a recurrent episode of depression. Further specify the severity of the episode and the presence of psychotic, melancholic, catatonic, or "atypical" features. *Melancholic* depressions account for 40 to 60% of all hospitalizations for depression (Klerman, 1984) and are characterized by *anhedonia* (lack of interest in life or the inability to experience life as pleasureable), excessive or inappropriate guilt, early morning awakening, anorexia, psychomotor disturbance, and diurnal variation in mood. The depressed melancholic patient may appear frantic, fearful, agitated, or alternately completely passive and withdrawn.

Psychotic depressions are characterized by the presence of delusions and/or hallucinations. Studies suggest that approximately 10 to 25% of patients hospitalized for major depression, especially geriatric patients, have psychotic symptoms (Schatzberg, 1992).

Atypical depressions denote neurovegetative symptoms that are generally opposite of what is seen in melancholia, such as hypersomnia, hyperphagia (sometimes with carbohydrate craving), mood reactivity (mood changes with environmental circumstances), plus a long-standing pattern of interpersonal rejection sensitivity. Patients with atypical depressions are also frequently reported to have an anxious or irritable mood rather than dysphoria (reviewed by Preskorn and Burke, 1992). These various subtypes of depression may have preferential responses to different treatment modalities. Thus identification of these subtypes can aid the clinician in determining the most appropriate treatment plan for the patient.

The prognoses of many diseases are worst among depressed patients (Simon et al, 1995, Von Korff et al, 1992) and depression may lead to significant psychosocial morbidity with diminished functioning in occupational or social roles (Agency for Health Care Policy and Research, 1993a). In the 15 months after the diagnosis of depression, mortality rates among affected patients are four times higher than in age-matched control subjects. Nearly 60% of all suicides are related to major depression, and 15% of depressed persons admitted to a psychiatric hospital eventually commit suicide (Agency for Health Care Policy and Research, 1993b).

Manic Episode

Mania is a mood disturbance characterized by a distinct period of abnormally elevated, expansive, or irritable mood. To diagnose a Manic Episode, in addition to the mood disturbance, a minimum of three associated symptoms (four associated symptoms if the primary mood disturbance is irritability) such as hyperactivity, pressured speech, racing thoughts, inflated self-esteem, decreased need for sleep, distractibility, and excessive involvement in potentially dangerous activity, must also be present. The manic patient may be hyperverbal, hyperactive, overconfident, adventuresome, disruptive, hostile, argumentative, and irrational. Speech is usually loud and/or rapid with circumstantial or tangential associations. Almost invariably there is a decreased need for sleep. Emotional liability (mood shifting from happy to irritable with little provocation) is frequently seen. Although not part of the diagnostic criteria, psychotic symptoms such as delusions and hallucinations may be seen in acutely manic patients and are not uncommon. Manic patients may be very paranoid. The mood disturbance and its associated symptoms must be present for at least 1 week (Table 7–3).

When euphoric, manics may be quite entertaining; however, angry and irritable manics are notorious for being verbally abusive and at times physically aggressive. The behavior of manic patients is usually so bizarre and their judgment is so impaired that they usually pose a danger to themselves or others. Unfortunately, the manic patient may have no insight into the severity of his condition. Manic patients are often forced into treatment by family or by the legal system. Mania is a psychiatric emergency often leading to involuntary hospitalization of the manic patient.

Mixed Episode

Some patients will develop symptoms meeting the diagnostic criteria for both a manic episode and a depressive episode at the *same time*. Traditionally, depression and mania were viewed as two opposite mood states in which the

---

Table 7–3 **Key Features of Bipolar Disorder: Manic Episode***

A distinct period of abnormally and persistently elevated, expansive, or irritable mood, lasting at least 1 week, of sufficient severity to cause marked impairment in social or occupational functioning.
During the period of the mood disturbance, at least three of the following (four if the mood is primarily irritable) symptoms are also present:
  a. gradiosity
  b. deceased need for sleep
  c. hyperverbal or pressured speech
  d. flight of ideas or racing thoughts
  e. distractibility
  f. increase in goal-directed activity or psychomotor agitation
  g. excessive involvement in pleasurable activities that have a high potential for painful consequences
There is no evidence of a physical or substance-induced etiology or the presence of another major mental disorder to account for the patient's symptoms.

* Summarized from DSM-IV. See DSM-IV (American Psychiatric Association, 1994) for specific diagnostic criteria.

---

explanation for the pathophysiology of one mood state would seem to preclude the existence of the other. It is now clear that both depression and mania can occur in the same individual at the same time. If the patient meets diagnostic criteria for both mania and depression every day for at least a 1-week period, the patient is diagnosed as being in a mixed state, sometimes called dysphoric or mixed mania. In mixed episodes, irritability is usually the predominant mood state. These mixed episodes tend to be more difficult to treat than either pure mania or pure depression. Like pure mania, a mixed episode is a psychiatric emergency. These patients are so emotionally unstable that they are at increased risk for self-injurious and dangerous behavior. Patients with mixed episodes tend to be female, have a higher lithium nonresponse rate, and tend to respond best when anticonvulsants are added to their medication regiment (McElroy et al, 1992).

Hypomanic Episode

In hypomania, many of the same features of mania are present but the mood disturbance is less severe. At times it may be difficult to differentiate severe hypomania from mania (Table 7–4). In mania, the mood disturbance is severe and causes marked impairment in social or occupational functioning. A manic-like syndrome not meeting this functional disability criteria should be called hypomania. Remember, if there are psychotic symptoms or if there is marked impairment in normal functioning such that hospitalization is necessary, the condition has progressed beyond hypomania into full-blown mania.

Table 7–4 **Key Features of Hypomanic Episodes***

A distinct period of sustained elevated, expansive, or irritable mood, lasting for at least 4 days, that is clearly different from the individual's nondepressed mood, yet does not cause marked impairment in social or occupational functioning such as in acute mania.

During the mood disturbance, at least three of the following symptoms are also present to a significant degree:
  a. inflated self-esteem or grandiosity
  b. decreased need for sleep
  c. more talkative than usual
  d. flight of ideas or racing thoughts
  e. distractibility
  f. increase in goal-directed activity or psychomotor agitation
  g. excessive involvement in pleasurable activities that have a high potential for painful consequences

The episode is not due to a physical or substance-induced etiology.

* Summarized from DSM-IV. See DSM-IV (American Psychiatric Association, 1994) for specific diagnostic criteria.

Epidemiology of Mood Disorders

Clearly, the mood disorders are a major public health concern. Different epidemiological studies have given various prevalence rates for these disorders. The 1980 Epidemiologic Catchment Area (ECA) Study, initiated by the National Institute of Mental Health, reported that the community-based lifetime prevalence rates for the major mood disorders in the United States are 3.5 to 5.8% for major depression, 2.1 to 4.7% for dysthymia, and 0.7 to 1.6% for bipolar disorders, (Robins and Regier, 1991; see below for definition of the major mood disorders). More recent data from the National Comorbidity Survey (NCS), however, suggest higher rates of depressive disorders than were previously reported. The NCS revealed that the lifetime prevalence of depressive disorders is 21 to 24% in women and 12 to 15% in men (Kessler et al, 1994; Regier et al, 1993). The NCS report noted that 13% of women and 8% of men are depressed in any 1-year period. The prevalence of dysthymia was also higher in the NCS report, with a lifetime prevalence rate of 8% in women and 5% in men and an annual prevalence rate of 3% for women and 2% for men (Kessler et al, 1994). While the prevalence of bipolar disorders is equal between sexes, both the ECA and the NCS found higher prevalence rates of depressive disorders in women.

Heritability and Mood Disorders

Genetic factors are undoubtedly important in the etiology of the major mood disorders. The relative risk of major depression is two to five times greater in the relatives of depressed patients than in the relatives of controls. The genetic evidence is even stronger for bipolar than for unipolar depression. First-degree relatives (parents, siblings, and offspring) of patients with bipolar disorders have been reported to be at least 24 times more likely to develop bipolar illness than relatives of control subjects. The incidence of both bipolar illness and unipolar depression is much higher in first-degree relatives of patients with bipolar illness than in the general population. First-degree relatives of patients with unipolar illness, on the other hand, have an increase only in the incidence of unipolar depression (Gold et al, 1988a; Willner, 1985).

Since familial aggregation may reflect a shared environmental precipitant, the increased incidence of mood disorders within families does not in itself establish that these illness are hereditary. Twin and adoption studies have attempted to address this issue. Twin studies compare the concordance rate for an illness in pairs of monozygotic twins with the rate of the illness in dizygotic twins and assume that both twins are exposed to the same environment. Due to identical genes, one would expect monozygotic twins to show a greater concordance for hereditary conditions than dizygotic twins. Twin studies have reported the concordance rate for bipolar illness to be approximately 79% in monozygotic twins, but only 19% in dizygotic twins. Adoption studies attempt to separate the contributions of nature and nurture by studying children raised away from their biological parents. Adoption studies have shown a greater prevalence of mood disorders among biological relatives of patients with bipolar illness, but not in adoptive relatives. Thus, there appears to be a strong genetic predisposition to the development of mood disorders, especially bipolar disorders. Advances in molecular genetic strategies are expected to reveal much more about the inheritance of mood disorders. Nonetheless, the most likely etiology of most mood disorders is multifactorial, with expression of the illness being secondary to a combination of various heredity traits and environmental factors (Berrettini, 1995; Pardes et al, 1989; Table 7–5).

Neurobiology of Mood Disorders

Sleep Abnormalities in Mood Disorders

The abnormal sleep of depressed patients was one of the earliest findings in biological psychiatry. Sleep may be monitored electroencephalographically and is divided into rapid eye movement (REM) and non-REM sleep (stages 1 to 4). The first REM period usually begins after a period of 70 to 100 minutes of non-REM sleep, followed by another three to five REM periods that usually occur in the latter part of the night. The REM periods generally increase in length as the night progresses (Gold et al, 1988b; see Chapter 22).

A number of sleep abnormalities distinguish endogenous ("biological") depressives from nonendogenous (reactive, situational, or characterological) depressives and normal subjects. Endogenous depressives tend to have prolonged sleep latency (the period of time between going to bed and falling asleep), shortened REM latency (the period of time from the onset of sleep to the first REM period), increased wakefulness, decreased arousal threshold, early morning awakening, and reduced stage 3 and 4 sleep (Coble et al, 1976; Gillin et al, 1979).

Table 7–5 **Genetics in Mood Disorders**

1. The relative risk of major depression is two to five times greater in the relatives of depressed patients than in the relatives of controls.
2. First-degree relatives of patients with bipolar illness are reported to be at least 24 times more likely to develop bipolar illness than relatives of control subjects.
3. The incidence of both bipolar illness and unipolar depression is much higher in first-degree relatives of patients with bipolar illness than in the general population.
4. The concordance rate for bipolar illness is approximately 19% in dizygotic twins but 79% in monozygotic twins
5. Adoption studies have shown a greater prevalence of mood disorders among biological relatives of patients with bipolar illness but not in their adoptive relatives.

Table 7–6 **Sleep Abnormalities in Depression**

Non-REM Changes in Depression
1. Prolonged sleep latency (the period of time between going to bed and falling asleep)
2. Shortened REM latency (the period of time from the onset of sleep to the first REM period)
3. Increased wakefulness
4. Decreased arousal threshold
5. Early morning awakening
6. Reduced stages 3 and 4 sleep

REM Sleep Changes in Depression
1. Shorter REM latency (i.e., 30 to 60 minutes instead of the normal average of 60–90 minutes)
2. A redistribution of REM sleep to the first half of the night, rather than the second half

With respect to REM sleep, in addition to a shorter REM latency (i.e., 30 to 60 minutes instead of 90 minutes), depressed patients may have a redistribution of REM sleep with most of the REM occurring in the first half of the night, rather than the second half (Reynolds and Kupfer, 1987; Table 7–6). These abnormal REM latencies tend to normalize with clinical recovery from depression (Kupfer and Thase, 1983).

Neuroendocrine Abnormalities in Mood Disorders

Secretion of hypothalamic hormones is modulated by many of the same neurotransmitters that are felt to be involved in the pathophysiology of mood disorders. Thus, neuroendocrine abnormalities reported in patients with mood disorders may reflect central neurotransmitter dysfunction (Table 7–7).

One of the most frequently reported biological abnormalities in patients with major depression is hyperactivity of the hypothalamic-pituitary-adrenal (HPA) axis. There are numerous reports documenting HPA axis hyperactivity in drug-free unipolar depressed and bipolar depressed patients (reviewed

Table 7–7 **Neuroendocrine Abnormalities in Depression**

1. Hyperactivity of the hypothalamic-pituitary-adrenal (HPA) axis, resulting in elevated plasma cortisol levels, nonsuppression of cortisol following dexamethasone (DST), hypersecretion of corticotrophin-releasing factor.
2. *Blunting** of the normally expected increase in plasma concentrations of thyroid stimulating hormone (TSH) following an infusion of thyrotropin-releasing hormone (TRH).
3. *Blunting* of the normally expected increase in plasma growth hormone induced by alpha-2 adrenergic receptor agonist stimulation.
4. *Blunting* of serotonin-mediated increases in plasma prolactin.

* The term "blunting" refers to deceased physiological responsiveness.

by Nathan et al, 1995). The dexamethasone suppression test (DST) is histor-ically the test most frequently used by clinicians to access the HPA axis (Arana et al, 1985). Dexamethasone is a synthetic corticosteroid that, when given orally, usually suppresses plasma adrenocorticotropic hormone (ACTH) and cortisol levels for at least 24 hours. In the evaluation of depres-sion, the DST is performed by giving 1 mg dexamethasone at 2300 hours and then drawing plasma cortisol levels at 1600 and 2300 hours the next day. Depressed patients may initially show a normal suppression of blood cortisol (below 5 mg/dl) following dexamethasone, but often escape from suppression significantly earlier than normal. Therefore, they may not show suppression when tested 17 to 24 hours later. This nonsuppression of cortisol 24 hours fol-lowing administration of dexamethasone appears to be more common in the melancholic subgroup (Carroll, 1982). It has also been observed that a patient who appears to have recovered from depression but fails to suppress cortisol after dexamethasone administration may be at higher risk for relapse (Holsboer et al, 1982). Unfortunately, nonsuppression is not specific or sen-sitive for depression, and there may be many false-positive, as well as false-negative results. Nonetheless, nonsuppression of the DST may be a helpful variable to consider when faced with difficult diagnostic and/or treatment decisions. DST nonsuppression, and many other measures of HPA axis hyper-activity in depressed patients, such as hypercortisolemia, hypersecretion of corticotrophin-releasing factor (CRF), blunting of the ACTH response to CRF, and adrenal gland hypertrophy, shift toward normal with resolution of the depressive episode (reviewed by Nathan et al, 1995).

Abnormalities in the hypothalamic-pituitary-thyroid axis have also been reported in both unipolar depressed and bipolar patients. Elevated concen-trations of cerebrospinal fluid (CSF) and thyrotropin-releasing hormone (TRH; reviewed by Nathan et al, 1995) and low levels of transthyretin, the thyroid transport globulin in the CSF, have been reported in depressed patients (Hatterer et al, 1993). Several studies have demonstrated that the normally expected increase in plasma concentrations of thyroid-stimulating hormone (TSH) following an infusion of TRH is blunted in approximately 25% of patients with major depression and tends to normalize with clinical recov-ery. However, some depressed patients, especially bipolar patients, may have an exaggerated TSH response to TRH (Loosen and Prange, 1982). It is unclear whether this exaggerated response identifies a unique neuro-endocrine abnormality in a subset of patients or whether these patients have primary thyroid disease (i.e., hypothyroidism) inducing or aggravating the mood disorder.

Other neuroendocrine abnormalities reported in depressed patients are blunting of the increase in plasma growth hormone induced by the alpha-2 adrenergic receptor agonist stimulation (reviewed by Siever et al, 1992; Willner, 1985) and blunting in the response of serotonin-mediated increases in plasma prolactin (reviewed by Lichtenberg et al, 1992; Shapira et al, 1992;

Table 7–7). It should be emphasized that none of these neuroendocrine abnormalities are true "biological markers" for depression, as many patients with a diagnosis of depression will have normal neuroendocrine measures. These abnormalities, found inconsistently, nevertheless point to some type of serious neuroendocrine dysfunction in major depression.

Neurotransmitter Hypothesis of Mood Disorders

Most of the biological literature on mood disorders has traditionally focused on the role of the classic monoamine neurotransmitters norepinephrine (NE), dopamine (DA), and serotonin [5-hydroxytryptamine (5-HT)] in the etiology of depression. NE and DA are catecholamines, while 5-HT is an indoleamine. The catecholamines are degraded by two enzymes, monoamine oxidase (MAO) and catechol-O-methyltransferase, which produce a variety of breakdown products. The degradation of 5-HT is simpler, with MAO producing 5-HT's sole breakdown product, 5-hydroxyindoleacetic acid (5-HIAA). The catecholamines and 5-HT are stored in synaptic vesicles and are released into the synapse when a nerve impulse invades the terminal. The major mechanism for clearing the released neurotransmitter from the synapse is presynaptic neuronal reuptake, not enzymatic degradation. Following reuptake, much of the neurotransmitter is recycled into the "functional pool" to be reused by the neuron (Willner, 1985).

Norepinephrine and the Catecholamine Hypothesis

The first major hypothesis to address the biological basis of depression emerged from the observation that approximately 15% of the patients who were treated for hypertension with the biogenic amine-depleting agent reserpine developed depression. Drugs that were known to enhance noradrenergic functioning, such as the MAO inhibitors, amphetamines, and cyclic antidepressants were noted to have antidepressant properties. These observations gave rise to the original catecholamine hypothesis of major depression, which stated that depression resulted from a functional deficit of NE in the central nervous system.

Although initially this theory seemed plausible, additional observations did not fully support the hypothesis. For example, drugs that interfere with noradrenergic transmission or block catecholamine synthesis do not regularly produce depression in most subjects (note that only 15% of reserpine-treated patients got depressed; Willner, 1985). Blockade of monoamine reuptake or MAO inhibition occurs within hours or days after administration of the antidepressant, yet the clinical effects do not usually appear until after 2 to 4 weeks of treatment.

To complicate matters further, attempts to demonstrate abnormalities in NE activity by measuring plasma, urine, and CSF concentrations of NE and its major metabolite, 3-methoxy-4-hydroxy-phenylglycol have produced conflicting data. Decreases, no change, and even increases in these noradrenergic parameters have been reported in depressed subjects (Davis and Bresnahan, 1987; Jimerson et al, 1983; Mass et al, 1987; Redmond et al, 1986; Roy et al, 1985). In short, these findings do not support the belief that depression is secondary to a generalized decrease in noradrenergic function (Table 7–8). Nonetheless, the catecholamine hypothesis has had a major impact on the field of psychiatry and has fostered a cascade of biological investigations into the etiology and treatment of psychiatric illnesses.

Drug-induced behaviors in humans suggest a possible role for the catecholamines in the pathophysiology of mania. The most striking pharmacological data are the consistent findings that direct or indirect NE and DA agonists (those drugs that stimulate noradrenergic or dopaminergic receptors or increase concentrations of these neurotransmitters in the brain, such as amphetamines and cocaine) can induce manic-like syndromes in subjects who do not appear to have an underlying vulnerability to develop a bipolar disorder. While an association between manic-like states in drug-induced hyperadrenergic and hyperdopaminergic conditions is firmly established (Potter et al, 1987), it is unclear whether a similar direct or indirect mechanism is responsible for the clinical symptoms of mania seen in bipolar disorders.

Indoleamine Hypothesis of Depression

Over the past three decades a burgeoning literature has accumulated implicating the importance of central serotonergic neurotransmission in both the pathophysiology of depression and the mechanism of action of antidepressant drugs (Table 7–9). Based on numerous studies, the serotonin system is thought to be functionally deficient in depressed patients. Findings include (1) decreases in brain concentrations of serotonin and decreases in CSF con-

---

Table 7–8 **Nonadrenergic Theory of Depression**

Data Supporting the Theory

1. Approximately 15% of patients treated for hypertension with reserpine develop depression.
2. Drugs that enhance nonadrenergic functioning (such as stimulants) are often found to have some antidepressant properties.

Data Against the Theory

1. Drugs that interfere with noradrenergic transmission, or block catecholamine synthesis, do not regularly produce depression in most subjects.
2. Blockade of norepinephrine reuptake or MAO inhibition by antidepressant drugs occurs within hours or a few days after administration of the antidepressant, but the clinical effects do not usually appear until after 2 to 4 weeks of treatment.
3. Attempts to demonstrate abnormalities in norepinephrine activity by measuring plasma, urine, and cerebrospinal fluid concentrations of norepinephrine and its major metabolite 3-methoxy-4-hydroxy-phenylglycol (MHPG) have produced conflicting data.

Table 7–9 **Data Supporting Serotonin Dysfunction in Major Depression**

1. Decreased concentrations of brain serotonin and CSF 5-HIAA in many depressed patients.
2. Most antidepressant agents have been shown to increase the efficacy of central serotonin neurotransmission.
3. Reduction in both central and peripheral 5-HT reuptake sites has been found in depressed subjects.
4. Neuroendocrine challenges have demonstrated that the postsynaptic serotonin-mediated stimulation of prolactin is blunted in depressed patients.

centrations of 5-HIAA in a sizable subgroup of depressed patients; (2) alterations in both presynaptic and postsynaptic central serotonergic receptors in depressed patients; (3) reduction in both central and peripheral 5-HT reuptake sites in many depressed patients; and (4) increased efficacy of central nervous system (CNS) serotonin neurotransmission by most antidepressant agents.

A subgroup of approximately 40% of depressed patients exhibits low concentrations of brain serotonin and its metabolite 5-HIAA (Gibbons and Davis, 1986). Depressed patients with low CSF concentrations of 5-HIAA are more likely to have attempted suicide than depressives with normal 5-HIAA levels (Asberg and Traskman, 1981; Banki and Arato, 1983). However, low 5-HIAA does not appear to be a phenomenon that accompanies an episode of depression, but rather is a state-independent marker that confers a predisposition to becoming depressed (Banki, 1977). When low CSF levels of 5-HIAA are observed in depressed patients, they usually remain low during periods of remission (Mendels et al, 1972; van Praag and DeHaan, 1979), and bipolar patients have been shown to have low CSF 5-HIAA levels even when they are in their manic phase (Cooper et al, 1972; Mendels et al, 1972).

Further support for the role of 5-HT in the pathophysiology of depression comes from the neuroendocrine literature. Serotonergic systems are involved in the regulation of a variety of neuroendocrine hormones including cortisol, prolactin, and growth hormone; as previously noted, these neuroendocrine measures have been reported to be abnormal in many depressed patients (see section on neuroendocrine abnormalities above). Collectively, the data support the hypothesis that abnormalities in serotonergic neurotransmission are associated with the clinical syndrome of depression.

Beyond the Monoamine Hypothesis

One thing is clear: a simple monoamine hypothesis for the etiology of depression or mania is inadequate. Both NE and 5-HT reuptake inhibitors are effective antidepressants, and both can induce manic symptoms. Apparently, by modifying neuronal activity, all antidepressants and mood stabilizers eventually induce some type of neuronal adaptation at the receptor or postreceptor level that is ultimately responsible for their therapeutic effects.

There are two major classes of neurotransmitter receptors in the brain, ligand-gated channels and G-protein-linked receptors. A ligand-gated channel is an ion channel that opens (gated) when a neurotransmitter binds to the ion channel's receptor, thereby modifying the action potential and thus the excitability of the neuron. G-protein-linked receptors transduce the neurotransmitter's signal into the interior of the cell by activating transmembrane G proteins. These activated G proteins can activate or suppress the generation of intracellular second messengers that regulate multiple biochemical functions within a cell. One of the most important classes of enzymes modified by G-protein-linked receptors are the protein kinases, the enzymes that catalyze protein phosphorylation. All receptor desensitization appears to be secondary to receptor phosphorylation. Phosphorylation also alters the responsiveness of ion channels, regulates enzymes that synthesize neurotransmitters, and controls a diverse number of biological functions within neurons. All of the known noradrenergic and DA receptors, and practically all known 5-HT receptors are G-protein-linked receptors.

Chronic treatment (2 to 3 weeks) with most antidepressants will induce downregulation of central adrenergic and serotonergic receptors (Banerjee et al, 1977; Gonzalez-Heydrich and Peroutka, 1990; Smith et al, 1981; Vetulani et al, 1976). Although we do not know the precise mechanism of action by which antidepressant drugs work, receptor downregulation tells us that various internal proteins have been modified through phosphorylation, and the neurons are now in an adapted state (Hyman, 1995). Although the mood-stabilizing drugs have not been shown to induce receptor downregulation, mood-stabilizing drugs in some way stabilize neuronal functioning to correct and/or prevent the pathophysiological activity responsible for the severe mood swings seen in bipolar disorders.

In summary, the catecholamines were initially identified as the major neurotransmitters underlying the pathophysiology of depression and mania. Following the introduction of the serotonin-reuptake inhibitors, the role of serotonin in the etiology of mood disorders and many other psychiatric conditions has taken center stage. Clearly, however, a simple monoamine hypothesis for the mood disorders is scientifically inadequate. Recent research has shifted from focusing on prereceptor and receptor activation to postreceptor mechanisms and a host of various intracellular second messenger systems.

Kindling-Sensitization Hypothesis of Mood Disorders

A model that attempts to account for many of the longitudinal features of mood disorders is the neurophysiological *kindling-sensitization* hypothesis advanced by Post and colleagues (Post et al, 1981). In this model, repeated exposures to stress and/or repeated neurochemical and neuroendocrine changes that accompany an episode of depression may sensitize key limbic substrates that integrate affective experiences (e.g., the induction of tearful affect). The potential neurobiological ravages of each new episode of severe depression, coupled with stress-induced or age-related changes, may permanently alter limbic and various central neurotransmitter systems. The resultant progressive sensitization of limbic substrates may account for many of the trends reported in mood disorders, including the predisposition to develop depression as a result of early stressful experiences, the gradual worsening of mood episodes after repeated recurrences, the progressively shorter latency between and episode's onset and its peak severity, the tendency for the frequency of bipolar mood swings to increase, and the gradual attainment of autonomy and spontaneity (lack of obvious stressors). The prophylactic efficacy of the anticonvulsants carbamazepine and valproic acid (which inhibit certain kindled seizures) in bipolar illness lends support to this model (Post, 1992; Thase, 1992).

DEPRESSIVE DISORDERS

Adjustment Disorder With Depressed Mood

Although not formally classified as a mood disorder in DSM-IV, an Adjustment Disorder With Depressed Mood is a frequent clinical depressive syndrome. An adjustment disorder is a psychiatric disorder that occurs following an identifiable psychosocial stressor (such as divorce, job loss, physical illness, natural disaster). The individual's response to that stressor is considered to be extreme or in excess of what would normally be expected or results in significant impairments in the individual's social, occupational, or interpersonal functioning (Table 7–10). It is assumed that the symptoms will remit in time, either when the stressor(s) resolve or when a new level of coping (or adaptation) is reached. Strictly defined, the symptoms should not persist for more than 6 months after termination of the precipitating stressor(s) (American Psychiatric Association, 1994). If the stressor persists for longer than 6 months, the adjustment disorder is specified as chronic, rather than acute. In adjustment disorders with depressed mood, the typical symptoms are sadness, social isolation, difficulty concentrating, preoccupation with stressful events, and sleep and appetite disturbances. Although it is expected to resolve in time, an adjustment disorder with depressed mood is not necessarily an inconsequential condition. Adjustment disorders may cause major disruptions in the patient's life and may be associated with severe dysphoria, despondency, and suicidal ideations.

There is no way to predict who will develop an adjustment disorder in the wake of adverse circumstances. The severity of the adjustment disorder does not always parallel the intensity of the precipitating event. The important factor appears to be the relevance or meaning of the event (stressor) to the individual and the ability of the individual to "cope" or manage the stress. Individuals with poor coping skills or inadequate social supports may be more prone to develop adjustment disorders than those with good coping skills and strong social supports.

Table 7–10 **Diagnostic Criteria for Adjustment Disorders***

A. The development of emotional or behavioral symptoms in response to an identifiable stressor(s) occurring within 3 months of the onset of the stressor(s).
B. These symptoms or behaviors are clinically significant as evidenced by either of the following:
  1. marked distress that is in excess of what would be expected from exposure to the stressor
  2. significant impairment in social or occupational (academic) functioning
C. The stress-related disturbance does not meet the criteria for another specific Axis I disorder and is not merely an exacerbation of a preexisting Axis I or Axis II disorder.
D. The symptoms do not represent bereavement.
E. Once the stressor (or its consequences) has terminated, the symptoms do not persist for more than an additional 6 months.
Specify if: **Acute:** if the disturbance lasts less than 6 months or
  Chronic: if the disturbance lasts for 6 months or longer.
Adjustment Disorders are coded based on the subtype, which is selected according to the predominant symptoms. The specific stressor(s) can be specified on Axis IV—with Depressed Mood; with Anxiety; with Mixed Anxiety and Depressed Mood; with Disturbance of Conduct; with Mixed Disturbance of Emotions and Conduct; unspecified.

* May present primarily as anxiety, depression, or mixed features. See DSM-IV (American Psychiatric Association, 1994) for specific diagnostic criteria.

In general, adjustment disorders with depressed mood are relatively transient and are not accompanied by the major cognitive symptoms seen in major depressions (see below). For example, patients with adjustment disorders feel bad about their situation, but do not necessarily feel bad about themselves. In addition, although adjustment disorders can generally be managed by the primary care provider, clergy, friend, or family member, the development of extreme withdrawal, hopelessness, suicidal ideations, or failure to improve as circumstances improve, is a clear indication for psychiatric referral. Treatment of adjustment disorders includes supportive psychotherapy, crisis-orientated psychosocial interventions, and occasionally time-limited pharmacotherapy to alleviate specific target symptoms (e.g., insomnia). Note that depressed mood is only one of the six types of maladaptive adjustment responses that may occur in response to a psychosocial stressor as defined by the DSM-IV. These episodes can nevertheless be extremely serious and result in suicide.

Major Depressive Disorder

The essential feature of a Major Depressive Disorder is the development of one or more major depressive episodes, without a history of mania or hypomania (American Psychiatric Association, 1994). The course or natural history of major depressive disorder is quite variable. While some will have only a single episode of depression with full recovery, many depressed patients will have multiple episodes. Some will have isolated episodes separated by many years of normal functioning; others will have clusters of episodes followed by periods of remission; while others will have increasingly frequent episodes as they grow older (American Psychiatric Association, 1993).

The National Institute of Mental Health (NIMH) Collaborative Program on the Psychobiology of Depression Study (Collaborative Depression Study [CDS]) reported that although most patients recovered following therapy, one-fourth of the patients who recovered during the first year of follow-up had relapses within 12 weeks of recovery. Fifty to 95% of individuals who suffer a major depressive episode will have multiple episodes (Goodwin and Jamison, 1990; NIMH Consensus Development Panel, 1985; Zis and Goodwin, 1979). The one very strong factor that predicted relapse was a history of three or more previous episodes of major depression (Keller and Baker, 1992). The risk of recurrence is approximately 70% after two depressive episodes and 90% after three episodes (Agency for Health Care Policy and Research, 1993a). Corollary clinical observations indicate that psychosocial stressors are often (but not always) identifiable before the first few affective episodes but become less contributory with later episodes. Hence, as the illness evolves, relapses appear to be more likely to occur independently of life events (reviewed by Gold et al, 1988a,b).

Depression used to be viewed as an episodic, time-limited condition with full interepisode recovery. Untreated major depressions resolve spontaneously approximately 40% of the time within 6 months to 1 year. In 20 to 30% of cases, resolution is incomplete, and subclinical depression may persist between episodes or chronically for years (Rush et al, 1991). In the remaining 40% of persons with major depression, symptoms continue longer than 1 year (DSM-IV). Furthermore, researchers and clinicians have become increasingly aware that some major depressions can become chronic conditions. In the ECA study, 20% of subjects diagnosed with depression on initial assessment were still depressed 1 year later (Katon and Schulberg, 1992). Data from the Collaborative Depression Study (Coryell et al, 1990; Keller et al, 1982a,b, 1984, 1986) revealed that 50% of the patients *had not* recovered from their major depressive episode after 1 year, and 21% of patients continued to suffer from depression for longer than 2 years. The Agency for Health Care Policy and Research (1993a) reported that 40% of individuals with major depression will continue to be depressed after 1 year, and an additional 17%, while improved, will continue to have significant residual symptoms. In short, every major epidemiological study reports high rates of chronicity and relapse in patients with major depression. It should be noted, however, that in the ECA study, a substantial number of patients who had poor outcomes (chronic or recurrent episodes) were not receiving adequate antidepressant therapy (Keller at al, 1982a).

Recognition of depression in geriatric populations may be more difficult than in nongeriatric populations. Depressed elderly persons are more apt to report somatic symptoms or anxiety and may actually deny feeling depressed. According to the ECA study, depressive symptoms occur in approximately 15% of community residents over 65 years of age (NIH Consensus Development Panel on Depression, 1992). In the elderly, both clinicians and patients may incorrectly assume that some depressive symptoms are expected with aging. For example, because of declining physical abilities, medical illnesses, and social and economic difficulties, it is easy to conclude that depression is a normal consequence of these problems. Remember that many of these problems may be a consequence of depression (or at least made worst by depression) rather than being the cause of depression per se. Though the elderly make up only 12% of the U.S. population, they account for 25% of U.S. suicides each year (De Leo and Diekstra, 1990). Clearly depression is a major problem in the elderly. All elderly depressed patients should be treated because the benefits of treatment greatly outweigh the risk of treatment.

A major depressive episode is a *syndrome* characterized by a mood disturbance, plus a variety of cognitive, psychological, somatic, and "vegetative" disturbances, which causes *significant impairments* in the individual's ability to function. While there are a variety of symptoms associated with the syndrome of depression, none (not even the compliant of "feeling depressed") is essential for the diagnosis! Depression is associated with high rates of relapse, chronicity, psychosocial and physical impairment, mortality, and morbidity.

Psychosocial Theories of Depression

A number of variables appear to put a person "at increased risk" for developing depression. These variables include recent stressors, the individual's social support system, history of early parental loss, gender, and family history of depression. Most clinicians agree that the likelihood of having an episode of depression is greatly increased following stressful "life events." In a study of nonmelancholic patients with recurrent depression, 73% of the depressive episodes were related to a distressing life event (Brown et al, 1994). However, the relationship between life events and depression is not consistent. While many episodes of depression occur during times of stress, only a minority of persons encountering such difficulties will develop a major depressive episode, suggesting that there are underlying biological vulnerability factors in those that do (Belsher and Costello, 1988).

The absence of a positive social support system predisposes an individual to depression (Aneshensel and Stone, 1982; Williams et al, 1981), and the belief that a solid social support system contributes to psychological well-being is generally well accepted. The status of childhood loss as a factor predisposing to depression is controversial. A review by Lloyd (1980) that specifically considered the effects of childhood bereavement concluded that parental loss in childhood, particularly maternal loss, was associated with a two- to threefold increase in the likelihood of developing an adult depression. Subsequent research, however, has indicated that the quality of home life in which the parent loss occurred is the most critical variable in determining vulnerability to psychiatric illness in later life (Brier et al, 1988).

In regard to gender and depression, women are generally reported to have a two- to threefold higher rate of depression than men (Boyd and Weissman, 1981; Hirschfeld and Cross, 1982). The reasons for this sex difference are not entirely clear. Some investigators have suggested that social or hormonal factors may contribute to the higher incidence of depression in women. Although there does not appear to be any single personality trait that is common among all depressives, one psychological attribute that does appear to predispose to depression is introversion, a personality trait associated with a decrease in social contacts and support (Akiskal et al, 1983).

According to *cognitive learning theories,* depressed patients have a cognitive style that focuses on what is wrong or negative, rather than what is right or positive. Beck (1974) described a cognitive triad in depression consisting of a person's (1) negative view of self, (2) negative interpretation of experiences, and (3) negative expectation of the future. Thus depression is secondary to negative cognitive constructs. According to Beck's cognitive theory, once a state of depression is established, information processing is biased in such a negative way that the negative mood is reinforced and maintained. Depressed patients tend to underestimate positives, overestimate negatives, and recall more unpleasant memories, and to have a decreased ability to experience pleasure and an increased sensitivity to adverse events. Low self-esteem may lead the depressed individual to see himself or herself as being unworthy of pleasure, praise, or reward. While Beck's model may explain the etiology of depressive symptoms in many patients with dysthymia or mild-to-moderate depressions, it does not account for the biological and autonomous nature of many severe, especially melancholic, major depressive episodes.

With 10 to 14 million people in the United States suffering from depression each year, it is one of the most common of the major psychiatric disorders (Keller and Hanks 1994). Even though most patients recover from a major depressive episode, there is a high probability of recurrence, and each new episode carries renewed risks of chronicity, psychosocial impairment, and suicide (Thase, 1992).

Dysthymic Disorder

The essential feature of Dysthymic Disorder is a chronically depressed mood (or possibly an irritable mood in children or adolescents) present for most of the day and occurring on more days than not, for at least 2 years (1 year for children or adolescents); however, the severity of the mood disturbance does not meet the criteria for major depression (see above). Brief periods of normal mood may be present within the 2-year diagnostic period for adults, but should not have lasted more than 2 months. In addition to a depressed mood, there must be some associated symptoms, such as low self-esteem, feelings of inadequacy, hopelessness, pessimism or guilt, social with-drawal, decreased productivity, low energy, and difficulty with concentration and memory (Table 7–11). The diagnosis is not made if there is clear evidence of a Major Depressive Episode during the first 2 years of the disturbance, if the disturbance is superimposed on another psychiatric disorder, or if it is judged to be induced by a concurrent medical problem or by medications. Dysthymia is designated as either early or late onset, based on the development of the illness before or after age 21 (American Psychiatric Association, 1994). After meeting diagnostic criteria for dysthymia (2 years of depressed mood), 60% of patients will continue to be dysthymic 1 year later, and it appears that approximately 26% will remain indefinitely dysthymic (Agency for Health Care Policy and Research, 1993a).

The differentiation of dysthymia from chronic major depression can be difficult (Table 7–12). In dysthymia the depressed mood is usually mild to moderate in severity, is chronic (at least 2 years), often without a clear onset,

Table 7–11 **Diagnostic Criteria for Dysthymic Disorder***

A. Depressed mood for most of the day, for more days than not, as indicated either by subjective account or observation by others, for at least 2 years. **Note:** In children and adolescents, mood can be irritable and duration must be at least 1 year.

B. Presence, while depressed, of two (or more) of the following: (1) poor appetite or overeating; (2) insomnia of hypersomnia; (3) low energy or fatigue; (4) low self-esteem; (5) poor concentration or difficulty making decisions; (6) feelings of hopelessness.

C. During the 2-year period (1 year for children or adolescents) of the disturbance, the person has never been without the symptoms in Criteria A and B for more than 2 months at a time.

D. No Major Depressive Episode has been present during the first 2 years of the disturbance (1 year for children and adolescents), i.e., the disturbance is not better accounted for by chronic Major Depressive Disorder, or Major Depressive Disorder, In Partial Remission.

E. There has never been a Manic Episode, a Mixed Episode, or a Hypomanic Episode, and criteria have never been met for Cyclothmic Disorder.

F. The disturbance does not occur exclusively during the course of a chronic Psychotic Disorder, such as Schizophrenia or Delusional Disorder.

G. The symptoms are not due to the direct physiological effects of a substance (e.g., a drug of abuse, a medication) or a general medical condition (e.g., hypothyroidism).

H. The symptoms cause clinically significant distress or impairment in social, occupational, or other important areas of functioning.

* DSM-IV (American Psychiatric Association, 1994).

Table 7–12 **Depressive Disorders**

	ADJUSTMENT DISORDER	DYSTHYMIA	MAJOR DEPRESSIVE EPISODE
Onset	Sudden	No clearly identifiable onset (no history of consistently sustained normal mood during adulthood)	Usually gradual onset (but periods of normal functioning during adulthood can be identified)
Precipitating event	Always	None	Occasionally
Duration	<6 months	At least 2 years	>2 weeks
Response to treatment	Good	Fair	Good to excellent

is relatively persistent (patient has only brief periods of relief from depression), and is not associated with psychotic symptoms. The mood disturbance in patients with chronic major depression may be mild, moderate, or severe, yet generally has a period of identifiable onset, is often episodic in nature (i.e., history of previous depressive episodes with periods of normal functioning between episodes), and may reach psychotic proportions. Although patients with dysthymia may be socially and occupationally impaired, the severity of their symptoms rarely warrants hospitalization. It should be noted, however, that approximately 10% of patients with dysthymia will develop a major depressive episode (Agency for Health Care Policy and Research, 1993a). This combination of dysthymia and major depression is often referred to as a *double depression* (Keller et al, 1983).

There is no universally accepted conceptual framework for the etiology of dysthymia. From a psychological and behavioral perspective, dysthymia may be secondary to poor self-esteem, which could have been caused by a lack of emotional or physical safety, nurturing, love, or acceptance during early childhood. Other developmental experiences thought to lead to dysthymia include early parental loss through death or divorce, neglect, sexual and/or physical abuse, and alcoholism and drug use in the home. (Many of these same developmental factors have been identified in patients with major depression as well). Excessive criticism from parents can be incorporated into the child's own conscience (superego) and cause the development of a personality marked by harsh self-criticism and low self-esteem. These individuals often feel inadequate, unlovable, and insecure and lack the ability to appreciate their value to others. In addition, dysthymics often experience problems in their interpersonal relationships. The combination of dysphoria, low self-esteem, and poor interpersonal relationships often places the dysthymic at an increased risk for substance abuse and suicide.

In some patients with dysthymia, depressive symptoms respond to antidepressant medications, *suggesting* a biological etiology for at least some of the symptoms. Therefore, treatment of the dysthymic patient may include insight-oriented psychotherapy, cognitive therapy, behavioral therapy, and a trial of pharmacotherapy.

Depressive Disorders not Otherwise Specified

A number of clinically significant depressive syndromes do not meet diagnostic criteria for Major Depression, Dysthymia, or Adjustment Disorder With Depressed Mood and are thus grouped under the general category of Depressive Disorders Not Otherwise Specified. Included under this category are Premenstrual Dysphoric Disorder, depressive disorders superimposed on other primary psychiatric conditions, various minor or brief depressive syndromes, and other depressive syndromes in which inadequate information exists to categorize the depressive disorder more specifically.

Premenstrual Dysphoric Disorder

Within the category of depressive disorders not otherwise specified, Premenstrual Dysphoric Disorder has been the best characterized and studied. This is a syndrome characterized by the repeated occurrence of a number of affective, cognitive, and behavioral symptoms during the luteal phase of the menstrual cycle. The diagnostic criteria for Premenstrual Dysphoric Syndrome are found in Table 7–13. While the presence of premenstrual symptoms is high (80% prevalence rate in women of reproductive age), only a relatively small number of women have symptoms of sufficient severity to warrant the formal diagnosis (Mortola, 1992). The patient must experience "functional impair-

Table 7–13 **Premenstrual Dysphoric Disorder**

Five or more of the following symptoms, occurring during most menstral cycles within the past year, which are most prominent during the last week of the luteal phase, begin to remit with menses, and are absent in the week postmenses, with at least one of the symptoms being either 1, 2, 3, or 4:
1. Depressed mood, hopelessness, self-deprecation
2. Marked anxiety or tension
3. Marked affective lability
4. Anger or irritability
5. Decreased interest in usual activities
6. Difficulty concentrating
7. Decreased energy
8. Marked change in appetite
9. Sleep disturbance
10. Sense of being overwhelmed or out of control
11. Physical symptoms generally associated with changes in the menstral cycle

Symptoms cause a marked disturbance in normal functioning and do not represent an exacerbation of another disorder.

ment" secondary to having these symptoms. The symptoms must have a characteristic pattern of occurrence: be present for most menstrual cycles over the past year, occur mostly over the last week of the luteal phase, and remit a few days after the onset of the follicular phase; no symptoms should be present in the week after menses.

Treatment should include education on the biology of the disorder, supportive psychotherapy, and in severe cases, pharmacotherapy. Pharmacological strategies that have been reported to be successful include benzodizepines, fluoxetine, and gonadotropin-releasing hormone agonist (reviewed by Mortola, 1992).

BIPOLAR DISORDERS

Bipolar I and II Disorders

The presence of mania or hypomania defines Bipolar Disorder (see Mood Episodes above). There are two major subtypes of bipolar disorder: Bipolar I and Bipolar II. Type I Bipolar Disorder requires documentation of at least one manic or mixed bipolar episode. A history of depression or hypomania may also be present in the Bipolar I patient, but neither of these conditions is essential for the diagnosis. Remember, documentation of a bona fide manic or mixed episode is all that is needed to make the diagnosis of Bipolar I disorder. In Bipolar II disorder, there is a history of hypomania and *at least* one major depressive episode, but *no* history of overt severe mania or mixed episodes. The category Bipolar Disorder Not Otherwise Specified is reserved for an array of bipolar spectrum illnesses that do not meet the criteria for Bipolar I, Bipolar II, or Cyclothymic Disorder (see below).

In general, the clinical presentations of unipolar and bipolar depressions do not appear to differ markedly in the quality or characteristics of their depressions. Antidepressants and electroconvulsive therapy (ECT) effectively treat both unipolar and bipolar depressions, and the prophylactic efficacy of lithium has been consistently demonstrated to be superior to placebo in both conditions. Thus, the distinction between unipolar and bipolar depression is based on the presence or absence of a past history of mania, hypomania, or a mixed manic episode. Given the genetic predisposition for bipolar illnesses (see below), a depression in a patient with a family history of bipolar illness is a strong indication that the patient has a bipolar disorder. Recognition that the patient has a bipolar disorder has important treatment implications for the depressed patient (see below: Treatment of Bipolar Illness).

Patients with untreated bipolar disorders frequently have multiple major mood disturbances throughout their lifetime. The cumulative probability of relapse after 1 year is approximately 50% and by 5 years between 80 and 90% (Keller et al, 1993; Tohen et al, 1990); however, recovery and relapse rates may differ among the subtypes of bipolar illnessess. The NIMH Collaborative Program on the Psychobiology of Depression 5-year follow-up revealed that patients with mixed episodes had the lowest recovery rates; after recovery, these mixed patients relapsed more quickly than patients with pure manic episodes. While *the numbers* of mood episodes in all bipolar patients during the first 5 years of follow-up were not correlated with the numbers of episodes in the last 5 years of follow-up (Coryell et al, 1992; Winokur et al, 1994), the *best predictor* of future episodes was *past* episodes. Bipolar patients were more likely to have had subsequent episodes if they had previous episodes prior to the study's index episode. Contrary to expectation, however, cycle lengths in the first 5 years of follow-up were similar to cycle lengths in the last 5 years of follow-up. The NIMH study also showed that rapid cyclers do not maintain their rapid cycling patterns over time. Nearly one in five (18.5%) bipolar patients who exhibited mania or hypomania during the first year of follow-up developed a rapid cycling course. The proportion of patients with rapid cycling decreased in the second year to only 6%. Rapid cycling was associated with a lower likelihood of recovery in the second year of follow-up, but not the third, fourth, or fifth. Furthermore, tricyclic antidepressants and monoamine oxidase inhibitors (MAOIs) did not appear to induce rapid cycling in this study, contrary to the impression of most psychiatrists. These findings from the NIMH CDS report are not consistent with the kindling hypothesis and are contrary to what is generally taught about the natural history of mood disorders. Clearly, further research into the natural history of mood disorders is warranted, and the results should be viewed with caution.

In contrast to notions that bipolar disorder has a good prognosis, the data seem to indicate otherwise, revealing not only high rates of recurrence, as noted above, but chronicity and significant subsyndromal morbidity in a significant number of patients. In the NIMH 5-year follow-up study, at the 2-year point 4% of manic, 15% of depressed, and 28% of mixed patients had not recovered. In a study by Winokur and colleagues (1993), 14% of acutely ill bipolar patients were unremitted after 2 years had elapsed, and 5% were unremitted after 5 years. Of 51 bipolar I manic patients, approximately 60% still experienced severe difficulty in at least one major area of functioning at their 4.5-year follow-up (Goldberg et al, 1995). Psychosocial impairments seen in bipolar patients include difficulties with educational pursuits, occupational functioning, marital relationships, interpersonal relationships, and the ability to reside independently.

Several factors negatively affect the course of bipolar illness. Substance abuse, psychotic features, subsyndromal symptoms, rapid cycling, mixed mania, and comorbid personality disorders all appear to increase relapse and chronicity.

Cyclothymia

Cyclothymia is a chronic mood disturbance of at least 2 years' duration involving numerous hypomanic and mild depressive episodes (which do not meet the criteria for mania or major depression), and with no periods of euthymia greater than 2 months. The mood disturbance is not severe enough to impair social or occupational functioning markedly (American Psychiatric Association, 1994). Cyclothymia can be conceptualized as a relatively less severe form of bipolar illness. The data indicate that approximately 30% of cyclothymics have a positive family history for bipolar illness; that the prevalence of cyclothymia in the relatives of bipolar patients is much higher than the prevalence of cyclothymia in patients with other psychiatric disorders; and that half of the cyclothymics report improvement while on lithium (Kaplan and Sadock, 1988).

THE SECONDARY MOOD DISORDERS

The essential feature of secondary mood disorders is evidence of a medical or drug-induced etiology for the symptoms. Numerous medical conditions, medications, or illicit drugs may induce mood disturbances (Cohen-Cole and Harpe, 1987). The possibility of a secondary mood disorder should always be considered. A basic history and physical exam, along with a medication review and/or appropriate laboratory screening tests, will rule out the majority of secondary mood disorders.

Mood Disorder Due to a General Medical Condition

The essential feature of a Mood Disorder Due to a General Medical Condition is that the mood disturbance is judged to be due to the physiological effects of a medical illness (American Psychiatric Association, 1994). While the mood disturbance may resemble that of any of the mood disorders (depressed, manic, mixed, or hypomanic), all the criteria for a mood disorder do not have to be met to make the diagnosis of a mood disorder due to a medical condition. The development of clinically significant mood symptoms is all that is required. The presenting symptoms are used to specify the subtype of mood disturbance caused by the general medical condition. There are four subtypes: With Depressive Features, With Major-Depression-Like Features, With Manic Features, and With Mixed Features. Medical conditions that may present as mood disorders include endocrinopathies, malignancies, and central and systemic infections. General medical conditions that cause mood disorders are discussed in Chapter 20 and have been briefly discussed in Chapter 1.

Substance-Induced Mood Disorder

The essential feature of a Substance-Induced Mood Disorder is that the mood disturbance is judged to be due to the physiological effects of a substance. While the mood disturbance may resemble that of any of the mood disorders (depressed, manic, mixed, or hypomanic), all the criteria for a mood disorder do not have to be met to make the diagnosis of a substance-induced mood disorder. The development of clinically significant mood symptoms is all that is required. The clinical symptoms are used to specify the subtype of mood disturbance induced by the substance. There are three subtypes: With Depressive Features, With Manic Features, and With Mixed Features. In addition, the substance-induced mood disorder can be further characterized based on whether the symptoms developed during intoxication or withdrawal. Drugs that have been implicated in inducing secondary mood disorders include steroids, reserpine, alpha-methyldopa, carbonic anhydrase inhibitors, stimulants, hallucinogens, alcohol, sedative–hypnotics, benzodiazepines, and narcotics.

SPECIAL CIRCUMSTANCES

Diagnosis and Treatment of Depression in the Medical Setting

Depressive symptoms are common in medical–surgical patients. In some instances, the depressive symptoms can be a consequence of the underlying medical illness, or they can be induced by medications. Feelings of helplessness, pain, injuries to self-esteem, and disruption in personal and occupational pursuits as a result of illness are just a few of the many factors that appear to be involved in the pathogenesis of depressive symptomatology in medically ill patients. If the physical illness is chronic and debilitating, progressive loss of health, independence, and financial stress may induce depressive reactions, especially if the patient begins to feel that he or she is now a burden to the family. In searching for the psychological precipitants of depression, the physician must look beyond the immediate circumstances of the patient's illness and evaluate the patient's general ability to "cope," the amount of family support available, the degree of financial and occupational strain, and other conflicts, pressures, or losses with which the patient may be struggling.

Most depressive reactions in medical–surgical patients do not meet the diagnostic criteria for a mood disorder. A decrease in mood is expected when one has to deal with unpleasant circumstances, and such reactions tend to resolve with stabilization of the medical condition. If significant disturbances in social, occupational, interpersonal, or psychological functioning occur, a diagnosis of an adjustment disorder can be made; however, if the depressive symptoms do not resolve with improvement in the medical condition, the continuation of symptoms should be considered a red flag and the diagnosis of a major depressive episode should be considered. Furthermore, cognitive expressions of decreased self-esteem, worthlessness, excessive guilt, "giving up," or wishing to die are not normal reactions to stress. When such cognitive symptoms are present, the physician should immediately suspect the development of a depressive disorder and request psychiatric consultation. Although it is "normal" to be sad in view of serious medical illness, it is not "normal" to be depressed. Depression is a serious medical condition.

The relationship between pain, particularly chronic pain, and depression is a frequent question that arises in medical–surgical patients. Chronic pain patients have a high frequency of depressive complaints (sleep disturbance, appetite changes, irritability, decreased libido, social withdrawal, and somatic preoccupation). Whether or not this symptom constellation constitutes true clinical depression independent of the patient's pain problem remains a matter of controversy. Arguments in this area soon become circular: chronic pain can cause significant reactive depression, or "masked" depressions can present as chronic pain syndromes. At any rate, the net result is the development of a patient who exhibits chronic pain behavior (focus of life is on pain complaints and obtaining relief from pain). Frequently, however, improvements in both the patient's mood and pain complaints are seen with antidepressant therapy.

In addition to pain complaints, somatic complaints attributable to almost every organ system have been reported by depressed patients in medical settings (such as weakness, dizziness, nausea, nervousness, tremor). Depressions presenting with somatic complaints (including pain) in the absence of an obviously depressed mood have been described as "masked depressions" or "somatizing depressions," and the symptoms considered "depressive equivalents." Indeed, a significant percentage of depressed patients in medical settings will present with these "masked depressions"! Thus, a caveat to bear in mind in evaluating depression is that some depressions may be "masked" by the patient being unaware of, denying, or having a limited ability to verbalize feelings. The physician should not accept denial of depression by the patient as excluding the diagnosis. After a medical workup has ruled out a physical or medical basis for the patient's complaints, a therapeutic trial of an antidepressant medication should be considered, along with further evaluation of the patient's psychosocial circumstances (Stoudemire, 1993).

Assessment of Suicide Risk

One of the myths surrounding assessment of suicidal risk in depressed patients is that asking about suicide ideation will bring the idea to the patient's mind or serve to "plant" the idea, and thus increase the chances that suicide will occur. In actuality, the opposite is true: bringing up the subject of suicide and allowing patients to ventilate is often a good way to "diffuse" a suicidal situation. Therefore, thorough questioning for suicidal ideation should be conducted in every depressed patient. Questioning the family is also important since the most lethal patient is one who may have already "made up their mind" and is determined that no one will be allowed to intervene. Patients who suddenly begin to "get their affairs in order," make out a will, or suddenly "get better" inexplicably (due to the idea that they now feel they have a way out of their intractable depressing situation) should be evaluated carefully.

Studies indicate that the rates of suicide in major depression are between 15 and 30% (reviewed by Gold et al, 1988a,b). In general, while women tend to attempt suicide more often, men complete the act successfully at a greater rate. A number of factors may help identify patients who are at higher risk for suicide, such as increasing age, living alone, recent major loss, chronic illness, and a previous history of depression and/or suicide attempts. Depressed patients with low self-esteem, excessive guilt, and feelings of helplessness and hopelessness may be extremely suicidal. Add alcohol or drugs to any of the above, and you have a particularly dangerous situation. If the patient appears to be a significant suicide risk, then psychiatric consultation should occur before the patient is allowed to go home. Management of suicidal patients is further discussed in Chapter 19.

TREATMENT OF DEPRESSIVE DISORDERS

Depressions are an etiologically heterogeneous group of disorders. Therefore, there is no one single treatment of choice for all cases of depression. In formulating a treatment plan for the depressed patient, first assess whether the patient meets the DSM-IV criteria for major depressive episode as the primary disorder. Rule out the presence of coexisting substance-abuse disorders and/or general medical conditions. Assess the psychosocial circumstances, the degree of impairment, the chronicity of the disturbance, and the presence of suicidal ideations. Patients with mild depressions or depressions secondary to environmental "stress" or interpersonal conflicts are best treated with counseling or psychotherapy (see below). Moderate-to-severe depressions will frequently benefit from antidepressant medication.

Recently there has been an expansion and refinement of the array of treatment modalities for depression. The pharmaceutical armentaterium of antidepressants include the cyclic antidepressants, MAOIs, selective serotonin-reuptake inhibitors (SSRIs), and lithium. All these agents are discussed here, as well as in the overview chapter on psychopharmacology in this text (see Chapter 18). No one medication can be recommended as optimal for all patients because of the substantial heterogeneity among patients and among the various antidepressants. There are, however, some general consensus statements that can be made.

Nonpsychotic *melancholia* responds well to most antidepressant medications; *atypical* depressions have a preferential response to MAOIs, patients with bipolar depressions should be treated with both an antidepressant and a mood stabilizer, and psychotically depressed individuals require a combination of an antidepressant and an antipsychotic, or ECT (Schatzberg, 1992). Thus, if it is determined that somatic treatment is warranted, the next step is to define the subtype of depression you will be treating. Besides the aforementioned clinical caveats, no convincing data suggest that one antidepressant is superior to any of the other antidepressants in regard to its ability to treat major depressions. Therefore, the choice of antidepressant in most cases is often predicated on other factors such as the patient's age, the side effect profile of the antidepressant, cost of the medication, and the patient's past personal or family history of antidepressant treatments. A personal history of prior response to an antidepressant or a favorable response by a family member is a good predictor of a favorable response to that same antidepressant again. The somatic or "vegetative" symptoms (i.e., sleep, appetite, and psychomotor disturbances) are relatively clear target symptoms for antidepressant medication and are usually the first symptoms to improve. The "cognitive" symptoms of depression (low self-esteem, guilt, uncertainty, pessimism, suicidal thoughts) tend to improve more slowly.

In general, a lag time of 2 to 4 weeks may be seen before a true mood-elevating effect is seen with the antidepressants, and patients should be warned not to expect results overnight. Significant antidepressant responses in elderly patients often occur later than in younger patients and require at least 6 to 12 weeks of therapy (NIH Consensus Development Panel on Depression in Late Life, 1992). Improvement in sleep disturbance, agitation, and anxiety may be seen early in the treatment and precede the onset of true antidepressant activity.

Traditionally, the cyclic antidepressants have been the first-line drugs in the treatment of depression, followed by the MAOIs if the patient failed to respond; however, more and more clinicians are using the newer generation antidepressants as their first choice in the treatment of depression.

Tricyclic Antidepressants and Related Compounds

The tricyclic antidepressants (TCAs) have been around for more than 30 years. Although maprotiline is a tetracyclic and amoxapine is a dibenzoxazepine, these two drugs are usually discussed with the TCAs because of their similar mechanism of action and side effect profiles (Table 7–14). The TCAs are relatively inexpensive and are considered the gold standard for comparing efficacy and side effect profiles of other antidepressant medications. Their mechanism of action is via inhibition of NE and/or 5-HT presynaptic reuptake in the central nervous system.

In general, the average dose range for most tricyclics is 100 mg/day up to a maximum of 300 mg/day. The most prominent exceptions are nortriptyline (50 to 150 mg/day), and protriptyline (10 to 60 mg/day). In general the

Table 7–14 **Selected Characteristics of Tricyclic Antidepressants**

	ADVERSE EFFECTS*			DRUG INTERACTIONS†	USUAL DAILY DOSE (MG/DAY)
	A	**S**	**OH**		
Tricyclics					
Amitriptyline	++++	++++	++	+++	150–300
Clomipramine	+++	+++	++	+++	150–250
Doxepin	++	+++	++	+++	150–300
Imipramine	++	++	+++	+++	50–300
Trimipramine	++	+++	++	+++	150–300
Desipramine	++	++	+	+++	75–300
Protriptyline	+++	+	+	++	15–60
Nortriptyline	++	++	+	+++	50–150
Related Tricyclics					
Amoxapine	+++	++	+	+++	150–400
Maprotiline	++	++	+	++	75–225

* A, anticholinergic; S, sedation; OH, orthostatic hypotension (scale from 0 = none to ++++ = very high).
† Significant drug interactions only.

Formulary/Source: Emile Risby, MD, Deane Donnigan, PharmD, BCPS, and Charles B. Nemeroff, MD, PhD

tricyclics should be started at low bedtime doses (25 to 50 mg/day) and gradually increased by 25 or 50 mg/day every third or fourth night over a 10- to 14-day period of time (with the exceptions as already noted). Elderly patients generally require lower doses than younger adults. (Start with 10 or 25 mg and build up the dose gradually, monitoring for side effects.) The half-life of most antidepressants is such that they can be administered once daily in the evening. This approach may facilitate both sleep induction and compliance.

The major TCA side effects are attributable to their blockade of neurotransmitter receptors, unrelated to their therapeutic mechanism of action. These side effects include anticholinergic effects (i.e., dry mouth, blurred vision, urinary retention, constipation, sinus tachycardia, and memory dysfunction) and orthostatic hypotension secondary to alpha-1 adrenergic receptor blockade. Orthostatic hypotension may precipitate falls, as well as cerebrovascular or cardiac events. The elderly are particularly sensitive to these side effects. Unfortunately, there is no tendency for the body to accommodate to these difficult to manage side effects. The demethylated or secondary tricyclics (i.e., desipramine, nortriptyline, protriptyline) are generally better tolerated and less likely to produce anticholinergic and orthostatic side effects. Tricyclic antidepressants may lower the seizure threshold in patients with seizure disorders, but the exacerbation of seizures is usually not a problem if therapeutic levels of anticonvulsants are maintained.

The use of tricyclics in patients with cardiovascular disease warrants some special concerns. In addition to orthostasis, the tricyclics tend to slow cardiac conduction and, as a group, tend to increase the P-R interval, QRS duration, and QTc time and to flatten T-waves on the electrocardiogram in patients with cardiac conduction disease (Stoudemire et al, 1993). Thus, patients with either bundle branch blocks or intraventricular conduction defects should be treated very carefully with TCAs. Interestingly, however, since the tricyclics have properties characteristic of Type 1A antiarrhythmic compounds (such as quinidine and procainamide), premature ventricular contractions may decrease when tricyclics are administered (Glassman and Bigger, 1981; Veith et al, 1982). Therefore, the combination of tricyclics and Type 1A antiarrhythmics should be avoided because of their additive effects on cardiac conduction. One advantage of the newer antidepressant agents such as the selective serotonin reuptake inhibitors (SSRI's) is that they have few, if any, effects on cardiac function in healthy adults. Although there are very few controlled studies assessing the effects of these newer agents in diseased hearts, it is widespread clinical practice to use these newer agents in patients with cardiac conditions.

Monitoring of tricyclic plasma drug levels may be helpful in selected patients, particularly in patients who are unresponsive to usual therapeutic doses. Cigarette smoking, oral contraceptives, alcohol, and barbiturates tend to lower plasma levels of antidepressants through hepatic enzyme induction; disulfiram (Antabuse), antipsychotics, and SSRIs tend to raise tricyclic levels. In evaluating drug levels, the clinician should strive to obtain levels under uniform conditions. A standard procedure is to draw levels in the morning, approximately 12 hours after the last dose of medication. (Glenn and Taska, 1984).

Monoamine Oxidase Inhibitors

Currently, only two MAOIs are available in the United States: phenelzine and tranylcypromine (Table 7–15). Both are irreversible inhibitors of the enzyme MAO. MAOIs are not widely prescribed because of their potential to produce a hypertensive crisis if the patient ingests a food source high in tyramine or a sympathomimetic drug. They are generally prescribed for those patients who are unresponsive to cyclic antidepressants, who develop intolerable side effects with cyclic antidepressants, or who give a history of previous response to MAOIs. However, MAOI's may be the drug of choice in patients with "atypical" depression (McGrath et al, 1992; Quitkin et al, 1979). The usual dosage range is 15 to 60 mg for phenelzine and 20 to 30 mg for tranylcypromine, given in divided doses. The most frequently reported side effects are orthostatic hypotension, weight gain, sexual dysfunction, and insomnia. Patients with congestive heart failure, liver disease, or pheochromocytoma should not receive MAOIs.

Table 7–15 **Selected Characteristics of MAOIs**

MAOI	ADVERSE EFFECTS*			DRUG INTERACTIONS[†]	USUAL DAILY DOSE (MG/DAY)
	A	S	OH		
Phenelzine	+	+	+	+++++	15–60
Tranylcy-promine	+	+	0	+++++	20–30

* A, anticholinergic; S, sedation; OH, orthostatic hypotension (scale from 0 = none to +++++ = highest).
† Significant drug interactions only.

Formulary/Source: Emile Risby, MD, Deane Donnigan, PharmD, BCPS, and Charles B. Nemeroff, MD, PhD

Foods rich in tyramine—aged cheese, yogurt, Chianti wine, foreign beer, liver, snails, pickled herring, chocolate, broad beans, soy sauce, and avocados—should be avoided during treatment with MAOIs. Patients should avoid medications containing sympathomimetic compounds such as amphetamines, diet pills, and most over-the-counter common cold preparations. MAOIs should not be used in combination with guanethedine, sympathomimetics of any kind, narcotics or serotonergic enhancing agents (such as the SSRIs, clomipramine, venlafaxine).

Selective Serotonin-Reuptake Inhibitors (SSRI's)

The SSRIs have become the most commonly prescribed antidepressants in the United States (Table 7–16). The SSRIs produce antidepressant response rates approaching 70%, which is comparable to the response rate of the tertiary TCAs (Bennie et al, 1995; Gattuz et al, 1995). While they are as effective as the cyclic antidepressants in the treatment of depression, they have some distinct tolerability and dosing advantages. The combination of clinical efficacy, safety, ease of administration, and favorable side effect profile is responsible for their rapid acceptance and widespread use. The SSRIs are potent inhibitors of presynaptic 5-HT reuptake, but have a low affinity for histaminic, cholinergic, and alpha-1 adrenergic receptors. Therefore, the SSRIs are without many of the TCA-like side effects that are frequently associated with noncompliance (Richelson, 1990), and usually can be safely given to elderly patients and patients who are medically compromised. Their therapeutic and starting doses are generally the same, so, unlike other classes of antidepressants, there is no "delay" between initiation of therapy and titration to a therapeutic dose. Overdoses with SSRIs only are generally not fatal. The SSRIs are not associated with any significant cardiotoxicity, sedation, or weight gain. Gastrointestinal symptoms (nausea and diarrhea), headache, insomnia, anxiety, nervousness,

Table 7–16 **Selected Characteristics of SSRIs**

SSRI	ADVERSE EFFECTS*			DRUG INTERACTIONS†	USUAL DAILY DOSE (MG/DAY)
	A	S	OH		
Fluoxetine	0/+	0/+	0/+	++	20–80
Fluvoxamine	0/+	0/+	0	++++	100–300
Paroxetine	0+	+	0	++	20–50
Sertraline	0	0/+	0	++	50–200

* A, anticholinergic; S, sedation; OH, orthostatic hypotension (scale from 0 = none to ++++ = very high).
† Significant drug interactions only.

Formulary/Source: Emile Risby, MD, Deane Donnigan, PharmD, BCPS, and Charles B. Nemeroff, MD, PhD

agitation, tremor, and sexual dysfunction (delayed ejaculation in men, anorgasmia in women) are among the most commonly reported side effects (Leonard, 1992; Rickels and Schweizer, 1990). Although the SSRIs share similar pharmacodynamic profiles (they all inhibit serotonin reuptake), structurally they are a heterogeneous group, resulting in different pharmacokinetic properties. Currently four SSRIs are available in the United States, fluoxetine, sertraline, paroxetine, and fluvoxamine, the last of which has Food and Drug Administration (FDA) approval for obsessive–compulsive disorder only at this time (Table 7–16).

Drug–drug interactions have been reported with the SSRIs. The most important is the interaction between the SSRIs and the MAOIs. This combination, or use within close temporal proximity to each other, has been associated with the serotonin syndrome, which is characterized by diaphoresis, shivering, tremor, hyperpyrexia, hypertension, seizures, and death (Sterinbach, 1991). Other drug interactions are largely secondary to the inhibition of the activity of one or more of the hepatic cytochrome P450 isoenzymes. A more extensive discussion of SSRI drug interactions is found in Chapter 18.

Most clinicians consider the SSRIs their first-line drug for the treatment of depression because of their documented clinical efficacy, once-a-day dosing, favorable side effect profile, and safety in overdose.

Atypical Antidepressants

Bupropion
Bupropion is a unicyclic antidepressant that differs chemically and pharmacologically from other currently available antidepressants. Although it exerts weak effects on NE, DA, and 5-HT reuptake, bupropion's mechanism of action remains obscure (Richelson, 1990). A number of controlled trials have shown bupropion to be as effective as tricyclics in the treatment of depression. Its side effect profile, however, is much more favorable than that of the tricyclics. It is

essentially devoid of anticholinergic, antihistaminic, and adrenergic side effects (Table 7–17). Side effects reported with bupropion include dizziness, agitation, insomnia, headache, and nausea. Bupropion is not associated with cognitive impairment, withdrawal phenomenon, sedation, or sexual dysfunction. Its most serious side effect is drug-induced seizures, especially in patients with bulimia nervosa. The seizure risk appears to be dose and titration related and can be minimized by gradually increasing the dose, not exceeding 150 mg for any one dose, and not exceeding 450 mg total daily dose. Bupropion is usually started at 75 or 150 mg/day and increased to 300 mg/day over several days (reviewed by Risby et al, 1997; Weisler, 1991). A long-acting form of the drug is now available. Buproprion has also been useful as a part of smoking cessation programs.

Combined Serotonin-Reuptake Inhibitors and Serotonin Agonists

The combined 5-HT reuptake/5-HT$_2$ agonist are structurally and pharmacologically different from the other classes of antidepressants. The net result of these two distinct pharmacological actions is increased serotonergic activity in the CNS. Currently, trazodone and nefazodone are the only combined 5-HT reuptake/5-HT$_2$ antagonists available in the United States.

Trazodone. The major side effects of trazodone include sedation, orthostatic hypotension, dizziness, headache, and nausea (Richelson, 1990). Because trazodone is quite sedating it is generally prescribed at bedtime with the initial dose of 50 to 100 mg and gradually increased to the recommended antidepressant dose of 300 to 600 mg/day. There have been only a few case reports of trazodone-induced cardiac arrhythmias both in patients with preexisting heart disease and in patients with apparently healthy cardiovascular functioning (Rudorfer and Potter, 1989). Trazodone-induced priapism, which on occasion has required surgical intervention, occurs in approximately 1 in 600 male

Table 7–17 Selected Characteristics of Atypical Antidepressants

AGENT	ADVERSE EFFECTS*			DRUG INTERACTIONS[†]	USUAL DAILY DOSE (MG/DAY)
	A	S	OH		
Bupropion	0	0	+	+	150–400
Trazodone	+	+++	+++	0	300–600
Nefazodone	0/+	++	+	+++	300–600
Venlafaxine	0	0	0	0	75–375
Mirtazapine	+/++	+++	++	+	15–45

* A, anticholinergic; S, sedation; OH, orthostatic hypotension (scale from 0 = none to ++++ = very high).
[†] Significant drug interactions only.

Formulary/Source: Emile Risby, MD, Deane Donnigan, PharmD, BCPS, and Charles B. Nemeroff, MD, PhD

patients (Warner et al, 1987). Trazodone has relatively few known drug–drug interactions. Although the combination of trazadone with MAOIs is discouraged because of the possibility of inducing the serotonin syndrome, trazodone is used by many clinicians to treat antidepressant-induced (including MAOI-induced) insomnia. Two significant advantages of trazodone are its lack of anticholinergic effects and its safety in overdose. Trazodone's sedative effects at therapeutic doses and the general clinical impression that it is not as efficacious as other antidepressants are its major disadvantages (Risby et al, 1997).

Nefazodone. The most commonly reported side effects of nefazodone include somnolence, dry mouth, nausea, dizziness, constipation, asthenia, light headedness, blurred or abnormal vision, and confusion. Nefazodone has no significant effects on cholinergic receptors; however, it does have weak alpha-1 adrenergic receptor blocking properties, which may be responsible for reports of postural hypotension in some subjects. Unlike trazodone, nefazodone reportedly does not cause priapism. The therapeutic dose range for nefazodone is 300 to 600 mg/day in divided doses. Treatment is usually initiated at 100 mg twice a day, increasing to 150 mg twice a day during the second week. Many patients, especially the elderly, should be treated initially with half the usually recommended dose, but the therapeutic dose range is the same for both nongeriatric and geriatric patients. Nefazodone is a potent inhibitor of the P450 IIIA4 isozyme. Therefore, coadministration of nefazodone with other drugs metabolized by this isoenzyme (such as terfenadine, astemizole, triazolam, midazolam, and alprazolam) is absolutely contradicted (for the first two drugs listed) or done with extreme caution. Currently, there are only rare reports of nefazodone causing sexual dysfunction in men or women, a major drawback of the SSRIs (Risby et al, 1997).

Combined Norepinephrine and Serotonin Reuptake Inhibitor

Venlafaxine. Venlafaxine is a potent 5-HT and NE reuptake inhibitor. Like most of the newer generation antidepressants, venlafaxine has virtually no affinity for muscarinic, histaminergic, or adrenergic receptors (Muth et al, 1986). Therefore, its side effect profile is similar to that of the SSRIs. The most frequently reported side effects include nausea, anorexia, insomnia, headache, mild elevations in blood pressure, and increased heart rate. The nausea associated with venlafaxine generally occurs at the initiation of therapy, and usually improves with time. Unlike the SSRIs, venlafaxine does not inhibit any of the cytochrome P450 isoenzymes in the doses used to treat depression; thus clinically significant pharmacokinetic drug interactions have not been reported with venlafaxine. Because of its 5-HT-enhancing properties, however, venlafaxine should not be coadministered with MAOIs. The therapeutic dose range for venlafaxine is between 75 and 375 mg/day. The manufacturer's recommended starting dose of venlafaxine is 75 mg/day in divided doses, taken with meals. However, because of the nausea, many clinicians will initiate therapy with venlafaxine at lower doses (12.5 to 37.5 mg/day) and gradually increase the dose every 3 to 4 days by 25 or 37.5 mg/day. One major advantage of venlafaxine is that it is effective in many patients with severe depression, including patients who have been reported to be refractory to other agents (Nierenberg et al, 1994; Schweizer et al, 1991). Age-related adjustments in venlafaxine dosing are generally not necessary; however, patients with renal or hepatic impairments should receive lower doses and be monitored more closely for adverse side effects. A long-acting form of this drug that will improve patient compliance has recently become available.

Combined Noradrenergic Antagonist and Serotonergic Antagonist

Mirtazapine (Remeron) is a tetracyclic, yet its pharmacological profile is distinctly different from that of other cyclic antidepressants. Mirtazapine has presynaptic alpha-2 receptor antagonist properties plus 5-HT$_2$ and 5-HT$_3$ receptor antagonist properties, which result in a net increase of both noradrenergic and serotonergic neurotransmission (Chow, 1996; de Boer and Ruigt, 1995). The adverse events most commonly reported with mirtazapine are somnolence, increased appetite, weight gain, and dizziness. The recommended starting dose is 15 mg/day, increasing by 7.5 or 15 mg every 1 to 2 weeks (depending on the patient's tolerance for the drug), to a maximum of 45 mg/day or until clinical response is achieved. Be aware that the clearance of mirtazapine is reduced in elderly patients and in patients with renal and hepatic disease. Experience with this drug remains limited in the general patient population.

Psychostimulants

Stimulants such as methylphenidate, amphetamine, and pemoline are sometimes used to treat depressed medically ill patients (especially patients with the acquired immunodeficiency syndrome). This strategy is usually employed as an augmentation strategy to standard antidepressants. Stimulants, however, may produce rebound depression, insomnia, restlessness, agitation, and even paranoid reactions. Their antidepressant action may be short lived, and they are not approved by the FDA for use as antidepressants. In addition, in some patients, they have great abuse potential. Nonetheless, in selected patients, stimulants can be a reasonable and effective option.

Electroconvulsive Therapy

Although a large armamentarium of clinically effective antidepressants is available to the clinician, both psychotic and melancholic depressions tend to respond most predictably to ECT (American Psychiatric Association, 1993). In fact, ECT is clearly the most effective treatment for all major depressions and should be considered in depressed patients who cannot tolerate the side effects of antidepressant medications or who are severely suicidal. Other indications for ECT include refractory depressions (usually defined as failure to respond to at least two different antidepressants given for 4 to 6 weeks at therapeutic doses), depressions in frail elderly patients, and in some cases of acute mania, schizoaffective disorders, or acute-onset psychotic episodes (including schizophrenia) presenting with a predominance of affective or catatonic symptoms. The only contraindications to electrotherapy are the presence of CNS mass lesions, recent myocardial infarction (usually defined as within 6 months), or a history of malignant ventricular arrhythmia.

Duration of Treatment in Depression

There are no clear indications as to how long antidepressant drugs should be continued once an antidepressant effect is achieved. Clearly, extended antidepressant treatment effectively reduces recurrences of depressive episodes (Frank et al, 1990). The need to continue treatment is underscored by studies showing that the risk of relapse after 1 year is about 60% for placebo and 25% for active treatment; after 2 years, it is approximately 75% for placebo, but remains about 25% for active treatment. Without question, rapid discontinuation of effective treatment is ill advised: relapse rates are considerably less among those who remain in active treatment over a period of several years (Greden, 1995–96). In general, antidepressant medications should be continued for an average of 9 to 12 months, and then a gradual taper can be attempted, closely watching for signs of relapse. If the patient has had multiple episodes of depression in the past, or has a strong family history of depression, he or she may well need to be maintained on antidepressants indefinitely. In conjunction with medication treatment, supportive psychotherapy (or some form of counseling to deal with conflicts, stressors, or other precipitants that may contribute to depression) is usually recommended (even if the therapy is relatively brief and confined to the early stages of treatment).

Psychotherapy in the Treatment of Depression

The Agency for Health Care Policy and Research (1993b) states that the goals of psychotherapy are symptom amelioration and elimination of functional impairment. Psychotherapy attempts to help the individual understand how certain relationships, events, or ways of thinking contribute to their clinical condition. A wide range of psychotherapeutic interventions may be useful in the treatment of depressive disorders.

Supportive psychotherapy generally consists of (1) helping the patient understand the nature of his/her symptoms; (2) providing ongoing education, knowledge, and feedback in regard to the patient's illness, prognosis, and treatment; (3) providing emotional support in dealing with difficult interpersonal relationships, work, and major life adjustments; (4) helping to bolster the patient's morale; (5) setting realistic goals; (6) being available in times of crisis; and (7) mobilizing and reinforcing sources of social support.

Insight-oriented psychotherapy focuses on gaining insight and understanding of concious and unconscious psychological conflicts. Once the forces causing or perpetuating are made conscious, future difficulties can be anticipated and mastered, or future conflicts can be neutralized through the process of insight (reviewed by American Psychiatric Association, 1993). It is the most common form of psychotherapy provided to depressed patients in psychiatric settings.

Interpersonal therapy seeks to recognize and explore depressive precipitants that involve interpersonal losses, role disputes, social isolation, or deficits in social skills (reviewed by American Psychiatric Association, 1993). Cognitive therapy approaches the patient's symptoms as being secondary to irrational beliefs and distorted attitudes towards self, the environment, and the future (see above: Cognitive Theory of Depression).

The efficacy of psychotherapy is difficult to ascertain because of the challenges in conducting research in this area and in evaluating the results. It is generally agreed that patients with situational depressions (adjustment disorders), mild depressions, or dysthymic disorders are most likely to benefit from a purely psychotherapeutic approach. In these conditions, behavioral, cognitive, and interpersonal psychotherapies have all shown efficacy rates of 40 to 50% (Agency for Health Care Policy and Research, 1993b). There is general consensus among experienced clinicians that the optimal treatment of major depression requires some form of somatic intervention coupled with some form of psychotherapeutic management. Psychotherapy can assist the patient in reversing the negative self-images, negative feelings about the future, and poor self-esteem that are ubiquitous features of depression. The establishment of a supportive therapeutic relationship is often crucial in the treatment of all psychiatric patients, regardless of their diagnosis (American Psychiatric Association, 1993).

PHARMACOLOGICAL TREATMENT OF BIPOLAR DISORDERS

Bipolar Depression

Clinically, unipolar depressions cannot be distinguished from bipolar depressions, yet this differentiation is important since antidepressants have been reported to precipitate manic episodes and possibly increase "cycling" in some bipolar patients. Hence, if the patient has a personal or family history of bipolar disorder, antidepressants (particularly TCAs) should be used cautiously. If a decision is made to give an antidepressant to a depressed bipolar patient, usually a mood stabilizer is also started to help prevent the induction of mania. Lithium itself has antidepressant properties, especially in bipolar patients and should be considered the sole *maintenance* agent (Glenn and Taska, 1984).

Bipolar Mania

Mania is a psychiatric emergency. Rapid control of manic symptoms is important. Lithium, valproate, and carbamazepine are the mood stabilizers generally used to treat manic episodes. More recently, the anticonvulsant lamotrigine has shown efficacy in bipolar disorder as well. While each of these mood stabilizers is effective in the treatment of acute mania, they have different pharmacokinetics, dosing strategies, and clinical side effects. To date, only lithium and divalproex (an enteric coated combination of sodium valproate and valproic acid) are approved by the FDA for the treatment of acute mania in the United States. In addition, benzodiazepines and antipsychotics are also often employed to achieve behavioral control of acutely manic patients. Traditionally, lithium has been the treatment of choice for acute and maintenance treatment of mania.

The phosphoinositide (PI) cycle has long been recognized as an important intracellular second messenger system. In this system, receptor recognition triggers the hydrolysis of membrane bound phosphatidyl-inositol-bis-phosphate, to form inositol triphosphate (IP_3) and diacylglycerol (DAG). IP_3 liberates intracellular calcium and DAG stimulates the enzyme protein kinase C, both actions are powerful intracellular catalyst that modify a multitude of intellular functions, including receptor sensitivity. At therapeutic blood levels, lithium inhibits the action of inositol phosphate, the enzyme responsible for replenishing PIP_2, thus decreasing the amount of IP_3 and DAG produced after receptor stimulation. This slowing of the PI cycle and resulting "down regulation" of receptor sensitivity may explain the perplexing ability of lithium to treat and be prophylactic in both depression and mania. Lithium may "slow down" any pathologic or dysregulated intracellular mechanisms responsible for these clinical syndromes.

Although the onset of lithium's therapeutic action is somewhat slow (5 to 10 days), 60 to 70% of manic patients will respond to therapeutic blood levels of lithium. Suppes and colleagues (1991) demonstrated that in 123 bipolar patients stabilized on lithium, when lithium treatment was discontinued, 50% developed a recurrence within 5 months. Renal function, electrolytes, and thyroid function should be evaluated prior to initiating lithium. Lithium has no metabolites and is excreted almost entirely by the kidney. The rates of renal excretion are affected by advancing age, medical conditions that impair renal blood flow, and sodium intake (because the two cations compete with each other for the same ion transport sites in the kidney). The possibility that lithium can produce clinically significant renal damage is controversial. Tubular atrophy, interstitial fibrosis, glomerulosclerosis, and full renal failure secondary to lithium-induced interstitial nephritis all have been reported after many years of use (Hestbach et al, 1977), yet the risk of clinically significant renal damage in patients treated with therapeutic concentrations of lithium appears to be very small (Scully et al, 1981). More commonly, lithium may suppress thyroid functioning and induce thyroid goiters and/or clinical hypothyroidism. The inhibition of thyroid function appears to be dose dependent and is readily reversible with cessation of lithium therapy. Lithium occasionally causes cardiac abnormalities such as inversion and flattening of T-waves on the electrocardiogram, sinus node dysfunction, SA block, and ventricular irritability (Glenn and Taska, 1984). Hypercalcemia has also been reported to be a complication of lithium therapy.

To begin inpatient treatment for acute mania, lithium carbonate can usually be started at 900 to 1,200 mg/day (depending on the size of the individual) in divided doses, increasing the dose by 300 mg/day every 3 to 4 days until a therapeutic blood level is achieved. Lower doses will be needed in patients who are elderly, have renal insufficiency, or who are otherwise medically compromised. The optimal serum blood level during an acute manic episode should be at the upper spectrum of the therapeutic range (between 1.0 and 1.5 mEq/L). Serum levels should be drawn in the morning before the morning lithium dose (approximately 12 hours after the last dose). Serum levels above 1.5 mEq/L often produce signs of toxicity, and levels of 5 mEq/L can be fatal. Since clinical response usually takes several days, antipsychotic or sedative medications are frequently needed during the initial treatment. Following the acute episode, the usually recommended maintenance lithium levels are between 0.6 and 1.2 mEq/L (Glenn and Taska, 1984).

It should be emphasized that close monitoring of side effects, not serum lithium concentrations, is the ultimate criterion for lithium toxicity. Signs and symptoms of lithium toxicity include tremor, weakness, ataxia, drowsiness, dysarthria, blurred vision, tinnitus, nausea, vomiting, hyperactive deep tendon reflexes, nystagmus, confusion, seizures, and coma. Some of these side effects (such as tremor, weakness, gastrointestinal complaints) are seen with therapeutic levels of lithium. The lithium-induced tremor can be alleviated by the addition of 20 to 60 mg of propranolol. Gastrointestinal disturbances can best be treated by dividing total dosage or switching to one of the slow-release formulations. Some patients develop marked polyuria and polydipsia, which may improve by lowering the lithium dose or by adding low doses of a thiazide diuretic. (NOTE: monitor for lithium toxicity if you add the diuretic.) If hypothyroidism develops (check TSH to find out), decrease the dose of lithium if possible, or treat with thyroid supplements (i.e., levothyroxine).

Women of child-bearing potential should be warned of reports of a possible increase in cardiovascular abnormalities in the offspring of lithium-treated mothers. Lithium should be used with caution in patients with unstable renal or cardiovascular disease or severe dehydration in patients receiving thiazide diuretics, angiotensin-converting enzymes, or nonsteriodal antiinflammatory agents. Although there have been some reports of neurotoxicity in patients being treated with a combination of lithium and neuroleptics (Cohen and Cohen, 1974), in general, the combination of lithium and neuroleptics is well tolerated.

Carbamazepine was the first anticonvulsant used to treat bipolar disorders (Post et al, 1989). The overall response rate for carbamazepine in acute mania is approximately 50% (Keck et al, 1992). The usual starting dose of carbamazepine is 200 mg twice a day with a gradual increase by 200 mg/day every 2 to 3 days until a plasma level of 4 to 12 μg/ml is achieved. Side effects most frequently reported with carbamazepine include diplopia, blurred vision, vertigo, psychomotor slowing, and ataxia. Transient leukopenia may occur in approximately 10% of patients and benign liver enzyme elevations in 5 to 15% of patients. Rarely, agranulocytosis, aplastic anemia, hepatic failure, and exfoliative dermatitis may also occur (McElroy and Keck, 1995). Carbamazepine has teratogenic effects and should be avoided during pregnancy. One major disadvantage of carbamazepine is that it has multiple drug–drug interactions and induces its own metabolism, which make it more complicated for the busy clinician and the medically complicated patient.

Divalproex has been shown to be an effective antimanic agent. One advantage of divalproex is that you can quickly get the patient to a therapeutic blood level by administering a loading dose. The patient is administered 20 mg/kg/day of divalproex in divided doses (Keck et al, 1993). This strategy is well tolerated by patients and generally results in significant clinical improvement within days. Valproate levels above 45 μg/ml are more likely to produce a clinical response, and the usually recommended plasma concentrations are between 50 and 150 μg/ml (Bowden et al, 1996). Divalproex is efficacious and safe in the treatment of elderly bipolar patients also, even in those with co-existing medical conditions (Kando et al, 1996). Side effects most frequently reported are gastrointestinal symptoms, benign hepatic transaminase elevations, tremors, sedation, transient hair thinning, and weight gain (McElroy and Keck, 1995). Valproate is supplanted to use of lithium in bipolar disorder.

The use of psychopharmacological agents in the treatment of mood disorders is more fully discussed in Chapter 18.

Nonpharmacological Treatment of Bipolar Disorders

Although medication predominates in the treatment of bipolar disorder, psychoeducation and psychosocial interventions are also helpful. Basic information about the disorder, the role of medications, knowledge of medication side effects, symptom identification, stress management, resource books, and financial management are all important areas of psychoeducation that should be a part of practically every bipolar patient's treatment plan. Common issues that arise in individual psychotherapy in bipolar patients include overcoming denial, dealing with guilt from actions done while manic, anger over having a disease, demoralization, hopelessness, and relationship, financial, and employment problems. Group psychotherapy should help to increase medication compliance, decrease denial regarding the illness, and increase awareness of stress factors that may lead to relapse by reviewing these factors in group members who may relapse. Family therapy must be tailored to the family. The issues are different for the older bipolar patient with a spouse and children, compared with the younger bipolar patient, who may be living with parents or attending college.

CLINICAL PEARLS

- Major depression is a syndrome, characterized by a mood disturbance, plus a variety of cognitive, psychological, and somatic symptoms.
- The subjective sense of "being depressed" may not be present in every patient who has a major depression. Some depressions may be "masked" by the patient being unaware of, in denial of, or having limited ability to verbalize feelings.
- Elderly patients may complain of anxiety, irritability, weakness, or multiple somatic complaints rather than verbalize complaints of depression per se.
- Somatic symptoms of depression can include pain, gastrointestinal complaints, a variety of neurological complaints, general fatigue, and lethargy.
- The development of extreme withdrawal, hopelessness, or suicidal ideations are clear indications for psychiatric referral.
- Major depressions, which were once thought to consist of discrete episodes followed by full recovery, may become chronic in some patients.
- There is a high recurrence rate for major depression.
- An adjustment disorder may occur following an identifiable psychosocial stressor and may be associated with severe dysphoria, despondency, and suicidal ideations and attempts.
- The essential feature of a dysthymic disorder is a chronic (minimum of 2 years) history of a mild-to-moderate depression, with only brief, if any, periods of euthymia.
- The presence of mania, hypomania, or mixed mania defines bipolar disorder.
- Bipolar patients with mixed mania have a higher lithium nonresponse rate and tend to respond best when antimanic anticonvulsants are used or added to their medication regimen.
- No one antidepressant can be recommended as optimal for all patients because of the substantial heterogeneity among patients and among the various antidepressants.
- In general, nonpsychotic depressions can be treated with any of the available antidepressants; depressions with atypical features have a preferential response to MAOIs; and psychotic depressions require a combination of an antidepressant and an antipsychotic, or ECT.
- The most common cause of "refractory" major depression is noncompliance or inadequate dosing of the antidepressant.
- In some cases, the efficacy of antidepressants can augmented by adding lithium to the antidepressant regimen.
- Traditionally, the cyclic antidepressants have been the first-line drugs in the treatment of depression. Now however, most clinicians use non-TCAs, such as the SSRI's, as their first-line treatment for depressive disorders.
- At therapeutic doses, anticholinergic effects, sedation, and weight gain are the most problematic side effects of the traditional cyclic antidepressants. The newer antidepressants have almost none of these problems.
- The half-life of most antidepressants is such that they can be administered once daily. This approach may facilitate both sleep and compliance.
- In addition to having a low incidence of anticholinergic, antihistaminic, and adrenergic side effects, the SSRIs have the dosing advantage of having their starting dose being the generally recommended therapeutic dose; thus there is usually no treatment delay because of having to titrate to a therapeutic dose.
- Antidepressant medications should be continued for an average of 9 to 12 months, and then a gradual taper can be attempted while watching for signs of relapse. If the patient has had multiple episodes of depression in the past or has a strong

family history of depression, he or she may well need to be maintained on anti-depressants indefinitely.

- When taking lithium, have the patient take it on a full stomach or use the slow-release preparations to decrease gastric irritation.
- The anticonvulsants carbamazepine and valproic acid are effective in the treatment of acute mania. These anticonvulsants appear to be the drugs of choice in patients presenting with mixed mania.
- Valproic acid has the dosing advantage over lithium and carbamazepine in that a loading dose can be administered to achieve therapeutic blood levels rapidly and quicker therapeutic response.
- Several medications may interfere with the excretion of lithium such as diuretics, nonsteroidal antiinflammatory agents and angiotensin-converting enzyme inhibitors. Watch for lithium toxicity if these medications are added to a stable lithium regimen.
- Acute psychotic mania may be indistinguishable from acute schizophrenic psychosis; consider both possibilities in evaluating the acutely psychotic patient.
- In a patient over 40 who develops psychotic symptoms for the first time, consider a mood disorder in addition to ruling out a neurological, metabolical, or substance-induced etiology, as new-onset schizophrenia is uncommon after age 40.

ANNOTATED BIBLIOGRAPHY

American Psychiatric Association: Practice Guideline for Major Depressive Disorder in Adults. Am J Psychiatry 150(suppl):1–26, 1993

> Reviews the American Psychiatric Association's recommended treatment guidelines for the management of major depression in adults. It also reviews the diagnosis, epidemiology, and natural history of the illness. It addresses both pharmacologic and psychotherapeutic strategies for the treatment of depression.

American Psychiatric Association: Practice Guidelines for the treatment of of patients with bipolar disorders. Am J Psychiatry 151(suppl):1–36

> Reviews the American Psychiatric Association's recommended treatment guidelines for the management of bipolar disorders. It also reviews the diagnosis, epidemiology, and natural history of the illness. It addresses both pharmacologic and psychotherapeutic strategies for the treatment of bipolar patients.

Management of Patients Who Are Nonresponders to or Nontolerators of Initial Antidepressant Therapy. J Clin Psychiatry, Monograph Series, Vol. 10, No. 1, May 1992

> This monograph contains a series of very practical, clinically oriented articles on the treatment of depressed patients.

Risby ED, Donnigan D, Nemeroff CB: Pharmacotherapeutic considerations for psychiatric disorders: Depression. Formulary 32:46–59, 1997

> Reviews the pharmacologic options for treating depression and addresses efficacy issues, side effects, dosing, and pharmacoeconomic considerations.

Shader RI, Greenblatt DJ (eds): Journal of Clinical Psychopharmacology Supplement 12(1): February 1992

> A collection of papers appears in this supplement of the journal that covers the differential diagnosis of bipolar disorders, mechanism of action of anticonvulsants in

mood disorders, pharmacokinetics of the anticonvulsants, and an algorithm for patient management of acute mania.

Stoudemire A: New Antidepressant Drugs and the Treatment of Depression in the Medically Ill Patient. Psychiatric Clinics of America, Vol. 19, 495–514, 1996.

Willner P: Depression: A Psychobiological Synthesis. New York, Wiley-Interscience Publication, 1985

A comprehensive review of the biological and cognitive theories of depression

REFERENCES

Agency for Health Care Policy and Research: Depression in Primary Care: Vol. 1. Detection and Diagnosis: Clinical Practice Guideline, No. 5. Washington, DC, US Department of Health and Human Services, USPHS publication No. 93-0551, 1993a

Agency for Health Care Policy and Research: Depression in Primary Care: Vol. 2. Treatment of Major Depression: Clinical Practice Guideline, No. 5. Washington, DC, US Department of Health and Human Services, USPHS publication No. 93-0551, 1993b

Akiskal HS, Hirschfeld RMA, Yerevanian BI: The relationship of personality to affective disorders: A critical review. Arch Gen Psychiatry 40:801–810, 1983

American Psychiatric Association: Practice Guideline for Major Depressive Disorder in Adults. Am J Psychiatry 150(suppl):1–26, 1993

American Psychiatric Association: Diagnostic and Statistic Manual of Mental Disorders, 4th ed. Washington, DC, American Psychiatric Association, 1994

Aneshensel CS, Stone JD: Stress and depression: a test of the buffering model of social support. Arch Gen Psychiatry 39:1392–1396, 1982

Arana GW, Baldessasini RJ, Ornsteen M: The dexamethasone suppression test for diagnosis and prognosis in psychiatry. Arch Gen Psychiatry 42:1193–1204, 1985

Asberg M, Traskman L: Studies of CSF 5–HIAA in depression and suicidal behavior. Adv Exp Med Biol 133:739–752, 1981

Banerjee SP, Kung CS, Riggi SJ, Chanda SK: Development of beta-adrenergic subsensitivity by antidepressants. Nature 268:455–456, 1977

Banki CM: Correlation of anxiety and related symptoms with cerebrospinal fluid 5-hydroxyindoleacetic acid in depressed women. J Neural Transm 41:135–143, 1977

Banki CM, Arato M: Amine metabolites and neuroendocrine responses related to depression and suicide. J Affect Disord 5:223–232, 1983

Beck AT: The development of depression: a cognitive model. In Friedman, Katz MM (eds): The Psychology of Depression: Contemporary Theory and Research, pp 3–20. New York, John Wiley & Sons, 1974

Belsher G, Costello CG: Relapse after recovery from unipolar depression: A critical review. Psychol Bull 104:84–96, 1988

Bennie EH, Mullin JM, Martindale JJ: A double-blind multicenter trial comparing sertraline and fluoxetine in outpatients with major depression. J Clin Psychiatry 56:229–237, 1995

Berrettini W. Diagnostic and genetic issues of depression and bipolar illness. Psychophamacotherapy 15:69S–75S, 1995

Bowden CL, Brugger AM, Swann AC, et al: Efficacy of divalproex versus lithium and placebo in the treatment of mania. The Depakote Mania Study Group. [Published erratum appears in JAMA 271:1830, 1994. See comments.] JAMA 271:918–924, 1994

Bowden CL, Janicak PG, Orsulak P, et al: Relation of serum valproate concentration to response in mania. Am J Psychiatry 153:765–770, 1996

Boyd JH, Weissman M: Epidemiology of affective disorder. A reexamination and future directions. Arch Gen Psychiatry 38:1039–1046, 1981

Breier A, Kelsoe JR, Kirwin PD, Beller SA, Wolkowitz OM, Pickar D: Early parental loss and development of adult psychopathology. Arch Gen Psychiatry 45:987–993, 1988

Brown GW, Harris TO, Hepworth C: Life events and endogenous depression: a puzzle reexamined. Arch Gen Psychiatry 51:525–534, 1994

Carroll BJ: The dexamethasone supresion test for melancholia. Br J Psychiatry 140:292–304, 1982

Chow MSS: Focus on mirtazapine: A new antidepressant with noradrenergic and specific serotonergic activity. Formulary 31:455–469, 1996

Coble P, Foster FG, Kupfer DJ: Electroencephalographic sleep diagnosis of primary depression. Arch Gen Psychiatry 33:1124–1127, 1976

Cohen-Cole S, Harpe C: Diagnostic Assessment of Depression in the Medically Ill. In Stoudemire A, Fogel BS (eds): Principles of Medical Psychiatry. Orlando, FL, Grune & Stratton, 1987

Copoper A, Prange AJ, Whybrow PC, Noguere R: Abnormalities of indoleamines in affective disorders. Arch Gen Psychiatry 26:474–478, 1972

Coryell W, Endicott J, Keller M: Outcome of patients with chronic affective disorder: a five year followup. Am J Psychiatry 147:1627–1633, 1990

Coryell W, Endicott J, Keller M: Rapidly cycling affective disorder: demographics, diagnosis, family history, and course. Arch Gen Psychiatry 49:126–1311, 1992

Davis JM, Bresnahan DB: Psychopharmacology in clinical psychiatry. In Holes R, Franes HJ (eds): Psychiatry Update, Vol. 6, pp 159–187. Washington, DC, American Psychiatric Association, 1987

de Boer T, Ruigt GSF: The selective alpha$_2$-adrenoreceptor antagonist mirtazapine (Org 3770) enhances noradrenergic and 5-HT$_{1A}$-mediated serotonergic neurotransmission. CNS Drugs 4(suppl 1):29–38, 1995

De Leo D, Diekstra RFW: Depression and Suicide in Late Life, pp. 177–197. Lewiston, NY, Hogrefe & Huber, 1990

Finkelstein SN, Berndt ER, Greenberg PE: Economics of Depression: A Summary and Review. Prepared for the National Depressive and Manic-Depressive Association-Sponsored Consensus Conference on the Undertreatment of Depression, January 17–18, 1996.

Frank E, Kupfer DJ, Perel JM, et al. Three-year outcomes for maintenance therapies in recurrent depression. Arch Gen Psychiatry 47:1093–1099, 1990

Gattuz WF, Vogel P, Kick H, Kohnen R: Moclobemide vs fluoxetine in the treatment of inpatients with major depression. J Clin Psychopharmacol 15(suppl 2):35S–40S, 1995

Gibbons RD, Davis JM: Consistent evidence for a biological subtype of depression characterized by low CSF monoamine levels. Acta Psychiatr Scand 74:8–12, 1986

Gillin JC, Duncan W, Pettigrew KD, Erakel BL, Snyder F: Successful separation of depressed, normal and insomniac subjects by EEG sleep data. Arch Gen Psychiatry 36:85–90, 1979

Glassman AH, Bigger JT: Cardiovascular effects of therapeutic doses of tricyclic antidepressants: a review. Arch Gen Psychiatry 38:815–820, 1981

Glenn M, Taska RJ: Antidepressants and lithium. In Karasu TB (ed): The Psychiatric Therapies. Washington, DC, American Psychiatric Association, 85–118, 1984

Gold PW, Goodwind FK, Chrousos GP: Clinical and biochemical manifestations of depression, part I: Relation to the neurobiology of stress. N Engl J Med 319:348–353, 1988a

Gold PW, Goodwin FK, Chrousos GP: Clinical and biochemical manifestations of depression, part II: Relation to the neurobiology of stress. N Engl J Med 319:413–420, 1988b

Goldberg JF, Harrow M, Grossman LS: Course and outcome in bipolar affective disorder: a longitudinal follow-up study. Am J Psychiatry 152:379–384, 1995

Gonzalez-Heydrich J, Peroutka SJ: Serotonin receptors and reuptake sites: pharmacologic significance. J Clin Psychiatry 51(suppl):5–12, 1990

Goodwin FK, Jamison KR: Course and outcome. In Goodwin FK, Jamison KR (eds): Manic–Depressive Illness, pp 127–156. New York, Oxford University Press, 1990

Greden J: Maintenance antidepressant treatment [Progress Notes]. Am Soc Clin Psychopharmacol 6:28–34, 1995–96

Greenburg PE, Stiglin LE, Finkelstein SN, Berndt ER: The economic burden of depression in 1990. J Clin Psychiatry 54(suppl 11):405–418, 1993

Hall RCW, Wise MG: The clinical and financial burden of mood disorders. Psychosomatics 36:S11–S18, 1995

Hatterer JA, Herbert J, Hidaka C, et al: CSF transthyretin in patients with depression. Am J Psychiatry 150:813–815, 1993

Hestbach J, Hansen HE, Amdisen A, Olsen S: Chronic renal lesions following long-term treatment with lithium. Kidney Int 12:205–213, 1977

Hirschfeld RM, Cross CC: Epidemiology of affective disorders: psychosocial risk factors. Arch Gen Psychiatry 39:35–47, 1982

Holsboer F, Liebl R, Hofschuster E: Repeated desmethasone suppression test during depressive illness: normalization of test result compared with clinical improvement. J Affect Disord 4:93–101, 1982

Hyman S: How antidepressants might work [Progress Notes]. Am Soc Clin Psychopharmacol 6:11–15, 1995–96

Jimerson DC, Insel TR, Reus VI, Kopin IW: Increased plasma MHPG in dexamethasone-resistant depressed patients. Arch Gen Psychiatry 40:173–176, 1983

Kando JC, Tohen M, Castillo J, Zarate CA: The use of valproate in an elderly population with affective symptoms. J Clin Psychiatry 57:238–240, 1996

Kaplan HI, Sadock BJ: Mood disorders. In Kaplin HI, Sadock BJ (eds): Synopsis of Psychiatry. Baltimore, Williams & Wilkins, 288–309, 1988

Katon W, Schulberg H: Epidemiology of depression in primary care. Gen Hosp Psychiatry 14:237–247, 1992

Keck PE, McElroy SL, Nemeroff CB: Anticonvulsants in the treatment of bipolar disorder. J Neuropsychiatry Clin Neurosci 4:395–405, 1992

Keck PE, McElroy SL, Tugrul KC, et al: Valproate oral; loading in the treatment of acute mania. J Clin Psychiatry 54:305–308, 1993

Keller MB, Baker LA: The clinical course of panic disorder and depression. J Clin Psychiatry 53(3, suppl)5–8, 1992

Keller MB, Hanks DL: The natural history and homogeneity of depressive disorders; implications for rational antidepressant therapy. J Clin Psychiatry 55(suppl):1–7, 1994

Keller MB, Klerman GL, Lavori PW, et al: Treament received by depressed patients. JAMA 248:1848–1855, 1982a

Keller MB, Shapiro RW, Lavori PW, et al: Recovery in major depressive disorder: analysis with the life table and regression models. Arch Gen Psychiatry 39:905–910, 1982b

Keller MB, Klerman GL, Lavori PW, et al: Longterm outcome of episodes of major depression. Clinical and public health significance. JAMA 252:788–792, 1984

Keller MB, Lavori LA, Coryell W, et al: Bipolar I: a five-year prospective follow-up. J Nerv Ment Dis 181:238–245, 1993

Keller MB, Lavori W, Rice J, et al: The consistent risk of chronicity in recurrent episodes of non-polar major depressive disorder: a prospective followup. Am J Psychiatry 143:24–28, 1986

Keller MB, Lavori PW, Endicott J: "Double depression." Two year follow-up. Am J Psychiatr 140:689–694, 1983

Kessler RC, McGonagle KA, Zhao S, et al: Lifetime and 12-month prevalence of DSM-III-R psychiatric disorders in the United States. Arch Gen Psychiatry 51:8–18, 1994

Klerman GL: History and developments of modern concepts of affective illness. In Post RM, Ballenger JC (eds): Neurobiology of Mood Disorders, pp 1–19. Baltimore, Williams & Wilkins, 1984

Kupfer DJ, Thase ME: The use of the sleep laboratory in the diagnosis of affective disorders. Psychiatr Clin North Am 6:3–25, 1983

Leonard BE: Pharmacological differences of serotonin reuptake inhibitors and possible clinical relevance. Drugs 43(suppl 2):3–10, 1992

Lichtenberg P, Shapira B, Gillon D, et al, Hormone responses to fenfluramine and placebo challenge in endogenous depression. Psychiatry Res 43:137–146, 1992

Lloyd C: Life events and depressive disorder reviewed, Part I: Events as predisposing factors. Arch Gen Psychiatry 37:529–535, 1980

Loosen PT, Prange AJ: Serum thyroptropin response to thyrotropin-releasing hormone in psychiatric patients: a review. Am J Psychiatry 139:405–416, 1982

Mass JW, Koslow SH, David J, Katz M, et al: Catecholamine metabolism and disposition in healthy depressed subjects. Arch Gen Psychiatry 44:337–344, 1987

McElroy SL, Keck PE: Antiepileptic drugs. In Schatzberg AF, Nemeroff CB (eds): Textbook of Psychopharmacology. Washington, DC, American Psychiatric Press, 351–375, 1995

McElroy SL, Keck PE, Pope HG, Hudson JI, Faedda GL, Swann AC: Dysphoric or mixed mania: clinical and research implications. Am J Psychiatry 149:1633–1644, 1992

McGrath RJ, Stewart JW, Harrison WM, et al: Predictive value of symptoms of atypical depression for differential drug treatment outcome. J Clin Psychopharmacol 12:197–202, 1992

Mendels J, Frazer A, Fitzgerald RG, Ramsey TA, Stokes KW: Biogenic amine metabolites in cerebrospinal fluid of depressed and manic patients. Science 175:1380–1382, 1972

Mortola, JF: Issues in the diagnosis and research of premenstral syndrome. Clin Obstet Gynecol 35:587–598, 1992

Muth EA, Haskins JT, Moyer JA, et al: Antidepressant biochemical profile of the novel bicyclic compound W4-45,030: an ethyl cyclohexamol derivative. Biochem Pharmacol 35:4493–4497, 1986

Nathan KI, Musselman DL, Schatzberg AF, Nemeroff CB: Biology of mood disorders. In Schatzberg AF, Nemeroff CB (eds): Textbook of Psychopharmacology. Washington, DC, American Psychiatric Press, 1995

Nierenberg AA, Feighner JP, Rudolph R, Cole JO, Sullivan J: Venlafaxine for treatment-resistant unipolar depression. J Clin Psychopharmacol 14:419–423, 1994

NIH Consensus Development Panel on Depression in Late Life: Diagnosis and treatment of depression in late life. JAMA 268:1018–1024, 1992

NIMH Consensus Development Panel: Mood disorders: pharmacologic prevention of recurrences. (NIMH/NIH Consensus Development Conference Statement). Am J Psychiatry 142:469–476, 1985

Pardes H, Kaufmann CA, Pincus HA, et al: Genetics and psychiatry: past discoveries, current dilemmas, and future directions. Am J Psychiatry 146:435–443, 1989

Post RM: The transduction of psychosocial stress into the neurobiology of recurrent affective disorder. Am J Psychiatry 149:999–1010, 1992

Post RM, Ballenger JC, Uhde TW, Putman TW, Bunney WE: Kindling and drug sensitization: implications for the progressive development of pychopathology and treatment with carbamazepine. In Sadler M (ed): The Psychopharmacology of Anticonvulsants, pp 27–53. Oxford, Oxford University Press, 1981

Post RM, Rubinow DH, Uhde TW, et al: Dysphoric mania: clinical and biological correlates. Arch Gen Psychiatry 46:353–358, 1989

Potter WZ, Rudorfer MV, Goodwin FK: Biological Findings in Bipolar Disorders. Annual Review, Vol. 6. Washington, DC, American Psychiatric Association, 1987

Preskorn SH, Burke M: Somatic therapy for major depressive disorder: selection of an antidepressant. J Clin Psychiatry 53(9, suppl):5–18, 1992

Quitkin F, Rifkin A, Klein DF: Monoamine oxidase inhibitors. Arch Gen Psychiatry 36:749–759, 1979

Redmond DE, Katz MM, Mass JW, Swann A, Casper R, David JM: Cerebrospinal fluid amine metabolites. Arch Gen Psychiatry 43:939–947, 1986

Regier DA, Narrow WE, Rae DS, et al: The de facto US Mental and Addictive Disorders Service System: Epidemiologic Catchment Area prospective 1-year prevalence rates of disorders and services. Arch Gen Psychiatry 50:84–94, 1993

Reynolds CF, Kupfer DJ: Sleep research in affective illness: state of the art circa 1987. Sleep 10:199–215, 1987

Richelson E: Antidepressants and brain neurochemistry. Mayo Clin Proc 65:1227–1236, 1990

Rickels K, Schweizer E: Clinical overview of serotonin reuptake inhibitors. J Clin Psychiatry 51(suppl B, 12):9–12, 1990

Risby ED, Donnigan D, Nemeroff CB: Pharmacotherapeutic considerations for psychiatric disorders: depression. Formulary 32:46–59, 1997

Risch SC, Nemeroff CB: Neurochemical alterations of serotonergic neuronal systems in depression. J Clin Psychiatry 53(10 suppl):3–7, 1992

Robins LN, Regier DA (eds): Psychiatric Disorders in America: The Epidemiologic Catchment Area Study. New York, The Free Press, 1991

Roy A, Pickar D, Linnoila M, Doran AR, Ninan P, Paul SM: Cerebrospinal fluid monoamine metabolite concentrations in melancholia. Psychiatry Res 15:281–292, 1985

Rudorfer MV, Potter, WZ: Antidepressants. A comparative review of the clinical pharmacology and therapeutic use of the 'newer' versus the 'older' drugs. Drugs 37:713–718, 1989

Rush AJ, Cain JW, Raese J, et al: Neurobiological basis for psychiatric disorders. In Rosenburg RN (ed): Comprehensive Neurology, pp 555–603. New York, Raven Press, 1991.

Schatzberg AF: Recent developments in the acute somatic treatment of major depression. J Clin Psychiatry 53(3, suppl):20–25, 1992

Schweizer E, Weise C, Clary C, et al: Placebo-controlled trial of venlafaxine for the treatment of major depression. J Clin Psychopharmacol 11:233–236, 1991

Scully RF, Galdabini JJ, McNely BV: Case records of the Massachusetts General Hospital. N Engl J Med 304:1025–1032, 1981

Shapira B, Yagmur MJ, Gropp C, Newman M, Lerer B: Effect of clomipramine and lithium on fenfluramine-induced hormone release in major depression. Biol Psychiatry 31:975–983, 1992

Siever LJ, Trestman RL, Coccaro EF, et al: The growth hormone response to clonidine in acute and remitted depressed male patients. Neuropsychopharmacology 6:165–177, 1992

Simon GE, Von Korff M, Barlow W: Health care cost of primary care patients with recognized depression. Arch Gen Psychiatry 52:850–856, 1995

Smith SB, Garcia-Sevilla JA, Hollingsworth PJ: Adrenoceptors in rat brain are decreased after long-term trycyclic antidepressant drug treatment. Brain Res 210:413–418, 1981

Snyder SH: Molecular Strategies in Neuropsychopharmacology: Old and New. In Meltzer HY (ed): Psychopharmacology. The Third Generation of Progress. New York, Raven Press, 17–22, 1987

Sterinbach H: The serotonin syndrome. Am J Psychiatry 148:705–713, 1991

Stoudemire GA, Fogel BS, Gulley LR, Moran MG: Psychopharmacology in the medical patient. In Stoudemire GA, Fogel BS (eds): Psychiatric Care of the Medical Patient, pp 155–206. New York, Oxford University Press, 1993

Suppes T, Baldessarini RJ, Faedda GL, et al. Risk of recurrence following discontinuation of lithium treatment in bipolar disorder. Arch Gen Psychiatry 48:1082–1088, 1991

Thase ME: Long-term treatment of recurrent depressive disorders. J Clin Psychiatry 53(suppl 9): 32–44, 1992

Tohen M, Waternaux CM, Tsuang MT: Outcome in mania: a 4-year prospective follow-up of 75 patients utilizing survial analysis. Arch Gen Psychiatry 47:1106–1111, 1990

Van Praag HM, DeHaan S: Central serotonin metabolism and frequency of depression. Psychiatr Res 1:219–224, 1979

Veith RC, Raskind MA, Caldwell JH: Cardiovascular effects of tricyclic antidepressants in depressed patients with chronic heart disease. N Engl J Med 306: 954–959, 1982

Vetulani J, Stawarz RJ, Dingell JV, Sulser F: A possible common mechanism of action of anti-depressant treatments: reduction in the sensitivity of the noradrenergic cycle AMP generating system in the rat limbic forearm. Naunyn-Schmiedebergs Arch Pharmacol 293:109–114, 1976

Von Korff M, Ormel J, Katon W, et al. Disability and depression among high utilizers of health care: a longitudinal analysis. Arch Gen Psychiatry 49:91–100, 1992

Warner MD, Peabody CA, Whiteford HA, Hollister LE: Trazadone and priapism. J Clin Psychiatry 48:244–245, 1987

Weisler RH: A Profile of bupropion: a nonserotonergic alternative. J Clin Psychiatry Monogr 9:29–35, 1991

Weissman MM, Klerman GL: Depression: Current understanding and changing trends. Annu Rev Publ Health 13:319–339, 1992

Williams AW, Ware JE, Donald CA: A model of mental health, life events, and social supports applicable to general populations. J Health Soc Behav 22:324–336, 1981

Willner P: Depression: A Psychobiological Synthesis. New York, Wiley-Interscience, 1985

Winokur G, Coryell W, Akiskal HS, Endicott J, Keller M, Mueller T: Manic-depresive (bipolar) disorder: the course in light of a prospective ten-year follow-up of 131 patients. Acta Psychiatr Scand 89:102–110, 1994

Winokur G, Coryell W, Keller M, et al: A prospective follow-up of patients with bipolar and primary unipolar affective disorder. Arch Gen Psychiatry 50:457–465, 1993

Zis AP, Goodwin FK: Major affective disorders as a recurrent illness: a critical review. Arch Gen Psychiatry 36:835–839, 1979

8 *Anxiety Disorders*

Linda M. Nagy,
Mickey R. Riggs,
John H. Krystal, and
Dennis S. Charney

The anxiety disorders discussed in this chapter are those included in the *Diagnostic and Statistical Manual of Mental Disorders,* 4th ed (DSM-IV): Panic Disorder and Agoraphobia, Social Phobia, Specific Phobia, Obsessive–Compulsive Disorder, Posttraumatic Stress Disorder, Generalized Anxiety Disorder, and Acute Stress Disorder (American Psychiatric Association, 1994). For each disorder, epidemiological data, a basic description of the syndrome, differential diagnosis, pathophysiology/etiological theories, and treatment approaches are reviewed. It is crucial for physicians to recognize anxiety disorders accurately and be aware of their appropriate treatments. These conditions are among the most common in the general population, lead to high utilization of healthcare services, and, when untreated, produce significant distress and disability. Common errors among physicians include failure to consider nonpsychiatric medical disorders and treatments as causative or contributing to the patient's symptoms, nonspecifically labeling the patient's problem as "anxiety" without making a specific anxiety disorder diagnosis, or referral to a specialist for assessment after medication (usually benzodiazepine) has already been prescribed, which hampers assessment and the patient's receptiveness regarding treatment recommendations. As discussed below, the category of Anxiety Disorders includes several distinct disorders that differ with respect to symptoms, epidemiology, pathophysiology, and treatment.

ADJUSTMENT DISORDER
WITH ANXIETY

The general category of *adjustment disorder* has been mentioned in Chapter 7 in reference to depressive reactions. In the context of anxiety, an adjustment disorder with anxiety would be defined as a *maladaptive* reaction to an identifiable environmental or psychosocial stress, accompanied predominantly by symptoms of anxiety, that interferes with the patient's functioning. Although the degree of anxiety-related stress can be disabling, the anxiety is expected to remit after the stress remits or an adaptation is made. Adjustment Disorder With Mixed Anxiety and Depressed Mood can be specified if symptoms of anxiety and depression appear enmeshed.

These types of stress-related reactions often bring patients to physicians' offices with a variety of physiological symptoms of their anxiety. Short-term use of low-dose benzodiazepines may be of benefit as long as the patient is helped to identify the stress that may have caused the symptoms and means of managing it more effectively are discussed. If the stress appears to be chronic or unmanagable by the patient, the patient may require further evaluation and possibly some form of psychotherapy. Referral for a thorough psychiatric evaluation should be made well before the long-term use of benzodiazepines becomes the only alternative for managing chronic anxiety.

PANIC DISORDER AND AGORAPHOBIA

Panic disorder is characterized by recurrent discrete attacks of anxiety accompanied by several somatic symptoms, such as palpitations, paresthesias, hyperventilation, diaphoresis, chest pain, dizziness, trembling, and dyspnea. Usually the condition is accompanied by agoraphobia, which consists of excessive fear (and often avoidance) of situations, such as driving, crowded places, stores, or being alone, in which escape or obtaining help would be difficult. Current DSM-IV classifications include Panic Disorder Without Agoraphobia, Panic Disorder With Agoraphobia, and Agoraphobia Without History of Panic Disorder.

Epidemiology

The Epidemiologic Catchment Area (ECA) Study reports prevalence estimates based on DSM-III diagnoses, which were separated into agoraphobia and panic disorder. Lifetime prevalence rates at the three sites varied between 7.8 and 23.3% for all phobias (including social and simple) and between 1.4 and 1.5% for panic disorder. Six-month prevalence rates were 2.7 to 5.8% for agoraphobia and 0.6 to 1.0% for panic disorder. The lifetime rate for females was 2.4 to 4.3 times greater than that for males for agoraphobia and 1.3 to

3.5 times greater for panic disorder; however, 6-month prevalence rates for panic disorder were either similar between sexes or increased in males (Myers et al, 1984; Robins et al, 1984). It is generally felt that there may be under-reporting of these disorders by men either due to reluctance to admit to having these symptoms or through disguise by alcoholism. Alternatively, there may be true higher rates in females because of hormonal, social, or other types of gender-related differences.

Age of onset is typically in the late teens to early thirties and is unusual after the age of 40 years. *The majority (78%) of patients describe the initial panic attack as spontaneous* (occurring without an environmental trigger). In the remainder the first attack is precipitated by confrontation with a phobic stimulus or use of a psychoactive drug. Onset of the disorder often follows within 6 months of a major stressful life event, such as marital separation, occupational change, or pregnancy (Breier et al, 1986).

These disorders appear to be less prevalent in the elderly, but there is at least preliminary new evidence that undiagnosed agoraphobia may contribute significantly to dysfunction in some people over 65. Both 6-month and lifetime rates are lower in the over-65 age group, suggesting possible under-reporting, decreased survival of those with the disorder, or a cohort effect, such that the frequency of the disorder is increased in the middle-age groups. Rates are generally similar for blacks and whites, and higher for non-college graduates and unmarried individuals. It is not yet established whether these differences reflect predisposing factors, noncausal associations, or consequences of the disorder. Panic disorder is increased among family members of those with the disorder (see Etiology, below). A history of childhood separation anxiety disorder is reported by 20 to 50% of patients. Preliminary findings of high rates of behavioral inhibition in the offspring of patients with panic disorder are consistent with the hypothesis that the disorder may have a biogenetically determined component and thus developmental antecedents. In addition, this hypothesis has been supported recently by more sophisticated longitudinal studies.

Description and Differential Diagnosis

Panic disorder usually begins with a spontaneous panic attack that often leads the individual to seek medical treatment, such as presenting to an emergency room believing that he or she is having a heart attack, stroke, losing his or her mind, or experiencing some other serious medical event (Table 8–1). Some time may pass before subsequent attacks, or the patient may continue to get frequent attacks. Patients may feel constantly fearful and anxious after the first attack, wondering what is wrong and fearing it will happen again. Some patients experience nocturnal attacks that awaken them from sleep. Usually patients gradually become fearful of situations (1) that they associate with the attacks, (2) in which they would be unable to flee if the attack occurred, (3) in

Table 8–1 **Symptoms of a Panic Attack***

A discrete period of intense fear or discomfort, in which at least four of the following symptoms developed abruptly and reached a peak within 10 minutes:
1. palpitations, pounding heart, or accelerated heart rate
2. sweating
3. trembling or shaking
4. sensations of shortness of breath or smothering
5. feeling of choking
6. chest pain or discomfort
7. nausea or abdominal distress
8. feeling dizzy, unsteady, lightheaded, or faint
9. derealization (feelings of unreality) or depersonalization (being detached from oneself)
10. fear of losing control or going crazy
11. fear of dying
12. paresthesias (numbness or tingling sensations)
13. chills or hot flushes

* Adapted from DSM-IV criteria (American Psychiatric Association, 1994).

which help would not be readily available, or (4) in which they would be embarrassed if others should notice they are experiencing an attack (although attacks are not usually evident to others). The symptoms of agoraphobia and the diagnostic criteria for panic disorder with agoraphobia are listed in Table 8–2. (It should be noted that panic disorder may occur with or without agoraphobia.) Less frequently, a history of phobia may precede the first panic attack. Before patients are educated about the symptoms of the disorder they believe they are suffering from a serious medical condition. They are often embarrassed about their symptoms and will try to hide them from others, often making excuses not to attend functions or enter phobic situations.

The differential diagnosis of panic disorder and agoraphobia includes anxiety disorders due to general medical conditions; anxiety due to substances such as caffeine, cocaine, or amphetamines; withdrawal from alcohol, sedative–hypnotics, and benzodiazepines; and other phobic conditions, generalized anxiety disorder, and psychosis. Medical illness that may produce symptoms similar to panic attacks must be excluded. Endocrine disturbances, such as pheochromocytoma, thyroid disorder, or hypoglycemia, may produce similar symptoms and can be excluded with appropriate clinical history and laboratory evaluations. When gastrointestinal symptoms of attacks are prominent one may need to exclude the diagnosis of colitis. Symptoms of tachycardia, palpitations, chest pain or pressure, and dyspnea may be confused with cardiac or respiratory conditions. Lightheadedness, faintness, dizziness, derealization, shaking, numbness, and tingling may suggest a neurological condition. The association between mitral valve prolapse and panic disorder is controversial. The presence of mitral valve prolapse in panic disorder patients does not

Table 8–2 **Symptoms of Agoraphobia and Diagnostic Criteria for Panic Disorder with Agoraphobia***

Symptoms of Agoraphobia

A. Anxiety about being in places or situations from which escape might be difficult (or embarassing) or in which help may not be available in the event of having an unexpected or situationally predisposed Panic Attack or paniclike symptoms. Agoraphobic fears typically involve characteristic clusters of situations that include being outside the home alone; being in a crowd or standing in a line; being on a bridge; and traveling in a bus, train, or automobile.
Note: Consider the diagnosis of Specific Phobia if the avoidance is limited to one or only a few specific situations, or Social Phobia if the avoidance is limited to social situations.

B. The situations are avoided (e.g., travel is restricted) or else are endured with marked distress or with anxiety about having a Panic Attack or paniclike symptoms, or require the presence of a companion.

C. The anxiety or phobic avoidance is not better accounted for by another mental disorder, such as Social Phobia.

Diagnostic Criteria for Panic Disorder with Agoraphobia

A. Both (1) and (2):
   (1) recurrent unexpected Panic Attacks
   (2) at least one of the attacks has been followed by 1 month (or more) of one (or more) of the following:
       (a) persistent concern about having additional attacks
       (b) worry about implications of the attack or its consequences (e.g., losing control, having a heart attack, "going crazy")
       (c) a significant change in behavior related to the attacks

B. The presence of Agoraphobia

C. The Panic Attacks are not due to the direct physiological effects of a substance (e.g., a drug of abuse, a medication) or a general medical condition (e.g., hyperthyroidism)

D. The Panic Attacks are not better accounted for by another mental disorder.

* Adapted from DSM-IV criteria (American Psychiatric Association, 1994).

---

appear to alter treatment response or course, so the diagnosis of panic disorder should be made independently of mitral valve prolapse.

Panic disorder differs from generalized anxiety disorder in that the panic attacks are distinguished by recurrent discrete, intense episodes of panic symptoms, although in both disorders anticipatory anxiety and generalized feelings of anxiety may be present. Although some of the same situations may be feared, agoraphobia differs from social and simple phobias in that the fear is related to feeling trapped or being unable to escape and that the fears often become generalized. Agoraphobics may additionally have a history of other phobias.

Panic disorder is frequently associated with major depression, other anxiety disorders, and alcohol and substance dependence. In clinical samples as many as two-thirds of panic patients report experiencing a major depressive episode at some time in their lives. Similarly, studies of patients seeking treatment for major depression report high rates of panic in these patients and their relatives. Once symptoms begin, patients often describe becoming demoralized as a result of fear related to the symptoms and imagined causes, as well as impairment when their activities are restricted by their agoraphobia. Unlike depressed patients, panic disorder patients usually lack vegetative symptoms and have a normal desire to engage in activities but avoid them because of their phobias.

The disorder may cause personality changes. Patients' premorbid personalities may be highly independent, outgoing, and active, but while symptoms are active they can become very dependent, passive, and overly agreeable, with an extreme need to please others, and may resist making appointments or social engagements. Patients typically are fearful of being alone.

Attempts to self-medicate the intolerable anxiety may increase the risk of alcoholism and substance abuse. Patients may require a drink before entering phobic situations. Approximately 20% of patients report a history of alcohol abuse, but the onset of alcoholism precedes the first attack in almost all patients. Alcoholism may also alter the course of the disorder. Preliminary data suggest that panic disorder precipitated by cocaine use may be less likely to respond well to the usual pharmacological treatments and may have less association with a family history of panic disorder.

Etiological/Pathophysiological Theories

Familial/Genetic Theories

Genetic epidemiological studies have consistently demonstrated increased rates of panic disorder among first- and second-degree relatives of panic disorder probands. This observation could result from genetic, nongenetic biological, and/or cultural factors shared by family members. The reported recurrence risk of illness in first-degree relatives of panic disorder probands is 15 to 18% by patient report versus 0 to 5% in controls, and is 20 to 50% by direct interview of relatives of panic probands versus 2 to 8% in relatives of controls. Segregation analysis indicates that the pattern of familial transmission is consistent with single-locus autosomal dominant transmission with incomplete penetrance, although a multifactorial mode of inheritance (additive effects of more than one gene) or genetic heterogeneity (different gene defects producing similar clinical syndromes) have not been excluded as possibilities. Comparison of concordance rates in monozygotic versus dizygotic twins is used to differentiate between genetic and environmental factors in families, since monozygotic twins share 100% of their genetic material and dizygotic twins on average share half. Concordance for anxiety disorder with panic attacks in 4 of 13 monozygotic and 0 of 16 dizygotic twin pairs. Other preliminary reports suggest identical HLA genotypes in sibling pairs concordant for panic disorder; genetic linkage studies thus far have been negative.

Studies of the genetics of panic disorder in general support the idea that panic disorder, while comorbid with major depressive disorder, is a distinct entity, and that panic disorder appears to be heterogeneous in origin. This heterogeneity, combined with the high comorbidity of major depression in patients with panic, may help to explain the variable estimates of the suicide rate in patients with panic disorder as well as the varying response to pharmacotherapy and other therapeutic modalities observed in those patients with panic disorder with and without comorbidity.

Other Biological Theories

Investigation of biological systems in panic disorder includes examination of adrenergic, benzodiazepine, serotonergic, and opiate neurotransmitter systems; anxiogenic response to caffeine, lactate, and CO_2; models of locus ceruleus involvement; and brain imaging studies. Yohimbine, an alpha-2 adrenergic receptor antagonist, produces greater increases in anxiety (resembling panic attacks), blood pressure, and plasma levels of the norepinephrine metabolite MHPG in panic disorder patients than in healthy subjects. This responsiveness appears to be specific to panic disorder patients; it is not observed in generalized anxiety disorder, obsessive–compulsive disorder, major depression, or schizophrenia. However, posttraumatic stress disorder patients have similar responses (see below). Panic patients exhibit panic attacks and a blunted heart rate response to isoproterenol, a beta-adrenergic agonist, as well as decreased lymphocyte beta-adrenergic receptors. It is hypothesized that downregulation of beta-adrenergic receptor function is due to chronic or episodically increased presynaptic noradrenergic activity.

The benzodiazepine inverse agonist FG-7142 precipitated severe anxiety states comparable to panic attacks in healthy individuals; this is consistent with animal studies in which beta-carboline produces an acute fear state. The benzodiazepine antagonist flumazenil precipitated a modest level of anxiety and panic attacks in some panic disorder patients. Further evidence for benzodiazepine system involvement is the finding of a blunted saccadic eye movement response in panic patients.

Preclinical studies have suggested possible serotonergic involvement in anxiety and in the mechanisms of action of medications used to treat anxiety. However, the prolactin response to the serotonin precursor tryptophan is not altered in panic disorder. The serotonin agonist m-chlorophenylpiperazine (MCPP) may elicit greater anxiety responses in panic disorder patients, but the response is not as pronounced or consistent as that observed with yohimbine or lactate. Fenfluramine (a serotonin release and reuptake blocker) can also produce panic in panic disorder patients.

Klein (1996) notes that panic disorder and agoraphobia have been thought to occur by mechanisms of catastrophic cognition and physiological dysfunction of fear responses in the noradradrenergic system. He proposes that the efficacy of the selective serotonin-reuptake inhibitors (SSRIs) may be related to the role of serotonin in a "suffocation false alarm system" that is symptomatically quite visible in children with panic. However efficacious the SSRIs may be in the treatment of the disorder, the role of serotonin dysregulation in panic is likely to be multiple and complicated, and more research is needed.

Neuropeptides are receiving increasing attention. The peptide hormone cholecystokinin (CCK) is anxiogenic in healthy controls as well as panic patients. Neuropeptide Y is anxiolytic in animals but has not been studied in panic patients. Interactions between opiate and adrenergic systems were studied using yohimbine and naloxone, an opiate antagonist. The combination produced a synergistic effect of increasing anxiety symptoms and plasma cortisol. This is postulated to occur through opiate-noradrenergic interactions in the locus ceruleus, amygdala, cerebral cortex, or hypothalamus.

Although provocation of panic attacks with sodium lactate is the best replicated of the provocation procedures in panic, the mechanism by which lactate causes panic attacks is not established. Effects on noradrenergic activity, calcium, and regulation of intracellular pH and ion channels have been explored. Panic patients also demonstrate an increased anxiogenic response to breathing a mixture of air and CO_2 compared with controls. Effective antianxiety medications appear to block lactate-, yohimbine-, or CO_2-induced attacks.

Caffeine produces significantly greater anxiety symptoms in panic disorder patients than in controls. Therefore, patients are usually advised to eliminate caffeine from their diet. The most likely mechanism of caffeine's anxiogenic effect is antagonism of central adenosine receptors, which have neuromodulatory effects on acetylcholine, norepinephrine, and firing rates of locus ceruleus and other neurons. In animal studies of the locus ceruleus, the major norepinephrine-containing nucleus in the brain, stimulation produces a marked fear and anxiety response and ablation diminishes fear response to threatening stimuli. Additionally, many drugs that increase locus ceruleus firing in animals are anxiogenic in humans, whereas several drugs that decrease locus ceruleus discharge are anxiolytic in humans.

Unlike major depression, nondepressed panic disorder patients fail to show nonsuppression of cortisol following dexamethasone and worsen rather than improve with sleep deprivation.

Behavioral Theories

Behavioral theories (learning theory) have mainly been applied to the development of agoraphobia. This involves contiguity learning, the paired association of events that have occurred together (e.g., a panic attack and driving over a bridge), together with instrumental learning or operant conditioning, the modification of behavior to avoid future negative events and invite future positive events (e.g., by avoiding bridges, avoid the discomfort of an attack). Stimulus generalization may occur or subsequent attacks may occur in different situations and become associated with those situations. Panic disorder has also been viewed as a phobia in which the feared stimuli are internal rather than external. Patients associate somatic sensations with immediate threat and respond with anxiety and fear. After the first panic attack, subsequent attacks begin with unexpected peripheral somatic sensations to which the patient responds with anxiety, resulting in additional somatic symptoms and a spiraling increase in anxiety and symptoms. This theory has led to the application of relaxation, cognitive, and exposure techniques to the treatment of the attacks themselves (see Barlow and Lehman, 1996).

Psychoanalytic Theories

Psychoanalytic theory stems from Freud's hypothesis that panic attacks result from incomplete repression of unacceptable impulses. Later he revised this theory to conceptualize anxiety as a signal to the ego that it is in a dangerous situation. The patient then develops neurotic symptoms to reduce the signal anxiety and avoid danger. In any case, unconscious psychological conflict is believed to be the root cause. Freud also felt agoraphobia was due to the recollection of an anxiety attack along with fear of a future attack occurring in a situation in which the patient believed he or she could not escape it. He observed constitutional variability in individuals' capacities to experience anxiety and predicted that the mechanisms of biological predispositions would be better elucidated with advancing knowledge of brain neurochemistry.

Treatment

Pharmacological Treatment

Imipramine is the most well-established medication for panic, but most tricyclic antidepressants (TCAs) probably have similar efficacy. Monoamine oxidase inhibitors (MAOIs) can be very effective medications for anxiety patients but are not necessarily the drugs of choice, because they necessitate a low-tyramine diet to minimize the risk of hypertensive crisis. Anxiety patients are especially fearful and need extra education and reassurance to take MAOIs. The SSRIs have become well-established treatments for panic disorder. Paroxetine received early recognition as an effective and safe drug in this category, but all of the newer SSRIs may also be effective. This class of medications, like the TCAs, may best be employed in conjunction with some form of behavioral therapy. Despite efficacy in depression, trazodone and buproprion appear to be ineffective in panic disorder.

With all TCAs, MAOIs, and SSRIs, roughly 20% of panic patients will experience a stimulant-like reaction (with jitteriness, insomnia, and possibly increased panic attacks) during initial treatment. We recommend the following: (1) explain to the patient that this may occur and they need not be alarmed, and encourage them to call to discuss problems (rather than abruptly and unnecessarily discontinue treatment); (2) start with the lowest available dose (e.g., 10 mg imipramine, 5 mg fluoxetine); (3) if activation occurs, decrease to the dose that was previously tolerated until symptoms subside, then increase slowly. Some patients will habituate to the activation syndrome, but symptoms may reemerge with each dose increment. As in depression, antipanic effects are delayed for 2 to 6 weeks after reaching a therapeutic dose. Extra reassurance and encouragement are often needed when treating patients with this disorder.

Although alprazolam is the best studied of the benzodiazepines in panic disorder, other benzodiazepines, including lorazepam, clonazepam, and diazepam, are also effective when adequate doses are used. Clonazepam has gradually supplanted alprazolam as the benzodiazepine of choice for panic disorder in many clinicians' practices. Onset of therapeutic effects is fairly rapid. Some respond to low doses (i.e., 0.25 mg t.i.d. of alprazolam or equivalent), but 3.0 to 6.0 mg/day in divided doses is common. Benzodiazepines are usually used after other treatments have failed for panic because of concerns about difficulty with discontinuation and withdrawal reactions. Benzodiazepines should be avoided in patients with a history of alcohol or substance-abuse problems or personality disorder. Benzodiazepines with an intermediate elimination half-life (see Table 8–11) are sometimes preferred due to the need for less frequent dosing. Very long acting benzodiazepines such as diazepam can lead to problems with dose accumulation, particularly in older or medically compromised patients.

To initiate pharmacological treatment, begin with a low dose and gradually increase to therapeutic range (see Table 8–3 and Chapters 7 and 18). Reduction of phobic symptoms in particular may require maximal dosages. Once remission is achieved (1 to 3 months), lower maintenance doses may be adequate (up to 8 to 12 months), during which time patients should consolidate treatment improvements and return to a normal lifestyle. Discontinuation of medication should be gradual for both pharmacological and psychological reasons. Symptoms may reemerge shortly after benzodiazepine discontinuation and up to 2 to 3 months after discontinuation of antidepressants. Benzodiazepine withdrawal symptoms can be minimized by tapering slowly (e.g., 0.25 to 0.5 mg alprazolam every 3 to 7 days) and even more gradually for the last 1.5 mg. Patients need to understand that they may be asked to tolerate mild-to-moderate symptoms that are not dangerous for 4 to 10 days and the doctor should be available for guidance and support through this period (Ballenger, 1992). If symptoms persist 3 weeks after a benzodiazepine is discontinued, additional treatment should be considered.

Despite its usefulness in treating generalized anxiety disorder, the nonbenzodiazepine anxiolytic buspirone is ineffective in treating panic. Beta-blockers may block symptoms of palpitations or tremor but generally are not as effective against panic attacks as TCAs, MAOIs, SSRIs, or benzodiazepines. Occasionally a combination of a TCA and benzodiazepine is required. If both medications are initiated together, there is some possibility that the benzodiazepine may block the therapeutic effect of the TCA, based on reemergence of symptoms on attempts to withdraw the benzodiazepine.

Table 8-3 Pharmacotherapy for Anxiety Disorders

	ALPRAZOLAM*‡/OTHER BENZODIAZEPINES	BUSPIRONE	IMIPRAMINE‡/TCA	PHENELZINE‡/MAOI	FLUOXETINE‡/SSRI
Main indications†	PD, GAD, SP(?)	GAD	PD, PTSD, GAD(?), SP(?)	PD, PTSD, SP, OCD(?)	OCD, PD, SP(?), noncombat PTSD
Starting dose	0.25–0.5 mg t.i.d.	5 mg t.i.d.	10 mg qhs	15 mg q a.m.	5–20 mg/day
Initial side effects	Sedation, ataxia, memory impairment	Dizziness, nausea, diarrhea, headache, nervousness	Sedation, orthostatic hypotension, dry mouth, anxiety	Orthostatic hypotension, stimulant, tyramine reaction	Gastrointestinal, anorexia, insomnia, anxiety, drowsiness
Onset of effect	Immediate	2–4 wk delay	2–4 wk delay	2–4 wk delay	3–6 wk delay
Common target dose	0.25–2.0 mg t.i.d.	5–20 mg t.i.d.	25–300 mg qhs (or divided dose)	15–30 mg t.i.d.	20–80 mg/day
Long-term side effects	Physical dependece	None known at this time	Weight gain	Tyramine reaction	Unknown
Rate of discontinuation	0.25 mg/wk	No need to taper	50 mg/1–2 wk	15–45 mg/wk	3 wk taper
Symptoms of abrupt discontinuation	Increased sensitivity to sound/light/touch, autonomic arousal, confusion, seizures	None known at this time	Flulike symptoms, anxiety, nightmares	Hypertension, anxiety, nightmares, autonomic arousal, psychosis	Dizziness, insomnia, fatigue, mood swings, nausea, headache, sensory

* Benzodiazepine dose equivalents: 1 mg alprazolam = 0.5 mg clonazepam = 2 mg lorazepam = 10 mg diazepam; intermediate-acting benzodiazepines may have advantages. See text regarding discontinuation guidelines.
† PD, panic disorder; SP, social phobia; OCD, obsessive-compulsive disorder; GAD, generalized anxiety disorder; PTSD, posttraumatic stress disorder.
‡ Alprazolam, imipramine, phenelzine, and fluoxetine are listed as prototypical drugs in their respective classes for purposes of dosage guidelines. Other drugs in the same class were also effective.
(Adapted from Kyrstal JH, Charney, DS: Advances in anxiety therapy. Internal Medicine for the Specialist 9:93–111, 1988)

An alternative explanation is that benzodiazepine discontinuation itself induces symptoms of panic. This factor can be diminished by using long-acting benzodiazepine, like clonazepum. The combination of pharmacological treatment with behavioral or supportive psychotherapy is very important, especially when phobias are present. Table 8–3 summarizes pharmacological approaches for panic disorder/agoraphobia.

Behavioral Treatment

Prolonged exposure in vivo (see behavioral therapies in Chapter 17) appears to be the most effective behavioral treatment for agoraphobia. The usual procedure is to develop a hierarchical list of phobias, gradually enter the least phobic situations repeatedly, and then work up the hierarchy to more strongly feared situations. Prolonged (2 hours), in vivo, and frequent (daily) exposure sessions are superior to brief (0.5 hour), imaginal, and spaced (weekly) exposure sessions. Good results can be achieved in groups, individually, or as a self-help or spouse-assisted program. Group therapy may have the additional advantages of being cost effective, providing the patient with coping models, and leading to fewer dropouts. It is not essential to evoke anxiety during exposure. Follow-up studies report enduring effects several years after treatment.

Cognitive therapy appears to reduce irrational beliefs but by itself may not reduce anxiety or avoidance. The focus is to identify distorted patterns of thinking, interrupt the thought with self-instruction to stop, and substitute either distraction or positive thoughts. There is some evidence favoring the combination of relaxation training and biofeedback with cognitive therapy in the treatment of panic attacks. A newer form of cognitive–behavioral therapy—panic control treatment (PCT), which is comprised of breathing retraining, cognitive restructuring, and exposure to somatic cues—can be effective for desensitizing to symptoms of panic attacks in patients with no or mild agoraphobia. A multicenter trial is under way comparing PCT with imipramine and combinations.

Assertiveness training can help with dependency, passivity, and suppressed anger, which commonly result from patients' attempts to deal with panic and phobias. Aggressive individuals can be taught to recognize their aggressive behavior and substitute assertiveness.

The use of behavioral techniques, whether alone or in combination with pharmacotherapy, is well established for control of panic in certain patients and has proved useful in dealing with the sequelae of panic attacks, such as phobic avoidance. Some studies show that behavioral techniques may be of greater efficacy initially and after extended periods in the treatment of panic disorder than either placebo or pharmacotherapy alone; others show little difference, and still others advocate a combined approach. Again, these variations in the literature are most likely due to the presence or absence of comorbidity and the heterogenous origin of the syndrome itself.

Psychoeducation plays a very important role in the management of these patients. Knowing their diagnosis is enormously reassuring to many patients, who tend to believe they have a rare, perhaps life-threatening condition that doctors have failed to recognize. It is important to emphasize that although they feel they will die, faint, lose control, or go crazy during attacks, this will not happen. They also should understand current theories of etiology and that, with treatment, the prognosis for a significant reduction in symptoms and improvement in functioning is very good. Also, *group treatment* is helpful for patients to recognize that others suffer from the same syndrome. These groups can provide very beneficial understanding, support, and encouragement from peers. Many communities have self-help groups for panic/agoraphobic patients.

Combinations of behavior therapies or medication together with behavior therapy are commonly employed. It is important to emphasize alternative treatments to patients expecting to receive only one form of treatment, such as individuals who are "phobic" of medications or patients expecting complete relief from a "magic pill." The possibility of noncompliance with treatment recommendations should be considered in treatment failure.

Psychodynamically oriented psychotherapy may be an important adjunctive treatment for individuals with significant interpersonal difficulties but has no proven specific effect in alleviating panic attacks or agoraphobia.

Role of the Nonpsychiatric Physician in Patient Management

Nonpsychiatric physicians play a crucial role in the initial evaluation and recognition of panic disorder since patients will most frequently present with symptoms of panic attacks in medical settings. Following a negative workup for medical pathology, it is insufficient to attribute the patient's symptoms to "anxiety" or "stress." As stated above, it is very important that patients receive the appropriate diagnosis and treatment.

In ongoing pharmacological treatment (especially with benzodiazepines), it is important to differentiate the patient's desire to alleviate symptoms with effective medication from the drug-seeking behavior of substance abusers. Once symptoms are relieved, panic patients usually do not request dose increases. On the contrary, they typically fear "addiction" and have the long-term goal of dose reduction or being medication free. However, due to the chronic nature of the disorder, and because medications provide treatment without necessarily a cure, prolonged pharmacological treatment or repeated courses of treatment may be necessary. Alcohol use needs to be closely monitored in these patients.

Indications for Psychiatric Consultation and Referral

In cases that are not straightforward, psychiatric evaluation can aid in establishing the diagnosis, comprehensively assessing comorbid disorders, and selecting appropriate treatments. When a patient's response to initial treatment is inadequate, psychiatrists experienced in treatment of panic and agoraphobia may facilitate a treatment response with dosage adjustment, management of side effects, addressing resistance to treatment recommendations, and ensuring the adequacy of nonpharmacological treatments.

CLINICAL PEARLS FOR PANIC DISORDER

- Suspect panic attacks in patients without physical pathology who present with somatic symptoms suggestive of cardiac, endocrine, and neurological disorders.
- In establishing the diagnosis of panic attacks, ask how quickly the symptoms reach their peak, not how long they last. Ask also if any attacks were unexpected.
- When using antidepressants be sure to warn patients about a possible initial "activation syndrome" and use small doses to begin treatment.
- Benzodiazepines may be required in higher dosages and for longer periods than indicated for other disorders; tricyclics, MAOIs, and SSRIs should be considered first lines of treatment.
- Be alert for coexisting anxiety disorders, major depression, alcoholism, and substance abuse, and address them as indicated.

SOCIAL PHOBIA

Social fears are commonly experienced by healthy individuals, especially in initial public-speaking experiences. For some people, fear of social or performance situations becomes persistent and overwhelming, limiting their social or occupational functioning because of intense anxiety and, often, avoidance. Social phobia has received more research attention in recent years, resulting in an increased understanding of the epidemiology and effective treatments, while at the same time raising more questions regarding biology.

Epidemiology

Lifetime and 1-month prevalence estimates in the National Comorbidity Study (NCS) are 13.3 and 4.5%, respectively, so this disorder is quite common (Magee et al, 1996). Onset is typically during childhood (median age 16), and rarely after age 25. The course tends to be chronic and unremitting. Social phobia is associated with lower education and income, persons who never married, students, the unemployed, and people who live with their parents. The association with comorbid disorders is highest for other phobic disorders (seven- to eightfold increased risk), followed by panic disorder and mania. The association with substance dependence is low, and nonsignificant for substance abuse. Most of these findings are consistent with other recent epidemiological studies.

Description and Differential Diagnosis

Social phobia is characterized by a persistent and exaggerated fear of humiliation or embarrassment in social or performance situations, leading to high levels of distress and possibly avoidance of those situations (Table 8–4). Patients may become fearful that their anxiety will be evident to others, which can intensify their symptoms or even produce a situational panic attack. The fear may be of speaking, meeting people, eating, or writing in public and relates to the fear of appearing nervous or foolish, making mistakes, being criticized, or being laughed at. Often physical symptoms of anxiety such as blushing, trembling, sweating, and tachycardia are triggered when the patient feels under evaluation or scrutiny. DSM-IV allows for specification of *generalized* subtype if the fear includes most social situations. The diagnosis requires interference with one's normal routine, academic, occupational, or social functioning, or marked distress about the phobia. In children, a 6-month duration is required. Two case vignettes of social phobia follow.

CASE 1

A 29-year-old single businessman stated that at age 12 his voice "cracked" during an audition and people laughed at him. A few years later he became very anxious when he had to speak in class.

Table 8–4 **Criteria for Social Phobia***

A. A marked and persistent fear of one or more social or performance situations in which the person is exposed to unfamiliar people or to possible scrutiny by others. They fear that they may act in a way that will be humiliating or embarrassing. Examples include being unable to continue talking while speaking in public, choking on food when eating in front of others, being unable to urinate in a public lavatory, hand-trembling when writing in the presence of others, and saying foolish things or not being able to answer questions in social situations.
B. Exposure to the feared social situation almost invariably provokes anxiety, which may take the form of a situationally bound panic attack.
C. The person recognizes that his or her fear is excessive or unreasonable.
D. The feared social or performance situations(s) is avoided, or else endured with intense anxiety or distress.
E. The avoidance, anxious anticipation, or distress in the feared social or performance situations interferes significantly with the person's normal routine, occupational (academic) functioning, or with social activities or relationships with others, or there is marked distress about having the phobia.
F. The fear or avoidance is not due to a Substance-Induced or Anxiety Disorder Due to a General Medical Condition, and is not better accounted for by Panic Disorder With or Without Agoraphobia, Separation Anxiety Disorder, Body Dysmorphic Disorder, a Pervasive Developmental Disorder, or Schizoid Personality Disorder.
G. If another nonanxiety condition is present (e.g., Stuttering, Parkinson's disease, or Anorexia Nervosa), anxiety about the social impact of the disorder is clearly in excess of that usually associated with the disorder.

* Adapted from DSM-IV criteria (American Psychiatric Association, 1994).

He gradually became very anxious or avoided any situation in which he might be called on or observed, even to answer a roll call. His avoidance of professional meetings was interfering with his work.

CASE 2

A 33-year-old single female chemist described how, during the rehearsal dinner for her best friend's wedding, she became very anxious and broke into a cold sweat. She began anticipating that she would perspire excessively when encountering people, which then would occur. She began avoiding any organized social event and was frustrated about this limitation on her life.

Probably the most difficult diagnostic distinctions are between social phobia and normal performance anxiety, or social phobia and panic disorder. Normal fear of public speaking usually diminishes as the individual is speaking or with additional experience, whereas in social phobia the anxiety may worsen or fail to attenuate with rehearsal. The degree of impairment or distress distinguishes a clinically significant disorder. Social phobics may experience situational panic attacks resulting from anticipation or exposure to the feared social situation. Some panic disorder/agoraphobia patients avoid social situations due to fear of embarrassment if a panic attack should occur, but usually their initial panic attack is unexpected (occurs in a situation they previously did not fear), and the subsequent development of phobias is generalized beyond social phobia situations. As above, social phobia and panic disorder sometimes coexist. Social phobia can be differentiated from specific phobias in that the latter do not involve social situations involving scrutiny, humiliation, or embarrassment. In major depression, social avoidance may develop from apathy rather than fear and resolves with remission of the depressive episode. In schizoid personality disorder, social isolation is due to lack of interest rather than fear. In avoidant personality disorder, the avoidance is of personal relationships; however, if the patient develops a marked anxiety about and avoidance of most social situations, the additional diagnosis of social phobia should be given. Posttraumatic stress disorder (PTSD) patients might appear to have social avoidance, but careful exploration of their symptoms more likely will reveal avoidance of trauma-related cues, loss of interest, or hypervigilance. DSM-IV criteria exclude fears related to another disorder, such as stuttering, tremor in Parkinson's disease, or abnormal eating behaviors in eating disorders. One must also exclude physiological effects of a substance (illicit or prescribed), other nonpsychiatric medical conditions, or symptoms better accounted for by another psychiatric disorder (e.g., panic/agoraphobia, separation anxiety disorder, body dysmorphic disorder, or schizoid personality disorder.)

Etiology

Familial/Genetic Theories

Animal studies demonstrate heritability of various fear, anxiety, exploratory, escape, or avoidant behaviors, often mediated by combinations of genes. These observations may be relevant to social phobia and other anxiety disorders. Human studies of general population samples have suggested some genetic heritability for traits such as fear of strangers, shyness, social introversion, and fear of social criticism. A twin study found greater monozygotic than dizygotic twin concordance for social phobic features such as discomfort when eating with strangers, or when being watched while eating, writing, working, or trembling. The strong heritability of blood-injury phobia has led to the hypothesis that blushing, for example, may be an autonomic response under genetic influence that is tied to social cues and might lead to social phobia. A family history study found familial aggregation of social phobia, and a direct-interview family study found that relatives of social phobics without other anxiety disorders had a threefold increased risk for social phobia but not for other anxiety disorders. A study of female twins found higher concordance for social phobia among monozygotic compared with dizygotic twins and support for the role of both genetic and random environmental factors.

Psychoanalytic Theories

Psychoanalytic theories do not differentiate between phobias and thus would explain social phobias in a manner similar to agoraphobia (see above). A number of traits have been observed in social phobia, such as rigid concepts of appropriate social behavior, an unrealistic tendency to experience others as critical or disapproving, increased awareness and fear of scrutiny by others, exaggerated awareness, and tendency to overreact to minimal somatic symptoms, but the relevance of these traits to social phobia and whether they cause or result from the disorder has not been studied. As adults, social phobia patients retrospectively rate their parents as less caring, more rejecting, and overprotective compared with healthy adults' perceptions of their parents; however, the accuracy of retrospective reporting and the specificity of this finding in social phobia are not established.

Behavioral Theories

It has been suggested that social phobia may result from a lack of social skills (skills-deficit model), faulty evaluation of one's performance in social situations (cognitive inhibition model), hypersensitivity to criticism or rejection, or early unpleasant social or performance experiences (conditioned-anxiety model). These models have led to application of various behavioral techniques to the treatment of social phobia (see below).

Biological Studies

The neurobiological literature of social phobia is characterized by the absence of definitive abnormalities. Many systems have been investigated, including adrenergic, dopaminergic, serotonergic, adenosine, hypothalamic-pituitary-thyroid, growth hormone, CCK, lactate, and CO_2. A variety of study designs, including phobic challenge paradigms, have been employed. For the most part, findings in social phobics have not differed from normals. A few exceptions include (1) a blunted growth hormone response to clonidine, similar to that observed in panic patients; (2) increased cortisol rise, but normal prolactin response, following fenfluramine, which was interpreted as evidence for postsynaptic 5-hydroxytryptamine (5-HT) receptor supersensitivity; (3) a modest anxiogenic response to caffeine (but the quality of the anxiety differed from that of their social anxiety); and (4) lower density of striatal dopamine reuptake sites in social phobics, which suggests that selective MAO-B blockers or dopamine reuptake inhibitors might be considered in treatment trials. A potential relationship between anxiety and short stature or growth disturbance resulted from the study of a group of children with short stature. Many had social phobia, panic disorder, or elective mutism and parents with social phobia or panic disorder. Furthermore, they experienced reduced anxiety during growth hormone therapy. Many of these findings require replication.

Treatment

Psychodynamic Treatments

Psychodynamic psychotherapy may be useful in social phobia, but systematic studies have not been conducted. Countertransference reactions to patients can interfere with recognizing and treating social phobia. Although aspects of social phobia are evident in patients described in the psychodynamic literature, this disorder has been largely neglected. Case examples are often given in psychodynamic literature, exploring issues of shame, aggression, trauma, and unresolved grief thought to be etiologically related to social phobia. Fuller integration of psychodynamic principles with pharmacological and cognitive–behavioral treatments may achieve greater efficacy in treating these patients.

Behavioral Treatment

A number of cognitive–behavioral treatments for this disorder have been investigated, such as various exposure treatments, cognitive approaches, social skills training, rational–emotive therapy, applied muscle relaxation, and combinations of these procedures. Controlled trials have used plausible but nonspecific "placebo" therapies and waiting-list controls. Many trials have assessed outcome not only after treatment, but also at various follow-up intervals.

The theory that social phobics have a deficit in social skills led to the development of social skills training, consisting of counterconditioning through behavioral rehearsal. Results of treatment trials have yielded mixed results, with marked improvement on self-report measures, but not behavioral performance ratings.

It is hypothesized that cognitive distortions are a central aspect of social phobia, thus the application of cognitive restructuring to social phobia treatment. In one trial, although behavioral ratings showed greatest improvement after cognitive therapy with exposure, exposure alone was superior on several other measures. Treatment differences were not apparent at follow-up.

So far, rational–emotive therapy does not seem to add any benefit to exposure, particularly at follow-up. Subjective outcome may be improved when anxiety management training is added to exposure, but not clinician ratings.

Cognitive–behavioral group therapy (CBGT) is clearly effective in treating social phobia and the most widely studied of the cognitive–behavioral treatments. The original format is 12 weekly group sessions lasting 2.5 hours. It consists of education regarding a cognitive–behavioral model of social phobia, cognitive restructuring exercises, exposure to simulated phobic situations in the group, application of cognitive restructuring to the simulated exposures, and homework assignments for exposure in vivo with self-administered cognitive restructuring procedures to use before and after exposure assignments. Several studies have demonstrated effectiveness that is superior to wait-list control or "treatment placebo." Comparison with exposure alone suggested short-term superiority of exposure on several measures, but similar long-term outcome. Comparisons with phenelzine (see below) suggested similar efficacy, with perhaps a slight advantage for phenelzine. Other strengths of CBTG include demonstration of sustained treatment effects after 5 years, effectiveness for both generalized and nongeneralized subtypes of social phobia, and successful use outside the center where it was developed. However, data are inconsistent regarding what components of the treatment are effective and whether their integration is necessary.

Pharmacological Treatment

The MAOIs are the most well-established pharmacological treatment for social phobia. They are effective for anxiety as well as avoidance in generalized social phobics. One trial demonstrated the superiority of phenelzine over atenolol. Although tranylcypromine is less well studied than phenelzine in controlled trials, open studies strongly support its efficacy. Studies using selective MAO-A inhibitors (also referred to as reversible inhibitors of monoamine oxidase-A) are limited. A placebo-controlled trial of brofaromine (not available in the U.S.) 150 mg/day demonstrated clear efficacy with a high response rate, reduction of social anxiety and depression, and progressive improvement over 9-month follow-up. In another trial, moclobemide had efficacy comparable to that of phenelzine, but improvement was slower.

Data regarding benzodiazepines are inconsistent. Investigations have focused on high-potency medications (alprazolam and clonazepam). One controlled trial of clonazepam found a high response rate, which was maintained despite a 50% dose decrease over the following year. However, alprazolam was found to have less efficacy than phenelzine and greater recurrence rates 2 months after discontinuation.

Initial controlled trials of SSRIs suggested moderate benefit for social anxiety, but not other aspects of the disorder, such as avoidance. The response rates using fluvoxamine (150 mg/day) or sertraline (50 to 200 mg/day) were 42 to 46%, roughly half that observed with phenelzine or CBGT, and similar to rates seen with "therapy placebo." For both SSRIs, improvement in social anxiety ratings was significant, but not other ratings. Open trials of fluoxetine, sertraline, and paroxetine reported higher response rates. It was noted that, unlike panic disorder, social phobia patients do not exhibit initial jitteriness/activation with these medications. Most studies used flexible dosing in the full range of doses considered therapeutic for depression, as well as treatment trials lasting 8 to 12 weeks.

Beta-blockers (p.r.n.) have been used for performance anxiety in nonclinical populations, such as musicians and public speakers. However, controlled investigations in social phobia have not been encouraging. It has been suggested that intermittent use of beta-blockers could be helpful for discrete social phobias, but this hypothesis has not been tested.

A variety of other medications have been tested in a single controlled study or uncontrolled reports. Initial open trials suggested moderate-to-marked improvement with buspirone. However, in two controlled trials, buspirone was no more effective than placebo. Ondansetron (a 5-HT-3 antagonist) was found to be superior to placebo in a preliminary analysis of a multisite trial. Case reports of tricyclics, including clomipramine and imipramine, have reported some efficacy; apparently, controlled trials are under way. There is a case report of benefit from bupropion, but no clinical trial data.

Much remains to be learned about the pharmacotherapy of this common disorder. For example, the pharmacological treatment of social phobia with comorbid major depression is not well studied. Several cognitive–behavioral trials have reported improvement in depression during treatments designed for social phobia, without specific treatment for depression.

Combined and Comparative Pharmacological/ Cognitive–Behavioral Studies

It is difficult to compare data from one study to the next due to the wide variation in subjects, assessments, and "responder" criteria. The most effective pharmacological and cognitive–behavioral treatments are reported to have 80% responder rates; however, it is difficult to know what this means without direct comparison, using the same study design and assessments.

To date, two trials have included both CBGT and phenelzine. One trial compared CBGT, phenelzine, alprazolam, and pill placebo; the three medication groups also received self-exposure instructions. Short-term outcome was similar between all groups, with some superiority of phenelzine on trait anxiety. However, at 2-month follow-up, the phenelzine and CBGT groups maintained treatment gains whereas the alprazolam and placebo groups demonstrated loss of effect. In a multicenter trial, phenelzine, CBGT, pill placebo, and "therapy placebo" (educational supportive group therapy) were compared. Both active treatments (phenelzine and CBGT) were highly efficacious, with similar response rates (70 to 80%). Another drug–therapy comparison included four treatment conditions: (1) buspirone, (2) CBT with buspirone, (3) CBT with pill placebo, and (4) pill placebo. The efficacy of buspirone was similar to that of placebo. Both CBT groups did well, with some superiority of the CBT with pill placebo group. In another trial, flooding was compared with atenolol and pill placebo; flooding was best on some measures.

Patient Management and Indications for Psychiatric Consultation and Referral

Consultation with a psychiatrist may help in establishing the diagnosis, especially when features of other psychiatric disorders are present. After identification of the disorder, a trial of an MAOI and/or CBGT should be considered. A circumscribed performance phobia might respond to a beta-blocker taken before the performance, but be sure the patient takes a test dose first.

CLINICAL PEARLS

- Social phobia is differentiated from normal social or performance anxiety by the degree of distress resulting from the fear or by the presence of social or occupational impairment. Anxiety often increases rather than attenuates in the phobic situation.
- As currently defined, social phobia patients have never experienced a spontaneous panic attack; situational panic attacks are confined to the social phobic situations.
- Consider phenelzine (MAOIs) as first-line treatment for social phobia; beta-blockers may help limited performance anxiety; initial reports suggest that benzodiazepines or SSRIs may have some benefit as well.
- Behavioral treatment with a combination of exposure and cognitive–restructuring techniques is effective and likely to result in continued improvement. Patients with poor social behavior may respond best to social skills training or group exposure therapy, whereas those with increased heart rate on exposure to their phobia respond to applied relaxation.

SPECIFIC PHOBIA

The previous name for this disorder, "simple phobia," was changed to Specific Phobia in DSM-IV, and differentiation from other anxiety disorders was emphasized in that the anxiety or avoidance is not better accounted for by obsessive–compulsive disorder, PTSD, panic disorder with agoraphobia, agoraphobia without history of panic disorder, or social phobia. Subtypes include: Animal, Natural Environment (e.g., storms, water, heights), Blood-Injection-Injury, Situational (e.g. airplanes, elevators, enclosed places), and Other.

Epidemiology

Six-month prevalence rates of simple phobia reported in the ECA Study were between 4.5 and 11.8%; rates were higher for females than for males. The NCS (using DSM-III-R criteria for simple phobia) reported 11.3% lifetime and 8.8% 12-month prevalence rates. The onset of animal phobia is usually in childhood. Blood-injury phobia usually begins in adolescence or early adulthood and can be associated with vasovagal fainting on exposure to the phobic stimulus. Age of onset may be more variable for other specific phobias. Many childhood-onset phobias remit spontaneously. Impairment depends on the extent to which the phobic object or situation is routinely encountered in the individual's life. Specific phobias may coexist with social phobia and panic disorder but are believed to be unrelated. An analysis of data from the Normative Aging Study suggested an association between higher levels of phobic anxiety, higher resting heart rate, and lower heart rate variability, which is considered a risk factor for sudden cardiac death. This potentially important finding requires further investigation.

Description and Differential Diagnosis

Specific Phobia is a circumscribed fear of a focal object or situation (Table 8–5). As for other phobias, the patient has a marked and persistent fear that he/she recognizes is excessive or unreasonable. Exposure to the phobic stimulus almost always produces an anxiety response, and the situation is either avoided or endured with intense distress. Unlike common minor fears, the avoidance, anticipatory anxiety, or distress when exposed to the phobic situation results in marked distress or some degree of impairment in activities or relationships. Unlike social phobia, the fear does not involve scrutiny or embarrassment and, unlike agoraphobia, the fear is not of being trapped or of having a panic attack. The nature of the fear is specific to the phobia, such as a fear of falling or loss of visual support in height phobia, or fear of crashing in a flying phobia. The fear is not related to a traumatic event, as in PTSD, or avoidance of school, as in Separation Anxiety Disorder of Childhood.

Table 8–5 **Features of Specific Phobia***

A. Marked and persistent fear that is excessive or unreasonable and is cued by the presence or anticipation of a specific object or situation (e.g., flying, heights, water, animals, receiving an injection, seeing blood).
B. Exposure to the phobic stimulus almost invariably provokes an immediate anxiety response, which may take the form of a situationally bound or predisposed panic attack.
C. The person recognizes that the fear they are experiencing is excessive or unreasonable.
D. The phobic situation(s) is avoided, or else endured with intense anxiety or distress.
E. The avoidance, anxious anticipation, or distress in the feared situation interferes significantly with the person's normal routine, occupational (academic) functioning, or social activities or relationships with others. The person experiences marked distress about having the phobia.
F. The anxiety, panic attacks, or phobic avoidance associated with the specific object or situation is not better accounted for by another mental disorder, such as Obsessive–Compulsive Disorder (e.g., fear of contamination), Posttraumatic Stress Disorder (e.g., avoidance of stimuli associated with a traumatic event), Separation Anxiety Disorder (e.g., avoidance of school), Social Phobia (e.g., avoidance of social situations because of fear of embarrassment), Panic Disorder with Agoraphobia, or Agoraphobia Without History of Panic Disorder.

* Adapted from DSM-IV criteria (American Psychiatric Association, 1994).

Etiology

A family study of specific (simple) phobia demonstrated a high degree of familial transmission of specific phobia, but not of subclinical fears, and supported separation from other anxiety disorders, including other phobic disorders. A study of female twins found higher monozygotic than dizygotic concordance for animal phobia. Blood-injury phobia has a strong family history; 68% of probands have relatives with blood phobia. Concordance rates were higher in monozygotic than dizygotic twins. When blood-injury phobics were exposed to their phobic stimuli, they exhibited a biphasic cardiovascular response with initial tachycardia followed by extreme bradycardia, which can produce syncope. It is presumed that this autonomic response is genetically determined and present at an early age. In other subtypes, phobic exposure caused increases in subjective anxiety, heart rate, blood pressure, plasma norepinephrine, and epinephrine. Preliminary imaging studies are under way to examine brain areas involved in phobic anxiety.

In behavior theory, the classic case study of Little Albert illustrates how operant learning may produce specific phobia. A 2-year-old boy experienced a loud noise while playing with a white rat and became fearful of rats and objects resembling rats. In this example, the loud noise is the unconditioned stimulus, and the fear reaction to the noise is the unconditioned response. The white rat, the conditioned stimulus, is paired with the loud noise and elicits a similar fear response, the conditioned response.

Freud's psychoanalytic theory of phobias is portrayed in the classic analytic study of Little Hans, a 5-year-old boy who developed a fear of horses. Freud hypothesized that the phobia was a symptom of an unresolved unconscious oedipal conflict in which the boy had sexual longings for his mother, but felt guilt and feared retribution from his father in the form of castration. The libidinal impulse was repressed into the unconscious and the threat of danger displaced onto the horse, an avoidable object. However, the love for and desire to marry one's opposite-sexed parent is also believed to be a normal developmental stage, and it is not clear why this dynamic might result in phobic symptoms in some individuals and not others.

Treatment

The standard treatment for specific phobias is exposure, to achieve habituation to or extinction of the fear response. The types of phobias in which efficacy is documented include height, darkness, animals, blood-injury, and claustrophobia. The treatment of different subtypes might require slight variations in the exposure procedure. For example, blood-injection-injury phobia involves the usual in vivo exposure to increasingly more feared stimuli, but, in addition, the patient performs whole-body muscle tension exercises during exposure to avoid hypotension. In a recent innovation, the entire hierarchy of feared stimuli was presented to patients during a single session, lasting 2 hours on average. Most patients were either much improved or fully recovered, and improvement was sustained at 4-year follow-up (see Barlow and Lehman, 1996 for review). Cognitive therapy has been attempted, but does not appear to add any benefit. There is some evidence supporting the use of applied relaxation techniques in patients with strong physiological reactions. When exposure to the phobic stimulus is infrequent, predictable, and difficult to practice repeatedly, such as in flying phobia, benzodiazepines on a p.r.n. basis may be considered. Self-medication with alcohol is common.

OBSESSIVE–COMPULSIVE DISORDER

Obsessions are recurrent distressing thoughts, ideas, or impulses experienced as unwanted and senseless, but irresistible. Compulsions are repetitive, purposeful, intentional behaviors, usually performed in response to an obsession, which are recognized as unrealistic or unreasonable, but again irresistible. What was considered a rare disorder with poor response to treatment has recently received more attention. Advances in treatment and exploration of the underlying etiology and pathophysiology have increased the importance of recognizing obsessive–compulsive disorder. Public awareness and decreased stigma have been fostered by the media, and advocacy for obsessive–compulsive disorder sufferers is accomplished through organizations such as the Obsessive–Compulsive Disorder Foundation and the National Alliance for the Mentally Ill.

Epidemiology

Obsessive–compulsive disorder was previously thought to be a rare disorder affecting only 0.05% of the population. However, with increased awareness and detection, recent estimates of population rates have been higher. The ECA Study found lifetime population prevalence rates of 2 to 3% and 6-month prevalence rates of 1.3 to 2.0%. Although there were problems with the accuracy of the ECA diagnosis, 1 to 2% prevalence rates have been confirmed in other surveys. Rates of obsessive–compulsive traits and disorder are increased in family members of patients (see Etiology, below). Age of onset is usually in childhood or early adulthood, but several years may pass between onset and when a patient first seeks treatment. Obsessive traits are commonly present before onset of the disorder. Most patients are unable to identify an environmental trigger as a precipitant to onset of the disorder, but once the disorder is established, many individuals experience an increase in symptoms with stressful life events.

The majority of obsessive–compulsive disorder patients report depressive symptoms after experiencing impairment from obsessive–compulsive disorder symptoms. Obsessive–compulsive disorder also can coexist with panic disorder in up to 15 to 20% of patients. Other co-occurring disorders include other anxiety disorders, eating disorders, schizophrenia, and Gilles de la Tourette's syndrome. Males are more likely to have comorbid tics, with more violent and aggressive obsessions and harm-avoidant compulsions than in OC without tics. Separation anxiety disorder in childhood also is occasionally reported by obsessive–compulsive disorder patients (see Chapter 16).

Description and Differential Diagnosis

Obsessive–compulsive disorder is defined as the presence of obsessions or compulsions that produce discomfort or impairment (Table 8–6). Obsessions are thoughts, impulses, or images that are recurrent, persistent, intrusive, and recognized as senseless (at least initially). Compulsions are behaviors (rituals) or mental acts (counting, praying) that are repetitive, purposeful, and intentional; are in response to an obsession; are performed in a stereotyped fashion or according to certain rules to prevent discomfort or a dreaded event; and

Table 8–6 **Diagnostic Criteria for Obsessive–Compulsive Disorder***

A. Either obsessions or compulsions:

Obsessions as defined by (1), (2), (3), and (4):
(1) recurrent and persistent thoughts, impulses, or images that are experienced, at some time during the disturbance, as intrusive and inappropriate and that cause marked anxiety or distress
(2) the thoughts, impulses, or images are not simply excessive worries about real-life problems
(3) the person attempts to ignore or suppress such thoughts, impulses, or images, or to neutralize them with some other thought or action
(4) the person recognizes that the obsessional thoughts, impulses, or images are a product of his or her own mind (not imposed from without as in thought insertion)

Compulsions as defined by (1) and (2):
(1) repetitive behaviors (e.g., hand washing, ordering, checking) or mental acts (e.g., praying, counting, repeating words silently) that the person feels driven to perform in response to an obsession, or according to rules that must be applied rigidly
(2) the behaviors or mental acts are aimed at preventing or reducing distress or preventing some dreaded event or situation; however, these behaviors or mental acts are either not connected in a realistic way with what they are designed to neutralize or prevent or are clearly excessive

B. At some point during the course of the disorder, the person has recognized that the obsessions or compulsions are excessive or unreasonable. *Note:* This does not apply to children.
C. The obsessions or compulsions cause marked distress, are time consuming (take more than 1 hour a day), or significantly interfere with the person's normal routine, occupational (or academic) functioning, or usual social activities or relationships.
D. If another Axis I disorder is present, the content of the obsessions or compulsions is not restricted to it (e.g., preoccupation with food in the presence of an Eating Disorder; hair pulling in the presence of Trichotillomania; concern with appearance in the presence of Body Dysmorphic Disorder; preoccupation with drugs in the presence of a Substance Use Disorder; preoccupation with having a serious illness in the presence of Hypochondriasis; preoccupation with sexual urges or fantasies in the presence of a Paraphilia; or guilty ruminations in the presence of Major Depressive Disorder).
E. The disturbance is not due to the direct physiological effects of a substance (e.g., a drug of abuse, a medication) or a general medical condition.

* DSM-IV criteria (American Psychiatric Association, 1994).

---

are initially recognized as excessive or unreasonable. Obsessions and compulsions are not in themselves pleasurable, and patients usually attempt to ignore, suppress, or neutralize obsessions. In clinical samples, both obsessions and compulsions are almost always present, and multiple obsessions and/or compulsions are common. To diagnose a "disorder," the symptoms should cause marked distress, consume at least an hour a day, or interfere with functioning. Changes in DSM-IV more clearly delineate obsessive–compulsive disorder from other disorders and include a specifier for poor insight (for patients who do not recognize their symptoms as excessive or unreasonable).

Patients are often reluctant to divulge their symptoms spontaneously, so these must be inquired about directly (e.g., one study found that unrecognized obsessive–compulsive disorder was common among patients presenting to a dermatology clinic with dermatitis; they did not reveal their obsessive–compulsive symptoms). Reasons for the patient's difficulty in discussing symptoms include embarrassment over content that is perceived as socially unacceptable, recognition of the strangeness of the thoughts and behaviors, fear of being viewed as "crazy," and content that is disturbing to the patient. It is also possible that cognitive brain factors are involved. Sometimes long-standing symptoms become incorporated into the patient's lifestyle and are no longer recognized as abnormal.

Obsessive thoughts may take the form of images of a child being killed, counting rituals, mental list-making that can occupy hours or entire days, or repeated thoughts of having sex with a dead person, which the patient finds disgusting and distressing, yet is unable to dismiss. Compulsive cleaners spend hours meticulously dusting, vacuuming, and so on. Compulsive hoarders are unable to discard useless objects, resulting in a home cluttered with mail, bags of used containers, dustballs, and so on. Some patients need to repeat tasks over and over to "get it right" or repeatedly rearrange objects so that they assume an exact pattern. Fear of contamination can result in avoidance of any contact with dirt or any object that might have come in contact with the feared contaminant or was sold in the same store as the contaminant. While driving, the thought that the patient hit someone may come to mind, followed by the need to return repeatedly to a location to check, despite the virtual certainty that no accident occurred. One individual feared losing his daughter, repeatedly checked billboards and envelopes for her presence, knew that this was absurd, yet was unable to pass a billboard or discard an envelope without repeated checking. Common obsessions and compulsions are listed in Table 8–7. Symptoms can result in lateness due to time spent repeating rituals or in chapped and thickened skin from repeated washing. The disorder can cause isolation and dependence on others; some patients make demands on family and treaters to decontaminate objects, check for them, and so on. Suicide risk must be considered since death may be perceived as the only escape from chronic symptoms.

In clinical samples, symptoms are present continuously from the time of onset until the patient seeks treatment. Occasionally, there is a chronic

Table 8–7 **Common Obsessions and Compulsions**

OBSESSIONS	COMPULSIONS
Contamination/illness	Checking
Violent images	Cleaning/washing
Fear of harming others/self	Counting
Perverse/forbidden sexual thoughts, images, or impulses	Hoarding/collecting
	Ordering/arranging
Symmetry/exactness	Repeating
Somatic	
Religious	

deterioration in which the obsessions and compulsions become more pronounced and more difficult to resist; they may consume all the individual's time so that he or she is unable to function outside of performing rituals. An episodic course of illness is uncommon (2%) in clinical samples, but may be more frequent in individuals who do not seek treatment (or go undiagnosed).

The differential diagnosis of obsessive–compulsive disorder may include schizophrenia, major depression, phobias, Tourette's syndrome, amphetamine intoxication, other neurological conditions, obsessive–compulsive personality, and normal thoughts and behavior. In obsessive–compulsive disorder, behavior can be bizarre and can have an impact on social and occupational functioning similar to schizophrenia. However, the behaviors are limited to the execution of compulsive rituals. When reality testing is lost, the loss is limited to convictions regarding obsessive ideas and does not extend to other areas of thinking. Occasionally, the depressive ruminations seen in major depressive episodes may be mistaken for obsessions, but depressive ruminations have a brooding, depressive, or guilty quality and resolve with recovery from the episode. Avoidance of contaminants or other objects and situations may resemble the avoidance seen in phobic disorders, but the fear is not of being trapped as in agoraphobia, or social embarrassment as in social phobia, but is directly related to the obsessional thought. It is distinguished from generalized anxiety disorder in that these patients worry excessively about realistic concerns, as opposed to the senseless and ego-dystonic nature of obsessions. The repetitive, irresistible movement or utterances of Tourette's syndrome may be difficult to differentiate from obsessive–compulsive disorder, and the disorders may coexist. The repetitive, stereotyped behavior seen in amphetamine (or cocaine) intoxication usually is mechanical, without the intellectual quality and intention of obsessive–compulsive disorder.

Obsessive–compulsive personality (see Chapter 6), although similar in name, consists of ego-syntonic attitudes and behaviors that are not resisted or experienced as intrusive. Such patients have increased risk for personality disorders in general, but interestingly do not have increased rates of obsessive–compulsive personality disorder. Other repetitive behaviors, such as gambling, addiction, sexual behavior, and eating, are to some degree inherently pleasurable, resisted only due to deleterious consequences, and lack the senseless, unrealistic nature of obsessive–compulsive disorder symptoms. Normal checking or meticulousness is not intrusive, senseless, distressing, difficult to resist, or time consuming to the extent of interference with usual activities.

The designation "obsessive–compulsive spectrum disorders" is used inconsistently. Some use "spectrum" to indicate inclusion of subjects who fall just short of the full diagnosis. Others use it to define a probably heterogeneous group of disorders with obsessional or compulsive features (e.g., trichotillomania, etc.), for which the relationship with obsessive–compulsive disorder remains to be determined.

Obsessive–compulsive behavior is present in a number of disorders affecting the basal ganglia (for differential diagnosis, see Cummings in Jenike, 1996). Such symptoms are treated in the same way as obsessive–compulsive disorder of other etiologies.

Etiology and Pathophysiology

Familial and Genetic Theories

Reports of the prevalence rates of obsessive–compulsive disorder in first-degree relatives of obsessive–compulsive disorder probands range from 0 to 37%; of obsessive–compulsive personality, from 3 to 33%; of mood disorder, from 3 to 11%; and of any psychiatric disorder, from 9 to 73%. Concordance rates summarized across three twin studies are 75% for monozygotic and 32% for dizygotic twin pairs. Only the two studies reporting obsessional features in cotwins of obsessive–compulsive disorder probands showed any concordance. The hypothesis that milder obsessional tendencies may be inherited is supported by the high proportion of the variance (45%) for obsessive traits and symptoms that is hereditary in normal twin pairs, as measured by the Leyton Obsessional Inventory. In probands with Tourette's syndrome (with or without obsessive–compulsive disorder), rates of both disorders are increased in biological relatives, suggesting that in these families, obsessive–compulsive disorder and Tourette's syndrome, which is more common in males, may be alternative phenotypic expressions of the same underlying genetic defect (a highly penetrant, sex-influenced, autosomal dominant trait). A recent family study compared relatives of patients with healthy controls and found approximately fivefold increased risk for full and subthreshold obsessive–compulsive disorder. They concluded that the condition is etiologically heterogeneous; some cases are familial and related to tics, some are familial and unrelated to tics, and others are nonfamilial.

Psychoanalytic Theories

Psychoanalytic theories of obsessive–compulsive disorder attribute symptoms to a disturbance in the anal–sadistic phase of development. A conflict (such as the oedipal–genital impulse) may lead to regression to use of earlier defenses, including isolation, undoing, displacement, and reaction formation, resulting in ambivalence and magical thinking.

Cognitive Theories

Obsessive–compulsive disorder patients appear to have a defect in their cognitive information-processing mechanism, with frequent mismatch between beliefs and sensory data (e.g., a patient may continue rinsing his hands because he feels the soap is not washed off or restack dishes because they do not appear to be straight).

Behavioral Theories

Psychiatrists working from a behavioral perspective have suggested a two-stage classical instrumental conditioning model of obsessive–compulsive disorder. Obsessions are thought to result from pairing mental stimuli with anxiety-provoking thoughts. Compulsions are neutral behaviors that have been associated with anxiety reduction and thereby reinforced. Avoidance of anxiogenic stimuli may also be reinforced, as in phobic disorders.

Neurobiological Theories

The predominant neurobiological hypothesis of the etiology of obsessive–compulsive disorder involves dysfunction of brain serotonin neuronal systems. These systems have been the subject of much investigation in obsessive–compulsive disorder since the potent 5-HT reuptake blocker clomipramine was found to have therapeutic efficacy. Clomipramine was found to have greater efficacy than other antidepressants having less serotonergic selectivity or potency, and its efficacy correlated with levels of the serotonergically selective compound clomipramine rather than with desmethylclomipramine, the noradrenergically active metabolite. In one study, higher baseline cerebrospinal fluid (CSF) 5-hydroxyindoleacetic acid (5-HIAA), a serotonin metabolite, and platelet 5-HT concentrations and greater drug-induced decreases of these measures correlated with treatment response. Other treatments with serotonergic effects (fluoxetine, sertraline, fluvoxamine, and L-tryptophan) have also been used to decrease obsessive–compulsive symptoms. Whole-blood 5-HT levels were decreased in obsessive–compulsive disorder patients in one study, whereas the opposite finding was reported in patients with a family history of obsessive–compulsive disorder in another study. Studies of peripheral 5-HT receptors have produced conflicting findings. Initial reports of elevated CSF 5-HIAA have not been confirmed thus far in a large replication study. The identification of several different 5-HT receptor subtypes has highlighted the need for greater sophistication in pharmacological studies. Obsessive–compulsive disorder patients may have a blunted neuroendocrine response and behavioral hypersensitivity to 5-HT agonists, but results are inconsistent.

The absence of robust or consistent findings, despite the number of studies of the 5-HT system, have led investigators to question whether changes seen in 5-HT function are compensatory rather than primary abnormalities in obsessive–compulsive disorder. The role of serotonin function in habituation has been explored in animal studies. Experimentally induced lesions of 5-HT systems in rats exacerbated amphetamine-induced preservative behavior, which may be analogous to compulsions. It appears that the mechanism of action of SSRIs in obsessive–compulsive disorder differs from that of major depression because patients who responded to SSRIs did not experience exacerbation of symptoms following tryptophan depletion, although depressive symptoms worsened (as was observed in patients treated for major depression). Neurobiological systems believed to be involved in other anxiety disorders have been examined in obsessive–compulsive disorder. Yohimbine, an alpha-2 antagonist, produced no consistent change in MHPG, cortisol, or behavior. Caffeine, lactate, and CO_2 did not produce anxiogenic responses such as those in panic disorder; however, reduced functional benzodiazepine receptor sensitivity in obsessive–compulsive disorder is similar to that seen in panic patients. Tests of opiate antagonists have produced conflicting results. These were based on the hypothesis that ruminative doubt and compulsive checking behavior in obsessive–compulsive disorder represent a cognitive deficit in reaching certainty, due to a deficit in opiate-mediated "drive reward reduction."

The possible involvement of dopamine and serotonin systems is implied by positron emission tomography findings of increased metabolic activity in the heads of the caudate nuclei and orbital gyri. It was hypothesized that in obsessive–compulsive disorder, functional activity in the cortex and orbital gyrus increased beyond the caudate's ability to maintain integrative function. Successful pharmacological or *behavioral* therapy (see below) is associated with decreased glucose metabolic rate in the caudate nucleus, as well as decreased correlation of brain activity between orbital gyri with both the head of the caudate and thalamus. The finding of changes in the brain as a result of behavioral therapy underscores the lack of dichotomy between "biological" and "psychological" processes. Brain imaging during obsessive–compulsive symptom provocation demonstrates increased blood flow in the orbitofrontal cortex bilaterally, the right caudate nucleus, and the anterior cingulate cortex. These findings are specific to obsessive–compulsive disorder, whereas other anxiety states show activation in the limbic and/or paralimbic system (for review, see Rauch in Jenike, 1996.) Brain imaging during obsessive–compulsive symptom provocation demonstrated increased activation of brain systems involved with both cognition and emotion. Another imaging study reported diffuse decrease in white matter, but some increase in cortex/white matter ratio; one explanation involves failure of normal programmed cell death or myelination during brain maturation, which corresponds to the age onset of obsessive–compulsive disorder. Inconsistencies between imaging studies might be explained by the heterogeneity of the condition.

Obsessive–compulsive symptoms occur in several diseases affecting the caudate nucleus (e.g., Tourette's syndrome, Sydenham's chorea, Parkinson's disease, Huntington's disease, neuroacathoscytosis, basal ganglia calcification, caudate ischemia, Rett's syndrome, Lesch–Nyhan syndrome) or globus pallidus (postencephalitic parkinsonism, manganese intoxication, pallidal ischemia, progressive supranuclear palsy). One model proposes that obsessive–compulsive disorder occurs with injury to the circuit projecting from the orbitofrontal cortex to the caudate nucleus, globus pallidus/substantia nigra, and thalamus. The corticocaudal and thalamocortical pathways are glutamatergic, whereas gamma-aminobutyric acid is the primary neurotransmitter between the basal ganglia. The main neuromodulatory neurotransmitters are dopamine, from substantia nigra to caudate/putamen, and serotonin, from raphe to globus pallidus.

It is thought that dopaminergic medications affect the motor circuit/parkinsonism, whereas serotonergic medications affect the orbitofrontal circuit and obsessive–compulsive disorder symptoms (see Cummings in Jenike, 1996).

Treatment

Psychodynamic Treatment

If psychotherapy is undertaken, caution may be advisable, as a searching, interpretive, in-depth approach may exacerbate introspective obsessional thinking. There are individual anecdotal reports of successful analytic treatment.

Behavioral Treatment

A variety of psychosocial techniques have been applied to obsessive–compulsive disorder; however, exposure and response prevention (ERP) is consistently the only treatment with evidence for effectiveness. The specific elements responsible for treatment efficacy are prolonged exposure to ritual-eliciting stimuli (e.g., contaminating substances, obsessional thoughts), together with prevention of the compulsive response (e.g., washing, checking). An "adequate trial" requires at least 15 to 30 hours of both exposure and response prevention. Although self-help books can be a helpful adjunct, current data indicate that therapist involvement is required. Around 75% of patients can be expected to respond with symptom reduction of at least 30%, and treatment gains are maintained at long-term (more than 2 years') followup. Prolonged rather than short exposure sessions and attention focusing instead of distraction improve outcome.

Behavior therapy may be enhanced by pharmacological treatment and assertiveness training. Obsessions appear less responsive to behavioral treatment, but prolonged exposure to obsessive material in imagination may have some benefit. Most improvement occurs in the first month of treatment, but improvement may continue with additional treatment for up to 6 months. Treatment gains have been maintained at 2- to 6-year follow-up. Earlier age of onset is associated with better long-term outcome; higher initial anxiety and depression are associated with poorer short-term, but similar long-term outcome (for review, see Barlow and Lehman, 1996).

Pharmacological Treatment

Clomipramine was the first medication discovered to have an effect on obsessive–compulsive disorder symptoms and is the best studied. It is believed that clomipramine's potent serotonergic effects are responsible for somewhat specific treatment for obsessive–compulsive disorder symptoms, since it has greater efficacy than antidepressants with less potent serotonergic activity. Other SSRIs also reduce obsessive–compulsive disorder symptoms. These include fluvoxamine, a selective and potent SSRI, fluoxetine, sertraline, and paroxetine.

Pharmacological treatment response in obsessive–compulsive disorder is characterized by delayed, gradual, and incomplete symptom reduction, as well as a response rate lower than that observed in major depressive disorder or panic disorder. Return of symptoms is common when effective medication is decreased or discontinued. Higher doses of SSRIs than typically used to treat depression may be required, but lower maintenance doses are often adequate.

A pharmacokinetic study of fluoxetine found no correlation between blood level and clinical response. Whereas fluoxetine continues to accumulate in the brain over several months, fluvoxamine, which has a shorter half-life, reaches steady state in the blood after 10 days at a consistent dose, and after 30 days in the brain. Steady-state brain concentrations of fluvoxamine are much higher than and strongly correlated with serum levels, but not with daily dose. More rapid achievement of steady state and clearance might offer clinical advantages, especially in women of child-bearing potential or elderly patients.

For nonresponders, there is no evidence thus far that switching to another SSRI or augmentation with a second drug is effective, so the best strategy is to maximize the initial drug trial and behavioral therapy. To optimize the initial medication trial, begin with low doses so side effects are tolerated, adjust doses slowly to allow time to respond, increase the dose to the maximum recommended or higher, and continue medication trials to 12 weeks (additional improvements have been reported up for to 28 weeks). Also, review the behavior therapy for compliance, adequate "dose," and duration (see above).

MAOIs are not well studied, but several case reports describe good response in individuals who failed initial treatment. MAOIs may be especially helpful in obsessive–compulsive disorder patients with a history of panic attacks. Current evidence does not support the use of neuroleptics alone in obsessive–compulsive disorder. However, controlled trials suggest that addition of a neuroleptic (e.g., pimozide, haloperidol, risperidone) to an SSRI may have benefit, especially for patients with tics (current, past, or family history of tics), schizotypal features, or delusions. An initial trial of inositol 6 g t.i.d. was effective in a minority of patients. Its use was based on data suggesting that the phosphatidylinositol cycle is a second messenger system for several serotonin receptor subtypes, the preclinical finding that inositol reverses desensitization of serotonin receptors, and observations of its effectiveness in depression and panic disorder. Clonazepam may reduce anxiety, but does not alleviate the core symptoms of the disorder. Despite encouraging case reports, placebo-controlled studies of augmentation of an SSRI with lithium or buspirone are disappointing. Adding an SSRI to clomipramine is not recommended, due to poor efficacy and potential serious drug interactions. Fenfluramine added to an SSRI can be helpful. Case reports of venlafaxine, carbamazepine, valproate, stimulants, tryptophan, and multiple infusions of i.v. clomipramine await confirmation in controlled trials.

Combination Treatment

Currently, the accepted standard treatment is a combination of ERP (see Behavioral Therapy, above) and an SSRI (see Pharmacological Treatment, above). Controlled multisite studies are needed to determine the comparative efficacy of behavioral therapy, medication, and the combination. Preliminary data from a study comparing ERP, clomipramine, both treatments, and pill placebo suggest that ERP has powerful and lasting effects.

Electroconvulsive Therapy

In general, electroconvulsive therapy is not effective in obsessive–compulsive disorder, unless the patient develops a concurrent psychotic depression, but symptom response is reported in individual cases.

Psychosurgical Treatment

In severe, debilitating cases that have failed all attempts at more conservative treatment, psychosurgical techniques such as cingulotomy, subcaudate tractotomy, stereotactic limbic leukotomy, or anterior capsulotomy can be beneficial. The effectiveness of these procedures is believed to be based on the disruption of efferent pathways from frontal cortex to basal ganglia.

Role of the Nonpsychiatric Physician in Patient Management

The most important role of primary care physicians is detection of the disorder, which has been difficult due to both physician recognition and patient concealment. Initial treatment of obsessive–compulsive disorder is usually best accomplished by psychiatrists who have familiarity and experience in treating this disorder. Supportive or behavioral psychotherapies are usually necessary in addition to pharmacotherapy. Once satisfactory treatment has been initiated, ongoing pharmacological treatment can at times be managed by a nonpsychiatric physician.

Indications for Psychiatric Consultation and Referral

Consultation with a psychiatrist can assist in establishing the diagnosis and in forming an appropriate treatment plan. In individuals with severe persistent symptoms who are unable to tolerate the distress resulting from their illness, or when concurrent depression is present, assessment of suicide potential and indications for hospitalization may require evaluation by a psychiatrist. Any patient requesting psychosurgery should have careful psychiatric evaluation to determine if less invasive treatment options have been exhausted. Obsessive–compulsive disorder patients also may benefit from involvement in support groups; the Obsessive–Compulsive Disorder Foundation (P.O. Box 9573, New Haven, CT 06535) is a useful resource that was formed by obsessive–compulsive disorder sufferers in 1987.

CLINICAL PEARLS FOR OBSESSIVE–COMPULSIVE DISORDER

- Recognition of obsessive–compulsive disorder can be difficult; if the specific obsessions or compulsions the patient experiences are not directly inquired about, the diagnosis can be missed. Therefore, when you suspect the disorder, question the individual or the family about each of the common obsessions or compulsions.
- The course of the illness is usually chronic and is exacerbated by stressful life events; treatment response is often gradual and incomplete.
- The combination of pharmacotherapy and behavioral therapy is considered optimal treatment. SSRIs are specifically effective for this disorder, whereas most other agents are ineffective. Behavioral therapy consisting of exposure to ritual-eliciting stimuli and prevention of the compulsive response is beneficial in most cases.
- Depression, panic attacks, schizotypal features, delusions, and Tourette's syndrome may coexist with obsessive–compulsive disorder symptoms.

POSTTRAUMATIC STRESS DISORDER

PTSD can be an immediate or delayed response to a catastrophic life event, characterized by reexperiencing the trauma, avoidance, emotional numbing, and symptoms of hyperarousal (Table 8–8). A rapid growth of information is increasing our understanding of complex issues regarding trauma, PTSD, and associated features, but also raising new questions.

Epidemiology

Although descriptions of the syndrome date at least to the Crimean and American Civil Wars, PTSD was not recognized as an independent diagnosis until the publication of DSM-III in 1980, largely due to efforts of Vietnam veterans. The ECA study estimated a population prevalence of 1 to 2%, which is well below more recent reports. In a remarkable epidemiological survey, the National Vietnam Veterans Readjustment Study (NVVRS; Kulka et al, 1990) examined PTSD in Vietnam veterans and matched civilian controls. The lifetime rate of PTSD in male Vietnam veterans was 31%, and 15% had current PTSD. Rates in women were 27% and 9%, respectively. There was a

Table 8–8 **Diagnostic Criteria for Posttraumatic Stress Disorder***

A. The person has been exposed to a traumatic event in which both of the following were present:
   (1) the person experienced, witnessed, or was confronted with an event or events that involved actual or threatened death or serious injury, or a threat to the physical integrity of self or others
   (2) the person's response involved intense fear, helplessness, or horror. *Note:* In children, this may be expressed instead by disorganized or agitated behavior.
B. The traumatic event is persistently reexperienced in one (or more) of the following ways:
   (1) recurrent and intrusive distressing recollections of the event, including images, thoughts, or perceptions. *Note:* In young children, repetitive play may occur in which themes or aspects of the trauma are expressed.
   (2) recurrent distressing dreams of the event. *Note:* In children, there may be frightening dreams without recognizable content.
   (3) acting or feeling as if the traumatic event were recurring (includes a sense of reliving the experience, illusions, hallucinations, and dissociative flashback episodes, including those that occur on awakening or when intoxicated). *Note:* In young children, trauma-specific reenactment may occur.
   (4) intense psychological distress at exposure to internal or external cues that symbolize or resemble an aspect of the traumatic event
   (5) physiological reactivity on exposure to internal or external cues that symbolize or resemble an aspect of the traumatic event
C. Persistent avoidance of stimuli associated with the trauma and numbing of general responsiveness (not present before the trauma), as indicated by three (or more) of the following:
   (1) efforts to avoid thoughts, feelings, or conversations associated with the trauma
   (2) efforts to avoid activities, places, or people that arouse recollections of the trauma
   (3) inability to recall an important aspect of the trauma
   (4) markedly diminished interest or participation in significant activities
   (5) feeling of detachment or estrangement from others
   (6) restricted range of affect (e.g., unable to have loving feelings)
   (7) sense of a foreshortened future (e.g., does not expect to have a career, marriage, children, or a normal life span)
D. Persistent symptoms of increased arousal (not present before the trauma), as indicated by two (or more) of the following:
   (1) difficulty falling or staying asleep
   (2) irritability or outbursts of anger
   (3) difficulty concentrating
   (4) hypervigilance
   (5) exaggerated startle response
E. Duration of the disturbance (symptoms in Criteria B, C, and D) is more than 1 month.
F. The disturbance causes clinically significant distress or impairment in social, occupational, or other important areas of functioning.

* DSM-IV criteria (American Psychiatric Association, 1994).

direct relationship between level of combat and risk for PTSD, even when premilitary factors were taken into account. Hispanic race also increased risk. Rates of most other psychiatric disorders were elevated among those with PTSD.

An epidemiological survey of adult women revealed alarmingly high rates of traumatic events, particularly being the victim of a crime; lifetime and current prevalence estimates of PTSD were 13 and 3%, respectively. Victims of sexual assault were at especially high risk for subsequent mental health problems and suicide. In a survey of 20- to 30-year-olds in a large HMO, 39% experienced a traumatic event, and the lifetime rate of PTSD in those exposed was 24% (i.e., lifetime population prevalence 9%). Risk factors for *exposure to traumatic events* included family history of any psychiatric disorder, history of conduct disorder symptoms, male sex, extroversion, and neuroticism. Risk factors for *PTSD following exposure to trauma* included separation from parents during childhood, family history of anxiety, preexisting anxiety or depression, family history of antisocial behavior, female sex, and neuroticism.

Data from the National Comorbidity Study (NCS) (Kessler et al, 1995) were largely consistent with the previous study. Diagnosis was based on DSM-III-R criteria, 12 types of trauma were assessed, and PTSD criteria were evaluated for only the "most upsetting" event for subjects with multiple events. The lifetime prevalence of PTSD was estimated to be 8% (a validation study indicated PTSD was underdiagnosed by approximately 10%). Estimates of exposure to a traumatic event were 61% in men and 51% in women, and exposure to multiple events was common. The most common events among men were witnessing a trauma (36%), accident (25%), and threat with a weapon (19%), and among women, fire (15%), witnessing a trauma (15%), and accident (14%). The events with the highest risk of producing PTSD in men were rape (62%), combat (39%), and serious neglect in childhood (24%); in women, they were childhood physical abuse (49%), rape (46%), and threat with a weapon (33%.) Men were more likely to experience at least one trauma, but women were more likely to experience a trauma that is highly associated with PTSD. Of all cases of PTSD, the highest proportions were related to rape, combat, witnessing a trauma, sexual molestation, accident, and childhood physical abuse. Comorbidity with other psychiatric disorders was high, consistent with previous studies. Affective and substance-use disorders often had a later onset, whereas anxiety disorders were more likely to predate the trauma. Retrospective analysis suggested that recovery was common (35 to 40%) in the first 12 months, more gradual from 1 to 6 years, and then leveled off, with approximately one-third becoming chronic. Treatment was associated with more rapid recovery in the first 6 years.

In a sample of postpartum women who were participants in a study of birth weight, lifetime prevalence of traumatic events was 40% and of PTSD was 14%. Events reported included assault (12%), witnessing (10%), accident (8%), rape (7%), and disaster (6%). Twenty-one percent of subjects reported two or more events, and 18% reported multiple episodes of PTSD to separate events. Age onset of PTSD was prior to age 15 for one-third of the sample, and age 25 or earlier for over 75%, suggesting that the highest period of risk was between ages 18 and 22. Risk factors for exposure to trauma included prior major depression, anxiety disorder, illicit substance use disorder, and urban environment. Risk factors for PTSD following trauma included prior depression and prior trauma. PTSD was associated with new-onset alcoholism and major depression. Trauma that did not result in PTSD did not appear to lead to increase of the other psychiatric disorders assessed.

Description and Differential Diagnosis

The mental status examination should routinely include questions about exposure to trauma, including abuse. Examples of traumatic events are listed in Table 8–9. DSM-IV criteria specify that the event must involve actual or threatened death or serious injury, and be experienced with intense fear, helplessness, or horror to be considered a traumatic event capable of leading to PTSD. The way questions are asked can influence whether an event is detected; for example, many sexual assault victims are uncertain whether their experience was a "rape" and, likewise, victims might not conceptualize childhood trauma as "abuse." Therefore, it is helpful if questions describe these events concretely, e.g., "were you ever made to have sex when you did not want to," or "did anyone ever touch your private parts" or "hit you so hard it left a mark." For patients too distressed to describe their trauma, ask if, without getting into details, they can just say what type of event occurred, then give examples, e.g., for combat, seeing a buddy killed, being under fire, being involved in something they wish they had not done, etc. If necessary, assist the patient to curtail the description to prevent "flooding" and distress in the initial evaluation.

The symptoms of PTSD are clustered into three categories: reexperiencing the trauma, psychic numbing or avoidance of stimuli associated with the trauma, and increased arousal (Table 8–8). Reexperiencing phenomena include intrusive memories, flashbacks, nightmares, and psychological or physiological distress in response to trauma reminders. Intrusive memories are spontaneous, unwanted, distressing recollections of the traumatic event.

Table 8–9 **Typical Traumatic Events In PTSD**

Physical assault (e.g., rape, physical or sexual abuse, mugging, torture)
Combat, other war or peacekeeping experiences
Serious accidents (e.g., crash, fire, explosion, etc.)
Natural disaster (e.g., tornado, hurricane, flood, earthquake, etc.)
Serious neglect in childhood
Other serious danger of death or severe injury to oneself
Witnessing the mutilation, serious injury, or violent death of another person
Receiving news of above in someone close to you

Note: Events can occur in childhood.

Repeated nightmares contain themes of the trauma or a highly accurate and detailed recreation of the actual event(s). Flashbacks are dissociative states in which the person feels as if he or she is actually reliving the event and loses contact with their current environment, usually for a few seconds or minutes. Reactivity to trauma-related stimuli can involve intense emotional distress or physical symptoms similar to those of a panic attack when exposed to sights, sounds, smells, or events that were present during the traumatic event. Avoidance can include thoughts, feelings, situations, or activities that are reminders of the trauma. Numbing might occur through amnesia for parts of the event, emotional detachment, restricted affect, or loss of interest in activities. Increased arousal can include insomnia, irritability, hypervigilance (exaggerated watchfulness, feeling on guard, checking for danger), increased startle response ("jumpiness"), or impaired concentration.

This disorder can have pervasive effects on an individual's interpersonal behavior and all spheres of her or his life. Since events of this magnitude are markedly distressing to most people and are commonly followed by transient PTSD symptoms, distinguishing between a normal reaction and clinically relevant symptoms can be difficult. The level of distress, the impairment, and the duration of the symptoms are key. Recent research suggests that a 3-month duration may be a threshold between "acute" and "chronic" PTSD. However, a 1-month duration is the threshold for diagnostic criteria at the time of this writing. Usually the disorder begins shortly after the trauma, but sometimes onset is delayed. Exacerbation or relapse can occur after a period of remission. The disorder can occur in childhood.

In adjustment disorder, the stressor is usually less severe, and the characteristic symptoms of PTSD, such as reexperiencing and avoiding, are not present. Avoidance of trauma-associated stimuli may resemble a phobia; however, in PTSD the avoidance is limited to reminders of the trauma. The physiological response to events symbolizing the trauma may resemble panic attacks, but in pure PTSD no spontaneous attacks occur, nor do attacks occur apart from trauma-related stimuli. Many of the symptoms resemble those of major depression. If a full depressive syndrome also exists, both diagnoses should be made; the same is true of coexisting anxiety disorders. The amnesia and impaired concentration may resemble a neurological disorder; if the trauma involved head injury, brain impairment should be considered. Checking behavior can be a manifestation of hypervigilance, but is clearly related to safety concerns connected with the traumatic event, distinguishing it from obsessive–compulsive disorder. Flashbacks are often mistaken for hallucinations, since auditory and visual aspects of the event can be re-experienced. PTSD patients were misdiagnosed as schizophrenics in the 1970s. Patients are frequently referred for medication to help with sleep. It is essential to inquire about nightmares and other trauma-related symptoms in order to recognize the underlying disorder and not mistake it for other causes of insomnia (see psychobiology and treatment, below).

Etiology

Psychodynamic Theories

PTSD is unique among psychiatric disorders in that a specific triggering event can be identified for the psychological, behavioral, and physiological symptoms that comprise this syndrome. Early psychodynamic theories focused on the function of traumatic experiences in reactivating latent conflicts originating in infancy. Subsequent theories suggest that PTSD is related to a failure to integrate the trauma with one's self-concept, world image, and meaning of life. A conflict between internal and external information is expressed through defenses, such as intrusion and avoidance symptoms.

Psychobiological Theories

A series of psychophysiological studies of PTSD found heightened autonomic or sympathetic nervous system arousal in response to trauma reminders. Other studies report dysregulation of sympathetic nervous system activity, including elevated urine norepinephrine excretion and decreased alpha-2 adrenergic receptor density. The alpha-2 antagonist yohimbine produced panic attacks and flashbacks in patients with combat PTSD, as well as heightened biochemical and cardiovascular responses, which could not be accounted for by comorbid panic disorder. Similarly, increased responsiveness to MCPP suggested serotonergic system dysregulation in combat veterans, and there appeared to be little overlap between yohimbine and MCPP responders. If replicated, this biological variation might be useful in predicting treatment response. Involvement of opiate systems was supported by finding that naloxone reversed the stress-induced analgesia from watching combat films in combat PTSD patients.

Abnormalities of the hypothalamic-pituitary-adrenal (HPA) axis suggested that central inhibition of corticotropin-releasing factor and adrenocorticotropic hormone (ACTH) was increased in PTSD, consistent with HPA adaptation to chronic stress in preclinical studies. HPA findings in PTSD are well replicated and in the reverse direction of those in major depression, namely, enhanced suppression (rather than nonsuppression) of cortisol following low-dose dexamethasone, decreased baseline cortisol, and increased number and sensitivity of glucocorticoid receptors. An augmented ACTH response to metyrapone suggested enhanced negative feedback sensitivity. It appeared that baseline increases in glucocorticoid receptors were associated with the severity of trauma exposure rather than PTSD, whereas cortisol hypersuppression was correlated with the presence and severity of PTSD. Investigators questioned whether neuroendocrine alterations were risk factors for PTSD rather than consequences of the traumatic event. A study that examined assault history in rape victims found that previous assault was associated with lower cortisol shortly after the index rape and with a much higher probability of subsequently developing PTSD. Women with no prior assault had higher acute cortisol levels, particularly following high-severity rapes.

Based on preclinical studies, it was hypothesized that processes involving the locus ceruleus, amygdala, hypothalamus, hippocampus, and prefrontal cortex were involved in the pathophysiology of PTSD. Several studies observed decreased hippocampal volume in PTSD patients. Similar to other findings, further work is needed to rule out confounding effects of substance abuse and other comorbid disorders and determine whether this finding is a preexisting risk factor or sequela of trauma/PTSD.

Preliminary evidence from family and twin studies suggested that genetic and familial factors may play a role in vulnerability to PTSD, which was consistent with preclinical data on genetic vulnerability to stress responses. A possible relationship with other anxiety disorders is being explored. Genetic factors may influence exposure to trauma as well.

As discussed above, sleep disturbance is often a chief complaint in PTSD patients. Clinically significant and subclinical sleep apnea and periodic limb movements were reported in a high proportion of PTSD patients, suggesting that many patients might benefit from sleep disorder assessment. In addition, decreased sleep efficiency, increased awake time, and microawakenings were more frequent in PTSD patients than controls. Further data are needed regarding sleep stages, gender, type of trauma, specificity for PTSD, and relationship to comorbid disorders and medications. A study of hurricane victims suggested that prior sleep disorder was a risk factor for PTSD.

Questions have arisen concerning the accuracy of memory/reporting of traumatic events (especially recovered memories of abuse in legal proceedings). PTSD also seems to be characterized by a maladaptive enhancement of trauma memory via intrusive memories, symptoms triggered by memory cues, flashbacks, and trauma nightmares.

The brain literature describes several memory systems involving a number of neuroanatomical structures which are sensitive to neurochemical influences, and alterations from stressful stimuli have been reported. Experimental, retrospective, and prospective clinical studies have examined memory following stressful or traumatic events.

Children appear to remember events well and memory improves with age at time of the event, stressfulness of event, and serial questioning. However, another study reported that rape was less well remembered than other intense experiences. Delayed recall of childhood sexual abuse was associated with threats, younger age at abuse onset, and less maternal support. Memories were highly accurate despite prior forgetting or a sense of vagueness. Recent recall was associated with high levels of PTSD symptoms. In Gulf War veterans, reporting more trauma over time was correlated with higher ratings of PTSD symptoms. Issues such as developmental stage of cognitive processes, possible dissociation or fragmentation during encoding of trauma memories, and recall problems unrelated to conscious suppression or blocking have been proposed. There is some evidence for increased organization of trauma memory and elaboration of thoughts and feelings during exposure therapy.

To improve our understanding of memory processes in relation to PTSD, we need a greater scientific understanding of encoding, recall, accuracy, distortion, stability over time, and factors affecting these processes. Further clarification of memory processes is needed for neutral, stressful, and traumatic events, and to determine whether traumatic memory differs between those with and without PTSD.

Behavioral Models

Two-factor learning theory has been applied to PTSD. Classical (aversive) conditioning, in which previously neutral stimuli are paired with reaction to the trauma, and higher order conditioning (additional stimuli become associated and produce anxiety) lead to instrumental learning, whereby behaviors are acquired to avoid anxiety from the conditioned stimuli. A number of factors may interfere with extinction occurring naturally. Specific behavioral models used to design cognitive–behavioral treatments are discussed below.

Treatment

Initiating assessment and treatment quickly after a trauma is hoped to prevent many of the complications and disability associated with prolonged PTSD. As with other anxiety disorders, treatment often is best accomplished with a combination of pharmacological and nonpharmacological therapies. It has been proposed that pharmacological treatment may be required to control the physiological symptoms so that the patient will be able to tolerate working through highly emotional material in psychotherapy. Treatment of PTSD is often complicated by comorbid disorders. If alcohol or substance abuse is present, these problems should be the initial focus of treatment. For many PTSD patients with comorbid depression, the course, biology, and treatment response are unlike that of classic major depression. Therefore, until additional data are available, we suggest that clinicians focus on treating PTSD (unless depression is endogenous or bipolar). For example, several behavioral therapies for PTSD have demonstrated a decrease in depression without specific treatment directed toward depression.

Psychotherapies

Controlled studies of cognitive–behavioral therapies have demonstrated significant clinical improvement. As for other some other anxiety disorders, the techniques have not been tested at multiple sites. The control groups were usually a wait-list sample or a less specific therapy. Variability between outcome ratings and description of results makes comparisons difficult.

Foa and associates (1991) compared Prolonged Exposure (PE), Stress Inoculation Training (SIT), Supportive Counseling (SC), and a Wait-List control (WL). Treatments consisted of nine biweekly 90-minute sessions. SIT included coping skills, relaxation training, cognitive techniques, modeling, and role-playing. In PE, patients described the event aloud in sessions, listened to a tape of the session daily, and completed exposure homework. In SC, patients were taught a general problem-solving technique, and then kept a diary of daily problems and their attempts at solving these problems. Short-term outcome was favorable with SIT and PE (up to 55% decrease in PTSD ratings), but at 3 month follow-up, there was a slight increase in PE efficacy and slight decrease in SIT, making PE the superior treatment. The WL controls had only 20% decrease of PTSD symptoms. Only a subset of the subjects participated in follow-up, so these data should be interpreted with caution.

Resick and Schnicke (1992) examined Cognitive Processing Therapy (CPT) versus a wait-list control in rape victims. CPT is based on the formulation that PTSD symptoms are related to conflicts between prior beliefs and aspects of the event. The procedure consisted of 12 individual or group sessions which included education about PTSD symptoms and information processing theory, exposure through writing and reading detailed accounts of the event, training to identify thoughts and emotions, techniques for challenging maladaptive beliefs, and modules for five belief areas (safety, trust, power, esteem, and intimacy) that seem to be disrupted by victimization. PTSD symptoms were reduced by 48 to 57%; depression also improved, and gains were maintained at 6-month follow-up. The control group did not change significantly, but PTSD scores were not cited. Anecdotally, after successful cognitive–behavioral treatment, a subsequent relapse due to a new trigger of traumatic memories can respond to another course of cognitive–behavioral therapy.

In early trials of systematic desensitization and flooding, reexperiencing and hyperarousal symptoms decreased, but not avoidant/numbing symptoms. One controlled study compared psychodynamic therapy, hypnotherapy, and systematic desensitization to waiting list controls. Hypnotherapy was similar to desensitization, with more improvement in reexperiencing symptoms and less improvement in avoidance, whereas psychodynamic therapy had a greater effect on avoidance than reexperiencing.

Unfortunately, specialized inpatient treatment for PTSD in the VA system was not successful. Alternative outpatient treatment models are being explored.

Psychopharmacotherapy

There are still very few controlled medication trials in PTSD. In a double-blind placebo-controlled trial of phenelzine and imipramine in Viet Nam veterans (Kosten et al, 1991), the mean decrease in PTSD symptoms of "intrusion" (reexperiencing) and avoidance (hyperarousal was not assessed) was 45% for phenelzine, 25% for imipramine, and 5% for placebo-treated patients. The completion rate was highest for phenelzine (79% versus 39% and 33% for imipramine and placebo, respectively), suggesting that it was well tolerated and effective. Usual dose ranges were 60 to 75 mg/day for phenelzine and 200 to 300 mg/day for imipramine. To date, phenelzine is the most effective of the medication treatments for combat PTSD. For reasons not yet understood, placebo-controlled trials of fluoxetine demonstrated efficacy for noncombat PTSD (45% symptom reduction, mainly in avoidance/numbing and hyperarousal), but no response in combat PTSD. The medication response in PTSD appears to be gradual and incomplete. Other controlled trials suggested equivocal results with amitriptyline and no efficacy for alprazolam, brofaramine, or desipramine. The lack of efficacy, together with a high rate of substance use disorders in PTSD, makes benzodiazepines a poor choice.

Open trials and case reports suggest efficacy for a variety of other medications, but controlled trials are needed to confirm these results. Open trials of fluvoxamine, sertraline, cabamazepine, and valproate were encouraging. Nalmefene (an opiate antagonist) was helpful for symptoms in all three clusters in almost half of a veteran sample. Clonidine 0.2 to 0.4 mg/day and propranolol 120 to 180 mg/day relieved startle, explosiveness, nightmares, and intrusive reexperiencing in some patients. Lithium decreased autonomic arousal, reexperiencing symptoms, and ethanol use in many patients. Case reports described benefits from buspirone for reexperiencing and hyperarousal, guanfacine (alpha-2 agonist) for nightmares, and naltrexone for flashbacks. Neuroleptics did not appear to be helpful for dissociative symptoms, and may not be effective for psychotic symptoms in PTSD patients.

CLINICAL PEARLS FOR POSTTRAUMATIC STRESS DISORDER

- Establish exposure to a traumatic event that (1) meets Criterion A (Table 8–8), (2) predates the onset of PTSD symptoms, and (3) is represented in the patient's reexperiencing symptoms.
- Multiple traumas are common. Attempt to clarify which event is most closely associated with PTSD symptoms, but recognize that past events can lower the threshold for PTSD.
- The high spontaneous recovery rate in the first 3 months after a trauma should be supported with psychotherapy and perhaps a beta-blocker; benzodiazepines should be avoided. Help the patient maximize social supports (see also Acute Stress Disorder).
- Preliminary controlled studies indicate efficacy for cognitive/exposure treatments, phenelzine (Nardil, an MAOI), imipramine (a TCA) and, for civilian but not combat trauma, fluoxetine (Prozac, an SSRI). Other treatments might also have some benefit.
- If a comorbid substance use disorder is present, it should be treated first. Trauma-focused work should be delayed until a period of stable abstinence.
- Comorbid psychiatric illnesses are common; however, some may not share etiology, pathophysiology, or treatment response characteristics with the nontraumatic form of the illness.

ACUTE STRESS DISORDER

A new disorder, acute stress disorder, was added to DSM-IV. Surveys of disaster victims (e.g., fire, earthquake, witnessing an execution) revealed acute symptoms that predicted subsequent PTSD. These acute symptoms were highly correlated with the severity of trauma exposure. Other than being a precursor for PTSD, little is known about this disorder. Initial data were based on anonymous surveys; a few studies have used clinical instruments. It is hoped that the identification of this disorder will facilitate early detection and treatment and reduce long-term complications.

A number of retrospective studies have explored risk factors for PTSD; however, the unreliability of retrospective memory makes prospective studies essential. Consecutive hospitalized patients with a physical injury due to trauma were assessed 1 week and 6 months after trauma. High initial severity on a PTSD symptom rating had high sensitivity, but low specificity for predicting subsequent PTSD. Dissociation at the time of the event was highly associated with the development of PTSD. Avoidance symptoms were low initially, but increased markedly in those who developed PTSD. In a study of survivors 1 month after a mass shooting, most who developed PTSD had no preexisting psychiatric disorder, but previous depression was a possible risk factor. Almost all persons experienced some PTSD symptoms, particularly intrusive memories, exaggerated startle, insomnia, and hypervigilance. Therefore, experiencing some of these symptoms after a trauma is the norm and should not be considered pathological. Regarding use of health services, 71% of those with PTSD and 50% of those without PTSD saw a physician or counselor. Medication was prescribed for 49% of those with PTSD, especially women, but only 7% of those without PTSD. Among Israeli evacuees during the Gulf War, very high rates of symptoms meeting criteria for PTSD (except duration) were reported within 1 week of evacuation. Follow-up data are needed to determine subsequent rates of PTSD and predictors.

As for PTSD, Criterion A for Acute Stress Disorder specifies that the individual must have been exposed to a traumatic event (Table 8–8). In addition, this syndrome is characterized by at least three of five numbing or dissociative symptoms during or after the event, such as numbing/lack of emotional responsiveness/detachment, decreased awareness of one's surroundings (e.g., "in a daze"), derealization, psychogenic amnesia, and depersonalization. Other symptoms are essentially those specified in the B, C, and D clusters of PTSD, but only one symptom per cluster is required, i.e., at least one reexperiencing symptom (Table 8–8, item B), avoidance of stimuli that provoke memories of the trauma, and symptoms of either hyperarousal (Table 8–8, Item D) or restlessness. The diagnosis of acute stress disorder is made when the level of distress is clinically significant, when there is impairment in functioning, or when the individual fails to pursue a necessary task, such as obtaining medical, legal, or social assistance. The duration of acute stress disorder is from 2 days to

4 weeks; if symptoms persist beyond 4 weeks after the trauma, consider the diagnosis of PTSD.

A review of the empirical literature on psychological reactions to trauma suggests that this pattern of dissociation, anxiety, and other symptoms has been described across many types of traumatic events. The authors postulate that this is an adaptation that limits painful thoughts and feelings and allows an individual to function in the immediate aftermath. However, if it becomes prolonged, it can lead to impairment. Therefore, it is important to identify this pattern, so appropriate intervention can be provided. Some interventions that have been reported to reduce acute symptoms include rituals consistent with the local culture, supportive psychotherapy, crisis intervention, more focused psychotherapies, and medication. However, it is unclear at this point if these interventions can affect the progression to PTSD.

Given the recent identification of Acute Stress Disorder, studies are just beginning. A preliminary report suggests that a brief prevention program within 2 weeks of an assault, consisting of four weekly 2-hour sessions of education, relaxation, exposure, and cognitive restructuring produced a significant decrease in PTSD symptoms after treatment and at 1-month follow-up. A group of acute interventions termed *critical incident stress debriefing* has been widely used, particularly with civilians in trauma-related occupations, but its efficacy is being hotly debated, and some claim it is actually detrimental.

An important study of recent trauma survivors (Gelpin et al, 1996) revealed that benzodiazepines, beginning the week after trauma, were ineffective both in the short-term and in preventing progression to PTSD. This finding is consistent with the evidence that alprazolam is ineffective for PTSD and with data suggesting that benzodiazepines interfere with learning processes felt to be necessary for adaptation following a trauma. Studies of memory in healthy volunteers suggest that beta-blockers might be helpful in the immediate posttrauma period. However, this theory needs to be confirmed in controlled trials.

GENERALIZED ANXIETY DISORDER

Generalized anxiety disorder (GAD) is characterized by chronic excessive and uncontrollable worry about multiple life circumstances accompanied by symptoms of restlessness, fatigue, concentration problems, irritability, muscle tension, and difficulty falling or staying asleep. The symptoms are present a majority of the time for at least 6 months and cause clinically significant distress or impairment. The anxiety is unrelated to panic attacks, phobic stimuli, obsessions, physical complaints, or traumatic events (in PTSD). One must rule out physiological effects of substances, medical conditions, and mood, psychotic, or pervasive developmental disorders. The diagnostic criteria for GAD have undergone considerable refinement between DSM revisions to correct problems with reliability and differentiation from other disorders. Uncontrollability of worry and somatic symptoms unlike those of other anxiety disorders have been identified as the key features of the disorder.

Epidemiology

Prevalence surveys based on DSM-III or Research Diagnostic Criteria (RDC) criteria reported rates of GAD around 4 to 7% lifetime and 1 to 6% current. The National Comorbidity Study (NCS), using DSM-III-R criteria, found a 5.1% lifetime and 1.6% 1-month prevalence. Rates were higher among females, in those older than 24, previously married, or unemployed, in homemakers, and in persons living in the Northeast. Comorbidity was highest for affective and panic disorders (10- to 12-fold increased risk). For only 20% of those affected, GAD was the first-onset disorder or the only lifetime disorder. A high proportion report impairment and help-seeking. A study of female twins found similar rates of comorbid disorders among those with GAD. Age at onset is variable, but is usually in the 20s to the 30s. GAD may begin as childhood overanxious disorder. In clinical samples, the prevalence in males and females appears to be equal, and the course tends to be chronic.

Description and Differential Diagnosis

The most common diagnostic error made by beginning students is to misdiagnose GAD when another anxiety disorder is present, which leads to inappropriate treatment decisions. The *symptom* of anxiety is prominent in a number of other psychiatric conditions, medical conditions (especially with dyspnea), medication side effects (e.g., sympathomimetic), and normal reactions to life circumstances; therefore, careful assessment is needed to differentiate between multiple causes of anxiety.

GAD is characterized by chronic excessive anxiety about life circumstances accompanied by symptoms of motor tension, vigilance, and scanning of the environment (Table 8–10). The individual often "awakens with" apprehension and unrealistic concern about future misfortune. One patient described experiencing the anxiety of a final exam with every task he was assigned at work. The current diagnostic criteria require a 6-month duration of symptoms to differentiate the disorder from more transient forms of anxiety, such as adjustment disorder with anxious mood. DSM-IV criteria emphasize that the worry is out of proportion to the likelihood or impact of the feared events, is pervasive (focused on many life circumstances), is difficult to control, is not related to hypochondriacal concerns or PTSD, and is not secondary to substances or medical etiologies. Tension or nervousness may be manifested by three of the following: restlessness, easily fatigued, feeling keyed up or on edge,

Table 8–10 **Diagnostic Criteria for Generalized Anxiety Disorder***

A. Excessive anxiety and worry (apprehensive expectation) occurring more days than not for at least 6 months, about a number of events or activities (such as work or school performance).
B. The person finds it difficult to control the worry.
C. The anxiety and worry are associated with three (or more) of the following six symptoms (with at least some symptoms present for more days than not for the past 6 months). **Note:** Only one item is required in children.
   (1) restlessness or feeling keyed up or on edge
   (2) being easily fatigued
   (3) difficulty concentrating or mind going blank
   (4) irritability
   (5) muscle tension
   (6) sleep disturbance (difficulty falling or staying asleep, or restless unsatisfying sleep)
D. The focus of the anxiety and worry is not confined to features of an Axis I disorder, e.g., the anxiety or worry is not about having a Panic Attack (as in Panic Disorder), being embarrassed in public (as in Social Phobia), being contaminated (as in Obsessive–Compulsive Disorder), being away from home or close relatives (as in Separation Anxiety Disorder), gaining weight (as in Anorexia Nervosa), having multiple physical complaints (as in Somatization Disorder), or having a serious illness (as in Hypochondriasis), and the anxiety and worry do not occur exclusively during Posttraumatic Stress Disorder.
E. The anxiety, worry, or physical symptoms cause clinically significant distress or impairment in social, occupational, or other important areas of functioning.
F. The disturbance is not due to the direct physiological effects of a substance (e.g., a drug of abuse, a medication) or a general medical condition (e.g., hyperthyroidism) and does not occur exclusively during a Mood Disorder, a Psychotic Disorder, or a Pervasive Developmental Disorder.

* DSM-IV criteria (American Psychiatric Association, 1994).

difficulty concentrating/ mind going blank, and irritability. In addition, significant functional impairment or marked distress is required for the diagnosis.

Persistent anxiety may develop between attacks in panic disorder, but usually it is apprehensive anxiety related to panic and phobias. GAD is not diagnosed if limited to episodes of depression; however, as discussed below, it may share etiological elements with depression. In patients with somatization disorder, the focus of worry is about health concerns and physical symptoms, rather than apprehensive worry about life circumstances.

As with panic disorder, medical conditions that may produce anxiety symptoms, such as hyperthyroidism or caffeinism, must be excluded. Careful research has shown that anxiety disorders are not increased among alcohol-dependent patients. Temporary, but sometimes severe, substance-induced anxiety syndromes can mimic GAD, panic, or social phobia, which will subside with sustained abstinence or require only short-term intervention. If anxiety disorder is present that does not fit the criteria for any of the anxiety disorders, somatization, psychoactive substance-related, or medical conditions, then the diagnosis of Anxiety Disorder Not Otherwise Specified may be considered. However, careful assessment will usually lead to a more specific diagnosis. If in doubt, obtain consultation from an anxiety disorders specialist.

Etiology

An early twin study found no evidence for genetic transmission of GAD. Diagnostic heterogeneity of GAD is suggested by the high frequency of nonanxiety psychiatric disorders in cotwins. However, a family study of GAD probands reported an increased rate of GAD, but not other anxiety disorders, in first-degree relatives, suggesting some degree of familial transmission and separation of GAD from panic disorder and agoraphobia. A study of disorders in the cotwins of probands with anxiety disorder versus probands without anxiety found that GAD was increased in the cotwins of probands with both GAD and mood disorder. Kendler and colleagues (1995) examined genetic and environmental contributions to risk for GAD, panic disorder, phobia, major depression, bulimia, and alcoholism in female twin pairs. They estimated the proportion of risk for GAD due to genetic and environmental factors as follows: genetic factors contributed 32%, with the largest portion shared with depression; environmental factors accounted for 66% of risk, with the largest proportion from nonfamilial environmental factors shared with depression, and a substantial proportion due to nonfamilial environmental factors specific to GAD. Family environmental factors were not significant. These findings are consistent with previous reports, suggesting some degree of genetic contribution to GAD and separation from panic disorder, and shared genetic factors with depression.

Psychodynamic theories are based on "neuroses," which do not directly correspond to current diagnostic classification. As stated above, unconscious conflict is felt to be the underlying cause of anxiety, which, as a symptom, is a "signal" to the ego of the danger of expressing unacceptable impulses.

Behavioral theories consider anxiety, like panic disorder, a conditioned response to a stimulus that the individual has come to associate with danger. However, in GAD, it is difficult to identify specific anxiogenic stimuli. There is some suggestion that the onset of GAD may be related to the cumulative effects of several stressful life events. It is of interest that patients with GAD respond to psychological stress with autonomic inflexibility, that is, with less variability in heart rate, skin conductance, etc., compared with healthy controls, in laboratory-based psychological challenges. However, laboratory measures of muscle tension are increased. An information-processing model proposes that anxiety is maintained by selective attention to potentially threatening information on a preconscious or subliminal level. In addition, patients perceive a lack of control over the threat. Excessive worry is considered the predominant way of coping to anticipate and avoid future catastrophes.

The biology of GAD is not well characterized. Factors that might contribute to the absence of consistent abnormalities in groups of GAD patients include changes in diagnostic criteria, the high comorbidity with other psychiatric disorders (80% lifetime), for which specific abnormalities have been demonstrated, and failure to demonstrate abnormalities in biological functions involved in normal anxiety. Catecholamine function appears to be normal at baseline, but GAD patients may have subtle abnormalities, such as reduced adrenergic receptor sensitivity. Although some alterations were found in peripheral benzodiazepine receptors, studies of central benzodiazepine receptors in GAD patients are unconvincing. Anxiolytic effects of compounds with effects on 5-HT-1A and 5-HT-2 receptors have stimulated interest in serotonin function in GAD. Preliminary investigations have cited increased anxiolytic and anger responses to MCPP, decreased CSF serotonin levels, and decreased platelet H_3-paroxetine binding. Studies of autonomic function are inconsistent, but some suggest a weak response to stress and slower recovery time than controls. Biological differentiation of GAD from panic disorder is supported by the absence of panic response to challenge paradigms. Nonsuppression of cortisol in response to dexamethasone was observed in 25 to 38% of GAD patients, suggesting possible involvement of the HPA axis. A challenge paradigm involving infusion of pentagastrin (CCK-B receptor agonist) resulted in a much higher rate of panic attacks in GAD subjects compared with normal controls. This finding requires replication; however, CCK is a neuromodulator of several systems relevant to anxiety. Imaging studies suggest potential regional alterations of CBF in GAD patients.

Treatment

Psychodynamic psychotherapy may be indicated for cases of GAD in which the clinician feels that unresolved unconscious conflict causes or perpetuates a patient's chronic anxiety (see Chapter 17).

Cognitive therapy involves identifying negative thoughts and then evaluating and modifying those thoughts by substituting more realistic thoughts. Behavioral therapy helps patients assess the validity of negative thoughts by exposure to real-life experiences. Additional specific components might include social skills training, problem-solving, or time management and goal setting. Relaxation training can demonstrate to patients that they have control over their symptoms. Preliminary studies of cognitive–behavioral treatment of GAD suggest that more highly specialized treatments, for example, targeting the worry associated with GAD, are more effective. Some of the elements of treatment include bringing the worry process under control, training to cope more effectively with anxiety, and problem-solving strategies to address sources of anxiety (interpersonal, time management, etc.). Of 12 cognitive–behavioral studies reviewed (Barlow and Lehman, 1996), 10 found improvement (40 to 60%), especially when compared with a different type of treatment. One study found no added benefit of diazepam, and significantly better outcome for cognitive–behavioral therapy alone versus diazepam alone. Thus far, these treatments have not been studied outside the center where they were developed. In addition, there is inadequate description of study samples regarding variables associated with severity and chronicity, which might influence treatment response.

The most commonly used pharmacological agents for GAD are benzodiazepines such as diazepam, alprazolam, lorazepam, and clonazepam (Table 8–11). Advantages include rapid onset of efficacy and long-term safety. Disadvantages include memory impairment, sedation, driving impairment, difficulty with discontinuation, dependence, and abuse potential. Antidepressant medications were believed to be ineffective in treating GAD, but some studies suggest that imipramine may be of some benefit.

Buspirone, a nonbenzodiazepine anxiolytic, may become the treatment of choice for GAD. The mechanism of action is not well established, but pharmacological activity includes decrease in serotonin and increase in dopamine and norepinephrine cell firing. In contrast to benzodiazepines, therapeutic effects are relatively slow in onset, taking from 1 to 4 weeks. Side effects are usually mild and transient but may include dizziness, nausea, diarrhea, headache, or nervousness and can be managed by reducing the dose and working upward to an effective range. Buspirone does not produce drowsiness or impair driving skill and lacks abuse potential or withdrawal symptoms with abrupt discontinuation. The drug is not sedating. Consider buspirone as the first-line treatment in patients with an alcohol or drug abuse history. In addition, buspirone has been shown to decrease drinking and anxiety in anxious alcoholics. It is important to note that buspirone does not block alcohol or benzodiazepine withdrawal symptoms, so in patients exposed to these agents, withdrawal symptoms should not be confused with lack of efficacy of anxiolytic therapy. Unlike the folklore that prior benzodiazepine treatment renders patients "immune" to buspirone, Delle Chiaie and colleagues blindly switched benzodiazepine-treated patients to buspirone (using a 2-week benzodiazepine taper and 15 mg/day buspirone) and found no rebound anxiety or benzodiazepine withdrawal (1995). In addition, buspirone was as

Table 8–11 **Commonly Used Benzodiazepines**

TYPE	PRIMARY ROUTE OF BIOTRANSFORMATION	ELIMINATION HALF-LIFE (HOURS)
Diazepam (Valium)	Oxidation	36–200
Flurazepam (Dalmane)	Oxidation	50–120
Halazepam (Praxipam)	Oxidation	36–200
Chlordiazepoxide (Librium)	Oxidation	30–90
Alprazolam (Xanax)	Oxidation	12–15
Triazolam (Halcion)	Oxidation	3–5
Clorazepate (Tranxene)	Oxidation	36–200
Prazepam (Centrax, Vestran)	Oxidation	36–200
Midazolam (Versed)*	Oxidation	2–4
Lorazepam (Ativan)	Conjugation	10–20
Temazepam (Restoril)	Conjugation	8–12
Oxazepam (Serax)	Conjugation	8–12
Clonazepam (Klonopin)	Nitroreduction	30–60

* IM or IV route only.
(Reprinted with permission from Stoudemire A, Fogel BS, Gulley LR, Moran MG: Psychopharmacology in the medical patient. In Stoudemire A, Fogel BS (eds): Psychiatric Care of the Medical Patient, p 188. New York, Oxford University Press, 1993)

effective as lorazepam, but caused fewer side effects. Ipsapirone (an azapirone with high specificity for the 5-HT-1A receptor) 5 mg t.i.d. was found to be effective in one trial. A preliminary report of adinazolam-SR demonstrated clear efficacy for GAD compared with placebo. There was no apparent difference in efficacy among doses of 30, 60, or 90 mg/day over 4 weeks. Other serotonergic agents and mixed agonist–antagonist benzodiazepines are being studied.

As with the other anxiety disorders, optimal treatment may involve a combination of psychotherapy, behavioral therapy, and/or pharmacotherapy. Comparative trials are needed to establish the relative efficacies of these treatment modalities or their combination.

Rickels and Schweizer (1990) reviewed long-term management of GAD. The chronicity of the disorder might lead to chronic treatment, making buspirone a good choice. They caution that long-term medication (especially with benzodiazepines) might interfere with the patient's learning of improved coping skills. They recommend periodic reassessment and anxiolytic-free intervals of several weeks to determine whether further anxiolytic therapy is indicated. It is suggested that patients learn to cope with small levels of anxiety and use medication only when overwhelmed by stress.

Role of the Physician in Patient Management and Indications for Psychiatric Consultation and Referral

Most GAD patients initially seek treatment in the primary care setting. Therefore, the recognition of this disorder by nonpsychiatric physicians is critical. The initial step in evaluating an anxious patient is to exclude medical conditions that produce anxiety syndromes. If another anxiety disorder (such as panic attacks or phobias) or another Axis I disorder (such as major depression or psychosis) is present, specific treatments are indicated for these disorders. Due to the high rate of comorbid psychiatric disorders and the importance of nonpharmacological therapies for GAD, psychiatric evaluation *prior* to initiating treatment is advisable.

CLINICAL PEARLS FOR GENERALIZED ANXIETY DISORDER

- Exclude medical conditions that cause anxiety.
- Exclude other psychiatric disorders, particularly other anxiety disorders.
- Inquire about use of ethanol or other substances, *especially* caffeine. If a history of substance abuse exists, avoid use of benzodiazepines.
- Consider buspirone, antidepressant medications, or benzodiazepines (at lowest effective dose and shortest duration necessary).
- Consider psychotherapy or behavioral therapy, alone or with medication.

ANXIETY DISORDERS DUE TO GENERAL MEDICAL CONDITIONS AND SUBSTANCE-INDUCED ANXIETY DISORDERS

Anxiety caused by general medical disorders (e.g., hyperthyroidism) and substances (such as caffeine) are frequently overlooked. A high index of suspicion, a rigorous history in regard to the use of medications and drugs, and a good physical evaluation will usually reveal the most common causes of anxiety syndromes caused by medical conditions and substances. Chapter 20 discusses general medical conditions that cause psychiatric symptoms including anxiety in more detail.

REFERENCES

American Psychiatric Association: Diagnostic and Statistical Manual of Mental Disorders, 4th Ed., Washington DC, American Psychiatric Association, 1994

Ballenger JC: Medication discontinuation in panic disorder: J Clin Psychiatr 53 (suppl3):31, 1992

Barlow DH, Lehman CL: Advances in the psychosocial treatment of anxiety disorders: implications for national health care. Arch Gen Psychiatry 53:727–735, 1996

Delle Chiaie R, Pancheri P, Casacchia M, Stratta P, Kotazalidis GD, Zibiellini M: Assessment of the efficacy of buspirone in patients affected by generalized anxiety disorder, shifting to buspirone from prior treatment with lorazepam: a placebo-controlled, double-blind study. J Clin Psychopharm 15(1):12–19, 1995

Foa EB, Rothbaum BO, Riggs DS, Murdock TB: Treatment of posttraumatic stress disorder in rape victims: a comparison between cognitive behavioral procedures and counseling. J Consult Clin Psychology 59:715–723, 1991

Gelpin E, Bonne O, Peri T, Brandes D, Shalev AY: Treatment of recent trauma survivors with benzodiazepines: a prospective study. J Clin Psychiatry 59:390–394, 1996

Jenike MA, chairperson. Recent developments in neurobiology of obsessive-compulsive disorder. J Clin Psychiatry 57:492–503, 1996

Kessler RC, Sonnega A, Bromet E, Hughes M, Nelson CB: Posttraumatic stress disorder in the National Comorbidity Survey. Arch Gen Psychiatry 52:1048–1060, 1995

Klein DF: Panic disorder and agoraphobia: hypothesis hothouse. J Clin Psychiatry 57 suppl 6; 21–27, 1996

Kosten TR, Frank JB, Dan E, McDougle CJ, Giller EL: Pharmacotherapy for posttraumatic stress disorder using phenelzine or imipramine. J Nerv Ment D 179:336, 1991

Kulka RA, Schlenger WE, Fairbank JA, Hough RL, Jordan BK, Marmar CR, Weiss DS: Trauma and the Vietnam War Generation. New York, Brunner/Mazel, 1990

Magee WJ, Eaton WW, Wittchen HU, McGonagle KA, Kessler RC: Agoraphobia, simple phobia, and social phobia in the National Comorbidity Survey. Arch Gen Psychiatry 53:159–168, 1996

Myers JK, Weissman MM, Tishler GL, et al: Six-month prevalence of psychiatric disorders in three communities 1980–1982. Arch Gen Psychiatry 41:959–967, 1984

Robbins LN, Helzer JE, Weisman MM, et al: Lifetime prevalence of specific psychiatric disorders in three sites. Arch Gen Psychiatry 441:949–958, 1984

Wittchen HU, Zhao S, Kessler RC, Eaton WW: DSM–III–R generalized anxiety disorder in the National Comorbidity Survey. Arch Gen Psyc 51(5):355–564, 1994

9 Somatoform Disorders, Factitious Disorders, and Malingering

David G. Folks,
Charles V. Ford,
and Carl A. Houck

Somatoform disorders, factitious disorders, and malingering represent various degrees of illness behavior characterized by the process of somatization. These distinct diagnostic categories are often conceptualized as a continuum of abnormal illness behavior. Particular attention is given to the question of whether symptoms are consciously or unconsciously produced. This chapter will cover many of the current concepts in the epidemiology, diagnosis, etiology, and clinical management of each diagnostic group. The management of chronic pain is not thoroughly covered in this chapter, which rather addresses aspects of pain relevant to somatization; the reader is referred to Chapter 23 by Drs. Boland and Goldberg for more extensive coverage of pain management.

THE PROCESS OF SOMATIZATION

Somatization is a process by which an individual consciously or unconsciously uses the body or bodily symptoms for psychological purposes or personal gain. The observed prevalence of abnormal illness behavior characterized by somatization varies according to the clinical setting and the medical specialty, with reported figures ranging between 5 and 40% of patient visits (Ford, 1983). Somatization is more prevalent among clinical populations presenting to primary care clinicians. Somatizing disorders undoubtedly result in increased use of medical services and significantly affect the cost of medical care. Conservative estimates indicate that at least 10% of all medical services are provided for patients who have no evidence of physical disease; these figures do not include services provided for patients with identified psychiatric syndromes (Smith et al, 1986).

Somatization is facilitated in cultures that accept physical disease as an excuse for disability but reject psychological symptoms as acceptable for entry into the "sick role." Similarly, governmental agencies, insurance companies, and other third-party payers may allow financial restitution for medical expenses, or approve disability payments for physical disease, but deny benefits for disturbances that are psychiatric. Thus, many somatizing individuals receive secondary gain for illness behavior. Ford (1986) has elucidated other specific motivations for somatization as follows: (1) the manipulation of interpersonal relationships; (2) the privileges of the sick role, including sanctioned dependency; (3) financial gain; (4) communication of ideas or feelings that are somehow blocked from verbal expression; and (5) the influence of intrapsychic defense mechanisms.

Perhaps the major conscious or unconscious motivation for somatization is the achievement of the *sick role.* The sick role, first examined by Parsons (1951), allows release from the normal and usual obligations of society while absolving the affected person from blame for the condition. When considering etiologic factors relevant to the process of somatization, one must also appreciate the distinction between the concepts of illness and disease (Eisenberg, 1977). *Disease* is defined as objectively measurable anatomic deformations and pathophysiologic states presumably caused by such varied factors as degenerative processes, trauma, toxins, and infectious agents. *Illness* refers to those experiences associated with disease that ultimately impact on an individual's state of being and social functioning. Therefore, illness takes into account the personal nature of suffering, alienation from one's usual gratifying activities, and a decreased capacity to participate in society, all of which significantly affect life quality.

Irrespective of the underlying motivation(s), all of the possible explanations for somatization encourage a thorough diagnostic investigation and therapeutic approach that focuses on the psychosocial history while formulating the extent of the patient's disease, the magnitude of the illness, and the degree to which the patient is suffering and unable to engage in his or her usual activities. Also worthy of consideration is the appropriateness of an individual's illness behavior in the context of existing disease and the extent to which a patient's symptoms could serve to resolve life problems or represent psychological conflicts. In this regard, Brodsky (1984) has identified family factors that predispose to somatization as follows: (1) growing up in a family of somatizers; (2) being raised by parents who were demanding and unrewarding when the child was well, but caring and loving when the child was ill; (3) experiencing an environment in which one or both parents suffered illness; (4) living in an environment in which other coping mechanisms for dealing with a psychosocial crisis are unavailable; (5) developing a repertoire of reactions used to withdraw from usual life activities or to engage or punish others; and (6) consciously feigning illness to obtain something or to avoid punishment, responsibility, or required duties.

One must also consider the possibility that somatization is primarily or secondarily associated with an underlying psychiatric syndrome, a coexisting personality disorder, or a psychosocial stressor that has diagnostic significance with respect to the interpersonal or intrapsychic features of the case (Miranda et al, 1991). For example, psychiatric disorders and medical symptoms are common in women with histories of severe childhood sexual abuse (Walker et al, 1992). Individuals with or without diagnosed psychiatric disorder and with panic anxiety are among the highest utilizers of ambulatory services for unexplained medical symptoms (Katon et al, 1992).

Psychiatric referral is infrequent with somatization, probably because cases are not recognized as such or these patients lack the psychological capacity and motivation to cooperate with a psychiatric consultant. Fortunately several recommendations have evolved regarding the general therapeutic approach outlined in Table 9–1.

Somatothymia and Psychological-Mindedness

Some individuals have a limited capacity to articulate their feelings and intrapsychic conflicts in psychologically based verbal language. Research has shown that the capability to use abstract psychological terms varies among cultures and individuals within a given culture. The ability to use psychological

Table 9–1 **Somatization: Principles of Clinical Management**

1. The clinical presentation is considered in the context of psychosocial factors, both current and past.
2. The diagnostic procedures and therapeutic interventions are based on objective findings.
3. A therapeutic alliance is fostered and maintained involving the primary care and/or psychiatric physician.
4. The social support system and relevant life quality domains* are carefully reviewed during each patient contact.
5. A regular appointment schedule is maintained for outpatients, irrespective of clinical course.
6. The patient dialogue and examination and the assessment of new symptoms or signs are engaged judiciously, and usually primarily address somatic rather than psychological concerns.
7. The need for psychiatric referral is recognized early, especially for cases involving chronic symptoms, severe psychosocial consequences, or morbid types of illness behavior.
8. Any associated, coexisting, or underlying psychiatric disturbance is assiduously evaluated and steadfastly treated.
9. The significance of personality features, addictive potential, and self-destructive risk is determined and addressed.
10. The patient's case is redefined in such a way that management rather than cure is the goal of treatment.

* Quality of life is an elusive concept but includes the psychosocial domains of occupation; leisure; family, marital, and health; and sexual and psychological functioning.

language (as defined by Western cultural standards) may be determined by a variety of developmental, familial, educational, and linguistic factors. In many non-Western cultures somatically or physically based terms are still the predominant mode of communicating emotional distress.

When examining the development of emotional language in children, it may be observed that children first appear to experience affective states such as anxiety and fear *physically* long *before* they have verbal language either to conceptualize or label these feelings and communicate them to others. It is only later in development that children "learn" to label their feelings and to communicate them to others in verbal terms. Even in our own culture, many individuals as adults may be observed to have a limited capacity to communicate their inner experience and feelings using abstract psychological language.

It is often the task of the astute physician to interpret physical symptoms (or psychosomatic illness) as the patient's characteristic means of expressing and communicating the presence of internal emotional distress. Some individuals may be able to recognize their physical distress as a manifestation of emotional distress, yet others may have limited insight to make such connections.

The phenomenon of communicating emotional distress in physical language has been termed *somatothymia* or *somatothymic language.* Some patients with somatoform disorders may be understood as using a somatic or somatothymic language in which their physical symptoms are a manifestation of emotional distress and intrapsychic conflict. Somatothymic language is the earliest form of affective communication in the developing human and in many cultures and, in some patients with somatoform disorders, remains the predominant mode of "psychological communication." The somatoform disorders may be, at least in part, understood as *clusters of behavior* in which the predominant language used by the patient is somatothymic (Stoudemire, 1991a, b). The concept of somatothymia is also discussed in Chapters 1 and 7.

SOMATOFORM DISORDERS

Somatoform disorders are characterized by physical complaints lacking a known medical basis or demonstrable physical findings in the presence of psychological factors judged to be etiologic or important in the initiation, exacerbation, or maintenance of the disturbance. A comparison of the individual subtypes of somatoform disorder is presented in Table 9–2. These clinical features are fundamentally important and serve to facilitate the discussion that follows.

Somatization Disorder

Formerly termed "hysteria" or Briquet's syndrome, somatization disorder represents a polysymptomatic disorder beginning in early life, affecting mostly

(text continues on page 350)

Table 9–2 **Somatoform, Factitious or Malingering: A Comparison of Clinical Features**

DIAGNOSTIC SUBTYPE	CLINICAL PRESENTATION	DEMOGRAPHIC EPIDEMIOLOGIC FEATURES	DIAGNOSTIC FEATURES	MANAGEMENT STRATEGY	PROGNOSTIC OUTLOOK	ASSOCIATED DISTURBANCES	PRIMARY DIFFERENTIAL PRESENTATION	PSYCHOLOGICAL PROCESSES CONTRIBUTING TO SYMPTOMS	MOTIVATION FOR SYMPTOM PRODUCTION
Somatoform Disorders									
Somatization disorder	Polysymptomatic Recurrent/ chronic "Sickly" by history	Younger age Female predominance 20 to 1 Familial pattern 5–10% incidence in primary care populations	Systems review profusely positive Multiple clinical contacts Polysurgical	· Therapeutic alliance · Regular appointments · Crisis intervention	Poor to fair	Personality disorder Sociopathy Substance/ alcohol use Many life problems Conversion	Physical disease Depression	Unconscious Cultural/ developmental	Unconscious psychological factors
Conversion disorder	Monosymptomatic Mostly acute Simulates disease	Highly prevalent Female predominance younger age Rural/lower social class Less educated psychologically unsophisticated	Simulaton incompatible with known psychological mechanisms or anatomy	· Suggestion and persuasion · Multiple techniques	Excellent except chronic conversion	Drug/alcohol dependence Sociopathy Somatization disorder Histrionic personality	Depression Schizophrenia Neurologic disease	Unconscious Psychological stress or conflict may be present	Unconscious psychological factors
Pain Disorder	Pain syndrome simulated or magnified by physiological factors	Female predominance 2 to 1 Older: 4th or 5th decade Familial pattern Up to 40% of pain populations	Simulation or intensity incompatible with known physiological mechanisms or anatomy	· Therapeutic alliance · Redefine goals of treatment · Antidepressant medications	Guarded variable	Depression Panic disorder Substance/ alcohol use Dependent/ histrionic personality	Depression Psychophysiological Physical disease Malingering/ disability syndrome	Unconscious Acute stressor/ developmental Physical trauma may predispose	Unconscious psychological factors

(continued)

Table 9-2 *(continued)*

DIAGNOSTIC SUBTYPE	CLINICAL PRESENTATION	DEMOGRAPHIC EPIDEMIOLOGIC FEATURES	DIAGNOSTIC FEATURES	MANAGEMENT STRATEGY	PROGNOSTIC OUTLOOK	ASSOCIATED DISTURBANCES	PRIMARY DIFFERENTIAL PRESENTATION	PSYCHOLOGICAL PROCESSES CONTRIBUTING TO SYMPTOMS	MOTIVATION FOR SYMPTOM PRODUCTION
Hypochondriasis	Disease concern or preoccupation	Previous physical disease Middle or older age Male/female ratio equal	Disease conviction amplifies symptoms Obsessional	· Document symptoms · Psychosocial review · Psychotherapeutic	Fair to good Waxes and wanes	Depression Panic disorder Obsessive-compulsive disorder	Depression Physical disease Personality disorder Delusional disorder	Unconscious Stress— bereavement Developmental factors ratio	Unconscious psychological factors
Body dysmorphic disorder	Subjective feelings of ugliness or concern with body defect	Adolescence or young adult ? Female predominance Largely unknown	Pervasive bodily concerns	· Therapeutic alliance · Stress management · Psychotherapies · Antidepressant medications	Fair to good	Obsessive-compulsive disorder Anorexia nervosa Psychosocial distress Avoidant/ compulsive personality disorder	Delusional psychosis Depression Somatization disorder	Unconscious Self-esteem factors	Unconscious psychological factors

Factitious Disorders

DIAGNOSTIC SUBTYPE	CLINICAL PRESENTATION	DEMOGRAPHIC EPIDEMIOLOGIC FEATURES	DIAGNOSTIC FEATURES	MANAGEMENT STRATEGY	PROGNOSTIC OUTLOOK	ASSOCIATED DISTURBANCES	PRIMARY DIFFERENTIAL PRESENTATION	PSYCHOLOGICAL PROCESSES CONTRIBUTING TO SYMPTOMS	MOTIVATION FOR SYMPTOM PRODUCTION
Factitious with predominantly physical symptoms	Feigned or simulated physical symptoms or signs or disease	Female, younger, socially conforming Employed in medical field Social supports often available	Feigned illness No external goal of simulation is obvious Organ mode of presentation varies but is physical	· Confront as appropriate · Redefine illness as psychiatric · Psychiatric referral	Fair to good except Munchausen's subtype	Depression Borderline or other personality disorder	Malingering Conversion disorder Hypochondriasis Depression Schizophrenia	Unconscious Developmental/ family factors Masochism, dependency, and mastery are utilized	Conscious effort to assume patients status

Factitious with predominantly psychological symptoms	Multiple hospitalizations	Female, younger, socially conforming Employed in medical field Social supports often available	Feigned illness No external goal of simulation is obvious Mode of presentation varies but is psychiatric	· Confront as appropriate · Redefine illness as psychiatric · Psychiatric referral	Fair to good except Munchausen's subtype	Schizophrenia Borderline or other personality disorder	Malingering Conversion disorder Hypochondriasis Depression Schizophrenia	Unconscious Developmental/family factors Masochism, dependency, and mastery are utilized	Conscious effort to assume patient status
Munchausen's syndrome	Multiple hospitalizations	Male, younger, socially nonconforming Social supports often unavailable	Feigned illness Pathologic liar Geographic wandering Antisocial features Frequently leaves against medical advice	· Recognize · Confront · Avoid invasive or iatrogenic procedures or treatments · Social work referral	Poor	Antisocial, histrionic, or borderline personality	Malingering Conversion disorder Hypochondriasis Depression Schizophrenia	Unconscious Developmental/family factors Masochism, dependency, and mastery are utilized	Conscious effort to assume patient status

Malingering

Malingering	Feigned or simulated with physical or psychological symptoms	? Male predominance Psychosocial stress or failure present	Feigned illness External incentives for disease present	· Confront · Consider psychiatric or psychosocial problems	N/A	Antisocial personality Substance abuse/dependence	Factitious disorder Personality disorder Ganser syndrome Munchausen syndrome Major psychosis Disability syndrome	Conscious but may display other psychopathology	Conscious response or external incentives

women, and characterized by recurrent, multiple somatic complaints reflected in a diffusely positive review of systems. Cases date back more than 3,000 years, with the first systematic evaluation being reported by Briquet, for whom the condition was originally named (Folks and Houck, 1993). Certain diagnostic aspects of the syndrome have been refined, resulting in the more reliable diagnostic criteria ultimately included in the DSM-IV nomenclature (American Psychiatric Association, 1994).

Epidemiology

Estimates from the Epidemiologic Catchment Area Study show an estimated lifetime prevalence of approximately 0.4% for somatization disorder (Swartz et al, 1986). Although accurate point prevalence figures are not readily available, 1 to 2% prevalence is suggested for women with a female-to-male predominance of approximately 20:1. Somatization disorder is more commonly observed in lower socioeconomic groups. Between 5 and 10% of a primary care ambulatory population will meet diagnostic criteria for somatization disorder, suggesting that somatization is the fourth most common diagnostic group seen in an ambulatory medical setting. A relationship between somatization disorder and polysurgery is also well documented. A familial pattern is observed affecting 10 to 20% of female first-degree biological relatives of females with somatization disorder; male relatives of females with this disorder show an increased risk of antisocial personality disorder and/or substance-use disorder (Bohman et al, 1984). Adoption studies have indicated that both genetic and environmental factors contribute to the risk for the disorder. Several investigators have reported the tendency for somatization disorder to be associated with sociopathy, alcoholism, and drug addiction. Although no specific data exist to establish the economic impact of somatization disorder, the prevalence and tendency to use surgery and advanced technology in diagnosis of treatment undoubtedly represents a significant cost.

Diagnosis and Differential Diagnosis

The most important diagnostic feature of somatization disorder is recurrent, multiple somatic complaints of several years' duration for which medical attention has been sought. The diagnostic criteria are summarized in Table 9–3. A specific pattern of complaints not fully explained by a known medical condition must include (1) pain symptoms (at least four) involving multiple sites or functions, (2) gastrointestinal symptoms (at least two), (3) sexual or reproductive symptoms other than pain (at least one), or (4) pseudoneurological symptoms (at least one) (American Psychiatric Association, 1994).

The diagnosis has been shown to possess criterion stability, with a high degree of reliability and validity. Liskow et al (1986) observed that the disorder is quite heterogeneous and that other psychiatric illness is likely to coexist. Personality disorders are more frequently associated and may appear in conjunction with an anxiety disorder or depressed mood, as well as a substance use disorder. Interestingly, avoidant, paranoid, and compulsive personality disorder

Table 9–3 **Diagnostic Criteria for Somatization Disorder***

A. A history of many physical complaints beginning before age 30 years that occur over a period of several years and result in treatment being sought or significant impairment in social, occupational, or other important areas of functioning.
B. Each of the following criteria must have been met, with individual symptoms occurring at any time during the course of the disturbance:
  1) *four pain symptoms:* a history of pain related to at least four different sites or functions (e.g., head, abdomen, back, joints, extremities, chest, rectum, during menstruation, during sexual intercourse, or during urination)
  2) *two gastrointestinal symptoms:* a history of at least two gastrointestinal symptoms other than pain (e.g., nausea, bloating, vomiting other than during pregnancy, diarrhea, or intolerance of several different foods)
  3) *one sexual symptom:* a history of at least one sexual or reproductive symptom other than pain (e.g., sexual indifference, erectile or ejaculatory dysfunction, irregular menses, excessive menstrual bleeding, vomiting throughout pregnancy)
  4) *one pseudoneurological symptom:* a history of at least one symptom or deficit suggesting a neurological condition not limited to pain (conversion symptoms such as impaired coordination or balance, paralysis or localized weakness, difficulty swallowing or lump in throat, aphonia, urinary retention, hallucinations, loss of touch or pain sensation, double vision, blindness, deafness, seizures; dissociative symptoms such as amnesia; or loss of consciousness other than fainting)
C. Either (1) or (2):
  1) after appropriate investigation, each of the symptoms in Criterion B cannot be fully explained by a known general medical condition or the direct effects of a substance (e.g., a drug of abuse, a medication)
  2) when there is a related general medical condition, the physical complaints or resulting social or occupational impairment are in excess of what would be expected from the history, physical examination, or laboratory findings
D. The symptoms are not intentionally produced or feigned (as in Factitious Disorder or Malingering)

* DSM-IV criteria (American Psychiatric Association, 1994).

occur with greater frequency than do histrionic or antisocial personality disorder (Rost et al, 1992). Panic disorder with and without agoraphobia, panic attacks, dissociative disorder, obsessive–compulsive disorder, depressive disorder, and alcohol dependence are the more frequently occurring Axis I comorbid conditions. Somatization disorder has been reported in 23% of women and 5% of men with panic disorder (Battaglia et al, 1995). Somatization disorder is also a frequent and serious comorbid disorder among patients with dissociative disorder. One controlled study found that 64% of the patients with dissociative disorders met diagnostic criteria for somatization disorder with an average of 12.4 somatic symptoms per case (Saxe et al, 1994). A significant correlation was found between the degree of dissociation and of somatization in patients with dissociative disorders. Conversion symptoms may also be a prominent clinical feature with somatization disorder (Folks et al, 1984). Antisocial behavior and occupational, interpersonal, or marital difficulties are frequently observed.

The differential diagnosis includes schizophrenia, panic disorder, conversion disorder, factitious disorder, and psychological factors affecting medical condition. Consideration must be given to medical disorders that present with confusing, vague somatic symptoms. Patients with somatization disorder may present in the context of acute general medical illness, psychophysiological symptoms, or other chronic medical conditions. A history of depression, panic, suicide attempt, and divorce is also common (Tomasson et al, 1991). Thus, a mix of primarily psychogenic and physical symptoms is the rule rather than the exception, making these cases extraordinarily challenging diagnostically.

Etiology and Pathogenesis

The etiologic foundations of somatization disorder are not readily discernible, although familial incidences and association with antisocial and histrionic personality disorder, as well as substance- and alcohol-use disorders, suggest a biologic predisposition. Undoubtedly, a learning model or behavioral theory is applicable, because the general use of somatizing behavior in the family of origin or culture may predispose to the syndrome (Brodsky, 1984). Furthermore, the disorder begins early in life (before age 30).

Clinical Management

The first step in the management of somatization disorder is simply to recognize the syndrome and initiate a therapeutic strategy in keeping with the principles outlined in Table 9–1. These patients see themselves as functionally disabled and readily use medical services even though no objective measures have determined that they are physically sick. The following case is illustrative:

A CASE STUDY

A 40-year-old woman presented to the emergency room with a complaint of chest pain. A preliminary evaluation revealed no obvious cause, but because she reported numerous symptoms in her systems review, she was admitted for a more complete evaluation. Her diagnostic workup ultimately included cardiac catheterization, which yielded totally normal results. The medical student involved in her case learned that her twin children, who had "always helped" her in illness, had recently left to attend college. Furthermore, a review of her complaints in view of the negative findings seemed to indicate that the patient was "psychosomatic." At this point a psychiatric consultant was asked to see the patient and obtained a thorough psychosocial history revealing that the patient had been sickly since about age 15, with numerous chronic symptoms arising in different organ systems; nausea, bloating, back pain, dysuria, pain in her knees, palpitations, dizziness, dyspnea, double vision, gait unsteadiness, weakness of her arms, trouble swallowing, dyspareunia, and dysmenorrhea were all mentioned at various times throughout the interview. She dramatically related that she was "tired of suffering" and was "frustrated" with her doctors, who had been unable to diagnose her case or explain the disabling symptoms satisfactorily.

The psychiatrist, who recognized her problem as somatization disorder, suggested psychotherapy as a means to help her cope with the rather obvious family stresses that had precipitated her pain, but she declined, saying that she preferred to see "a real doctor who can understand me better."

As represented in the case above, many patients are highly resistant to psychiatric referral; thus the recommendations for treatment must first consider the general principles outlined in Table 9–1. A collaborative care model involving the psychiatric consultant as part of the team can effectively address many psychiatric issues. The development of a combined treatment plan has been shown to provide both symptomatic relief and improved physical functioning in somatizers who were previously "highly impaired" (Rost et al, 1994). In addition, several studies have indicated that overall costs of care and health care utilization are reduced in comparison with the typical somatization disorder case that does not receive psychiatric intervention (Smith et al, 1986, 1995). The psychiatric consultant's role also involves crisis intervention or attention to comorbid conditions with key therapeutic interventions resulting from a well-developed therapeutic relationship between the patient and the primary clinician. A cure is seldom achieved, but recurrent debilitating symptoms can be relinquished and perhaps exchanged for controlled dependence on a clinic or physician.

Conversion Disorder

Conversion symptoms have been described since antiquity and may represent a type of somatoform disorder. One or more symptoms or deficits affecting sensory or motor function occur in which there is a loss or alteration in physical functioning. The physical disorder, however, cannot be explained on the basis of known physiological mechanisms. Conversion disorder is usually seen in ambulatory settings or emergency departments, and frequently runs a rather short-lived course, eventually responding to nearly any therapeutic modality that offers a suggestion of cure.

Epidemiology

Conversion symptoms are exceedingly common in medical practice; estimates of 20 to 25% prevalence are given for patients admitted to a general medical setting (Ford, 1983). General hospital patients have consistently shown conversion symptoms in 5 to 14% of all psychiatric consultations (Folks et al, 1984). Conversion symptoms are also ubiquitous among randomly selected psychiatric clinic patients and are prevalent among patients with drug dependence, sociopathy, alcoholism, and somatization disorder or "hysteria." The disorder more typically occurs in women. In men the disorder tends to be associated with a history of industrial accidents or in association with military duty. Conversion disorder reportedly encompasses ages ranging from early childhood into the ninth decade. The disorder appears more frequently in lower socioeconomic groups and in rural or less psychologically sophisticated populations. The more primitive and grossly nonphysiological conversion symptoms are observed in patients of rural background; by contrast, conversion symptoms observed in better educated populations will more closely simulate known disease.

Diagnosis and Differential Diagnosis

Diagnostic descriptions and terminology relating to conversion phenomena have changed markedly over the past four decades. Diagnostic criteria are depicted in Table 9–4. The diagnosis is unique, implying that specific psychological factors account for the disturbance. In contrast to somatization disorder, which is chronic and polysymptomatic, involving many organ systems, conversion disorder is generally sporadic and monosymptomatic with a symbolic relationship between the underlying psychological conflict and the disturbance in physical functioning. *A number of traditional clinical features previously associated with conversion—for example, secondary gain, histrionic personality, and* la belle *indifference (a "happy" lack of concern about the symptoms)—appear to have no diagnostic significance; these are regarded as "soft signs," supportive of the diagnosis but having no firm diagnostic validity.* The diagnosis of conversion must ultimately rest on positive clinical findings clearly indicating that the symptom does not derive from physical disease. Common examples of conversion symptoms include paralysis, abnormal movements, aphonia, blindness, deafness, or pseudoseizures, the last of which is illustrated by a case vignette.

Table 9–4 **Diagnostic Criteria for Conversion Disorder***

A. One or more symptoms or deficits affecting voluntary motor or sensory function that suggest a neurological or other general medical condition.
B. Psychological factors are judged to be associated with the symptom or deficit because the initiation or exacerbation of the symptom or deficit is preceded by conflicts or other stressors.
C. The symptom or deficit is not intentionally produced or feigned (as in Factitious Disorder or Malingering).
D. The symptom or deficit cannot, after appropriate investigation, be fully explained by a general medical condition, or by the direct effects of a substance, or as a culturally sanctioned behavior or experience.
E. The symptom or deficit causes clinically significant distress or impairment in social, occupational, or other important areas of functioning or warrants medical evaluation.
F. The symptom or deficit is not limited to pain or sexual dysfunction, does not occur exclusively during the course of Somatization Disorder, and is not better accounted for by another mental disorder.

Specify type of symptom or deficit: with Motor Symptom or Deficit; with Sensory Symptom or Deficit; with Seizures or Convulsions; with Mixed Presentation

* DSM-IV criteria (American Psychiatric Association, 1994)

A CASE STUDY

*A 42-year-old woman was admitted to the neurology service for
evaluation of seizures beginning 1 month earlier. The seizures
consisted of gradual onset of tonic-clonic movements, lasting about
10 minutes and involving weeping, vocalizations, alternating
movements of the head, and pelvic thrusting. The seizures resolved
abruptly, with no postictal confusion or diminished consciousness.
An intensive neurological evaluation revealed no abnormal physical findings; laboratory screen, magnetic resonance imaging of the
brain, lumbar puncture, and routine electroencephalogram (EEG)
were all normal. The patient was then monitored continuously with
video telemetry and showed no abnormal EEG patterns despite the
occurrence of several "seizure" episodes. A psychiatric consultant
was called in who learned that the seizure activity—now thought to
represent a conversion disorder—began within a week of learning
that her husband had been unfaithful. An amobarbital interview
revealed that the patient had been considering a divorce although
such an alternative was unacceptable to her or her family of origin's
value system.*

As suggested by the case, conversion symptoms will usually conform to
the *patient's* concept of disease rather than to typical pathophysiological
mechanisms or anatomical patterns. When the symptom occurs in isolation, it
is appropriate to assign a diagnosis of conversion disorder; however, conversion symptoms may also occur as a part of other major syndromes, such as
somatization disorder, schizophrenia, depression, and even general medical or
neurological disease.

Approximately one in five cases diagnosed initially as conversion disorder are later found to be somatization disorder (Kent et al, 1995). Common
comorbid diagnoses with conversion disorder include dissociative disorders
(especially with pseudoseizures), mood and anxiety disorders, and personality disorders. Posttraumatic stress disorder commonly occurs in association
with history of sexual abuse, physical abuse, or other significant traumas
(Bowman and Markand, 1996; Nemiah, 1991; Saxe et al, 1994; Tomasson et al,
1991).

Etiology and Pathogenesis

Clinical descriptions of conversion phenomena date back to at least 1900
BC, at which time the Egyptian papyri attributed symptoms to "wandering of
the uterus." Conversion symptoms result from stressful events acting on the
affective part of the brain in predisposed individuals. Some patients' symptoms
conform to Freud's concept of "conversion" in reference to the concept that
conversion results from the *substitution* of a somatic symptom for a repressed

idea or psychological conflict. Conversion may also be a means of expressing forbidden feelings or ideas, as a kind of communication via pantomime or mimicry when direct verbal communication is blocked, or may simply serve as an acceptable means of enacting the sick role or as an acute entry into illness behavior. The individual with conversion avoids certain responsibilities or noxious situations and is frequently able to control or manipulate the behavior of others. Classical conditioning paradigms have provided other possible explanations for conversion phenomena. Learned symptoms of illness are then later used as a means of coping with particularly stressful situations. More recent theories have proposed social, communication, and sophisticated neurophysiological mechanisms (Folks et al, 1984).

Pseudoseizures (also called hysterical seizures, psychogenic seizures, and nonepileptic seizures) are most likely a somatic form of communication involving conversion *and* dissociative mechanisms (Nash, 1995). These cases are frequently linked to prior or current abuse as illustrated in the above case (Bowman, 1996). Approximately two-thirds of the cases are found with comorbidity—both Axis I and Axis II. As with other conversion subtypes, seizure cases represent reactions to a specific event, or expression of dependence, or need for control (Couprie et al, 1995).

Clinical Management

A wide variety of treatment techniques have been successfully used for conversion disorder. Brief psychotherapy focusing on stress and coping, and suggestive therapy—sometimes using hypnosis or amobarbital interviews that focus on symptom removal—are commonly employed with amazing efficacy. A short hospital admission may also be helpful, particularly when symptoms are disabling or alarming. Full or partial hospitalization may serve to remove the patient from the stressful situation, demonstrate to the family that the matter is important, or facilitate resolution of the psychological trauma.

Many patients experience spontaneous remission of symptoms or demonstrate marked or complete recovery after a brief therapeutic intervention. In fact, prompt recovery is the rule, and few patients will need long-term management. For example, one case seen involved a healthy 29-year-old man who experienced acute blindness when confronted with a mortgage foreclosure notice and was ultimately "cured" with saline drops. The psychiatric consultant merely told the patient that the "special" eye drops had "cured several others in a matter of days."

Regarding patients with pseudoseizures, a single counseling session that includes appropriate presentation of the diagnosis may suffice (Lesser, 1996). Psychotherapy (either psychodynamic or cognitive behavioral) works equally well. Most therapeutic approaches involve a combination of dynamic, behavioral, and educational strategies together with techniques that begin with the diagnostic interview (Nash, 1995). As with somatization disorder, psychiatric intervention is found to reduce subsequent health care costs and utilization

(Smith et al, 1995). Unfortunately, chronic conversion disorder carries a poorer prognosis and is notoriously difficult to treat, resembling somatization disorder. Behavior modification can be used in the approach to recalcitrant conversion symptoms maintained by secondary gain. The therapeutic principles outlined in Table 9–1 are particularly relevant to these chronic cases, and psychiatric consultants are often required.

Pain Disorder Associated with Psychological Factors

The general category of Pain Disorder in DSM-IV involves clinically significant pain in one or more anatomical sites. Psychological factors appear to be etiological or contribute significantly to the pain. Pain syndromes in which psychological factors are believed to have a primary role in the onset, severity, exacerbation, or maintenance of a patient's pain complaints are distinguished from other pain syndromes. If the patient has a general medical condition, that condition should not have a major role in the manifestation of pain if this diagnosis is assigned. In many situations, however, the patient may have a bona fide physical illness (such as lumbar disk disease), but psychological factors appear to magnify their clinical pain symptoms. If the medical disorder appears to be present and playing a significant role in the patient's pain complaints, and these complaints are magnified in severity by psychological factors, then the patient may be diagnosed with "pain disorder associated with *both* psychological factors *and* a general medical condition."

This section will primarily focus on pain syndromes in which psychological factors appear to predominate, with minimal contributions from bona fide medical and neurological factors. (The treatment of more routine pain syndromes not complicated by major psychological factors is discussed by Drs. Boland and Goldberg in Chapter 23.) As noted above, this discussion is primarily in reference to "pain disorders associated with psychological factors." Multidisciplinary pain clinics have developed in which patients can be effectively evaluated and treated by consultants from a variety of disciplines—anesthesia, neurology, neurosurgery, orthopedics, psychiatry, psychology, and social work. Various diagnostic categories of pain are encountered. This chapter is confined to the diagnosis and clinical management of certain aspects of pain associated with psychological factors.

Epidemiology

As much as 40% of pain patients exhibit pain that is psychological in origin (Stoudemire and Sandhu, 1987). Pain typically presents in the fourth or fifth decade, usually as acute pain increasing in severity over time. Pain that is associated with prominent psychological features is diagnosed in women twice as frequently as in men. Evidence exists to suggest a familial pattern, with first-degree biological relatives being at higher risk for developing the disorder. A known familial pattern that includes a history of anxiety, depression, or alcohol dependence occurs at a greater frequency than might be expected within the general population.

Diagnosis and Differential Diagnosis

Pain disorder associated with psychological factors may involve one or more anatomic sites and cause significant. DSM-IV (American Psychiatric Association, 1994) criteria are more descriptive and "less divisive" than previous terminology (Eisendrath, 1995). The terms psychogenic or somatoform have been eliminated from their diagnostic category as outlined in Table 9–5. Patients with pain associated with psychological factors actually perceive pain—the pain is "real." Essentially, the pain represents a conversion disorder, perhaps most commonly in developed societies (Merskey, 1986). Usually a significant relationship is found with a role model, or else a history of physical or sexual abuse, prior hypochondriacal complaints, or severe guilt is identified as shown by the following case (Eisendrath et al, 1986).

Table 9–5 **Diagnostic Criteria for Pain Disorder**[*,†]

A. Pain in one or more anatomical sites is the predominant focus of the clinical presentation and is of sufficient severity to warrant clinical attention.
B. The pain causes clinically significant distress or impairment in social, occupational, or other important areas of functioning.
C. Psychological factors are judged to have an important role in the onset, severity, exacerbation, or maintenance of the pain.
D. The symptom or deficit is not intentionally produced or feigned (as in Factitious Disorder or Malingering).
E. The pain is not better accounted for by a Mood, Anxiety, or Psychotic Disorder and does not meet criteria for Dyspareunia.

Code as follows: **Pain Disorder Associated with Psychological Factors:** psychological factors are judged to have the major role in the onset, severity, exacerbation, or maintenance of the pain. (If a general medical condition is present, it does not have a major role in the onset, severity, exacerbation, or maintenance of the pain.) This type of Pain Disorder is not diagnosed if criteria are also met for Somatization Disorder.
Specify if: **Acute:** duration of less than 6 months; **Chronic:** duration of 6 months or longer

Pain Disorder Associated With Both Psychological Factors and a General Medical Condition: both psychological factors and a general medical condition are judged to have important roles in the onset, severity, exacerbation, or maintenance of the pain. The associated general medical condition or anatomical site of the pain (see below) is coded on Axis III.
Specify if: **Acute:** duration of less than 6 months; **Chronic:** duration of 6 months or longer

[*] Pain per se may be associated with psychological factors and/or a general medical condition; it may be acute with a duration of less than 6 months or chronic. The anatomical site(s) is coded Axis III of DSM-IV.
[†] DSM-IV criteria (American Psychiatric Association, 1994).

A CASE STUDY

A 29-year-old man complained to his family physician of constant abdominal pain so severe he had used all his sick leave and was having to consider resigning his prestigious new position. An admission to the hospital led to a comprehensive but fruitless evaluation of the pain, culminating in an unremarkable exploratory laparotomy. On learning that the surgery was unrevealing, the patient appeared surprised, frustrated, and distraught, proclaiming that he was "afraid" he would be unable to return to work with his boss, the division chief, who happened to be his father.

The differential diagnosis of pain must take into consideration other psychiatric syndromes, such as somatization disorder, depressive disorder, or schizophrenia, in which complaints of pain are common. Of course, a significant minority of these patients are ultimately found to have factitious disorder or malingering (as discussed below), and the symptoms are manifest for the sole purpose of obtaining an obviously explainable or recognizable goal, or the patients are motivated to secure narcotic analgesics or other substances. Another important differential diagnosis is psychophysiological disorders, such as muscle contraction headache, muscular spasm back pain, proctalgia fugax affecting the musculature of the anus, or other syndromes that may involve a clear pathophysiological mechanism that reasonably accounts for the pain syndrome.

Comorbid conditions may include illness-affirming disorders such as conversion disorder, somatization disorder, and hypochondriasis. Other conditions that coexist include depressive disorder, anxiety disorder—especially panic and posttraumatic stress—and delusional disorder. Anxiety or depressive symptoms may represent either an underlying or coexisting disorder (Smith, 1992). The changes in mood and in personality that accompany chronic pain are also frequently seen in depression. Indeed, all pain patients seem to report symptoms or changes in their physiological response, with the emergence of vegetative symptoms similar or identical to those that accompany anxiety or depression. The observed personality disorders that most frequently accompany somatoform pain are histrionic and dependent (Reich et al, 1983). For a discussion of more specific pain syndromes, the reader is referred to Ford (1983), who discusses clinical features of psychogenic aspects of pelvic pain, phantom pain, low back pain, and atypical facial pain.

Etiology and Pathogenesis

Pain disorders are sometimes diagnosed only on the basis of psychosocial features identified by history: evidence of past somatization, the presence of a symptom model, prominent guilt, or a history of physical or psychogenic abuse by either a parent or a spouse. However, these "soft" findings together with negative physical or laboratory or radiographic findings do not necessarily imply that pain is attributable to psychological factors. Despite agreement that significant comorbidity exists between pain and depression, debate continues as to which condition initiates the other. Perhaps a shared mechanism exists involving similar biological underpinnings (Eisendrath, 1995). Similarly, posttraumatic stress disorder may also be a predisposing factor or share biologic mechanisms that affect pain perception. Certainly a number of general medical diseases commonly coexist with pain—perhaps these conditions amplify pain perception and also contribute to the pain disorder itself. Moreover, as with all forms of somatization, a complete separation of etiology into physical or psychogenic factors may be difficult and in some ways unnecessary. Full appreciation of the etiological factors involved in any form of pain that appears to be exacerbated by psychological factors is complicated, since the clinician must account for the economy of secondary gain or reinforcement, understand abnormal illness behavior, and evaluate the role of unconscious motivations and primary gain.

Individuals receiving financial compensation are prone to confound their management; compensation neurosis or disability syndromes (not covered in this chapter) are perhaps the best studied etiological and consequential factors resulting in patients with pain syndromes. Psychological tests, most popularly the Minnesota Multiphasic Personality Inventory (MMPI), are used routinely in pain clinics to identify psychological factors. An elevation of scores on the three scales labeled hypochondriasis (Hs), depression (D), and hysteria (Hy), referred to as the *conversion V profile,* purportedly provides evidence that the patients are "neurotic," representing themselves as physically ill and obtaining appreciable secondary gain from their symptoms. These psychological tests should not be carried out or interpreted in a vacuum and are unlikely to be useful diagnostically without other means of supporting data. In short, correlations do *not* distinguish organic from nonorganic patients for whom "conversion" or psychogenic forces are assumed to account for the pain.

Clinical Management

A multiplicity of treatments for pain syndromes influenced or magnified by psychological factors have been suggested in the literature (Eisendrath, 1995; Stoudemire and Sandhu, 1987). Generally, a systems approach and a variety of therapeutic techniques are necessary. The therapeutic strategy is to minimize the doctor-shopping and other interpersonal "games" initially while establishing a strong therapeutic alliance and assuring the patient that complete relief is unlikely. The therapeutic principles outlined in Table 9–1 are effective. A major task is to convince patients that they must work to modify their therapeutic expectations and attempt to manage to live with their pain. A therapeutic contract can usually be initiated and the clinician quickly discerns whether the patient is really motivated to "get better." Because stress and psychological problems are always a component of pain cases, the psychiatric consultant is an invaluable participant in the psychological treatment and should be involved early. Moreover, the possible role of psychosocial or psychological factors and the impact of stress are better considered during the initial evaluation process. Specifically, many experienced clinicians recommend involving the psychiatric consultant at the outset of the diagnostic evaluation to minimize any feelings of rejection or abandonment that may otherwise emerge when psychiatric consultation is deemed necessary.

A number of nonpharmacological treatments are useful in pain patients: transcutaneous nerve stimulation, nerve blocks, accupuncture, biofeedback, and other forms of behavioral or psychotherapy. Irrespective of the selected intervention, attention must be given to the patient's psychosocial, marital, and family situation, and to the meaning and significance of the pain itself. Regarding pharmacological modalities, narcotics or other addicting substances are rarely indicated, but the psychotropics may serve as adjuvants. The cyclic antidepressants often afford pain relief (i.e., 50 to 75 mg daily of nortriptyline). Monoamine oxidase (MAO) inhibitors have been suggested as reasonable when combined with some of the aforementioned nonpharmacological therapies. Selective serotonin-reuptake inhibitors and newer antidepressants, especially those with serotonergic properties, such as fluoxetine and sertraline, may also be beneficial—especially in cases with comorbidity, e.g., depression, anxiety, migraine, and fibromyalgia. Obviously, the selection of a pharmacological agent will depend on the individual case presentation.

Hypochondriasis

Epidemiology

The actual prevalence of hypochondriasis as a disorder distinct from other somatoform disorders is unknown, with estimates varying with culture and diagnostic criteria. Only a few twin studies have been reported, and inadequate evidence exists for conclusions about the importance of genetic factors. Developmental or other predisposing factors include parental attitudes toward disease, previous physical disease, lower social class, and culturally acquired attitudes relevant to the epidemiology and etiology of the disorder. Hypochondriasis typically begins in middle or older age and is equally common in men and women—features that serve to distinguish it from somatization and conversion disorder.

Diagnosis and Differential Diagnosis

Pilowsky (1970) defines hypochondriasis as "a concern with health or disease in one's self which is present for the major part of the time." The preoccupation must be unjustified by the amount of physical pathology and must not respond more than temporarily to clear reassurance given after a thorough examination. The core features of hypochondriasis appear to consist of a complex of attitudes: disease fear, disease conviction, and bodily preoccupation associated with multiple somatic complaints. These diagnostic features are reflected in Table 9–6. On presentation, the medical history is often related in

Table 9–6 **Diagnostic Criteria for Hypochondriasis***

A. Preoccupation with fears of having, or the idea that one has, a serious disease based on the person's misinterpretation of bodily symptoms.
B. The preoccupation persists despite appropriate medical evaluation and reassurance.
C. The belief in Criterion A is not of delusional intensity (as in Delusional Disorder, Somatic Type) and is not restricted to a circumscribed concern about appearance (as in Body Dysmorphic Disorder).
D. The preoccupation causes clinically significant distress or impairment in social, occupational, or other important areas of functioning.
E. The duration of the disturbance is at least 6 months.
F. The preoccupation is not better accounted for by Generalized Anxiety Disorder, Obsessive–Compulsive Disorder, Panic Disorder, a Major Depressive Episode, Separation Anxiety, or another Somatoform Disorder.

Specify if: **With Poor Insight:** if, for most of the time during the current episode, the person does not recognize that the concern about having a serious illness is excessive or unreasonable.[†]

* DSM-IV criteria (American Psychiatric Association, 1994).
† The patient's level of insight is of prognostic significance and may be specified.

---

great detail in the context of doctor-shopping, deteriorating doctor–patient relationships, and associated feelings of frustration and anger. Anxiety, depression, and obsessive personality features are frequently encountered. The clinical course is chronic with waxing and waning of symptoms. Complications may arise secondary to numerous exposures to medical care and the dangers of repeated diagnostic procedures. The possible evolution of this pattern is illustrated by the following case.

A CASE STUDY

A 35-year-old accountant presented to a gastroenterologist with a request to be "checked for colon cancer." The patient stated that, in contrast to his usual pattern of daily bowel movements, he had been constipated for the past 3 weeks. He also stated that 6 months previously, he had been constipated and an evaluation had revealed nothing wrong. However, a family history of colon cancer and fears relating to his dietary habits were elaborated. The current episode was not associated with rectal bleeding, abdominal pain, or other symptoms. Subsequently, a thorough outpatient evaluation, including digital rectal exam, flexible sigmoidoscopy, and barium enema revealed no significant abnormalities. While exploring psychological possibilities, a personal history revealed some occupational distress related to his not yet becoming a full partner in the accounting firm, which in the same breath was compared with the rather glowing career of his brother, recently promoted to vice president at the local bank. The patient seemed quite irritated by the questions pertaining to his personal life and emotional well-being. Reluctantly he stated that he would "just have to accept the fact that everything's okay" but proceeded to question the doctor's credentials and the diagnostic validity of the completed procedures. Within 2 weeks, a letter from a gastroenterology colleague across town requested the patient's records, implying that the same complaints had been offered with a request for a "more thorough evaluation."

The most important step in the differential diagnosis of hypochondriasis is the exclusion of physical disease. A number of medical disorders can be difficult to identify in their early course, including myasthenia gravis, multiple sclerosis, slowly deteriorating degenerative diseases of the neurological system, endocrinopathies, or systemic diseases such as systemic lupus erythematosus or occult neoplastic disorders. However, the diagnosis should not be one of exclusion; a positive diagnosis can be made by careful history in the absence of objective physical findings and on recognition that an emotional component contributes to the symptoms.

Among psychiatric diagnoses, the most important are anxiety disorders or major depression: patients with comorbid panic or depression represent the good prognosis case versus those with generalized anxiety and somatization disorder symptoms (Barsky et al, 1994). One must also carefully consider the existence of other somatoform disorders, factitious disorders, or malingering, and of psychotic disorders for cases manifesting hypochondriacal delusions. Investigators have consistently reported syndromes of hypochondriasis that qualify as a delusional state.

Patients with hypochondriasis seem to perceive their bodily functions more acutely than others. Barsky's (1979) suggested term "amplifying somatic style" emphasizes that these individuals selectively perceive bodily functions and attribute their symptoms to physical disease; *why* patients develop this type of behavior is unknown. Worry about disease and absorption in their health can be a powerful motive for attending selectively to a bodily sensation. Anxiety escalates and further serves as a motive for selective perception. Depression or dysphoria exists since the patient suffers and feels helpless or hopeless as the illness evolves. Anger may also arise as a result of unmitigated distress, conflicting diagnoses, ineffective treatments, and experiences of encountering impatient, rejecting, or hostile physicians. These emotions are compounded by doctor-shopping, medication problems, conflicting opinions from physicians, and iatrogenic phenomena, as well as the specific personality features in any individual case (Kellner, 1987).

Clinical Management

The most crucial management technique in caring for the hypochondriacal patient is the inclusion of a legible psychosocial history in a prominent place in the patient's record. The general therapeutic principles described in Table 9–1 are applicable to the vast majority of cases. The effective therapeutic strategy is to appreciate the obsessional features and understand the fascinating displacement of psychodynamics involved in the symptom formation while appreciating the psychosocial history.

Generally, effective treatment takes place in the context of collaboration by a consulting psychiatrist and the primary physician, who continues to offer regular appointments to the patient. The possibility of concurrent medical disease or intercurrent illness exists—indeed, these will eventually occur as life progresses. Adequate physical examination on a regular basis is helpful, and the judicious and coordinated use of other medical consultants is also appropriate to evaluate new or justifiable physical complaints. Hypochondriacal patients are best managed in a primary care or medical setting. Psychiatric consultation should be considered when the patient requests adjunctive psychiatric treatment—usually for anxiety, depression, or psychosocial distress—or with concern about suicide or overt symptoms of depression. Effective management requires recognition of interpersonal and psychological contributors to the symptoms, with a shift toward assisting the patient to cope with their symptoms. Cognitive educational approaches seem to work best (Barsky, 1996). Surprisingly, the prognosis for hypochondriasis is good in a substantial portion of patients. More severe symptoms, longer duration of illness, and coexisting psychiatric illness are predictive of a worse outcome (Noyes et al, 1994).

Body Dysmorphic Disorder

Body dysmorphic disorder, or dysmorphophobia, has been included as a separate disorder in the DSM-IV nomenclature. This syndrome had been regarded as a hypochondriacal subtype or unspecified somatoform syndrome in past literature.

Epidemiology

Because the vast majority of references involve case reports, descriptive accounts of body dysmorphic disorder offer little substantial information regarding epidemiological or etiological factors. Onset typically occurs in adolescence, but the initial presentation can be as late as the third decade. The condition can persist for years and significantly affect social or occupational functioning. Polysurgery or unnecessary surgical procedures complicate these cases. Body dysmorphic disorder is associated with a high rate of psychiatric hospitalization and suicide (Phillips, 1996). The male to female ratio appears to be equal, but epidemiological data is lacking.

Diagnosis and Differential Diagnosis

The fundamental diagnostic feature is primarily a pervasive subjective feeling of ugliness or physical defect; the patient genuinely feels that changes are readily apparent to others. The diagnostic criteria for body dysmorphic disorder are outlined in Table 9–7. Commonly, the symptoms of body dysmorphic

Table 9–7 **Diagnostic Criteria for Body Dysmorphic Disorder***

A. Preoccupation with an imagined defect in appearance. If a slight physical anomaly is present, the person's concern is markedly excessive.
B. The preoccupation causes clinically significant distress or impairment in social, occupational, or other important areas of functioning.
C. The preoccupation is not better accounted for by another mental disorder (e.g., dissatisfaction with body shape and size in Anorexia Nervosa).

* DSM-IV criteria (American Psychiatric Association, 1994).

disorder involve facial flaws such as wrinkles; spots on the skin; excessive facial hair; the shape of the nose, mouth, jaw, or eyebrows; and swelling of the face. Complaints may involve the feet, hands, breasts, genitals, back, or some other body part. A slight physical defect may actually be present, but the concern expressed is grossly in excess of what might be considered appropriate. Most patients engage in repetitive behaviors such as mirror checking, skin picking, or reassurance seeking. Insight is poor and some cases involve delusional thoughts (Phillips, 1996). This disorder is characterized by much distress but is not to be confused with those transient feelings commonly experienced by adolescents. A case illustration can better distinguish the pathologic state:

A CASE STUDY

A 19-year-old college student approached her campus physician with a request for him to "remove some of the bone" from her nose. She described the end of her nose as "too large," and believed that she could not attract a date because her nose was "repugnant." She conceded that perhaps her nose was really not too excessively large, but continued to worry about its impact on her social life and presented again and again wanting it "fixed." She was reluctantly referred to a plastic surgeon, who concurred that indeed no appreciable defect existed and that a surgical procedure was not justifiable. However, the surgeon was familiar with such presentations and suggested that a psychiatric colleague could "help her cope with her distress." The patient, who was somewhat compulsive, felt obliged to accept psychiatric referral. She was evaluated and ultimately became involved in group cognitive psychotherapy, which was therapeutic in helping her correct her distorted self-perceptions.

The differential diagnoses entertained with hypochondriasis are equally applicable to body dysmorphic disorder. However, the differential diagnosis must also consider phobias; personality disorders, especially avoidant and compulsive types; major depression; delusional disorder (somatic subtype); and the other somatoform disorders.

Body dysmorphic disorder may also accompany anorexia nervosa and transsexualism, in which the patient displays unfounded beliefs about body weight and/or gender-related physical characteristics. Comorbidity also includes major depressive disorder, social phobia, and obsessive–compulsive disorder. An earlier onset of these comorbid conditions has been reported with body dysmorphic disorder (Mintzer et al, 1995; Phillips et al, 1993).

Etiology and Pathogenesis

Individuals with body dysmorphic disorder who indeed appear normal develop a low sense of aesthetic perception, whereas those who are somewhat abnormal regard their appearance in the context of a high sense of aesthetic perception. Avoidance of social or occupational situations due to anxiety or apprehension about the defect is the rule. Clinical features are similar to social phobia. Thus, a "neurotic" syndrome is operating with secondary features of anxiety and depression. Many cases involve hypersensitivity and mood reactivity similar to that seen in atypical depression. The belief in the physical defect of appearance can sometimes be delusional. The delusional variant of body dysmorphic disorder may be a more severe form of the disorder.

Clinical Management

Persons with body dysmorphic disorder frequently visit primary care physicians, dermatologists, or plastic surgeons repeatedly in an effort to correct the defect; depressive and obsessive personality traits and psychosocial distress frequently coexist with the disorder and require treatment. Psychiatric consultation may be useful in identifying and treating depression, anxiety, and other disturbances that require pharmacological or psychotherapeutic intervention. Patients with persistent anxiety or depressive symptoms may be started on a trial of antidepressant therapy, either a cyclic antidepressant with serotonin-active properties or an MAO inhibitor. Similarly, patients have been shown to be responsive to the selective serotonin-reuptake inhibitors, especially with underlying anxiety, e.g., obsessive–compulsive disorder (Phillips, 1996). The antipsychotic drug pimozide has also produced startling and sustained improvement, particularly in patients whose preoccupation has become delusional. However, no other antipsychotic or other pharmacological agents have proved as effective in the treatment of this disorder. As illustrated in the above case, psychiatric intervention with individual or group cognitive therapy may be useful, focusing on psychosocial functions and body image complaints.

Undifferentiated Somatization Disorder (Somatoform Disorders not Otherwise Specified)

DSM-IV includes an undifferentiated somatoform disorder category for clinical presentations that do not meet the full symptom picture of somatization disorder or one of the other somatizing syndromes. Autonomic arousal disorders or psychophysiological disturbances involving the cardiorespiratory, gastrointestinal, or urogenital systems, or the skin are being considered as specific types or subtypes. In these cases, psychological factors contribute to symptomatology and/or the disturbance cannot be explained by a known nonpsychiatric medical condition or known pathophysiologic mechanism, e.g., effects of medication, substances, or injury (American Psychiatric Association 1994). Also, neurasthenia has traditionally been considered a distinct diagnostic entity. This disturbance is characterized by persistent complaints of mental fatigue, physical fatigue, or body weakness or exhaustion after performing daily activities. The individual does not recover with rest or leisure. Symptoms include dizziness, muscular aches, headache, irritability, sleep disturbance, and gastrointestinal complaints. The diagnostic criteria for undifferentiated somatization disorder are illustrated in Table 9–8. This newly added diagnosis was recently assigned in the following case.

A CASE STUDY

A 68-year-old woman presented to her family physician for an evaluation of dysuria and fatigue. She had experienced the symptoms for many years. Complete evaluation produced no evidence of a physical disease to account for her symptoms. Further questioning revealed no other physical symptoms and she did not display a depressive or associated psychiatric disorder. A consulting psychiatrist subsequently learned that the patient lost her parents, both at 65 years of age, due to cancer—leukemia in her father and renal cell carcinoma in her mother.

Table 9–8 Diagnostic Criteria for Undifferentiated Somatoform Disorder*

A. One or more physical complaints (e.g., fatigue, loss of appetite, gastrointestinal or urinary complaints).
B. Either (1) or (2):
  (1) after appropriate investigation, the symptoms cannot be fully explained by a known general medical condition or the direct effects of a substance (e.g., a drug of abuse, a medication)
  (2) when there is a related general medical condition, the physical complaints or resulting social or occupational impairment is in excess of what would be expected from the history, physical examination, or laboratory findings
C. The symptoms cause clinically significant distress or impairment in social, occupational, or other areas of functioning.
D. The duration of the disturbance is at least 6 months.
E. The disturbance is not better accounted for by another mental disorder (e.g., another Somatoform Disorder, Sexual Dysfunction, Mood Disorder, Anxiety Disorder, Sleep Disorder, or Psychotic Disorder).
F. The symptom is not intentionally produced or feigned (as in Factitious Disorder or Malingering).

* DSM-IV criteria (American Psychiatric Association, 1994).

As illustrated, these disorders involve a single, circumscribed condition that is not explainable on the basis of demonstrable physical findings or known pathophysiological mechanisms. In keeping with somatoform disorders, the presentation is apparently linked with psychological factors. The circumscribed symptoms are of 6 months' duration or longer and, of course, not a part of another type of somatoform disorder, sexual dysfunction disorder, mood disorder, anxiety disorder, sleep disorder, or one of the other major psychotic syndromes important in differential diagnosis. A diagnosis of somatoform disorder that cannot be otherwise specified is assigned for somatoform symptoms that are of less than 6 months' duration, hypochondriacal in nature, nonpsychotic, or presenting with non-stress-related physical complaints.

FACTITIOUS DISORDER

Most clinicians will at some point in their career encounter a case of factitious disorder. These somatizing states are essentially characterized by the voluntary production of signs, symptoms, or disease for no apparent goal other than to achieve the role of being a patient. By contrast, the somatoform disorders are collectively viewed as having symptoms that are manifested unconsciously. *Munchausen's syndrome*, the most extreme type of factitious disorder, is characterized by a triad of features involving simulation of disease, pathological lying, and wandering. These types of cases frequently involve men of lower socioeconomic class who have had a lifelong pattern of social maladjustment. Several other clinical features of the Munchausen type are depicted in Table 9–9. However, most authorities concur that the vast majority of factitious disorders involve socially conforming young women of a higher socioeconomic class who are intelligent, educated, and frequently employed in a medically related field. Thus, one will rarely encounter the socially nonconforming "wanderers" who satisfy the Munchausen's syndrome criteria listed in Table 9–9.

Epidemiology

The available literature provides only a few indications of the incidence of factitious illness. These disorders appear to be far more common than was once generally believed, perhaps because of the progress in medical technology and the popular medical journalism that is readily available to the lay public. The paucity of systematic studies and disproportionate number of case reports on the Munchausen syndrome have resulted in contradictory data on the age and sex ratio. Patient age averages approximately 30 years and ranges from adolescence to old age. The available epidemiographical data on factitious disorders are inadequate, but again strongly suggest a preponderance of young adults, the majority of whom are female and likely to be employed in the health professions.

Table 9–9 **Munchausen's Syndrome: Diagnostic Features***

Essential Features
Pathologic lying (pseudologia fantastica)
Peregrination (traveling or wandering)
Recurrent, feigned, or simulated illness

Supporting Features†
Borderline and/or antisocial personality traits
Deprived in childhood
Equanimity for diagnostic procedures
Equanimity for treatments or operations
Evidence of self-induced physical signs
Knowledge of or experience in a medical field
Most likely to be male
Multiple hospitalizations
Multiple scars (usually abdominal)
Police record
Unusual or dramatic presentation

---

* Patients will meet criteria for a chronic factitious disorder or an atypical factitious disorder.
† May also support the diagnosis of other factitious disorders.
(Reprinted with permission from Folks DG, Freeman AM: Munchausen's syndrome and other factitious illness. Psychiatr Clin North Am 8:263–278, 1985)

Differential Diagnosis

Factitious illness is not real, genuine, or natural. Thus, physical or psychological symptoms are under voluntary control and are simulated to deceive the physician, although the manifestation of symptoms possesses a rather compulsive quality. The characteristic presenting modes and organ system subtypes of factitious disorder are listed in Table 9–10. Clinical presentation may involve physical or psychological symptoms or both. Factitious disorder with predominantly physical symptoms is the most common subtype. Diagnostic criteria are shown in Table 9–11. A dramatic presentation with a history of multiple hospitalizations and, of course, the primary goal of assuming the patient role are the pertinent diagnostic features. Eisendrath (1984) suggests that factitious presentation may be manifested at one of three levels of enactment: (1) a fictitious history, (2) a simulated disease, or (3) the presence of verifiable pathophysiology. The last is illustrated by the following case vignette.

A CASE STUDY

A 32-year-old psychiatric nurse was hospitalized for uncontrolled diabetes mellitus. During her hospitalization, her serum glucose levels fluctuated markedly despite diligent efforts to regulate her insulin dosage requirements. On the fourth hospital day, the patient suggested that perhaps she needed further diagnostic testing to

Table 9–10 **Commonly Presenting Features of Chronic Factitious Illnesses**

ORGAN SYSTEM SUBTYPES	DEMEANOR OR BEHAVIOR
Abdominal*	Bizarre
Cardiac	Demanding
Dermatological†	Dramatic
Genitourinary	Evasive
Hematological*,†	Medically sophisticated
Infectious	Self-mutilating
Neurological*	Unruly
Psychiatric	
Self-medication*,‡	

* Original subtypes identified.
† Recently reported to be more common.
‡ Especially insulin, thyroid, vitamins, diuretics, and laxatives.
(Reprinted with permission from Folks DG, Freeman AM: Munchausen's syndrome and other factitious illness. Psychiatr Clin North Am 8:263–278, 1985)

determine whether any other unrecognized problems might be present. Her physician discouraged further testing. The next morning the ward nurse found the patient lying comatose in her bed. A stat blood sugar showed severe hypoglycemia. During the emergency evaluation, a medical student found a used syringe and a bottle of regular insulin lying behind the patient's nightstand. When the patient recovered and was confronted with the discovery of the covert insulin, she became highly indignant and left the hospital against medical advice.

A diagnosis of inclusion, not exclusion, factitious disorder with either predominantly physical or psychological symptoms or both requires a high index of suspicion and clinical perseverance once the diagnosis is established. In addition to the possibility that a true disease exists and accounts for the presentation, malingering, pseudomalingering, conversion disorder, and hypochondriasis are the leading differential diagnoses. Diagnostic criteria for

Table 9–11 **Key Features of Factitious Disorder*,†**

- Intentional production of clinical signs or symtoms.
- Primary intent is to assume the sick role.
- The patient does not benefit from or have external incentives for the production of signs or symptoms.

* Factitious disorder may occur predominantly with psychological and/or physical signs and symptoms.
† Summarized from DSM-IV (American Psychiatric Association, 1994)

factitious disorder are depicted in Table 9–11. Cases involving psychological presentations of factitious illness include factitious mourning or grief, or feigned psychosis or posttraumatic stress disorder.

Cases seen in psychiatric consultation may have already been misdiagnosed as a range of psychiatric disorders, including conversion disorder, somatization disorder, malingering, schizophrenia, or other major psychoses. Histrionic, schizotypal, borderline, antisocial, and masochistic personality disorders often, if not always, are concurrently diagnosed on Axis II; borderline personality disorder is the most common type of personality disorder observed. Understanding the relationship between personality disorders and response styles are helpful to the treatment planning process. Poorly defined distinctions between factitious disorder, somatization disorder, and malingering have probably contributed to the diversity of diagnoses included in the differential diagnosis of factitious disorder. Factitious disorder not otherwise specified is an appropriate diagnosis for patients who do not seek hospital admission and for atypical cases involving simulated illness, such as dermatitis artifacta.

Factitious disorder by proxy has received increased attention as a focus of clinical attention. Factitious disorder by proxy, more popularly known as Munchausen's syndrome by proxy, involves a parent or caregiver who creates and induces an illness in a child. The range has been reported from 7 weeks of age to 14 years of age, but cases usually involve infants. Similar to factitious disorder, the motivation for the perpetrator's behavior is a psychological need to have the child assume the sick role, indirectly in this case. Mothers tend to be young, in their early 20s, and married, and are predominantly articulate, middle class individ-uals with pathological attachments to their children. Psychological profiles of the mothers include personality disorder, somatizing behaviors, and significant family dysfunction. Interestingly, a small number of fathers have been described as the perpetrators. Clinical presentations generally follow two patterns. Apnea, seizures, and cyanosis comprise the first pattern, more often seen in infants. The second pattern involves cases with diarrhea and vomiting, more commonly observed among older children. Other frequent complaints include headache, nausea, cyanosis, and bone and joint problem. Infants may present with significant failure to thrive or recurrent otitis media, or may have history of multiple hospitalizations and repeated thorough medical workups. Neurological symptoms often include ataxia, hyperactivity, chorea, weakness, inability to walk, lassitude, headache, and limb paralysis.

Etiology and Pathogenesis

Any attempt to understand the etiology of factitious disorder requires careful consideration of any developmental disturbance, personal history, and current life stressors and an appreciation of primary psychodynamic mechanisms—masochism, dependency, and mastery. The desire to be the center of interest and attention; a grudge against physicians and hospitals that is somehow satisfied by frustrating and deceiving the staff; a desire for drugs; a desire to escape the police; and a desire to obtain free room and board while tolerating the consequences of various therapeutic investigations and treatment are some of the more frequently listed reasons that might possibly motivate the self-destructive behaviors of patients with a factitious disorder.

Although patients often possess borderline personality traits, one can often obtain a history of childhood emotional insecurity; excluding or rejecting parents; and broken homes leading to foster home placement or adoption and subsequent delinquency, antisocial behavior, or failure in psychosexual development. The possible enactment of past or present developmental disturbances within the medical setting should also be considered. In essence it seems that these patients, through their illness, also may primarily seek to compensate for developmental traumas and secondarily escape from and make up for stressful life situations. Psychodynamic explanations suggest that the factitiously disordered patients experience satisfaction from manipulating as many aspects of their own medical and surgical care as possible (mastery), receive strong sexual gratification from diagnostic and therapeutic procedures (masochism), and enjoy the warm and personal but ambivalent care inherent in the doctor–patient relationship (dependency), culminating in the excitement of the hospital experience. These features are associated with a poor consolidated sense of self and difficulty regarding emotional experience as real.

Clinical Management

The general therapeutic approach outlined in Table 9–1 is applicable to cases of factitious disorder, and a comparison with the somatoform disorders is presented in Table 9–2. The initial clinical approach also requires a clear recognition of the syndrome or a high index of suspicion that a factitious disorder is indeed present. Psychiatric consultation should be requested for all cases, and if confrontation is advisable, the primary physician (as opposed to the consultant) should confront the patient in a nonpunitive manner (Hollender and Hersh, 1970). Patients are usually less difficult to confront than might be expected and do not show the intense anger, impulsivity, or instability of interpersonal relationships that is commonly reported with the more extreme cases representing Munchausen's syndrome (Reich and Gottfried, 1983). If confronted with the factitious nature of the illness, the patient may deny it, refuse psychiatric intervention, and resume the same behavior; may admit that the factitious illness is present but refuse psychiatric intervention; or may acknowledge the factitial nature of the illness and cooperate with psychiatric intervention (Ford, 1983; Hollender and Hersh, 1970).

Confrontation is not necessarily appropriate for all cases; the psychiatrist may simply attempt to build rapport with the patient while the primary physician continues any necessary noninvasive medical treatment. Confrontation is more often favored in the hospitalized patient who has the intelligence, psychosocial supports, and personal attributes necessary for a more mature adaptation. A psychotherapeutic approach that validates the patient's subjective experience may lead to reduced factitious behavior. Family members can be especially therapeutic in providing pertinent history or assisting the medical staff in maintaining acceptable limits on the illness behavior. Treatable psychopathology such as anxiety disorders, depressive syndromes, conversion symptoms, and major psychoses should be assiduously evaluated and steadfastly treated.

The prognosis for factitious illness has generally been considered poor. However, careful exclusion of malingerers, severe borderline personalities, wandering patients with Munchausen's syndrome, and the chronic medically ill can result in a subgroup of potentially treatable patients (Table 9–12). The prognosis is better for patients with an underlying depression than for those merely possessing a personality disorder. Reich and associates observed that once the diagnosis was established, even some of the more severe and chronic cases responded quite well to a combined medical and psychiatric approach (Reich and Gottfried, 1983). Finally, as noted with other forms of somatization, the possibility of coexisting physical disease or intercurrent illness should be appreciated in all diagnostic and therapeutic endeavors.

MALINGERING

The essential clinical feature of malingering is the intentional production of illness or grossly exaggerated physical or psychological symptoms that is motivated by external incentives such as avoiding military duty,

Table 9–12 **Aspects of Factitious Illness Potentially Amenable to Treatment**

1. Presence of treatable psychiatric syndromes, including:
   Mood disorders
   Anxiety disorders
   Psychotic disorders
   Conversion disorders
   Substance abuse disorders
   Neuropsychiatric disorders
2. Personality organization closer to compulsive, depressive, or histrionic rather than borderline, narcissistic, or antisocial
3. Stability in psychosocial support system as manifested by marriage, stable occupation, and family ties, as opposed to the single, unemployed wanderer
4. Ability to cope with confrontation or some redefinition of the illness behavior
5. Capability of establishing and maintaining rapport with the treating clinicians

(Reprinted with permission from Folks DG, Freeman AM: Munchausen's syndrome and other factitious illness. Psychiatr Clin North Am 8:263–278, 1985)

obtaining financial compensation through litigation or disability, evading criminal prosecution, obtaining drugs, or simply securing better living conditions (Gorman, 1982). Clinical reports suggest that malingering should be strongly suspected in the following circumstances: (1) a medical/legal context overshadows the presentation, (2) a marked discrepancy exists between the clinical presentation and the objective findings, (3) a lack of cooperation is experienced with diagnostic efforts or in compliance with medical regimen, and/or (4) the psychosocial history suggests the presence of an antisocial personality disorder. Responses or personality tests such as the MMPI and Rorschach may be helpful in the evaluation of feigned illness (see Chapter 3). Malingerers typically give responses that are overly dramatic, less emotionally restrained, and exaggerated. However, no consensus exists as to the utility or reliability of these measures in making a "diagnosis" of malingering (Fruech and Kinder, 1994; Ganellen et al, 1996).

Malingering can be fundamentally viewed as a feigning of illness: the fraudulent simulation or exaggeration of physical or mental disease or defect consciously produced to achieve a specific goal. The reasons for the illness behavior in the individual circumstances can be readily understood by an objective observer. Unlike the patient with factitious disorder, who merely wishes to assume the patient role, a malingering individual has as more clearly external motivation, and the illness behavior is intentional and consciously produced to achieve a consciously desired goal. This distinction is represented in Table 9–2 and illustrated by the following case.

A CASE STUDY

A 57-year-old man appearing thin and disheveled presented to the emergency room one cold wintry night at 2:00 a.m. complaining of chest pain. He stated that he had a history of angina; he stated that only intravenous morphine could alleviate his pain. The emergency physician, in obtaining a history of the pain, noted that it did not seem to fit the pattern of any of the common causes of chest pain; routine physical exam, laboratory screen, arterial blood gases, and electrocardiogram were surprisingly normal. However, as a precaution, the patient was admitted for further observation and evaluation. The next day, the chest pain persisted and the patient still requested narcotics. A medical student ascertained that no relatives were available and that the patient had no reasonable plan for how he might manage following hospital discharge. On afternoon rounds, the patient, after being informed that he would be given no narcotics, reported that his pain had disappeared, and despite the physician's willingness to search further for the cause, he insisted on leaving the hospital.

Malingering may sometimes be adaptive (arguable in the case just presented) and is, to a lesser degree, observed in apparently normal children, students, test subjects, and employees; thus malingering behavior does not always represent a maladaptive or malignant form. A few clinicians have promulgated the theory that pure malingering is a mental disease worthy of a therapeutic response. Malingering has also been conceptualized as occurring on a continuum with conversion disorder (Ford, 1986). Briefly, the conscious effort to falsify symptoms may in some cases include rather complex motivations, originating in part from the unconscious. Malingering is also likely to arise in individuals with antisocial personality disorder or other various forms of feigned illness, such as Ganser's syndrome, or as a component of a psychiatric disorder. Coexisting disturbances are the focus of evaluation and treatment for these "mentally ill" malingerers.

Irrespective of one's views on malingering, some basic legal principles should be considered in examining for the presence or absence of malingering. In particular, before reporting malingering one should steadfastly follow the basic rules of confidentiality and privilege. Another important aspect of malingering concerns the way in which physicians perceive such behavior and their moral judgment of it. As a case in point, situations certainly exist in which this extreme form of somatization is regarded as acceptable, constructive, or even praiseworthy, as in the case of the prisoner of war who malingers to protect his or her country's interests. Therefore, a professional and therapeutic posture in approaching the malingering patient must initially include an examination of one's own feelings of anger, disgust, or humiliation, recognizing that the malingering behavior often threatens the very foundations of the doctor–patient relationship. Frank, nonjudgmental communication between the physician and the malingerer and awareness that the behavior may be an ongoing reaction to stress or due to a psychiatric disorder may lead to an open discussion of the patient's needs—which may, in turn, provide a basis for an adequate therapeutic alliance or a solution to the problem (Lande, 1989; Mark et al, 1987).

Finally, a number of authors have described simulation among persons seeking compensation for work-related injuries or disease (Weighill, 1983). However, the psychological difficulties in these cases vary greatly, and the physician must be able to appreciate and assess a number of background factors, such as severity of injury, preexisting personality traits, developmental characteristics, social class, attitudinal response, and the pertinent family, social, and employment factors, as well as the actual progress of the physical condition or legal process of settlement. Unfortunately, these disability syndromes are beyond the scope of this chapter.

As a final note, a number of clinical pearls and suggested readings will serve to expand upon the material presented in this chapter. A thorough review of Tables 9–1 and 9–2 in conjunction with the Clinical Pearls section will aid in the diagnostic and therapeutic approach to each diagnostic type.

CLINICAL PEARLS

General Points

Somatoform disorders, factitious disorders, and malingering represent illness behavior, whether symptoms are consciously or unconsciously produced and whether the motivations for the production of symptoms are conscious or unconscious will determine what particular diagnostic category is assigned.

- Somatization is a process by which an individual consciously or unconsciously uses the body or bodily symptoms for psychological purposes or personal gain.
- Somatizing individuals are primarily motivated and secondarily receive gain for illness behavior, including the privileges of the sick role and sanctioned dependency.
- The presence of somatization encourages a thorough diagnostic investigation and therapeutic approach that focuses on psychosocial history and illness behavior in the context of existing disease, life problems, and psychological conflicts.
- Somatization may be primarily or secondarily associated with an underlying psychiatric syndrome, coexisting personality disorder, or psychosocial stressor of diagnostic significance.
- Some individuals may lack the ability to verbalize their feelings and intrapsychic conflicts in psychological terms. Somatothymia, or somatothymic language, describes the use of physically based language terms to communicate emotional distress.

Somatization Disorder

Somatization disorder is a polysymptomatic disorder that begins in early life, affects mostly women, and is characterized by recurrent multiple somatic complaints and a profusely positive review of systems.

- The disorder is commonly associated with sociopathy, alcoholism, and drug abuse.
- The disorder is heterogeneous and likely to coexist with a psychiatric disturbance or personality disorder.
- Management includes a therapeutic alliance with an empathic primary care physician, regularly scheduled patient visits, appreciation of the psychological significance of symptoms, use of diagnostic or therapeutic procedures or medications based on objective findings, and use of psychiatric consultation for complications, coexisting disturbances, or crisis intervention.

Conversion Disorder

Conversion symptoms are ubiquitous among psychiatric patients with schizophrenia, somatization disorder, alcoholism, sociopathy, and drug use.

- Conversion disorder typically occurs in women who are of lower socioeconomic class, psychologically unsophisticated, or of rural background.
- The diagnosis of conversion disorder must ultimately rest on positive clinical findings clearly indicating that the symptom does not derive from physical disease or is a part of another psychiatric disorder.
- Conversion symptoms often accompany degenerative neurological syndromes such as multiple sclerosis, amyotrophic lateral sclerosis, and so on. These and other disorders need to be carefully considered and ruled out before making the diagnosis.
- Acute conversion disorder can usually be etiologically related to psychological conflict, allows an individual to avoid certain responsibilities or noxious situations, and secondarily enables control or manipulation of the behavior of others (i.e., secondary gain).

- Treatment usually includes supportive and suppressive approaches that include some element of suggestion or persuasion using the therapeutic principles outlined in Table 9–1; a multitude of treatments have proved successful.

Pain Disorder Associated with Psychological Factors

In as many as 40% of patients presenting with pain, the pain will be considered psychogenic or idiopathic.

- Pain disorder with psychological factors is diagnosed when psychological factors are believed by the clinician to have a significant role in the outset, severity, exacerbation, or perpetuation of pain syndromes.
- Psychological factors must be appreciated and may include any of the following:
  identified precipitants by history
  avoidance of an activity or responsibility that is unacceptable or noxious
  acquisition of significant psychosocial support that would not otherwise be forthcoming
- Major depression or anxiety, e.g., obsessive–compulsive or panic disorder, is often present and may be a component of the pain syndrome or represent a coexisting disorder.
- The best therapeutic strategy is to limit doctor-shopping and modify the patient's therapeutic expectations from "cure" to "management" of the pain, while attempting to appreciate the role of psychosocial or psychological factors and the impact of stress on the case, using psychiatric consultation as appropriate.

Hypochondriasis

Hypochondriasis is characterized by a concern or preoccupation with health or disease in oneself that is present most of the time and is not justified by the physical pathology.

- The core features include disease fear, disease conviction, and bodily preoccupation associated with multiple amplified somatic complaints.
- As with pain, the possibility of an underlying or secondary anxiety or depression should be strongly considered, and physical disease should be excluded.
- Treatment is most effective when there is collaboration between a primary physician who continues regular appointments and a consulting psychiatrist who focuses on coping with the pain syndrome and treats symptoms of anxiety, depression, or psychosocial distress.

Body Dysmorphic Disorder

Body dysmorphic disorder typically occurs in adolescence or young adulthood, persists for years, and significantly affects social and occupational functioning.

- The fundamental diagnostic feature is a pervasive feeling of ugliness or physical defect that the patient feels is readily apparent to others.
- Patients frequently consult primary care physicians, dermatologists, and plastic surgeons in an effort to correct the defect.
- Depressive and anxious symptoms, obsessive personality traits, and psychosocial distress frequently coexist with the disorder and provide a basis and rationale for psychiatric consultation.
- Individual therapy that focuses on psychosocial distress and group or family cognitive therapy as appropriate are the primary interventions, in keeping with the principles outlined in Table 9–1.

Factitious Disorders

Factitious disorders usually involve socially conforming young women of a higher socioeconomic class who are intelligent, educated, and frequently employed in a medically related field.

- A distinction can be drawn between "wanderers," who frequently safisfy the Munchausen's syndrome criteria, and "nonwanderers," who do not. The latter (the majority) are amenable to treatment.
- As opposed to somatoform disorders, factitious disorders are characterized by psychological and/or physical symptoms that are *consciously* produced (or induced by proxy) with the goal of assuming the patient role; thus a patient (or caregiver) may be confronted about the illness behavior. However, unconscious motivations are responsible for the clinical presentation and must be addressed as such (see below).
- The primary therapeutic approach involves an attempt to understand the etiology, including consideration of developmental disturbances, personal history, and current life stressors; appreciation of primary psychodynamic mechanisms (masochism, dependency, and mastery); and an appreciation of any personality disorders that might complicate treatment planning. Usually a borderline personality disorder is involved.
- Clinical management includes confrontation by the primary physician and/or referral to a psychiatric consultant who redefines the illness as primarily psychiatric and offers a psychotherapeutic approach to those patients who do not represent the Munchausen's syndrome.
- The possibility of intercurrent illness or coexisting physical disease should be appreciated in all diagnostic and therapeutic endeavors. Careful follow-up by the primary physician is essential.

Malingering

The essential feature of malingering is the intentional production of illness consciously motivated by external incentives such as avoiding military duty, obtaining financial compensation through litigation or disability, evading criminal prosecution, obtaining drugs, or securing better living conditions.

- Malingering should be suspected when a medical/legal context overshadows the presentation, a marked discrepancy exists between clinical presentation and objective findings, a lack of cooperation is experienced with diagnostic efforts or in compliance with medical regimen, and possibly when the psychosocial history suggests the presence of an antisocial personality disorder.
- The malingering should be confronted in a confidential and empathic but firm manner that leaves an opportunity for constructive dialogue and appreciation of any psychological or psychosocial problems.

ANNOTATED BIBLIOGRAPHY

Barsky AJ: Hypochondriasis: medical management and psychiatric treatment. Psychosomatics 3748–56, 1996

> An overview of somatization disorder and management strategy in terms of the specific problems encountered in the doctor–patient relationship and in developing a therapeutic alliance.

Eisendrath SJ: Psychiatric aspects of chronic pain. Neurology 45 (Suppl 9):S26–S34, 1995

> A comprehensive article that reviews the various pain syndromes encountered in clinical practice with special attention to psychogenic or somatoform pain and its evaluation and treatment.

Folks DG: Munchausen syndrome and other factitious disorders. Neurol Clin 13:267–281, 1995

> A thorough review of the factitious disorders, distinguishing those that are potentially treatable from Munchausen syndrome and other more refractory factitial syndromes. Includes a section covering Munchausen by proxy encountered in practice.

Ford CV: The somatizing disorders. Psychosomatics 27:327–337, 1986

> Includes an excellent overview of the process of somatization illustrating somatizing behaviors, sociocultural and interactional influences on somatization, and the specific diagnostic categories relevant to the process of somatization.

Ford CV, Folks DG: Conversion disorders: an overview. Psychosomatics 26:371–383, 1985

> An excellent overview of conversion disorder that includes a detailed discussion of its etiology and pathogenesis as well as a review of the diagnostic and treatment approaches.

Gorman WF: Defining malingering. J Forensic Sci 27:401–407, 1982

> An excellent overview that conceptualizes malingering on a continuum from normal to the abnormal to the pathologic forms. Provides the reader with a pragmatic conceptualization for approaching malingers therapeutically.

Kellner R: Hypochondriasis and somatization. JAMA 258:2718–2722, 1987

> A superb discussion of hypochondriasis and of how those affected use somatization in their clinical presentation. An excellent review follows outlining caveats in the management of hypochondriasis.

Phillips KA, McElroy SL, Keck PE: Body dysmorphic disorder: 30 cases of imagined ugliness. Am J Psychiatry 150:302–308, 1993

> An excellent review of body dysmorphic disorder including clinical descriptions, management, and prognosis.

REFERENCES

American Psychiatric Association: Diagnostic and Statistical Manual of Mental Disorders, 4th ed. Washington, DC, American Psychiatric Association, 1994

Barsky AJ: Patients who amplify bodily sensations. Ann Intern Med 91:63–70, 1979

Barsky A J: Hypochondriasis: Medical management and psychiatric treatment. Psychosomatics 37:48–56, 1996

Barsky AJ, Barnett MC, Cleary PD: Hypochondriasis and panic disorder: boundary and overlap. Arch Gen Psychiatry 51:918–925, 1994

Battaglia M, Bernardeschi L, Politi E, et al: Comorbidity of panic and somatization disorder: A genetic-epidemiological approach. Compr Psychiatry 36:411–420, 1995

Bohman M, Cloninger R, Von Knorring A-L, et al: An adoption study of somatoform disorders: III. Cross-fostering analysis and genetic relationship to alcoholism and criminality. Arch Gen Psychiatry 41:872–878, 1984

Bowman ES, Markand ON: Psychodynamics and psychiatric diagnosis of pseudoseizure subjects. Am J Psychiatry 153:57–63, 1996

Brodsky CM: Sociocultural and interactional influences on somatization. Psychosomatics 25:673–680, 1984

Couprie W, Wijdicks EFM, Rooijmans HGM, et al: Outcome in conversion disorder: a follow up study. J Neurol Neurosurg Psychiatry 58:750–752, 1995

Eisenberg L: Disease and illness: Distinctions between professional and popular ideas of sickness. Cult Med Psychiatr 1:9–23, 1977

Eisendrath SJ: Factitious illness: A clarification. Psychosomatics 25:110–116, 1984

Eisendrath SJ: Psychiatric aspects of chronic pain. Neurology 45(suppl 9):S26–S34, 1995

Eisendrath SJ, Way LW, Ostroff JW, et al: Identification of psychogenic abdominal pain. Psychosomatics 27:705–7111, 1986.

Folks DG, Ford CV, Regan WM: Conversion symptoms in a general hospital. Psychosomatics 25:285–295, 1984

Folks DG, Freeman AM: Munchausen's syndrome and other factitious illness. Psychiatr Clin North Am 8:263–278, 1985

Folks DG, Houck CA: Somatoform Disorders, Factitious Disorders and Malingering. In Stoudemire A, Fogel BS (eds): Psychiatric Care of the Medical Patient, pp 267–287. New York, Oxford University Press, 1993

Ford CV: The Somatizing Disorders: Illness as a Way of Life. New York, Elsevier, 1983

Ford CV: The somatizing disorders. Psychosomatics 27:327–337, 1986

Ford CV, Folks DG: Conversion disorders: an overview. Psychosomatics 26:371–383, 1985

Fruech BC, Kinder BN: The susceptibility of the Rorschach inkblot test to malingering of combat-related PTSD. J Pers Assess 62:280–298, 1994

Ganellen RJ, Wasyliw OE, Haywood TW, et al: Can psychosis be malingered on the Rorschach? An empirical study. J Pers Assess 66:65–80, 1996

Gorman WF: Defining malingering. J Forensic Sci 27:401–407, 1982

Hollender MH, Hersh SP: Impossible consultation made possible. Arch Gen Psychiatry 23:343–345, 1970

Katon WJ, Von-Korff M, Lin E: Panic disorder: relationship to high medical utilization. Am J Med 92:7S–11S, 1992

Kellner R: Hypochondriasis and somatization. JAMA 258:2718–2722, 1987

Kent DA, Tomasson K, Coryell W: Course and outcome of conversion and somatization disorders. Psychosomatics 36:138–144, 1995

Lande RG: Malingering. J Am Osteopath Assoc 89:483–488, 1989

Lesser RP: Psychogenic seizures. Neurology 46:1499–1507, 1996

Liskow B, Othmer E, Penick EC, et al: Is Briquet's syndrome a heterogeneous disorder? Am J Psychiatry 143:626–629, 1986

Mark M, Rabinowitz S. Zimran A, et al: Malingering in the military: understanding and treatment of the behavior. Milit Med 152:260–262, 1987

Mersky H: Psychiatry and Pain. In Sternback RA (ed): The Psychology of Pain, 2nd ed, pp 97–120. New York, Raven Press, 1986

Mintzer O, Lydiard RB, Phillips KA: Body dysmorphic disorder in patients with anxiety disorders and major depression: a comorbidity study. Am J Psychiatry 152:1665–1667, 1995

Miranda J, Perez-Stable EJ, Munoz RF, et al: Somatization, psychiatric disorder, and stress in utilization of ambulatory medical services. Health Psychol 10:46–51, 1991

Nash JL: Pseudoseizures: an update. Compr Ther 21:486–491, 1995

Nemiah JC: Dissociation, conversion and somatization. In Tasman A, Goldfinder SM (eds): American Psychiatric Association Review of Psychiatry, Vol. 10, pp 248–260. Washington DC, American Psychiatric Press, 1991

Noyes R, Kathol RG, Fisher MM, et al: One-year follow-up of medical outpatients with hypochondriasis. Psychosomatics 35:533–545, 1994

Parsons T: Social structure and dynamic process: the case of modern medical practice. In Parsons T(ed): The Social System, pp 428–479. New York, Free Press, 1951

Phillips KA: Body dysmorphic disorder: diagnosis and treatment of imagined ugliness. J Clin Psychiatry 57(suppl 8):61–65, 1996

Phillips KA, McElroy SL, Keck PE: Body dysmorphic disorder: 30 cases of imagined ugliness. Am J Psychiatry 150:2:302–308, 1993

Pilowsky I: Primary and secondary hypochondriasis. Acta Psychiatr Scand 46:273–285, 1970

Reich P, Gottfried LA: Factitious disorders in a training hospital. Ann Intern Med 99:240–247, 1983

Reich J, Tupin JP, Abramowitz SI: Psychiatric diagnosis of chronic pain patients. Am J Psychiatry 140:1495–1498, 1983

Rost KM, Akins RN, Brown FW, Smith GR: The comorbidity of DSM-III-R personality disorders in somatization disorder. Gen Hosp Psychiatry 14:322–326, 1992

Rost K, Kashner TM, Smith GR: Effectiveness of psychiatric intervention with somatization disorder patients: improved outcomes at reduced costs. Gen Hosp Psychiatry 16:381–387, 1994

Saxe GN, Chinman G, Berkowitz MD, et al: Somatization in patients with dissociative disorders. Am J Psychiatry 151:1329–1334, 1994

Smith GR: The epidemiology and treatment of depression when it coexists with somatoform disorders, somatization, or pain. Gen Hosp Psychiatry 14:265–272, 1992

Smith GR Jr, Monson RA, Ray DC: Psychiatric consultation in somatization disorder a randomized controlled study. N Engl J Med 314:1407–1413, 1986

Smith GR, Rost K, Kashner TM: A trial of the effect of a standardized psychiatric consultation on health outcomes and costs in somatizing patients. Arch Gen Psychiatry 52:238–243, 1995

Stoudemire A: Somatothymia: Part I. Psychosomatics 32:365–370, 1991a

Stoudemire A: Somatothymia: Part II. Psychosomatics 32:371–381, 1991b

Stoudemire A, Sandhu J: Psychogenic/idiopathic pain syndromes. Gen Hosp Psychiatry 9:79–86, 1987

Swartz M, Hughes D, George L, et al: Developing a screening index for community studies of somatization disorder. J Psychiatr Res 20:335–343, 1986

Tomasson K, Kent D, Coryell W: Somatization and conversion disorders: comorbidity and demographics at presentation. Acta Psychiatr Scand 84:288–293, 1991

Walker EA, Katon WJ, Hansom J, et al: Medical and psychiatric symptoms in women with childhood sexual abuse. Psychosom Med 54:658–654, 1992

Weighill VE: "Compensation neurosis": a review of the literature. J Psychosom Res 27:97–104, 1983

10 Alcoholism and Substance Abuse

Robert M. Swift

Throughout history, men and women have used psychoactive substances for medicinal, social, recreational, and religious purposes. Today, psychoactive substances continue to be widely used for similar socially sanctioned purposes. Population surveys suggest that approximately 90% of the American population use at least some alcohol, 80% use caffeine-containing beverages or medications, and 25% use tobacco products. The 1988 National Household Survey of Drug Abuse estimated that 72.4 million Americans age 12 or older (37% of the population) have used an illicit psychoactive drug at least once in their lifetime. Although the use of illicit drugs appears to have declined over the previous decade, 14.5 million Americans (7% of the population) are estimated to have used at least one illicit psychoactive substance over the month prior to the survey.

Many people use psychoactive substances to excess, in an uncontrolled fashion, in situations that are not socially approved, or in circumstances in which there are deleterious effects on health or behavior. Such individuals are considered to have a substance-use disorder. The causes of substance use problems are complex and involve contributions of social, psychological, genetic, and pharmacological factors.

SOCIAL AND ECONOMIC ASPECTS OF SUBSTANCE USE

The impact of substance-use disorders on society is considerable. The total economic losses to the United States were estimated to be $85.8 billion from alcohol abuse and $58.3 billion from drug abuse (Rice, 1990). Substance-use disorders are a major contributing factor to injuries and medical and psychiatric illnesses. Each year, alcoholism is estimated to cause 100,000 deaths; illicit drug abuse, 19,000 excess deaths; and tobacco, 400,000 excess deaths (McGinnis and Foege, 1993). It has been estimated that 25 to 50% of patients admitted to general or psychiatric hospitals or in outpatient settings are habitual users of psychotropic substances. Alcohol use is highly correlated with suicide and homicide. A major epidemiological study found high associations between alcohol use and anxiety disorders, depression, and schizophrenia (Regier et al, 1990). Other studies have found associations between cocaine, opioid, or nicotine use and depressive disorders. Substance use and eating disorders are related, especially in women. The comorbidity of substance use and psychiatric illness is called *dual diagnosis* and is a major complication in the successful treatment of these patients. Alcohol and drugs are major causes of family dysfunction, including domestic violence and child abuse.

Over the past decade, the costs of addiction treatment and who pays for it have become major factors in determining the treatment that is available for patients. Frequently, addiction treatment requires administrative approval by third-party payers, such as insurance companies or managed care programs, and cost is a major consideration. It is important, therefore, to act as the patient's advocate and to negotiate for the most effective, optimal treatment, consistent with the patient's coverage. Treatment standards, such as those developed by the American Society of Addiction Medicine (ASAM), can assist the clinician in matching the intensity of treatment to the severity of the substance-use disorder and the medical and psychiatric condition (ASAM, 1993). The so called ASAM Criteria for determination of treatment placement have been widely adopted and accepted by many third-party payers.

RECOGNITION OF SUBSTANCE USE

The best way to reduce the medical, social, and economic impact of substance abuse and dependence is through prevention and treatment, yet physicians often fail to diagnose substance use and to treat substance use properly in their patients (Holden, 1985; Samet et al, 1996). To recognize and treat substance abuse and dependence, physicians must:

1. know the pharmacokinetics and pharmacodynamics of alcohol and other psychoactive substances
2. be able to identify the presence of substance abuse or dependence in the patient, despite efforts of the patients to deny or conceal use
3. have knowledge about therapies for the acute management of intoxication and withdrawal of specific psychoactive substances

4. have knowledge about options for long-term rehabilitation and treatment of patients

5. be aware of one's own attitudes and biases toward the subject of substance use and toward such patients.

This chapter will provide basic information on the etiology and nosology of substance-use disorders and on the identification and treatment of substance-abuse disorders in medical and psychiatric patients. Management of specific drug intoxications and emergencies is discussed in Chapter 19.

CLINICAL PHARMACOLOGY OF PSYCHOACTIVE SUBSTANCES

For a drug to have psychoactive effects, it must be present in a high enough concentration as a free drug at its active site in the brain. Usually, only a small amount of the total administered drug is delivered to the site of action. The rest of the drug may be bound to serum or tissue proteins, metabolized or excreted, or otherwise unavailable. Since brain capillaries prevent the passage of many polar molecules into the brain (blood-brain barrier), most psychoactive substances are lipid soluble.

Figure 10–1 illustrates the competing pharmacokinetic processes that determine the availability of active drug. The *potency, duration,* and *mode of*

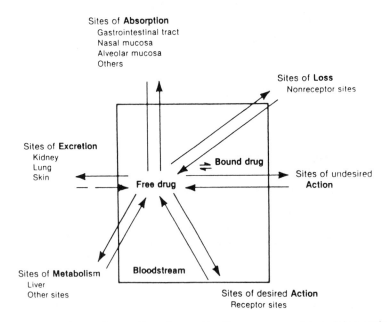

Figure 10–1. *Competing pharmokinetic processes determining active drug availability.*

administration of a drug can be predicted by understanding its *pharmacokinetics.* For example, differences in potency of cocaine hydrochloride and freebase cocaine can be explained by the slower absorption of the hydrochloride from the nasal mucosa and the rapid absorption of freebase from the alveolar mucosa. The rapid absorption of alcohol from the gastric mucosa accounts for its preferred oral administration.

To have psychoactive effects, a drug also must affect some neuronal process. The manner in which drugs act at the active receptor site is known as *pharmacodynamics.* Many psychoactive substances, such as stimulants, sedatives, anxiolytics, and hallucinogens bind to a specific cellular component such as a receptor. Receptors have now been identified for the site of action of caffeine (adenosine receptors), cannabis (THC receptor), hallucinogens (serotonin and N-methyl-D-aspartate [NMDA] receptors), nicotine (nicotinic cholinergic receptors), opioids (opioid receptors), phencyclidine (NMDA receptor), sedatives (benzodiazepine, barbiturate-binding sites associated with the gamma-aminobutyric [GABA] receptor-chloride channel). Cocaine and other stimulants appear to bind to specific neurotransmitter transporters. Alcohol and inhalant solvents may nonspecifically dissolve in cell membranes and disrupt cellular functions. Ethyl alcohol has been demonstrated to have significant effects on several brain neurotransmitter systems. Receptors associated with ion channels, including the NMDA, GABA, and serotonin-3 receptors are particularly sensitive to the action of alcohol. Alcohol also modifies the activity of beta-adrenergic and adenosine neurotransmitter receptors linked to adenylate cyclase through membrane-bound G proteins.

THE NEUROBIOLOGY OF SUBSTANCE-USE DISORDERS

Over the past decade, much has been learned about the brain mechanisms that mediate drug and alcohol use. A dopaminergic pathway from the *ventral tegmental area* to the *nucleus accumbens* is activated by drugs such as cocaine, opioids, nicotine, and alcohol. The activation of this dopamine pathway stimulates locomotor behavior and mediates drug reward. The psychomotor stimulant theory of drug dependence hypothesizes that the dependence-producing properties of all drugs of abuse are mediated through a common mechanism involving dopamine-mediated reinforcement in the brain (Wise and Bozarth, 1987). With repeated drug use, the system becomes increasingly sensitized to the effects of the drug (Robinson and Berridge, 1993). Stimuli associated with drug use, such as behaviors or locations, can also release dopamine in the nucleus accumbens and may act as a "primer," facilitating more drug or alcohol use.

In addition to the positive reinforcing stimulant effects of drugs, the chronic use of many drugs induces negatively reinforcing, withdrawal effects.

It has been suggested that these withdrawal effects may account for drug dependence, in that people will continue drug use to avoid this negative state. The negatively reinforcing effects of many drugs (withdrawal reactions) may be mediated by a neuronal system involving the locus ceruleus (LC) and other structures (Nestler et al, 1994).

Advances in molecular neurobiology are leading to an understanding of how drug and alcohol use leads to the development of tolerance, dependence, and withdrawal. In the LC, opiates inhibit noradrenergic neurons through a cyclic adenosine monophosphate (AMP) pathway. Chronic opiate treatment increases levels of adenylate cyclase, cyclic AMP-dependent protein kinases, and several phosphoproteins in this brain region, by altering gene expression (Nestler et al, 1994). It is hypothesized that this altered gene expression leads to upregulation of the cyclic AMP system in these neurons and contributes to opioid tolerance, dependence, and withdrawal. Researchers have identified similar changes in gene expression in neurons in the nucleus accumbens, the LC, and other brain structures, due to exposure to different psychoactive substances. These findings suggest commonalities in the molecular neurobiological mechanisms underlying the development of addiction.

IDENTIFYING RISK FACTORS FOR THE DEVELOPMENT OF SUBSTANCE ABUSE AND DEPENDENCE

The factors that determine susceptibility of an individual to a substance-use disorder are not well understood. Studies of populations with substance abuse or at risk for developing substance abuse have identified many factors that foster the development and continuance of substance use. These influences are genetic, familial, environmental, occupational, socioeconomic, cultural, personality, life stress, psychiatric comorbidity, biological, social learning, behavioral, and conditioning. The relative contributions of any of these factors will vary from individual to individual, and no single factor appears to account for the risk entirely.

The influence of genetic factors has been best studied for alcohol. It is now well established that alcoholism is a familial disorder. Children of alcoholics (especially males) are several times more likely to become alcoholic than are the children of nonalcoholics (Cloninger, 1987). The increased risk of alcoholism exists regardless of whether children are raised by their biological parents or by nonalcoholic foster parents, suggesting that genetic factors are important. A genetic predisposition for alcoholism is also supported by differences in alcoholism rates between identical and fraternal twins (70 versus 35%); however, environmental influences must have influences, as 30% of identical twins of alcoholics do not become alcoholic. Children of alcoholics are also more susceptible to other drug dependence.

Factors proposed to account for the genetic predisposition for alcoholism include genetic variations in the metabolism of ethanol and acetaldehyde; differences in brain electrophysiology; differential sensitivity to the intoxicating effects of alcohol; and altered neurotransmitter receptors (Schuckit and Smith, 1996). The identification of specific genes that predispose to alcoholism is an active area of investigation. Some genetic marker studies have suggested that alcoholism is associated with a certain subtype of the dopamine D_2 receptor; other studies suggest associations with genes controlling serotonergic systems (Goldman, 1995).

CRITERIA FOR THE DIAGNOSIS OF SUBSTANCE USE

The description of substance-use disorders is complicated by the ambiguity of the language used to describe substance use and by basic questions of whether use of psychoactive substances constitutes a medical or a moral condition. In addressing these issues, organizations such as the World Health Organization and the American Psychiatric Association (APA) consider problem use of psychoactive substances to be a medical disorder and have formally defined criteria to determine *when* the use of psychoactive substances constitutes a medical disorder.

In a strict pharmacological sense, *dependence* is often defined as a state in which a syndrome of drug-specific withdrawal signs and syndromes follows reduction or cessation of drug use. *Tolerance* refers to (1) the state in which the physiological or behavioral effects of a constant dose of a psychoactive substance decreases over time or (2) when a greater dose of a drug is necessary to achieve the same effect. *Withdrawal* describes a physiological state that follows cessation or reduction in the amount of drug. In general, the behavioral effects of withdrawal are opposite to effects produced by the drug (i.e., withdrawal from depressants produces psychomotor activation; withdrawal from stimulants produces psychomotor slowing).

Nosology of Addictive Disorders

In its *Diagnostic and Statistical Manual of Mental Disorders* (DSM-IV), the APA (1994) classifies the acute and chronic effects of psychoactive substances under two major categories: Substance-Use Disorders (Substance Dependence and Substance Abuse) and Substance-Induced Disorders. The various disorders are described in Table 10–1 and the criteria for diagnosing dependence in Table 10–2.

Eleven distinct classes of psychoactive substances are designated by DSM-IV: alcohol, amphetamine, or related substances; caffeine; cannabis; cocaine; hallucinogens; inhalants; opioids; nicotine; phencyclidine or related

Table 10–1 **Classification of Substance-Use and Substance-Induced Disorders***

A. Substance-Use Disorders

(1) *Substance Dependence:* A maladaptive pattern of substance use with adverse clinical consequences. The DSM-IV has widened the concept of dependence to include the association of substance use with uncontrolled use or with use in spite of adverse consequences (see Table 10–2).

(2) *Substance Abuse:* A maladaptive pattern of substance use that causes clinically significant impairment, not meeting dependence criteria. This may include impairments in social, family, or occupational functioning, in the presence of a psychological or physical problem, or in situations in which use of the substance is physically hazardous, such as driving while intoxicated.

B. Substance-Induced Disorders

(1) *Substance Intoxication:* Reversible, substance-specific physiological and behavioral changes due to recent exposure to a psychoactive substance. Produced by all substances.

(2) *Substance Withdrawal:* A substance-specific syndrome that develops following cessation of or reduction in dosage of a regularly used substance. Occurs with chronic use of all substances, except perhaps cannabis and hallucinogens.

(3) *Substance-Induced Delirium* (confusion, psychosis): Occurs with overdose of many substances.

(4) *Substance-Induced Psychotic Disorder* (psychosis): May occur with phenylcyclidine (PCP) and hallucinogens, stimulants, cannabis, and alcohol.

(5) *Substance-Induced Mood Disorder* (depression, mania), also **Anxiety:** Common with many substances, especially alcohol and stimulants. Disorder must be distinguished from primary psychiatric disorder that preceded drug use.

(6) *Substance-Induced Sleep Disorder:* A sleep disturbance attributable to acute or chronic substance use. Common with alcohol, sedatives, and stimulants.

(7) *Substance-Induced Sexual Dysfunction:* Alcohol, benzodiazepines, and opioids commonly reduce sexual responsiveness and performance.

(8) *Substance-Induced Persisting Disorders:* Substance-specific syndromes that persist long after drug use ceases (e.g., hallucinogen "flashbacks," memory impairments, or dementia).

* DSM-IV criteria (American Psychiatric Association, 1994).

Table 10–2 **Diagnosing Substance Dependence***

At least *three* of the following conditions occurring over a 12-month period:

Tolerance: The need for increased amounts of the substance to achieve intoxication or other desired effect; or markedly diminished effect with use of the same amount of substance

Characteristic *withdrawal* symptoms, or the use of the substance (or a closely related substitute) to relieve or avoid withdrawal [may not apply to cannabis, hallucinogens, or phenylcyclidine (PCP)]

Substance taken in larger amounts or over a longer period of time than the person intended

Persistent desire or one or more unsuccessful attempts to cut down or control substance use

A great deal of time spent in activities necessary to get the substance (e.g., theft), taking the substance (e.g., chain smoking), or recovering from its effects

Important social, occupational, or recreational activities given up or reduced because of substance use

Continued substance use despite knowledge of having a persistent or recurrent social, psychological, or physical problem that is caused by or exacerbated by use of the substance

* Adapted in part from DSM-IV criteria (American Psychiatric Association, 1994).

substances; and sedatives, hypnotics, or anxiolytics. Under the category of Substance-Use Disorders, all classes (except nicotine and caffeine) are associated with abuse *and* dependence. Dependence *only* is defined for nicotine.

Polysubstance dependence is defined as using three or more categories of substances. The category Other Substance Use Disorders includes use of anabolic steroids, anticholinergic agents, and other psychoactive substances. Ingenious "underground" chemists are continually developing new, synthetic psychotropic chemicals, known as *designer drugs.* Usually these substances can be related to one of the classes, based on effects and chemical structure. A good example is flunitrazepam (also known as the "date rape" drug or "roofies"), a benzodiazepine not legally available in the United States that has been a focus of current media attention.

EVALUATING SUBSTANCE USE

The physician's tasks in evaluating a patient for substance use or dependence is not only to detect and confirm the diagnosis, but also to establish an effective therapeutic relationship. In the context of this relationship, the physician should conduct a detailed alcohol and drug history as well as a physical and mental status examination, order and interpret necessary laboratory tests, and meet with family or significant others to obtain additional information and to facilitate their involvement in the diagnostic and treatment process.

Assessing and treating patients who have *both* a psychiatric disorder and a substance-use disorder (dual diagnosis) is particularly complex. The physical, psychological, and behavioral effects of psychoactive substances *may be similar to* symptoms of a psychiatric disorder or alternatively, *may mask* the symptoms of a psychiatric disorder. The physical, psychological, and social consequences of substance use may impair treatment of other illnesses as well. An important general clinical rule is to defer making definitive psychiatric diagnoses until the role of the substance use is clarified and the patient is detoxified. Most authorities would also agree that substance-use disorders must receive *high priority* in the treatment process if more than one Axis I diagnosis is identified.

The Interview

As discussed in Chapters 1 and 2, the patient interview remains the *single most important component* of the diagnostic and assessment process. In a well-conducted interview, the physician may not only obtain information relevant to the diagnosis and etiology of substance-use disorders in a patient, but may also set the tone for further treatment of that patient. Empathy and concern are necessary to instill trust. This may be difficult, as interviewers often have negative feelings about substance users or about their prognosis. Judgmental attitudes and pejorative statements may severely limit the interviewer's ability to gather information and to initiate treatment.

In obtaining information about a patient's alcohol and drug use, the most *effective interview strategy* focuses on whether the patient has experienced *negative consequences* from use of psychoactive substances, has poor control of use, or has been criticized by others about substance use. Quantity and frequency questions such as "how much?" and "how often"? are not especially effective in detecting substance use. Knowing the quantity of substance consumed does not by itself make the diagnosis; knowing the effects of that substance on the individual's *functioning* is more important.

Several formalized interviews are well validated in their ability to discriminate alcoholism. The CAGE questionnaire (Ewing, 1984), is a highly sensitive four-item test using the letters C, A, G, and E as a mnemonic:

> Have you ever felt the need to *Cut* down on drinking (or drug use)?
> Have you ever felt *Annoyed* by criticisms of drinking (or drug use)?
> Have you ever had *Guilty* feelings about drinking (or drug use)?
> Have you ever taken a morning *Eye* opener (or used drugs to get going in the a.m.)?

A "yes" answer to *two or more* of the questions suggests alcohol abuse. The CAGE may be a better predictor of alcoholism in medical patients than laboratory tests (Beresford et al, 1990) and is often adapted to include other drug use as well.

Another reliable screen for heavy alcohol use is the Michigan Alcohol Screening Test (MAST). This 25-item scale identifies abnormal drinking through its social and behavioral consequences with sensitivity of 90 to 98% (Selzer, 1971). A shortened 10-item test, the Brief MAST, has been shown to have similar efficacy.

Although less documentation exists regarding the optimal interview for assessing a drug-abusing patient, the same considerations apply: *it is more effective to ask the patient and family about the behavioral consequences of drug abuse than to question the quantity and frequency of use.*

Even under the best of interviewing circumstances, some patients who use psychoactive substances are reluctant to report the full extent of their drug and alcohol use. In addition, the patient's family, friends, and colleagues collude in the denial of problems with substance use. Getting through denial requires that the patient and/or the family be confronted with the evidence of substance use, yet the confrontation needs to be conducted in the context of a supportive, concerned, and empathic interaction.

Obviously, patients who are experiencing an altered mental status due to intoxication or withdrawal from a psychoactive substance may be incapable of providing an accurate history. In these circumstances, it is important to interview family or acquaintances. It is also helpful to examine pill bottles or medications in the patient's possession.

The Physical Examination

The physical examination of the patient provides important information about substance use and its medical manifestations. Physical findings of interest include the cutaneous abscesses and track marks of intravenous drug abuse, nasal lesions from cocaine abuse, peripheral neuropathy from alcohol use or solvent inhalation, and signs of liver disease from alcoholic or infectious hepatitis. Intravenous drug use should be suspected in any patient who is seropositive for hepatitis B or the human immunodeficiency virus (HIV) or who presents with signs and symptoms of the acquired immunodeficiency syndrome (AIDS; Stein, 1990). Substance use disorders should be considered in all patients who present with accidents or signs of repeated trauma, especially to the head.

The physical examination of the alcoholic often shows telangiectasis of the facial region, facial edema, and parotid gland enlargement. Hepatic enlargement, dilated abdominal veins, and hemorrhoids may be present with those with cirrhosis. Neurological abnormalities include peripheral neuropathies, cerebellar dysfunction, and dementias. Because of complex effects on endocrine functioning, male alcoholics also may experience "feminization" effects such as testicular atrophy.

A complete mental status examination should also be performed, including tests of memory, concentration, abstract reasoning, affect, mood, and form and content of thought (see Chapter 1).

Laboratory Testing

Laboratory abnormalities associated with substance-use disorders are diverse and may be related to end organ damage, vitamin deficiencies, and generalized malnutrition. In alcoholism, abnormalities observed on hematological screening include leukopenia, thrombocytopenia, macrocytic anemia, and target cells. Opioid users may have abnormal liver function tests and positive serology for hepatitis B, hepatitis C, or HIV.

Serum and urine toxicological screens have an important role in the assessment and treatment of patients with substance-use disorders. However, it is important that such testing be properly conducted and the results of the testing be properly interpreted. Informed consent should be obtained for all drug testing. As with all laboratory tests, both false-positive and false-negative results may be obtained; the test result may be affected by methods of sample collection and accuracy of the laboratory. To minimize collection errors, all samples for toxicological analysis should be obtained under direct observation. Both serum and urine samples should be obtained, as substances may be differentially distributed in body fluids. Because compounds in foods or medications may mimic illicit drugs in some analyses, positive test results should be confirmed by a second test using a different analytical method on the same sample. For example, eating poppy seed bagels has been reported to yield a positive urine test for opioids. A positive toxicological screen may indicate past exposure to a psychoactive substance, but it may not indicate the extent of the exposure, when it occurred, or whether there was behavioral impairment.

Abnormal values on diagnostic laboratory tests are sometimes used to screen for alcohol use, but they are not absolutely reliable or specific (Litten et al, 1995). In heavy users of alcohol, liver function tests such as aspartate aminotransferase and gamma glutamyl transferase may be abnormal; however, a significant number of heavy drinkers may have normal test values. Carbohydrate-deficient transferrin has been found to be quite effective in discriminating heavy drinking. The test is based on the observation that alcohol inhibits the addition of sialic acid to glycoproteins, such as serum transferrin.

TREATMENT

To provide optimal treatment of substance use and dependence, the physician must know about therapies for the acute management of intoxicated or withdrawing patients and also about options for long-term treatment and rehabilitation. A treatment plan should be practical, economical, and based on sound principles.

Treatment for substance abuse and dependence ranges from very low cost, less intensive methods (e.g., brief advice to stop drinking or drug use and self-help programs), to higher cost, more intensive methods (e.g., inpatient detoxification and rehabilitation programs). There are also many different orientations toward treatment, ranging from the medical/biological to the spiritual/religious, and from total abstinence to controlled drinking, which are utilized to varying extent by different programs. For patients with *substance dependence*, the goals of treatment usually include the establishment of a drug- or alcohol-free state. If total abstinence is not obtainable, a significant reduction in harmful drug or alcohol use will still be of some benefit. For patients with *substance abuse*, the goal should be a reduction in harmful drug or alcohol use. Using a number of treatment strategies that include brief interventions, counseling, pharmacotherapy, and referral to specialized treatment and other community programs, all physicians should be able to assist patients who are identified as having potential alcohol and drug disorders,

For all patients, treatment goals should include psychological, medical, family, and social interventions to reduce or eliminate the harmful effects of drugs and alcohol. Changes in living situation, work situation, or friendships may be necessary to decrease drug availability and to reduce social pressure to use drugs. Individual and group psychotherapy can be useful in helping the patient to understand the role of the drug in his or her life, improve self-esteem, and relieve psychological distress. The adequate treatment of underlying psychiatric symptoms, medical illness, and pain is important, as this may reduce the need for self-medication. Although most treatment can be provided in an outpatient setting, halfway houses, therapeutic communities, and other residential treatment situations may be necessary to ensure a drug-free environment. Self-help groups, such as Alcoholics Anonymous (AA), Narcotics Anonymous (NA), Al-Anon, and Rational Recovery (RR) provide effective treatment, education, emotional support, and hope to patients and their families (Emrick, 1987).

When a patient is referred to a specialized addiction treatment program or an addiction treatment professional, it is important for the referring physician to remain in contact with the patient, the family and the other clinicians, so as to maintain continuity of care and to help coordinate treatment.

The Role of the Family and Significant Others in Treatment

Many patients presenting for treatment do so in the context of a family structure, which is also experiencing dysfunction; therefore, substance dependence should be considered a chronic disorder that involves the entire family system. Although family influences may motivate an individual to seek treatment for substance use, more often family members "enable" or facilitate substance use on the part of the patient and may not be aware of their contribution. Substance use in the family may serve to maintain a pathological equilibrium; eliminating the substance use may lead to intrapersonal conflicts and loss of family integrity. It is therefore important for the clinician to be aware of family dynamics and family dysfunction and to recognize the denial, defensiveness, and hostility (as well as the strengths) present in family members.

Spouses and children may experience considerable physical or emotional abuse due to the substance use within the family. The clinician should recommend psychological or social treatment for other family members when appropriate. Self-help organizations such as Al-Anon, Narc-Anon, and Alateen may provide valuable emotional support and education for family members.

Confronting the Patient and Family: The Initial Intervention

Effectively confronting patients with their alcohol or drug problem and then getting them into treatment requires special skills and techniques. Historically, physicians have felt poorly prepared to contend with addictive disorders (Holden, 1985). In the past decade, several methods have been developed to help physicians intervene successfully (Samet et al, 1996). *The Physician's Guide to Helping Patients with Alcohol Problems,* recently released by the National Institute on Alcohol Abuse and Alcoholism (NIAAA), presents several useful intervention methods (NIAAA, 1995).

Brief interventions conducted in a supportive manner are extremely effective in enhancing entrance into alcoholism treatment. Brief interventions consist of one or more sessions in the physician's office, during which education about substance use and dependence is provided and a plan for cutting down or eliminating substance use is negotiated. Some authorities argue that presenting the substance-use problem to the patient and family as a *disease* with a genetic basis is most effective. In this model, the patient is told that the use of alcohol and drugs poses a serious threat to his or her health and well-being; the evidence (historical or medical data) is presented in an objective and nonjudgmental manner. The physician can explain that alcohol (or drugs) has affected the brain and central nervous system to the extent that the patient can no longer control its use and may have lost sight of the negative effects. Emphasis should be placed on the effects the substance has had on the patient's health, behavior, family, employment, etc. and not on the amount consumed. During the intervention, the physician should be prepared for initial denials, excuses, and insincere promises to stop.

Blame for the problem should be placed on the alcohol or drug, *not* on the patient; however, the physician should point out that even though the disease may not be the patient's fault, now that he or she is advised of the illness, getting effective treatment for the illness is his/her responsibility. The patient and physician together should develop a contract, preferably written, defining the treatment and intervention plan. A formal means of assessment of effectiveness and follow-up should be part of the plan. Involvement of the patient's spouse, family, significant others, and employers may be helpful in bringing an individual into treatment. Should this type of presentation not be effective in getting the patient to agree to treatment, then consultation with a specially trained addictive disorders specialist is recommended.

Detoxification and Treatment of Withdrawal

There are four objectives of initial treatment: (1) relief of distress and discomfort due to intoxication or withdrawal; (2) prevention of and/or treatment of serious complications of substance intoxication, withdrawal, or dependence; (3) establishment of a drug- or alcohol-free state; and (4) preparation for and referral to longer term treatment or rehabilitation.

The object of detoxification is the achievement of a drug-free state and the minimization of any morbidity associated with withdrawal. *Withdrawal* is a physiological and behavioral state that follows cessation or reduction in the amount of drug used. In general, the signs and symptoms of withdrawal are the opposite of those that the drug produces (i.e., withdrawal from depressants produces excitation). The proposed neurobiological mechanism for withdrawal is a change in the number of postsynaptic neurotransmitter receptors or change in receptor sensitivity with chronic drug use. It should be emphasized that withdrawal is not specific to addictive substances; chronic use of beta-adrenergic blockers, antihistamines, antiarrhythmics, and antidepressants may be associated with mild withdrawal reactions upon drug discontinuation. Several methods for minimizing withdrawal signs and symptoms are described in Table 10–3.

Ideally, patients with substance dependence should undergo a supervised detoxification. This may be accomplished in an outpatient, inpatient, or residential setting depending on the drug used, the level of physiologic and psychologic dependence, and the presence of coexisting medical and psychiatric problems.

During detoxification, patients should develop a long-term treatment or rehabilitation plan. The objectives of this longer term treatment should be: (1) persistence of the alcohol- or drug-free state; and (2) psychological, family, and vocational interventions to ensure its persistence. The following sections will describe treatment of specific substance intoxication and dependence. Treatment of specific drug overdose is covered in Chapter 19.

TREATMENT OF SPECIFIC SUBSTANCES

Alcohol

The word "alcoholism" has many definitions and encompasses a number of alcohol-related behaviors. Generally defined, it is a condition in which there is a repetitive, but inconsistent and sometimes unpredictable *loss of control* of drinking that produces symptoms of serious personal dysfunction or disability. Alcohol withdrawal, alcohol dependence, and alcohol abuse are medical diagnoses of the DSM-IV. It is estimated that 7 to 10% of adult Americans have alcoholism. Chronic use of alcohol is associated with the cognitive and memory deficits of *alcohol dementia* and the more restrictive memory deficits of *alcohol amnestic syndrome.* Alcohol use may also produce *alcohol hallucinosis,* which is characterized by isolated auditory and visual hallucinations; *alcohol paranoia,* characterized by suspiciousness and single or multiple delusions; and *alcohol withdrawal delirium.*

Heavy maternal alcohol intake has adverse consequences on the fetus and infant. The constellation of physical and behavioral abnormalities is known

---

Table 10–3 **General Methods of Detoxification**

1. Controlled administration of the drug, with a slow taper in the daily drug dose (example: tapering nicotine gum or patch in nicotine dependence)
2. Administration of a cross-tolerant agent that is slowly tapered over time (example: chlordiazepoxide in alcohol withdrawal, methadone in opioid withdrawal)
3. Administration of an alternate agent to suppress signs and symptoms of withdrawal (example: clonidine in opioid withdrawal, atenolol in alcohol withdrawal)
4. Nonpharmacological detoxification, with supportive care (example: social setting detox in alcohol dependence)

as *fetal alcohol syndrome* (Randall, 1987). Affected infants are smaller in length, and most fall below the third percentile for head circumference. They are also notable by the presence of palpebral fissures and epicanthal folds, maxillary hypoplasia, thin vermilion of the upper lip, micrognathia, cleft palate, dislocation of the hips, flexion abnormalities of a number of joints, abnormal external genitalia, and capillary hemangiomata. Infants with this syndrome exhibit poor sucking and sleeping behavior and are often irritable, tremulous, and hyperactive. Studies suggest that these infants have learning disabilities and are prone to a variety of behavioral abnormalities in later childhood.

Although alcohol is a drug that does not act through a single receptor, alcohol has effects on several neurotransmitter systems in the brain. GABA is the major inhibitory neurotransmitter in the central nervous system (CNS). Alcohol, at physiologically relevant concentrations, facilitates GABA-induced inhibition (Hunt, 1983). Benzodiazepines bind to a neuronal "receptor" associated with the GABA receptor and facilitate GABA binding. Other sedative medications and drugs also act at the GABA–chloride channel complex. The existence of a common mechanism for the actions of alcohol and sedative–hypnotics accounts for the cross-tolerance between these substances.

Glutamate is the major excitatory neurotransmitter in the CNS. When glutamate binds to its receptors, an ion channel opens and stimulates the neuron or makes it more likely to fire. Low doses of alcohol are strongly inhibitory to the glutamate receptor and inhibit neurons (Tsai et al, 1995). Thus, the combined effect of alcohol on these two neurotransmitter systems is to inhibit neurons and produce sedation.

Alcohol Intoxication and Withdrawal

Patients who present for alcohol treatment may show various types of impairment. Particularly frustrating to both clinician and patient is the alcoholic who has profound social needs, who is not eligible for medical treatment, or who refuses medical treatment. In this case, referral to social agencies may assist the patient, but there are many instances in which no assistance can be obtained.

Acute *alcohol intoxication* results in behaviors ranging from coma to a hyperactive state with affective lability. Large ingestions of alcohol may be fatal. Treatment of alcohol intoxication is essentially supportive and consists of maintaining physiological homeostasis through support of vital functions, as described in Chapter 19.

Patients who present with the *alcohol withdrawal syndrome* require evaluation of the severity of their withdrawal and may need behavioral or pharmacological intervention. The consequences of withdrawal may be minimal or may include autonomic hyperactivity, seizures, and *withdrawal delirium*. The severity of withdrawal depends on the amount and length of alcohol exposure, the presence of medical complications, and the psychological state of the patient. In addition, chronic alcohol ingestion is associated with poor nutrition, poor hygiene, and general debilitation. Current data suggest that less than 5%

of individuals undergoing detoxification develop severe withdrawal delirium, with a mortality of 1 to 2%.

The administration of over 100 different pharmacological agents can reduce the signs and symptoms of the withdrawal syndrome. Such agents include adrenergic blocking agents, antidepressants, antihistamines, barbiturates, benzodiazepines, chloral derivatives, lithium, neuroleptics, and paraldehyde (Liskow and Goodwin, 1987). Today, benzodiazepine derivatives are the treatment of choice. Their efficacy is well established by double-blind controlled studies. Benzodiazepines are minimally toxic and have anticonvulsant activity. A withdrawal scale such as the Clinical Institute Withdrawal Assessment for Alcohol (CIWA-A) Scale can be used to titrate the medication according to the severity of withdrawal symptoms (Foy et al, 1988). To treat withdrawal, patients receive an initial oral or intravenous dose of a long-half-life benzodiazepine (10 to 20 mg diazepam or 25 to 100 mg chlordiazepoxide) repeated every hour until the patient is sedated, or until withdrawal signs and symptoms are significantly decreased. A short-acting benzodiazepine such as lorazepam may be used and is indicated when elimination time for benzodiazepines is prolonged, e.g., when significant liver disease is present or in the elderly. Most patients show marked reduction in withdrawal signs and symptoms after several doses of medication. Patients administered long-half-life benzodiazepines usually require little or no additional medication after medication loading; however, patients with heavy sedative dependence or polysubstance dependence may require additional medication to suppress withdrawal. Elderly patients and patients with medical illnesses require close observation to prevent overmedication. In patients receiving calcium channel blockers and adrenergic blockers, some signs of withdrawal such as hypertension, tachycardia, and tremor may be obscured.

Other medications, such as beta-adrenergic blocking drugs, anticonvulsants, and antipsychotics, often are administered to control symptoms. Anticonvulsants, such as carbamazepine and valproic acid, appear effective in reducing most signs and symptoms of alcohol withdrawal and are widely used in European countries. In using anticonvulsants, patients are rapidly titrated to the blood levels that are therapeutic for seizures. It is useful to add benzodiazepines for breakthrough symptoms. Beta-adrenergic blockers, such as propranolol and atenolol, have been used as primary agents in the treatment of alcohol withdrawal, but are most effective in reducing peripheral autonomic signs of withdrawal, and less so for CNS signs such as withdrawal delirium. Adrenergic blocking drugs are particularly useful for controlling tachycardia and hypertension in patients with coronary disease. Neuroleptics, such as haloperidol, are useful for treatment of hallucinosis and paranoid symptoms associated with withdrawal.

Alcoholics commonly suffer from poor nutrition and deficiencies in vitamins and minerals. To prevent the development of the ataxia, nystagmus, ophthalmoplegia, and mental status changes that characterize the *Wernicke-Korsakoff syndrome,* oral or parenteral thiamin should be administered to all alcohol users as soon as possible, and *prior to the administration of glucose.*

Low magnesium is often present in alcoholics and may intensify withdrawal and predispose to seizures. Magnesium levels should be obtained and deficits replaced with oral or intramuscular magnesium sulfate. Multivitamin supplements also are commonly administered, as well as folic acid.

Recent studies suggest that many alcohol-dependent patients may not require pharmacologically assisted detoxification. "Social setting detoxification," a nondrug method, is used with excellent results by many alcohol-treatment facilities. This method utilizes intensive peer and group support in a nonmedical environment; it reduces withdrawal signs and symptoms without increasing medical complications. Even within a medical setting, many patients respond to "supportive care" and require little or no pharmacological intervention; however, those patients with a history of delirium tremens or seizures or the presence of medical or psychiatric comorbidities require inpatient detoxification and pharmacotherapy. Some authorities have expressed concerns that repeated, untreated alcohol withdrawal may worsen subsequent episodes, due to kindling effects, and have suggested that all symptomatic withdrawing patients receive pharmacological treatment.

There is an association between alcoholism and affective illness and anxiety disorders (Helzer and Pyrzbeck, 1988). Often these mood disturbances are directly related to alcohol and will resolve soon after detoxification. Mood symptoms persisting beyond this time should be treated with psychotherapy, antidepressants, or electroconvulsive therapy (ECT), in severe cases of depression. Also, patients known to have recurrent mood disorders or a strong family history of a mood disorder should be treated immediately after detoxification if mood symptoms are severe.

Long-Term Treatment

The goals of long-term treatment include maintaining a state of abstinence from alcohol, as well as psychological, family, and social interventions to maintain recovery. These goals are best achieved through the patient's participation in a comprehensive treatment program, beginning after discharge from the acute care setting.

AA is an independent organization, founded in 1939. Its only goal is to help individuals maintain a state of total abstinence from alcohol and other addictive substances through group and individual interactions between alcoholics in various stages of recovery. While there are a paucity of objective outcome data on the efficacy of self-help groups (Emrick, 1987), self-help groups are useful for many individuals. Often, hospitals are used as meeting sites by local AA groups, and psychiatric or medical inpatients may easily attend meetings. If the spirituality emphasis of AA is not consistent with the patient's beliefs, other self-help organizations, including RR and Secular Organization for Sobriety (SOS), should be considered.

As mentioned above, family involvement is extremely important in alcohol treatment. Alcohol use causes many family problems, due to the financial and emotional stress created by drinking. Educating and counseling other family members about their role(s) in the patient's alcohol use and treatment are important in avoiding enabling and denial. Often, it is necessary to treat emotional distress, psychopathology, or substance use in other family members, as well. Valuable emotional support and education for spouses and children may be provided by self-help organizations such as Al-Anon and Alateen.

Medications to Reduce Alcohol Consumption

Several pharmacological agents have shown efficacy as adjuncts in the treatment of alcohol dependence, in decreasing drinking, and in reducing relapse in patients in treatment. Pharmacological agents should always be used as adjuncts in treatment, as part of a comprehensive treatment program that addresses the psychological, social, and spiritual needs of the patient.

Aversive Therapy: Disulfiram

Disulfiram (Antabuse) is an irreversible inhibitor of the enzyme acetaldehyde dehydrogenase and is used as an adjunctive treatment in selected alcoholics (Brewer, 1993). If alcohol is consumed in the presence of disulfiram, the toxic metabolite acetaldehyde accumulates in the body and produces tachycardia, skin flushing, diaphoresis, dyspnea, nausea, and vomiting. Hypotension and death may occur if large amounts of alcohol are consumed. This unpleasant reaction provides a strong deterrent to the consumption of alcohol.

The typical dose of disulfiram is 250 mg once daily. Daily doses of 125 to 500 mg are sometimes used, depending on side effects and patient response. The optimal duration of treatment is unknown. Most patients use the medication for brief periods of high risk of relapse; however, some patients use the medication continuously for years. Patients using disulfiram must be able to understand its benefits and risks. Alcohol present in foods, shaving lotion, mouthwashes, or over-the-counter medications may produce a disulfiram reaction. Disulfiram may have interactions with other medications, notably anticoagulants and phenytoin. Patients with liver disease require close monitoring. A complete blood count and liver function tests should be monitored prior to starting disulfiram and periodically thereafter. Monitoring patients for disulfiram compliance improves treatment success.

Medications to Reduce Alcohol Craving

The opioid neurotransmitter system has been strongly implicated in mediating alcohol consumption. In clinical trials with recently abstinent human alcoholics, subjects treated with the opioid antagonist naltrexone (ReVia) had lower rates of relapse to heavy drinking and more total abstinence than did a placebo group (O'Malley et al, 1992; Volpicelli et al, 1992). Subjects receiving naltrexone also report decreased "craving" and decreased "high" from alcohol.

The usual dose of naltrexone is 50 mg/day, with a range of 25 to 150 mg/day. The most common side effects include anxiety, sedation, and nausea in approximately 10% of patients. High doses of naltrexone (300 mg/day) have been associated with hepatotoxicity. Although little hepatic toxicity is observed at a 50-mg daily dose, naltrexone should probably be avoided in patients with hepatitis or severe liver disease. It is recommended that liver functions be monitored prior to naltrexone treatment and at 1 month and periodically thereafter. Naltrexone should only be used in the context of a comprehensive alcoholism treatment program, which includes counseling and other psychosocial therapies.

Buspirone (Buspar) is a nonbenzodiazepine anxiolytic medication that has partial agonist activity at the 5-hydroxytryptamine (5-HT)-1a receptor and dopamine receptor antagonist activity. Buspirone reduces alcohol consumption and improves the psychological status of alcoholics experiencing significant anxiety (Kranzler et al, 1994).

Selective serotonin-reuptake inhibitors such as fluoxetine (Prozac), sertraline (Zoloft), and fluvoxamine (Luvox), which augment serotonergic function, also appear to reduce overall alcohol consumption modestly by 15 to 20%. The effective daily doses were somewhat higher than those used typically in depression (e.g., 60 mg fluoxetine, 200 mg sertraline).

Acamprosate (calcium acetylhomotaurine) is a structural analog of GABA and has agonist effects at GABA receptors and inhibitory effects at NMDA receptors. In clinical trials with alcoholics, acamprosate reduced relapse drinking and craving for alcohol and had minimal side effects (Sass et al, 1996). The medication has been approved in several European countries for the prevention of alcoholic relapse and is currently under clinical testing in the United States. All of these drugs should be considered adjunctive therapies to comprehensive psychosocial treatment plans and not sole treatment modalities.

AMPHETAMINES AND SIMILARLY ACTING SYMPATHOMIMETIC AMINES

Drugs of this class are structurally related to the catecholamine neurotransmitters norepinephrine, epinephrine, and dopamine. They release catecholamines from nerve endings and are catecholamine agonists in the peripheral autonomic and central nervous systems. Intoxication with amphetamines, methylphenidate, or other sympathomimetics produces euphoria, improved concentration, and sympathetic and behavioral hyperactivity (Gawin and Ellinwood, 1988). Severe hypertension is seen in overdose and may be treated with alpha-adrenergic blockade.

Chronic users of amphetamines typically engage in a pattern of use of escalating doses of the drug for a period of several days, followed by a period of abstinence. A paranoid psychosis that is diagnostically similar to schizophrenia, with manifestations of agitation, paranoia, delusions, and hallucinosis, may occur with chronic use and even persist following cessation of stimulant use. Antipsychotic medication such as haloperidol is useful in the treatment of stimulant psychoses; however, such patients may frequently require psychiatric hospitalization. Withdrawal from amphetamines may cause marked dysphoria, fatigue, and restlessness. Stimulant users may also suffer from underlying psychiatric disorders, such as mood disorders, and a comprehensive psychiatric evaluation is necessary for all patients.

The use of over-the-counter sympathomimetic amines such as ephedrine and phenylpropanolamine as stimulants has increased dramatically. These medications are frequently sold for their effects on suppressing appetite, or as decongestants of bronchodilators. Signs of intoxication are similar to those of amphetamines, although there tends to be less CNS stimulation and greater autonomic effects. Hypertensive crises have resulted from the use of these drugs.

CAFFEINE

Caffeine and the related methylxanthines theophylline and theobromine are ubiquitous drugs in our society. These agents are consumed in beverages such as coffee, tea, cola, and other carbonated drinks by more than 80% of the population (Dews, 1982). Caffeine is present in chocolate and in many prescribed and over-the-counter medications including stimulants (NoDoze) appetite suppressants (Dexatrim), analgesics (Anacin, APC tablets), and cold and sinus preparations.

Methylxanthines produce cardiac stimulation, diuresis, bronchodilation, and CNS stimulation through several mechanisms. They inhibit the enzyme cyclic AMP phosphodiesterase and increase intracellular levels of cyclic AMP, thereby augmenting the action of many hormones and neurotransmitters, such as norepinephrine and epinephrine. They also have direct inhibitory effects on adenosine receptors.

The CNS effects of caffeine include psychomotor stimulation, increased attention and concentration, and suppression of the need for sleep. Even at low or moderate doses, caffeine exacerbates the symptoms of anxiety disorders and increases requirements for neuroleptic or sedative medications. At high doses and in sensitive individuals, methylxanthines produce tolerance and behavioral symptoms of tremor, insomnia, jitteriness, and agitation. In moderate-to-heavy users, a withdrawal syndrome characterized by lethargy, hypersomnia, irritability, and severe headache follows cessation of use. Significant caffeine withdrawal symptoms are commonly observed in even low-to-moderate users (Hughes et al, 1991) and may occur with reduced caffeine intake during an illness or hospitalization. The duration of withdrawal is usually 24 to 72 hours.

Treatment of caffeine dependence consists of limiting consumption of caffeine-containing foods, medications, and beverages. Decaffeinated forms of the beverage should be substituted for beverages such as coffee or cola. Patients require education about the extent of their caffeine consumption and the caffeine content of consumables.

COCAINE

Cocaine use has undergone an epidemic increase. Based on the 1985 National Survey of Drug Abuse, 22 million Americans had tried cocaine at least once, and 12 million had used it during the preceding year. Along with an increase in use, the manner of cocaine use has changed from intranasal "snorting" of cocaine powder to smoking or intravenous injection of the more potent cocaine "freebase." Freebase cocaine is inexpensive and widely available as "crack."

Cocaine is an alkaloid extracted from the leaves of the plant *Erythroxylon coca,* native to South America. It is a local anesthetic that blocks the initiation and propagation of nerve impulses by affecting the sodium conductance of cell membranes. It is a potent sympathomimetic agent that potentiates the actions of catecholamines in the autonomic nervous system, causing tachycardia, hypertension, and vasoconstriction. In addition, cocaine is a CNS stimulant, which increases arousal and produces mood elevation and psychomotor activation.

Cocaine intoxication is characterized by elation, euphoria, excitement, pressured speech, restlessness, stereotyped movements, and bruxism. Sympathetic stimulation, including tachycardia, mydriasis, and sweating, also occurs. Paranoia, suspiciousness, and psychosis may occur with prolonged use. Overdosage produces hyperpyrexia, hyperreflexia, seizures, coma, and respiratory arrest.

Cocaine has a rather short plasma half-life of 1 to 2 hours, which correlates with its behavioral effects. Along with the decline in plasma levels, users experience a period of dysphoria or "crash," which often leads to additional cocaine use within a short period. The dysphoria of the "crash" is intensified and prolonged following repeated use.

Treatment

The optimal treatment of the chronic cocaine user is still not established. Although cessation of cocaine use is not followed by a physiological withdrawal syndrome of the magnitude of that seen with opioids or alcohol, the dysphoria, depression, and drug craving that follow chronic cocaine use are often intense and make abstinence difficult. Psychotherapy, group therapy, and behavior modification have been found to be useful in maintaining abstinence (Higgins et al, 1994).

The efficacy of pharmacotherapy for the treatment of cocaine abuse and dependence remains an open question. Clinical studies comparing placebo with the antidepressant desipramine in the treatment of cocaine dependence found that desipramine was no better than placebo in keeping patients in treatment; however, for those who remain in treatment, desipramine may be helpful in maintaining abstinence. Dopamine agonists, such as bromocriptine and amantadine, have been inconsistently reported to block cocaine craving. A recent review of studies on the pharmacotherapy of cocaine points out that the discrepant findings between various cocaine treatment studies may result from poor experimental design and implementation of some of the studies (Meyer, 1992).

Many psychiatric and drug hospitals now offer short-term inpatient treatment of the cocaine user. Intensive psychological treatment and drug education in a drug-free environment is provided. For recidivists, long-term residential drug-free programs, including therapeutic communities, may be efficacious. Self-help groups such as NA may be useful both as a primary treatment modality for cocaine dependence and as an adjunct to other treatment.

Certain psychiatric disorders, such as depression and attention deficit disorder, may be common in cocaine users. Recognition and treatment of these underlying disorders may be necessary to stop cocaine use. In addition, many cocaine users also use alcohol or other drugs, particularly sedatives and heroin, and may require treatment for these substances as well.

CANNABIS

Cannabis sativa, also called marijuana or hemp, is a plant indigenous to India, but now grown worldwide. The leaves, flowers, and seeds of the plant contain many biologically active compounds, the most important of which are the lipophilic cannabinoids, especially Δ-9-tetrahydrocannabinol (THC). The biologically active substances are administered by smoking or ingesting dried plant parts (marijuana, bhang, ganja), the resin from the plant (hashish), or extracts of the resin (THC or hash oil). After inhalation or ingestion, THC rapidly enters the CNS. It has a biphasic elimination with a short initial half-life (1 to 2 hours) reflecting redistribution and a second half-life of days to weeks. Recent research has demonstrated that the biological activity of THC and its analogs is due to stimulation of cannabinoid receptors on brain cells. The receptor is linked to a G protein and inhibits adenylate cyclase in neurons (Musty et al, 1995).

Cannabis intoxication is characterized by tachycardia, muscle relaxation, euphoria, and a sense of well-being. Time sense is altered and emotional lability, with inappropriate laughter, may be seen. There is impaired performance on psychomotor tasks, including driving (Klonoff, 1974). Marijuana has antiemetic effects and reduces intraocular pressure and has been used medically for these effects. High doses of this drug can cause depersonalization, paranoia, and anxiety. Although tolerance to the effects of cannabis occurs with chronic use, cessation of use does not produce significant withdrawal phenomena. Chronic use of cannabis has been associated with an apathetic amotivational state that improves on discontinuation of the drug. In males a feminization effect has been well-described with chronic use.

In spite of its mostly illicit status, a high percentage of the American population has used marijuana. In 1982, 64.1% of young adults (18 to 25) had used marijuana. Although such use appears to be declining, millions of individuals continue to use marijuana regularly.

Treatment

Treatment of cannabis dependence is similar to treatment of other drug dependencies. As part of the initial assessment, all patients should undergo complete psychiatric and medical examinations. Short-term goals should focus on reducing or stopping cannabis use and on interventions to ensure compliance. Inpatient treatment may be necessary to achieve an abstinent state. Since many patients with cannabis dependence are adolescents or young adults, involvement of the family in assessment and treatment is critically important.

Long-term treatment should involve behavioral and psychological interventions to maintain an abstinent state. Often a change in social situation is necessary to decrease drug availability and reduce peer pressure to use drugs. Individual and group psychotherapy may be useful in helping patients understand the role of the drug in their lives, in improving self-esteem, and in providing alternate methods of relieving psychosocial distress. Self-help groups such as NA can provide group and individual support.

HALLUCINOGENS

Many drugs may be used for their hallucinogenic or psychotomimetic effects. These include psychedelics, such as lysergic acid diethylamide (LSD), mescaline, psilocybin, and dimethyltryptamine (DMT); hallucinogenic amphetamines, such as methylenedioxymethamphetamine (MDMA, or ecstasy), and methylenedioxyamphetamine (MDA); and anticholinergics, such as scopolamine. All are capable of causing hallucinosis, affective changes, and delusions.

The mechanism of action of hallucinogens is thought to involve stimulation of CNS dopamine or inhibition of serotonin (Abraham et al, 1996). The administration of hallucinogenic amphetamines to animals produces persistent depletions of brain monoamines, which is consistent with a neurotoxic effect of these substances. Whether neurotoxicity also occurs in humans is not yet established.

Hallucinogens are primarily used by young adults on an intermittent basis. Chronic daily use of hallucinogens is not common. In 1982, 21.1% of 18 to 25 year olds reported use of hallucinogens at some time during their life, although more recent statistics report a decrease in use.

The differential diagnosis of hallucinogen-induced psychosis includes schizophrenia, bipolar disorder, delusional disorder, and cognitive impairment disorders. Disorders, such as encephalitis and brain tumor, and other toxic ingestions should be considered. Psychoses, including those that are drug-induced, produce an analgesic state, and medical problems such as pain may be obscured.

Treatment of hallucinogen intoxication includes measures to reduce agitation and psychosis, to prevent patients from harming themselves or others, and to maintain vital functions. Agitation and psychosis usually respond to verbal reassurance and decreased sensory stimulation, but sometimes require treatment with benzodiazepines or high-potency neuroleptics. Most hallucinogen intoxications are short lived (several hours), although prolonged drug-induced psychoses may occur, particularly in persons predisposed to psychiatric illness. Many individuals experience brief recurrences of the psychomimetic state (flashbacks) following a drug-free interval.

INHALANTS

Inhalants are volatile organic compounds inhaled for their psychotropic effects. Substances in this class include organic solvents such as gasoline, toluene, ethyl ether, fluorocarbons, and volatile nitrates, including nitrous oxide and butyl nitrate. Inhalants are ubiquitous and readily available in most households and places of employment. At low doses, inhalants produce mood changes and ataxia; at high doses, they may produce dissociative states and hallucinosis. Dangers of organic solvent use include suffocation and organ damage, especially hepatotoxicity and neurotoxicity in the central and peripheral nervous systems (Watson, 1982). Cardiac arrhythmias and sudden death may occur. Inhaled nitrates may produce hypotension and methemaglobinemia.

The typical user of inhalants is adolescent and male. According to the National Household Survey on Drug Abuse, 9.1% of 12 to 17 year olds and 12.8% of 18 to 25 year olds have tried an inhalant at least once.

Optimal treatment of the inhalant user is not well established. Since most users are adolescents, treatment must involve the family. Long-term residential treatment may be helpful in the treatment of heavy users.

NICOTINE

Nicotine is an alkaloid drug present in the leaves of the tobacco plant, *Nicotiana tabacum*. The plant is indigenous to the New World and has been used for centuries by American Indians in ceremonies and rituals and as a medicinal herb. Since its discovery by Europeans, tobacco use has spread worldwide, and today nicotine is the most prevalent psychoactive drug in use. Over 50 million persons in the United States are daily users of cigarettes, with another 10 million using another form of tobacco. Since the publication of the

Surgeon General's Report on Smoking and Health in 1964, there has been a gradual decline in smoking in the United States. Most of this decline has occurred in men. The numbers of young women who smoke and the use of other tobacco products such as smokeless tobacco have increased.

To maximize the absorption of nicotine, tobacco products are usually smoked in pipe tobacco, cigars, or cigarettes, or instilled intranasally or intra-orally as snuff or "smokeless tobacco." Following absorption, nicotine levels peak rapidly and then decline with a half-life of 30 to 60 minutes.

Nicotine affects the peripheral autonomic and central nervous systems. It is a "nicotinic" cholinergic agonist and stimulates autonomic ganglia in the parasympathetic and sympathetic nervous systems, producing salivation, increased gastric motility and acid secretion, and increased catecholamine release. In the brain, nicotine acts as a mild psychomotor stimulant, increasing alertness, attention, and concentration and suppressing appetite. The fact that tobacco use can prevent weight gain makes the drug attractive, particularly to young women.

Repeated use of nicotine produces tolerance and dependence. The degree of dependence is considerable, as over 70% of dependent individuals relapse within 1 year of stopping use. The nicotine withdrawal syndrome is character-ized by increased irritability, decreased attention and concentration, an intense craving, and preoccupation with nicotine. Frequently, there is increased appetite and a significant weight gain. Withdrawal symptoms may begin within several hours of cessation of use or reduction in dosage and typically last about a week. Craving and weight gain may, however, persist for weeks.

The morbidity and mortality resulting from use of nicotine includes car-diovascular and respiratory disease and cancers, particularly of the lung and oropharynx. Most of the deleterious effects of tobacco are not due to nicotine but to other toxic and carcinogenic compounds present in tobacco extract or smoke. There is a strong association between cigarette and alcohol use. Although the overall prevalence rate of alcoholism is approximately 15% in the general population, 85% of alcoholics smoke cigarettes. Moreover, combined alcohol and tobacco use increases the risk of several of types of cancer, e.g., lung, oropharyngeal, and gastrointestinal.

Treatment

The treatment of nicotine dependence should follow the principles of treatment common to all addictive substances. Short-term goals should consist of reduction or cessation of tobacco use. Few patients are able to reduce tobacco use on their own. The use of smoking cessation treatment is usually necessary to stop (Greene et al, 1988). Brief education and advice on smoking cessation provided by physicians has been shown to be effective in helping patients stop smoking. The most successful treatment programs use cognitive–

behavioral techniques to educate patients about the health hazards of tobacco and to provide patients with behavioral methods of coping with urges. Some programs use gradual reduction in tobacco use over days to weeks (nicotine fading); others suggest abrupt discontinuation (cold turkey).

Nicotine replacement therapy is increasingly popular in the treatment of nicotine dependence. The principle of replacement therapy is to provide the patient with nicotine in a form not associated with the carcinogenic elements in tobacco products. Two methods of nicotine administration have been approved: nicotine gum and the transdermal nicotine patch. Both of these methods are now available over the counter. A third method, intranasal nicotine, is under consideration by government agencies. While nicotine replacement has been used primarily for detoxification and relief of withdrawal symptoms during smoking cessation, some patients use nicotine replacement in a maintenance fashion. The most successful treatment of nicotine dependence occurs with interventions that combine pharmacological and behavioral therapies.

Nicotine gum consists of a sweet, flavored resin containing 2 mg of nicotine that is released slowly when chewed. Nicotine is absorbed across the buccal mucosa. The gum is chewed whenever the individual feels the need for tobacco. When tingling of the mouth or tongue is perceived, chewing should cease for a short period of time, while still holding the gum in the mouth. Rapid chewing releases excess nicotine and may cause nausea and other side effects. The gum is chewed for 20 to 30 minutes and then discarded. This method reduces tobacco craving and withdrawal discomfort through nicotine blood levels that rise and fall, mimicking smoking. (Schneider, 1984).

A schedule for tapering gum use is planned after the daily maintenance dose is established. For example, a patient using 15 pieces of gum each day during the first week of treatment gradually reduces the number to 10 a day by the end of the first month and 5 a day by the end of the second month. Patients are typically able to discontinue nicotine gum after 3 to 6 months of treatment.

Nicotine transdermal patches consist of various doses of nicotine (7, 14, and 21 mg) impregnated into an adhesive patch for transdermal administration. Nicotine patches deliver a steady and predictable amount of nicotine. After stopping tobacco use, one patch is applied to uncovered skin during each 24-hour period, and the previous patch is discarded. Some individuals wear patches during the daytime only and remove them while asleep. Typical nicotine patch treatment involves application of a high-dose patch for 1 to 2 weeks, an intermediate dose patch for 1 to 2 weeks, and then the smallest dose patch for 1 to 2 weeks. Side effects include irritation from the patch and nicotine effects (nausea, cardiac effects, etc.). It is important that patients not use tobacco products while using the patch, as toxic nicotine blood levels may occur.

Other Medications for Smoking Cessation

Several clinical studies have shown a high incidence of major depression occurring within days to weeks following smoking cessation and nicotine withdrawal. Patients with a personal or family history of affective illness appear to be at most risk for depression. Antidepressants have been shown to reduce the prevalence of depression and to improve the chances of remaining abstinent from nicotine. Antidepressants reported to be effective include desipramine, doxepin, and bupropion (Wellbutrin). A sustained-release formulation of bupropion (Zyban) was recently approved by the Food and Drug Administration in the United States as an adjunct in smoking cessation. The dose of antidepressant is similar to that used for depression.

Clonidine, an alpha-2-receptor agonist, has also been reported to be efficacious in reducing nicotine withdrawal symptoms (Glassman et al, 1988). The doses used are similar to those for the treatment of mild hypertension. Clonidine is available in oral and transdermal preparations. Side effects include hypotension and sedation. Clonidine is usually prescribed for a period of 3 to 4 weeks, with the dose gradually reduced over the detoxification period. As with other forms of treatment for nicotine addiction, clonidine should be used in conjunction with a behavioral recovery program.

OPIOIDS

Opioid abuse and dependence are significant sociological and medical problems in the United States, with an estimated opioid addict population of approximately 500,000. These patients are frequent users of medical and surgical services because of the multiple medical sequelae of intravenous drug use and its associated lifestyle. Intravenous opioid users now constitute the second largest group of persons with AIDS.

Opiate drugs have physiological effects, due to stimulation of receptors for endogenous hormones, enkephalins, endorphins, and dynorphins. There exist at least four distinct opioid receptors, which are designated by the Greek letters mu, kappa, delta, and epsilon (Jaffe and Martin, 1985). Morphine, heroin, and methadone act primarily through mu receptors and produce analgesia, euphoria, and respiratory depression. Drugs that appear to be mediated through the kappa receptor include the so-called mixed agonist–antagonists, butorphanol and pentazocine, which produce analgesia, but less respiratory depression. The delta receptor binds endogenous opioid peptides.

Treatment

Opioid overdose is a life-threatening emergency and should be suspected in any patient who presents with coma and respiratory suppression. Treatment of suspected overdose includes emergency support of respiration and cardiovascular functions. Parenteral administration of the opioid antagonists naloxone 0.4 to 0.8 mg or nalmefene 0.5 to 1.0 mg will rapidly reverse coma and respiratory suppression, but will not affect depression caused by other sedatives, such as alcohol or barbiturates. Naloxone and nalmefene can precipitate opioid withdrawal, causing one whose life was just saved to be extremely ungrateful.

The opioid withdrawal syndrome is unpleasant but not life threatening. It is characterized by increased sympathetic nervous system activity, coupled with gastrointestinal symptoms of nausea, vomiting, cramps, and diarrhea. Patients may also report myalgias and arthralgias. There is increased restlessness, increased anxiety, insomnia, and an intense craving for opioids. Treatment for withdrawal consists of minimizing signs and symptoms.

Opioid detoxifications are performed by readministering an opioid until withdrawal symptoms cease and then gradually decreasing the dose of opioid over a period of up to 21 days, as specified by federal law. Although any opioid could be used for detoxification, methadone is most used, due to its long half-life and once-daily oral administration. Initially, patients should be given 10 to 20 mg of methadone orally every 2 to 4 hours until withdrawal symptoms are suppressed. The total initial dose is typically 20 to 40 mg for heroin addicts. This dose is then tapered over time.

The alpha-2-adrenergic agonist clonidine hydrochloride may also be used to suppress many of the signs and symptoms of opioid withdrawal. Clonidine acts at presynaptic noradrenergic nerve endings in the locus ceruleus of the brain and blocks the adrenergic discharge produced by opioid withdrawal (Gold et al, 1979; Washton and Resnick, 1981). Clonidine suppresses approximately 75% of opioid withdrawal signs and symptoms, especially autonomic hyperactivity, anxiety, and gastrointestinal symptoms. Withdrawal symptoms that are not significantly ameliorated by clonidine include drug craving, insomnia, and arthralgias and myalgias. Insomnia may be treated with a short-acting hypnotic such as chloral hydrate, and pain may respond to nonnarcotic analgesics such as ibuprofen or acetaminophen. Clonidine may cause dry mouth, sedation, and orthostatic hypotension. It should be used cautiously in hypotensive patients and in those receiving antihypertensives, antidepressants, or antipsychotics.

Methadone Maintenance

Since its introduction in 1965, methadone maintenance has become a major modality of long-term treatment of opioid abuse and dependence. Currently, over 100,000 individuals are maintained on methadone in the United States. The demand for treatment exceeds the availability, and many programs have waiting lists; however, it is possible for a physician to apply to the Drug Enforcement Administration to maintain a patient on methadone outside of an established methadone program.

In a typical methadone program, patients receive a daily dose of oral methadone, coupled with behavioral and psychologically oriented therapy as well as periodic toxicological analysis of urine to ensure compliance. Patients may receive methadone for various periods, often for years.

Methadone maintenance is clearly effective in reducing illicit drug use and criminality and in improving social and psychological health in many heroin users (Newman, 1987; Senay, 1985). Methadone maintenance also reduces the chances of HIV seroconversion. There are several theories to explain the efficacy of methadone maintenance, including decreasing illicit opioid use by increasing tolerance, treating an endorphin deficiency, and inducing addicts to enter a structured, rehabilitation-oriented treatment.

A recent national survey of methadone programs about treatment practices found wide variations in length of treatment and wide differences in the methadone doses among the programs (D'Aunno and Vaughn, 1992). Many programs emphasized short periods of treatment and low doses of methadone. The authors point out that these practices are counter to evidence on the effectiveness of methadone, showing that the longer patients remain in treatment, the more likely they are to remain abstinent from other drugs and that treatment with higher doses of methadone (80 mg or more daily) is more likely to retain patients in treatment.

If hospitalized in a psychiatric or medical facility, patients who are clients of a methadone maintenance program can have their daily dose of methadone continued in the hospital, as long as the facility has a license to prescribe methadone. If methadone is to be administered, it is important to communicate with the methadone program to determine the daily methadone dose, for the program to suspend dispensing while the patient is in the hospital, and to resume methadone dispensing after discharge from the hospital. If analgesia is needed, patients should receive additional opioids of a different class, such as meperidine or oxycodone, rather than methadone. This differentiates between the use of opioids for analgesia and for maintenance and does not change the dose of methadone.

l-Alpha-acetylmethodol acetate (LAAM) is a long-acting, orally active opiate with pharmacological properties similar to those of methadone. Studies on LAAM have shown it to be equal or superior to methadone maintenance in reducing intravenous drug use, when used in the context of a structured maintenance treatment program (Ling et al, 1994). The advantages of LAAM include a slower onset of effects and a longer duration of action than methadone. This allows LAAM to be administered only 3 times a week and potentially reduces the use of take-home medications that may be diverted to illegal uses. Patients treated with LAAM should be started on 20 mg administered three times weekly, with the dose increased weekly in 10-mg increments, as necessary. Doses of up to 80 mg three times weekly are safe and effective.

Buprenorphine is a partial agonist opiate medication (mixed agonist–antagonist), originally used medically as an analgesic. The agonist properties predominate at lower doses, and the antagonist properties predominate at higher doses. In the setting of a structured treatment program, daily dosing of buprenorphine is effective in the maintenance treatment of narcotics addicts (Compton et al, 1996). Buprenorphine may also reduce cocaine use.

Buprenorphine doses usually range from 4 mg/day to up to 16 mg/day, administered sublingually, since the medication is not effective orally. Advantages of buprenorphine include a milder withdrawal syndrome upon discontinuation and less potential for abuse, as agonist effects diminish at higher doses. Opioid-dependent patients may be started on 2 to 4 mg buprenorphine immediately after opiates are discontinued, and the dose of buprenorphine titrated to 8 to 16 mg over several days.

Opioid Antagonist Therapy

Opioid antagonist therapy reduces the use of illicit drugs by blocking the effect of the drugs at neurotransmitter receptors, leading to decreased use. There is some evidence that opiate antagonists may block the craving for opiates as well. Naltrexone (ReVia) is a long-acting orally active opioid antagonist that, when taken regularly, entirely blocks mu-opioid receptors and thus blocks the euphoric, analgesic, and sedative properties of opioids (Resnick et al, 1980). Naltrexone is administered either daily to detoxified opioid users at a dose of 50 mg or three times weekly at doses of 100, 100, and 150 mg. The drug appears to be most effective in motivated individuals with good social support and appears to be less helpful for heroin addicts. Although naltrexone may be prescribed by any physician, it is most effective as part of a comprehensive rehabilitative plan.

Drug-Free Treatment

Drug-free treatment modalities are also efficacious in the treatment of the opioid abuser (Bale et al, 1984). These emphasize total abstinence from opioids, alcohol, and other drugs, as well as social and psychological rehabilitation. Programs differ widely in their intensity and their theoretical orientation. Therapeutic community programs usually require a long-term treatment commitment of at least several months, during which the addict is sequestered away from his or her usual environment and involved in intensive psychological and behavioral individual and group therapy. Long-term residential treatment may be most useful for the chronic opioid abuser who requires a change in lifestyle.

Self-help groups such as NA may be useful either as a primary treatment modality for opioid dependence or as an adjunct to other treatment. NA, like AA, utilizes the 12-step philosophy and the idea of total abstinence. Each NA group often has its own individual orientation, and thus patients should be encouraged to visit several groups to increase the chances that they will find a compatible group.

PHENCYCLIDINE AND SIMILARLY ACTING ARYLCYCLOHEXYLAMINES

Phencyclidine (PCP) and similarly acting arylcyclohexylamines, such as ketamine, are used as anesthetic agents in veterinary medicine and in pediatrics (ketamine). The mechanism of action of this group of drugs is not well understood, although recently this class of drugs has been shown to bind to the so-called sigma opioid receptor in the brain

PCP intoxication has several definitive features. The agents produce an amnestic, euphoric, and hallucinatory state, although the effects may be unpredictable, and a prolonged, agitated psychosis with violence directed at self or at others may occur (Peterson and Stillman, 1979). Vertical and horizontal nystagmus, myoclonus, ataxia, and autonomic instability are common.

As with the hallucinogens, treatment of PCP or similarly acting arylcyclohexylamine intoxication includes maintaining cardiovascular and respiratory functions, amelioration of psychotic symptoms, and supportive measures to prevent patients from harming themselves or others. Both haloperidol and benzodiazepines have been described as useful for decreasing agitation and psychosis. Psychiatric hospitalization may be necessary in prolonged psychosis.

SEDATIVES, HYPNOTICS, AND ANXIOLYTICS

Sedative medications are among the most prescribed medications and are routinely used for their anxiolytic and hypnotic effects; however, they are also a major source of drug overdoses and of adverse drug reactions. Medications in this group include barbiturates, such as secobarbital, butalbital, and phenobarbital; benzodiazepines, such as alprazolam and diazepam; and nonbarbiturate sedative–hypnotics, such as chloral derivatives, ethchlorvynol, glutethimide, meprobamate, and methaqualone. Patients who become dependent on sedative and anxiolytic medications often obtain them by prescription from physicians who are unaware of an abuse problem. Sedatives are commonly used by adolescents and young adults for their acute intoxicating effects, often in combination with alcohol and other drugs ("partying," "raves"). Hypnotic medications used in Europe, but illegal in the United States, including gamma-hydroxybutyrate (GHB) and the benzodiazepine flunitrezepam (Rohypnol, roofies), have been used to intoxicate unsuspecting individuals acutely for nefarious purposes, such as "date rape."

The effects of most sedative–hypnotic and anxiolytic drugs are mediated through interactions with the GABA–chloride channel receptor complex. In the case of benzodiazepines, there exists a neuronal binding site linked to the

GABA receptor in both location and function. Binding of benzodiazepines to nerve cell membranes facilitates binding of GABA to its receptors and augments GABA inhibition of nerve cells (Hunt, 1983). Barbiturates, anticonvulsants, and other sedative–hypnotic drugs also have discrete binding sites closely associated with the chloride channel and affect the transport of chloride and inhibition of neurons.

Assessment of the sedative user begins with the history, which should include drug and alcohol use, psychiatric illness, and medical history. Toxicological screens may be useful in assessing the type of medications used.

Treatment

Treatment of acute sedative intoxication or overdose includes support of vital functions until the drug effect wears off. Because of the respiratory supression produced by sedatives, all patients should be closely monitored and may require intubation and respiratory support. Flumazenil (Mazicon) is a benzodiazepine antagonist approved for the treatment of benzodiazepine overdose and the reversal of benzodiazepine oversedation. Flumazenil binds competitively and reversibly to the GABA–benzodiazepine receptor complex and inhibits the effects of benzodiazepines. It has minimal effects on nonbenzodiazepine sedatives. Also, flumazenil may not fully reverse the inhibitory effects of benzodiazepines on the hypoxic respiratory drive; hence, respiration monitoring is essential. Flumazenil also has a short duration of action and may need to be repeatedly administered to antagonize long-acting benzodiazepines, such as diazepam. The drug may induce seizures in patients who are prone to seizures or epilepsy.

Treatment of the sedative-dependent patient occurs in two stages, detoxification and long-term rehabilitation. Pharmacological detoxification is usually necessary, as the withdrawal syndrome that follows cessation of drug use may be severe and include seizures, cardiac arrhythmias, and death. The *pentobarbital challenge test* is useful for predicting the need for pharmacologically assisted detoxification to prevent severe withdrawal in heavy users (Wesson and Smith, 1977). Pentobarbital 200 mg is administered orally and the patient observed 1 hour later. The patient's condition after the test dose will range from no effect to sleep. If the patient develops drowsiness or nystagmus on a 200-mg dose, the patient is not barbiturate dependent. If 200 mg has no effect, the dose should be repeated hourly until nystagmus or drowsiness develop. The total dosage administered approximates the patient's daily sedative habit. The barbiturate dose should be tapered over 10 days, with approximately a 10% reduction each day. Long-acting benzodiazepines such as diazepam or clonazepam are sometimes used in the detoxification of shorter acting benzodiazepines such as alprazolam.

Anticonvulsants such as carbamazepine or valproic acid also are used for the treatment of sedative and benzodiazepine withdrawal (Klein et al, 1986).

Patients are loaded with the anticonvulsants to produce therapeutic blood levels. The levels are maintained for 7 to 14 days and then tapered.

Long-term treatments should be individualized to the patient but may include residential drug-free programs and self-help groups such as AA or NA. A certain number of patients may be found to have an underlying psychiatric disorder, such as an anxiety disorder or depression. If pharmacological treatment is deemed necessary, antidepressants or non-dependence-producing anxiolytics such as buspirone should be utilized.

ANABOLIC STEROIDS

The use of anabolic steroids, once found predominantly in fanatical athletes, has now become a relatively common problem in adolescents. A recent study found that 6.5% of adolescent boys and 1.9% of adolescent girls reported using anabolic steroids without a doctor's prescription (DuRant et al, 1993). The use of anabolic steroids is associated with the use of other substances, including cocaine, alcohol, injectable drugs, marijuana, and cigarettes.

Medical complications of anabolic steroid use include myocardial infarction, stroke, and hepatic disease. HIV infection has been associated with shared needle use in steroid injectors. Psychiatric symptoms associated with anabolic steroid use include severe depression, psychotic (paranoid) symptoms, aggressive behavior, homicidal impulses, euphoria, irritability, anxiety, and hyperactivity (Pope and Katz, 1988). Although most of these symptoms will gradually abate with drug discontinuation, depression, fatigue, decreased sex drive, insomnia, anorexia, and dissatisfaction with body image may continue.

The treatment of anabolic steroid dependence should be within the same general model of other addictions, with due consideration to the high likelihood of dependency on other drugs, particularly in adolescents. Psychiatric management of drug-induced mood and paranoid syndromes is necessary. Issues regarding narcissistic body image are often present in certain athletes and body builders and should be considered in the psychotherapy of such individuals.

SUMMARY

Substance-use disorders are chronic disorders that involve individuals and their families. Identification and treatment of the disorders involves several skills on the part of the physician, including knowledge of the biological, psychological, and social substrates of substance use; an ability to interview patients and to take a substance use history; knowledge of acute and long-term treatment modalities for intoxication, dependence, and withdrawal; and an awareness of medical and community resources available for specialized treatment. The treatment process involves identification of the problem, making the patient and family aware of it, and motivating them to seek help. The process is best conducted in the context of a supportive and empathic relationship.

ANNOTATED BIBLIOGRAPHY

Institute of Medicine: Broadening the Basis of Treatment of Alcoholism. Washington, DC, National Academy Press, 1991

> An excellent review of the etiology and treatment of alcoholism, with an emphasis on social policy aspects.

Jaffe JE: Drug addiction and drug abuse. In Gilman AG, Goodman LS, Gilman A (eds): The Pharmacological Basis of Therapeutics, 6th ed., pp 535–585. New York, Macmillan, 1980

> This book is an extremely comprehensive and detailed description of the clinical and behavioral pharmacology of psychoactive substances, with emphasis on chemistry and pharmacology. It is "The Bible" on drugs for medical students.

Lowinson JH, Ruiz P, Millman RB, Langrod JG (eds): Substance Abuse: A Comprehensive Textbook, 3rd ed. Baltimore, MD, Williams & Wilkins, 1997

> This detailed and comprehensive book contains chapters authored by many of the experts in the field of substance abuse and dependence.

Miller N (ed): Principles and Practice of Addictions in Psychiatry. Philadelphia, WB Saunders, 1997

> A multiauthored text covering addictions from a psychiatric perspective.

Nestler EJ: Molecular mechanisms of drug addiction. J Neurosci 12:2439–2450, 1992

> An excellent review of substance dependence, intoxication, and withdrawal from a neurobiological perspective.

Samet JH, Rollnick S, Barnes H: Beyond CAGE. A brief clinical approach after detection of substance abuse. Arch Intern Med 156:2287–2293, 1996

> This paper provides an excellent overview of identification and treatment of the patient with substance abuse and dependence. It is directed at primary care physicians.

Senay E: Methadone maintenance treatment. Int J Addictions 20:803–821, 1985

> This paper provides an excellent review of the principles and practice of the use of methadone for the treatment of opioid dependence.

US Department of Health and Human Services: The Health Consequences of Smoking: Nicotine Addiction. A Report of the Surgeon General. DHHS Publication No. (CDC 88-8406), Washington, DC, 1988

> The controversial Surgeon General's report on smoking, which has excellent sections on the clinical and behavioral pharmacology of nicotine and which presents the thesis that nicotine dependence is an "addiction."

REFERENCES

Abraham HD, Aldridge AM, Gogia P: The psychopharmacology of hallucinogens. Neuropsychopharmacology 14:285–298, 1996

American Psychiatric Association: Diagnostic and Statistical Manual of Mental Disorders, 4th ed. Washington, DC, American Psychiatric Association Press, 1994

American Society of Addiction Medicine: ASAM Patient Placement Criteria, Psychoactive Substance Use Disorders, Chevy Chase, MD, 1993

Bale RN, Zarcone VP, Van Stone WW: Three therapeutic communities. A prospective controlled study of narcotic addiction treatment process and follow up results. Arch Gen Psychiatry 41:185–191, 1984

Beresford TP, Blow KC, Singer K, Lucey, MR: Clinical practice: comparison of CAGE questionnaire and computer assisted laboratory profiles in screening for covert alcoholism. Lancet 336:482–485, 1990

Brewer C: Recent developments in disulfiram treatment. Alcohol Alcoholism 28:383–395, 1993

Cloninger CR: Neurogenetic adaptive mechanisms in alcoholism. Science 236:410–416, 1987

Compton PA, Wesson DR, Charuvastra VC, Ling W: Buprenorphine as a pharmacotherapy for opiate addiction. Am J Addictions 5:220–230, 1996

D'Aunno T, Vaughn TE: Variations in methadone treatment practices. JAMA 267:253–258, 1992

Dews PB: Caffeine. Annu Rev Nutr 2:323–341, 1982

DuRant RH, Rickert VI, Ashworth CS et al: The use of multiple drugs among adolescents who use anabolic steroids. N Engl J Med 328:922–926, 1993

Emrick CD: Alcoholics Anonymous: affiliation processes and effectiveness as treatment. Alcoholism 11:416–423, 1987

Ewing JA: Detecting alcoholism: the CAGE questionnaire. JAMA 252:1905–1907, 1984

Foy A, March S, Drinkwater V: Use of an objective clinical scale in the assessment and management of alcohol withdrawal in a large general hospital. Alcoholism Clin Exp Res 12:360–364, 1988

Gawin FH, Ellinwood EHJ: Cocaine and other stimulants. Actions, abuse and treatment. N Engl J Med 318:1173–1182, 1988

Glassman AH, Stetner F, Walsh BT, Raizman PS: Heavy smokers, smoking cessation and clonidine. Results of a double-blind, randomized trial. JAMA 259:2863–2866, 1988

Gold MS, Pottash AC, Sweeney DR, Kleber HD: Opiate withdrawal using clonidine: a safe, effective, and rapid non-opiate treatment. JAMA 234:343–344, 1979

Goldman D: Identifying alcoholism vulnerability alleles. Alcohol Clin Exp Res 19:824–831, 1995

Greene HL, Goldberg R, Ockene JK: Cigarette smoking: the physician's role in cessation and maintenance. J Gen Intern Med 3:75–87, 1988

Helzer JE, Pyrzbeck TR: The co-occurrence of alcoholism with other psychiatric disorders. J Stud Alcohol 49:219–224, 1988

Higgins ST, Budney AJ, Bickel WK: Applying behavioral concepts and principles to the treatment of cocaine dependence. Drug Alcohol Depend 34:87–97, 1994

Holden C: The neglected disease in medical education. Science 229:741–742, 1985

Hughes JR, Higgins, ST, Bickel WK, Hunt WK, Gulliver S: Caffeine self-administration, withdrawal and adverse effects among coffee drinkers. Arch Gen Psychiatry 48:611–617, 1991

Hunt WA: The effect of ethanol on GABAergic transmission. Neurosci Biobehav Rev 7:87–95, 1983

Jaffe JH, Martin WR: Opioid analgesics and antagonists. In Gilman AC, Goodman LS, Rall TW, (eds): Pharmacological Basis of Therapeutics. New York, Macmillan, 494–534, 1985

Klein E, Uhde T, Post RM: Preliminary evidence for the utility of carabamazepine in alprazolam withdrawal. Am J Psychiatry 143:235–236, 1986

Klonoff H: Marihuana and driving in real-life situations. Science 186:317–324, 1974

Kranzler HR, Burleson JA, Del Boca FK, et al: Buspirone treatment of anxious alcoholics. A placebo-controlled trial. Arch Gen Psychiatry 51:720–731, 1994

Ling W, Rawson RA, Compton PA: Substitution pharmacotherapies for opioid addiction: from methadone to LAAM and buprenorphine. J Psychoactive Drugs 26:119–128, 1994

Liskow BI, Goodwin DW: Pharmacological treatment of alcohol intoxication, withdrawal and dependence: a critical review. J Stud Alcohol 48:356–370, 1987

Litten RZ, Allen JP, Fertig JB: Gamma-glutamyltranspeptidase and carbohydrate deficient transferrin: alternative measures of excessive alcohol consumption. Alcohol Clin Exp Res 19:1541–1546, 1995

McGinnis JM, Foege WH: Actual causes of death in the United States. JAMA 270:2201–2212, 1993

Meyer RE: New pharmacotherapies for cocaine dependence . . . revisited. Arch Gen Psychiatry 49:900–904, 1992

Musty RE, Reggio P, Consroe P: A review of recent advances in cannabinoid research and the 1994 International Symposium on Cannabis and the Cannabinoids. Life Sci 56:1933–1940, 1995

Nestler EJ, Alreja M, Aghajanian, GK: Molecular and cellular mechanisms of opiate action: studies in the rat locus coeruleus. Brain Res Bull 35:521–528, 1994

Newman RG: Methadone treatment. Defining and evaluating success. N Engl J Med 317:447–450, 1987

NIAAA: The Physician's Guide to Helping Patients With Alcohol Problems. Rockville, MD, NIAAA, 1995

O'Malley SS, Jaffe AJ, Chang G, Schottenfeld RS, Meyer RE, Rounsaville B: Naltrexone and coping skills therapy for alcohol dependence. Arch Gen Psychiatry 49:881–887, 1992

Peterson CA, Stillman RC: PCP (Phencyclidine) Abuse: An Appraisal. Washington, DC, US Government Printing Office, 1979

Pope HG, Katz DA: Affective and psychotic symptoms associated with anabolic steroid use. Am J Psychiatry 145:487–490, 1988

Randall CL: Alcohol as a teratogen: a decade of research in review. Alcoholism Clin Exp Res 1(suppl):125–132, 1987

Regier DA, Farmer ME, Rao DS: Comorbidity of mental disorders with alcohol and other drug abuse. JAMA 264:2511–2518, 1990

Resnick RB, Schuyten-Resnick E, Washton AM: Assessment of narcotic antagonists in the treatment of opioid dependence. Annu Rev Pharmacol Toxicol 20:463–470, 1980

Rice DP: The economic cost of alcohol abuse and alcohol dependence. Alcohol Health Res World 17:10–11, 1990

Robinson TE, Berridge KC: The neural basis of drug craving: an incentive-sensitization theory of addiction. Brain Res Rev 18:247–291, 1993

Samet JH, Rollnick S, Barnes H: Beyond CAGE. A brief clinical approach after detection of substance abuse. Arch Intern Med 156:2287–2293, 1996

Sass H, Soyka M, Mann K, Zieglgänsberger W: Relapse prevention by acamprosate: results from a placebo-controlled study on alcohol dependence. Arch Gen Psychiatry 53:673–680, 1996

Schneider NG: Nicotine vs placebo gum in the allieviation of withdrawal during smoking cessation. Addictive Behav 9:149–156, 1984

Schuckit MA, Smith TL: An 8-year follow-up of 450 sons of alcoholic and control subjects. Arch Gen Psychiatry 53:202–210, 1996

Selzer ML: The Michigan Alcoholism Screening Test: the quest for a new diagnostic instrument. Am J Psychiatry 127:89–84, 1971

Senay E: Methadone maintenance treatment. Int J Addictions 20:803–821, 1985

Stein M: Medical consequences of intravenous drug abuse. J Gen Intern Med 5:249–257, 1990

Tsai G, Gastfriend DR, Cyle JT: The glutamatergic basis of human alcoholism. Am J Psychiatry 152:332–340, 1995

Volpicelli JR, Alterman AI, Hayashida M, O'Brien CP: Naltrexone in the treatment of alcohol dependence. Arch Gen Psychiatry 49:876–880, 1992

Washton AM, Resnick RB: Clonidine for opiate detoxification: outpatient clinical trials. J Clin Psychiatry 43:39–41, 1981

Watson JM: Solvent abuse: presentation and clinical diagnosis. Hum Toxicol 1:249–256, 1982

Wesson DR, Smith DE: A new method for the treatment of barbiturate dependence. JAMA 231:294–295, 1977

Wise RA, Bozarth MA: A psychomotor stimulant theory of addiction. Psychol Rev 94:469–492, 1987

By the turn of the century, it is estimated that one in five Americans (about 50 million people) will be over 55 years of age, and 13% will be over 65 years of age. Estimates reaching to the year 2050 place 22% of Americans over the age of 65 and 5% over 85 years of age. The elderly are at increased risk for social stressors, including retirement, widowhood, and physical infirmity.

Aging individuals thus bring to their physicians problems that occur in a multilayered context. The features of clinical syndromes are often different in older patients, and therapy frequently requires modification. The examination of geriatric psychopathology and its treatment begins best with a perspective on normal aging.

AGING AND THE LIFE CYCLE

Most early developmental theorists felt that psychological development stopped at an early age. According to them, the basic psychological structure was formed during childhood and refined during adolescence. This structure determined how the adult would perceive, interpret, and react to internal drives and the external circumstances of life. Erik Erickson (1959) proposed that psychological development continued throughout life in a series of predictable life crises (Table 11–1). In his outline, young adulthood is the time when people confront their ability to maintain intimate emotional relationships while in the crisis of *intimacy versus isolation.* Middle-aged adults struggle with *generativity versus self-absorption,* trying on the one hand to raise and

Table 11–1 **Erikson's Stages of Human Development**

STAGE	LIFE CRISIS	AGE	DEVELOPMENTAL TASK
I	Basic trust versus basic mistrust	First year	Knowledge that world and self are trustworthy
II	Autonomy versus shame and doubt	1–3 years	Confidence in own physical and mental capacities
III	Initiative versus guilt	4–6 years	Socially appropriate curiosity and strivings
IV	Industry versus inferiority	6–12 years	Healthy competition with peers
V	Identity versus identity diffusion	Adolescence	Self-definition and differentiation from parents
VI	Intimacy versus isolation	Young adulthood	Sexual, emotional, and spiritual maturity and social responsibility
VII	Generativity versus self-absorption	Middle age	Establishment, guiding, and nurturing of subsequent generations
VIII	Integrity versus despair	Late life	Acceptance of mortality, satisfaction with one's meaning in the world

nurture future generations, and on the other, to satisfy self-centered goals. Finally, elderly adults have to deal with *integrity versus despair.* Their struggle is to reevaluate their lives and to accept their roles during life (and the meaning of their relationships with others). They learn to own responsibility for their actions and to accept the things that might not be pleasant, but that cannot be changed. If they cannot do so, they are left with the despair of knowing that the unacceptable aspects of their lives cannot be undone.

The range of life stressors confronting the aging individual is broad. Friends and relatives become ill and die, children grow up and move away, retirement is often mandatory, and physical health may fail. To deal with such a wide array of stressors, one must mobilize a multitude of coping strategies. These strategies, known in psychodynamic terminology as *defense mechanisms,* are the ways that people process the data from the environment so as to maintain emotional stability. Such mechanisms may include taking control of and mastering a situation, retreating into fantasy in the face of overwhelming stress, or allowing oneself to ask for and receive necessary help. The individual whose earlier life has allowed him or her to adopt many kinds of defense mechanisms is better able to weather these stressors without psychological symptoms than one who has come to use only a narrow range of coping skills. In dealing with the death of a spouse, for example, some degree of denial and retreat into fantasy may be adaptive if elements of mastery and control are also utilized (Bienenfeld, 1990).

COGNITION AND AGING

Cognitive functioning can be divided into learning, memory, and intelligence. Age affects each of these areas differently. Learning is the ability to gain new skills and information. The elderly can continue to learn throughout their life; however, it appears that they tend to learn at a slower rate than younger individuals. This slowing becomes particularly evident in verbal learning. The total amount that can be learned is probably unchanged, but this learning takes longer.

Memory can be divided into immediate and short- and long-term memory. Immediate memory, such as repeating words within seconds of hearing them, appears to be largely unaffected by healthy aging. Short-term memory—repeating those same words 5 minutes later—is also largely undiminished in the healthy elderly person. However, short-term memory is related to attention, and aging individuals are more prone to distraction than younger ones.

Long-term memory, in which information is stored for anywhere from minutes to decades, seems to be the area most seriously affected by aging. Although the total amount of stored information is probably unchanged, the retrieval of this information appears to be less efficient. The elderly often require more cues to remember learned objects. Frequently, patients or family members will comment that the elderly seem to remember distant events quite well, but have considerable difficulty with more recent happenings. This phenomenon is probably more apparent than real. The elderly will tend to remember those events that are emotionally charged or in other ways significant. Since they have lived longer, they are more likely to have experienced these events in the more distant past, and they will tend to remember these events preferentially over more recent but less significant events.

The third major component of cognition is intelligence, which can be defined as the ability to use information in an adaptive way or to apply knowledge to specific circumstances. Intelligence can be further divided into crystallized and fluid intelligence. Crystallized intelligence includes areas such as vocabulary, verbal skills, and general information. With proper intellectual stimulation, crystallized intelligence can continue to increase throughout life. Fluid intelligence consists of recognizing new patterns and creative problem-solving. This form of intelligence tends to peak in adolescence and declines gradually throughout the rest of life. The decline of fluid intelligence leads people to attempt to maintain constancy so as to minimize the necessity for major cognitive or attitudinal adjustments. This effort to maintain constancy is often perceived as intellectual "rigidity" on the part of elders.

Older individuals often complain about cognitive decline, but the correlation of these subjective complaints with objective measures has repeatedly been found to be weak. On the other hand, aging is associated with certain cognitive difficulties that do not interfere substantially with daily functioning. These problems include forgetting names, misplacing items, and experiencing difficulty with complex problem-solving. This cluster of complaints has been proposed as a nonpathological entity called *aging-associated cognitive decline.*

EVALUATION

Although much of the psychiatric evaluation of the elderly is similar to any psychiatric evaluation, some features require special consideration. The evaluation needs to take place in a private area that is quiet, well lit, and free from distractions. The physician should ensure that he or she will have the time to perform a complete evaluation. Because of the breadth of the evaluation and the slower response time of some elderly patients, it may often last over an hour. The physician also must be flexible enough to conduct the interview in stages if it becomes clear that the patient cannot tolerate an extended interview.

Because geriatric patients are often referred to physicians by family members or other health professionals, collateral information is essential. This information should be obtained in a timely, efficient manner and should include facts about the patient's recent functional baseline and any changes in behavior, cognition, or personality. Family members often can detail changes in behavior that are not otherwise available. This history should include known information about the patient's medical and psychiatric history, as well as current medications.

Because geriatric patients have had a different exposure to mental health concepts from that of the (usually) younger examining clinicians, it is useful to ask older patients for their ideas about what the psychiatric examination might be like. When history and experience have bred misperceptions, examiners can correct them and explain that they are medical specialists who deal with emotional difficulties such as those the patient has described. Reassurance of ongoing communication and cooperation with the patient's primary physician is often helpful. The patient's wishes concerning family involvement in the therapy also must be determined early in the evaluation.

To understand current problems in a developmental context, it is beneficial to conduct a historical review. Not only do examiners ask the patient about past psychiatric symptoms, they also inquire about expectable life stressors and transitions, e.g., marriage, departure of children from the home, and retirement. Knowing the types of coping skills mobilized in these transitions allows the clinician to assess the potential coping skills brought by the patient to the current situation.

It is a principle in all of medicine that diagnosis is only the first step in evaluating a patient. Assessment must follow. Knowing that a patient meets criteria for a major depressive episode does not by itself dictate the appropriate therapy. It is further essential to determine the effect the illness has had on the patient's life and the resources that can be brought to bear in the service of treatment.

Finally, the clinician should present a formulation to the patient for the latter's comment, correction, or endorsement. The clinician recaps the presenting symptoms, the relevant stressors, the social environment that surrounds the patient, and the historical context of the current distress. The physician then presents a clinical opinion of the syndrome diagnosis in terms comprehensible to the patient, as well as a dynamic formulation explaining the relationship of the chief complaint to this individual's past and present. Once there is concurrence with the patient about the target of the therapy and its meaning to the patient, the physician outlines a treatment plan that follows logically from the biopsychosocial formulation that has been shared.

PSYCHIATRIC DISORDERS IN THE ELDERLY

Although the diagnostic criteria for adult mental disorders do not rely on age, clinical diagnosis in geriatric psychiatry entails some particular features. The physician who deals with the elderly confronts presentations of common disorders that change over the course of life, as well as disorders that increase in incidence with age.

Dementia and Other Cognitive Disorders

Dementia is a common problem among the elderly. International measures of the prevalence of dementia find rates of 2.2 to 8.4% in all those over age 65, 10.5 to 16.0% after age 75, and 15.2 to 38.9% after age 85 (Rockwood and Stadnyk, 1994). This rate then seems to level off without notable increase after about age 90 or 95 (Ritchie and Kildea, 1995). Although Alzheimer's disease may be the most common single entity causing dementia, it would be a mistake to dismiss all dementia in the elderly as Alzheimer's disease.

A review that looked at nearly 3,000 elderly with dementia (with a mean age of 72.3 years) found that 57% suffered from Alzheimer's disease, 13% from vascular dementia, and 4% from alcoholism. About 10 to 15% of cases represent a combination of more than one of those three diagnoses. Drug use and depression were also found to be commonly listed as causes of the dementia (Clarfield, 1988). The specific causes and diagnostic criteria for dementia are discussed in Chapter 4. The elderly also are quite susceptible to numerous central nervous system insults that can lead to delirium.

Mood Disorders

Depression

Depressive symptoms and disorders are endemic in the elderly. They account for 50% of all admissions of older adults to acute psychiatric hospitals. Prominent depressive symptoms may exist in 30% of adults over age 60, although some studies put that figure as high as 60%. Prevalence of depressive symptoms and major depression varies with setting and health status. Among community-dwelling, healthy elders, depressive symptoms are present in about 10% on a given day, and about half of those will meet criteria for major depression. Among cognitively intact nursing home residents, the prevalence is about six times that high for both symptoms and disease (Fig. 11–1; Borson, 1995). Depressed elders are functionally disabled by their mood disorder and use significantly more primary care medical resources than their nondepressed cohort. For individuals with almost any medical condition, the presence of depressive symptoms is associated with significantly reduced survival.

Beside the discomfort and disability caused by the depressive symptoms alone, the risk of suicide also increases greatly in those with depression. For those over age 65, the risk of death by suicide is about twice what it is for the population as a whole. The rate for suicide in males climbs from about age 65 with no plateau; for women, it peaks between 50 and 65 years of age. Part of this increase is attributable to the increased lethality of the elderly person's suicide attempt. Before the age of 50, only one in eight (13%) who attempts suicide actually kills him/herself with the attempt. After age 65, that completion rate approaches one in two (50%!). The elderly suicide tends to use more lethal means, communicates the intent less frequently, and less often than younger persons uses suicide threats and gestures as tools for manipulating others (Bienenfeld, 1990).

Depressive disorders, including major depression and dysthymic disorder, are not always obvious in the elderly because the clinical presentations

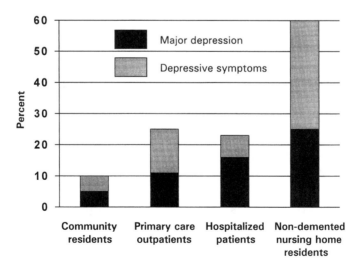

Figure 11–1. *Prevalence of late-life depression by setting and health status.*

may change with age. Whereas epidemiological surveys find that about one in four patients in primary care settings suffer from depression, primary care physicians only recognize the condition in about 2 to 6% of their patients. It is fairly rare, for example, that an elderly patient will give as a chief complaint, "I'm depressed." Much more commonly, the patient will describe vague somatic complaints, decreased energy, sleep difficulties, memory disturbances, anxiety, or "nerves." Somatic complaints, in fact, are the predominant way in which elderly patients present their depression or anxiety. Pain, weakness, and gastrointestinal disturbances are the most frequent avenues of presentation. Often, there will be complaints by the patient or others that the elderly individual is becoming regressed and more dependent or is not eating properly. Even someone with numerous neurovegetative complaints may deny depression or sadness, but admit to feeling "down" or "blue."

A wide variety of cardiovascular, pulmonary, endocrine, and neurological diseases, most of which increase in prevalence with aging, can present with depressive symptoms such as fatigue, anorexia, and decreased functioning. Depression also can be induced or mimicked by numerous medications commonly used in the elderly, including antihypertensives, benzodiazepines, corticosteroids, and cimetidine. It is equally hazardous to attribute problems in appetite, energy, sleep, or concentration to either depression or medical causes alone. An appropriate evaluation should be conducted to assess accurately the physical status of the depressed patient in regard to medical illness, including relevant aspects of the history, physical examination, laboratory tests, and radiological procedures.

The prognosis for elderly patients diagnosed with depression may not be as good as for their younger counterparts. Whereas 20% of a mixed population will remain depressed for more than 18 months, upwards of 30% of elderly patients will remain depressed for that long (Alexopoulos and Chester, 1992). A significant number of geriatric patients with major depression will also develop delusions. These delusions are most often persecutory or hypochondriacal in nature and can occur in 3% of community-dwelling depressed patients and in 20 to 45% of those elderly depressed patients who require hospitalization (Meyers, 1992). Patients with delusions tend to be less responsive to traditional antidepressant therapy. The addition of an antipsychotic or the use of electroconvulsive therapy greatly increases the patient's response. At least one study has indicated a very poor prognosis in psychotic depression, with only 10% of elderly patients recovered and well 1 year after the onset of their depression. Other studies (Baldwin and Jolley, 1986; Murphy, 1983) found no significant difference between the outcomes of depressed patients with or without delusions.

Bereavement

Although uncomplicated bereavement (normal grieving) is not a psychopathological condition, it can display many of the features of depressive disorders, and it is important to recognize grief for the purposes of differential diagnosis. Grieving individuals may experience, transiently, such symptoms as anorexia and insomnia in the context of their situational sadness. Normal grieving generally starts with a period of *shock* that lasts a few weeks or less, characterized by emotional numbing and even brief episodes of denial. Next comes a period of *preoccupation* with thoughts of the lost loved one; symptoms including crying, fatigue, and withdrawal. This phase may easily last a year or much longer in older widows and widowers and may recur on the lost person's birthday, the wedding anniversary, or the anniversary of the death. Finally, preoccupation gives way to *resolution,* as somatic and depressive symptoms diminish and the survivor regains interest in social and individual activities (see Chapter 20). These phases are similar at all ages, but in the elderly, somatic symptoms are often predominant expressions of the emotional distress, and the phases may take much longer to progress and resolve than at younger ages.

Mania

While bipolar disorder usually begins in the third or fourth decade of life, episodes usually persist into old age. Additionally, first onset of mania in the sixth or even seventh decade may be observed. Compared with younger manic patients, older individuals are more likely to be *irritable* than euphoric and *paranoid* rather than grandiose. Older patients are more likely than younger ones to present with *dysphoric mania* ("miserable mania"), a constellation in which there is pressure of speech, flight of ideas, and hyperactivity, but thought content is as morbid and pessimistic as that of a patient with typical major depression.

Psychotic Disorders

Schizophrenia

Most elderly schizophrenics developed their illness between ages 20 and 40. Only 7% of schizophrenias are first diagnosed after age 60, and only 3% after age 70 (Harris and Jeste, 1988). Aging affects the clinical appearance of schizophrenia, particularly producing a blunting of the "positive" symptoms, such as delusions and hallucinations. Residual delusions and hallucinations become less bizarre and more monotonous. The "negative" symptoms, including social withdrawal, apathy, and blunted affect, become more apparent (Cohen, 1990).

Although the numbers are small, some individuals do develop schizophrenia after their 50s and into their 60s, a condition formerly labeled *paraphrenia.* These individuals are more likely to be women than men. The clinical presentation usually centers on persecutory delusions and generally does not include a formal thought disorder. Treated with antipsychotic agents, at least 48% of late-onset schizophrenic patients experience a resolution of symptoms (Pearlson et al, 1989).

Delusional Disorders

Delusional disorders generally present in mid- to late life. These patients are generally brought in by concerned family members as the patients themselves see nothing wrong with their ideas. In the elderly, the delusions most often involve persecutory or somatic themes. Delusions appear to be more common in immigrants and are more common in those with a sensory deficit since sensory deficits are also correlated with delusional disorders. In a community-based study, 78% of elders with persecutory ideation had visual impairment, and 58% had hearing deficits, compared with 51 and 37% of age-matched controls without paranoia (Christenson and Blazer, 1984). Medications are only marginally successful at stopping the delusions, but do tend to decrease their intensity and lessen the chance of the patient's acting on them. Psychotherapy generally does not produce good results, since the beliefs are unshakably true to the patient, who sees little motivation for therapy.

Anxiety and Somatoform Disorders

Anxiety

As a symptom and diagnosis, anxiety is common in the elderly. Ten to 20% of the elderly complain of anxiety severe enough to warrant a visit to a physician. On self-rating scales, 27% of individuals in their 60s and 29% above the age of 70 report significant anxiety symptoms. Individuals over 65 years of age are five times more likely to be regular users of anxiolytics than are younger individuals. Fifteen percent of those individuals who chronically use anxiolytics are over the age of 65 (Bienenfeld, 1990).

There is a broad differential for anxiety in the elderly. One of the first diagnoses that must be considered is depression. Upward of 70% of elderly individuals with major depression will also experience considerable anxiety. Situational anxiety originating from any one of the many psychosocial changes experienced by the elderly can manifest as an adjustment disorder with predominant anxiety symptoms. Numerous medical illnesses also can cause anxiety symptoms (Table 11–2).

Although anxiety is a common complaint in the elderly, new-onset anxiety disorders are not frequently diagnosed. A disorder such as obsessive–compulsive disorder may be present for many years, but not reveal itself to others until later in life.

Disorders such as generalized anxiety disorder (GAD), obsessive–compulsive disorder, and panic disorder, while not uncommon in the elderly (up to 7% of the elderly may have GAD), rarely begin in old age. Most patients begin to develop their symptoms within the first three or four decades of life. Posttraumatic stress disorder can be common in specific cohorts, such as concentration-camp survivors, and might develop de novo following the traumatic death of a spouse. The exception to this rule may be specific phobias, which may be experienced by 7% of men and 14% of women older than age 65 within a 6-month period. The most common phobia in the elderly who seek psychi-

Table 11–2 **Medical Causes of Anxiety Symptoms in the Elderly**

Cardiopulmonary

Anemia
Angina pectoris
Arrhythmias
Chronic obstructive lung disease
Pulmonary infections
Pulmonary embolus
Valvular heart disease

Endocrine and Metabolic

Hyperthyroidism
Hypocalcemia
Hypoglycemia
Hypoparathyroidism
Vitamin deficiencies (B_{12}, folate)

Neurological

Encephalopathies (infectious, metabolic, toxic)
Delirium

Substance related

Stimulants
  Caffeine
  Nicotine
Prescription and over-the-counter drugs
  Antihypertensives
  Decongestants
  Digitalis
  Theophylline
Withdrawal syndromes
  Alcohol
  Narcotics
  Sedative hypnotics

atric help is agoraphobia, which can often worsen the social isolation to which the elderly are prone. When elderly patients complain of anxiety, depression should be at the top of the clinician's differential diagnosis. The same may be said when elderly patients complain of insomnia.

Somatoform Disorders

Like those with primary anxiety disorders, most patients with somatoform disorders begin to experience them well before late life. While somatizing behavior, including the expression of anxious and depressive symptoms as somatic complaints, may increase with aging, new-onset somatoform disorders are uncommon in old age. Delusional disorders with predominately somatic symptoms occur in the elderly, but in these conditions, the complaints are more bizarre and lack the initial plausibility of those voiced in somatoform disorders. In those individuals with persistent somatoform disorders that started earlier in life, the particular complaints, especially in somatization disorder and hypochondriasis, may change over the course of middle age and late life. Elderly patients with somatization disorder will focus less on sexual function and more on gastrointestinal distress. Elderly hypochondriacs may voice the unfounded conviction that they have a dementia (see also Chapter 9). Hypochondriacal complaints are extremely common as secondary symptoms of depression in the elderly.

Substance Abuse

Alcoholism

Although alcoholism has no clear definition in any age group, it is clear that alcohol abuse is a common problem in the elderly. Five percent of the elderly population in the community may meet the criteria for alcohol dependence, and twice as many drink alcohol in an abusive fashion. According to self-reports, 10 to 20% of the elderly drink daily, up to 25% have five to seven drinks a week, and 7 to 8% have between 12 and 21 drinks a week. One-fifth of elderly medical and psychiatric patients may be problem drinkers, as are as many as 45% of patients admitted to acute geriatric psychiatric units (Liberto et al, 1992).

Despite this evidence of continued problem drinking throughout life, the actual incidence in cross-sectional studies declines sharply after the age of 70. Possible reasons for this decrease include an increased mortality in problem drinkers at ages younger than 70 or a cohort effect, since many of those who are currently in their 70s and 80s grew up during the Prohibition era and may have always had a lower prevalence of problem drinking.

Because of the alterations in ethanol metabolism that accompany aging, a given amount of alcohol will produce a higher blood alcohol level in an older person than in a younger one. Additionally, the brain and other organs become increasingly sensitive to the effects of alcohol. As a result, it is fairly common for a person to maintain a constant level of alcohol consumption over many years and only begin to have problems such as confusion, depression, or hepatic dysfunction after age 60.

Confounding the recognition of alcoholism in the elderly is the fact that many of the diagnostic criteria for alcohol abuse and dependence involve features that may not apply to aging individuals. Largely because of retirement, the elderly are not likely to suffer occupational problems due to their drinking. They are also less likely to suffer legal consequences. Changes in their behavior such as confusion, self-neglect, malnutrition, and depression may be improperly dismissed as "normal" aging (Bienenfeld, 1990). Using standardized screening tests also may be ineffective. Tests that identify 60% of subjects under the age of 60 as alcohol abusers identify only 37% of those over the age of 60 who abuse alcohol (Liberto et al, 1992).

There are, nonetheless, serious medical, social, and psychiatric complications from alcohol abuse in the elderly. Compared with elderly subjects who do not abuse alcohol, those who do are more likely to commit suicide, live alone, and have serious health problems such as hepatic, pulmonary, and cardiovascular diseases. Fifteen percent of those elderly who present to emergency rooms with depression or confusion develop these conditions as a result of alcohol use.

Four out of five geriatric patients who abuse alcohol and have evidence of depression are experiencing a depression due to their alcohol use. Up to 60% of older alcoholics will fit the criteria for dementia. They suffer difficulty because of the direct toxic effects of alcohol on the central nervous system or exacerbations of other causes of dementia. Alcohol can exacerbate the changes in sleep and sexual function that normally accompany aging. It can also interact with over 150 prescribed medications, including anticoagulants, phenytoin, sedatives, and antidepressants (Bienenfeld, 1990).

Treatment of elderly alcoholics is similar to the treatment of their younger counterparts with only slight differences. Detoxification will more frequently require hospitalization because of concern for autonomic and cardiovascular instability. Because of the particular risk of delirium, it is also generally recommended that they not receive prophylactic benzodiazepines unless they have a history of complicated alcohol withdrawal. If these agents are required, lorazepam and oxazepam are generally preferred because of their rapid hepatic oxidation. Disulfiram, which can be used to discourage alcohol consumption in younger patients, is not recommended in the elderly because it may react with numerous drugs besides alcohol, and the elderly can experience severe and even life-threatening reactions.

Abuse of Other Substances

The use of illicit drugs such as narcotics and hallucinogens is not generally a significant problem in the elderly. Much more common is the abuse of prescription and over-the-counter medications. The average American senior citizen receives 3.6 prescriptions a year for psychotropic medications alone. Sixty-two percent of the elderly use at least one prescription medication daily. The elderly often will have multiple providers who are not fully aware of what other medications are being prescribed. Since some elderly individuals tend to hoard pills, trade medications, and take their medications in a nonprescribed manner, the situation is ripe for abuse.

Over-the-counter medications also represent a problem for the elderly. Sixty-nine percent of people over 65 take at least one over-the-counter medication a day. Many of these can interact with alcohol or other medications that the patient is taking. Since these medications are not prescribed, many people do not consider them drugs and will not volunteer them when asked about medications. Over-the-counter cold remedies often include ingredients that can induce delirium (such as sleeping pills that have anticholinergic effects), as can nonsteroidal antiinflammatory drugs. Laxatives, which are taken weekly by one-third of the population over 65, can result in diarrhea, malabsorption, and even hypokalemia. The practitioner is thus well advised to inquire about over-the-counter medications in evaluating the elderly patient (Bienenfeld, 1990). Always ask about the contents of the patient's medicine chest, cabinet, or pill box.

Personality Disorders

The basic characteristics of individuals with personality disorders are evident early in adult life and are manifest in long-standing patterns of maladaptive perception, communication, and behavior. People do not develop personality disorders in late life, but the characteristic features of these disorders do change over time within individuals. In general, the behavior of individuals with narcissistic, borderline, and histrionic personality disorders becomes less intense with age. Some belated maturation may occur, impulsive actions may become incompatible with the geriatric lifestyle, and early mortality from hazardous behaviors may eliminate those with the most severe personality pathology.

Before making a new diagnosis of a personality disorder in an older patient, one should assess carefully and treat aggressively Axis I disorders, particularly depressive disorders and substance abuse. The influence of a hostile environment in which the patient may live might temper the clinician's interpretation of ideas that sound unusually suspicious. Psychotherapy (see below) is the optimal treatment for personality disorders at any age; in late life, it is particularly important to make sure the therapeutic goals of the therapy are matched to the patient's resources and life circumstances.

TREATMENT

Pharmacotherapy

Although caution must be used whenever medications are prescribed, there are some special considerations in the use of psychotropic medications in the elderly. Because most elderly psychiatric patients will already be receiving some medication for somatic disorders, their drug regimens may become quite confusing, and the clinician must carefully consider the possible drug interactions and additive side effects of any proposed new medication. Additionally, noncompliance becomes a problem when the reasons for the medication and the prescribed dosing schedule are poorly understood. Cognitive impairment may mandate that a third party set up or administer the medications.

Certain alterations in metabolism and sensitivity occur with aging. There is a decrease in the lean body mass and total body water along with an increase in body fat. These changes decrease the volume of distribution of hydrophilic drugs such as alcohol and increase the volume of distribution of lipophilic drugs such as benzodiazepines, accounting for the relative increase in blood alcohol content and the decreased clearance of benzodiazepines in the elderly user. Hepatic metabolism decreases, in general, with age, as does the production of albumin. The former effect results in a generalized slowing of hepatic clearance, and the latter effect can cause a relative increase in the free fraction of drugs such as tricyclic antidepressants, which are largely protein bound. Receptor sensitivity seems to change with age, causing older patients to be more sensitive to the therapeutic and adverse effects of medications.

Drugs for Psychosis

Antipsychotics such as the phenothiazines remain the drugs of choice for psychosis of virtually any etiology. As no one class of antipsychotics appears more effective than the others, they are generally selected on the basis of their side-effect profile. The high-potency drugs such as haloperidol are widely used in aged patients because of their relatively low anticholinergic and antiadrenergic effects. Antipsychotics seem to be equally effective throughout life, but the risks of extrapyramidal symptoms such as akathisia and parkinsonism increase with age. Lower potency agents, such as thioridazine, minimize the risk of extrapyramidal effects, but are potently anticholinergic, producing constipation, postural hypotension, and cognitive impairment. Medium-potency agents, such as perphenazine, provide a reasonable compromise, allowing the clinician to modify the regimen according to observed effects, moving to a higher potency drug if anticholinergic or sedative effects predominate or to a lower potency drug if parkinsonian symptoms appear.

The atypical antipsychotics have found some use in aging patients. Because older patients with chronic psychotic conditions frequently exhibit tardive dyskinesia, clozapine has proved to be of some value because it does not exacerbate tardive dyskinesia and may even improve movement symptoms. It is quite sedating and highly anticholinergic; it also carries a risk of agranulocytosis. Olanzapine is slightly less sedating and anticholinergic, with no particular risk of blood dyscrasia, and its efficacy in tardive dyskinesia is comparable to that of clozapine. Risperidone has little sedation or anticholinergic effect; in doses under 4 mg/day, it does not cause parkinsonian side effects. Experience with newer atypical antipsychotics, such as quetiepine and sertindole, in the elderly is as of yet limited. Sertindole has been reported to prolong the QT_c interval on the EKG, making use of this drug in elderly cardiac patients potentially problematic.

Drugs for Mood Disorders

For depression in the elderly, the selective serotonin-reuptake inhibitors (SSRIs) have assumed a place as the first-line agents. Fluoxetine, sertraline, and paroxetine appear to be nearly as effective as the tricyclic antidepressants (see below) and, with the exception of paroxetine, have almost no anticholinergic or cardiovascular side effects. In general, they are well tolerated by the elderly. Fluoxetine may produce agitation and anorexia and has an active metabolite with a half-life of 10 to 14 days. The slightly stimulating effects of the SSRIs may be desirable in the patient with a retarded depression. Sertraline and paroxetine have half-lives of 24 hours or less. Sertraline produces little or no sedation. Paroxetine is mildly sedating and moderately anticholinergic.

The tricyclic antidepressants have been traditional choices for geriatric depression and are probably more effective than the SSRIs in hospitalized elders with agitated melancholic depressions (Roose et al, 1994). Secondary amines, such as desipramine and nortriptyline, are equally effective and have fewer toxic side effects than the older tertiary amines, such as imipramine and amitriptyline. The latter category of tricyclic antidepressants produce anticholinergic effects and orthostatic hypotension that may outweigh their therapeutic benefit. Although average therapeutic doses of antidepressants decrease with age, the range of therapeutic plasma levels does not. Once therapeutic plasma levels are attained, therapy may need to be maintained for 4 to 8 weeks before maximum clinical benefit is observed.

Although it has been traditional to reduce the dose of antidepressant for maintenance after remission of an acute depressive episode, there is no empirical support for this practice. The effective acute antidepressant dose is also the effective maintenance dose (Frank, 1994). For a first episode of major depression, therapy should be continued for at least one year or longer before a taper is considered. Indications for longer term maintenance treatment (i.e., 1 year to lifetime) are listed in Table 11–3 (Depression Guideline Panel, 1993).

Of the many tricyclic antidepressant side effects that occur in the elderly, two of the more troubling are confusion, which often is related to the anticholinergic effect, and hypotension due to antiadrenergic effects, which can result in dangerous and even life-threatening falls. Cognitive impairment can develop in up to 35% of patients over the age of 40 who are placed on tertiary amines. In comparison, a study that looked at nortriptyline in the elderly over a 7-week trial found no cognitive changes. In general, the tertiary amines are the most likely to cause orthostatic hypotension, whereas nortriptyline is the least likely. Even nortriptyline, however, caused an average decrease of systolic blood pressure of 9 mm Hg in elderly patients. This orthostasis seems to develop within the first week of therapy and does not correlate well with plasma levels of medication or symptomatic complaints. Tricyclic blood levels also can be altered by many medications. Concurrent use of antipsychotics, fluoxetine, paroxetine, cimetidine, methylphenidate, thiazide diuretics, estrogen, and erythromycin tend to increase serum levels; anticonvulsants, barbiturates, vitamin C, and doxycycline tend to decrease levels. For all these reasons, tri-

Table 11–3 **Indications for Maintenance Antidepressant Therapy**

1. Three or more lifetime episodes of major depression
2. Two or more episodes of major depression and one of:
   a. Family history of bipolar disorder
   b. History of recurrence within 1 year or less after previously effective antidepressant was discontinued
   c. Family history of recurrent major depression
   d. First episode before age 20
   e. Both episodes were severe, sudden, or life threatening in the past 3 years

(From Depression Guideline Panel: Depression in Primary Care, Vol. 2. Treatment of Major Depression. Rockville, MD, US Department of Health and Human Services, 1993)

cyclic antidepressants and their side effects need to be closely monitored in the elderly (McCue, 1992).

Trazodone (a heterocyclic antidepressant) has little anticholinergic effect, moderate antiadrenergic effect, and significant sedative effects. It can be useful in the depressed patient with significant agitation, anxiety, or insomnia. Most clinicians view trazodone as a relatively "weak" antidepressant in which high doses, which elderly patients may not tolerate, are needed to achieve a therapeutic response. Monoamine oxidase inhibitors (MAOIs) are used with elderly patients on occasion and appear to be particularly effective in those who complain of decreased energy or motivation or who are less severely depressed. Caution must be exercised in their use, however, as they can agitate demented patients and can cause autonomic instability. Patients often will have difficulty with orthostatic hypotension while on MAOIs. Compliance with the tyramine-restricted diet required for MAOI therapy may be difficult for the cognitively impaired elder or for someone who depends on others to provide meals.

Psychostimulants such as dextroamphetamine and methylphenidate are used by some physicians in the treatment of their elderly depressed patients. These medications can be used to treat those patients who have prominent medical illnesses and cannot tolerate tricyclic antidepressants or who display prominent lethargy and apathy. One of the great benefits of these medicines is the rapidity of their therapeutic activity. Although stimulants improve depressive symptoms quickly in many individuals, their effect on the core depressive illness has never been demonstrated, and their long-term usefulness is controversial. The antidepressant bupropion, which has stimulant properties, should be used first if psychostimulants are being considered for long-term treatment (see Chapter 18). Bupropion has almost no cardiovascular side effects.

Aging bipolar patients continue to require treatment as they can experience both manic and depressive episodes throughout their life. Lithium may be used for acute manic episodes and for prophylaxis, although intolerance of lithium's side effects increase with age. The elderly are more sensitive to the effects of lithium, but can often be managed with serum levels of 0.4 to 0.7 mEq/L. The decrease in renal functioning that occurs with aging slows the elimination of lithium, increasing its half-life from 18 hours at age 20 to 36 hours by age 70 (Jenike, 1989). As a result, the serum lithium levels of an elderly patient can be two or even three times higher than a younger patient's after taking equal doses of the medication. The elderly are more sensitive to the toxic effects of lithium and can experience difficulty with doses that are considered routine in younger patients. Patients should be periodically assessed for tremor, nausea, diarrhea, and memory deficits. Numerous drugs that the elderly commonly use, such as nonsteroidal antiinflammatory drugs and thiazide diuretics, can also raise the serum lithium level and induce lithium toxicity.

Since lithium can be so problematic to use in the elderly, and since the likelihood of symptomatic breakthrough increases with the duration of bipolar illness, anticonvulsants, such as vulproate, have become increasingly accepted agents for mania in the elderly. Available information suggests that these drugs may be useful in those elderly patients who cannot tolerate lithium or for whom lithium has lost some of its prophylactic benefit (Alexopoulos, 1996). Generally, valproate is much better tolerated than carbamazepine and is more likely to maintain its benefit without breakthrough symptoms of mania.

Drugs for Anxiety

Benzodiazepines have traditionally been overprescribed for the elderly, and care needs to be taken that these medications are prescribed only when truly indicated. For adjustment disorders that manifest with anxiety, they typically should be prescribed for only 1 to 2 months and then tapered off and discontinued. Long-term therapy with benzodiazepines is indicated only when there are clear chronic symptoms. Drugs with long half-lives and active metabolites such as diazepam and chlordiazepoxide should be avoided. These medications tend to accumulate and cause oversedation and confusion, which is very slow to clear. The very high potency, short half-life drugs such as alprazolam and triazolam also should be avoided as their use has been related to cognitive impairment. The shorter half-life of these drugs also leaves the elderly patient prone to experience withdrawal when discontinuation is attempted. Drugs such as lorazepam and oxazepam, which are more rapidly and simply metabolized, are generally the drugs of choice in the elderly. Even with these agents, the elderly are more prone to side effects such as sedation, confusion, and memory disturbance.

Buspirone is a nonbenzodiazepine anxiolytic that has demonstrated safety and efficacy in the elderly. It differs from the benzodiazepines clinically in that it may take 3 to 6 weeks of therapy before the patient's anxiety diminishes. Elderly patients appear to require the same dosages of buspirone as younger patients, approximately 15 to 40 mg a day given in divided doses (Fernandez et al, 1995).

Psychotherapy

For much of the early history of psychiatry, elderly patients were not considered appropriate candidates for psychotherapy. During that time, psychoanalysis was essentially the only method available and individuals over the age of 40 were seen as too close to death and too rigid in their personality structure to benefit. As the scope of psychotherapy has broadened, the prospect of treating elderly patients has been reexamined. In fact, the aging process brings about a number of challenges and issues that could be best dealt with by psychotherapy.

The aging person needs to deal with the changing environment around her or him and shifting societal expectations. Retirement, changes in financial status, the loss of loved ones, and decreased social support can threaten the elderly person. The patient also may experience changes in the family role as parent, grandparent, and spouse or widow/widower. Those who obtained self-esteem from their work roles or their roles as parents must begin to find other sources for this esteem. Dependency issues begin to surface as aging individuals find themselves less able to control the environment. Failing health and approaching death also are universal issues that will need to be dealt with in some way. In addition, advancing age can bring an increased awareness of abilities that were not utilized, goals that were not actively pursued, or personality features that were left underdeveloped.

Grief and loss are central issues in much of the psychotherapy of older persons. From a psychodynamic perspective, the therapeutic task is to identify the particular meaning of the loss to the individual and to find less distressing ways to cope. For example, a man who is embittered in his retirement may come to discover through therapy that he had tied his entire sense of self-worth to his business accomplishments. He then can use the psychotherapy as a forum for exploring other sources of self-esteem. From a more behavioral perspective, the objective is to redirect energy and activity to pursuits more likely to foster emotional recovery so that the same retiree might be encouraged to participate in church activities or to engage regularly with his grandchildren.

Group therapy directly lessens the elder's sense of isolation. The patient is encouraged to practice social and communicative skills in a nonthreatening environment. Feedback concerning communication and behavior is received from peers and not just from the therapist, who might be significantly younger than the patient. The group environment also tends to increase self-esteem by allowing the patient to help others with their problems. To be an appropriate member, the patient must be able to make meaningful relationships, be motivated to participate in the group, and be cognitively able to follow the conversation and group interactions.

Despite the increased mobility of our society, families continue to play a pivotal role in the life of the elderly. Almost 10% of American homes contain family members from three generations, and 82% of geriatric Americans live within 30 minutes of one of their children. Over half of elderly Americans have contact with their families more than twice a week, and families provide more than 80% of social support services for their elderly members. Families thus can be a part of the therapy and more than just sources of information. The clinician helps the family identify and clarify the problems and frame them into managable terms. A statement such as "My children don't care for me" may be reformulated as "I wish you would visit me more often." Solutions then are crafted in measurable dimensions to address the mutually identified problem.

Typically, too, children overcome the loss of parents more quickly than elders recover from the loss of spouses. There may come a period months after a death when the adult children avoid contact with the still grieving parent or make comments such as "You should be over that by now." Education to families about the time course of grieving in later life can prevent the mourning from becoming complicated by guilt and isolation from family.

CLINICAL PEARLS

- Any acute or subacute change in cognition is pathological and needs to be evaluated carefully, not dismissed as just "normal aging."
- Major depression and anxiety in the elderly are frequently secondary to physical illness, drug effects, and alcoholism. These disorders must be sought carefully when evaluating an elderly individual with depression or anxiety.
- Although the new onset of schizophrenia in the elderly is uncommon, persistence of schizophrenic signs and symptoms is very common.
- The elderly with sensory impairment are more prone to experience delusional disorders.
- Because of alterations in metabolism and increased sensitivity to the therapeutic and side effects of medication, the elderly generally require less medication for the same symptoms, but dosage must be judged on an individual basis.
- The dose of antidepressant that gets the patient well is the dose that keeps the patient well.
- A person who has not changed a lifelong pattern of alcohol use may first begin to have alcohol-related problems, including depression and cognitive impairment, in later life.

ANNOTATED BIBLIOGRAPHY

Bienenfeld D (ed): Verwoerdt's Clinical Geropsychiatry, 3rd ed. Baltimore, Williams & Wilkins, 1990

This book provides comprehensive and readable chapters on most of the major areas in geriatric psychiatry. In particular, the chapters on the psychology of aging, the evaluation of the elderly patient, psychopharmacology, and substance abuse in the elderly are of interest for those who will deal with the elderly on a regular basis, regardless of specialty.

Copeland JRM, Abou-Saleh MT, Blazer DG (eds): Principles and Practice of Geriatric Psychiatry. New York, John Wiley & Sons, 1994

Written from a more international perspective than most texts in the United States, this voluminous work features 148 chapters examining the field of geriatric psychiatry in both depth and breadth. The style varies from enjoyable to turgid, but few references are as informative as this one.

Fernandez F, Levy JK, Lachar BL, Small GW: The management of depression and anxiety in the elderly. J Clin Psychiatry 56(suppl 2):20–29, 1995

In a brief yet thorough review, the authors cover the two most common emotional disorders in geriatric psychiatry. The material is useful for nonpsychiatrists.

Sadavoy J, Lazarus LW, Jarvik LF, Grossberg GT (eds): Comprehensive Review of Geriatric Psychiatry—II. Washington, DC, American Psychiatric Press, 1996

This volume is a useful reference book, featuring 37 chapters on the most important aspects of the field, presented in a factual style by the nation's leading authorities. Self-assessment questions complete the cycle of learning.

Stoudemire A, Fogul BF (eds): Psychopharmacology in the Medically Ill in Psychiatric Cure of the Medical Patient. New York, Oxford University Press, 1993

A comprehensive review of the use of psychotropic drugs in the medically ill, including geriatric patients.

Tran-Johnson TK, Krull AJ, Jeste DV: Late life schizophrenia and its treatment: pharmacologic issues in older schizophrenic patients. Clin Geriatr Med 8:401–410, 1992

> A useful overview of schizophrenia in older patients, including late-onset schizophrenia, which also discusses some of the pharmacokinetic and pharmacodynamic changes that accompany aging.

REFERENCES

Alexopoulos GS: Affective disorders. In J Sadavoy, LW Lazarus, LF Jarvik, GT Grossberg (eds): Comprehensive Review of Geriatric Psychiatry—II, pp 563–592. Washington, DC, American Psychiatric Press, 1996

Alexopoulos GS, Chester JG: Outcomes of geriatric depression. Clin Geriatr Med 8:363–376, 1992

Baldwin R, Jolley D: The prognosis of depression in old age. Br J Psychiatry 149:574–583, 1986

Bienenfeld D (ed): Verwoerdt's Clinical Geropsychiatry, 3rd ed. Baltimore, Williams & Wilkins, 1990

Borson S: Psychiatric problems in the medically ill elderly. In HI Kaplan, BJ Sadock (eds): Comprehensive Textbook of Psychiatry, 6th ed. Vol. 2, p 2586. Baltimore, Williams & Wilkins, 1995

Christenson R, Blazer D: Epidemiology of persecutory ideation in an elderly population in the community. Am J Psychiatry 141:1088–1091, 1984

Clarfield AM: The reversible dementias: do they reverse? Ann Intern Med 109:476–486, 1988

Cohen CI: Outcome of schizophrenia into later life: an overview. Gerontologist 30:790–797, 1990

Depression Guideline Panel: Depression in Primary Care, Vol. 2, Treatment of Major Depression. Public Health Service Agency for Health Care Policy and Research, AHCPR publication no. 93-0551. Rockville, MD, US Department of Health and Human Services, 1993

Erikson EH: Identity and the Life Cycle. New York, International Universities Press, 1959

Fernandez F, Levy JK, Lachar BL, Small GW: The management of depression and anxiety in the elderly. J Clin Psychiatry 56(suppl 2):20–29, 1995

Finch EJL, Ramsay R, Kalona CLE: Depression and physical illness in the elderly. Clin Geriatr Med 8:275–287, 1992

Frank E: Long-term prevention of recurrences in elderly patients. In LS Schnieder, CF Reynolds, BD Lebowitz et al. (eds): Diagnosis and Treatment of Depression in Late Life, pp 317–329. Washington, DC, American Psychiatric Press, 1994

Harris MJ, Jeste DV: Late onset schizophrenia: an overview. Schizophr Bull 14:39–55, 1988

Jenike MA: Geriatric Psychiatry and Psychopharmacology: A Clinical Approach. Chicago, Year Book Medical Publishers, 1989

Liberto JG, Oslin DW, Ruskin PE: Alcoholism in older persons: a review of the literature. Hosp Community Psychiatry 43:975–984, 1992

McCue RE: Using tricyclic antidepressants in the elderly. Clin Geriatr Med 8:323–334, 1992

Meyers BS: Geriatric delusional depression. Clin Geriatr Med 8:299–308, 1992

Murphy E: The prognosis of depression in old age. Br J Psychiatry 142:111–119, 1983

Pearlson GD, Kreger L, Rabins PV, et al: A chart review study of late-onset and early-onset schizophrenia. Am J Psychiatry 146:1568–1574, 1989

Ritchie K, Kildea D: Is senile dementia "age-related" or "ageing-related"?—evidence from meta-analysis of dementia prevalence in the oldest old. Lancet 346:931–934, 1995

Rockwood K, Stadnyk K: The prevalence of dementia in the elderly: a review. Can J Psychiatry 39:253–257, 1994

Roose SP, Glassman AH, Attia E, et al: Comparative efficacy of selective serotonin reuptake inhibitors and tricyclics in the treatment of melancholia. Am J Psychiatry 151:1735–1739, 1994

Skoog I, Nilsson L, Palmertz B, Andreasson L, Svanborg A: A population-based study of dementia in 85-year-olds. N Engl J Med 328:153–158, 1993

Steiner D, Marcopulos B: Depression in the elderly. Nursing Clin North Am 26:585–600, 1991

Tran-Johnson TK, Krull AJ, Jeste DV: Late life schizophrenia and its treatment: pharmacologic issues in older schizophrenic patients. Clin Geriatr Med 8:401–410, 1992

Winstead DK, Mielke DH, O'Neill PT: Diagnosis and treatment of depression in the elderly: a review. Psychiatr Med 8:85–98, 1990

Young RC: Geriatric mania. Clin Geriatr Med 8:387–399, 1992

12 *Eating Disorders*

Joel Yager

Cases of women who starved themselves have been reported for hundreds of years, including cases of *anorexia mirabilis* in sainted women of the Middle Ages and of notorious "fasting girls" of the 16th through 19th centuries. Anorexia nervosa, as we now recognize it, was first described in the late 1870s; interest in the eating disorders has grown considerably over the past two decades. The death of the 1970s popular singer Karen Carpenter from anorexia nervosa in 1983 resulted in a flood of television programs and magazine articles that brought considerable attention to the eating disorders. After popular magazines featured articles suggesting that several female idols, including Jane Fonda, Olympic gymnast Cathy Rigby, and even the tragically deceased Princess Diana of England, may have suffered from anorexia nervosa and/or bulimia nervosa, virtually every female in the United States became aware of the existence of these disorders and their attendant dangers. Binge eating disorder, similar in many respects to what has been often referred to as "compulsive overeating," has been added to the *Diagnostic and Statistical Manual,* 4th ed. (DSM-IV; American Psychiatric Association 1994) as a potential diagnosis worthy of additional study. Many patients seen in practice who may not meet the strict diagnostic criteria for any single one of these disorders, but who present with variations of the psychological and behavioral signs and symptoms described below, are considered to have Eating Disorders Not Otherwise Specified. These patients merit careful assessment and, depending on their specific problems and impairments, management consisting of strategies used for the other disorders.

EPIDEMIOLOGY

Current studies suggest that among adolescent and young adult women in certain high school and college settings, the prevalence of clinically significant eating disorders is about 4% and for more broadly defined syndromes may be as high as 8% (Kendler et al, 1991). Individual symptoms of eating disorders are relatively common and include body image distortion; extreme fear of being fat out of line with health concerns; the desire to reduce body fat to levels below those ordinarily considered healthy; restrictive and fad dieting; amphetamine and cocaine use for anorectic effects; purging by means of vomiting, laxative abuse, or diuretic abuse; and excessive or compulsive exercise among normal-weight and even underweight individuals (Drewnowski et al, 1988). Some of these general symptoms may even be seen in the majority of certain subgroups of the female population, as in select college sororities or among female dance majors.

Males with anorexia nervosa and bulimia form the minority of cases. Ninety to 95% of cases are female. The age of onset is most typically in the teenage and early adult years, but cases with prepubertal onset and with onset in the 40s and older have been reported. Although these disorders were previously associated primarily with the upper and upper-middle social classes and almost exclusively with Caucasians, more recent data suggest that these disorders are now well represented among middle- and lower-middle-class women, including nonwhites.

Binge eating disorder has been reported in 1 to 4% of nonpatient community samples. Although, as with other eating disorders, binge eating disorder is more common among females, males constitute about 35% of sufferers, a higher percentage than in other eating disorders. Binge eating disorder is quite common among overweight individuals seeking treatment. It has been estimated that about 70% of participants in Overeaters Anonymous and 30% of participants in weight loss programs suffer from binge eating disorder (Devlin, 1996; de Zwann et al, 1992).

DESCRIPTION, DIAGNOSTIC CRITERIA, AND DIFFERENTIAL DIAGNOSIS

Diagnostic criteria for the eating disorders have been the subject of much discussion and are shown in Table 12–1 (American Psychiatric Association, 1994). Primary symptoms for both *anorexia nervosa* and *bulimia nervosa* are a preoccupation with weight and the desire to be thinner. The two disorders are *not* mutually exclusive, and there appears to be a continuum among patients of the two symptom complexes of self-starvation and the binge–purge cycle: about 50% of patients with anorexia nervosa will also have bulimia nervosa, and many patients with bulimia nervosa may previously have had at least a subclinical form of anorexia nervosa.

Table 12–1 **Diagnostic Criteria for Anorexia Nervosa and Bulimia Nervosa***

Anorexia Nervosa

A. Refusal to maintain body weight at or above a minimally normal weight for age and height (e.g., weight loss leading to maintenance of body weight less than 85% of that expected; or failure to make expected weight gain during the period of growth, leading to body weight less than 85% of that expected).

B. Intense fear of gaining weight or becoming fat, even though underweight.

C. Disturbance in the way in which one's body weight or shape is experienced; undue influence of body weight or shape on self-evaluation, or denial of the seriousness of the current low body weight.

D. In postmenstrual females, amenorrhea, i.e., the absence of at least three consecutive menstrual cycles. (A woman is considered to have amenorrhea if periods occur only following hormone, e.g., estrogen, administration.)

Specify type:

Restricting Type: during the current episode of Anorexia Nervosa, the person has not regularly engaged in binge eating or purging behavior (i.e., self-induced vomiting or the misuse of laxatives, diuretics, or enemas)

Binge Eating/Purging Type: during the current episode of Anorexia Nervosa, the person has regularly engaged in binge eating or purging behavior (i.e., self-induced vomiting or the misuse of laxatives, diuretics, or enemas)

Bulimia Nervosa

A. Recurrent episodes of binge eating. An episode of binge eating is characterized by both of the following:

(1) eating, in a discrete period of time (e.g., within any 2-hour period), an amount of food that is definitely larger than most people would eat during a similar period of time and under similar circumstances

(2) a sense of lack of control over eating during the episode (e.g., a feeling that one cannot stop eating or control what or how much one is eating)

B. Recurrent inappropriate compensatory behavior in order to prevent weight gain, such as self-induced vomiting; misuse of laxatives, diuretics, enemas, or other medications; fasting; or excessive exercise.

C. The binge eating and inappropriate compensatory behaviors both occur, on average, at least twice a week for 3 months.

D. Self-evaluation is unduly influenced by body shape and weight.

E. The disturbance does not occur exclusively during episodes of Anorexia Nervosa.

Specify type:

Purging Type: during the current episode of Bulimia Nervosa, the patient has regularly engaged in self-induced vomiting or the misuse of laxatives, diuretics, or enemas

Nonpurging Type: during the current episode of Bulimia Nervosa, the person has used other inappropriate compensatory behaviors, such as fasting or excessive exercise, but has not regularly engaged in self-induced vomiting or the misuse of laxatives, diuretics, or enemas

* DSM-IV criteria (American Psychiatric Association, 1994).

Anorexia Nervosa

Although the diagnosis of anorexia nervosa requires a loss of weight of at least 15% below normal, many patients have lost considerably more by the time they come to medical attention. Patients engage in a variety of behaviors designed to lose weight. In addition to markedly reduced caloric intake—

usually in the range of 300 to 600 KCalories/day—strange dietary rituals include the refusal to eat in front of others, avoidance of entire classes of food, and unusual spice and flavoring practices (such as putting huge quantities of pepper or lemon juice on all foods). Some exercise compulsively for hours each day; non-eating-related compulsions such as cleaning and counting rituals are not uncommon. Although patients may initially seem cheerful and energetic, about half will develop an accompanying major depression, and all will become moody and irritable. A lifetime prevalence of obsessive–compulsive disorder of 25% has been reported in anorexia nervosa (Halmi et al, 1991). Many complain of having no real sense of themselves apart from the anorexia nervosa. Weight losses of 30 to 40% below normal are not unusual. Accompanying these losses are signs and symptoms indicative of the physical complications of starvation: depletion of fat, muscle wasting (including cardiac muscle loss in severe cases), bradycardia and other arrhythmias, constipation, abdominal pains, leukopenia, hypercortisolemia, osteoporosis, and in extreme cases the development of cachexia and lanugo (fine baby-like hair over the body). Metabolic alterations that conserve energy are seen in thyroid function (low T3 syndrome) and reproductive function, with a marked drop or halt in luteinizing hormone (LH) and follicle-stimulating hormone (FSH) secretion. All female patients stop menstruating; up to a third stop menstruating even before losing sufficient body fat to account for the onset of amenorrhea. Osteopenia is often noted after only 6 months of amenorrhea. Since anorexia nervosa often begins in the early to midteens, during the peak age of bone formation, the risk of osteoporosis is significant. Anorexia nervosa patients in their mid-20s have seven times the rate of pathological stress fractures as age-matched controls (Rigotti et al, 1984, 1991).

Anorexia nervosa appears in two general varieties, the *restricting* and *binge eating/purging* subtypes, although these occasionally may alternate in the same patient. The *restricter* tends to exert maximal self-control regarding food intake and tends to be socially avoidant, withdrawn, and isolated, with an obsessional thinking style and ritualistic behavior in nonfood areas. By contrast, the *bulimic* subtype is unable to restrain herself from frequent food binges and then purges by means of vomiting or ingesting extremely large quantities of laxatives and/or diuretics to further weight loss; the bulimic subtype is also commonly depressed and self-destructive; often displays the emotional, dramatic, and erratic personality cluster; and not infrequently abuses alcohol and drugs.

Full recovery within a few years is seen in 30 to 50% of patients. Younger onset patients and those with the restricter rather than bulimic subtype appear to have a better prognosis. Death from starvation, sudden cardiac arrhythmias, and suicide occurs in 5 to 10% of patients within 10 years and in almost 20% of patients within 20 years of onset (Hsu, 1987; Steinhausen et al, 1991). The death rate for anorexia nervosa has been estimated to be 12 times higher than for age-matched comparison groups of females in the community, and twice as high as for other aged matched groups of female psychiatric patients (Sullivan, 1995).

A CASE STUDY

A 24-year-old graduate student was brought in by her husband at a weight of 76 pounds because she was fainting repeatedly and would not permit herself to eat in spite of his pleas and concerns for her safety. Her height was 5 feet 4 inches, and she had never weighed more than 90 pounds over the past 4 years; she had not had a menstrual period since age 16. She permitted herself to eat only tiny bits of white-colored food and only from someone else's plate. Her exercise pattern included 200 push-ups and sit-ups each morning; if she lost count, she was obliged to start at the beginning. In addition, she swam 32 laps each day in the university's pool. On days when she permitted herself an extra morsel and thereby considered herself to have been "bad" with respect to eating, she would force herself to swim an additional even number of laps in multiples of four, or she would take handfuls of laxatives to induce severe cramps and diarrhea, both as a punishment and to ensure that she lost additional weight. In spite of these limitations, she was able to carry out complex and demanding intellectual assignments in her courses. Under duress, she finally agreed to gain weight, but could do so only by means of an extremely ritualistic diet of carefully measured amounts of cheese and ice cream.

Bulimia Nervosa

This disorder occurs predominantly in weight-preoccupied females (90 to 95%) who engage in marked eating binges and purging episodes at least twice a week for 3 consecutive months. According to the DSM-IV, two subtypes can be distinguished: the *purging type* uses self-induced vomiting or misuses laxatives or diuretics, and the *nonpurging type* uses other inappropriate compensatory behaviors, such as excessive exercise or fasting, but does not ordinarily self-induce vomiting or misuse laxatives or diuretics. Although most patients with bulimia nervosa appear never to have had frank anorexia nervosa, a past history of the disorder or many of its individual features is not uncommon. Patients frequently consume between 5,000 and 10,000 calories per binge, and binge–purge cycles may occur as frequently as several times a day. The patients always feel as if their eating is out of control, feel so ashamed that they're often secretive about their problem, and have a concurrent major depression or anxiety disorder in up to 75% of cases (Johnson and Connors, 1987). Substantially increased rates of anxiety disorders, chemical dependency disorders, and personality disorders have also been reported among bulimia nervosa patients (American Psychiatric Association, 1993).

All patients with a known or suspected eating disorder need a thorough medical evaluation, as well as an assessment of other medical disorders that may cause gastrointestinal symptoms (Table 12–2).

Physical complications of binge–purge cycles include fluid and electrolyte abnormalities with hypochloremic hypokalemic alkalosis, esophageal and gastric irritation and bleeding, large bowel abnormalities due to laxative abuse, marked erosion of dental enamel with accompanying decay, and parotid and salivary gland hypertrophy (squirrel face) with hyperamylasemia of about 25 to 40% over normal values (Mitchell et al, 1987). The medical complications of eating disorders are summarized in Table 12–3.

The disorder is often chronic when untreated, lasting years to decades, but may tend toward slight spontaneous improvement in symptoms (Yager et al, 1988b). Other aspects of outcome are discussed in the treatment section.

A CASE STUDY

An 18-year-old athletically built college freshman had been bulimic since the age of 15, gorging an estimated 5,000 to 20,000 calories of junk food each evening after her family went to bed and vomiting repeatedly when she felt painfully full. The disorder began at a time when her mother became seriously depressed about the deteriorating health of her own alcoholic mother. In addition to feeling out of control and despondent about her eating, the patient had been sexually promiscuous since the age of 16, and since starting college,

---

Table 12–2 **Differential Diagnosis of Binge Eating and Vomiting**

Binge Eating

Bulimia Nervosa
Binge Eating Disorder (in obese or nonobese)
Central nervous system lesions (e.g., Kleine-Levin syndrome, seizures, and rarely tumors)
Appetite increases due to metabolic conditions or drugs
Other psychiatric disorders such as schizophrenia and atypical depression

Vomiting

Self-induced purging in Bulimia Nervosa
Central nervous system causes (e.g., increased intracranial pressure, tumor or seizure disorder)
Gastrointestinal causes (e.g., mechanical obstruction, infections, toxins, metabolic, allergic, "functional")
Migraine
Instrumental (goal-directed) vomiting (e.g., wrestlers before a match to reduce weight)
Endocrine causes (e.g., early pregnancy with "morning sickness," hyperemesis gravidarum)
Psychogenic causes (e.g., other psychiatric disorders such as anxiety, conversion disorders)

Table 12–3 **Medical Complications of Eating Disorders**

Related to Weight Loss

Cachexia: loss of fat, muscle mass, reduced thyroid metabolism (low T3 syndrome), cold intolerance, and difficulty maintaining core body temperature

Cardiac: loss of cardiac muscle, small heart, cardiac arrhythmias including atrial and ventricular premature contractions, prolonged His bundle transmission (prolonged Q-T interval), bradycardia, ventricular tachycardia, sudden death

Digestive/gastrointestinal: delayed gastric emptying, bloating, constipation, abdominal pain

Reproductive: amenorrhea, infertility, low levels of luteinizing hormone (LH) and follicle-stimulating hormone (FSH)

Dermatologic: lanugo (fine babylike hair over body), edema

Hematologic: leukopenia

Neuropsychiatric: abnormal taste sensation (zinc deficiency?), apathetic depression, irritability, obsessional thinking, compulsive behaviors, mild cognitive dysfunction

Skeletal: osteoporosis

Related to Purging (Vomiting and Laxative Abuse)

Metabolic: electrolyte abnormalities, particularly hypokalemic, hypochloremic alkalosis; hypomagnesemia

Digestive/gastrointestinal: salivary gland and pancreatic inflammation and enlargement with increase in serum amylase, esophageal and gastric erosion, dysfunctional bowel with haustral dilitation

Dental: erosion of dental enamel (perimyolysis), particularly of front teeth, with corresponding decay

Neuropsychiatric: seizures (related to large fluid shifts and electrolyte disturbances), mild neuropathies, fatigue and weakness, mild degrees of cognitive dysfunction

---

had been drinking heavily and using cocaine whenever it was available. Treatment ultimately required programs that addressed her substance-abuse problems, as well as the eating and mood disorders.

Binge Eating Disorder

Patients with binge eating disorder typically manifest all the psychological and behavioral aspects of patients with bulimia nervosa, but usually without employing the compensatory behaviors such as vomiting or use of laxatives. Consequently, they tend to be obese, since they do not subject themselves to the self-damaging methods of purging. As the condition is currently construed, binge eating must occur at least twice a week for at least a 6-month period. Eating binges are triggered by dysphoric feelings of tension or distress, boredom, habit, or attempts to diet excessively. Some individuals describe eating to numb themselves emotionally. In comparison with others of similar weight who do not display these patterns, including obese people who are not binge eaters, those with binge eating disorders ordinarily have more self-loathing, depression, anxiety, and interpersonal sensitivity. Onset is usually in the teens or 20s, often occurring after strict attempts to diet. Patients with binge eating disorders are more likely to have comorbid depressive substance abuse and personality disorders than comparison groups of non-binge eating disordered obese persons, but may be less likely to have these comorbid problems than patients with bulimia nervosa (Spitzer et al, 1992, 1993). Suggested research diagnostic criteria are shown in Table 12–4 (American Psychiatric Association, 1994).

A CASE STUDY

A 44-year-old married woman, 5'5" and weighing 150 pounds, complained of being a compulsive overeater for more than 20 years, since shortly after the birth of her first child. Although she weighed only 125 pounds when she got married, she gained 60 pounds during her first pregnancy and was never able to return to her earlier weight in spite of multiple diets using everything from Weight Watchers to very low calorie diets to diet pills. She found herself compulsively eating large quantities of chocolate and pastries, "my downfall," several times a week, whenever she was alone in the house, particularly when she felt stressed or irritable. She felt defeated and demoralized, and had considerable self-hate in relation to her appearance. Although her husband had been generally sup-

---

Table 12–4 Research Criteria for Binge Eating Disorder*

A. Recurrent episodes of binge eating. An episode of binge eating is characterized by both of the following:
  (1) eating, in a discrete period of time (e.g., within any 2-hour period), an amount of food that is definitely larger than most people would eat in a similar period of time under similar circumstances
  (2) a sense of lack of control over eating during the episode (e.g., a feeling that one cannot stop eating or control what or how much one is eating)
B. The binge eating episodes are associated with three (or more) of the following:
  (1) eating much more rapidly than normal
  (2) eating until feeling uncomfortably full
  (3) eating large amounts of food when not feeling physically hungry
  (4) eating alone because of being embarrassed by how much one is eating
  (5) feeling disgusted with oneself, depressed, or very guilty after overeating
C. Marked distress regarding binge eating is present
D. The binge eating occurs, on average, at least 2 days a week for 6 months
  Note: The method of determining frequency differs from that used for Bulimia Nervosa; future research should address whether the preferred method of setting a frequency threshold is counting the number of days on which binges occur or counting the number of episodes of binge eating.
E. The binge eating is not associated with the regular use of inappropriate compensatory behaviors (e.g., purging, fasting, excessive exercise) and does not occur exclusively during the course of Anorexia Nervosa or Bulimia Nervosa.

* DSM-IV criteria (Appendix B, American Psychiatric Association, 1994).

portive, she felt that he was starting to make snide remarks about her figure and her "inability to control yourself," and she feared for her marriage.

ETIOLOGY AND PATHOGENESIS

Theories regarding the etiology and pathogenesis of the eating disorders have implicated virtually every level of biopsychosocial organization.

Biological Theories

Several biological causes have been proposed. One popular theory posits the presence of a hypothalamic or suprahypothalamic abnormality to account for the profound disturbances seen in eating disorder patients in the secretion of LH, FSH, cortisol, and arginine-vasopressin, among other hormones and peptides, and for abnormalities in opioid and catecholamine metabolism (Fava et al, 1989). Although this possibility may ultimately prove to be at least partly valid, the theory suffers from being based exclusively on data obtained from patients who are already starving or nutritionally unbalanced; no firm support for this theory is as yet available from potentially predisposed but unaffected patients, such as unaffected twins or younger sisters of affected patients. Biological data obtained from patients who have recovered and who have been allowed to stabilize for long enough periods of time virtually always show a return to normal values.

Another theory suggests that some eating disorders, particularly bulimic syndromes, may be variants of mood disorders. Supporting arguments include the frequent comorbidity of affective disturbance with eating disorders, an increased prevalence of mood disturbance in first-degree relatives of bulimic patients, and responses of bulimic patients to antidepressant medications.

Genetically transmitted vulnerability cannot be ruled out, although exactly what the vulnerability might be is obscure. Eating disorders have a familial pattern of transmission, but such patterns do not necessarily suggest genetic as opposed to environmental influences (Yager, 1982). However, the largest series of twins for both anorexia nervosa and bulimia nervosa shows much higher concordance for both monozygotic (about 50%) than dizygotic (about 14%) twins (Crisp et al, 1985; Kendler et al, 1991), suggesting that some genetic influences may be important. Genetic vulnerability to obesity may play a role in predisposing to bulimia nervosa and binge eating disorders.

Still another theory suggests that the process of dieting and exercise produces an "autointoxication" with endogenous opioids, essentially an altered state of consciousness as a consequence of the starvation state, and that at a certain point this autointoxication creates an autoaddiction to internally generated opioids. According to this theory, the subsequent starvation and exercise are maintained in the effort to continue to generate adequate amounts of endogenous opioid to sustain the good feelings initially produced (Marrazzi and Luby, 1986).

Aside from these speculative theories, the primary biological influences in the pathogenesis of eating disorder symptoms are those related to starvation and malnutrition per se. Studies with starving normal volunteers have demonstrated that many of the psychopathological as well as physical signs and symptoms of eating disorders are attributable to starvation. Of course, starvation produces all the organ wasting and laboratory findings described above (Garfinkel and Garner, 1982). More interesting from the point of view of the pathogenesis of psychopathology is the observation that starved normal volunteers become food preoccupied, depressed, and irritable, hoard food, develop abnormal taste preferences, and binge eat when food is readily available. Furthermore, in one study in which previously normal volunteers were starved over a period of several months to 25% below their usual, healthy weights, full psychological recovery didn't occur until 6 months to a year *after* the subjects had regained all their lost weight. In other words, many of the strange and bizarre psychological symptoms, including compulsive rituals and markedly disturbed personality traits, may *result* from, rather than cause, the severe starvation. Many other psychopathological features of patients with severe anorexia nervosa, such as immature cognitive capacity as evidenced by decreases in the ability to verbalize feelings, the complexity of cognition, and the use of fantasy, also appear related to weight loss rather than to premorbid immaturity; these symptoms improve with weight gain unrelated to psychotherapy. Of course, there do seem to be psychopathological features that antedate the severe weight loss, as well.

Psychological Theories

Hypotheses regarding possible psychological factors in etiology and pathogenesis have been derived from classical, operant, cognitive, and social learning theories; psychodynamic schools, including classical psychoanalysis, ego psychology, object relations, and self-psychology theories; existential psychology; and several schools of family theory (Garner and Garfinkel, 1997). Accordingly, it is thought that eating disorders may result from the following (not necessarily mutually exclusive) processes:

1. Maladaptive learned responses (based on classical or operant conditioning principles) that reduce anxiety. In the patient with anorexia nervosa, these responses may take the form of food and/or weight phobias. In the patient with bulimia nervosa, inner tension states may be relieved by excessive eating. (In many families children at a very young age learn, and may be actively taught, to use food for stress reduction.)

Immediately thereafter, the anxiety generated by the shame, guilt, and loss of self-control brought about by the eating binge is in turn relieved by purging.

2. Cognitive distortions that develop in efforts to reduce and manage anxiety in socially awkward and sensitive adolescents (as well as in others). These misguided and erroneous self-statements tend to confound self-worth with physical appearance. The self-statements are constantly repeated as preconscious inner thoughts, cycled over and over again in a ruminative fashion, and have a self-reinforcing quality, so that they become overlearned shibboleths. The thinking distortions include tendencies to overgeneralize, to magnify horrible things (making a mountain out of a molehill), to think in "all or none" and black-and-white terms, to take everything personally, and to think superstitiously. Examples include such self statements as, "If I gain one pound, everyone will notice how fat and ugly I am"; "If I only had thinner thighs, I'd be much more popular and attractive"; "Any bite I take will immediately turn to fat"; "I am special only if I'm thin"; and "I just can't control myself. If I eat one chip, I'll never be able to stop, and I'll eat the whole bag.

3. Distortions of perceptions and interoceptions. Experiments with photographs, distorting mirrors, and videotape recordings, while not all in agreement, generally tend to support the idea that patients with eating disorders have a greater tendency to distort and misperceive their body widths, seeing themselves as much wider than they are. Although many women without eating disorders also have this tendency, the extent and degree of this distortion is much greater among women with the disorders. Patients with eating disorders also have greater difficulty than others in clearly identifying inner states such as hunger and satiety (interocepts) and in clearly identifying some of their own emotional states, as well.

4. Several authorities have suggested that children who will be predisposed to eating disorders suffer developmentally from a weak sense of self and from low self-worth. As patients, they display a pervasive sense of ineffectiveness (Bruch, 1973). According to one view, these weaknesses may stem from the failure of the parents to treat the child as a legitimate and authentic person in her own right. Instead, such parents are thought to take their child for granted and to value the child primarily for behaving well (so that the parents don't have to be bothered) and for satisfying the parents' own needs to feel valuable and to show off. The child satisfied the parents' own narcissistic needs by means of various achievements and

accomplishments, which may have had little intrinsic satisfaction for the child; hence, some pre-anorexia nervosa children have been characterized as "the best little girl in the world." Sometimes the inner weakness in the sense of self is very evident, as in the overly timid and anxious child who always clings to the mother and who has a hard time advancing and emancipating at each step of psychosocial development; this character structure may result from constitutional factors, as well as from parenting style. Sometimes the weakness is well hidden, at least superficially, by a defensive superficial personality shell and an outer facade that may appear to be strong, willful, and determined, but that lacks the adaptive flexibility of a truly strong personality structure.

5. Conflicts over adolescent development and the tasks of psychosexual maturity. Since anorexia nervosa resembles both psychological and physiological regression from the healthy adolescent state to prepubertal structures, the idea that patients may develop the disorder as a way of putting off the tasks of adolescence has had considerable appeal. In this view, patients may avoid the difficult tasks of establishing a separate identity, value system, and life plan, separating from their families, and contending with heterosexual urges and peer pressures.

6. Family factors. To start, we must stress that a family cause for eating disorders has not been proved; that a reasonable number of patients seem to come from families that are, for all intents and purposes, "normal"; and that many normal adults grow up in families that manifest the presumed pathogenetic patterns to be described. Therefore, indiscriminate "parent-bashing," i.e., the practice of laying excessive, often undue blame on parents for their children's psychiatric disorders—an all too common practice among health workers—is insupportable. Even when family problems are evident, it is far too easy to attribute the eating disorders erroneously to the family's problems; even in such instances, the disorders may result from entirely different factors (Yager, 1982).

With this caveat in mind, it can be said that some families are thought to be more likely than others to produce a child with an eating disorder. Several of the hypothesized and observed parental characteristics were described above. These family patterns are not idiosyncratic for eating disorders; they are also believed to produce other types of problems and possibly to exacerbate the course of illness for children with other diseases that may have "psychosomatic components," such as asthma and juvenile diabetes mellitus.

Families believed more likely to produce children with eating disorders include those in which (1) a parent is enmeshed with a child (i.e., overinvolved to the point of being unable to distinguish the parent's needs and wishes from the child's); (2) overt conflict between the parents or between parent and child is studiously avoided; and (3) rules about how family members communicate with one another are so rigid that it may be impermissible to address the sources and even the existence of tensions in the family (Minuchin et al, 1978). Patterns of childhood physical and sexual abuse and other forms of parental "boundary violations" have been cited as contributing factors. A family pattern characterized by "negative expressed emotion" has been empirically linked to poorer outcome for anorexia nervosa (and other psychiatric disorders such as schizophrenia and mood disorders). In this pattern, a family member, usually a parent, is highly emotional and unrelentingly critical of the patient, often blaming the patient for bringing on the disorder and for using it to harm everyone else in the family. Finally, families in which food is used as a salve for emotional problems to distract from or relieve tensions related to family dysfunctions and other sources may contribute to the subsequent appearance of binge eating during times of distress.

Social and Cultural Factors

Several factors suggest strong social and cultural influences in the appearance of eating disorders. First, *the prevalence of these disorders seems to have increased dramatically over the past several decades.* The prevalence of eating disorders parallels society's attitudes about beauty and fashion. A previous increase in eating disorders was observed in the mid-1920s at the height of the "flapper" era when women's fashion promoted a slim, boyish look. The current increase in the prevalence of eating disorders also has occurred concurrent with changing cultural standards of beauty, as documented by steadily decreasing weights for height over the past two decades among fashion models, *Playboy* magazine centerfolds, and Miss America beauty pageant winners. From the beginning of the 1960s, with the exception of Barbara Bush, the first ladies of America have also been much slimmer than they were previously.

Social–feminist theorists have suggested that anorexia nervosa may signify the unconscious hunger strikes of women who have been demeaned by society; and the highly skewed sex distribution, with a roughly 9 to 1 preponderance of females to males, has also been interpreted as due to cultural influences. Other factors may be at work, however, including the fact that psychosexual maturation occurs about 2 years earlier in females than in males, forcing them to face the associated urges and peer pressures at a younger age and perhaps rendering females more vulnerable to maturational conflicts than males. Also, males who develop anorexia nervosa may have more conflicts over sexual identity and even a higher prevalence of homosexual behavior than others. Homosexual male college students' attitudes toward their bodies and food fall midway between those of other college student males and females (Yager et al, 1988a). Once again, such a finding may be due to cultural and/or biological influences.

Given the complexity and diversity of human nature, upbringing, and family life, suffice it to say that although no one theory seems to be universally true, many of the theories of etiology and pathogenesis described above find some support in clinical observations, and each has been the basis of some form of intervention.

TREATMENT

Treatment planning for eating disorders must be based on a comprehensive assessment that includes attention to physical status; psychological and behavioral aspects of the eating disorders; associated psychological problems, such as substance abuse and mood and personality disturbances; and the family (American Psychiatric Association, 1993). Each patient's problem list will have unique aspects, and treatment components should be targeted to each specific problem. Treatment usually includes attention to weight normalization; symptom reduction through cognitive and behavioral therapy programs, supportive nursing care, dietary management, and counseling; individual and family psychological counseling through individual, group, and family psychotherapies; and psychopharmacological interventions for some mood disturbances and some eating-disorder symptoms. As is true for many types of disorders, some self-help programs may be useful. At the present time, the best treatment approach combines elements pragmatically. The following discussion is organized around the management of specific eating-disorder-related problems.

Anorexia Nervosa

Low Weight

Most controlled studies have dealt with short-term weight restoration rather than long-term treatment, and in current practice, initial attention to weight restoration is followed closely by individual and family psychotherapies (Agras, 1987).

There is general, but not universal, agreement that weight restoration should be a central and early goal of treatment of the emaciated patient. Weight restoration per se may bring about many psychological benefits, including a reduction in obsessional thinking and mood and personality disturbance. Although some underweight patients may be treated successfully outside of the hospital—up to 50% in some series (Garfinkel and Garner, 1982)—such a program usually requires a highly motivated patient, a cooperative family, and good prognostic features, such as younger age and brief duration of symptoms. The large majority of severely emaciated patients (25 to 50% below recommended weight) require inpatient treatment in a psychiatric unit, a competently staffed general hospital unit, or a specialized eating-disorder unit. The problem is how to encourage, persuade, or, in the case of the preterminal recalcitrant patient, benevolently coerce the patient into gaining weight. Unfortunately, although many clinicians employ supplemental estrogens, calcium, and vitamin D to combat osteopenia and early osteoporosis, these interventions have not been shown to be effective in reversing these conditions in anorexia nervosa (Rigotti et al, 1991). Experimental treatments are now being studied.

Carefully designed studies have demonstrated that behavioral programs can reliably encourage weight gain (Agras, 1987). Programs that combine informational feedback regarding weight gain and caloric intake, large meals, and a behavioral program that includes both positive reinforcers (such as praise and desired visits) and negative reinforcers (such as bed rest, room and activity restrictions, and prolonged hospital stays) have the best therapeutic effects on eating and weight gain. Such programs usually require a minimum of several weeks and sometimes several months in the hospital or possibly in a suitable alternative, such as an intensive outpatient day hospital.

Compared with programs that use medications or psychotherapy as the principal forms of therapy, programs including behavior therapy programs are at least more efficient, in that lengths of hospital stays are generally shorter for those treated with behavior therapy. However, they have not yet been shown to be necessarily any more effective in the long run. Nasogastric tube feeding and total parenteral nutrition programs are rarely necessary, but may sometimes be lifesaving.

Psychotherapies. The role of individual and family psychotherapy in bringing about weight gain per se is difficult to evaluate. To the extent that a patient's motivation to change may be increased through such therapies, they may be valuable. Families can benefit from family therapy and counseling as soon as the problems are identified. In any event, patients often appear to make the best use of these therapies to deal with their own and their families' long-standing psychological problems after they have regained some weight and are better able to think more clearly.

Psychopharmacological Approaches. Many authorities avoid medications in severely malnourished patients with anorexia nervosa because such patients may be especially prone to serious side effects and because no one has yet demonstrated that medication approaches to gaining and sustaining weight have any convincing long-term advantages over nonmedication programs. In one controlled study, cyproheptadine in doses of up to 32 mg/day showed some, although by no means striking, benefit for lower weight nonbulimic patients (Halmi et al, 1986). The drug's mechanism of action in this situation is uncertain, but it does seem to increase hunger; paradoxically, this makes it unacceptable to many patients. Low doses of neuroleptics or of antianxiety drugs are sometimes prescribed, but existing studies do not support their general use. In one controlled trial, fluoxetine has been helpful in maintaining weight gain for a year following initial weight gain (Kaye et al, 1991). Thus far, aside from small case series (Gwirtsman et al, 1990), the value of selective serotonin-reuptake inhibitors (SSRIs) or other antidepressant medications for weight gain per se is unproved (Garfinkel and Garner, 1987). Studies are underway to more carefully assess the potential value of SSRIs in promoting weight gain in anorexia nervosa. Medical regimens are sometimes required for patients with laxative abuse, severe constipation and other abdominal symptoms, and associated problems.

Psychological Problems

Psychotherapeutic Approaches. For anorexia nervosa, most authorities suggest that individual psychotherapy using a highly empathic and nurturant reality-based perspective is most useful in helping the patient to examine and confront the many psychological distortions and developmental issues described above. Sessions are frequently scheduled weekly or twice weekly. The value of family therapy following hospital discharge has also been demonstrated in controlled studies of younger patients with anorexia nervosa (Russell et al, 1987).

Psychopharmacological Approaches. Antidepressant medication is often used for depression that persists following weight gain and sometimes for depression in the still underweight patient. However, the efficacy of this approach in the still seriously underweight patient is questionable, and such patients may be more prone to the cardiotoxic side effects of tricyclic antidepressants. Although little justification exists by way of controlled trials, many clinicians have started to use SSRIs to treat both depressive and obsessive–compulsive symptoms in low-weight anorexics who are not responding to psychotherapeutic or behavioral interventions alone. Low-dose neuroleptics or antianxiety drugs are sometimes used for specific target symptoms such as psychotic thinking and severe anxiety in patients with anorexia nervosa, but their use in this fashion is based solely on clinical impressions of their occasional value (Garfinkel and Garner, 1987).

Bulimia Nervosa

Binge Eating and Purging

Although with few exceptions psychotherapeutic and psychopharmacological interventions have thus far been evaluated separately from each other, in practice, the various approaches are frequently combined, depending on the individual's needs.

Psychotherapeutic Approaches. Many controlled studies have shown the value of individual and group cognitive–behavioral psychotherapies in particular, although other approaches including interpersonal psychotherapy

(Fairburn, 1995) and focal psychodynamic psychotherapy may be of value as well (Hartmann et al, 1992).

A *cognitive–behavioral* approach includes several stages, each consisting of several weeks or more of weekly or biweekly individual and/or group sessions. The *first* stage emphasizes the establishment of control over eating by using behavioral techniques such as self-monitoring (e.g., keeping a detailed symptom-relevant diary) and response prevention (e.g., eating until satiated without being allowed to vomit), the prescription of a pattern of regular eating, and stimulus-control measures (e.g., avoidance of situations most likely to stimulate an eating binge). Patients are actively educated about weight regulation, dieting, and the adverse consequences of bulimia. The *second* stage focuses on attempts to restructure the patient's unrealistic cognitions (e.g., assumptions and expectations) and instill more effective modes of problem solving. The *third* stage emphasizes maintaining the gains and preventing relapse and often provides 6 months to a year of weekly sessions to provide close follow-up during the time that patients are most likely to relapse (Fairburn, 1981; Johnson and Connors, 1987). Intensive outpatient programs for bulimia also have been employed in which patients start their programs by attending various group programs several hours each day for several weeks. The overall success rate of these methods varies considerably. For those completing the programs, about 50 to 90% experience a substantial reduction in binging and purging rates, averaging about 70%, and about one-third of patients stop these symptoms entirely (the dropout problem is considerable, however, in many groups). Available follow-up reports, generally for less than 3 years, indicate that many of the gains are maintained, although some recidivism is seen, particularly at times of severe stress. Recent studies show that many patients can benefit from self-guided cognitive–behavior therapies provided through structured manuals (Treasure et al, 1994).

Psychodynamic Psychotherapy. In a controlled comparison with a 3-year follow-up, interpersonal psychotherapy proved in many respects to be as or more effective than cognitive–behavior therapy for treating bulimia nervosa (Fairburn, 1995). This approach focuses on issues of losses, grief, interpersonal conflicts, and interpersonal deficits (i.e., personality problems). Although long-term psychodynamic psychotherapy often has been employed in the treatment of bulimia, no controlled studies of its effectiveness in comparison with other modalities are available. Most cognitive–behavioral programs utilize important interpersonal and psychodynamically derived therapy principles, and most psychodynamically oriented therapists who treat patients with bulimia nervosa often effectively employ cognitive–behavioral and interpersonal strategies or work concurrently with other therapists who do.

Psychopharmacological Approaches. Controlled studies indicate that tricyclic antidepressants (particularly imipramine and desipramine), fluoxetine, monoamine oxidase inhibitors (MAOIs) (particularly phenelzine) and other antidepressants are useful in reducing binge eating and purging in bulimia nervosa (Agras et al, 1992; Levine et al, 1992; Walsh et al, 1991), although they are not by themselves an adequate treatment program, and often more than one type will have to be tried before the best one for the patient is found. Common problems include medication compliance and maintaining good blood levels in the face of persistent vomiting.

Fluoxetine and the tricyclic antidepressants imipramine and desipramine have been best studied in double-blind placebo-controlled trials and are used most frequently; they are effective in patients with or without concurrent major depression. Whereas effective doses of the tricyclic antidepressants for bulimia nervosa are similar to those used to treat depression, controlled trials have shown that higher doses of fluoxetine than those used for depression are necessary for optimal response (e.g., 60 mg/day rather than the usual antidepressant dose of 20 mg/day; Goldbloom et al, 1995). Open trials have shown that other SSRIs such as fluvoxamine (50 to 150 mg/day) can also be useful (Ayuso-Gutierrez et al, 1994). In the case of MAOIs, patients are very prone to side effects and may have a hard time following a tyramine-free diet. Results of medication treatment are similar to those with cognitive–behavioral psychotherapies, and many patients who do not respond to psychological treatment alone benefit from medication; symptoms are reduced in 70 to 90% of patients, and about one-third are reported to become abstinent (Garfinkel and Garner, 1987). Some evidence suggests that combining medication and cognitive–behavioral psychotherapy is better than either treatment alone (Agras et al, 1992). In practice, many clinicians utilize a combined approach, particularly for patients who do not respond to available psychotherapeutic and educational interventions within a brief period.

Hospitalization. Hospitalization is rarely indicated for uncomplicated bulimia nervosa. Indications include failure to respond to adequate outpatient treatment trials, worrisome medical complications not managable in the outpatient setting, and a severe mood disorder with suicidality.

Binge Eating Disorder

Relatively few good studies have been published concerning the treatment of binge eating disorders, and many clinicians use information and experience gleaned from the treatment of bulimia nervosa to guide their clinical decision making. In addition to binge eating episodes, target symptoms often include weight loss for the obese binge eaters.

Binge Eating and Purging

Substantial reductions in the frequency of binge eating and purging have been obtained with cognitive–behavioral therapy in individual and group settings, in highly structured programs using intensive self-monitoring, nutritional and behavioral counseling, cognitive restructuring, and relapse prevention. Self-guided manuals employing these techniques may be helpful (Treasure et al, 1994). Psychotherapy alone does not appear to be effective. Medication trials have yielded mixed results. Gains made on medication almost all disappear once medication is stopped (Devlin, 1996). Some studies have shown that desipramine may help obese binge eaters decrease the frequency of their episodes. In one study, 100 mg/day of fluvoxamine was no better than placebo for binge eating (de Zwaan et al, 1992), although the dose may have been too low to be optimal, since, in another open-label study, patients were helped by 200 mg/day (Gardiner et al, 1993). Finally, in a group of patients carefully screened to eliminate early placebo responders, dexfenfluramine was shown to be superior to placebo in reducing binge eating symptoms, but these effects disappeared after medication was discontinued (Stunkard et al, 1996). Due to serious cardiac side effects, dexfenfluramine was removed from the market by the FDA in 1997.

Weight Loss

Results have been mixed regarding weight loss among obese binge eaters. When cognitive–behavioral programs are employed specifically to help obese binge eaters lose weight, patients are more likely to lose weight compared with patients who receive cognitive–behavior therapy aimed solely at reducing binge eating episodes. This weight loss often has been maintained in follow-ups lasting a year or more. However, obese binge eaters are no more likely to lose weight in such programs than non-binge eating obese patients. Furthermore, other studies of obese patients reveal that substantial numbers will regain much of their lost weight within 2 to 5 years following such treatments.

Pharmacological treatments for weight loss among binge-eating and non-binge eating obese persons is a matter of considerable interest and some controversy (National Task Force, 1996). In patients with degrees of obesity considered to place them at high risk for medical problems, treatment studies lasting several years using combinations of the anorexant phentermine (chemically related to the amphetamines) and the satiety-promoting agent fenfluramine (a serotonin agonist) yielded sustained weight loss, but only for as long as the medications were continued (during which time the large amount of weight initially lost had a tendency to creep back). Due to serious cardiac side effects, fenfluramine was removed from the market in 1997. In shorter term studies, high doses of fluoxetine have been superior to placebo in facilitating weight loss, again lasting only while medication is taken.

ROLE OF THE NONPSYCHIATRIC PHYSICIAN IN PATIENT MANAGEMENT

The nonpsychiatric physician should play a major role in the prevention, detection, and management of patients with eating disorders. Pediatricians and family physicians should be alert to excessive concerns about dieting and appearance in preteens and their families and educate them about healthy nutrition and the dangers of unrealistic appearance-oriented dieting and eating disorders. Because the prevalence of subclinical and full-blown forms of these disorders is so high, physicians should routinely question young female patients about what they desire to weigh; their dietary, dieting, and exercise practices; and their use of laxatives. Psychological problems in young women should stimulate attention to eating-disorder symptoms, as well as to problems with mood, substance abuse, sexual behavior, etc. Gynecologists, internists, gastroenterologists, and dentists also are likely to encounter large numbers of eating-disorder patients in their practices.

Once an eating disorder is detected, patients merit a full physical exam; screening laboratory tests, including electrolytes, complete blood count, thyroid, calcium, magnesium, and amylase studies; and, for the very thin patient, an electrocardiogram or rhythm strip. The physician should work together with a registered dietician and mental health worker knowledgable about eating disorders to see if the problems can be ameliorated in outpatient care. With motivated patients, this multidisciplinary team approach can be highly successful. The physician's role is to educate and monitor the patient's weight and laboratory tests. For the anorexia nervosa patient, monitoring should include weekly or twice weekly visits to the office for nonclothed postvoiding weights (with care taken that the patient has not imbibed large quantities of fluid just prior to being weighed) and for ongoing monitoring of any physiological abnormalities of concern.

For young adults, the physician should also be able to prescribe and monitor a course of antidepressant medication for patients with bulimia nervosa and mood or anxiety disorders associated with an eating disorder. The extent to which the physician is willing and/or able to assume a more intense involvement with the psychological and family issues varies considerably.

Patients with binge eating disorders should be referred for cognitive–behavioral and dietary counseling. If depression or anxiety symptoms are severe, treatment with tricyclic antidepressants or an SSRI should be considered. For morbidly obese patients, i.e., those who are at least 100 pounds overweight, for whom more conventional treatments fail, surgical approaches such as gastroplasties with banding should be considered and may be lifesaving.

INDICATIONS FOR PSYCHIATRIC CONSULTATION AND REFERRAL

Every patient with a serious eating disorder warrants consultation with a psychiatrist knowledgable about eating disorders for guidance to the patient, family, and referring physician about the nature, severity, and prognosis of the disorder and available treatment options. The physician can expect specific guidelines for psychosocial and medical management.

Specific indications for mandatory consultation include failure of the patient to respond to attempts at management in the physician's setting with deteriorating status, severe depression with suicidality, or marked family problems.

CLINICAL PEARLS

A high index of suspicion is warranted with all female adolescents and young adults. Most want to weigh too little.

- Alerting signs include menstrual irregularities, infertility, desire to weigh 10 to 15 pounds less than reasonable for habitus, overconcern with weight or physical appearance, vague gastrointestinal complaints, overuse of laxatives or diuretics, and mood disturbance.
- Signs of self-induced vomiting include puffy cheeks, scars on the knuckles, and decay of the front teeth.
- Alerting laboratory signs include mild disturbances in serum electrolytes, magnesium, and amylase.
- Patients with anorexia nervosa often are devious in providing information and in getting weighed (e.g., drinking large quantities of fluids or putting weights in their clothing). Alternative informants such as family members are always required.
- Clinicians should suspect osteopenia and early osteoporosis in patients amenorrheic for as little as 6 months. Bone densiometry may be indicated to educate the patient about the objective seriousness of her condition.

ANNOTATED BIBLIOGRAPHY

American Psychiatric Association Practice Guidelines for Eating Disorders. Am J Psychiatry 150:207–228, 1993

> A thorough overview and synthesis with authoritative treatment guidelines.

Fairburn CG. Overcoming Binge Eating New York, Guilford Press, 1995

> Well written, intended for lay audiences, includes a self-guided and therapist-assisted treatment manual.

Fairburn CG, Wilson GT (eds): Binge Eating: Nature, Assessment, and Treatment. New York, Guilford Press, 1993

> Excellent analysis of all aspects of binge eating, with added bonus of outstanding cognitive–behavioral treatment manual.

Garner DM, Garfinkel PE (eds): Handbook of Psychotherapy for Anorexia Nervosa and Bulimia, 2nd ed. New York, Guilford Press, 1997

> A major collection of articles from leading experts describing the rationale and methods for diverse psychotherapeutic approaches including cognitive, behavioral, psychoeducational, and psychodynamic approaches to individual, group, and family therapy in the outpatient and inpatient setting.

Hsu LKG: Eating Disorders. New York, Guilford Press, 1990

> A concise and comprehensive textbook dealing with all aspects from phenomenology through treatment and prognosis.

Rock CL, Yager J: Nutrition and eating disorders: a primer for clinicians. Int J Eating Disord 6:267–280, 1987

> An assessment of basic nutritional contributions to the pathogenesis of eating disorders, with corresponding nutrition-related treatment recommendations.

Russell GFM, Szmukler GI, Dare C, Eisler I: An evaluation of family therapy in anorexia nervosa and bulimia nervosa. Arch Gen Psychiatry 44:1047–1056, 1987

> A sophisticated research study of 80 patients.

Wadden TA, Van Itallie TB: Treatment of the Seriously Obese Patient. New York, Guilford Press, 1992

> An excellent compendium covering all aspects of serious obesity, from the basic biological through the psychosocial. Strong focus on treatment and treatment outcomes.

Yager J (ed): Eating Disorders. Psychiatr Clin North Am 19(4), 1996

> Updates, appraisals, and critiques of major clinical areas by a panel of experts, with special attention to strategies for complex assessment and treatment issues.

REFERENCES

Agras WS: Eating Disorders: Management of Obesity, Bulimia and Anorexia Nervosa. Oxford, Pergamon, 1987

Agras WS, Rossiter EM, Arnow B, et al: Pharmacologic and cognitive–behavioral treatment for bulimia nervosa: a controlled comparison. Am J Psychiatry 149:82–87, 1992

American Psychiatric Association: Practice guideline for eating disorders. Am J Psychiatry 150:207–228, 1993

American Psychiatric Association: Diagnostic and Statistical Manual, 4th ed. Washington, DC, American Psychiatric Association, 1994

Ayuso-Gutierrez JL, Palazon M, Ayuso-Mateos JL: Open trial of fluvoxamine in the treatment of bulimia nervosa. Int J Eating Disord 15:245–249, 1994

Bruch H: Eating Disorders: Obesity, Anorexia Nervosa and the Person Within. New York, Basic Books, 1973

Crisp AH, Hall A, Holland AJ: Nature and nurture in anorexia nervosa: a study of 34 pairs of twins, one pair of triplets and an adoptive family. Int J Eating Disord 4:5–29, 1985

Devlin M: Assessment and treatment of binge eating disorder. Psychiatr Clin North Am 19:761–772, 1996

de Zwaan M, Nutziger DO, Schoenbeck G: Binge eating in overweight women. Compr Psychiatry 33:256–261, 1992

Drewnowski A, Hopkins SA, Kessler RC: The prevalence of bulimia nervosa in the US college student population. Am J Public Health 78:1322–1325, 1988

Fairburn CG: A cognitive behavioral approach to the treatment of bulimia. Psychol Med 11:707–711, 1981

Fairburn CG, Norman PA, Welch SL, et al: A prospective study of outcome in bulimia nervosa and the long-term effects of three psychological treatments. Arch Gen Psychiatry 52:304–312, 1995

Fava M, Copeland P, Schweiger U, Herzog D: Neurochemical abnormalities of anorexia nervosa and bulimia nervosa. Am J Psychiatry 146:963–971, 1989

Gardiner HM, Freeman CPL, Jesinger DK, et al: Fluvoxamine: an open pilot study in moderately obese female patients suffering from atypical eating disorders and episodes of bingeing. Int J Obesity 17:301–305, 1993

Garfinkel PE, Garner DM: Anorexia Nervosa: A Multidimensional Perspective. New York, Brunner/Mazel, 1982

Garfinkel PE, Garner DM (eds): The Role of Drug Treatments for Eating Disorders. New York, Brunner/Mazel, 1987

Goldbloom DJ, Wilson MG, Thompson VL, et al: Fluoxetine Bulimia Nervosa Research Group. Long-term fluoxetine treatment of bulimia nervosa. Br J Psychiatry 166:660–666, 1995

Gwirtsman HE, Guze BH, Yager J, et al. Treatment of anorexia nervosa with fluoxetine: an open clinical trial. J Clin Psychiatry 51:378–382, 1990

Halmi KA, Eckert E, LaDu TJ, et al: Anorexia nervosa: treatment efficacy of cyproheptadine and amitriptyline. Arch Gen Psychiatry 43:177–181, 1986

Halmi KA, Eckert E, Marchi P, Sampugnaro V, Apple R, Cohen J: Comorbidity of psychiatric diagnosis in anorexia nervosa. Arch Gen Psychiatry 48:712–718, 1991

Hartmann A, Herzog T, Drinkmann A: Psychotherapy of bulimia nervosa: what is effective? A meta-analysis. J Psychosom Res 36:159–167, 1992

Hsu LKG: Outcome and treatment effects. In Beumont PJV, Burrows BD, Casper RC (eds): Handbook of Eating Disorders, Part I. Amsterdam, Elsevier, 1987

Johnson C, Connors ME: The Etiology and Treatment of Bulimia Nervosa. New York, Basic Books, 1987

Kaye WH, Weltzin TW, Hsu LKG, Bulick C: An open trial of fluoxetine in patients with anorexia nervosa. J Clin Psychiatry 52:464–471, 1991

Kendler KS, MacLean C, Neale M, Kessler R, Heath A, Eaves L: The genetic epidemiology of bulimia nervosa. Am J Psychiatry 148:1627–1637, 1991

Levine L, et al (Fluoxetine Bulimia Nervosa Collaborative Study Group): Fluoxetine in the treatment of bulimia nervosa: a multicenter, placebo-controlled, double-blind trial. Arch Gen Psychiatry 49:139–147, 1992

Marrazzi MA, Luby ED: An auto-addiction opioid model of chronic anorexia nervosa. Int J Eating Disord 5:191–208, 1986

Minuchin S, Rosman BL, Baker L: Psychosomatic Families: Anorexia Nervosa in Context. Cambridge, Harvard University Press, 1978

Mitchell JE, Seim HC, Colon E, et al: Medical complications and medical management of bulimia. Ann Intern Med 107:71–77, 1987

National Task Force on the Prevention and Treatment of Obesity: Long-term pharmacotherapy in the management of obesity. JAMA 276:1907–1915, 1996

Rigotti NA, Neer RM, Skates SJ, et al: The clinical course of osteoporosis in anorexia nervosa: a longitudinal study of cortical bone mass. JAMA 265:1133–1138, 1991

Rigotti NA, Nussbaum SR, Herzog DB, et al: Osteoporosis in women with anorexia nervosa. N Engl J Med 311:1601–1606, 1984

Russell GFM, Szmukler GI, Dare C, et al: An evaluation of family therapy in anorexia nervosa and bulimia nervosa. Arch Gen Psychiatry 44:1047–1056, 1987

Spitzer RL, Devlin MC, Walsh BT, et al: Binge eating disorder: a multisite field trial of the diagnostic criteria. Int J Eating Disord 11:191–203, 1992

Spitzer RL, Yanovski S, Wadden T, et al: Binge eating disorder: its further validation in a multisite study. Int J Eating Disord 13:137–153, 1993

Steinhausen H-Ch, Rauss-Mason C, Seidel R: Follow-up studies of anorexia nervosa: a review of four decades of outcome research. Psychol Med 21:447–454, 1991

Stunkard A, Berkowitz R, Tanrikut C, et al: d-Fenfluramine treatment of binge eating disorder. Am J Psychiatry 153: 1455–1459, 1996

Sullivan PF: Mortality in anorexia nervosa. Am J Psychiatry 152:1073–1074, 1995

Treasure J, Schmidt U, Troop N, et al: First Step in Managing Bulimia Nervosa: Controlled Trial of Therapeutic Manual. BMJ 308:686–689, 1994

Walsh BT, Hadigan CM, Devlin MJ, Gladis M, Roose SP: Long-term outcome of antidepressant treatment for bulimia nervosa. Am J Psychiatry 148:1206–1212, 1991

Yager J: Family issues in the pathogenesis of anorexia nervosa. Psychosom Med 44:43–60, 1982

Yager J, Kurtsman F, Landsverk J, et al: Behaviors and attitudes related to eating disorders in homosexual male college students. Am J Psychiatry 145:495–497, 1988a

Yager J, Landsverk J, Edelstein CK: A 20-month follow-up study of 628 women with eating disorders, Part I: Course and severity. Am J Psychiatry 144:1172–1177, 1988b

13 *Dissociative Disorders*

George K. Ganaway,
Mark E. James,
and Steven T. Levy

The diagnostic grouping *dissociative disorders* refers to a group of clinical conditions with the common feature of a disturbance of the integration of consciousness, memory, or identity. The disorders in the category are listed in Table 13–1. These disturbances may be sudden or gradual, transient or chronic. If memory for a significant period of time is lost in the absence of a neurological disorder, a diagnosis of *dissociative amnesia* is made. If an individual loses memory for his or her entire previous identity and a new identity is assumed along with travel to a new location, the diagnosis is *dissociative fugue*. If more than one distinct identity or personality state dominates consciousness and behavior at different times in any individual, a diagnosis of *dissociative identity disorder* (formerly multiple personality disorder) is made. If an individual experiences him- or herself as unreal, strange, or changed in some way, yet remains in contact with reality in the absence of any gross change in identity, the diagnosis is *depersonalization disorder* as long as these symptoms are not part of any other known psychiatric disorder.

This grouping of psychiatric disorders is based both on the similarity of clinical manifestations seen in each, and on a presumed underlying psychological process: the phenomenon of *dissociation*. Dissociation is an activity of the mind that results in a "separation of mental structures or content that were previously connected or associatively linked" (Counts, 1990). All individuals are capable of experiencing variable degrees of dissociative alterations of consciousness, information processing, and memory storage and retrieval. Such dissociative experiences of everyday life include "spacing out" during a

Table 13–1 **Dissociative Disorders**

Dissociative Amnesia
Dissociative Fugue
Dissociative Identity Disorder (Multiple Personality Disorder)
Depersonalization Disorder
Dissociative Disorder Not Otherwise Specified

conversation or lecture; daydreaming; becoming immersed in a movie; or doing something automatically, such as driving a car "on autopilot" with little memory of part of the trip. Other phenomena in which dissociative processes play a role include hypnosis, meditation, and other trance phenomena; states of religious fervor and ecstasy; and, in some cultures, states of spirit possession. When dissociation becomes extreme and causes significant distress or impairment of functioning, psychiatric diagnosis and intervention become warranted.

By virtue of their dramatic character, the dissociative disorders have long been of interest to psychiatrists. Explanations of dissociation play an important role in the history of modern psychiatry (Putnam, 1989; Nemiah, 1995). Early attempts to explore the process of dissociation did not link it exclusively with those disorders now grouped together in the *Diagnostic and Statistical Manual,* 4th edition (DSM-IV; American Psychiatric Association, 1994) as the dissociative dis-orders. Early investigators thought that a variety of other clinical entities, including hysteria and somnambulism, involved dissociative mechanisms (Abse, 1974).

Pierre Janet is given credit for first using the term *dissociation* in relation to mental disorders. He viewed dissociation as a pathological process in which traumatic memories could not be integrated into preexisting cognitive structures and instead were split off to form "subconscious fixed ideas" that existed outside of an individual's usual conscious experience and continued to exert an effect on behavior (van der Kolk and van der Hart, 1989). According to Janet, dissociation might occur when an individual's mind was weakened, either because of constitutional factors or due to acute states of fatigue, illness, intoxication, or extreme emotional arousal. Josef Breuer (Breuer and Freud, 1893–1895) agreed that pathogenic ideas may be split off from normal conscious awareness in the context of extreme emotional arousal, but added that this may also occur in individuals who enter into abnormal "hypnoid states." Sigmund Freud came to understand the process of the splitting of consciousness differently. In his work with patients, he noticed that certain thoughts were actively kept outside conscious awareness by defensive processes designed to ward off painful feelings resulting from conflict between wishful and prohibited thoughts. This idea that certain mental content can be banned from consciousness (repression) by being unacceptable to the individual became a cornerstone of dynamic psychiatry.

As a part of our modern diagnostic system, dissociative disorders are distinguished by both their clinical manifestations and a presumed common underlying psychological mechanism. This is a departure from diagnostic criteria used in other DSM-IV syndromes, which are diagnosed only on the basis of observable signs and symptoms or known neurological factors.

Since these early explorations of dissociative processes, various other explanations have been hypothesized. For example, neurobiological investigators have suggested that the disturbances of cognitive integration and memory function seen in dissociative disorders may reflect an underlying pathology of temporal lobe functioning. Patients in dissociated states may demonstrate alterations of brain physiology (electroencephalogram patterns, visual evoked responses, cerebral blood flow), autonomic functioning, dominant handedness, allergic sensitivities, visual acuity, and visual fields, as well as different responses to medications; how these differences come about remains unclear and speculative. Because these disorders are relatively rare, it has been difficult to study them in a systematic and longitudinal manner.

The capacity for gross alterations in conscious experience, such as is present in patients with dissociative disorders, represents a profound disturbance in mental life. When it does occur, it is usually in the face of overwhelmingly traumatic experiences or memories, or ambivalently viewed sexual and aggressive wishes and urges. Clinical manifestations vary from the mild disturbances seen in many patients with transient depersonalization experiences to episodic and short-lived dramatic episodes of amnesia and fugue to lifelong patterns of disturbance of the greatest severity in certain patients with dissociative identity disorder. The various dissociative disorders will be discussed individually in terms of description, etiology, and treatment, with common or linking trends emphasized where appropriate.

DISSOCIATIVE AMNESIA

The following often cited case of dissociative amnesia in colonial America was described by Benjamin Rush, "the father of American psychiatry," in his lectures (Carlson, 1981). A man named William Tenent, who was preparing for an examination for the Presbyterian ministry, developed an illness with chest pain, intermittent fever, and severe emaciation. He eventually collapsed and was believed dead. Funeral preparations were forestalled by his physician, who believed he felt a slight warmth in Tenent's body. After 3 days, the presumed corpse "opened its eyes, gave a dreadful groan, and sunk again into apparent death." This occurred again two more times, but after the last, he regained consciousness.

He gradually recovered fully during the next year, but was completely amnestic for his entire life before the deathlike state. Because he also lost his ability to read or write, his brother began teaching him these skills. One day during a Latin lesson, he suddenly felt a shock in his head. He remembered reading the book before. More recollections occurred, and he eventually recovered all memories of his life. He also described an experience during a 3-day coma in which he was "transported by a superior being to a place of ineffable glory." He remained healthy for the next 45 years. He became a minister, married, and had three sons.

Description

Dissociative amnesia is characterized by an inability to recall significant personal information beyond what could be explained by ordinary forgetfulness. The most common presentation of dissociative amnesia is a localized or circumscribed disturbance of recall, that is, the patient cannot recall any events that occurred during a certain period, usually the first few hours after a severely upsetting event of a stressful or traumatic nature (Fig. 13–1). Less common is selective amnesia, in which certain but not all events within a specified period are not remembered. On rare occasions, a patient may develop generalized amnesia (in which the patient cannot recall any information about his or her entire preceding life) or continuous amnesia (in which the patient cannot remember anything following a specific event and continuing to the immediate present). In the case above, William Tenent's amnesia was most likely the generalized type. Whether it was psychogenic or caused by his illness is open to speculation.

An episode of dissociative amnesia is usually precipitated by a particularly intense psychological trauma or stressor, either some threat of harm or death, an intolerable and/or inescapable life situation, or a morally unacceptable impulse or act. In some individuals, the amnesia may be preceded by a headache or some alteration of consciousness experienced as sleepiness or dizziness. Occasionally, an amnestic patient may wander aimlessly until the police eventually bring her or him to an emergency room. Some affected individuals may be unaware of their memory disturbance until confronted by another person. Some feel distressed by the amnesia, others seem indifferent, and some may make up information to fill in what is missing.

Epidemiology

The epidemiology of dissociative amnesia is poorly understood. It is believed to be most common in adolescent and young adult females and is most rare in the elderly. There is no information on familial transmission. During war, dissociative amnesia may occur in as many as 5 to 8% of combat soldiers. The incidence is believed to rise during disasters.

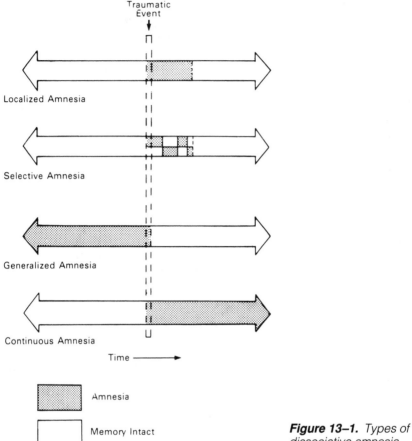

Figure 13–1. *Types of dissociative amnesia.*

Etiology

The precise psychological and/or neurological mechanisms of dissociative amnesia are unknown. One hypothetical model suggests that, in the face of overwhelming psychological trauma, mental mechanisms that interfere with the normal retrieval of stored, anxiety-provoking information are activated in susceptible individuals. The person can then function relatively adaptively compared with the cognitive disequilibrium that might result if the trauma continued to be experienced consciously (as occurs in patients with acute posttraumatic stress disorders). Obviously, the amnesia itself can become disabling or maladaptive.

How memories are sequestered outside of awareness is unclear. One possibility is that a neurologically based retrieval deficit or faulty encoding and storage of information may cause dissociative amnesia since these dysfunctions also cause other types of amnesia. However, dissociated memories often can be recovered by using hypnosis or a sodium amobarbital interview, so some capacity for storage and retrieval must remain intact on some level. The psychoanalytic model describes amnesia as unconsciously motivated. If a memory or thought is sufficiently conflict laden or traumatic so that conscious awareness of it is accompanied by significant anxiety, the mind will activate defense mechanisms such as repression and dissociation to keep the memory or thought outside of conscious awareness. The state-dependent learning model suggests that information storage and retrieval depends on the person's state of consciousness. If memories are stored under extreme emotional turmoil, they may not be accessible in other emotional states, and amnesia results.

Differential Diagnosis

Any of several neurological etiologies of amnesia should be ruled out by careful medical–neurological evaluation, particularly central nervous system disease, intoxication, and metabolic derangement (Table 13–2). The classic substance-induced amnesia is the "alcoholic blackout." Chronic alcohol use also may result in anterograde memory disturbances. Postconcussion amnesia may occur after head trauma. Epileptic seizures usually are accompanied by a period of amnesia. If a patient in legal trouble stands to gain by forgetting a period of time, malingering or feigned amnesia should be considered. The short-acting benzodiazepine triazolam may cause anterograde amnesia and thus has fallen into disfavor among many clinicians.

Diagnostic Evaluation

For all dissociative syndromes, evaluation should begin with a thorough, comprehensive history. Physical examination should include a complete neurological examination. The physician should look especially for evidence of head injury, intoxication, or focal neurological deficits. Findings on the mental

---

Table 13–2 **Medical and Neurological Disorders Causing Dissociative Symptoms**

Alcohol intoxication—blackout
Alcohol amnestic disorder
Postconcussion amnesia
Complex partial seizures
Migraine syndromes
Transient global amnesia
Carbon monoxide poisoning
Hypoglycemia
Hallucinogen intoxication
Hallucinogen persisting perception disorder (flashback)

status examination that would point toward a neurologic cause of dissociative syndromes would include clouding of consciousness, impaired attention, disorientation, slurred speech, blunted or labile affect, disorganized flow of thought associations, visual, olfactory or gustatory hallucinations, difficulty with complex mental tasks, impaired cognition beyond specific memory losses, inability to learn new things, and confabulation (Kopelman, 1987).

Laboratory assessment of glucose, electrolytes, CO_2, erythrocyte sedimentation rate, vitamin B_{12}, folate, thyroid, renal and hepatic functioning, and blood-alcohol level, as well as a urine drug screen, will help to rule out toxic, metabolic, infectious, and autoimmune encephalopathies. Additional findings on history and physical may justify human immunodeficiency virus serology or a urine heavy metal screen. Serial electro-encephalograms or a 24-hour ambulatory recording may be useful to assess for altered sensorium, temporal lobe dysfunction, epileptiform discharges, and sleep dysfunction. Typically, high-voltage activity will occur in stupor and low-voltage fast activity will be seen during excitement; in functional nonorganic cases (e.g., dissociative states), alpha activity, which responds to auditory and visual stimuli, will be present in the background. Skull X-ray, computed tomography, or magnetic resonance imaging may be indicated to rule out structural brain pathology. Sophisticated neuropsychological testing may help illuminate the type and severity of cognitive disturbance, as well as its specific location in the brain (see Chapters 3 and 4).

Treatment

Therapy involves two general principles: first, to remove the patient from the threatening circumstances (by hospitalization, if necessary); second, to explore his or her distress through psychotherapy. Some recommend an approach designed to retrieve the blocked memories as rapidly as possible, either through free association, hypnosis, or amobarbital interviews. Others believe this approach may be deleterious and advise, instead, a more cautious exploration of the patient's life situation and any psychological conflicts that may have resulted in the onset of amnesia under the given circumstances.

Psychotropic medications (except for amobarbital interviews) seldom are useful in treating dissociative amnesia. Small doses of benzodiazepines may provide symptomatic relief for anxiety reactions to awareness of lost time. During therapy, the amnesia often clears rapidly, sometimes completely.

DISSOCIATIVE FUGUE

William James described a famous case of dissociative fugue in *Principles of Psychology* (1918): Ansel Bourne, a 60-year-old evangelist, disappeared from Providence, Rhode Island. About 2 weeks thereafter, a man named A.J.

Brown opened a small shop in Norristown, Pennsylvania. He conducted business in a quiet and orderly fashion. Six weeks later, he woke up in a frightened state. He said his name was Ansel Bourne, asked to know where he was, and said he had no knowledge of Norristown or shopkeeping. His last memory was of conducting some personal business in Providence, and he could not believe that 2 months had passed. He returned home and maintained complete amnesia for the interval. James later examined Bourne under hypnosis, evoking the personality of A.J. Brown, who recounted the events in Norristown. James could never facilitate Bourne's recall of any of Brown's memories.

Description

During a classic dissociative fugue, a person suddenly and unexpectedly travels away from his or her home or workplace; is unable to recall the past; and is confused about his or her identity or may assume a new identity. During a fugue state, a person may appear perplexed or disoriented. After recovery from the fugue, there is no recall of events that took place during the episode. Patients typically present for help after the fugue, wanting to recall what happened.

Only occasionally will a fugue manifest the more dramatic and classical presentation in which a quiet, ordinary person suddenly assumes a more gregarious, uninhibited manner, travels thousands of miles, and carries on a new, complex social existence for months with a different name and a well-integrated new identity before ultimately shifting back into the former identity with no memory of the interval. More typically, the episode is less elaborate. The affected person engages in brief and apparently purposeful travel, but the new identity is less complete and socialization with others may be minimal. Most episodes of dissociative fugue last several hours to a few days (Reither and Stoudemire, 1988).

Occurrence

As with dissociative amnesia, the occurrence of dissociative fugue increases during wartime or natural disasters. Many cases reported are of soldiers in combat who wandered away from duty. The age of onset is variable. Little information exists about sex ratio or familial incidence.

Etiology

The pathological cause of fugue states is unknown. The same dissociative mental mechanism discussed under dissociative amnesia applies to dissociative fugue, but in fugue states, there is partial or complete loss of identity, and a new identity often is created. This phenomenon appears to be precipitated by severe psychological stress.

Differential Diagnosis and Treatment

As mentioned, evaluation and treatment is usually sought after the fugue has resolved. As with amnesia, the differential diagnosis must include the same list of disorders. Dissociative identity disorder should also be ruled out. Treatment of dissociative fugue involves the same principles discussed under dissociative amnesia.

DISSOCIATIVE IDENTITY DISORDER

Description

Dissociative identity disorder (formerly known as multiple personality disorder) is distinguished by the presence of two or more identities or personality states, each having a persistent and predictable pattern of perception, thought, and manner of relating to the environment and self. Additionally, at least two of these identities or states recurrently take control of the person's behavior, and there must be some degree of dissociative amnesia present to make the diagnosis. The personality part presenting for treatment typically is unaware of the existence of the other identities or states. The patient may report periods of "lost time," disremembered behaviors, or finding clothing and other possessions he or she does not recall purchasing. The patient may report hearing voices inside the head arguing, commanding, or threatening to take control of the mind and body. Affected individuals also often experience depression, nightmares, suicidal ideations and gestures, severe anxiety and phobias, rapid mood shifts, depersonalization and derealization, and headaches (Bliss, 1984; Kluft, 1987; Nemiah, 1995).

As diagnostic evaluation and treatment proceed, various personality parts may recurrently manifest, typically when exploring affectively charged, conflict-laden material. These alternate identities or personality states may appear normal or severely pathological (for example, psychotic or self-mutilating); they may vary in age, sex, race, and habits; and they may prefer different social circles. Each may have different mannerisms, speech, cognitive styles, patterns of affect, and behavior, even differing in dominant handedness. Patients may manifest nonhuman entities such as animals, mermaids, angels, and robots. The number, variety, and configuration of internal "parts" in the patient's fantasied internal "landscape" are limited only by his or her imagination and particular defensive needs. Authorities continue to debate the importance of the therapist's expectations and fascination with the phenomenology of "multiplicity" as shaping and reifying influences in this patient population (Ganaway, 1994); however, few disagree that interpersonal and sociocultural factors should be taken into account when assessing the overall clinical picture (Ganaway, 1995b).

There are often significant differences in psychological test profiles and psychophysiological characteristics among personality parts. Many studies over the years have replicated the finding of differential skin conductance (galvanic skin response) between personality states. Other measures of autonomic nervous system activity also differ, such as heart rate and muscle tone (Putnam et al, 1990). Optical differences also have been found, including altered visual acuity, visual fields, color vision, and measures of ocular physiology and eye muscle balance across personalities (Miller et al, 1991). Allergic sensitivities and response to medication may vary. Studies of brain physiology suggest different electroencephalographic (EEG) patterns, evoked responses, and regional cerebral blood flow among personalities; however, most of these findings can be duplicated in normal high hypnotizable subjects, so additional, larger studies using high hypnotizable subjects as controls are needed to replicate and verify these observations.

Illustrative Case

One of the most famous cases of multiple personality disorder was Sally Beauchamp, described by Morton Prince in *The Dissociation of a Personality* (1906). Her various personalities had "different trains of thought, . . . different views, beliefs, ideals, and temperament, and . . . different acquisitions, tastes, habits, experiences, and memories." She presented for treatment as a conscientious, well-educated young woman who appeared to be an "extreme neurasthenic." She was easily fatigued and had numerous physical complaints. Additionally, she was impressionable and emotional, suggesting the diagnosis of hysteria.

Her developmental history indicated that her parents had an unhappy marriage. Her father had a violent temper, and she felt disliked by her mother, who either ignored her or reprimanded her. Miss Beauchamp tended to idealize her mother and blamed herself. She kept feelings to herself and withdrew into fantasy. When she was 7, a brother was born, but died soon after. When she was 13, her mother died of a postpartum infection. During the next 3 years with her father, she suffered "continual mental shocks and strains." She had frequent headaches, nightmares, and fatigue. She had "attacks of somnambulism" and would go into trancelike states. At age 16, she ran away from home. Five years prior to seeking treatment, she became increasingly agitated and nervous and underwent a gradual change of character.

Dr. Prince began treatment with hypnotherapy. Soon, during a hypnotic trance, there emerged a second personality, which the doctor and patient eventually named "Sally." This personality was physically healthy with considerable stamina. She was lively, bold, amoral, and adventurous. She played mischievous pranks on Miss Beauchamp, such as causing automatisms, telling lies, or going on long walks that caused Miss Beauchamp to feel very fatigued.

Over a year into the treatment, a third personality emerged. She had more "womanly" traits and was vivacious, stubborn, ambitious, confident, and self-centered. She had more self-control, courage, and less reserve than Miss Beauchamp and was more "normal" in many respects. This personality remained unnamed, although the patient sometimes referred to her as "the idiot." Dr. Prince came to think of the three personalities as "the saint, the woman, and the devil." He eventually concluded that the patient's original "true" personality had dissociated into her presenting (Miss Beauchamp) personality and the third (unnamed) personality. Sally represented a dissociated state that would come and go. During the 6 years of treatment the first and third personalities were reintegrated, and the patient felt healthier and functioned better. Sally persisted and continued to "act up."

Occurrence

Dissociative identity disorder was previously believed to be rare, with only about 200 reported cases in the literature prior to 1980; however, increased interest sparked by the best selling book *Sybil* (Schreiber, 1973) and several other high-profile case reports in the late 1970s led to the founding in 1984 of the International Society for the Study of Multiple Personality and Dissociation, whose strongly attended annual scientific meetings spawned dozens of local and regional workshops and study groups. The result has been an explosion of reports (numbering in the thousands) of newly diagnosed cases. Investigators who have actively looked for dissociative disorders report a prevalence of multiple personality in approximately 2 to 5% of individuals screened. There is controversy in this area, however. At one end are investigators who believe dissociation and multiple personality are common and have been historically underdiagnosed or misdiagnosed (Kluft, 1987; Ross et al, 1991). At the other end are investigators who believe that the spontaneous occurrence of multiple personality is rare and that it may be produced iatrogenically in the clinical setting by suggestion (hypnotic or otherwise) or by behavioral shaping in suggestible hysterical patients who are eager to please the doctor (Merskey, 1992). More research is necessary to resolve this debate. Dissociative identity disorder is thought to originate in childhood, but individuals often do not come to clinical attention until adolescence or adulthood. It is more common in women than men (9:1) and is more common in first-degree relatives of probands than in the general population.

Etiology

Almost all recently diagnosed patients eventually report histories of exposure to overwhelming childhood trauma, usually in the form of severe physical, sexual, or emotional abuse; however, a linear causal relationship between childhood trauma and dissociative identity disorder has not yet been proved (Putnam, 1989). An alternative explanation suggests that when adult patients with a dissociative symptom cluster are diagnosed as having this disorder, they may unconsciously fabricate elaborate abuse histories to confirm the therapist's belief that such hidden memories must be there to account for the presenting symptoms (Ganaway, 1995b). Despite the ongoing controversy regarding etiology, authorities agree that affected individuals seem to have an increased tendency or ability to enter dissociative states using autohypnosis as the primary vehicle. Hypothetically, during extreme childhood abuse or trauma, this mechanism may protect the patient from being overwhelmed or incapacitated; however, if the dissociation is acquired through learning or conditioning as a coping strategy, information processed during different states of consciousness may be encoded and stored in different "circuits" inaccessible to one another, which eventually results in the development of different state-dependent "personalities." On a biological level, repeated experiences of traumatization may induce an alteration in temporal–limbic circuits analogous to the phenomenon of kindling seen in epilepsy. This may have the result of permanent alterations in the integration of sensory inputs, affects, memories, and cognition. These etiological explanations remain speculative and will require further study to validate.

Some have noted a similarity between multiple personality disorder and borderline personality disorder (Ganaway, 1994, 1995b). Patients with either disorder often suffer from depression, anxiety, emotional instability, interpersonal turmoil, and self-destructive behavior. Both groups use "primitive" defense mechanisms, including splitting, denial, dissociation, and projection. Both may report a history of abuse during childhood. Whether or not the two groups have any etiological connection is uncertain.

Differential Diagnosis

These patients may be diagnosed as having other psychiatric disorders, particularly schizophrenia, because of the possible history of hearing voices, believing themselves to be influenced by some unknown force, expressing strange ideas, and shifting patterns of identity. As mentioned, comorbidity may include anxiety disorders, depression, and personality disorders. Dissociative amnesia and dissociative fugue also should be considered. As with amnesia and fugue, any medical or neurological conditions that cause distubances of memory or consciousness should be ruled out, such as drug or alcohol intoxication or withdrawal, various other toxic, metabolic, infectious, and autoimmune disturbances, space-occupying intracranial lesions, and complex partial seizures. Malingering and factitious disorder with psychological symptoms presenting as dissociative identity disorder should also be included in the differential diagnosis.

The diagnosis of "multiple personalities" often brings with it something verging on celebrity status to the patient among psychiatrists and other mental health workers, who may be fascinated by the patient's symptoms. The physician must maintain a high index of suspicion for malingering or elaboration of symptoms in a patient with symptoms of dissociative identity disorder who is involved in a criminal justice proceeding and may be seeking a psychiatric defense.

Treatment

Various psychotropic medications may be indicated for relief of specific target symptoms if a patient with dissociative identity disorder shows evidence of severe depression, psychosis, or anxiety. If EEG findings are suggestive of temporal lobe pathology, an anticonvulsant such as carbamazepine may be of benefit to the patient (Fichtner et al, 1990). Psychotherapy can be used in an attempt to examine and ideally to change the use of dissociation and other pathological defense mechanisms by these patients. Some clinicians advocate using hypnosis to elicit the various personalities and eventually to reintegrate therapeutically the dissociated or split-off aspects of experience (Kluft, 1987; Putnam, 1989). Others believe this technique may reinforce the use of auto-hypnotic dissociation by patients (Merskey, 1992; Ganaway, 1994, 1995b). In therapy, the patient's perceived past traumas and current stressors and conflicts may be explored supportively to facilitate insight and to improve adaptation. In view of the suggestible and fantasy-prone nature of these individuals, however, the therapist should resist the temptation to use gratuitous validation of the patient's internal reality as a primary therapeutic tool.

An unfortunate byproduct of the hypothesized link between severe child abuse and adult dissociative disorders has been the spawning of a host of scientifically unsound self-help books, workshops, and seminars implicating child abuse as the primary cause of more common psychiatric disorders such as anxiety, depression, phobias, eating disorders, addictions, and severe character disorders (Ganaway, 1995a; Yapko, 1994). Ignoring the benefits of a century of methodical clinical and experimental research, a small but vocal group of self-styled "recovered memory therapists" combine simplistic distortions of early psychoanalytic concepts and techniques with hypnotherapy in a regressive experiential treatment setting to identify actively and ferret out specific "hidden memories" of alleged abuse in patients with no previous awareness of such memories. This has resulted in an epidemic of families divided by accusations of heinous sexual abuse crimes ranging from incest to forced participation in satanic human sacrifices and cannibalism. Responding to allegations arising from these therapies, in 1992 a group of accused families formed a consumer protection organization called the False Memory Syndrome Foundation (FMSF) to combat scientifically unsound forms of psychotherapy. With the assistance of an invited scientific advisory board of respected memory, hypnosis, and psychotherapy researchers and clinicians, the FMSF brought to the attention of the mental health profession the witch-hunt mentality of the "recovered memory therapies" and the need to police itself more carefully to prevent such unsound practices. On the negative side, the organization recently has begun to attract some antipsychiatry zealots keen on tarring traditional psychoanalytically oriented psychotherapies with the same brush. Care must be taken to protect the public from unsound theories and potentially harmful techniques, but at the same time, society must be careful not to "throw the baby out with the bath water."

DEPERSONALIZATION DISORDER

Description

Depersonalization is an alteration of experience in which a person feels detached from, or like an outside observer of, his or her body or mental processes. It often is accompanied by a dreamlike state. During a depersonalization episode, the person maintains intact reality testing and is generally distressed by the experience.

The symptom of depersonalization occurs in a number of disorders, including posttraumatic stress disorder, panic disorder, agoraphobia, anxiety disorders due to substances and general medical conditions, hallucinogen intoxication or hallucinogen persisting perception disorder (e.g., LSD flashbacks), severe depression, and schizophrenia (Table 13–3). Patients with seizure disorders, particularly complex partial seizures (especially those of temporal lobe origin) and other brain diseases, may experience depersonalization. Finally, depersonalization can occur in normal people as a result of stress, fatigue, or sleep deprivation. When depersonalization occurs recurrently or persistently in the absence of any of the disorders listed, a diagnosis of depersonalization disorder is made (Nemiah, 1995).

Depersonalization may be accompanied by derealization, which involves a sense of the unreality of objects in the external world (as opposed to the alteration of perception of one's self that occurs in depersonalization). Patients with depersonalization disorder may also complain of depression, anxiety, dizziness, obsessional thoughts, somatic worries, and a fear of going insane.

Table 13–3 **Other Psychiatric Disorders Presenting with Symptoms of Dissociation**

Drug intoxication or withdrawal
Schizophrenia and other psychotic disorders
Depression
Panic disorder
Agoraphobia
Anxiety disorder due to general medical conditions or substances
Posttraumatic stress disorder
Borderline personality disorder
Factitious disorder
Malingering

This condition is usually chronic with exacerbations and remissions. Patient impairment is widely variable. Some may develop secondary to alcohol or drug dependence or hypochondriasis.

Occurrence

Although single episodes of depersonalization occur in the majority of the population, the prevalence, sex ratio, and familial occurrence of depersonalization disorder are unknown.

Etiology

As with the other dissociative disorders, the etiology of depersonalization disorder is unclear. Intensely traumatic events such as military combat or physical assault may contribute to onset of the disorder. Psychoanalytic theories have viewed depersonalization as a defense against forbidden impulses, as a symptom of defective ego functioning, as a consequence of violation of one's ideals or conscience under abnormal circumstances, and as a response to interpersonal invalidation by significant others. The induction of depersonalization by hallucinogens indicates some neurological substrate for the symptoms of this disorder.

Treatment

Psychopharmacological interventions may be used for accompanying symptoms such as anxiety, depression, or obsessions, but the value of medication for depersonalization itself is unknown. Antipsychotics seem to make the condition worse.

The value of psychotherapy is also unknown, but a useful approach would generically include providing support, exploring ongoing stressors, examining the events and thoughts related to the onset of depersonalization experiences, and working to modify psychological defenses and intrapsychic conflicts.

DISSOCIATIVE DISORDER NOT OTHERWISE SPECIFIED

This category includes any disorders in which a dissociative symptom predominates but does not meet criteria for a particular specific dissociative disorder. Examples include cases resembling dissociative identity disorder in which other personality states are indistinct or amnesia does not occur; derealization experiences without depersonalization; dissociative states occurring in individuals subjected to "brainwashing" or indoctrination while held captive by cultists or terrorists; stupor, coma, or loss of consciousness not due to a general medical condition; and trance or possession states occurring in particular cultures. In many of the world's societies and cultures, dissociative phenomena manifest most often as states of possession by a spirit, demon, power, or another person, or as experiences of entering trance states beyond one's control. Some have proposed the term, "dissociative trance disorder," as a separate diagnostic classification for these collective phenomena.

ROLE OF THE NONPSYCHIATRIC PHYSICIAN AND INDICATIONS FOR PSYCHIATRIC CONSULTATION AND REFERRAL

Most patients with dissociative disorders will present for medical evaluation or treatment with complaints of amnesia, alteration of consciousness, or deteriorating psychosocial functioning. The nonpsychiatrist should be able to recognize these disorders clinically and formulate a differential diagnosis, including both neuropsychiatric and medical diagnoses. All patients with dissociative disorders should be referred for psychiatric intervention since these conditions are complex and require specialized management. The nonpsychiatrist should not leap to the conclusion that patients with dissociative symptoms should be referred elsewhere without first conducting a thorough medical–neurological evaluation to rule out the various illnesses that cause dissociative symptoms.

The dissociative disorders are dramatic clinical entities. Stirring the interest of early psychodynamic investigators, they led to the formulation of concepts such as intrapsychic conflict, altered states of consciousness, mechanisms of defense, and unconscious mental content, all of which play roles in the process described as dissociation. These dynamic mental phenomena have become part of our understanding of mental life in general and of various kinds of psychopathology. The dissociative disorders remain poorly understood manifestations of the complexity of mental life.

Patients with such disorders come to the attention of psychiatrists less often than those with more familiar clinical entities. By virtue of their dramatic presentation, such patients are often thought to be feigning their symptoms and are regularly treated with suspicion, mistrust, and even derision. Clinicians are challenged to maintain a professionally appropriate, unbiased, and technically neutral stance in attempting to understand the distress of these perplexing patients. Treatment planning must be flexible and innovative. When confronted with bizarre and somewhat theatrical behaviors, the clinician must persistently strive to be empathic, supportive, and vigorously objective. Many patients may be victims of severe past and present traumas and are reluctant to engage in any self-exploration. A negative attitude by the clinician further alienates the patient and makes a collaborative exploratory effort even less likely.

Dissociative mechanisms are particularly anxiety provoking for physicians because, despite their bizarre appearance, they occur in patients who appear in other respects in touch with reality and thus not radically different from those providing them with psychiatric care. Such mechanisms represent extreme instances of psychological processes that are constantly active in all individuals. Therefore, they continue to hold our scientific interest. Ideally, more systematic investigation will lead to a better understanding of them and subsequent improved responsiveness to treatment interventions.

CLINICAL PEARLS

The dissociative disorders should be considered in the differential diagnosis of any patient presenting with alteration of consciousness, amnesia, "spells," disturbance of identity, or alteration of feelings of reality.

- A complete medical–neurological evaluation should be conducted on these patients to rule out the multiple neurological causes of dissociative symptoms.
- The etiology of dissociative disorders remains poorly understood. Modern theories reflect the thinking of the early pioneers, including Janet, James, Prince, Breuer, and Freud. All include the theory that some pathogenic mental content is split off from conscious awareness, but continues to exert an influence on emotions, thought, and behavior. This splitting of the mind is thought to arise from state-dependent memory storage (Janet), autohypnotic phenomena (Breuer), and repression and other defense mechanisms occurring in the context of conflicting forces in the mind (Freud). Neurobiological theory also suggests a role of pathological temporal–limbic functioning that causes a disordered integration of the storage and retrieval of memories.
- Psychological trauma is thought to play an important pathogenic role in the development of most dissociative disorders. Dissociative identity disorder (multiple personality disorder) in particular is associated with self-reports of severe childhood physical and sexual abuse; however, a linear causal relationship has not been proved.
- Although certain medications may help with symptoms of anxiety, depression, or violent behavior in some patients with dissociative disorders, the treatment of choice continues to be psychotherapy.

ANNOTATED BIBLIOGRAPHY

Bliss EL: Multiple Personality, Allied Disorders, and Hypnosis. New York, Oxford University Press, 1986

> This book discusses the theory and practice of hypnosis and goes on to describe multiple personality and other dissociative disorders and their relationship to autohypnotic phenomena.

Braun BG: Treatment of Multiple Personality Disorder. Washington, DC, American Psychiatric Press, 1986

> The chapters of this book discuss different therapeutic approaches including psychotherapy, medication, group therapy, psychoanalysis, and social interventions; however, many of the techniques described here have come under heavy scrutiny and criticism from investigators who are concerned about iatrogenicity.

Breuer J, Freud S: Studies on Hysteria. In The Standard Edition of the Complete Psychological Works of Sigmund Freud, Vol. 2, 1893–1895. London, Hogarth Press, 1955

> This monumental work depicts Breuer and Freud's differing conceptions of the pathogenesis of hysterical phenomena, including both conversion and dissociative mechanisms. Freud goes on to describe the psychological treatment of hysteria.

Fisher C: Amnesic states in war neuroses: the psychogenesis of fugues. Psychoanal Q 14:437–468, 1945

> This classic paper discusses the psychodynamic processes involved in dissociation, with emphasis on amnesia and fugue.

Kenny MG: The Passion of Ansel Bourne: Multiple Personality in American Culture. Washington, DC, Smithsonian Institution Press, 1986

> This book describes the work of pioneering investigators, including William James and Morton Prince in America, and Charcot, Janet, and Freud in Europe, and elaborates on many of the famous cases described by the Americans. It provides a rich historical perspective on the theories of dissociation.

Lynn SJ, Rhue JW (eds): Dissociation: Clinical and Theoretical Perspectives. New York, Guilford, 1994

> This is a scientifically authoritative reference on all the major aspects of dissociation, including critiques of theoretical models, diagnostic and treatment approaches, research, and conceptual issues. The contributing authors address controversies and debates in a rational and even-handed manner.

Nemiah JC: Dissociative disorders. In Kaplan HI, Sadock BJ (eds): Comprehensive Textbook of Psychiatry/VI, 6th ed. Baltimore, Williams & Wilkins, 1995

> This textbook chapter by an eminent psychiatrist offers an excellent review of the concepts of hysteria, dissociation, and the dissociative disorders.

Putnam FW: Diagnosis and Treatment of Multiple Personality Disorder. New York, Guilford Press, 1989

> The author provides a historical perspective on dissociative experiences and describes his views of multiple personality disorder. His approaches to diagnosis and treatment are considered controversial by some authorities (see Lynn and Rhue).

Yapko MD: Suggestions of Abuse: True and False Memories of Childhood Sexual Trauma. New York, Simon & Schuster, 1994

> A clinical psychologist with extensive experience in both hypnotherapy and treatment of families involved with issues of child abuse provides an intelligent, sensitive assessment of the "false memory" debate and offers advice to therapists, patients, and families on how to avoid psychotherapeutic misadventures.

REFERENCES

Abse DW: Hysterical conversion and dissociative syndromes and the hysterical character. In Arieti S, Brody EB (eds): American Handbook of Psychiatry, 2nd ed, Vol. 3. New York, Basic Books, 1974

American Psychiatric Association, Diagnostic and Statistical Manual of Mental Disorders, 4th ed. Washington, DC, 1994

Bliss EL: A symptom profile of patients with multiple personalities, including MMPI results. J Nerv Ment Dis 172:197–201, 1984

Breuer J, Freud S: Studies on Hysteria. In The Standard Edition of the Complete Psychological Works of Sigmund Freud, Vol. 2, 1893–1895. London, Hogarth Press, 1955

Carlson ET: The history of multiple personality in the United States: I. The beginnings. Am J Psychiatry 138:666–668, 1981

Counts RM: The concept of dissociation. J Am Acad Psychoanal 18:460–479, 1990

Fichtner CG, Kuhlman DT, Gruenfeld MJ, et al: Decreased episodic violence and increased control of dissociation in a carbamazepine-treated case of multiple personality. Biol Psychiatry 27:1045–1052, 1990

Ganaway GK: Transference and countertransference shaping influences on dissociative syndromes. In Lynn SJ, Rhue JW (eds): Dissociation: Clinical and Theoretical Perspectives. New York, Guilford, 1994

Ganaway GK: Recovered memories may mislead therapists. Menninger Lett January:4–6, 1995a

Ganaway GK: Hypnosis, childhood trauma, and dissociative identity disorder: toward an integrative theory. Int J Clin Exp Hypn 18:127–144, 1995b

James W: The Principles of Psychology. New York, Dover, 1918

Kluft RP: An update on multiple personality disorder. Hosp Community Psychiatry 38:363–373, 1987

Kopelman MD: Amnesia: organic and psychogenic. Br J Psychiatry 150:428–442, 1987

Merskey H: The manufacture of personalities: the production of multiple personality disorder. Br J Psychiatry 160:327–340, 1992

Miller SD, Blackbum T, Scholes G, et al: Optical differences in multiple personality disorder: a second look. J Nerv Ment Dis 179:132–135, 1991

Nemiah JC: Dissociative disorders. In Kaplan HI, Sadock BJ (eds): Comprehensive Textbook of Psychiatry/VI, 6th ed. Baltimore, Williams & Wilkins, 1995

Prince M: The Dissociation of a Personality. New York, Longmans Green, 1906

Putnam FW: Diagnosis and Treatment of Multiple Personality Disorder. New York, Guilford Press, 1989

Putnam FW, Zahn TP, Post RM: Differential autonomic nervous system activity in multiple personality disorder. Psychiatr Res 31:251–260, 1990

Riether AM, Stoudemire A: Psychogenic fugue states: a review. South Med J 81:568–571, 1988

Ross CA, Joshi S, Currie R: Dissociative experiences in the general population: a factor analysis. Hosp Community Psychiatry 42:297–301, 1991

Schreiber FR: Sybil. Chicago, Henry Regnery, 1973

van der Kolk BA, van der Hart O: Pierre Janet and the breakdown of adaptation in psychological trauma. Am J Psychiatry 146:1530–1540, 1989

Yapko MD: Suggestions of Abuse: True and False Memories of Childhood Sexual Trauma. New York, Simon & Schuster, 1994

14 Psychosexual Disorders

Peter J. Fagan
and Chester W. Schmidt, Jr.

Sexual dysfunction is a subclass of sexual disorders in which the essential feature is inhibition in sexual interest or psychophysiological disturbances in the sexual response cycle. Sexual dysfunction is distinguished from the other sexual disorder group, paraphilia, in which there is generally no impairment in sexual function. A third category of disorders closely related to sexuality is disorders of gender identity. Readers who wish to learn more about this diagnostic group might consult Blanchard and Steiner (1990).

Sexual dysfunction is not a life-threatening condition, but the negative effects it can have on a patient's self-esteem or relationship should not be underestimated. Given the multiple biological, psychological, and social aspects of human sexual behavior, sexual dysfunction requires a careful and thorough diagnostic evaluation. Because sexuality is so central to self-esteem and the ability to relate to others, a person with a sexual dysfunction deserves skillful and sensitive therapy.

EPIDEMIOLOGY

The most adequate demographic survey of the incidence and prevalence of sexual dysfunction in the general adult (18–59 years) population of the United States is in the National Health and Social Life Survey (Laumann et al, 1994) (Table 14–1).

Among those with medical illnesses or postsurgical conditions, the prevalence of sexual dysfunction due to contributing psychogenic factors has been

Table 14–1 **Percentage of Sexual Problems in General Population of Adults (18-59 Years) by Gender**

SEXUAL PROBLEM	MEN	WOMEN
Lack of interest in having sex	15.7	33.4
Unable to climax	8.2	24.1
Climax too quickly	28.5	10.3
Physical pain during intercourse	3.0	14.4
Sex not pleasurable	8.1	21.2
Anxious about performance	17.0	11.5
Arousal (erection/lubrication)	10.4	18.8

(From Laumann et al 1994)

understandably difficult to establish because of the covarying effects of the medical illness. While sample sizes of studies of specific medical conditions are generally too small for epidemiological purposes, and specific psychogenic factors are usually not identified, sexual dysfunction is in general clearly highly prevalent among the medically ill (Schover and Jensen, 1988). There is an increase in orgasmic and erectile dysfunction among the medically ill and a decrease in the incidence of premature ejaculation (Spector and Carey, 1990).

About 30% of sexually dysfunctional individuals also have an additional (Axis I) psychiatric disorder that is not a primary etiological agent in the sexual dysfunction (e.g., major depression) (Fagan et al, 1988).

DESCRIPTION

Sexual dysfunctions have traditionally been understood as deviations from the normal human sexual response cycle, as described by Masters and Johnson (1966). This has been adapted and amplified in Figure 14–1 to display both the normal physiological arousal pattern (increased heart rate and blood pressure, myotonia) and the particular sexual disorders that may appear in each particular phase.

One of the problems with accepting the Masters and Johnson model of human sexual response uncritically is the possible denial in this model of the cultural factors that are developed and expressed. Since the 1960s, this model has been the dominant paradigm of sexual response in Western cultures. There is growing criticism of total reliance on such a simple physiological model to describe human sexual functioning. The social constructionist school argues that the meaning of sexual behavior (what makes it "unnatural" or "dysfunctional" or "pathological") is constructed from the dominant culture beliefs (Laquer, 1990; Tiefer, 1991). Social constructionists hold that individual deviations from this response pattern might be viewed not as dysfunction, but as

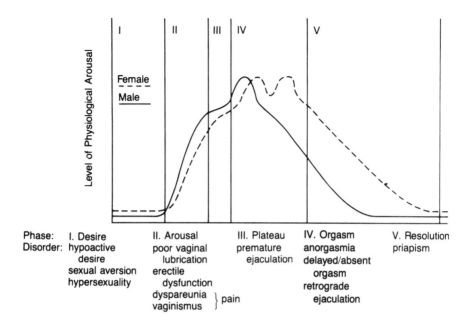

Figure 14–1. *Levels of physiological arousal and sexual disorders in men and women according to phases of sexual response. (Adapted from Masters and Johnson, 1966; and Fagan and Schmidt, 1987)*

cultural or experienced–learned differences, e.g., multiorgasmic men and nonorgasmic women. Uncritical dependence on traditional sex therapy (based on the Masters and Johnson sensate focus model) might pose obstacles for successful treatment of individuals from non-Western cultures.

However, with this caveat in mind, the human sexual response cycle provides clinicians with a relative norm with which they can obtain a clear phenomenology of the specific nature of the sexual dysfunction. This can be done during an elaboration of the presenting problem by asking patients to describe their last attempt at sexual intercourse or sexual activity. Particular attention should be paid to quantifying both time (e.g., in foreplay) and physiological response (e.g., vaginal lubrication). These data should then be compared with the human sexual response cycle described by Masters and Johnson (1966) and further elaborated in DSM-IV (American Psychiatric Association, 1994). When there appears to be more than one sexual dysfunction, the clinician must determine which disorder was historically first and, therefore, may be etiologically connected to the secondary condition. For example, a man distressed by premature ejaculation may develop secondary erectile dysfunction.

The DSM-IV groupings of the psychosexual dysfunctions are disorders of desire, arousal, orgasm, and pain. Categories for dysfunctions due to general medical conditions or induced by a substance (drug or medicine) have been added to DSM-IV. A diagnostic category, "sexual dysfunction not otherwise specified," provides for patients whose symptoms elude existing diagnostic taxonomy.

Disorders of Desire

DSM-IV lists two disorders of sexual desire: "hypoactive sexual desire disorder" and "sexual aversion disorder." Hypoactive sexual desire is a condition in which the patient reports usually a global lack of cognitive, emotional, and physiological readiness to initiate or take part in sexual activity. Compared with others of the same age, sex, health status, and availability of a sexual partner, a person with hypoactive sexual desire has fewer sexual fantasies and lower orgasmic frequency (through masturbation or intercourse). If the condition is acquired, the distress shown by the patient about the low sexual desire may range from preoccupation (e.g., in the "macho" male) to indifference (e.g., in the mother of multiple preschool children). In situations of long-standing hypoactive sexual desire, the condition may be quite ego-syntonic (i.e., not troublesome to the patient).

This disorder does not imply an inability to function sexually. Once activity is initiated, usually by the partner, the individual becomes aroused and, unless there is a separate dysfunction, is orgasmic. The hallmark of this disorder is that the baseline of sexual desire (libido) remains significantly low.

Sexual aversion disorder was a new diagnostic category in DSM-III-R. Conceptualized by Helen Singer Kaplan (1991), the disorder is the aversion to and avoidance of genital sexual activity with a partner. Sexual desire may be normal with fantasy and masturbation frequencies appropriate for age and sex. The patient may avoid intercourse completely or may participate only infrequently out of a sense of duty to the partner. Central to the disorder is a pattern of avoidance that results in infrequent intercourse. When experienced, intercourse is merely tolerated. A sense of enjoyment, satisfaction, and collaboration is usually minimal or absent. Poor body image, especially regarding breasts and genitals, is common; nudity is avoided. While disorders of desire may cause marked distress in the individual with hypoactive desire or sexual aversion, it is far more likely that the reason for seeking treatment is the distress of the partner and the resultant interpersonal difficulties.

Disorders of Arousal

Disorders of arousal pertain to an inability to achieve sufficient physiological or cognitive/emotional arousal during sexual activity. In women, the disorder is called Female Sexual Arousal Disorder; in men, the disorder is Male Erectile Disorder. Insufficient physiological arousal for women consists of failure to attain or maintain adequate lubrication-swelling response of the vagina and labia for the completion of sexual activity. Intercourse may be performed, but vaginal dryness will cause pain on initial penetration or throughout coitus. In men, the failure to attain or maintain erection until the completion of sexual activity is the criteria for arousal disorder. In most cases, it makes intravaginal penetration and ejaculation rare. In others, ejaculation is purposefully rushed after penetration to precede penile detumescence.

In addition to the insufficient peripheral response of the genitals, a disorder of arousal exists when the disturbance causes marked distress or interpersonal difficulty (DSM-IV).

Orgasm Disorders

Female orgasmic disorder is marked by the persistent or recurrent delay in, or absence of, orgasm following a normal sexual excitement phase (DSM-IV). The clinician judges that an orgasm disorder is present in a woman when there is less orgasmic capacity "than would be reasonable for her age, sexual experience, and the adequacy of sexual stimulation she receives" (DSM-IV). Many women do not experience vaginal (as distinct from clitoral) orgasm. During intercourse, there may generally be less clitoral stimulation than is necessary for them to achieve orgasm. For them, orgasm is achieved during the sexual experience by manual or oral stimulation of the clitoris. This phenomenon is a variant of the normal female sexual response cycle and should not be considered a sexual dysfunction. The coital anorgasmia may be etiologically related to constitutional sensory thresholds, rather than psychosexual conflicts (Derogatis et al, 1986).

Male orgasmic disorder is likewise the persistent or recurrent delay in, or absence of, orgasm following a normal excitement phase during sexual activity that is adequate in focus, intensity, and duration (DSM-IV). It is important to specify whether the orgasm disorder is present in all sexually stimulating situations (very rare for psychogenic dysfunction) or only in specific situations, e.g., interpersonal sex.

When evaluating a male patient with an orgasm disorder, the clinician should bear in mind the following clinical conditions. Men may ejaculate without a sense of orgasmic pleasure; this should be designated as Sexual Dysfunction Not Otherwise Specified (NOS). Others may have orgasm without the emission of ejaculate (e.g., retrograde ejaculation following surgery disrupting enervation of the bladder sphincter muscle); this is not an orgasm disorder. Finally, orgasm and ejaculation may occur without full penile tumescence. This is a disorder of arousal if maximum tumescence has been obtained after sufficient stimulation.

Premature ejaculation occurs persistently with "minimal sexual stimulation or before, upon, or shortly after penetration and before the person wishes it" (DSM-IV). Premature ejaculation may occur with partial or full tumescence and is usually a condition that has been present since the male was sexually active with a partner. While no reduction in orgasmic pleasure is reported, a man with premature ejaculation is usually distressed that he cannot last long enough for his female partner to have a satisfying sexual experience. As anorgasmia in women may be related to constitutional sensory thresholds, similarly, a relatively low threshold to physical sexual stimuli may be in some men a constitutional "vulnerability" to premature ejaculation (Strassberg et al, 1990). It is classified as a dysfunction only because of the effects of the behavior during interpersonal sexual activity.

Sexual Pain Disorders

There are two sexual pain disorders, Dyspareunia and Vaginismus. Dyspareunia in a man or woman is "recurrent or persistent genital pain . . . before, during or after sexual intercourse" (DSM-IV). To assign this diagnosis in women, the dyspareunia should not be caused by a lack of lubrication (Female Sexual Arousal Disorder) or be secondary to vaginismus. In both men and women, the pain is not caused by a medical condition or drugs.

Vaginismus is "recurrent or persistent involuntary spasm of the musculature of the outer third of the vagina that interferes with coitus" (DSM-IV). Although frequently secondary to genital or sexual trauma, the disorder is not caused *exclusively* by a physical disorder. The spasms of vaginismus are reflex spasms and not voluntary responses on the woman's part; her male partner often does not appreciate this fact and feels that his sexual advances are being willfully rejected. The condition is frequently generalized to interfere with a pelvic examination or, in rare cases, the insertion of a tampon.

ETIOLOGY

Human sexual behavior is motivated behavior in which physiological drives are expressed bodily, are experienced by a sentient person, and, if only in fantasy, are nearly always in an erotic relationship with another person (or object surrogate such as a fetish). When sexual behavior fails despite efforts that are appropriate for the desired end, then sexual dysfunction has occurred. The etiology of the dysfunction can be biogenic or psychogenic or a combination of the two.

Biogenic Causes

Biogenic sexual dysfunction is determined by a careful review of systems, as well as by physical examination (Table 14–2) (Buvat et al, 1990). A family history of chronic diseases should also be obtained. Symptomatology or history of endocrine, vascular, or neurological diseases deserves special attention. Table 14–3 elaborates some of the more common medical and surgical causes of sexual dysfunction in men and women.

Drugs are commonly a principal agent in sexual dysfunction and often contribute to the disorder in a patient whose body has already been compro-

Table 14–2 **Components of Physical Examination of Sexually Dysfunctional Patients**

ORGAN SYSTEM	PHYSICAL EXAMINATION
Endocrine system	
	Hair distribution
	Gynecomastia
	Testes
	Thyroid gland
Vascular system	
	Peripheral pulses
Gastrointestinal System	
	Hepatomegaly, or atrophic liver with peripheral neuropathy due to alcoholism
Genitourinary system	
	Prostate (in male)
	Pelvic examination (in female)
Nervous system	
Sacral innervation	
S1–S2	Mobility of small muscles of the foot
S2–S4	Internal, external anal sphincter tone
	Bulbocavernosus reflex (in male)
S2–S5	Perianal sensation
Peripheral sensation	
Deep tendon reflexes	
Long tract signs	

(Adapted from Wise TN, Schmidt CW: Diagnostic approaches to sexuality in the medically ill. In Hall RC, Beresford TP (eds): Handbook of Psychiatric Diagnostic Procedures, Vol 2. New York, Spectrum, 1985)

mised by disease. Table 14–4 lists many drugs reported to affect sexual response. Alcohol and drug abuse, beta-adrenergic blockers, centrally acting antihypertensives, and antiandrogens are commonly reported drugs implicated in sexual dysfunction (Fagan and Schmidt, 1993). Selective serotonin-reuptake inhibitors (SSRIs) have sexual dysfunction effects, mainly in the orgasmic/ejaculation phases, that are routinely experienced.

Referrals to allied medical specialties can be used to determine biogenic factors of sexual dysfunction. A urological examination for erectile dysfunction includes Doppler studies of penile blood flow and measurement of the penile-brachial index (PBI), the ratio of penile systolic pressure to brachial systolic pressure. A PBI less than 0.60 suggests vascular etiology for erectile dysfunction. Referral to urology should be had when there is no or inconsistent history of erection in noncoital situations, e.g., sleep, masturbation. Similarly, a referral to a gynecologist who is experienced in treating vulvar or vaginal pain

Table 14–3 **Medical Factors that May Affect Sexual Response in Men and Women**

MEN	WOMEN	BOTH
Peyronie's disease	Atrophic vaginitis	Chronic systemic disease in-
Urethral infections	Infections of the vagina	cluding endocrine disorders
Testicular disease	Cystitis, urethritis	Chronic pain
Hypogonadal androgen-	Endometriosis	Diabetes millitus
deficient states	Episiotomy, scars, tears	Angina pectoris
Hydrocele	Uterine prolapse	Hypertension
Lumbar sympathectomy	Infections of external	Multiple sclerosis
Radical perineal	genitalia	Hyperprolactinemia
prostatectomy	Androgen deficient	Spinal cord lesions
Sleep Apnea	states	Alcoholism
		Substance abuse

(Adapted and reprinted with permission from Schmidt CW Jr: Sexual disorders. In Harvey AM, Owens A Jr, McKusick A (eds): Principles and Practice of Medicine, p 1149, 16.10–1. East Norwalk, CT: Appleton & Lange, 1988)

should be made when these conditions are present—even when a previous physician could find no biogenic cause for the pain.

Endocrine studies of patients with suspected hormonal etiology should include measurement of fasting blood sugar and assays of follicle-stimulating hormone, luteinizing hormone, testosterone, and prolactin, as well as a general survey (e.g., SMA-18) for liver and renal disease. The level of free (bioavailable) testosterone may be more predictive of endocrine deficiency in male sexual response than the level of serum testosterone (Carani et al, 1990).

Neurological assessment of the motor, sensory, and autonomic nervous system should pay special attention to the lumbosacral spinal pathways (Table 14–2 and Fig. 14–2). A cystometrogram or urinary flow studies can grossly define autonomic function in this area. The nerve-sparing technique for retropubic prostatectomy means that such patients should not be considered a priori surgically impotent (Walsh et al, 1983).

Nocturnal penile tumescence (NPT) studies monitor the duration, frequency, and amount of penile tumescence during rapid eye movement sleep. NPT studies can also determine the relationship between penile blood flow and bulbocavernosus and ischiocavernosus muscle activity. In many centers, there is also a rigidity challenge in which the buckling force of the erection is measured by a technician with a handheld mercury strain gauge. While NPT is the most complete evaluation of nocturnal erections, research with normal volunteers (Schiavi, 1990) invites further exploration of the relationship between nocturnal erections and those sought or attained while awake.

When a sexual dysfunction has been linked with a medical illness or treatment, DSM-IV provides for the diagnoses of Sexual Dysfunction Due to General Medical Conditions, e.g., Painful Intercourse With Vestibular Adenitis, or Sexual

Table 14–4 **Medications that May Affect Sexual Response**

DRUG	SEXUAL RESPONSES
Antihypertensives	
1. Diuretics	
Bendroflumethazide (10 mg/day)	Libido, erectile, ejaculation problems
Chlorothiazide (100 mg/day)	Libido, erectile, ejaculation problems
Indapamide (2.5 mg/day)	No reports of impotence
Spironolactone (400 mg/day)	Erectile and libido problems
2. Adrenergic inhibitors—beta-adrenergic blockers	
Atenolol (50–100 mg/day)	Few reports of dysfunction
Bisopropol (5 mg/day)	No sexual dysfunction reported
Metoprolol (200 mg/day)	Few reports of dysfunction
Nadolol (40–240 mg/day)	Few reports of dysfunction
Pindolol (15 mg/day)	Few reports of dysfunction
Propranolol (dose related)	Libido, erectile problems
Timolol (ocular)	Libido, erectile, low ejaculate problems
3. Central-acting adrenergic inhibitors	
Clonidine (0.2–4.8 mg/day)	Libido, erectile problems
Guanabenz (4–64 mg/day)	<1% libido, erectile problems
Methyldopa (1–3 gm/day)	Libido, erectile, ejaculation problems
4. Peripheral-acting adrenergic antagonists	
Guanadrel + hydrochlorothiazide	Libido, erectile, ejaculation problems
Guanadrel + chlorothiazide	Libido, erectile, ejaculation problems
Guanethidine (>25 mg/day)	Libido, erectile, emission/ejaculation problems
Reserpine (0.1 mg/day)	Libido, erectile problems
5. Alpha-adrenergic blockers	
Phenoxybenzamine (5–70 mg/day)	Emission problems
Prazosin (3–20 mg/day)	Low incidence of sexual dysfunction
Terazosin (1–40 mg/day)	Low incidence of sexual dysfunction
6. Combined alpha- and beta-adrenergic blockers	
Labetalol (200–1,000 mg/day)	Erection, ejaculation, delayed detumescence problems
7. Vasodilators	
Hydralazine (35–50 mg/day)	No sexual dysfunction
Minoxidil	No sexual dysfunction
8. Angiotensin-converting enzyme inhibitors	
Captopril (100 mg/day)	19% had worsening of sexual dysfunction
9. Slow channel calcium-entry blocking agents	
Verapamil	No reports when used alone
Psychopharmacological Agents	
1. Antidepressants	
Amitriptyline (50–200 mg/day)	Libido, arousal, and orgasm problems
Amoxapine (126–210 mg/day)	Libido, arousal, and orgasm problems
Buproprion (300–600 mg/day)	No reports of sexual dysfunction
Clomipramine (25–75 mg/day)	Libido, arousal, and orgasm problems
Desipramine (75–300 mg/day)	Libido, arousal, and orgasm problems
Fluoxetine (20–80 mg/day)	Anorgasmia, delayed ejaculation
Fluvoxamine	Abnormal ejaculation (8%) in clinical trials
Imipramine (25–225 mg/day)	Libido, arousal, and orgasm problems

(continued)

Table 14–4 *(continued)*

DRUG	SEXUAL RESPONSES
Psychopharmacological Agents	
Maprotiline (150 mg/day)	Libido, arousal, and orgasm problems
Mirtazapine	Breast pain; impotence
Nortriptyline (125–200 mg/day)	Libido, arousal, and orgasm problems
Paroxetine	Ejaculatory disturbance (13%); other male genital disorders (10%) in clinical trials
Protriptyline (20–60 mg/day)	Libido, arousal, and orgasm problems
Sertraline	15% male, 2% female sexual dysfunction (anorgasmia and delayed ejaculation)
Trazodone (50–600 mg/day)	Priapism
Trimipramine	Libido, arousal, and orgasm problems
Venlafaxine	Abnormal ejaculation/orgasm (12%); impotence (6%) in clinical trials
2. Monoamine oxidase inhibitors	
Phenelzine (30–90 mg/day)	Arousal and orgasm problems
Tranylcypromine (20 mg/day)	Arousal and orgasm problems
3. Mood stabilizers	
Lithium	Libido and erectile problems
Carbamazepine	Decreased libido or erectile problems (13%)
4. Antipsychotics	
Butaperazine (40–160 mg/day)	Libido, erectile, ejaculation problems
Chlopromazine (1200 mg/day)	Libido, erectile, ejaculation problems, priapism
Chlorprothixine (300 mg/day)	Libido, erectile, ejaculation problems
Fluphenazine	Arousal, ejaculation, (painful) orgasm problems
Haloperidol (5 mg/day)	Libido, erectile, ejaculation problems
Mesoridazine (300–400 mg/day)	Libido, erectile, ejaculation problems, priapism
Perphenazine (24 mg/day)	Libido, erectile ejaculation problems
Pimozide (16 mg/day)	Libido, erectile, ejaculation problems
Risperidone	Erectile dysfunction
Thioridazine (30–600 mg/day)	Arousal, ejaculation, (painful) orgasm problems, priapism
Thiothixene (20 mg/day)	Libido, erectile, ejaculation problems
Trifluoperazine (20 mg/day)	Libido, erectile, ejaculation problems
5 Anxiolytics	
Alprazolam (3–10 mg/day)	Libido, erectile, ejaculation problems, anorgasmia
Buspirone	No reported sexual dysfunction
Diazepam (15–40 mg/day)	Libido, erectile, ejaculation problems in males No negative impact on female sexual function
Lorazepam (1–3 mg/day)	Libido, ejaculation problems
6. Stimulants	
Dextroamphetamine	Impotence, changes in libido
Exogenous Hormones	
1. Androgens	
Anabolic steroids	Libido decrease, impotence, testicular atrophy, azoospermia
Testosterone	No negative effect on sexual function
2. Estrogens	Decreased vaginal atrophy; decreased libido in males
Cancer Chemotherapy Agents	
1. Alkylating agents	Gonadal dysfunction in males and females
Busulphan	
Chlorambucil	

(continued)

Table 14–4 *(continued)*

DRUG	SEXUAL RESPONSES
Cancer Chemotherapy Agents	
Cyclophosphamide	
Melphalan	
2. Other agents	
Cytosine arabinoside	Gonadal dysfunction in males and females
Ketaconazole (400 mg t.i.d)	Supresses testicular and adrenal androgen synthesis
Procarbazine	Gonadal dysfunction in males and females
Vinblastine	Gonadal dysfunction in males and females
Carbonic Anhydrase Inhibitors	
Acetazolamide (1 gm/day)	Libido, erectile problems
Dichlorophenamide (100–200 mg/day)	Libido, erectile problems
Methazolamide (100–200 mg/day)	Libido, erectile problems
Antiepileptic Drugs	
Carbamazepine	13% decreased libido or erectile problems
Phenobarbital	16% decreased libido or erectile problems
Primadone	22% decreased libido or erectile problems
Phenytoin	11% male libido or erectile problems

(Adapted from Buffum J: Prescription drugs and sexual function. Psychiatric Med 10:181–198, 1992)

Dysfunction Induced by Either Drugs or Medications. These two diagnostic categories are new to the DSM series and should be entered on Axis I with the medical condition noted on Axis III and the drug/medication specified in the diagnostic code on Axis I.

Psychogenic Causes

To ascertain the psychogenic causes of sexual dysfunction, a complete psychosocial and psychosexual history should be taken. Table 14–5 lists the data particularly important for the sexual development and behavior of an individual. To obtain the sexual data, the clinician should establish an atmosphere of candor and relative comfort. The physician should ask every and any question that may be relevant to the diagnosis and treatment of the sexual dysfunction. If the clinician is confident that the information being obtained may be important, then this attitude will be conveyed to the patient, and a condition of relative comfort will exist between them.

Watching experienced clinicians take histories of both sexes will help the novice clinician learn the art of taking a sexual history. It is normal for medical students to be somewhat embarrassed in the initial stages of taking sexual histories, especially with patients of the opposite sex. In obtaining a sexual history, the clinician must be aware of and able to confront issues of sexuality in his or her own life. The discomfort or embarrassment should diminish fairly rapidly with experience. If it persists, the clinician should consult her or his clinical

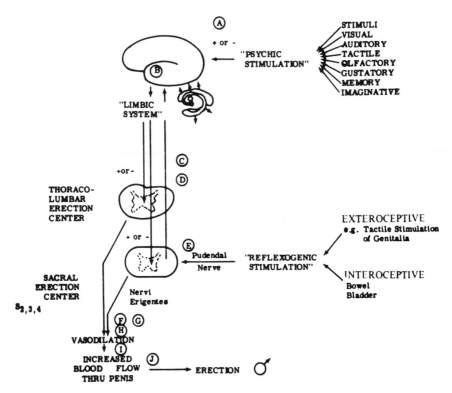

Figure 14–2. *Neurological pathways involved in human penile erection. A–J, sites where lesions could cause sexual dysfunction. (Reproduced with permission from Weiss HD:The physiology of human erection. Ann Intern Med 16:793–799, 1972)*

supervisor for assistance. Conversely, if the clinician feels absolutely no twinge of discomfort when initially taking sexual histories, he or she may lack sufficient sensitivity to the emotional issues connected with sexuality. This absence of any sort of feeling might also be discussed with a supervisor.

If the sexual history follows the lifeline and developmental stages (as suggested in Table 14–5), the patient has a schema of what to expect. This format helps to reduce the anxiety that would be generated if the patient felt that a set of completely random questions were being asked about his or her sexual behavior in symptom checklist fashion.

To learn about the phenomenology of the sexual dysfunction, it is helpful to ask patients to describe their most recent attempt at sexual experience. Questions should focus on the person's mental/emotional reactions to the sexual experience (e.g., "Did you think about what you were doing or were you thinking about something or someone else?"), as well as on the patient's physiological responses (e.g., "Were you lubricated when penetration was attempted?"). Thoughts and feelings about self and partner convey the emotional reactions.

Table 14–5 **Data Covered for a Complete Sexual History**

Childhood

First sex play with peers
Family sleeping arrangements
Sex play with siblings
Sexual abuse, incest, or molestation
Parental attitudes toward sex
Sources of sexual knowledge

Pubertal

Menarche or first ejaculation: subjective reaction
Secondary sex characteristics: subjective reaction
Body image
Masturbation fantasies and frequency
Homoerotic fantasies and behavior
Dating experiences (physical intimacies)
Intercourse
   Age at first occurrence
   Reaction to first intercourse

Young Adult

Lengthy or live-in relationships
Pattern of sexual activities with others
Paraphilic behaviors
Previous marriages
   Courtship
   Parental attitudes toward spouse
   Sexual activity (dysfunction?)
   Reasons for termination of marriage
Venereal diseases, including HIV exposure

Adult

Present Primary Sexual Relationship
Development of relationship
Significant nonsexual problems (e.g., money, alcohol, in-laws)
Infertility; contraceptive practices
Children (problems?)
Sexual Behaviors
Extramarital affairs
Intercourse frequency during relationship
Variety of sexual behaviors (e.g., oral-genital, masturbation)
Previous dysfunction (in either partner)
Elaboration of onset and history of present problem (without
   partner present)
Perception of partner's reaction to problem
Homosexual activity
Possible exposure to human immunodeficiency virus

(Reprinted with permission from Fagan PJ, Schmidt CW Jr: Sexual dysfunction in the
medically ill. In Stoudemire A, Fogel BS (eds): Psychiatric Care of the Medical Patient,
p 311. New York, Oxford University Press, 1993)

The human sexual response cycle serves as the framework for appreciating the physiological response of the patient. Even with a complete history, however, the multiple determinants of the dysfunction may not become apparent until the person or couple has been in psychotherapy for several sessions. For example, the role of imagery and positive sexual fantasy may be a sufficient component for sexual response in some individuals, but the nature and quality of such may not emerge until several therapy sessions have established adequate trust.

Psychogenic causes of sexual dysfunction are cognitions or emotions that either ignore (repress) nearly all sexual stimuli in disorders of sexual desire or, in the other sexual disorders, lead to a "fight-or-flight" physiological reaction in which excessive adrenergic effects inhibit the normal human sexual response cycle. The most common example is performance anxiety, in which (usually) the man is so concerned about his sexual functioning that the anxiety itself becomes a self-fulfilling prophecy.

The etiology of these cognitions or emotions that cause sexual dysfunction can be understood from a variety of theoretical frameworks, but none totally explains the etiology of all sexual dysfunction. The major systems that have addressed sexual behavior (and by extension, sexual dysfunction) are psychoanalytic theory, behaviorism, cognitive theory, and social learning theory. What follows is a brief statement about each theory, with a clinical example of the etiology of a sexual dysfunction, as explained by that theory.

A *psychoanalytic* approach to sexuality (Person, 1987) and to sexual dysfunction (Meyer et al, 1986) most often explains the disorder as a symptom of an underlying psychological conflict. As such, the dysfunction serves as a psychosomatic symbol of an unconscious conflict and a protection (defense) against consciously experiencing the anxiety of that primary conflict (e.g., separation from a loved object). For example, most sexual dysfunction promotes sexual estrangement, in which physical intimacy is reduced. One with an arousal disorder, therefore, reduces her or his exposure to the possibility of rejection by a lover. A psychoanalytic therapist might also suspect that this fear of rejection is rooted in an infantile experience of rejection by the mother or father. In the analytic tradition, but from the object relations viewpoint, *The Sexual Relationship* by David Scharf (1982) is an excellent description of psychosexual development throughout the life span.

Behaviorism explains sexual behavior as it does all behavior: as a response to environmental stimuli. In classical conditioning, an object becomes paired with a stimulus so that it can provoke the same response in the organism. In operant conditioning, the organism learns to interact with the environment so that a favorable reward is obtained or a negative result avoided. Sexual pleasure is a reward; sexual pain is a negative result. If sexual intercourse has become paired with pain, including emotional pain, then any approach to it will be avoided. This is commonly seen in sexual aversion disorder. In more extreme cases, the trauma of rape or incest results in aversion disorder or vaginismus.

Social learning theory stresses the role of learning by imitating others (McConaghy, 1987). A person learns how to be sexual with others by observing how others, especially those of the same gender, act sexually. The importance of parental and familial role models in sexual development is crucial. The attitude toward sexuality, the expression of affection, and communication skills in the family of origin are precursors to later adult attitudes and the manner of expressing affection and sexuality. Conflicts about sex role (e.g., insecurity about being able to act like a "real" man or woman) or sex stereotyping can result in sexual dysfunction.

If the parents believe that sex is bad and must be controlled at all costs, then the child as an adult is likely to find it difficult to accept sexual pleasure without emotional conflict. If one "learns" early that sex can be a controlling or manipulating force over others, then sexual activity as an adult will be colored by tones of a power struggle. Sex that is used mainly as an instrument of power usually results in sexual dysfunction in one of the partners unless a primarily sadomasochistic sexual relationship has been established.

Cognitive theory stresses the importance of cognitions or beliefs that determine emotional responses and behaviors in sexual activity (Walen and Roth, 1987). In many ways, it is similar to social learning theory, except that it places less stress on early childhood experiences. It is more concerned with the cognitions that are held here and now, and less with their etiology. If an individual believes, for example, that the opposite sex seeks to control, emotionally engulf, or dominate others, then those beliefs (often unrecognized) will influence the emotions the person has during sexual intimacy. Examples are a woman who is anorgasmic because she fears loss of control or a man who gets in and out of a "dangerous" situation with premature ejaculation.

Allied to cognitive etiology of sexual dysfunction are those cases in which a lack of sexual information causes dysfunction. Examples are an older man who expects to achieve an erection (as he did as a youth) without any direct penile stimulation or a menopausal woman who does not realize she may need a vaginal lubricant.

In conclusion, sexual dysfunctions that are psychogenic cannot be directly and universally related to any one specific etiological event or psychodynamic structure. It is never a case of "This is premature ejaculation; therefore, X must have caused it." Taking a careful history, further elaborating the patient's psychological constitution in therapy, and testing etiological hypotheses in therapeutic approaches are necessary to confirm the psychogenic factors for a particular patient.

TREATMENT

General Principles

Because patients often have difficulty discussing sexual problems, their presentation of the chief sexual complaint and the history of the present illness may be imprecise. It is therefore necessary to set aside enough time to evaluate the problem; more than one session may be necessary to complete the task.

With a patient whose sexual dysfunction involves a partner or a spouse, the evaluation ideally should include the partner's view of the problem. Finally, asking patients about their notions concerning the etiology of their sexual disorder and their expectations for treatment are helpful in understanding important patient cognitions.

The eventual development of a treatment plan depends on the specifics of each case, including several important favorable prognostic factors. Those factors include recent onset of symptoms, mild-to-moderate severity of dysfunction, prior history of good sexual function, identifiable situational stress factors, good mental health, absence of paraphilia, and a spouse or partner who is cooperative with the evaluation and willing to participate in treatment. Although evaluation often reveals that sexual dysfunctions may be secondary to marital or relational discord, the sexual complaint is the ticket of entry into the care system, and treatment should be provided on the basis of the presenting complaint. Once treatment has begun, relational issues may obtain priority and redirect the goals of treatment.

When patients do not require referral, the PLISSIT model developed by Annon and Robinson (1978) is very useful for evaluation and office counseling. The clinician gives *permission* (P) to the patient to discuss his or her sexual concerns and apprehensions by initiating discussion with appropriate questions. In response to the questions the patient may have about the sexual problem, the clinician provides *limited information* (LI) (i.e., enough information to enable informed decisions), without overloading the patient with accurate but excessive detail. As rapport is established between the clinician and patient, the clinician, gives *specific suggestions* (SS) about how to maximize sexual function (taking into account the circumstances of the current relationship and other psychological stressors). Patients who do not respond are referred for *intensive therapy* (IT).

MEDICAL DISORDERS

Sexual disorders that are secondary to chronic illness, chronic pain, or the side effects of medications may be reversed by medical interventions. Improvement of the patient's overall physical condition and relief of pain may restore sexual function. Drug holidays, a change of medication, or discontinuance of medication may reverse dysfunctions. Dysfunction secondary to the acute side effects of substance abuse or alcoholism will often remit once the abuse is controlled. Prolactin-secreting microadenomas (which cause loss of desire and arousal disorders) may be treated by surgical resection or medically by administering bromocriptine. Inhibited desire in men and/or male arousal disorders secondary to hypogonadism are responsive to intramuscular administration of exogenous testosterone, providing there is no evidence of prostatic carcinoma.

Sexual dysfunction irreversibly impaired by trauma, disease, or the sequelae of surgery is treatable by using the principles of rehabilitation medicine: quantify the loss of function, establish realistic rehabilitative goals, and develop training techniques to maximize residual functional capacities. Patients who suffer irreversible damage can be taught sexual techniques that enable them to maintain sexual relationships, a great psychological benefit to both the patient and the partner. Patients should also be referred to self-help associations (e.g., multiple sclerosis, ostomy, and cardiac support groups), which hold group meetings and provide literature on sexual function. Dysfunctions secondary to estrogen deficiency are responsive to estrogen replacement (providing no medical contraindications exist), largely by effecting an improved sense of well-being and by increasing the ability to lubricate vaginally.

Postmenopausal women may experience problems with adequate vaginal lubrication due to reduced circulating estrogen. Hormonal replacement of estrogen will reduce vaginal atrophy and improve lubrication during sexual stimulation (Walling et al, 1990). There is also indication that among younger surgically menopausal women, the administration of androgens may improve general sexual functioning (Sherwin, 1991). Postmenopausal women for whom hormone replacement therapy is contraindicated should be informed about over-the-counter vaginal lubricants.

There are several methods of treatment for medically based erectile dysfunction or dysfunction that is recalcitrant to psychotherapy. The noninvasive method is an external vacuum device that utilizes an elastic band to contain blood in the engorged penis. This method has had a fairly high satisfaction and continued utilization rate (Turner et al, 1991). The main disincentives of the vacuum device are the mastery of the mechanics of the pump and the likelihood of ejaculation not occurring intravaginally if conception is desired.

Yohimbine is an oral medication that acts as a likely alpha-1 and alpha-2 adrenergic antagonist with antidopaminergic properties. While it is widely employed as a first-line medical treatment of erectile dysfunction, it has yet to prove itself as a robust treatment of the impotence among biogenic patients (Mann et al, 1996).

Intracavernosal injections are an alternative medical treatment for erectile dysfunction and require intact tissue responsive to vasodilating substances (papaverine, phentolamine, prostaglandin E_1). The treatment involves injecting small amounts of the vasodilators into the corpora of the penis. Within minutes and with some stimulation, an erection is produced that may last fcr 60 to 90 minutes. Contraindications are priapism, fibrotic plaque from repeated needle sticks, and some abnormal liver function values (Althof et al, 1991; Turner et al, 1989).

There are two new methods of medically treating erectile dysfunction that may greatly add to treatment choice in the near future. First, transurethral administration of alprostadil (prostaglandin E_1), by which a medicated pellet is inserted with an applicator into the urethra, has been shown to be an effective method of treating men with chronic erectile dysfunction (Padma-Nathan et al, 1997). Second, an oral medication, sildenafil, has been found to be effective among men with no organic etiology for erectile dysfunction in the United Kingdom (Boolell et al, 1996). Sildenafil, a type-5-specific phosphodiesterase inhibitor, is currently in clinical trials by Pfizer Pharmaceuticals. In men for whom the above, less invasive interventions are not effective or are contraindicated, penile prostheses may be implanted. These are either silastic rods or inflatable devices. It is recommended that the man's partner be involved in the choice of this or other medical and mechanical treatments of erectile failure.

Lastly, both for the well as for the ill, appropriate exercise programs that improve individual fitness will probably have a beneficial effect upon overall sexual functioning (White et al, 1990).

PSYCHOSEXUAL DISORDERS

Desire Disorders

Loss of sexual desire is often associated with depressive disorders, which should be treated with antidepressants, psychotherapy, or both. Marital discord is a common psychogenic cause of loss of desire. Chronic discord leads to anger, and although the partners may be aware of their anger, they fail to connect their loss of sexual interest in each other with their anger toward each other.

Physicians and patients (through self-medication) sometimes try to treat loss of sexual desire with medications such as testosterone, alcohol, antianxiety compounds, or stimulants. Except for confirmed male hypogonadal states, when testosterone is useful, and for the treatment of hyperprolactinemia with bromocriptine, these strategies are rarely successful.

Patients suffering from sexual aversion disorders usually have experienced their dysfunction since beginning adult sexual activity. Aversion disorders exist on a spectrum: at one end is the patient who simply lacks desire to initiate sexual activity but can engage in it with reasonable gratification, and on the other end is the patient who experiences panic attacks when faced with a sexual opportunity. This reaction is clearly a more severe form of the disorder and requires aggressive treatment with chemotherapy and psychotherapy. Panic attacks are responsive to antidepressants, including the cyclic antidepressants, the monoamine oxidase MAO inhibitors, and benzodiazepines. Counseling patients with the less severe form of aversion disorder is directed toward helping the unaffected partner to be more assertive in initiating sexual experiences so that the affected partner is drawn into more frequent participation in sexual relations.

Sexual Arousal Disorder

In both sexes, the inability to develop and maintain levels of sexual excitement may be the result of internal psychological events that interfere with the ability to focus on the stimuli causing sexual excitement. A common psychological distraction is preoccupation with sexual performance. This can become a powerful distraction: as concern about performance becomes more and more absorbing, the psychological activity of worrying about performance crowds out the capacity to attend to sexual stimuli and eventually results in the loss of arousal. What occurs is performance anxiety and spectatoring. Other common psychological interferences are worry about stressful life situations and marital discord.

Office counseling is effective for patients who present with the already described prognostic factors. The goal of counseling is to eliminate the distracting psychological event(s) so that the patient can focus on sexual stimuli. This is accomplished by first illustrating the process (i.e., spectatoring) to the patient and then teaching him or her to focus on sexual stimuli by practicing touching exercises in private. The sensate focus exercises are described by Masters and Johnson (1970). Prescribing small amounts of alcohol or anti-anxiety medications has not proved to be a successful method of chemically inducing relaxation to block the process of spectatoring.

ORGASM DISORDERS

The most common presentation of orgasm disorder is delayed or inhibited orgasm due to antidepressants, especially SSRIs. The first course in reestablishing sexual function is to consider replacing the drug with an antidepressant drug not usually associated with sexual dysfunction, e.g. buproprion or nefazodone. Second, if an SSRI is necessary for the alleviation of depressive symptoms, switching to a shorter half-life SSRI (e.g. sertaline or paroxetine) and instituting a drug holiday, e.g., weekend dosages, may stop sexual dysfunction without relapsing into depression. If the particular SSRI must be used for the treatment of depression, several adjunctive drugs have been employed to restore orgasmic function. Among the drugs for whom case studies have indicated an effectiveness are amantidine 100 mg 5 to 6 hours prior to intercourse (Balon, 1996a,b); methylphenidate 15 mg and dextroamphetamine sublingually 5 mg (Bartlik et al, 1995); yohimbine 5.4 to 16.2 mg 2 to 4 hours prior to sex (Price and Grunhaus, 1990; Hollander and McCarley, 1992) or cyproheptadine 9 to 12 mg 1 to 2 hours prior to sex (Riley and Riley, 1986). Bethanecol 5 to 10 mg has also been shown to be effective in cases with tricyclic antidepressant-induced sexual dysfunction (Segraves, 1995).

Men who experience delay or absence of orgasm are usually found to have personality traits that require referral for evaluation and treatment. As noted earlier, inhibited orgasm must be differentiated from retrograde ejaculation. Retrograde ejaculation has been reported as a side effect of some medications, including thioridazine (Mellaril).

Women experiencing delay or absence of orgasm who give evidence of the favorable prognostic factors described above, including a past history of orgasmic response, are candidates for office counseling. A recent loss of orgasmic response may often be traced to recent sexual experiences during which the patient could not experience orgasm because of a psychological distraction (the process described above). Counseling is used to resolve the stress and then to shift the patient's focus of attention from her concern about orgasm to enjoyment of the total sexual experience. Again, the touching exercises (sensate focus) are prescribed to the patient and her partner.

Single patients and those women with primary anorgasmia are typically instructed to practice focusing on sexual stimuli during masturbation, with the expectation that a positive response (i.e., orgasm) will generalize to sexual experiences with a partner. Many women may enjoy sex completely without achieving orgasm and derive sufficient pleasure during the plateau stage. Concern about achieving orgasm varies among women, as does the need for specific treatment.

PREMATURE EJACULATION

Typically, the patient presents with a history of reaching orgasm as he is attempting to penetrate, just as he has penetrated, or within several pelvic thrusts after penetration. He often reports experiencing premature ejaculation since he became sexually active during late adolescence or early adulthood. Men with this dysfunction usually seek help only when their partners become exasperated with the chronic sexual frustration associated with the disorder. Single patients seek assistance when relationships fail as a result of the dysfunction.

There are two behavioral methods for treating premature ejaculation that effectively teach the patient an awareness of his progression through the sexual response cycle and help him control the timing of that progression. These goals are readily achieved when the patient has a regular sexual partner who will participate in the treatment program. Both the "squeeze" and the "stop-and-go" techniques have been used successfully. With the squeeze technique, the female partner places her thumb and first two fingers around the coronal ridge of the penis and presses firmly for 10 seconds. The pressure results in a 10 to 25% loss of erection and a decrease in the subjective sense of arousal. The stop-and-go technique is practiced by alternately stimulating the penis and resting without touching. Either technique is introduced as an exercise following initial practice with the sensate focus exercises. Control over the pacing of the sexual experience is achieved by practicing the exercises and by using one of these techniques throughout all phases of the response cycle.

Behavioral counseling of this sort can be done in an office setting, but it requires therapist training and experience. Treatment is often complicated by the anger typically experienced and expressed by the female partner and repressed by the patient, necessitating marital therapy in addition to sexually focused treatment.

There has been a recent report of the treatment of premature ejaculation by physiokinestherapy, which sought to strengthen the pelvic musculature and develop fuller self-awareness of the preejaculatory sensations in men (LaPera and Nicastro, 1996). We await further replications and development of this form of physical therapy.

Medical treatment of premature ejaculation (Balon, 1996) uses drugs that have been found to have had the effect of delaying ejaculation and/or orgasm: clomipramine, 25 mg., 12 to 24 hours before anticipated sexual activity (Althof et al, 1995; Haensel et al, 1996); fluoxetine, 20 mg/day to every other day (Graziottin, 1995); paroxetine, less than 40 mg/day (Waldinger et al, 1994); or sertraline, 100 to 150 mg/day (Mendels et al, 1995). Taking into account drug side effects and the cost of the medication, one should seek the lowest possible dosage that achieves the desired effect on ejacualtion. A combination of medication and cognitive–behavioral therapy should be sought, at least in initial stages of treatment.

SEXUAL PAIN DISORDERS

Dyspareunia

Psychogenic dyspareunia is rare, and the diagnosis should be made only after all possible medical causes of pain have been ruled out. Patients subject to psychogenic dyspareunia are likely to have personality traits that support the disorder (e.g., the tendency to somaticize conflict) or be conflicted about the sexual activity itself (Kaplan, 1991). Depending on the outcome of the evaluation, the type of treatment may be individual, group, or behavioral. For some patients, it may incorporate treatment principles associated with the management of chronic pain.

Vaginismus

The diagnosis of functional vaginismus is often made when a physician attempting a pelvic examination cannot pass a finger or the smallest speculum into the vagina because of contraction of the musculature around the vaginal outlet. Some women, however, will tolerate a pelvic examination, but have vaginal spasms only prior to sexual penetration. Successful treatment is based on behavioral methods that desensitize the patient to the experience of penetration. For some women, the desensitization process must begin with individual behavioral exercises. When she is comfortable with vaginal touching and penetration by herself, the transition is then made to couple exercises. The couple is instructed to create a relaxing milieu by taking a bath together, followed by touching exercises (sensate focus). Next, they are asked to repeat the general touching, but to include the genitals, avoiding touching that is overtly sexually stimulating. Having mastered the two sets of exercises, they are asked to repeat the bath, the general body touching, and genital touching, and then to pass a small dilator into the vagina. On subsequent days, the size of the dilator is increased until the dilator approximates the circumference of a penis. The penis is then substituted for the dilator. Patients without partners can be treated in a similar manner with the dilators self-applied; however, it is important to note that the acceptance of the dilators may not generalize to a shared sexual experience. Should this be the case, treatment should be delayed until the patient is in a relationship of sufficient commitment to permit including the partner in the treatment program.

ROLE OF THE NONPSYCHIATRIC PHYSICIAN IN PATIENT MANAGEMENT

Physicians in all specialities can expect to be approached by patients about sexual problems. Internists, obstetricians, gynecologists, and pediatricians are frequently questioned by patients about sexual issues; however, regardless of specialty, each physician must decide whether to evaluate the patient's complaint or make a referral. When the choice is to do an evaluation, the physician should schedule at least 30 minutes to complete an initial evaluation. Additional sessions may be necessary to complete the evaluation, to develop a diagnostic formulation, and to design a treatment strategy.

Counseling methods and techniques have been described in each subsection for those physicians interested in the office management of psychosexual dysfunction. The physician should contract with the patient or the couple for a specific number of sessions (about five), for a defined amount of time per session (30 to 60 minutes), and a regular meeting date (i.e., Thursday, 2 p.m.). The scheduling details are important components of the therapeutic framework. Patients who do not respond to office counseling should be referred for further treatment.

Once the decision to refer has been made, there are several issues to consider: Should a patient be referred to a general psychiatrist or psychologist or to someone specializing in the treatment of sexual disorders? How can a physician evaluate the credentials of therapists who state they are expert in evaluating and treating sexual disorders? Patients with sexual complaints that are secondary to major psychiatric disorders (i.e., schizophrenia, bipolar disorder, major depression) should be referred to a general psychiatrist for the necessary psychotropic medication, as well as psychotherapy. When a patient with a sexual dysfunction has a comorbid anxiety disorder or substance-use disorder, the latter conditions should receive prompt attention from a psychiatrist, psychologist, or clinical facility that specializes in the treatment of such dis-orders. In some cases, the sexual dysfunction can be treated concurrently, but generally, the anxiety disorder or substance abuse must be treated first.

Individuals or couples whose major problem is their inability to relate to others (in other words, sex is just one of several issues) need couple/marital therapy provided they are willing to work on general relationship issues rather than narrowly focused sexual problems. Patients whose Axis I diagnosis is a psychosexual disorder are the best candidates for sexually focused treatment. Because sexually focused treatment methods ultimately include relational issues, most therapists expert in the techniques of sexual therapy are also experienced in marital therapies and the relational issues associated with personality disorders. This combination of skills is important and useful because patients often need a course of treatment that includes several methods used in sequence.

The question of credentials may be approached in several ways. The certified generalist with the more advanced degree is likely to be better trained (for psychiatrists, board certified; for psychologists, Ph.D, or Psy.D. and licensed). Since most states do not license or certify sexual therapists, the professional should have trained for at least a year in a sexual disorders program; the best of such programs are associated with medical schools. If the referring physician has difficulty identifying a source for referral, the closest medical school is usually a good resource for sexual disorder programs and therapists. Several national organizations, such as the Society for Sex Therapy and Research, keep a list of members, listed geographically. The website htt://www.jagnut.com/~dgotlib/meanstreets.htm may be of assistance in identifying resources.

Sexual dysfunctions are moderately prevalent among medical patients and, to a lesser extent, in the general population. Whether the etiology is psychogenic, biogenic, or both, the physician should take time to ascertain the nature of the disorder and the extent to which the patient is distressed. For some dysfunctions, the physician can make effective office interventions; other patients require additional evaluation and treatment. In either instance, therapeutic attention should be given to the person with sexual dysfunction.

CLINICAL PEARLS

- Most patients are not comfortable talking about sexual problems. It is incumbent on the physician to create an atmosphere of comfort and trust that allows the patient to explore his or her sexual difficulties. The physician must be comfortable with issues concerning human sexuality and must speak in language that is respectful of the topic, but not too technical. In most cases, vulgar sexual terminology is alienating to the patient.

- When a patient is in a committed relationship, it is very helpful for the physician to have the partner's view of the problem in order to understand the whole story. Occasionally, a sexually functional partner will seek help to gain support for obtaining the evaluation of a dysfunctional partner; it is unusual for both partners to present with sexual dysfunctions. However, once treatment has begun, in at least 30% of the cases, a sexual dysfunction will be discovered in the partner who supposedly is sexually functional.
- When evaluating or treating couples with sexual problems, extramarital relationships are sometimes uncovered. It is the responsibility of the involved partner to decide whether to reveal such a relationship. The physician should not automatically view the extramarital relationship as a threat to the primary relationship; numerous relationships have survived extramarital affairs. Until the dynamics of the relationships are well understood by the physician, it is prudent to withhold recommendations about such affairs or to defer such decisions to a psychiatrist or psychologist.

ANNOTATED BIBLIOGRAPHY

Crenshaw TL, Goldberg JP: Sexual Pharmacology: Drugs that Affect Sexual Function. New York, WW Norton, 1996

> This is a compendium of information on the effects of drugs on sexual function: hormonal therapies, substance use and abuse, plus the medical and psychiatric medications and their effects.

Friedman RC: Normal sexuality and introduction to sexual disorders. In Michels R et al (eds): Psychiatry. Philadelphia, JB Lippincott, 1991

> This chapter provides basic information about biopsychosocial aspects of human sexuality and contains information with which the reader of this chapter is presumed to be familiar. There is also a lengthy treatment of the history of homosexuality as a diagnostic category and of present clinical issues regarding sexual orientation.

Kaplan HS: Psychosexual dysfunctions. In Michels R et al (eds): Psychiatry. Philadelphia, JB Lippincott, 1991

> Dr. Kaplan provides rich clinical descriptions of sexual dysfunctions and stresses an integrated treatment of them, combining behavioral, psychodynamic, and psychopharmacological modalities and interventions.

Schover LR, Jensen SB: Sexuality and Chronic Illness. New York, Guilford, 1988

> This book provides clinicians with a comprehensive approach to the evaluation and treatment of sexual problems among individuals with chronic illnesses and disabilities. It is a practical text that draws its usefulness from abundant case discussions; it should be on a physician's bookshelf.

REFERENCES

Althof SE, Levine SB, Corty EW, et al: A double-blind crossover trial of clomipramine for rapid ejaculation in 15 couples. J Clin Psychiatry 56:402–407, 1995

Althof SE, Turner LA, Levine SB, et al: Sexual, psychological and marital impact of self-injection of papaverine and phentolamine: a long-term prospective study. J Sex Marital Ther 17:101–112, 1991

American Psychiatric Association: Diagnostic and Statistical Manual, 4th ed. Washington, DC, American Psychiatric Association, 1994

Annon JS, Robinson CH: The use of vicarious learning in the treatment of sexual concerns. In LoPiccolo J, LoPiccolo L (eds): Handbook of Sex Therapy. New York, Plenum Press, 1978

Balon R: Antidepressants in the treatment of premature ejaculation. J Sex Marital Ther 22:85–96, 1996a

Balon R: Intermittent amantidine for fluoxetine-induced amorgasmia. J Sex Marital Ther 22:290–292, 1996b

Bartlik BD, Kaplan P, Kaplan HS: Psychostimulants apparently reverse sexual dysfunction secondary to selective serotonin re-uptake inhibitors. J Sex Marital Ther 21:264–271, 1995

Blanchard R, Steiner BW (eds): Clinical Management of Gender Identity Disorders in Children and Adults. Washington, DC, American Psychiatric Press, 1990

Boolell M, Gepi-Attee S, Gingell JC, Allen MJ: Sildenafil, a novel effective oral therapy for male erectile dysfunction. Br J Urol 78:257–261, 1996

Buffum J: Prescription drugs and sexual function. Psychiatr Med 10:181–198, 1992

Buvat J, Buvat-Herbaut A, Lemaire A, et al: Recent developments in the clinical assessment and diagnosis of erectile dysfunction. Annu Sex Res 1:265–308, 1990

Carani C, Zini D, Baldini A, et al: Effects of androgen treatment in impotent men with normal and low levels of free testosterone. Arch Sex Behav 19:223–234, 1990

Derogatis LR, Fagan PJ, Schmidt CW, et al: Psychological subtypes of anorgasmia: a marker variable approach. J Sex Marital Ther 12:197–210, 1986

Fagan PJ, Schmidt CW Jr: Sexual dysfunction in the medically ill. In Stoudemire A, Fogel BS (eds): Psychiatric Care of the Medical Patient, pp 307–322. New York, Oxford University Press, 1993

Fagan PJ, Schmidt CW Jr, Wise TN, et al: Sexual dysfunction and dual psychiatric diagnoses. Compr Psychiatry 29:278–284, 1988

Graziottin A: Prozac in the treatment of premature ejaculation. Presented at the 1995 Annual Meeting of the American Urological Association, Las Vegas, 1995

Haensel SM, Rowland DL, Kallan KT, Slob AK: Clomipramine and sexual function in men with premature ejaculation and controls. J Urol 156:1310–1315, 1996

Hollander E, McCarley A: Yohimbine treatment of sexual side effects induced by serotonin re-uptake blockers. J Clin Psychiat 53:207–209, 1992

LaPera G, Nicastro A: A new treatment for premature ejaculation: the rehabilitation of the pelvic floor. J Sex Marital Ther, 22:22–26, 1996

Laquer T: Making of Sex: Body and Gender from the Greeks to Freud. Cambridge, Harvard University Press, 1990

Laumann EO, Gagnon JH, Michael RT, Michaels S: The Social Organization of Sexuality: Sexual Practices in the United States. Chicago, University of Chicago Press, 1994

Mann K, Klinger T, Noe S, Roschke J, Muller S, Benkert O: Effects of yohimbine on sexual experiences and nocturnal penile tumescence and rigidity in erectile dysfunction. Arch Sex Behav 25:1–16, 1996

Masters WH, Johnson VE: Human Sexual Response. Boston, Little, Brown, 1966

Masters WH, Johnson VE: Human Sexual Inadequacy. Boston, Little, Brown, 1970

McConaghy N: A learning approach. In Geer JH, O'Donohue WT (eds): Theories of Human Sexuality. New York, Plenum Press, 1987

Mendels J, Camera A, Sikes C: Sertraline treatment for premature ejaculation. J Clin Psychopharmacol 15:341–344, 1995

Meyer JK, Schmidt CW Jr, Wise TN (eds): Clinical Management of Sexual Disorders, 2nd ed. Washington, DC, American Psychiatric Press, 1986

Padma-Nathan H, Hellstrom JG, Kaiser FE, et al: Treatment of men with erectile dysfunction with transurethral alprostadil. N Engl J Med 336:1–7, 1997

Person ES: A psychoanalytical approach. In Geer JH, O'Donohue WT (eds): Theories of Human Sexuality. New York, Plenum Press, 1987

Price J, Grunhaus LJ: Treatment of clomipramine-induced anorgasmia with yohimbine: a case report. J Clin Psychiatry 51:32–33, 1990

Riley AJ, Riley EJ: Cyproheptadine and antidepressant-induced anorgasmia (letter). Br J Psychiatry 148:217–218, 1986

Scharf DE: The Sexual Relationship: An Object Relations View of Sex and the Family. Boston, Routledge & Kegan Paul, 1982

Schiavi RC: Sexuality and aging in men. Annu Rev Sex Res 1:227–249, 1990

Schmidt CW Jr: Sexual disorders. In Harvey AM, Owens AH Jr, McKusick VA et al (eds): Principles and Practice of Medicine. Norwalk, CT, Appleton & Lange, 1988

Schover LR, Jensen SB: Sexuality and Chronic Illness. New York, Guilford, 1988

Segraves RT: Antidepressant-induced orgasm disorder. J Sex Marital Ther 21:192–201, 1995

Sherwin BB: The psychoendocrinology of aging and female sexuality. Annu Rev Sex Res 2:181–198, 1991

Spector HP, Carey MP: Incidence and prevalence of the sexual dysfunctions: a critical review of the empirical literature. Arch Sex Behav 19:389–408, 1990

Strassberg DS, Mahoney JM, Schaugaard M, et al: The role of anxiety in premature ejaculation: a psychophysiological model. Arch Sex Behav 19:251–257, 1990

Tiefer L: Historical, scientific, clinical and feminist criticisms of "the human sexual response cycle" model. Annu Rev Sex Res 2:1–23, 1991

Turner LA, Althof SE, Levine SB, et al: Self-injection of papaverine and phentolamine in the treatment of psychogenic impotence. J Sex Marital Ther 15:163–176, 1989

Turner LA, Althof SE, Levine SB, et al: External vacuum devices in the treatment of erectile dysfunction: a one-year study of sexual and psychosocial impact. J Sex Marital Ther 17:81–93, 1991

Waldinger MD, Hengeveld MW, Zinderman AH: Paroxetine treatment of premature ejaculation: a double-blind, randomized, placebo-controlled study. Am J Psychiatry 151:1377–1379, 1994

Walen SR, Roth D: A cognitive approach. In Geer JH, O'Donohue WT (eds): Theories of Human Sexuality. New York, Plenum Press, 1987

Walling M, Andersen BL, Johnson SR: Hormonal replacement therapy for postmenopausal women: a review of sexual outcomes and related gynecologic effects. Arch Sex Behav 19:119–137, 1990

Walsh PC, Lepor H, Eggleston JC: Radical prostatectomy with preservation of sexual function: anatomical and pathological considerations. Prostate 4:473–485, 1983

Weiss HD: The physiology of human erection. Ann Intern Med 76:793–799, 1972

White JR, Case DA, McWhirter D, Mattison AM: Enhanced sexual behavior in exercising men. Arch Sex Behav 19:193–209, 1990

15 *Paraphilias*

William D. Murphy
and Elizabeth D. Schwarz

Paraphilias, or sexual deviations, have provoked both curiosity and abhorrence in laypersons and professionals alike. The paraphilias as described in the *Diagnostic and Statistical Manual,* 4th edition (DSM-IV; American Psychiatric Association, 1994) are a group of disorders whose essential features are recurrent, intense sexual urges and sexually arousing fantasies generally involving either nonhuman objects or suffering or humiliation of one's self or partner (not merely simulated) or children or other nonconsenting persons.

Unlike many disorders described in this text, paraphilias represent not only psychiatric or psychological problems: many are illegal and can cause significant emotional and sometimes physical damage to victims (Finkelhor, 1986). Therefore, in many instances, the physician must be concerned not only about the presenting problem of the patient, but also about past victims and future danger. For example, in every state, a physician must report to the local child protection agency any incident of known or suspected child sexual abuse. Many times, the clinician who elects to treat a paraphilic patient who is involved in illegal acts assumes responsibility not only for the patient's behavior, but also for the protection of society.

Although most nonpsychiatric physicians will not provide direct psychological treatment to such patients, this chapter will serve to increase physician awareness of the extent of these disorders and to provide a better understanding of the characteristics of paraphilias, thus allowing physicians to serve victims and family members of paraphiliacs better and make appropriate referrals. Because knowledge in this area is based largely on paraphiliacs whose behavior is illegal and causes harm to others, this chapter will focus most heavily on this particular group of patients.

EPIDEMIOLOGY

Little is known about the true prevalence of various paraphilic disorders or other demographic factors, although knowledge is increasing, at least in the area of the victimization of children. Finkelhor (1994) has extensively reviewed surveys of prevalence rates in community samples of adult women. Results vary widely: studies have found victimization prevalence rates ranging from 2 to 62% for females (average 20 to 25%) and from 3 to 16% for males (average 8 to 10%). The variation in rates can be partly explained by three factors: the definition of sexual abuse used (offenses involving touching versus offenses involving hands-off experiences such as exhibitionism); the sample used; and, more importantly, the data collection method used (trained interviewers asking multiple questions provided higher rates than self-administered questionnaires with only one or two questions about sexual abuse). Although reporting rates may have increased, active rates of abuse may actually be somewhat lower today than among women born around World War II; however, differences are quite small, and there does not appear to have been any great increase in the last 20 years (Finkelhor, 1994).

Studies of adolescent sex offenders have suggested a 1-year prevalence rate of 1.5 to 3.5/1,000 for those offenders identified by the criminal justice system (James and Neil, 1996). This, however, would only represent a small percentage of actual offenders.

Although not as extensive, survey data exist for women who have been the victims of exhibitionists. Rates range from 32% in a female college sample (Cox and McMahon, 1978) to 44% of a group of British nurses (Gittleson et al, 1978). Moser and Levitt (1987) have reviewed similar survey studies for individuals engaging in sadomasochistic fantasies and behavior. As an example, Hunt (1974) found in a sample of 2,026 respondents that 4.8% of men and 2.1% of women reported having obtained pleasure from inflicting pain; 2.5% of men and 4.6% of women reported pleasure from receiving pain; however, it is highly likely that a much smaller percentage of these individuals would meet diagnostic criteria for sexual sadism or sexual masochism.

Although the above data cause concern and clearly indicate the extent of the problem of child sexual abuse, they do not provide us with clear evidence of the number of individuals who perpetrate such abuse and how many would actually meet the criteria for a paraphilic diagnosis. For example, Abel et al (1987) found that pedophiles with male targets averaged about 150 victims, while those with female targets averaged about 20 victims. Exhibitionism and voyeurism averaged 513 and 429 victims, respectively.

The disorder is seldom diagnosed in females, except in the area of sexual masochism. Although there is evidence that a small percentage of children are sexually abused by females (Finkelhor and Russell, 1984), it seems evident that the paraphilias are primarily male disorders. There is no evidence to suggest that the rates of paraphilias differ between ethnic groups or between geographical areas. There is clear evidence in many paraphiliacs that the onset of the disorder is in adolescence. Abel and Rouleau (1990), in a study of 561 male paraphiliacs, found that approximately 53% had the onset of their interest prior to age 18. The need for early intervention, before the pattern becomes fixed, is becoming increasingly recognized.

DESCRIPTION

Table 15–1 lists the major paraphilias and their general diagnostic criteria (American Psychiatric Association, 1994). All the paraphilias require at least that the patient (1) have recurrent, intense sexual urges and sexual fantasies regarding the specific paraphilia, and (2) have acted on these urges or be markedly disturbed by them.

Much of our knowledge is based on subject populations that are either apprehended for a sexual crime or that sought treatment. The extent to which characteristics of this population parallel other paraphiliacs who have not been caught or who have not sought treatment is unknown. Paraphiliacs are heterogeneous; many people have multiple paraphilias, and no one characteristic will apply to all individuals. In the literature, paraphiliacs are many times described as shy, inhibited, nonassertive individuals who have difficulty managing anger. When these characteristics are evaluated objectively, they are found to apply only to a certain percentage of paraphiliacs; no one personality profile would characterize any one paraphilia.

Exhibitionists obtain sexual pleasure from exposing their genitals to unsuspecting strangers; however, at times, an exhibitionist may also expose himself to neighbors or to children he knows. During the act, he may or may not have an erection and may or may not masturbate. Some exhibitionists leave the exhibitionistic situation and masturbate to the fantasy of exposing themselves. The vast majority of exhibitionists expose themselves to females, although we have seen some cases of exposure to males. Targets can be adults, adolescents, or children, and generally the exhibitionist does not attempt any further contact with the victim; however, for those individuals who expose to prepubescent children, the physician should rule out that the exposure is not a prelude to more active sexual involvement with the child. In general, the exhibitionist is looking for some reaction from the victim, such as shock or surprise; some may perceive, at least in fantasy, that their victim is sexually aroused by the behavior. We have also seen some exhibitionists whose arousal is increased when the victim shows fear.

The *voyeur's* behavior involves looking at individuals either undressing, nude, or engaging in sexual activities. In voyeurism, the behavior involves

Table 15–1 **Major Paraphilias***

Exhibitionism

Has had over the last 6 months recurrent sexual urges and sexually arousing fantasies to expose one's genitals to strangers and has either acted on these urges or is distressed by them.

Fetishism

Has had over the last 6 months recurrent sexual urges and/or arousing fantasies that involve the use of nonliving objects as sexual stimuli (e.g., female underwear) and has either acted on these or is distressed by them. The diagnosis should not be made if the fetish objects are only female clothing used in cross-dressing or devices designed specifically for sexual arousal (e.g., vibrators).

Frotteurism

Has had over the last 6 months recurrent sexual urges that involve rubbing against or touching a nonconsenting person and has either acted on these urges or is distressed by them. The touching and rubbing itself is sexually exciting, not the aggressive nature of the act.

Pedophilia

Has had over the last 6 months recurrent sexual urges and arousing fantasies that involve sexual interactions with a prepubescent child (generally younger than 13) and has either acted on these urges or is distressed by them. In addition, the patient should be at least 16 years old and at least 5 years older than the victim.

Sexual masochism

Has had over the last 6 months recurrent sexual urges and arousing fantasies that involve the act (not a simulation of the act) of being made to suffer, being humiliated, beaten, or bound and has either acted on these or is markedly distressed by them.

Sexual sadism

Has had over the last 6 months recurrent sexual urges and arousing fantasies that involve acts (not simulated acts) in which suffering, either physical or psychological, that includes humiliation is found to be sexually arousing by the person and the person has either acted on these or is distressed by them.

Transvestic Fetishism

A heterosexual male who over the last 6 months has had recurrent sexual urges and arousing fantasies that involve cross-dressing; the person has acted on or is markedly distressed by these urges and fantasies. The individual should not meet the criteria for gender identity disorder of adolescence or adulthood (nontranssexual type) or transsexualism.

Voyeurism

Has had over the last 6 months recurrent sexual urges and arousing fantasies that involve observing an unsuspecting person who is either naked, disrobing, or engaged in sexual behavior, and has acted on these or is distressed by them.

Paraphilia Not Otherwise Specified

Includes paraphilias that do not fit any of the above specific categories, such as telephone scatalogia (lewdness), necrophilia (corpses), etc.

* Adapted from DSM-IV criteria (American Psychiatric Association 1994).

people who are *unaware* that they are being watched; the diagnosis is *not* made for individuals who may watch filmed or live pornography, since in such cases, the individuals are aware that they are being seen. Clinicians should also be aware that a history of voyeurism is sometimes seen in rapists, and it is important to rule out that the voyeur does not have an aggressive sexual arousal pattern. At times, an individual may be arrested for voyeurism while in actuality he was peeping in a window with the intent of raping the victim.

The *fetishist* obtains sexual arousal from a nonliving object, commonly women's underwear, shoes, boots, or other apparel. The individual will usually masturbate while rubbing, holding, or smelling the object. The person may engage in this behavior alone or ask a partner to wear the object. Sometimes, an individual will steal the fetish object, such as underwear, or both steal and destroy it. In such cases, it is important to consider whether there is a sadistic component to the person's arousal pattern.

If a fetish object is limited to female clothes used in cross-dressing, the appropriate diagnosis is transvestic fetishism. Cross-dressing in women's clothes may be limited to single articles, such as underwear, or may involve total cross-dressing, including a wig and makeup. The transvestite may engage in this behavior alone or with a partner. Many transvestites are heterosexual, and cross-dressing is often part of sadomasochistic activity.

Frotteurs' sexual arousal arises from rubbing against or touching non-consenting individuals. This behavior usually occurs in crowded places, such as on public transportation, and may involve such things as rubbing their genitals against the buttocks of an unsuspecting woman, grabbing the woman's breasts, or grabbing the woman's genital area.

Pedophiles have sexual attraction to children and, along with exhibition-ists, are probably the *most frequent* paraphilias seen by mental health profes-sionals. In diagnosing pedophilia, it is important to state whether the attraction is to the same sex, opposite sex, or both; whether is limited to incest; and whether it is exclusive (only attracted to children) or nonexclusive. These fac-tors are related to the risk of recidivism since it has been found that males who molest young males have a high recidivism rate, while incest cases have the lowest recidivism rate.

Pedophiles may report sexual attraction to only one sex and to a limited age range (6 to 8 years old), although some may show attraction to all pre-pubescent children and either sex. Also, the age of the victim may not reflect the pedophile's true age preference, but merely the victim's availability. The behavior may be limited to fondling or may include other sexual behaviors such as oral–genital contact, digital penetration, insertion of objects in the vagina or anus, and intercourse. Pedophiles may use force, although many are quite adept at manipulating children into sexual activity. They may be very attentive to children's needs and may be involved in social activities or occupations that give them ready access to children (such as becoming the leader of youth groups). Pedophiles use numerous excuses to justify their behavior, such as, "it was educational for the child," "the child initiated the activity," and "the child got pleasure from the activity."

Sadists gain sexual pleasure from causing psychological or physical pain to their victims. In addition to pain, however, an integral part of the sadistic arousal pattern is the humiliation, degradation, and domination of the victim. The sadist may force nonconsenting victims or may engage in sadistic behavior with a consenting partner (a sexual masochist). In consenting relationships, unwritten rules usually govern how far the behavior is allowed to progress. Some sadists show progressive behavior, that is, an escalation in the degree of violence and force used. Behaviors may range from those meant to humiliate and degrade the victim (i.e., verbal abuse, locking in a cage, dressing the victim in diapers or in women's clothes, or urinating and defecating on the victim) to behaviors geared toward eliciting pain (spanking, pinching, burning, strangling, piercing with pins or needles, torture, mutilation, and murder).

Sexual masochism is seen as the opposite of sexual sadism, although at times, sadism and masochism occur in the same individual, who may engage in both roles in sadomasochistic activity. The person may engage in the behavior alone or with a partner. Again, with a partner, limits are many times agreed on as to how far the behavior is allowed to progress. A dangerous form of this behavior is autoerotic asphyxiation or hypoxiphilia (increasing sexual arousal by oxygen deprivation, obtained through such methods as placing a plastic bag over the head, strangling with a noose, or using chemicals such as nitrates). A number of deaths have been reported in the literature as a result of this behavior.

DIFFERENTIAL DIAGNOSIS

In diagnosing paraphilias, there are several factors to keep in mind. First, many paraphilias may meet the criteria for a number of the paraphilic disorders (Abel et al, 1987). If a patient presents complaining of one paraphilia, it is important to ask specifically about each other possible paraphilia in language understandable to the patient. Patients do not always volunteer this information spontaneously. Second, the paraphilic fantasies, urges, and behaviors may be continuous or episodic; in some patients, they may occur only during periods of stress or interpersonal conflict, and in other patients, they are always necessary for sexual arousal.

Differential diagnosis is less complicated by an overlap in symptomatology between disorders than by the patient's failure to provide honest details of his history. At times, paraphilic behavior is seen in other diagnostic categories, such as schizophrenia, mania, neuropsychiatric disorders, and mental retardation, but clinical experience suggests it is unlikely that another disorder is primarily responsible for the aberrant behavior. However, in transvestism and fetishism, it is important to rule out temporal lobe complex partial seizures (Blumer, 1969); numerous reports have suggested a relationship of these paraphilias to temporal lobe disorders, and more recently, a relationship between pedophilia and temporal lobe dysfunction has been reported (Langevin, 1990). However, most patients with temporal lobe disorders are not paraphiliacs, and probably most paraphiliacs do not have temporal lobe disorders. It is important that these diagnoses be assessed and appropriate treatment given if another disorder is diagnosed.

It is important to continue assessing for the presence of paraphilia, even when acute psychotic episodes or other disorders have been resolved. For example, our group saw one patient with clear evidence of paranoid schizophrenia. Following appropriate and reasonably successful pharmacological treatment, this patient continued to have recurrent and intense pedophilic urges that required specific treatment in and of themselves. Similar observations have been made in patients with mental retardation and substance-abuse disorders.

Criteria for the diagnosis of paraphilia are based largely on the patient's self-report. Paraphiliacs (especially those whose behavior is illegal) often provide very unreliable histories; specialists in the area have turned to other sources to assist in adequate treatment formulation and diagnosis. As part of the evaluation, extensive use is made of victims' statements, police reports, and interviews with significant others to get a clearer picture of the extent and nature of the patient's problem. Many clinical and research facilities use penile plethysmography as a means of direct assessment of sexual arousal to assist in diagnosis of sexual preference (Murphy et al, 1991).

ETIOLOGY

Data are limited about the etiology of the development of paraphilias. Therefore, the information reviewed in this area should be considered speculative. Traditional theories regarding etiology follow standard psychiatric theorizing (that is, from psychoanalytic, behavior, biological, or family systems perspectives). Some descriptive factors, however, warrant special attention.

First, clinical reports reveal that pedophiles appear to have been victimized themselves sexually as children at a higher rate than one would expect in normals (Groth et al, 1982). More recent data suggest, however, that this rate is not as high as previously thought. Hanson and Slater (1988), in reviewing a large number of studies, found that with large sample studies, the rate of sexual abuse in offenders was approximately 30%. In addition, given the large number of males who appear to have been abused in the general population, it would appear that most young males who are sexually abused do not become sex offenders. Although being sexually abused may be a risk factor for the development of pedophilia, it would appear that other, unidentified factors lead to the development of pedophilia. A number of factors could be proposed, such as whether the abuse had ever been disclosed, whether the young victim ever received treatment, adult reaction to disclosure of the abuse, and general family stability. To date, few of these factors have been investigated, although such knowledge would allow more appropriate early interventions in individuals at risk for sexual abuse. Recent data suggest that pedophiles who have been abused may experience more psychological disturbance and more severe paraphilias (Cooper et al, 1996).

A second factor about paraphiliacs is that the vast majority are male. Although this factor might raise both biological and genetic explanations, it also brings into question the role of male enculturation in the development of paraphilic behavior. Feminist writers (Brownmiller, 1975) and researchers (Stermac et al, 1990) have described various aspects of male social learning that may relate to sexual aggression against adult women. Such factors include males' need for dominance, perceptions of women as objects, society's reinforcement of rape myths, and various sex role stereotypes that, at least in the past, were culturally accepted. For pedophiles, such factors might include the masculine requirement to be dominant and powerful in sexual relationships, erotic portrayal of children in advertising, male tendencies to sexualize emotional needs, and repressive norms about sexuality (Finkelhor, 1984).

Psychoanalytic theories predominated early thinking regarding paraphilias, and early writings tended to follow directly Freud's theories of infantile sexuality. Although most individuals reach adult heterosexual orientation through adequate resolution of the Oedipal complex, paraphiliacs, because of extreme castration anxiety, express their infantile sexual desires through their paraphilic fantasies and acts. Hammer and Glueck (1957) proposed that the various paraphilias allow the individual to resolve in unconscious ways his castration anxiety and fears of adult women. The pedophile tends to choose children, who are less threatening than mature adult women; the exhibitionist displays his genitals, therefore provoking reactions from females and proving the existence of his penis; and the transvestic fetishist may use his cross-dressing to identify with the mother figure as a defense against his castration anxiety (Blair and Lanyon, 1981; Hammer and Glueck, 1957; Wise, 1985). Although there is little empirical support for analytic theories, there has been theoretical speculation regarding the application of *attachment theory* to the development of paraphilias (Ward et al, 1995).

Attachment theory, like psychoanalytic theory, places significant importance on the bond developed between the child and the caretaker; however, unlike psychoanalytic theory, attachment theory is much more grounded in empirical developmental research and established child development. Ward et al (1995) propose that sex offenders, because of early severe abuse and neglect, developed impaired attachment styles that led to loneliness and difficulties in establishing meaningful adult relationships. Such impairments leave the individual at risk for paraphilic acts and behaviors. To date, limited data support this theory, although it does hold promise for understanding at least some subsets of paraphiliacs and leads to more testable hypotheses than traditional analytic theory.

Early behaviorist writers, rather than focusing on early relationship with parental figures, have instead focused on early sexual experiences and the integration of such experiences into masturbatory fantasies. The basic tenet is that paraphilic arousal patterns are conditioned by the pairing of masturbatory fantasies with the paraphilic stimuli (McGuire et al, 1965; Rachman, 1966; Rachman and Hodgson, 1968). Later behavioral theories included other factors that at least might maintain or assist in the development of paraphilic behavior. For example, a lack of social skills or significant heterosexual anxiety might make it difficult for the individual to develop sexual relationships with appropriate sexual partners and leave the paraphilic outlet as the only means of sexual gratification (Barlow and Abel, 1976; Murphy and Smith, 1996). A number of cognitively oriented behavior therapists have focused on the role of what are called cognitive distortions (that is, the justifications paraphiliacs use to legitimize their behavior) in the maintenance of deviant sexual behavior (Conte, 1986; Murphy, 1990).

Throughout the literature on paraphilias, various case reports have associated the onset of paraphilic behaviors with neurological or other biological abnormalities. For example, Regestein and Reich (1978) described four cases of onset of pedophilia after illness that led to substantial cognitive impairment. Also, Berlin (1983) reported 34 cases of paraphilias (the majority pedophilic) with a variety of associated biological abnormalities, including elevated testosterone levels, schizophrenia, childhood dyslexia, Klinefelter's syndrome, and cortical atrophy. Also, as noted, temporal lobe epilepsy has been associated with fetishism and transvestite fetishism (Blumer, 1969), and more recently temporal lobe disorders have been noted among some pedophiles (Langevin, 1990).

None of these studies were based on random samples of either paraphiliacs or individuals suffering from the various biological abnormalities. Therefore, it is unclear what percentage of patients with such neurological or biological findings develop paraphilias and what percentage of paraphiliacs show such abnormalities. It cannot be assumed from studies that a biological abnormality is the factor leading to the development of paraphilia. At the clinical level, however, these case reports do suggest that the clinician needs to consider that individual paraphiliacs may have additional neurological disorders; the clinician should try to determine whether the neurological disorder has any relationship to the paraphilia. Because of the well-documented role that the temporal lobe and associated limbic structures play in regulating sexual behavior, further studies of temporal lobe disorders in paraphilias seem warranted.

Family interactions have also been implicated, at least within the subset of pedophiles involved in incest (Alexander, 1985; Larson and Maddock, 1986). Such theories have focused on factors such as the family's isolation, role confusion in the family, daughters who assume the mother's role, and a general emotional enmeshment among family members. Although it is clear to any clinician working with these families that many are quite dysfunctional, it is not clear whether the dysfunction is causative or secondary to the abusive behavior (Conte, 1986).

Although a number of factors have been implicated as in the etiology of the paraphilias, none have produced sufficient evidence to be considered predominant. We will probably find that paraphilias, like many psychiatric disorders, are multiply determined by an interaction of biological, psychological, and social/cultural variables. It is also likely that as our diagnostic abilities improve, we will be able to develop clearer subtypes of paraphiliacs and also to determine the role and importance of the various etiological factors in these subtypes.

TREATMENT

In this section, we will attempt to review the current general framework of paraphilic treatment as well as treatment issues addressed in sex-offender-specific programs. Recent biological approaches will also be integrated. There has been an increased use of the antiandrogen drug Depo-Provera (medroxyprogesterone acetate [MPA]) and recent clinical reports of the use of selective serotonin-reuptake inhibitors, such as fluoxetine, with this population.

Treatment in general focuses heavily on the specific paraphilic behavior or sex offense and the factors surrounding the offense, usually from a cognitive–behavioral framework. Less attention is given to early childhood experiences; therefore, psychodynamic or traditional psychotherapy approaches are usually not considered primary treatment modalities (Knopp, 1984). Most specialized programs use group therapy approaches with other paraphiliacs as the primary treatment modality and also male/female cotherapy teams.

In treating sex offenders, the therapist needs to be more directive and to set limits more clearly on patients' behaviors (such as having no contact with children) than in a traditional therapeutic setting. The treatment plan includes having patients waive confidentiality so that treatment failure and noncompliance can be reported to appropriate agencies. Most programs work closely with the courts, parole, probation, and child protection agencies; these systems are considered active members of the treatment team rather than agencies that interfere with the therapeutic relationship. Finally, offenders are clearly told that there is no "cure" and that the techniques learned in treatment should be employed on a lifelong basis.

The rest of this section will focus on specific components of treatment found in a number of treatment programs (Murphy and Smith, 1996).

Reducing Denial

Until an offender admits to the paraphilic behavior and provides specific details of the behaviors and factors surrounding the behaviors, it is difficult for treatment to progress. Therefore, one of the initial goals of treatment is to challenge the patient's denial. Denial is sometimes total ("I don't do it") or partial ("I didn't do everything he/she said I did"). Therapeutic approaches to reduce denial rely heavily on group approaches, including education, the use of victims' statements, and results of psychophysiological assessment of sexual arousal (Abel et al, 1983; Schlank and Shaw, 1996).

Sexual Arousal

By definition, paraphiliacs experience fantasies of and recurrent urges to engage in paraphilic behaviors. Therefore, most programs use some specific behavioral procedure to reduce such urges or to at least give the patient methods for controlling such urges. Mild electrical stimulation aversive techniques were frequently used in early treatment studies (Quinsey, 1977); a number of alternative procedures are now employed.

In *covert sensitization* (Cautela and Wisocki, 1971), the patient is taught to imagine a graphic picture of his paraphilic behavior and to link it with an equally graphic description of an aversive consequence, such as going to jail or losing his family (Brownell and Barlow, 1976; Brownell et al, 1977). In another technique that is used either in conjunction with covert sensitization (Maletzky, 1991) or alone (Laws and Osborn, 1983), the paraphilic stimulus or fantasy is linked with a noxious odor, such as spirits of ammonia or valeric acid. Also, many programs use some form of masturbatory or verbal satiation that requires patients to verbalize their deviant fantasies for long periods of time (30 to 45 minutes) without ejaculating (Laws and Osborn, 1983; Marshall, 1979). This leads to a reduction in the reinforcing value of the fantasies.

A number of biologically oriented approaches have also been used to reduce sexual arousal, although these are not specific to deviant sexual arousal and are geared to reducing libido in general (Berlin, 1983; Bradford, 1985). The two primary antiandrogen drugs are cyproterone acetate (CPA), which is available only in Canada and Europe, and MPA (Depo-Provera), which has been used in the United States (Berlin, 1983; Bradford, 1985). Although CPA has been used on a larger number of sex offenders, because it is unavailable in the United States we will focus on MPA.

According to Bradford (1985), MPA reduces testosterone through a number of mechanisms, primarily by inducing A-ring reductase inhibition in the liver and therefore increasing testosterone metabolism. Berlin (1983) recommends a starting dose of 500 mg/week of the 100 mg/ml solution, with no more than 250 ml given in a single injection site. Blood levels are taken periodically to assess whether testosterone levels have been suppressed, and the drug is then titrated so as not to cause total impotence; thus it is not feminizing. Optimal drug levels have not yet been determined. Common side effects of MPA include weight gain, mild lethargy, cold sweats, nightmares, hot flashes, and hypertension.

Berlin (1983) reported on a series of 20 chronic paraphiliacs, treated with MPA. While on the drug, only three relapsed (or only three were known to relapse); however, nine subjects dropped out of treatment, and eight of the nine recidivated while off the drug. Similar dropout problems have been reported by Meyer et al (1992) and Hucker et al (1988). Further studies are needed on increasing the acceptability of this drug to patients and on ways of increasing compliance. At the current time, Depo-Provera should be seen as a potential component of a comprehensive treatment program but should not be viewed as a treatment that can stand alone.

In addition to Depo-Provera, there have been recent clinical reports of the use of other pharmacological agents in the treatment of paraphilic and other compulsive sexual behaviors, such as compulsive masturbation. Because of the clinical observation that some individuals with paraphilias are quite compulsive in their behavior, there has been a specific interest in serotonin-reuptake inhibitors such as clomipramine and fluoxetine. In two open-label trials (10 and 20 subjects, respectively), Kafka (1991) and Kafka and Prentky (1992) reported significant results in subjects with a mixture of paraphilic behavior and nonparaphilic sexual compulsions with comorbid affective disorders. Most of these patients were treated with fluoxetine. Stein et al (1992) reported on a series of 13 patients, again mixed; some had paraphilic and others compulsive sexual behaviors, and many had comorbid obsessive–compulsive disorders. All the patients in the series were treated with either fluoxetine or clomipramine, and the results were much more mixed; none of the patients with paraphilias showed any significant changes. Finally, Kruesi et al (1992) reported on a double-blind crossover comparison of clomipramine versus desipramine with an initial placebo phase (using only eight subjects). There were no differences between clomipramine and desipramine, although both were superior to placebo.

At the current time, no firm conclusions can be drawn regarding the efficacy of serotonin-reuptake inhibitors. This is because of the small sample sizes, heterogeneity of populations studied, and variety of comorbid disorders within the studies to date; however, even the moderate improvements observed warrant further investigations of these agents, which have much fewer side effects than Depo-Provera.

Identifying Antecedents to Sexual Abuse and Increasing Social Competence

Paraphilic behavior is at times influenced by certain environmental stimuli or emotional events (Pithers et al, 1983). Many paraphiliacs have trouble managing various emotional states and difficulty with appropriate assertiveness and social skills. Therefore, programs provide a variety of structured social competency programs as part of treatment, such as stress management, anger management, interpersonal skills training, and assertiveness training.

Cognitive Distortions and Victim Empathy

Paraphiliacs whose behavior harms others tend to show limited empathy for their victims. We have hypothesized (Murphy, 1990) that one reason for the lack of empathy is that patients engage in a number of distortions that they use to reduce the guilt they feel about the behavior. These distortions include blaming the victim ("she asked for it"), denying the impact on the victim ("she/he liked it," "I didn't hurt her"), or attempting to make the behavior socially acceptable ("I was only providing sex education to the child"). Methods of challenging such belief systems involve educating the patient regarding victim impact, directly confronting the distortions, and teaching patients to identify the distortions themselves. Treatment programs commonly use books or articles written by victims or movies presented from a victim's standpoint; some programs use actual confrontations of the offender by the victim's therapist or by survivors of sexual abuse.

Other Treatment Issues

Several other issues need to be addressed with paraphilic patients. For example, offenders with alcohol and drug problems or with other concurrent psychiatric problems may need treatment for those problems. Alcohol and drug issues must be addressed, and appropriate medication is warranted for patients with major affective disorders or schizophrenic disorders. Similarly, marital therapy, family therapy, or sexual dysfunction therapy may be required for paraphiliacs with partners and for incest families that plan on reuniting.

ROLE OF THE NONPSYCHIATRIC PHYSICIAN IN PATIENT MANAGEMENT AND INDICATIONS FOR PSYCHIATRIC CONSULTATION AND REFERRAL

The vast majority of patients who present to physicians (victims or perpetrators) will require referral to an appropriate mental health professional. In all states, professionals are required by law and provided legal immunity to report to the proper authorities reasonable suspicion or evidence of child abuse, sexual or otherwise.

Physicians may encounter individuals who engage in paraphilic behavior or who have paraphilic urges that are not likely to harm others, the patient, or society (fetishism and transvestism, for example), and whose urges do not distress the patient. In such cases, depending on the physician's own moral beliefs and ethical standards, the physician might feel comfortable counseling the patient about the wide variety of sexual behaviors people engage in and letting the patient decide whether he needs to consult a specialist. Whenever a patient's fantasies and/or behavior involve either harming others or infringing on others' rights, more specialized services are required. The physician should remember that many paraphiliacs are not forthcoming with all their fantasy material or urges. In addition, as we have noted previously, many paraphiliacs have multiple paraphilias, and even though the one being presented may not seem to be of serious harm to others, there may be other issues the patient has not addressed. Even when the paraphilia does no physical harm, such as exhibitionism or voyeurism, many such patients also have other paraphilias that might be more directly harmful. Also, these paraphilias in and of themselves do infringe on the privacy of others. The physician faced with such a patient should maintain a nonjudgmental stance and should encourage the patient to disclose further material.

In making referrals, the physician should realize that not all mental health professionals (psychiatrists, psychologists, and social workers) have specialized training in treating paraphilic patients; in fact, they may have very little experience with this specific diagnostic category. Many times, district attorneys, parole and probation officers, and child protection workers may have the best knowledge of individuals who specialize in the treatment of paraphiliacs in the community.

Physicians can play an important role in prevention. Most primary care physicians who provide medical care to children on a regular basis can provide their patients with information on child sexual abuse in the same way they provide them with pamphlets and brochures on a variety of medical problems. Also, the physician, regardless of specialty, should continually be aware of the high frequency of sexual abuse in the population. Many patients being treated by physicians for a variety of disorders may have been sexually abused, and sometimes the physical complaints can be directly tied to the abuse. The physician should keep this in mind and should not be afraid to ask patients routinely about past or present traumatic sexual experiences as part of their diagnostic workup.

CLINICAL PEARLS

- Many paraphilic behaviors are both a psychiatric disorder and a crime. The patient's risk to society must always be considered.
- Patients may have multiple paraphilias, and these should always be considered during the evaluation.
- When evaluating a paraphiliac, especially one whose behavior harms others, the clinician should never rely solely on the patient's self-report and should seek collaborative information.
- Treatment of paraphilias is specialized. Not all mental health professionals have adequate training with this diagnostic group. When possible, referrals should be made to individuals with training in this area.
- Physicians should remember that victimization occurs frequently in our society. Physicians can play a key role in identifying victims and in prevention.

ANNOTATED BIBLIOGRAPHY

Blair CD, Lanyon RI: Exhibitionism: etiology and treatment. Psychol Bull 89:439–463, 1981

A good overall review of exhibitionism both clinically and theoretically. Provides an excellent description of the theoretical approach to understanding exhibitionism and common treatment techniques.

Bradford, JMW: Pharmacological treatment of the paraphilias. In Oldham JM, Riba MB (eds): American Psychiatric Press Review of Psychiatry, Vol. 14. Washington, American Psychiatric Press, 1995

A good overview of current pharmacological treatment of paraphiliacs.

Briere J, Berliner L, Bulkley JA, Jenny C, Reid T (eds): The APSAC Handbook on Child Maltreatment. Thousand Oaks, CA, Sage, 1996

The most up-to-date source for information regarding child maltreatment; includes medical, psychological, and legal perspectives.

Gelder M, Gath D, Mayou R: Oxford Textbook of Psychiatry. Oxford, Oxford University Press, 1983

Includes a brief description of the major paraphilias, with some attention to etiology and a cursory outline of treatment.

Kaplan HI, Saddock B: Comprehensive Textbook of Psychiatry, 4th ed. Baltimore, Williams & Williams, 1985

Contains a good overview of paraphilias and their proposed etiologies including environmental, biological, and analytic formulations and highlighting clinical features, differential diagnosis, and a very brief discussion of treatment.

Marshall WL, Laws DR, Barbaree HE: Handbook of Sexual Assault: Issues, Theories, and Treatment of the Offender. New York, Plenum Press, 1990

A most comprehensive review of sexual aggression against women and children. Includes information on the psychological, sociological, and biological aspects of this disorder plus clinical approaches.

REFERENCES

Abel GG, Becker JV, Mittelman M, et al: Self-reported sex crimes of nonincarcerated paraphiliacs. J Interpers Viol 2:3–25, 1987

Abel GG, Cunningham-Rathner J, Becker JV, McHugh J: Motivating sex offenders for treatment with feedback of their psychophysiologic assessment. Presented at the World Congress of Behavior Therapy, Washington, DC, December 1983

Abel GG, Rouleau JL: The nature and extent of sexual assault. In Marshall WL, Laws DR, Barbaree HE (eds): Handbook of Sexual Assault: Issues, Theories, and Treatment of the Offender. New York, Plenum Press, 1990

Alexander PC: A systems theory conceptualization of incest. Fam Process 24:79–88, 1985

American Psychiatric Association: Diagnostic and Statistical Manual of the Mental Disorders, 4th ed. Washington, DC, American Psychiatric Association, 1994

Barlow DH, Abel GG: Recent developments in assessment and treatment of sexual deviation. In Craighead WE, Kazdin AE, Mahoney MJ (eds): Behavior Modification Principles, Issues, and Applications. Boston, Houghton Mifflin, 1976

Berlin FS: Sex Offenders: A biomedical perspective and a status report on biomedical treatment. In Greer JG, Stuart IR (eds): The Sexual Aggressor: Current Perspectives on Treatment. New York, Van Nostrand Reinhold, 1983

Blair CD, Lanyon RI: Exhibitionism: etiology and treatment. Psychol Bull 89:439–463, 1981

Blumer D: Transsexualism, sexual dysfunction, and temporal lobe disorder. In Green R, Money J (eds): Transsexualism and Sex Reassignment. Baltimore, Johns Hopkins, 1969

Bradford JMW: Organic treatment for the male sexual offender. Behav Sci Law 3:355–375, 1985

Brownell KD, Barlow DH: Measurement and treatment of two sexual deviations in one person. J Behav Ther Exp Psychiatry 7:349–354, 1976

Brownell KD, Hayes SC, Barlow DH: Patterns of appropriate and deviant sexual arousal: the behavioral treatment of multiple sexual deviations. J Consult Clin Psychol 45:1144–1155, 1977

Brownmiller S: Against Our Will: Men, Women and Rape. New York, Simon and Schuster, 1975

Cautela JR, Wisocki PA: Covert sensitization for the treatment of sexual deviations. Psychol Rec 21:37–48, 1971

Conte JR: Sexual abuse and the family: A critical analysis. In Trepper TS, Barrett MJ (eds): Treating Incest: A Multimodal Systems Perspective. New York, Haworth, 1986

Cooper CL, Murphy WD, Haynes MR: Characteristics of abused and nonabused adolescent sexual offenders. Sexual Abuse: A J Res & Tr 8:105–119, 1996

Cox DJ, McMahon B: Incidence of male exhibitionism in the United States as reported by victimized female college students. Int J Law Psychiatry 1:453–457, 1978

Finkelhor D: Child Sexual Abuse: New Theory and Research. New York, Free Press, 1984

Finkelhor D: A Sourcebook on Child Sexual Abuse. Beverly Hills, Sage, 1986

Finkelhor D: Current information on the scope and nature of child sexual abuse. The Future of Children: Sexual Abuse of Children 4:31–53, 1994

Finkelhor D, Russell D: Women as perpetrators: review of the evidence. In Finkelhor D (ed): Child Sexual Abuse: New Theory and Research. New York, Free Press, 1984

Gittleson NL, Eacott ST, Mehta BM: Victims of indecent exposure. Br J Psychiatry 132:61–66, 1978

Groth AN, Hobson WF, Gary TS: The child molester: clinical observations. Soc Work Hum Sexuality 1:129–144, 1982

Hammer RF, Glueck BC Jr: Psychodynamic patterns in sex offenders: a four-factor theory. Psychiatr Q 31:325–345, 1957

Hanson RK, Slater S: Sexual victimization in the history of sexual abusers: a review. Annu Sex Res 1:485–499, 1988

Hunt M: Sexual Behavior in the 1970s. Chicago, Playboy Press, 1974

Hucker S, Langevin R, Bain J: A double-blind trial of sex drive reducing medication in pedophiles. Annu Sex Res 1:227–242, 1988

James AC, Neil P: Juvenile sexual offending: one-year period prevalence study within Oxfordshire. Child Abuse Negl 20:477–485, 1996

Kafka MP: Successful antidepressant treatment of nonparaphilic sexual addictions and paraphilias in men. J Clin Psychiatry 52:60–65, 1991

Kafka MP, Prentky R: Fluoxetine treatment of nonparaphilic sexual addictions and paraphilias in men. J Clin Psychiatry 53:351–358, 1992

Knopp FH: Retraining Adult Sex Offenders: Methods and Models. Syracuse, NY, Safer Society Press, 1984

Kruesi MJP, Fine S, Valladares L, et al: Paraphilias: a double-blind cross-over comparison of clomipramine versus desipramine. Arch Sex Behav 21:587–593, 1992

Langevin R: Sexual anomalies and the brain. In Marshall WL, Laws DR, Barbaree HE (eds): Handbook of Sexual Assault: Issues, Theories, and Treatment of the Offender. New York, Plenum Press, 1990

Larson NR, Maddock JW: Structural and functional variables in incest family systems: implications for assessment and treatment. In Trepper TS, Barrett MJ (eds): Treating Incest: A Multimodal Systems Perspective. New York, Haworth Press, 1986

Laws DR, Osborn CA: How to build and operate a behavioral laboratory to evaluate and treat sexual deviates. In Green JG, Stuart IR (eds): The Sexual Aggressor: Current Perspectives on Treatment. New York, Van Nostrand Reinhold, 1983

Maletzky BM: Treating the Sexual Offender. Newbury Park, CA, Sage, 1991

Marshall WL: Satiation therapy: a procedure for reducing sexual arousal. J Appl Behav Anal 12:10–22, 1979

McGuire RJ, Carlisle JM, Young BG: Sexual deviations as conditioned behavior: a hypothesis. Behav Res Ther 2:185–190, 1965

Meyer WJ, Cole C, Emory E: Depo-Provera treatment for sex offending behavior: an evaluation of outcome. Bull Am Acad Psychiatry Law 20:249–259, 1992

Moser CC, Levitt EE: An exploratory-descriptive study of a sadomasochistically oriented sample. J Sex Res 23:322–337, 1987

Murphy WD: Assessment and modification of cognitive distortions in sex offenders. In Marshall WL, Laws DR, Barbaree HE (eds): Handbook of Sexual Assault: Issues, Theories, and Treatment of the Offender. New York, Plenum Press, 1990

Murphy WD, Haynes MR, Worley PJ: Assessment of adult sexual interest. In Hollin CR, Howells K (eds): Clinical Approaches to Sex Offenders and Their Victims. West Sussex, England, John Wiley & Sons, 1991

Murphy WD, Smith TA: Sex offenders against children: empirical and clinical issues. In Briere J, Berliner L, Bulkley JA, Jenny C, Reid T (eds): The APSAC Handbook on Child Maltreatment. Thousand Oaks, CA, Sage, 1996

Pithers WD, Marques JK, Gibat CC, et al: Relapse prevention with sexual aggressives: a self-control model of treatment and maintenance of change. In Greer JG, Stuart IR (eds): The Sexual Aggressor: Current: Perspectives on Treatment. New York, Van Nostrand Reinhold, 1983

Quinsey VL: The assessment and treatment of child molesters: a review. Can Psychol Rev 18:204–220, 1977

Rachman S: Sexual fetishism: an experimental analogue. Psychol Rec 16:293–296, 1966

Rachman S, Hodgson R: Experimentally induced "sexual fetishism:" replication and development. Psychol Rec 18:25–27, 1968

Regestein QR, Reich P: Pedophilia occurring after onset of cognitive impairment. J Nerv Ment Dis 166:794–798, 1978

Schlank AM, Shaw T: Treating sexual offenders who deny their guilt: a pilot study. Sex Abuse 8:17–23, 1996

Stein DJ, Hollander E, Anthony DT, et al: Serotonergic medications for sexual obsessions, sexual addictions, and paraphilias. J Clin Psychiatry 53:267–271, 1992

Stermac LE, Segal ZV, Gillis R: Social and cultural factors in sexual assault. In Marshall WL, Laws DR, Barbaree HE (eds): Handbook of Sexual Assault: Issues, Theories, and Treatment of the Offender. New York, Plenum Press, 1990

Ward T, Hudson SM, Marshall WL, Siegert R: Attachment style and intimacy deficits in sexual offenders: a theoretical framework. Sex Abuse 7:317–335, 1995

Wise TN: Fetishism—etiology and treatment. A review from multiple perspectives. Compr Psychiatry 26:249–257, 1985

16 *Psychiatric Disorders of Childhood and Adolescence*

Arden D. Dingle
and Mina K. Dulcan

This chapter addresses the identification, evaluation, and treatment of psychiatric disorders as they occur in children and adolescents. Approximately 20% of children and adolescents in the general population have diagnosable psychiatric disorders, with 4 to 8% being considered severely emotionally disturbed (Costello et al, 1996a, b). As in adults, psychiatric disorders are diagnosed using the criteria described in the *Diagnostic and Statistical Manual of Mental Disorders,* 4th edition (DSM-IV; American Pyschiatric Association, 1994). The DSM-IV has a section that details the disorders that most commonly present in childhood and adolescence (Table 16–1). Although developmental characteristics may influence symptom presentations at various ages, children and adolescents may be diagnosed with any psychiatric disorder for which they meet criteria. They may have significant symptoms yet not meet criteria for any specific disorder. In general, personality disorder diagnoses are used sparingly for patients younger than 18 years old because personality development is not considered to be completed until adulthood. This chapter highlights the *differences* between adult and childhood forms of psychiatric illness in clinical manifestations, evaluation, and treatment, as well as discussing symptoms and problems frequently encountered in primary medical settings.

PSYCHIATRIC EVALUATION

A primary goal of assessment is to acquire information about an individual's type, extent, and severity of psychiatric symptoms, as well as the level of impairment (Table 16–2). For children and adolescents, this process usually

Table 16–1 **Disorders Usually First Diagnosed in Infancy, Childhood, or Adolescence***

Attention-Deficit Hyperactivity Disorder
Conduct Disorder
Oppositional Defiant Disorder
Separation Anxiety Disorder
Rumination Disorder
Enuresis
Encopresis
Tic Disorders
Mental Retardation
Pervasive Developmental Disorders
Learning Disorders
Communication Disorders

* Adapted from DSM-IV (American Psychiatric Association, 1994).

requires developing a sense of the child or adolescent in a variety of environments by collecting data from several adult sources, such as the parents, school staff, and others, in addition to the child or adolescent. Informants vary in accuracy and perspectives. Generally, children and adolescents are often better reporters about their internalized states, such as feelings of anxiety and depression, while their parents are more disclosing about conduct (externalizing) problems such as stealing, truancy, and/or difficulty with the legal system. Children, adolescents, and families of different cultures, races, and socioeconomic status may vary in their understanding and acceptance of the need for psychiatric services.

The importance of a thorough knowledge of normal development cannot be overemphasized. The symptoms of many psychiatric disorders in childhood and adolescence are characteristic of normal children at earlier developmental

Table 16–2 **Psychiatric Evaluation of a Child or Adolescent**

Biopsychosocial history (see Table 16–3)
    Information from caretakers, child or adolescent, teachers, other
      involved adults
    Supplemental self-report measures
Clinical interview of child and adolescent
    Developmental level
    Mental Status Exam
Medical history and examination
    Additional medical evaluation and laboratory testing as indicated
Psychological testing if appropriate
Observation of child or adolescent in an usual environment
    (i.e., school) if appropriate

Dell and Dulcan, 1998

stages (such as bed wetting or tantrums) or appear occasionally in many normal children (for example, lying, stealing, or short attention span). Psychopathology is determined by the pattern of symptoms, as well as their severity, intensity, frequency, and duration, and by the child's degree of impairment in functioning.

When evaluating a child or adolescent, a great deal of the history is gathered from the parents or guardians (Table 16–3); however, information always should be obtained from the child or adolescent, also. Standardized questionnaires often are used to supplement information from interviews. An excellent example is the Child Behavior Checklist, a self-report form that has been standardized on a general American population. It comes in several different versions to be completed by the parents, teachers, and the child or adolescent (Achenbach, 1991a–c).

When interviewing the child or adolescent, important information is gathered by direct questioning and by observation of appearance, affect, and behavior. Above the age of 5 years, children and adolescents should be seen individually for at least part of the interview. This focus is particularly important for older children and adolescents who may be reluctant or fearful to discuss or disclose information in front of their caretakers. For younger children, often the issue is relational, and separation from the involved adult may not be

---

Table 16–3 **Biopsychosocial History of a Child or Adolescent**

Chief complaint
History of present illness
   Development of the symptoms
   Attitudes toward the symptoms
   Effects on the child and family
   Stressors
   Prior psychiatric treatment and results
      Psychotherapy: type, frequency, duration
      Medication: doses, schedule, benefits, side effects
      Environmental changes
Past history
   Medical
   Psychiatric
   Physical or sexual abuse
Substance abuse
Medical review of symptoms
Review of psychological symptoms
Developmental history (milestones)
Social history
Family history
   Medical
   Psychiatric
   Developmental
   Social

optimal or as necessary. The interview must be adapted for the age and maturity of the patient. Younger and less verbal children may need to be involved in another activity (i.e., drawing, playing) while talking, and this endeavor may be as or more informative than the child's utterances. Most adolescents should be able to participate adequately in a primarily verbal interview. Children and adolescents vary in their capability to understand and discuss their difficulties and the roles of emotions, cognition, and other factors. Some individuals are able to discuss such issues early in the interview, while others require careful preparation. It is important to start with open-ended questions; however, many children and adolescents will require additional help (i.e., supplemental, more specific questions; explanations and examples of terms; and discussion of less threatening subjects first). A full mental status exam should be done on all children and adolescents above the age of 5. Questions about sexual and physical abuse should be included. Additionally, adolescents routinely should be asked about drug and alcohol use, sexual activity, and legal system involvement. Children, adolescents, and their families can tolerate very personal and intrusive questions if the interviewer is empathic, clear about the relevance of these topics, and assures complete confidentiality.

Children and adolescents commonly present with somatic symptoms. A physical examination should be performed to search for medical causes of symptoms and to discover any unrelated but coexisting medical disorders. Increasingly, genetic factors have been implicated as etiological agents in a variety of childhood psychiatric disorders (Lombroso et al, 1994). The decision to conduct additional medical evaluation, such as a neurological examination or laboratory tests, is made based on the findings of the medical history and physical examination (see Chapter 1 by Drs. Yates, Kathol, and Carter). Anticipated pharmacological treatment may require additional studies to establish baseline values and to rule out contraindications to a particular medication. While not particularly useful clinically, neuroimaging has been utilized to delineate abnormalities of brain structure and function in some of the childhood neuropsychiatric disorders. Structural and/or metabolic differences have been documented in schizophrenia, depression, mania, obsessive–compulsive disorder, Tourette's disorder, attention deficit–hyperactivity disorder (ADHD), dyslexia, and autism (Botteron et al, 1995; Jacobsen et al, 1996; Peterson, 1995; Piven et al, 1996; Steingard et al, 1996).

Information from the school is always useful and is essential when there is concern about learning, behavior in school, or functioning with peers. With parental consent, the clinician may interview teachers; obtain records of testing, grades, and attendance; and have school personnel complete a standardized rating form, such as the Teacher's Report Form of the Child Behavior Checklist (Achenbach, 1991c). Ideally, a visit to the school is arranged to observe the youngster in the classroom and on the playground. The clinician also may want to obtain information from other agencies with which the child or adolescent may be involved (i.e., after-school, foster care system, court).

Psychological testing, including individually administered intelligence tests and achievement tests, is obtained when there are questions about learning and IQ. More extensive testing for specific learning disabilities is conducted as indicated by school reports and the results of initial tests (Table 16–4 and Chapter 3 by Drs. Kaslow and Farber). Additionally, psychological testing (projective testing) can be performed to evaluate thought processes.

In a typical pediatric clinic, 15 to 20% of the children suffer from an emotional or behavior problem of sufficient severity to warrant mental health care (Costello and Pantino, 1987). Parents and children, however, often do not spontaneously report their concerns about behavior, development, and/or emotional problems because they perceive physicians as "too busy," not interested, or unable to help with "nonmedical" problems (Costello and Pantino, 1987). In medical settings, parents should be asked specifically if they have any worries about the child's development, school performance, emotions, or behavior. Children and adolescents are asked if they have been feeling depressed or sad or worried or nervous. The primary care physician should be prepared to detect physical or sexual abuse, neglect, and substance abuse and to provide anticipatory guidance regarding parenting, development, and/or sexuality.

Table 16–4 **Psychoeducational Test Instruments**

INSTRUMENT	AGE
Cognitive Development (Young Children)	
Bayley Scales of Development	3 to 30 months
Intelligence	
Kaufman Assessment Battery for Children (K-ABC) (less dependent on culturally based information and schooling)	2½ to 12½ years
Peabody Picture Vocabulary Test (PPVT-R) (brief test of receptive language abilities, often used as a screening IQ measure)	
Stanford-Binet Intelligence Scale, 4th ed. (heavily language based)	2 years to adulthood
Wechsler Preschool and Primary Scale of Intelligence (WPPSI)	4 to 6½ years
Weschler Intelligence Scale for Children, revised, 3rd ed. (WISC-IIIR)	6 to 16 years
Weschler Adult Intelligence Scale (WAIS)	16 years and older
Academic Achievement	
Peabody Individual Achievement Test (PIAT)	
Wide Range Achievement Test (WRAT)	
Woodcock Reading Mastery Tests	
Developmental Level of Adaptive Functioning	
Vineland Adaptive Behavior Scales	

Indications for specialty mental health consultation with a child and adolescent psychiatrist after the initial screening assessment include:

Physical symptoms with unexplained etiology or severity
Noncompliance with medical treatment
Developmental delays
Observation or report of depression, anxiety, or hyperactive behavior
Impaired school performance
Problems with peer or family relationships
Suspected substance abuse
Parental difficulties with child rearing

GENERAL PRINCIPLES OF TREATMENT PLANNING

The initial treatment plan is based on the diagnosis, target symptoms, and strengths and weaknesses of the patient and the family. The child's environment, including school, neighborhood, and social support network, also influence the choice of treatment strategy. Children and adolescents are usually best served by a combination of treatment modalities (Table 16–5). An essential aspect of treatment planning is obtaining parental understanding and consent, as well as patient understanding and assent. It is important to provide information about the probable course of the disorder if untreated, describe available treatments, and estimate the potential benefits and risks for their child. The child or adolescent patient should be included in this discussion, as appropriate. With only a few exceptions, all of the treatments used for adults may be used for children and adolescents, with modifications for the patient's developmental status. In most cases, coordination with the parents, school, pediatrician, child welfare agency, courts, and/or recreation leader will be part of the treatment plan.

Table 16–5 **General Treatment Modalities**

Psychotherapy: psychoanalytic, psychodynamic, or supportive
  Individual
  Family
  Group
Behavior modification
Cognitive–behavioral therapy
Psychopharmacology
Adjunctive treatments
  Educational placement
  Extracurricular programming
  Community services

Families of children and adolescents with psychiatric or learning problems need and deserve education in the nature of their child's disorder and in managing difficult behaviors. Caretakers spend far more time with their children than the therapist does, and parents can powerfully assist or impede the process of treatment. Treatment planning is an ongoing process, with reevaluations done as interventions are attempted and as additional information about the child and family comes to light.

Psychotherapeutic Treatment

For children and adolescents with psychiatric disorders, some type of psychotherapeutic intervention generally is considered essential. Indications for treatment include symptom reduction, promoting normal development, fostering autonomy and self-reliance, and aiming for positive change in the environment. Therapy may be individual, geared towards the child or adolescent or more global (i.e., family). Types of psychotherapy include psychoanalytic, psychodynamic, supportive, behavioral, cognitive, group, and family. It is important to remember that, regardless of the type of psychotherapy, working with children and adolescents means some ongoing involvement with and participation by the caretakers and other involved adults. Although clinicians believe that psychotherapeutic approaches are effective and useful clinically, there have been significant difficulties obtaining adequate scientific data about outcomes of mental health care for children and adolescents (Jensen, et al, 1996). In general, however, treatment appears more effective than no treatment.

Pharmacologic Treatment

When using psychopharmacological agents with children and adolescents, important general principles include minimizing the use of multiple medications and *rarely using medication as the only form of treatment.* Medications target specific symptoms and seldom eradicate problematic feelings, thoughts, and actions. Children, adolescents, and their families require additional interventions to help alleviate and prevent persistent symptoms and associated difficulties. Additionally, the physician must consider the potential meaning of medication to the child, family, school, and the child's peer group. It is important to educate the family regarding the medication; resources are available to assist in this process (Dulcan, in press).

In considering a specific medication treatment for a child or adolescent, the physician has a special responsibility to consider the risk/benefit ratio. Both therapeutic and side effects of the medication must be actively evaluated, seeking information from the child, parent, and other relevant adults such as teachers. There is a need to balance the potential risks of the medication with the prognosis of the untreated disorder and with what is known about the relative efficacy of medication. Nearly all psychopharmacological agents and indications lack pediatric labeling and are unapproved (off-label) for children as a consequence of the paucity of adequate research in child and adolescent psychopharmacology. The U.S. Food and Drug Administration (FDA) guidelines as published in the *Physicians Desk Reference* (PDR) cannot be relied upon for appropriate indications, ages, or doses for children. The clinician should therefore rely on the scientific literature rather than the PDR. Lack of approval for an age group or a disorder does not imply improper or illegal use, but clinicians should inform families of this fact, as well as discuss the relevant research and clinical data (Dulcan, 1992; Green, 1995; Werry and Aman, 1993; Laughren, 1996).

Adjunctive Treatments

Modified school programs are indicated for those children and adolescents who cannot perform satisfactorily in regular classrooms and who need additional structure, supervision, or specialized teaching techniques to reach their academic potential, maintain appropriate behavior, and/or achieve acceptable interactions and social relationships with peers and others. Educational systems are required by law to provide educational opportunities for all, regardless of their needs, in the most mainstream environment that is appropriate (federal law PL 94-142). Specialized educational services are determined on a local level with federal and state mandates describing minimum standards. For such a placement, children and adolescents require an evaluation coordinated and performed (or accepted) by school personnel. It generally includes IQ testing, achievement levels, social and psychological history, and functional status (daily living skills). If the child is determined to meet educational criteria (not the same as psychiatric criteria), the educational system is obligated to meet the educational needs of the child or adolescent in the least restrictive setting.

Although children and adolescents spend a substantial portion of their days in school, they also have considerable extracurricular time. Many benefit from participating in supervised and structured activities that provide constructive and meaningful activity, as well as the opportunity to have positive interactions and role modeling with both peers and adults. Additional advantages may include developing new skills, exposure to different adult interactional styles, and consolidation of learning. Developing a sport or hobby may be an especially important adjunct in the treatment of children and adolescents who lack positive relationships with peers or adults and/or have difficulty filling their time productively and appropriately. A relationship with an adult such as a Big Brother or Sister or a YMCA counselor or an opportunity to attend a camp may improve self-esteem and peer relationships.

Some children, adolescents, and families require additional community services because of an inability to manage at home. Most of these services are provided on a local level with community, city, county, state, and/or federal funding. Access to these resources is determined by the level of need; this type of aid includes out-of-home placement and intensive in-home help, as well as vocational and educational support. Children and adolescents may be removed from their homes and families if it has been determined that the child or adolescent is not managable at home or is in danger from neglect or abuse. Most of these youths are removed temporarily and eventually return to a family member. Placements include foster homes, group homes, emergency shelters, psychiatric facilities, and juvenile justice institutions. Decisions regarding type of placement are based on the psychopathology of the child and adolescent, the individual's and family's strengths, and the available resources in the environment.

DISRUPTIVE BEHAVIOR DISORDERS

Children and adolescents diagnosed with disorders in this category have externalizing symptoms and have been identified because their behavior has been problematic for others at home, school, and in the community. These individuals can have difficulty understanding and accepting not only the existence of problems, but also their own contribution to their problems. Rarely is the presenting reason for evaluation and treatment distress or concern on the part of the child or adolescent.

Attention-Deficit Hyperactivity Disorder

Children who have problems at home and school because they are inattentive, impulsive, fidgety, restless, and often overactive are considered to have ADHD (Table 16–6). In the past, these children and adolescent have been described with a variety of other disorders, such as minimal brain damage or dysfunction, hyperactivity, hyperkinetic reaction or syndrome of childhood, or attention-deficit disorder with or without hyperactivity. There has been some difficulty comparing research in this area, since the studies have been conducted using a variety of diagnostic systems. Currently, there are three subtypes: attention deficits only (inattentive type); hyperactive and impulsive type; and both groups of symptoms (combined type).

Epidemiology
Between 14 and 20% of preschool and kindergarten boys and approximately a third as many girls have ADHD (Campbell, 1985). In elementary schools, 3 to 10% of students have ADHD symptoms. Many overactive, inattentive, and impulsive children can be identified by parents and teachers, but have not been diagnosed or treated. A 1987 survey in Baltimore County, Maryland, found 6% of all public elementary school students, 3.7% of middle school

Table 16–6 **Attention-Deficit/Hyperactivity Disorder**

Characteristics
Inattention
Impulsiveness
Overactivity (some individuals)

Diagnosis
Onset prior to age 7
Duration at least 6 months
Pattern of behavior excessive for age and intelligence

Epidemiology
Up to 10% of school age population
Boys greater than girls
Associated with other psychiatric diagnoses and learning disabilities
Continued symptoms into adolescence and adulthood

Treatment
Medication: stimulants, antidepressants, alpha-adrenergic agents
Psychotherapy: supportive, family
Behavior modification
Educational placement and modification

students, and 0.4% of high school students to be receiving stimulant treatment for ADHD (Safer and Krager, 1988). Boys outnumber girls in the prevalence of ADHD more dramatically in clinical settings than in school populations.

Description

Diagnostic criteria for ADHD require a pattern of behavior that appears before than the age of 7 years, has been present for at least 6 months, and is excessive for age and intelligence (at least six symptoms in one category). The symptoms are divided into categories of inattention and hyperactivity–impulsiveness and must be present often, although not necessarily all the time or in every situation (American Psychiatric Association, 1994). Common presenting behaviors include restlessness, inability to stay seated, impulsive speech, difficulty following instructions, short attention span at work and play, forgetfulness, and difficulty with organizing.

Potentially dangerous impulsive behavior may also occur. Variability of symptoms from time to time and in different situations is a hallmark of ADHD. Many youngsters with ADHD can pay attention for an hour or more to a highly engaging activity of their own choosing, such as television or a computer game.

Teachers complain that children with ADHD are frequently "off task" and disturb others by fidgeting, making noises, or talking. Their written work is often messy and characterized by poor handwriting and impulsive, careless errors. Virtually all youngsters with ADHD have deficits in learning, achievement, or completion of school work by the time the diagnosis is made.

Hyperactive behavior per se is no longer considered the key or even a necessary feature of this disorder, although the term is often used as shorthand for ADHD. Douglas (1983) proposes as primary deficits:

1. Lack of investment, organization, and maintenance of attention and effort in completing tasks
2. Inability to inhibit impulsive action
3. Lack of modulation of arousal levels to meet the demands of the situation
4. Unusually strong inclination to seek immediate reinforcement

Commonly associated features of ADHD are low self-esteem, feelings of depression and demoralization, and lack of ability to take responsibility for one's actions. In social situations, these youngsters tend to be immature, bossy, intrusive, loud, uncooperative, out of synchrony with situational expectations, and irritating to both adults and peers. As a result, they may have few friends and prefer to play with older or younger children.

Research has demonstrated various associations between ADHD and neurological soft signs, minor physical anomalies, and electroencephalographic (EEG) abnormalities; however, these findings are not generally applicable clinically to specific children because they are not always present in ADHD and because many normal children and those with other psychiatric diagnoses have such findings (Rutter, 1982).

In adolescence, symptom patterns may change and appear to improve or remit, although from 50 to 80% of children with ADHD continue to show symptoms of hyperactivity, impulsiveness, and inattention during adolescence. The persistence of these symptoms frequently results in academic failure and/or school behavioral problems, depressed mood, low self-esteem, family conflict, and poor peer relationships. *In young adulthood, two-thirds of grown-up ADHD children continue to show at least some symptoms of restlessness, poor concentration, impulsiveness, and/or explosiveness, with resulting impairments in academic, vocational, and social functioning.*

In clinical settings, *at least two-thirds of patients with ADHD also have oppositional defiant disorder (ODD) or conduct disorder.* (These disorders are discussed later.) Youngsters with coexisting attention and conduct disorders tend to have an earlier age of onset, exhibit a greater total number of antisocial behaviors, and display more physical aggression. Of all children with ADHD, those with comorbid conduct disorder are virtually the only ones at risk for antisocial behavior and drug use as adults.

Differential Diagnosis
Inexperience or overly critical parents or teachers may confuse *normal age-appropriate overactivity* with ADHD. Onset of symptoms after age 7 or a duration of less than 6 months may indicate an *adjustment disorder,* especially if there is an identifiable stressor in the child's life. Children who are

fidgety and preoccupied may have an *anxiety disorder* instead of (or in addition to) ADHD.

Prepubertal children with *bipolar disorder* may manifest a chronic mixed affective state marked by irritability, overactivity, and difficulty concentrating. Family history may be helpful in differentiating this from ADHD, but long-term follow-up may provide the only conclusive answer.

Children who are restless and inattentive only at school may have *mental retardation* or a *specific developmental disorder* rather than ADHD. ADHD can be diagnosed *in addition to* mental retardation if symptoms are excessive for the child's *mental* age. Delays in specific learning skills, such as reading, math, and language, are commonly associated with ADHD.

Symptoms resembling ADHD can be caused by *drugs* such as phenobarbital (prescribed as an anticonvulsant) or theophylline (for asthma). *Hyper- or hypothyroidism* can be differentiated from ADHD by the presence of physical signs and by laboratory measures.

Etiology
Familial factors have been strongly implicated, although teasing out genetic from environmental influences is difficult. Children with ADHD alone have an elevated rate of first-degree relatives with ADHD. Children who have both ADHD and conduct disorder tend to come from families with an increased rate of ADHD, conduct disorder, ODD, and antisocial personality disorder (Biederman et al, 1986).

Neurotransmitter abnormalities in ADHD have been suggested, but have not been consistently documented. Quantitative EEG differences have been reported in ADHD children (Kuperman et al, 1996). Recent imaging studies suggest delayed or abnormal maturation of the frontal lobes of the brain. Biological insults associated with some cases of ADHD include complications of pregnancy, maternal alcohol use or smoking, postmaturity, long labor, health problems or malnutrition in infancy, lead poisoning, phenylketonuria, and glucose-6-phosphate dehydrogenase deficiency.

Evaluation
Reports should be obtained from multiple sources and should always include the teacher's report, preferably incorporating rating scales with standardized norms such as the Child Behavior Checklist for parents (Achenbach, 1991a) and the Teacher's Report Form (Achenbach, 1991c). Children often do not demonstrate problem behaviors in the doctor's office, but may be overactive, impulsive, and inattentive in the waiting room. Psychological testing is nearly always needed to evaluate the IQ and academic achievement and to search for specific developmental disorders. Motor or vocal tics should be sought in both the patient and family because patients with Tourette's disorder commonly have coexisting ADHD.

Treatment

The child or adolescent with ADHD either alone or in combination with other disorders is best served by multimodality therapy tailored to the youth and family. Medication often is a mainstay of treatment, but is not always required (Dulcan and Benson, 1997). The most common approaches for these disorders have been supportive psychotherapy, family therapy, group therapy, behavioral or cognitive–behavioral treatment, medication, and environmental manipulation.

Psychotherapy. Supportive psychotherapy may be helpful in addressing low self-esteem and demoralization resulting from the parent, teacher, and peer reactions to the ADHD child's behavior, or in resolving the effects of a parental divorce or other stressor. Family therapy can address problems caused by living with a difficult child or other marital or family dynamics that may interfere with consistent management. Group therapy is useful in improving social skills and peer relations.

Behavior Modification. Behavior modification can improve both academic achievement and behavioral compliance if they are specifically targeted (Barkley, 1990). Both nonphysical punishment (time out and response cost) and reward components are required. Behavioral techniques, including the teaching of specific social skills, can improve peer interactions. Behavior modification addresses symptoms that stimulants do not, but more cooperation from parents and teachers is required, and generalization and maintenance are elusive. Many youngsters require programs that are intensive and prolonged for months to years. The most effective behavioral treatment programs target specific behaviors at both home and school.

Classroom behavior modification techniques include explicit class rules, token economies, attention to positive behavior, and response cost programs (withdrawal of reinforcers following undesirable behavior; Abramowitz and O'Leary, 1991). Reinforcers such as praise, stars on a chart, or privileges may be dispensed by the teacher or by parents through the use of daily report cards.

Cognitive–Behavioral or Problem-Solving Therapy. This form of treatment combines behavior modification techniques, such as contingent reinforcement and modeling, with instruction in cognitive strategies, such as stepwise problem-solving and self-monitoring. It was developed in an attempt to improve the generalization and durability of behavior modification techniques and directly addresses presumed deficits in the control of impulsiveness and problem-solving (Kendall and Braswell, 1985). Unfortunately, most empirical studies have shown limited efficacy in the treatment of ADHD.

Psychopharmacological Treatment. The decision to use medication for ADHD is based on symptoms (not due to another treatable cause) of inattention, impulsiveness, and often hyperactivity that are persistent and of sufficient severity to cause functional impairment at school and, usually, at home and with peers. Parents must be willing to monitor the medication and to attend appointments.

Measures from both home and school of baseline symptoms and progress are essential in monitoring response to treatment. Prior to starting medication, the child, family, and teacher should be educated about the use and possible positive and negative effects of the medication. It is helpful to debunk common myths about treatment. The physician should work closely with parents on dose adjustments and obtain frequent reports from teachers and annual academic testing.

Unfortunately, every study of pharmacological treatment of hyperactivity that has used more than one outcome measure has shown that even children who respond positively continue to show deficits in some areas. Adjunctive treatments can focus on target symptoms remaining even after medication is optimized.

Stimulants. Stimulants, which include methylphenidate (Ritalin), dextro-amphetamine (Dexedrine), and pemoline (Cylert), are the most commonly used medications in the treatment of ADHD. One theory regarding their mechanism of action suggests that stimulants act by canalizing or reducing the excessive, poorly synchronized variability in the various dimensions of arousal and reactivity seen in ADHD (Evans et al, 1986). Contrary to previous belief, normal and hyperactive children, adolescents, and adults have similar cognitive and behavioral responses to comparable doses of stimulants, although children do not report euphoria. Stimulants do *not* have a paradoxical sedative action; they do *not* lead to drug abuse or addiction; and many adolescents with ADHD continue to require and benefit from their use. There are no predictors of which stimulant will be best for a particular child or adolescent; a substantial number will respond to one stimulant but not another.

Up to 96% of children with ADHD have at least some positive behavioral response to methylphenidate and/or dextroamphetamine, although side effects limit efficacy or require discontinuation of medication in some children (Elia et al, 1991). Both preschool children and adolescents may require lower weight-adjusted doses than school-aged children and may have greater likelihood of side effects and somewhat lower therapeutic efficacy (Varley, 1983). Up to 25% of children who respond poorly to one stimulant medication have a positive response to another. Stimulants reliably decrease physical activity, especially during times when children are expected to be less active (such as during school, but not during free play). They decrease vocalization, noise, and disruption in the classroom and improve handwriting. Stimulants consistently reduce off-task behavior and improve compliance to adult commands.

Stimulants produce improvement on cognitive laboratory tasks measuring sustained attention, distractibility, impulsiveness, and short-term memory. Cognitive learning strategies that the child typically uses are enhanced. Stimulants increase productivity and decrease errors in tests of arithmetic, reading comprehension, sight vocabulary, and spelling, and increase the percentage of assigned seat work completed (Pelham and Hoza, 1987).

Methylphenidate and behavior modification at home and school have been shown to be additive in effect on motor, attention, and social measures for many ADHD children (Pelham and Murphy, 1986). Stimulant medication and behavior modification can be synergistic in improving classroom behavior. Intensive behavior modification plus a low dose of medication yields a benefit equivalent to a higher dose of medication alone (Carlson et al, 1992).

Stimulant medication should be initiated with a low dose and titrated weekly, according to response and side effects (Tables 16–7 and 16–8). Weight-corrected doses provide an approximate range. Stimulants should be given after meals to reduce anorexia. The need for medication after school or on weekends is individually determined. Stimulants should be used cautiously in patients with a history of tics in themselves or their families, as stimulants may precipitate or aggravate motor tics in those predisposed to them. If target symptoms are not too severe, stimulants are discontinued for an annual drug-free trial for at least 2 weeks in the summer. If school functioning is stable, a trial off the medication in the middle of the school year is useful to assess whether it is still needed.

Tolerance has been reported occasionally, but compliance is often irregular, and missed doses should be the first possibility considered when medication appears to lose its effect. It is not wise for children to be responsible for their own medication. Alternate reasons for apparent decreased drug effect are a reaction to a change at home or school or decreased efficiency of a generic preparation.

Recent data suggest that the long-acting stimulant formulations—Ritalin Sustained Release (S-R) and Dexedrine Spansule—are more effective than previously thought, although there may be a delay in the onset of action and increased variability from day to day (Pelham et al, 1987). For some children, Dexedrine Spansule appears to be more consistently efficacious than other stimulant preparations (Pelham et al, 1990). The longer acting formulations are especially useful when the short-acting forms last only 2.5 to 3 hours or cause severe rebound symptoms or when medication cannot be administered at school. Highly individualized regimens combining short- and long-acting forms may be best for some children. Unpredictably high doses may result if a child chews a long-acting tablet instead of swallowing it.

Pemoline is a longer acting, mild central nervous system stimulant structurally dissimilar to methylphenidate and dextroamphetamine. Pemoline may be able to be given once a day, although absorption and metabolism vary widely, and some children need twice-daily doses. It tends to be used as a second-line drug, due to its potential side effects (liver toxicity) and required clinical and lab monitoring.

Stimulant side effects are listed in Table 16–8. There is no evidence that stimulants produce a decrease in the seizure threshold or clinically significant growth retardation (Spencer et al, 1996). Sleep problems and rebound effects

Table 16–7 **Clinical Use of Medications to Treat ADHD in Prepubertal Children**

	METHYLPHENIDATE (RITALIN)	DEXTROAMPHETAMINE (DEXEDRINE)	PEMOLINE (CYLERT)	CLONIDINE (CATAPRES)	IMIPRAMINE (TOFRANIL)
Doses (mg)	5, 10, 20 (tablet) 20 (sustained release)	5, 10 (tablet) 5 mg/ml (elixir) 5, 10, 15 (spanules)	18.75, 37.5, 75	0.1 (tablet)	10, 25, 50, 75, 100, 125, 150
Single dose range	0.3–0.8 mg/kg/dose	0.15–0.5 mg/kg/dose	0.5–2.5 mg/kg/dose	0.05–0.1 mg/dose	10–100 mg/dose
Daily dose (mg/kg/day)	0.6–2	0.3–1.25	0.5–3	0.003–0.006	1–5
Range (mg/day)	10–60	5–40	37.5–112.5	0.15–0.30	
Initial dose (mg)	5/day or b.i.d.	2.5–5/day	18.75–37.5/day	0.05–0.1/day	10–25 mg
Maintenance	2–4 doses/day	2–4 doses/day	1–2 doses/day	3–4 doses/day	2–3 doses/day
Monitor	Pulse Blood pressure Growth Dysphoria Tics	Pulse Blood pressure Growth Dysphoria Tics	Pulse Blood pressure Growth Dysphoria Tics Liver functions	Blood pressure Electrocardiograph Fasting glucose Sedation Dysphoria	Electrocardiograph Blood pressure

Table 16–8 **Side Effects of Stimulants**

Common Initial (try dose reduction)

Anorexia
Weight loss
Irritability
Abdominal pain
Headaches
Emotional oversensivity, easy crying

Less Common

Insomnia
Dysphoria
Social withdrawal
Rebound overactivity and irritability (add small dose in late after-
  noon/early evening; try sustained release form)
Impaired cognitive test performance (especially at high doses)
Less than expected weight gain
Anxiety
Nervous habits (picking at skin, hair twisting/pulling)
Allergic rash or hives

Withdrawal Effects

Insomnia
Rebound ADHD symptoms
Depression (rare)

Rare Potentially Serious

Motor or vocal tics
Tourette's disorder (exacerbation or precipitation)
Depression
Growth retardation (reversible when drug stopped)
Tachycardia
Hypertension
Psychosis (with hallucinations)
Stereotyped activities or compulsions

More Common in Preschool Children*

Sadness
Irritability
Clinginess
Insomnia
Anorexia

With Pemoline Only**

Choreiform movements
Dyskinesias
Night terrors
Lip licking or biting
Chemical hepatitis (rare)

* Campbell, 1985.
** McDaniel, 1986.

may be managed through different dosing strategies. Stimulants may be used in conjunction with other medications, either to treat different disorders (i.e., the addition of a selective serotonin-reuptake inhibitor [SSRI] for depression) or to target residual ADHD symptoms (i.e., the addition of clonidine). Stimulants alone at a dose that is tolerated may not provide adequate symptom relief. The combination of methylphenidate and the tricyclic imipramine has been associated with a syndrome of confusion, affective lability, marked aggression, and severe agitation in children (Grob and Coyle, 1986). Four deaths have been reported to the FDA of children who had been on both methylphenidate and clonidine; however, the evidence linking these deaths to the drugs is tenuous (Fenichel, 1995). Extra caution is advised when treating children with cardiac or cardiovascular disease.

Bupropion. Bupropion (Wellbutrin) may improve overactivity and aggression, as well as enhance the cognitive performance of children with ADHD and conduct disorder. One controlled study found bupropion to be statistically equal to methlyphenidate in improving behavioral and cognitive symptoms of ADHD (Barrickman et al, 1995). Potential difficulties/side effects include relatively common allergic reactions (rash, urticaria, and rare serum sickness), drowsiness, fatigue, nausea, anorexia, dizziness, tic exacerbation, and "spaciness" (Simeon et al, 1990). Seizures are possible at daily doses above 450 mg. The clinical history should include information on seizures and possible predisposing factors (e.g., head trauma, other central nervous system pathology, other drugs that lower the seizure threshold, eating disorders). An EEG may be indicated prior to initiating this medication. Bupropion is administered in 2 or 3 daily doses to a usual maximum of 250 mg/day (300 to 400 mg/day in adolescent). A single dose should not exceed 150 mg. Blood levels do not appear to be clinically useful (Berrickman et al, 1995; Conners et al, 1996).

Alpha-Adrenergic Agonists. Clonidine (Catapres) and guanfacine (Tenex) are employed as adjuncts to stimulants or as third-line drugs. Clonidine (Table 16–7) is useful for a subgroup of children with ADHD, including those with tics or a family history of Tourette's disorder or when a stimulant is only partially effective (Hunt et al, 1990). Clonidine is particularly useful in decreasing hyperactivity, impulsiveness, defiance, emotional lability, and temper tantrums and in improving frustration tolerance and the ability to fall asleep at night. Maximum therapeutic effect may not be seen for several months. Although clonidine is not helpful in improving attention per se, its effects may potentiate and complement those of a stimulant. It is most helpful in combination when the stimulant response is only partial or the stimulant dose is limited by side effects. Vital signs, complete blood count, fasting glucose, and urinalysis should be obtained before starting clonidine. A thorough cardiovascular history should be taken with a recent clinical cardiac examination; some clinicians recommend electrocardiogram (ECG). Relative contraindications include a history of syncope and ECG changes such as bradycardia or heart block. The most troublesome side effect of clonidine is sedation, although it tends to decrease after several weeks. Hypotension and dizziness may occur at high doses. Dry mouth, photophobia, dysphoria, bradycardia, and abnormal glucose tolerance have been reported. The transdermal form may produce a pruritic skin rash. Depression may occur, most often in children or adolescents with personal or family histories of depressive symptoms. Clonidine is started at a low dose of 0.05 mg at bedtime or 0.025 mg q.i.d. The dose is then titrated over several weeks to 0.15 to 0.3 mg/day (0.003 to 0.006 mg/kg/day) in three or four divided doses. Children younger than 7 years of age may require lower initial and maintenance doses. This medication has a slow onset of action, and significant clinical response may not be seen for as long as a month, with maximum results taking several months. Clonidine should be tapered rather than stopped suddenly to avoid a withdrawal syndrome consisting of increased blood pressure, elevated pulse, and motor restlessness (Leckman et al, 1986).

Guanfacine is similar to clonidine but has a longer half-life and more favorable side effect profile (less sedation and hypotension). It recently has been used for similar indications as clonidine for patients who cannot tolerate an adequate dose of clonidine due to side effects. Data from only open trials are available (Chappell et al, 1995; Horrigan and Barnhill, 1995). It is typically given in divided doses b.i.d. or t.i.d., starting with 0.5 mg in the morning or at bedtime. The daily dose is increased by 0.5 mg every 3 to 4 days, with a maximum dose of 3 mg/day. One milligram of guanfacine is equivalent to 0.1 mg of clonidine.

Tricyclic Antidepressants. Tricyclic antidepressants (TCAs) may be employed in the treatment of ADHD but are considered second- or third-line drugs because of their safety and side effect profiles. Generally, a TCA is considered when stimulants exacerbate tics or Tourette's disorder, when there is concern about abuse or reselling of stimulants, when stimulants are ineffective, or when stimulant side effects are intolerable. TCAs produce improvement in ADHD symptoms that exceed placebo effects, but are less effective than stimulants (Biederman et al, 1989). Currently, nortriptyline (Pamelor), and imipramine (Tofranil) are most commonly used. Desipramine (Norpramin) is occasionally used, especially in older adolescents. Drawbacks to using tricyclics such as desipramine include potentially serious cardiac side effects, especially in prepubertal children, the danger of accidental or intentional overdose, and bothersome anticholinergic and sedating side effects. TCAs have a longer duration of action than methylphenidate, so a dose at school is not needed, and rebound is not generally a problem. Prepubertal children should be given three divided doses to avoid excessive peaks and valleys in blood levels. Imipramine is begun at 10 or 25 mg/day and gradually titrated to a maximum dose of 2 to 5 mg/kg/day (Table 16–7). The use of tricyclics in children is discussed further in the section on childhood mood disorders. A number of sudden deaths have been attributed to the use of desipramine in children and thus clinicians have become wary about its use in this population.

Selective Serotonin-Reuptake Inhibitors. Despite considerable clinical interest in the use of the SSRIs in the treatment of ADHD, only anecdotal data are available. These medications do not appear to be effective for the core symptoms of ADHD, but may be useful as adjuncts for secondary or comorbid mood and behavioral disorders. The use of SSRIs in children and adolescents is discussed further in the section on childhood mood disorders.

Environmental Interventions for ADHD

Academic deficits, learning disabilities, and/or behavior problems may necessitate specific situational interventions at school, home, and elsewhere. Children and adolescents with ADHD may require educational services such as tutoring, reduced class size, or specialized classes and/or schools. Affected individuals may need supplemental programs for after school time and holidays. Recreational or camp programs are often useful. Families may have to reorganize their schedules and increase the structure of family life.

Many parents ask about special diets to treat childhood behavior problems. At most, 5% of hyperactive children show minimal behavioral or cognitive improvement on the so-called Feingold or Kaiser-Permanente diet (Wender, 1986). Inducing the child to comply is extremely difficult. Controlled studies have been unable to demonstrate consistently that ingestion of sugar has any effect on the behavior or cognitive performance of normal or hyperactive children, even those identified by their parents as sugar responsive (Milich et al, 1986; Wolraich et al, 1995).

Role of the Primary Care Physician

The pediatrician or family physician is likely to be the first to be approached by parents concerned about the possibility of ADHD; often, families have been referred by the child's or adolescent's school. Milder, uncomplicated cases of ADHD can be managed by the primary care physician in close collaboration with a psychologist to perform testing to identify intellectual deficits and learning disabilities, and a child and adolescent psychiatrist or psychologist to provide psychotherapeutic interventions as needed. Cases with psychiatric comorbidity or those that do not respond to simple stimulant regimens should be referred to a child and adolescent psychiatrist. Primary care physicians should not treat ADHD with concurrent psychological or psychiatric collaboration.

Conduct Disorders

The diagnosis of conduct disorder describes children and adolescents with a pattern of disruptive, willfully disobedient, and antisocial behaviors that can be categorized as aggression, property destruction, deceitfulness/theft, and serious violations of rules (Table 16–9).

Epidemiology

The prevalence of conduct disorder in children and adolescents has been estimated at 3 to 7%. Males predominate, especially in aggressive conduct

Table 16–9 **Conduct Disorder**

Characteristics
Repetitive and persistent pattern of behavior
Violates basic rights of others and age-appropriate rules of society
Lasts at least a year

Diagnosis
At least three symptoms from the categories of
    Aggression to people or animals
    Destruction of property
    Deceitfulness or theft
    Serious violations of rules
Childhood or adolescent onset
Variable severity

Epidemiology
Prevalence of 3 to 7%
Predominance of males but number of females increasing
Associated with chaotic and impaired families
Comorbid psychiatric disorders common

Treatment
Identification and treatment of any comorbid psychiatric disorders
Development of adequate structure and supervision for the child
  or adolescent
Psychotherapy for associated psychological issues/symptoms
Family work to help develop adaptive and constructive methods
  of management
Behavior management
Consideration of medication for explosive, aggressive behavior

disorders, but the prevalence in females is rising. *Conduct problems are the most common complaint in referrals to child and adolescent psychiatric clinics and hospitals.*

Description

    This diagnosis requires a repetitive and persistent pattern of behavior that violates the basic rights of others or age-appropriate rules of society, lasts a year, and is manifested by at least three of a list of specific behaviors, which include stealing, running away from home, staying out after dark without permission, lying in order to "con" people, deliberate fire-setting, repeated truancy (beginning before age 13), vandalism, cruelty to animals, bullying, physical aggression, and forcing someone into sexual activity (American Psychiatric Association, 1994). Subtypes exist for age of onset (childhood, adolescent) and severity (mild, moderate, severe).

    Conduct disorder is a purely descriptive label for a heterogeneous group of children and adolescents. It is important to remember that all conduct-disordered individuals are not the same and that it is essential to evaluate the type and severity of offenses, as well as the situational factors. Often, the families of these children and adolescents are chaotic and have significant difficulties. Many patients seem to lack appropriate responses of guilt or remorse, empathy for others, and feelings of responsibility for their own behavior. Irritability, tantrums, cheating, low frustration tolerance, inability to delay gratification, and provocative behavior are common. Precocious and promiscuous sexual activity is often seen. Social skills are poor with both peers and adults.

This is a potentially serious disorder because a substantial minority of patients will develop antisocial personality disorder or alcoholism in adulthood. The severity of prognosis increases with the number, variety, and frequency of problem behaviors. Among young children, the strongest predictors of adolescent delinquency are aggression, drug use, stealing, truancy, lying, and low educational achievement (Loeber, 1990). The combination of ADHD and conduct disorder results in a high risk of later delinquency.

Differential Diagnosis

Rule-violating behavior should be considered on a continuum. The least severe is the *normal* occasional lying and stealing seen in children less than 6 years old. A single occurrence of serious misconduct would be diagnosed as Childhood or Adolescent Antisocial Behavior. Behavior problems that are not as severe as those seen in conduct disorder and that are less persistent than in ODD are diagnosed as Adjustment Disorder With Disturbance of Conduct if there is an identifiable stressor. A significant number of those with conduct disorder will have one or more comorbid psychiatric disorders.

Etiology

A number of causal factors have been implicated, but there is no known single cause, and all factors are not present in each case. ADHD and/or ODD often precede the development of conduct disorder. Conduct disorder symptoms may result from depression (Puig-Antich, 1982), mania, or psychosis. Mentally retarded youth may be led into antisocial acts by peers, or their lack of more adaptive coping strategies may result in aggression or stealing.

Conduct disorder appears to result from an interaction among the following factors (selection differs from child to child):

1. *Temperament* characterized by an initial resistance to child rearing, poor adaptability to change, high activity level, intense reactivity, and low threshold of responsiveness.
2. *Parents who provide attention to problem behavior and ignore good behavior,* who tend toward prolonged negative interactions with the child, who do not provide adequate supervision, and whose discipline is inconsistent, ineffective, and either lax or extremely severe and even abusive. One or more generations of parental irritability and explosive discipline lead

to the poor socialization of children and inadequate parenting skills as adults. Children develop noncompliant and poorly controlled behaviors and lack social and academic survival skills. The results include rejection by normal peers and school failure (Patterson et al, 1989).

3. *Association with a delinquent peer group*
4. *Parental modeling* of impulsiveness and rule-breaking behavior
5. Genetic predisposition
6. Parental marital conflict
7. Placement outside of the home as an infant or toddler
8. Poverty
9. Low IQ or brain damage (especially in violent delinquents)

Evaluation

Reports from both parent and child, and often community sources, are required to assess the severity of the behavior accurately. A search should be made for the common concurrent diagnoses, especially ADHD, anxiety and mood disorders, substance abuse, specific developmental disorders (especially developmental reading disorder and expressive language disorder), and mental retardation. Because of the high frequency of brain damage in patients with violent conduct disorders, the physician should conduct a careful search for symptoms suggestive of complex partial seizures.

Treatment

An essential aspect of treatment is the development and implementation of an adequate level of structure and supervision for the child or adolescent. Therapy aimed at just the child or adolescent is rarely successful; family work and environmental restructuring are required. Often, the legal system has to mandate that these individuals and their families participate.

Psychotherapy. Multisystemic therapy (Henggeler and Borduin, 1990) is a comprehensive treatment model of documented efficacy that includes the combination of systemic family therapy with behavior modification techniques, the use of social service agencies, and active outreach to influence the youth's teachers and peer group. Individual psychotherapy based on a supportive therapeutic relationship using cognitive–behavioral, self-control, or social skills training may be included, as may individual or marital therapy with parents.

Conduct disorders are generally treated more effectively in family or group therapy. Dynamically oriented individual therapy can be helpful as an adjunct to address specific symptoms associated with adverse events such as abuse, family discord, and trauma. A recently developed model of individual supportive–expressive play psychotherapy based on object relations theory that is often combined with parent training and/or play group psychotherapy has been demonstrated to be effective in treating children with ODD or mild-to-moderate conduct disorder, as long as the child has the capability for social bonding and for appropriate degrees of guilt (Kernberg and Chazan, 1991).

Behavior Modification. Several effective parent management training programs, based on social learning theory, exist for parents of noncompliant oppositional and aggressive children (Forehand and McMahon, 1981; Patterson, 1975). Parents are taught to use clear and consistent rules, to reinforce good behavior positively, and to use appropriate discipline (limit setting and consequences other than physical punishment) effectively. One frequently used negative contingency is the "time out," so called because it puts the child in a quiet, boring area, where there is a time out from whatever positive reinforcement he or she may be receiving for the problem behavior. Treatment is more effective the earlier it is begun, with adolescents being particularly resistant.

Cognitive behavior modification (CBM) is a technique that combines training in problem-solving skills with behavior modification. Children are taught to delay action and to consider alternative ways of resolving conflict. Both CBM and parent management training in behavior modification have been demonstrated to decrease aggressive and delinquent behavior and increase positive social skills in preadolescent conduct-disordered children. The combination of the two treatments is more effective than either alone in improving child behavior and in reducing parental stress and depression (Kazdin et al, 1992).

Psychopharmacological Treatment. Multiple drugs have been utilized to treat aggression with variable and inconsistent results. For conduct-disordered individuals, the most effective strategy is to evaluate carefully for comorbid disorders and to focus psychopharmacological treatment on these disorders first, since many of them tend to be more responsive than aggressive and antisocial behaviors.

Lithium may be considered in the treatment of severe impulsive aggression, especially when accompanied by explosive affect (Campbell and Cueva, 1995b). Efficacy has been demonstrated for some hospitalized prepubertal, explosively aggressive children with conduct disorder in a double-blind placebo-controlled trial (Campbell et al, 1985, 1995; see section on mood disorders for more details on lithium use as well as Chapter 18).

Of the *anticonvulsants,* carbamazepine may benefit patients who have severe impulsive aggression accompanied by emotional lability and irritability and who have an abnormal EEG or a strong clinical suggestion of epileptic phenomena (even though deliberate aggression is rarely part of a seizure) (Evans et al, 1987). Some preliminary data suggest efficacy in children under 12 with severe explosive aggression, even in the absence of neurological findings (Kafantaris et al, 1992); however, effectiveness was not demonstrated in a placebo-controlled trial with hospitalized (DSM-III-R) conduct-disordered children (Cueva et al, 1996). Medical and behavioral side effects of carbamazepine are similar to those seen in adults (Evans et al, 1987; Herskowitz, 1987; Pleak et al, 1988; see Chapter 17). Valproic acid has been used, but there are no systematic data on its efficacy.

Propranolol, a beta-adrenergic blocker, may be useful in patients with otherwise uncontrollable rage reactions and impulsive aggression, especially those with evidence of neurological dysfunction (Williams et al, 1982); however, organic etiology does not appear to be required for effectiveness (Grizenko and Vida, 1988).

Neuroleptics historically have been used to control aggression, but given the risk of cognitive dulling and tardive dyskinesia, they should be low on the list of medication options. Neuroleptics may reduce aggression, hostility, negativism, and explosiveness in severely aggressive children (Campbell et al, 1985; Greenhill et al, 1985; see the section on schizophrenia for more detail on the use of neuroleptics.)

Other medications (buproprion, trazodone, clonidine, venlafaxine, and the atypical antipsychotic risperidone) have been investigated and observed to decrease aggression, even without co-existing ADHD (Derivan et al, 1995; Fras and Major, 1995; Ghaziuddin and Alessi, 1992; Kemph et al, 1993; Simeon et al, 1995).

If the conduct disorder is secondary to a major depression, successful treatment with *antidepressants* leads to remission of the conduct symptoms (Puig-Antich, 1982). In cases with coexisting ADHD, *stimulant* treatment may decrease impulsive conduct symptoms and defiance, as well as over activity and inattention.

Environmental Interventions. Community-based recreation programs or a Big Brother or Sister may be helpful. A special education placement may be needed to manage behavior, remediate learning disabilities and academic deficits, and provide vocational training. Hospitalization or a structured milieu such as a residential treatment center may be required for severely aggressive youth. Effective residential treatment programs use close supervision and a strict token economy, which are combined with instruction in adaptive social and educational skills. Legal sanctions may be necessary to enforce cooperation with treatment. Long-term treatment is necessary to prevent relapse. A significant number of these adolescents end up in the juvenile justice system; those who commit more serious crimes may be tried and incarcerated as adults.

Role of the Primary Care Physician

These children and adolescents are at high risk for injuries and accidents. The result is frequent hospitalizations and emergency room visits. They are exposed to considerable psychological and physical trauma. The primary care physician must be alert to possible medical complications, such as sexually transmitted diseases, pregnancy, and sequelae of drug abuse.

Oppositional Defiant Disorder

This relatively new diagnostic category was intended to describe *milder forms of chronic behavior problems than those seen in conduct disorder.* Children diagnosed with ODD are at risk for developing a conduct disorder. The diagnoses of conduct disorder and ODD cannot be given simultaneously to the same individual.

Epidemiology

From 6 to 10% of youth have ODD, with boys outnumbering girls from two to three to one (Anderson et al, 1987). This disorder is extremely common among children referred to psychiatric services.

Description

Children with ODD display a chronic pattern of stubborn, negativistic, provocative, hostile, and defiant behavior *without* serious violation of the rights of others. They are often irritable, resentful, and quick to take offense. These children are usually most difficult to manage at home, but problems can extend to school and peers. They often continue to resist compliance, even when cooperation would be in their own best interest. Specific diagnostic criteria include loss of temper, arguments with adults, noncompliance (refusal to follow commands, directions, or minor rules), blaming others, and vindictiveness (American Psychiatric Association, 1994).

Differential Diagnosis

ODD must be distinguished from milder forms of *stubbornness.* Negativity and tantrums are *normal* prior to 3 years of age, as are early adolescent arguments with adults and resistance to rules. Intentional and provocative noncompliance characteristic of ODD should be differentiated from the noncompliance resulting from impulsiveness and inattention in ADHD, although both disorders are often present. In that case, both should be diagnosed. Oppositional behavior that is limited to school may be a result of *mental retardation* or a *specific developmental disorder.*

Etiology

Hypothesized factors include an inherited predisposition (perhaps mediated by difficult temperament), modeling of parental oppositional and defiant behavior, and parental inability to reward positive behavior or to set firm, fair, and consistent limits.

Evaluation

Symptoms are more prominent when the patient is with familiar people. Behavior may not seem abnormal in a diagnostic interview, especially if few demands are placed on the child. Parent and teacher reports are important. Psychological testing may be needed to discover low IQ or learning disabilities.

Treatment

Behavior Modification. An operant approach, using environmental positive and negative contingencies to increase or decrease the frequency of behaviors, is the most useful. A token economy is one type of operant approach in which points, stars, or tokens can be earned for desirable behaviors (and lost for problem behaviors) and exchanged for backup reinforcers such as money, food, toys, privileges, or time with an adult in a pleasant activity. Techniques can be taught to parents (Forehand and McMahon, 1981) and can be used by teachers in classrooms. It is especially helpful if parents and teachers can learn to structure situations to provide the child with appropriate choices and to avoid power struggles (similar to the strategies used with toddlers in the "terrible twos").

Psychopharmacology. In children with coexisting ADHD and ODD, stimulant medication may reduce oppositional behavior and improve compliance, as well as address inattention, impulsiveness, and hyperactivity.

ANXIETY DISORDERS

Anxiety symptoms are common in children and adolescents; diagnoses can include those that also affect adults, as well as some that usually present in childhood. Separation anxiety generally occurs in childhood. So does selective mutism, which (although not classified as an anxiety disorder in the DSM-IV) is considered by some to be related to social phobia. Children also can have generalized anxiety disorder (formerly described as overanxious disorder in DSM-III-R), phobias, obsessive–compulsive disorder, panic disorder, and post-traumatic stress disorder. These disorders and their treatments will be reviewed briefly with more detail on separation anxiety and posttraumatic disorders (Table 16–10).

Epidemiology

The prevalence of anxiety disorders in children and adolescents has been estimated to be from 2 to 15%, depending on severity. There is considerable overlap among anxiety disorders and between anxiety and depressive disorders (Kashani and Orvaschel, 1990; Last et al, 1987). After puberty, anxiety disorders are more common in girls than boys. There is substantial continuity in anxiety disorders, both from generation to generation and in the childhood histories of adult patients with anxiety disorders. In contrast to common notions that anxiety disorders are of minor importance, overanxious disorder (generalized anxiety disorder) and separation anxiety disorder can be chronic, relapsing, and result in considerable social and academic impairment Also, children with anxiety disorders may be at higher risk of developing other psychiatric disorders, even if their anxiety disorder remits (Last et al, 1996).

Table 16–10 **Anxiety Disorders**

Characteristics
Generalized or specific anxieties or fears
Can be chronic, relapsing
Overlap with depression
Can have significant impairment

Diagnoses
Separation Anxiety Disorder
Generalized Anxiety Disorder
Obsessive–Compulsive Disorder
Panic Disorder
Posttraumatic Stress Disorder
Phobias (social, simple)

Epidemiology
Estimated prevalence of 2 to 15%
Strong association with familial factors
More common in girls after puberty

Treatment
Psychotherapy
Behavioral modification
Medication: benzodiazipines, SSRIs, TCAs, antihistamines*

* SSRI, selective serotonin-reuptake inhibitor; TCA, tricyclic antidepressant.

Etiology

Familial factors are strongly implicated, although sorting out genetic predisposition from family dynamic factors and imitation of a fearful parent is difficult. In patients with separation anxiety disorder seen in a clinical setting, 83% of the mothers had an anxiety disorder and 63% had a mood disorder (Last et al, 1987).

Children identified at age 2 as extremely inhibited, quiet, and restrained in unfamiliar situations tend to remain shy and socially avoidant at age 7 years. They have greater sympathetic reactivity than outgoing children, as measured by heart rate acceleration and early morning salivary cortisol levels. Two year olds who are uninhibited tend to remain fearless and outgoing (Kagan et al, 1988). Certain medications, such as propranolol (for headache) and haloperidol (for Tourette's disorder) may produce symptoms of separation anxiety and school refusal.

Evaluation

Techniques of assessment are similar for all of the anxiety disorders in children and adolescents. Children who are anxious about being interviewed or who are having difficulty separating from their parents may be helped by being seen together with the parent initially. The clinical interview with the young person is especially important because parents usually underreport the child's phobic, anxiety, and mood symptoms. A detailed history of school experiences should be taken. Family history should focus particularly on anxiety and mood disorders. A medical history and physical exam will generally rule out a medical cause for somatic complaints such as headaches, abdominal pain, nausea, or vomiting. In *separation anxiety disorder,* somatic symptoms are worst on evenings and mornings before school and absent on weekends and holidays, except the night before school starts. Extensive medical evaluations should be avoided unless there are clear indications for them. Information should be sought regarding any possible advantage or "secondary gain" that result from the patient's symptoms.

Treatment

A variety of treatment techniques are applicable to several of the anxiety disorders in children and adolescents. Primary interventions include family therapy, collaboration with school personnel, and behavior modification using contingencies and systematic desensitization (American Academy of Child and Adolescent Psychiatry, 1993).

Psychotheraphy. Individual psychotherapy may be useful, with special attention to the child's relationship to the therapist and to separations that occur in the therapy. Supportive psychotherapy may permit children to deal with their anxiety in a more adaptive way. The goal of insight-oriented psychodynamic individual psychotherapy, using verbal and play techniques, is to resolve the underlying psychological conflicts and promote more functional intrapsychic defenses to deal with anxiety. Cognitive therapy techniques aim to reduce anxiety and improve coping skills by using specific training to change the patient's maladaptive, self-defeating thoughts to ones that describe the child or adolescent as competent (Ollendick and Francis, 1988). Family therapy may be valuable to reduce parental modeling or subtle encouragement of fearful behavior.

Behavior Modification. Behavioral techniques used to treat anxiety disorders include relaxation training, systematic desensitization, assertiveness training, shaping, and operant conditioning (Ollendick and Francis, 1988).

Psychopharmacological Treatment. Unfortunately, few controlled trials exist, except for obsessive–compulsive disorder (OCD), and the establishment of effectiveness has been confounded by extensive comorbidity and high placebo response rates.

Benzodiazipines may be used in short-term treatment of children and adolescents with severe anticipatory anxiety (Pfefferbaum et al, 1987). Infants and children absorb diazepam (Valium) faster and metabolize it more quickly than adults (Simeon and Ferguson, 1985). Some studies indicate that alprazolam (0.03 mg/kg or 0.5 to 6.0 mg/day) may be useful for separation anxiety disorder (SAD) or school phobia (Bernstein et al, 1990; Kutcher et al, 1992), but a recent double-blind study found no benefit over placebo when alprazolam was combined with an intensive treatment program (Simeon et al, 1992). A double-blind placebo-controlled study of clonazepam (up to 2 mg/day)in children with SAD and comorbid anxiety and behavior disorders demonstrated improvement in some children, but the results were not statistically significant. Two children exhibited significant disinhibition with irritability, tantrums, aggression, and attempted self-injury (Graae et al, 1994). Dosage schedules depend on age of the child or adolescent and the specific drug (Coffey, 1990). Side effects are similar to those seen in adults.

Imipramine, a TCA has been utilized to treat school refusal secondary to SAD, but its efficacy is controversial. It may be tried for children or adolescents who do not respond to psychological treatments such as family therapy, behavior therapy, and modification of the school situation. Clear guidelines for use do not exist. Typically, the starting dose is low, with a gradual increase. Responses may take up to 6 to 8 weeks.

SSRIs have been utilized in the treatment of anxiety disorders with some success. In several open clinical trials, fluoxetine (mean dose 25.7 mg/day) for children and adolescents with overanxious disorder, social phobia, or separation disorder produced moderate to marked improvement in the majority of individuals, although symptom remission did not begin until after 6 to 8 weeks of treatment (Birmaher et al, 1994). Fluoxetine (0.6 mg/kg/day) demonstrated modest efficacy over placebo (parent ratings only) in the treatment of selective mutism (Black and Uhde, 1994).

As to *other medications,* in a small trial, the nonbenzodiazepine anxiolytic *buspirone* was noted to improve anxiety, mood, and behavioral symptoms in children and adolescents with a variety of anxiety disorders, some of which were comorbid with other anxiety disorders or ADHD (Simeon et al, 1994). *Antihistamines* are commonly prescribed, but no empirical data on their use exist.

Separation Anxiety Disorder

Description
SAD is characterized by excessive anxiety for the patient's age—lasting for at least 4 weeks—concerning separation from parents (or others to whom the child is attached). Specific criteria include severe and persistent worries that something terrible will happen to the child on his or her parents that will keep them apart, reluctance or refusal to go to school because of fear of separation, refusal to sleep alone or away from home, avoidance of being alone, nightmares about separation, and excessive distress and/or physical symptoms in anticipation of or during separation from parents (American Psychiatric Association, 1994). In the past, this disorder was considered synonymous with "school phobia."

Differential Diagnosis

Normal age-appropriate separation anxiety may transiently worsen under stress, especially in children under 6 years of age. Avoidance of school may be due to SAD or to a number of other causes. In *truancy,* the child stays away from home and the parents are not usually aware, unless told by the school. Some families may keep a child home from school to help with family tasks. The child may have a *realistic fear* (for example, of a bully), a *simple phobia* of something in the school enviroment, or a *social phobia.* Anxiety may be precipitated by unreasonable demands for academic performance at school or an undiagnosed *specific developmental disorder.* Social withdrawal and lack of energy secondary to *major depression* may lead to avoidance of school.

Role of the Primary Care Physician

The primary care physician is in a position to distinguish the temperamentally shy, but normal child from the one whose anxiety results in impairment in school or with peers. Every effort should be made to get the child back to school as soon as possible.

Mild cases of school avoidance secondary to SAD can be managed by the primary care physician with encouragement to the child, family, and school. The child should be sent to school unless there are objective signs of illness, such as a fever. If the child stays home, she or he should rest in bed and not be allowed to engage in activities that are fun. If significant school refusal persists for more than a week, immediate referral for psychiatric evaluation and treatment should be made because the longer the child is out of school, the more difficult treatment becomes.

The primary physician can use a contingency management program for young children whose separation anxiety is manifested primarily by refusal to sleep in their own bed. The program includes an explanation to child and parents, support for the parents in insisting the child stay in his or her own room, help with devising a schedule of rewards for successful performance, and efforts to increase the child's motivation by the physician's own encouragement for sleeping alone.

Generalized Anxiety Disorder

The child or adolescent with *generalized anxiety disorder* suffers from and verbalizes excessive or unrealistic worry in multiple areas. Specific characteristics include worry about future events, past behavior, and the child's own competence; somatic complaints; self-consciousness; excessive need for reassurance; and marked feelings of tension. Associated features may include such habits as nail biting, thumb sucking, and hair pulling or twisting. This diagnosis includes the former category of overanxious disorder.

Phobias

A *phobia* is defined as a persistent, specific fear that is out of proportion to the actual danger and that leads to impairment in social and/or academic functioning because of the need to avoid the feared object or situation.

Normal fears are common in children. Specific fears vary with age. For example, infants react with fear to loss of physical support, loud noises, and rapidly approaching large objects. Fear of strangers develops around 7 months of age. Toddlers (age 1 to 3 years) are frightened by loud noises, storms, some animals, the dark, and separation from their parents. These fears continue to be prevalent among 3 to 5 year olds and are joined by fears of monsters and ghosts. All these fears tend to decline after age 6. Common fears observed in school-age children (6 to 12 years) are those relating to bodily injury, burglars, being kidnapped, being sent to the principal, being punished, and failure. Fears of tests in school and of social embarrassment take the lead from puberty through adolescence (Ollendick and Francis, 1988). Girls generally report more fears than boys, although it is not clear whether they actually *have* more fears or are simply more willing to report them.

Traditional Freudian theory proposed that phobias result from unconscious defenses against unacceptable wishes and feelings, as described in the classic case of "Little Hans." Oedipal dynamics were thought to be prominent in childhood phobias.

According to classical conditioning (behavioral) theory, phobias are learned by the generalization of fears to other objects or situations that are similar or that are coincident in time or place. Phobias persist because avoiding the feared object reduces anxiety. This removal of an aversive stimulus strengthens the preceding behavior (the phobic avoidance).

Behavioral treatments are generally the treatment of choice for children with one or two phobias. Symptom substitution (the appearance of a new symptom if the phobia is removed without addressing the presumed underlying conflicts) is not a problem if attention is paid to removal of secondary gain and to ensuring that the child has the skills and the opportunities to deal with the problem situation in other ways.

Children and adolescents with a *social phobia* fear one or more situations in which they will be observed by others and where their actions may lead to humiliation or embarrassment. Answering questions or speaking in front of the class is commonly feared. The result is impaired grades in school, despite adequate learning. If severe, the phobia may lead to an avoidance of school altogether or "school phobia."

Obsessive–Compulsive Disorder

This serious and difficult-to-treat illness can begin in childhood or adolescence (see Chapter 8). In community samples, the point prevalence is 3 to

4% (Flament et al, 1988; Valleni-Basile et al, 1994; Zohar et al. 1992) with reports of subclinical symptomatology in approximately 8% of adolescents (Apter et al, 1996; Valleni-Basile et al, 1996). Many cases go undetected and untreated until adulthood. Diagnostic criteria are the same as in adults: the clinical phenomena are remarkably similar at all ages, although rituals are more common in children than obsessions. Frequency, severity, chronicity, bizarre characteristics, and interference with daily life distinguish obsessions and compulsions from typical childhood worries, rituals, and superstitious habits. Recently, several case studies have reported the occurrence of OCD in children who have had a group A beta-hemolytic streptococci infection; investigators hypothesize that an autoimmune response was involved in the development of the OCD symptoms (Allen et al, 1995). As in adults, clomipramine, fluoxetine, and fluvoxamine may reduce the force of obsessions and compulsions sufficiently to improve quality of life. Those with childhood onset often have a weaker response to medication (Ackerman et al, 1994). Supplemental behavior modification and/or psychotherapy are often necessary. Cognitive–behavioral programs (March et al, 1994), often in conjunction with medication, have been reported to be effective for children and adolescents with OCD. Treatment usually is necessary for years, with a high likelihood of relapse with discontinuation of medication.

Panic Disorder

The existence of panic disorder in youth has been controversial, but recent data document its presence in children and adolescents who have a parent with panic disorder and/or depression and thus suggests genetic or behavioral modeling etiologic contributions. There are few studies of the treatment of panic in children and adolescents, but preliminary evidence suggests that alprazolam, imipramine, or clonazepam may be useful (Kutcher et al, 1992; Reiter et al, 1992). Supportive individual and family psychotherapy with an educational focus and the encouragement of exposure to feared situations may be helpful (see also Chapter 8).

Posttraumatic Stress Disorder

Using the same criteria as in adults, children and adolescents can be diagnosed with this disorder. This approach can be problematic, given the developmental variation in symptoms. In the DSM-IV, the diagnosis of Acute Stress Disorder was added and may be used when an individual has been symptomatic for less than a month.

Description
Posttraumatic stress disorder (PTSD) is characterized by the development of specific, long-lasting emotional and behavioral symptoms, precipitated

by a shocking, unexpected event that is outside the range of usual human experience. During the event, the individual felt intensely fearful and helpless (see Chapter 8). Trauma may be chronic rather than acute, as in repeated sexual or physical abuse, when the stress is exacerbated by dread of the next episode. Symptoms include reexperiencing the traumatic event, avoidance of reminders of the event, and increased arousal. The precipitant may be experienced directly, by observation (as it occurs to another person), or vicariously after learning about a traumatic event or a severe threat to a close friend or relative.

The clinical phenomena of PTSD seen in children differ in some ways from those seen in adults (Terr, 1983 and 1987a). Immediate effects include fear of separation from parent(s), fear of death, and fear of further fear. Children withdraw from new experiences. Perceptual distortions occur most commonly in time sense and in vision, but auditory, touch, and olfactory misperceptions have been described. Many details of the experience are accurately remembered, but sequencing and/or duration of events is often altered.

In children, reexperiencing the event is likely to occur in the form of nightmares, daydreams, and/or repetitive and potentially dangerous reenactment in symbolic play or in actual behavior. Despite obvious similarities between the reenactments and the original event, most children are unaware of the connection. Even children younger than age 3 demonstrate through play and/or dreams memories of traumatic events that they cannot describe verbally.

A variety of fears of repetition of the experience and of other situations develop that may involve separation or danger or remind them of the event. Children may experience somatic symptoms, such as headaches and stomachaches. Later, many traumatized children develop a sense of pessimism and hopelessness about the future. As long as 4 to 5 years after the event, children remain deeply ashamed of their helplessness in the face of danger. Children with PTSD most often demonstrate increased arousal by sleep disturbances that may add to functional impairment in other areas (Pynoos et al, 1987). Children commonly regress (show behaviors characteristic of a previous developmental stage).

Associated symptoms may include anxiety and/or depression. Impulsivity, difficulty concentrating, and decreased motivation may interfere with school performance. Guilt due to surviving and/or to perceived or actual deficiencies in attempts to save others is common. The normal cognitive egocentricity and magical thinking of children may contribute to a false belief that their thought or action somehow caused the traumatic event.

Etiology

Children with preexisting stressors, anxiety, or depression, or children who have experienced a previous loss, are at risk for more severe and prolonged symptoms. A sufficiently severe stressor, however, may produce the disorder without any predisposition. The degree of exposure to a life-threatening situation is directly related to severity of PTSD (Pynoos et al, 1987). The changes in living circumstance caused by disasters, such as the loss of the family home, isolation from usual social supports, and even the death of parents or other family members, can exacerbate PTSD (Lyons, 1987). Symptoms may be partially ameliorated by a stable, cohesive, supportive family.

Evaluation

PTSD should be suspected in any child or adolescent who has had a significant change in behavior. A clinical interview technique for child and adolescent victims begins with the use of play and fantasy, using a projective drawing and storytelling task. The interviewer then structures a detailed recounting of the traumatic event, including affective responses and fantasies of revenge. The concluding stage includes a review of the child's current life concerns, a reassessment of the traumatic experience, anticipatory guidance regarding reactions that the child may experience, and efforts to support the child's self-esteem (Pynoos and Eth, 1986).

Treatment

Individual insight-oriented play and verbal psychotherapy is the most commonly used modality (Terr, 1987b). Time-limited focal psychotherapy may be effective in some cases (Pynoos and Eth, 1986). Group therapy organized in schools or in the community with victims who have been exposed to the same event may be helpful in decreasing distortions and reducing the spread of posttraumatic fears and symptoms. On the other hand, mixed groups of victims who have experienced different events (such as rape or incest) may actually lead to contagion of fears (Terr, 1987b). Supportive therapy for parents and siblings can provide information about the child's symptoms and their cause, as well as deal with vicarious trauma experienced by family members and reduce contagion.

The use of psychopharmacological agents for PTSD in children and adolescents has not been assessed systematically. Anecdotal reports suggest that propranolol may be effective in the treatment of agitated, hyperaroused children and adolescents with PTSD (Famularo et al, 1988). Case reports have indicated that carbamazepine (Looff et al, 1995) or guanfacine (Horrigan and Barnhill, 1995) may be helpful.

ELIMINATION DISORDERS

One of the most common developmental problems seen by primary care physicians is the child who has not attained or who has lost bladder or bowel control. Although these disorders are called "functional" enuresis and encopresis to differentiate them from medically caused incontinence, they have significant physiological components.

Enuresis

Epidemiology

Most children achieve urinary control between 2 and 3 years of age. Virtually all are dry in the daytime by age 4, but nocturnal control may lag behind. On average, boys are slower in achieving continence than girls. Among 5 year olds, 14% of boys and girls wet at least once a month. Approximately 10% of first graders are still nocturnally enuretic. By age 14, 1% of boys and 0.5% of girls remain enuretic (almost exclusively nocturnal). The spontaneous remission rate is high (Table 16–11).

Description

Enuresis is defined as a pattern of involuntary or intentional voiding of urine into bed or clothes after age 5 years. The diagnostic criteria require a frequency of at least twice a week for at least 3 consecutive months or marked impairment or distress (American Psychiatric Association, 1994). *Diurnal* is used to describe wetting in the daytime and *nocturnal* for wetting only during sleep, by far the more common form. Enuresis may unfortunately result in family conflict and punitive treatment or shaming of the child, teasing by peers, restriction of social activities due to peer rejection and fear of embarassment, and low self-esteem.

Table 16–11 **Enuresis**

Characteristics

Common in school-aged children
Runs in families
Some associated psychological symptoms often related to environmental responses

Diagnosis

Pattern of involuntary/intentional voiding of urine after age 5 years
At least twice a week for 3 months or marked impairment
Primary (no period of continence) or secondary (after period of continence)

Epidemiology

Approximately 10% of 1st graders have nocturnal enuresis
More common in boys
High spontaneous remission rate
Strong genetic component

Treatment

Behavior modification
Medication: TCAs, DDAVP*
Psychotherapy for associated psychological symptoms

* TCA, tricyclic antidepressant; DDAVP, desmopressin.

Differential Diagnosis

Transient loss of urinary control is common in young children when physically or psychologically stressed. Some children are careless in wiping or leave the toilet before urination is complete. The appearance of enuresis, is the result. Specific medical causes of urinary incontinence include:

Urethritis secondary to use of bubble bath
Urinary tract infections
Diabetes mellitus
Diabetes insipidus
Sickle cell anemia
Seizure disorders
Neurogenic bladder (e.g., secondary to spina bifida)
Genitourinary tract malfunction, malformation, or obstruction
Pelvic masses

Etiology

Enuresis has a strong genetic component. Seventy-five percent of enuretic youths have a first-degree relative with a history of enuresis. Nocturnal enuresis in younger children is largely a consequence of delayed maturation of bladder control mechanisms. General neuromaturational delay, small bladder capacity, and lack of systematic toilet training may contribute to enuresis. Constipation also has been implicated as a causative factor (O'Regan et al, 1986). Common physiological causes of diurnal enuresis in girls are vaginal reflux of urine, bladder spasm when frightened or laughing, and urgency incontinence.

Enuresis is occasionally related to other psychiatric disorders. In young children, it may be a symptom of an *adjustment disorder* or a regressive response to a stressor (i.e., hospitalization, moves). *Anxious* children may experience urinary frequency, which leads to incontinence if toilet facilities are not immediately available. Children with *ODD* may refuse to use the toilet as part of their battle for control. Many children with *ADHD* wait until the last minute to use the bathroom and may lose control on the way. Avoidance of dirty, dangerous, or insufficiently private toilet facilities in school may also lead to incontinence. Recent research does *not* show a relationship between enuresis and specific sleep stages for children with or without other psychiatric diagnoses.

Evaluation

The history includes details of wetting, including time of occurrence, amount, frequency, precipitants, details of toilet training, family history of enuresis, and family's and individual's reactions. A careful medical history, physical including neurological examination, and urinalysis are indicated in all cases. Urine cultures should be obtained in girls. Radiological studies or instrumentation of the genitourinary tract are not indicated unless there are specific indications of abnormality on the history or physical exam.

Treatment

Once medical causes have been eliminated, the main focus of treatment is to help the child and family manage this problem constructively.

Environmental Interventions. Nocturnal enuresis in children younger than 7 years old should be treated with patience while waiting for the child to mature. Secondary symptoms should be minimized by encouraging the parents not to punish or ridicule the child. To deal with this problem, the child and family should develop a routine that can be incorporated into their daily activities. Older children can be taught to change their own beds to reduce negative reactions from parents. Measures such as restricting fluids and waking the child during the night to urinate are not notably successful. Exercises to increase bladder capacity may reduce nocturnal enuresis, and start-and-stop exercises may strengthen the bladder sphincter muscles and improve control.

Behavior Modification. If treatment of uncomplicated enuresis is necessary, behavioral methods are the first choice, although parent and child motivation and participation are required. The first step is a simple monitoring and reward procedure using a chart with stars (for dry days or nights) to be exchanged for rewards. For children and adolescents who do not respond to simple interventions, more elaborate behavioral programs or a urine alarm device (available for about $50) may be used.

Children who are secondarily enuretic (having previously been dry) and those who have accompanying psychiatric problems are more difficult to treat. Referral to a child and adolescent psychiatrist for specialized evaluation and treatment may be necessary.

Psychotherapy. Individual or family psychotherapy may be indicated to deal with secondary effects of the enuresis or with coexisting psychiatric disorders that may be exacerbating the problem.

Psychopharmacological Treatment. Medication has been found to be effective, but it is not curative. It usually reduces symptoms rather than eliminates them; relapse often occurs once the medication is discontinued. Prior to starting medication, baseline frequency of wet and dry days or nights is recorded. Daily charting is then used to monitor the child's progress. If medication is used chronically, the child or adolescent should have a drug-free trial at least every 6 months to see if medication is still required.

Low doses of the tricyclic antidepressants (TCAs) imipramine, amitriptyline, desipramine, and nortriptyline are partially effective in the treatment of nocturnal enuresis. The mechanism remains unclear, but they do not seem to work by altering sleep architecture, treating depression, or increasing peripheral anticholinergic activity. Wetting usually returns when the drug is discontinued. Tolerance to the medication may develop and necessitate a dose increase. In some children, tricyclics lose their effect entirely. Parents must take special precautions to avoid overdoses by the patient or siblings. Imipramine may be useful on a short-term basis or for special occasions (such as camp).

Desmopressin (DDAVP), an analog of antidiuretic hormone, can be administered as a nasal spray to treat nocturnal enuresis. Onset of action is within several days. Few patients become completely dry, however, and relapse occurs when the medication is stopped (Klauber, 1989). In patients with normal electrolyte regulation, side effects are minimal (headache and rare nasal mucosa dryness or irritation). Because excessive water intake can result in hyponatremic seizures, fluids should be limited during the evening and night (Beach et al, 1992). A major drawback of DDAVP is its expense.

Encopresis

Epidemiology

Bowel control is usually achieved between 30 months and 4 years of age. The prevalence of encopresis is approximately 1.5% after age 5 and decreases with age. In late adolescence, it is almost nonexistent in the absence of severe mental retardation, psychosis, or conduct disorder. Boys outnumber girls six to one. Encopresis is slightly more common in poor children. Encopresis is less often an isolated symptom than enuresis is. Twenty-five percent of encopretics seen in psychiatric settings are also enuretic.

Description

This disorder is characterized by repeated involuntary (or, rarely, voluntary) passage of feces into clothing or other places other than the toilet (such as the floor or closets) at least once a month for at least 3 months after the age of 4 years (American Psychiatric Association, 1994). Encopresis rarely occurs during sleep. The older the child, the more resistant to treatment and the more negative the prognosis. Rejection by peers, school, and family increases with age. Families of affected individuals often have significant difficulties providing adequate supervision and structure.

Differential Diagnosis

Transient loss of continence may follow a stressor such as hospitalization or parental divorce. Medical causes of fecal incontinence include:

Metabolic factors
    Hypothyroidism
    Hypercalcemia
Dietary factors
    Lactase deficiency
    Overeating of fatty foods
Lower gastrointestinal tract
    Congenital aganglionic megacolon (Hirschsprung's disease)

Anal fissure
Rectal stenosis
Inflammatory bowel disease
Neurological factors, e.g., myelodysplasia

Etiology

Children with functional encopresis may be divided into three groups according to etiology. In all cases, predisposing subtle abnormalities in colon motility and sphincter function are likely. Familial factors are suggested by the 15% rate of childhood encopresis in fathers of encopretic children. The first group includes children who have never been systematically toilet trained, who are retarded, or who have neuromaturational delays. The second group is characterized by chronic severe constipation. This may be involuntary (due to dietary factors or pain on defecation caused by a skin rash or an anal fissure) or a result of a lack of opportunity to use the toilet. Voluntary stool withholding may result from punitive toilet training, improper management of common toilet-related fears, or environmental interference with normal toilet habits (unsafe or dirty bathrooms or lack of privacy). As a result of the constipation, the child develops impaired colon motility and contraction patterns, stretching and thinning of the walls of the colon (functional megacolon), and decreased sensation or perception of the urge to defecate or of actual passage of stool. Impaction results, with leakage of loose stool around the obstruction (overflow incontinence). The child becomes habituated to the smell and often does not know when he or she has soiled (a fact difficult for adults to believe). In the third group, encopresis is secondary to a psychiatric disorder such as ODD, ADHD, conduct disorder, psychosis, phobia, or adjustment disorder.

Evaluation

A complete medical history, a physical examination, and routine laboratory tests are indicated. A detailed history is needed to distinguish between passage of full bowel movements (likely to be volitional), overflow of loose stool around an impaction, or staining of underwear due to careless wiping after toileting. A history of toilet training and bathroom environments is needed. An X-ray of the abdomen or a barium enema may be required to assess fecal impaction. Urinalysis will detect an associated urinary tract infection (common in encopretic girls).

Treatment

Children and adolescents with this disorder generally require a comprehensive treatment plan that encompasses several approaches.

Psychotherapy. Traditional individual psychotherapy may be used in addition to other treatments. Children with encopresis are often angry and may benefit from improving their ability to express their emotions verbally.

Psychotherapy may also be useful in improving self-esteem. Behavioral treatments and bowel retraining programs are essential in most cases. Parents should be helped to avoid hostile or punitive responses to the child's incontinence and should be cautioned that relapses may occur.

Role of the Primary Care Physician

Medical treatment is essential for children with chronic constipation and resulting functional megacolon. Children and parents are educated in the physiology and anatomy of the lower bowel. Enemas and suppositories are used to evacuate the bowel. A bowel "retraining" program follows, using orally administered mineral oil, a high roughage diet, development of a regular toileting routine, and a mild suppository (such as Dulcolax), if necessary. Routine administration of enemas by parents is contraindicated as that alone does not improve bowel function and is toxic to the parent–child relationship.

Because children with encopresis more commonly have associated psychiatric disorders than those with enuresis, psychiatric consultation is indicated for most encopretic children older than 6 years of age.

MOOD DISORDERS

Mood disorders in children and adolescents are potentially serious, long-lasting, and recurrent (Kovacs et al, 1984a, b) (Table 16–12). This section will focus on age-related differences from mood disorders in adults (covered in Chapter 7).

Epidemiology

The incidence of mood disorders has increased in children and adolescents (Ryan et al, 1992) as the age of onset of both unipolar depression and bipolar disorder have declined, with the recognition that these disorders can occur at young ages. The prevalence of major depression has been estimated at 2% in prepubertal children and 5% in adolescents. Dysthymic disorder without coexisting major depression is found in 3.3% of adolescents (Kashani et al, 1987). Prior to puberty, depression is more common in boys than girls, with a change to the adult sex ratios (females greater than males) in adolescence. Mania is rare prior to puberty and often presents a confusing diagnostic picture. In late adolescence, the incidence approaches 20% of the adult rate.

Description

Diagnostic criteria are essentially the same for children as for adults, except that mood can be irritable instead of depressed, and failure to make expected weight gain can be seen instead of weight loss. The behaviors may manifest in different ways, appropriate for developmental level. Reduction in school performance and activities with friends or complaints of boredom or

Table 16–12 **Mood Disorders**

Characteristics

Same symptoms as adults except
  Irritability may be more pronounced than sadness
  Mania, especially in younger children, may appear similar to ADHD*
Potentially serious, long-lasting, recurrent
Increasing incidence with increased recognition and decreased age of onset

Diagnosis

Frequent somatic complaints
Fewer neurovegetative signs of depression compared with adults
Lack of cyclical vegetative symptoms in manic children

Epidemiology

Estimated prevalence of major depression of 2% in prepubertal children and 5% in
  adolescents
Incidence of adolescent mania approaches 20% of adult rate
After puberty, more common in girls

Treatment

Psychotherapy
Medication: SSRIs, TCAs, lithium, anticonvulsants[†]
Education of family and school

[*] ADHD, attention deficit–hyperactivity disorder.
[†] SSRI, selective serotonin-reuptake inhibitor; TCA, tricyclic antidepressant.

aches and pains may be key indicators of depression in young people. Young depressed patients are less likely than adults to show anhedonia, diurnal variation, psychomotor retardation, delusions (Carlson and Kashani, 1988), insomnia, or the classic vegetative signs of depression (Kutcher and Marton, 1989).

Among adolescents with major depression, subsequent bipolarity is predicted by precipitous onset of symptoms, psychomotor retardation, psychotic features, pharmacologically precipitated hypomania, and a family history of bipolar disorder (Strober and Carlson, 1982). Children with bipolar disorder can be difficult to identify (Weller et al, 1995).

Differential Diagnosis

Adolescent mania is frequently misdiagnosed as *schizophrenia* because of the psychotic manifestations and regression common to both. Because of the lack of cyclical vegetative symptoms in prepubertal children, mania often resembles *ADHD.* Belligerence, poor judgment, and impaired impulse control in mania (stealing, sexual activity) may be confused with *conduct disorder.* Secondary mania may result from prescribed (steroids, carbamazepine, tricyclic antidepressants) or abused (cocaine, amphetamines) *drugs, metabolic abnormalities, neoplasm* or *epilepsy.*

Children younger than 4 years of age may develop a clinical picture similar to major depression when separated from their parents. Children suffering from *reactive attachment disorder* secondary to parental abuse or neglect who present with lethargy, apathy, and withdrawal may appear depressed. In a subgroup of children with *conduct disorder,* a major depression precedes the development of the conduct problems (Marriage et al, 1986; Puig-Antich, 1982).

Evaluation

Since both depressive and manic symptoms can be caused and/or influenced by organic abnormalities, in addition to a thorough psychiatric evaluation, children and adolescents with mood symptoms should have an adequate medical evaluation. Vital signs, physical examination, and baseline laboratory tests (complete blood count [CBC] with differential, electrolytes, thyroid function tests, blood urea nitrogen [BUN], and creatinine) should be done. Depending on the symptoms, history, and findings, additional tests may be appropriate, such as EEG or neuroimaging.

Children can be asked direct questions related to their behavior, mood, and feelings, although the wording must be adjusted for their level of cognitive and emotional development. Young children have more difficulty recognizing and verbalizing their feelings and may use idiosyncratic words such as "bored" to describe dysphoria or anhedonia. "Cranky" may be more understandable to a child than "irritable." Although some children report their mood states more accurately than their parents can, observation of depressed affect by a trained clinician is often essential. Manic behavior may be described as overactive, "hyper," or "impossible to manage." Longitudinal course and family history are important.

It is crucial to assess the degree of suicidality. Children can be questioned regarding ideation, plans, and attempts. This questioning will *not* increase the likelihood of self-destructive behavior. If a child or adolescent is seen following a suicide attempt, a detailed evaluation should be made of the circumstances preceding and following the attempt, history of substance abuse or impulsive behavior, wishes to die or to influence others at the time of the attempt and at the time of evaluation, whether a friend or family member has committed suicide, and coping skills and supports in the patient and family. A careful search should be made for frequent comorbid conditions, such as anxiety disorders, ADHD, conduct disorders, and alcohol or drug abuse.

Treatment

Treatment approaches should be comprehensive, with attention focused on the family and school, as well as the child and adolescent. Education of school personnel and other involved individuals is essential.

Psychotherapy. Individual and family psychotherapy are cornerstones of the management of depression in childhood and adolescence; various types of therapy (psychodynamic, supportive, cognitive–behavioral) have been noted to be helpful. Even after successful treatment with medication, impaired interpersonal relations with peers and family members may require individual, group, or family therapy to address developmental deficits or the sequelae of the depression (Puig-Antich et al, 1985). Cognitive therapy techniques developed for the treatment of depression in adults, such as interpersonal therapy, are being adapted for use with children and adolescents (Emery et al, 1983; Mufson et al, 1993).

Behavior Modification. Behavior therapy techniques, such as social skills training or contingency management to reduce withdrawal and maintain activity, may be useful adjunctive treatments.

Psychopharmacological Treatment. The evidence for efficacy is less than in adults, and drugs should be used in conjunction with other treatments. For nonpsychotic depression, psychotherapy should be the first step, with medication added if there is no improvement in 4 to 6 weeks. Published algorithms based on clinical experience and extrapolation from adults exist for depression, but there is no consensus among the experts (Ambrosini et al, 1995; Johnston and Frehling, 1994). Selection usually is based on target symptoms, comorbidity, risk of impulsive behavior, family history (disorder and drug response), and side effect profile. There are few empirical data to guide therapeutic choices. A similar state exists for information on appropriate medication management for bipolar disorder in children and adolescents. Generally, clinicians base their therapies on current adult psychopharmacological treatment.

TCAs may be useful in the treatment of children and adolescents with major depression. These drugs have been the most studied antidepressants in children and adolescents. In open trials, 75% of patients treated with TCAs have responded positively. Only one double-blind study demonstrated an advantage of imipramine over placebo, however (Preskorn et al, 1987). In adolescents, there are no double-blind investigations that show the benefit of TCAs over placebo.

Tricyclic pharmacokinetics differ before and after puberty, with children having a faster metabolism and thus a shorter drug half-life. As a result, prepubertal children generally need a higher milligram per kilogram dose than adults and are prone to rapid, dramatic swings in blood levels from toxic to ineffective. Medication should be divided into three daily doses to produce more stable levels (Ryan, 1992). There are wide variations in plasma levels at a given fixed dose. Tricyclics may be given once or twice daily in adolescents.

TCAs have a quinidinelike effect and may slow cardiac conduction time and repolarization. Children and adolescents may develop mildly increased pulse and blood pressure, as well as small, statistically significant, but usually clinically benign, ECG changes (intraventricular conduction defects—first degree heart block, QRS complex widening) especially at doses equivalent to greater than 3 mg/kg/day of imipramine or desipramine (Bartels et al, 1991; Biederman et al, 1993; Leonard et al, 1995). Prolongation of the QTc interval may be a sensitive indicator of cardiac effect (Wilens et al, 1996). Approximately 5% of the population has a genetic defect in TCA metabolism, causing "slow hydroxylation" and increased risk of toxicity (Table 16–13).

There have been five reported deaths of youth (three prepubertal, two early adolescents) on desipramine as of 1995 (Popper and Zimnitzky, 1995; Riddle et al, 1993). A causal relationship between these deaths and the medication has not been established. The data suggest that desipramine treatment in the usual doses is associated with only a slightly added risk of dying suddenly beyond the natural hazard (Biederman et al, 1991 and 1995); however, desipramine may present a greater risk than the other TCAs. Due to these issues, clinicians often choose an SSRI as a first-line drug for depression; frequently, among the TCAs, nortriptyline or imipramine are utilized preferentially.

Prior to the start of TCA treatment, a thorough history and physical examination should occur, including vital signs. Particular attention should be paid to potential cardiac symptoms or signs in either the patient or family (Liberthson, 1996). An ECG should be done as well as baseline laboratory tests (CBC with differential, BUN, creatinine clearance, and thyroid function tests). Further tests, such as an EEG, maybe indicated in the presence of head trauma or seizures since TCAs lower the seizure threshold. Vital signs and the ECG should be periodically monitored during treatment and after any increases in dose (see Table 16–13 for titration parameters). Some recommend following plasma levels to ensure compliance and avoid toxicity. Parents must be reminded to supervise administration of medication closely and to keep pills in a safe place to prevent intentional overdose or accidental poisoning not only by the patient, but by other family members, especially young children.

Table 16–13 **Guidelines for TCA Use in Children and Adolescents**

	ONCE THESE PARAMETERS ARE REACHED, THE DOSE OF TCA SHOULD BE REDUCED OR DISCONTINUED:	
	Children	**Adolescents**
Electrocardiograph		
PR (sec)	0.2	0.2
QRS (sec)	0.12 130% of baseline	0.12
QTc (sec)	0.48	0.48
Vital signs		
Resting heart rate (bpm)	110–130	110–120
Chronic blood pressure (mmHg)	120/80	140/90

(From Wilens TE, Biederman J, Baldessarini R et al: Cardiovascular effects of therapeutic doses of tricyclic antidepressants in children and adolescents. J Am Acad Child Adolesc Psychiatry 35:1491–1501, 1996)

The starting dose of imipramine, amitriptyline, and desipramine is 1.5 mg/kg/day, which may be increased every 4 days by 1 mg/kg/day to a maximum dose of 5 mg/kg/day. Plasma levels may be helpful in patients who fail to respond to usual doses (possibly low levels) or those who have severe side effects at usual doses (possibly very high levels) (Geller et al, 1986). Anticholinergic side effects are similar to those in adults (Herskowitz, 1987), but less common. Behavioral toxicity that may be mistaken for a worsening of the original depression is manifested by irritability, psychotic symptoms, agitation, anger, aggression, nightmares, forgetfulness or confusion. Depressed children who are withdrawn and nonverbal may show a transient apparent worsening of sadness, crying, irritability, and aggression as their depression responds to medication. Side effects may be managed by decreasing the dose, changing to another medication (another TCA or different type of drug), addition of other drugs (i.e., laxative for constipation), and/or developing coping strategies to manage the dry mouth or orthostatic hypotension.

Sudden withdrawal of moderate or higher doses results in a flulike gastrointestinal syndrome with nausea, cramps, vomiting, headaches, and muscle pains. Other manifestations of tricyclic withdrawal may include social withdrawal, hyperactivity, depression, agitation, and insomnia (Ryan, 1990). Tricyclics should therefore be tapered over a 2- to 3-week period, rather than being abruptly discontinued. The short half-life of tricyclics in prepubertal children may produce daily withdrawal symptoms if medication is given only once a day or if a dose is missed (Ryan, 1992).

SSRIs have been increasingly utilized to treat depression and other disorders in children and adolescents, due to their demonstrated effectiveness in adults and more benign side effect profile—absence of cardiac side effects and relative safety in overdose (DeVane and Sallee, 1996). There is no information on their long-term effects on growing children. Fluoxetine has exhibited efficacy for both children and adolescents in open trials, as well as one double-blind placebo-controlled trial (Emslie et al, 1995). Children have relatively few somatic side effects (anorexia, weight loss, headaches, nausea, tremor, vomiting), but behavioral toxicity is more common with restlessness, insomnia, social disinhibition, agitation, and mania (Riddle et al, 1990/1991; Venkataraman et al, 1992). Other symptoms such as suicidal ideation, self-destructive behavior, aggression, and psychosis have been reported, but many of these children had preexisting risk factors for the development of these problems (King et al, 1991; Leonard et al, 1997; Riddle et al, 1995; Schuster et al, 1986). Fluoxetine may interfere with sleep architecture and thereby produce daytime sleepiness. Sertraline also reduced depressive symptoms in adolescents in an open trial (McConville et al, 1996)

Lithium carbonate may be considered in the treatment of children and adolescents with bipolar disorder, whether mixed or manic. It is the medication most commonly used to stabilize mood in children; manic children and adolescents demonstrate improvement on lithium, but rarely show the very positive response that can be seen in adults. Lithium should not be prescribed unless the family is willing and able to comply with regular multiple daily doses and with lithium levels. The medical workup is the same as in adults. Growth and thyroid and kidney function (serum creatinine and morning urine specific gravity) should be monitored every 3 to 6 months.

Therapeutic lithium blood levels are the same as for adults, 0.6 to 1.2 mEq/lt, which can usually be attained with 900 to 1,200 mg/day, in divided doses, although daily doses of up to 2,000 mg may be required (Campbell et al, 1985).

Since lithium excretion occurs primarily through the kidney and most children have more efficient renal function than adults, they may require higher doses for body weight than adults (Ryan, 1992; Weller et al, 1986). Lithium should be taken with food to minimize gastrointestinal distress. Children are at risk for the same side effects as adults, but may experience them at lower serum levels (Campbell et al, 1991). In growing children, the consequences of hypothyroidism are potentially more severe than in adults. *Because of its teratogenic potential, lithium is contraindicated in sexually active girls.* Lithium's tendency to aggravate acne may also be of particular clinical significance in adolescents.

Adequate salt and fluid intake is necessary to prevent lithium levels from rising into the toxic range. The family should be instructed in the importance of preventing dehydration from heat or exercise and in the need to stop the lithium and contact the physician if the child or adolescent develops an illness with fever, vomiting, diarrhea, and/or decreased fluid intake. Erratic consumption of large amounts of salty snack foods may cause fluctuations in lithium levels (Herskowitz, 1987).

Lithium also has been utilized to augment TCA treatment of depression; reports from open trials and case reports have been positive (Ryan et al, 1988a; Strober et al, 1992; Dulcan et al, 1997).

Carbamazepine may be useful in the treatment of mania that is resistant to lithium and neuroleptics or rapidly cycling (see Chapter 18). There are no systematic studies; however, anecdotal reports suggest that it can be useful.

Valproic acid, or valproate, increasingly has been employed to treat bipolar children and adolescents based on anecdotal clinical experience (West et al, 1994) and extrapolation from the treatment of adults.

Monoamine oxidase inhibitors rarely have been used to treat children and adolescents, due to concern about poor compliance with the dietary restrictions producing potentially severe side effects. Evidence exists that these drugs can be useful in carefully selected treatment-resistant depressed children and adolescents without significant problems with the diet (Ryan et al, 1988b).

Other medications have been used to treat mood disorders in children and adolescents. *Bupropion* demonstrated promising results in an open trial of adolescents with major depression (Arredondo et al, 1993).

SCHIZOPHRENIA

Schizophrenia in adults is covered in Chapter 5. The presentation of schizophrenia in adolescence is similar to that in adulthood, but clinical features in children are somewhat different. It is important to remember that there are other types of psychoses and that children and adolescents can have isolated psychotic symptoms (particularly in association with trauma) without having a psychotic disorder.

Epidemiology
Childhood schizophrenia has been estimated to be present at a rate of 0.5/1,000. The prevalence increases after puberty and approaches adult levels in late adolescence (Table 16–14).

Description
Diagnostic criteria are the same as for adults, with the exception that failure to reach expected levels of adaptive functioning may be seen instead of regression. Schizophrenic children are characterized by markedly uneven development and the insidious onset of symptoms. Language and social behavior are usually delayed and are qualitatively different from normal children at any developmental stage. Visual hallucinations are more common in children than in adults.

Table 16–14 **Childhood Schizophrenia**

Characteristics
Negative symptoms can be more prominent than positive
Uneven development
Insidious onset of symptoms

Diagnosis
Same criteria as adult except
    May have failure to reach developmental levels rather than
        regression
Usually associated with significant language and social delays

Epidemiology
Rate of 0.5/1000 in children
Approaches adult levels after puberty
All psychotic symptoms that occur in children are not schizophrenia

Treatment
Medication: neuroleptics
Increased structure and supervision
Educational placement
Education and support of family and school

Differential Diagnosis

Acute hallucinations are not uncommon in children and can result from *acute phobic reactions, physical illness* with fever or metabolic aberration, or *medications/drugs.* Some schizophrenic children younger than age 6 years have symptoms characteristic of *autistic disorder* prior to the development of the core symptoms of schizophrenia (delusions, hallucinations, formal thought disorder) (McKenna, 1994; Watkins et al, 1988).

Evaluation

During their initial episode of psychosis, all children and adolescents should receive a comprehensive medical assessment that includes a medical history, physical examination, vital signs, baseline laboratory tests (CBC with differential, electrolytes, BUN, creatinine, thyroid function tests, and rheumatological, toxic, and infection screens). The affected individual also should have an EEG and computed tomogram or magnetic resonance image of the brain. In addition, information should be obtained on the psychiatric symptoms (onset, course, content) of the child or adolescent, as well as any in the family. A full mental status exam should be done, if possible; often, it is helpful to have children and adolescents describe TV shows or movies as a way of determining their ability to organize and synthesize information. The child's level of function at both school and home should be ascertained. Often, these children present with predominant negative symptoms and the diagnosis can be difficult to make.

Treatment

These children and adolescents require intensive and comprehensive treatment that addresses their psychiatric problems, need for structure and supervision, developmental and educational deficits, difficulties with relationships, and the considerable demands on their caretakers.

Psychotherapy. Individual psychotherapy may be useful as a part of a comprehensive treatment plan for schizophrenic children (Cantor and Kestenbaum, 1986). Family psychoeducational treatment (Anderson et al, 1980) may also prove beneficial. Token economies may be useful in shaping adaptive behavior and reducing inappropriate behaviors.

Psychopharmacological Treatment. Neuroleptics (also called major tranquilizers) can ameliorate psychotic symptoms, but are less effective in adolescents than in adults and least effective in children. Even with a positive response, children often continue to have significant symptoms and impairment. Neuroleptics should be used only as part of a comprehensive treatment program. Target symptoms that may respond include overactivity, aggression, agitation, stereotyped movements, delusions, and hallucinations. In general, higher potency agents, such as haloperidol, are considered first due to the potential of a greater degree of problematic side effects (sedation, cognitive dulling, memory deficits) with the low potency compounds, such as chlorpromazine; however, the higher risks of dyskinesia and extrapyramidal symptoms with the high-potency drugs, especially with long-term use, are of concern. The development of new antipsychotic medications with potentially lesser side effects has been exciting. Clozapine in a double-blind trial was found to be superior to haloperidol for both positive and negative symptoms for children and adolescents with early-onset schizophrenia (Kumra et al, 1996). Risperidone increasingly has been used to treat these children and adolescents, with small case series reports indicating positive responses (Quintana and Keshavan, 1995; Simeon et al, 1995), although children appear to be more sensitive than adults to developing extrapyramidal symptoms (Mandoki, 1995).

The dose range for haloperidol in children is 0.5 to 16 mg/day (0.02 to 0.2 mg/kg/day; Campbell et al, 1985). Medication should be started at a low dose and gradually increased. Common doses are 0.25 to 6 mg of haloperidol or 10 to 200 mg of chlorpromazine a day, with older adolescents possibly requiring more. An initial trial of about 4 weeks is needed to assess efficacy, and a full response may take months. Laboratory studies should be monitored at regular intervals. Neutropenia and seizures at a higher rate than in adults may limit the usefulness of clozapine. A drug-free trial after 4 to 6 months of stability may be useful in assessing the continued need for medication.

Acute extrapyramidal side effects occur as in adults and may be treated with oral or intramuscular diphenhydramine (25 to 50 mg), depending on age. Chronic extrapyramidal side effects in adolescents can be treated with diphenhydramine or the anticholinergic drug benztropine—1 to 2 mg/day—in divided doses. Adolescent boys seem to be more vulnerable to acute dystonic reactions than adult patients, so prophylactic antiparkinsonian medication may be indicated. In children, reduction of neuroleptic dose is preferable to the use of antiparkinsonian agents (Campbell et al, 1985). Clonazepam (0.5 mg/day) may alleviate neuroleptic-induced akathisia (Kutcher et al, 1987) in adolescents.

Tardive or withdrawal dyskinesias—some transient, but others irreversible—are seen in 8 to 51% of neuroleptic-treated children and adolescents (Campbell et al, 1985) and are one of the major reasons why these drugs should not be used casually. Tardive dyskinesia (TD) has been documented in children and adolescents after as brief a period of treatment as 5 months (Herskowitz, 1987). Chronic neuroleptic treatment during development may have a higher risk of TD than treatment that begins in adulthood. A careful examination for abnormal movements using a scale such as the Abnormal Involuntary Movements Scale should be conducted before placing the patient on a neuroleptic and periodically reused thereafter. Parents and patients (as they are able) should receive regular explanations of the risk of movement disorders.

Potentially fatal neuroleptic malignant syndrome (NMS) has been reported in children and adolescents, with a presentation similar to that seen in adults (Latz and McCracken, 1992). Adolescents may present with serious medical complications or have NMS without fever (Hynes and Vickar, 1996; Peterson et al, 1995). The most common side effects of the neuroleptics are sedation, weight gain, and hypersalivation. Weight gain may be problematic with the long-term use of the low-potency neuroleptic risperidone. Abnormal laboratory findings are less often reported in children than in adults, but the clinician should be alert to the possibility of blood dyscrasias and hepatic dysfunction. If an acute febrile illness occurs, medication should be withheld and a CBC (with differential) and liver enzyme tests performed (Campbell et al, 1985). Abdominal pain may occur, especially early in treatment. Enuresis has been reported (Realmuto et al, 1984). Photosensitivity due to chlorpromazine may be a problem when youngsters play outside.

Of particular concern is behavioral toxicity, manifested as the worsening of preexisting symptoms or development of new symptoms such as hyper- or hypoactivity, irritability, apathy, withdrawal, stereotypies, tics, or hallucinations (Campbell et al, 1985). The so-called low-potency antipsychotic drugs such as chlorpromazine and thioridazine can produce cognitive dulling and sedation, interfering with the ability to benefit from school (Campbell et al, 1985) and are probably best avoided. Children and adolescents are more sensitive to sedation than are adults (Realmuto et al, 1984).

Environmental Interventions. The best outcome is obtained with an intensive school-based treatment program that incorporates multiple methods of intervention. Hospitalization or long-term residential treatment may be needed. Families and school systems often require ongoing education about the disorder and its manifestations at different developmental stages. Caretakers can benefit from participation in mental health advocacy and support groups.

EATING DISORDERS

Problematic eating habits and disorders can occur throughout childhood and adolescence, as discussed in Chapter 12. About 25 to 40% of infants and toddlers exhibit feeding problems that require pediatric intervention. Types of problems include mismatch between the feeding styles of the child and caretaker, difficulty adjusting to the child's increased independence and assertion of preferences, and changes in normal growth rate with age and development for children. It is estimated that approximately 25% of nonreferred adolescents have a eating disorder (anorexia nervosa, bulimia, or obesity), with many more having subclinical syndromes. By kindergarten, most children demonstrate aversion to pictures of chubby children. They choose thinness in girls and muscles in boys as measures of popularity. Studies of school-aged children reveal that a significant proportion desire to be thinner and have already attempted to diet. When surveyed, a significant number of adolescent girls wish to weigh less, with only approximately 14% being satisfied with their weight. Many indicate that their ideal body image is smaller and thinner than their current body image. Although adolescent boys show an aversion to being overweight, they are not as concerned as the girls are.

Often, eating behaviors are complicated and difficult to describe, classify, and understand. Several classification systems exist, and disorders vary on whether they are considered primarily psychiatric or medical. The DSM-IV includes three eating disorders of early childhood (pica, feeding disorder of infancy or early childhood, and rumination disorder); failure to thrive (FTT) and obesity are considered medical disorders. Eating disorders of later childhood and adolescent include anorexia nervosa and bulimia nervosa (Table 16–15).

FTT is a disorder characterized by poor weight gain accompanied by problems with social and emotional development in the first 3 years of life. It is associated with increased risk for chronic deficits in growth, cognition, and socioeconomic functioning. Its etiology is multifactorial with both organic and psychosocial components. Both feeding disorder of infancy or early childhood and rumination disorder can be associated with FTT. There is little information about feeding disorder since it is a new diagnostic category in DSM-IV.

Table 16–15 **Eating Disorders**

Characteristics
Inappropriate feeding/eating behaviors and amounts
Abnormal social interactions around eating

Diagnosis
Early childhood: pica, feeding disorder, rumination disorder
Later childhood and adolescence: anorexia nervosa and bulimia nervosa
Both childhood and adolescence: obesity (not psychiatric disorder in DSM-IV)

Epidemiology
Approximately 25–40% of infants and toddlers need pediatric intervention around feeding behavior
Estimated that 25% of adolescents have undiagnosed eating disorder (obesity, anorexia, bulimia)
Only 14% of adolescent girls are satisfied with their weight

Treatment
Identification and treatment of comorbid psychiatric disorders
Behavior management
Psychotherapy for associated relational and/or psychological symptoms
Environmental interventions

Rumination Disorder of Infancy

This potentially fatal disorder is one of the key differential diagnoses in the evaluation of children seen in pediatric services with FTT. It is relatively rare.

Epidemiology

Rumination appears in infants between 3 months and 1 year of age and in persons with moderate or severe mental retardation. In both groups, males predominate five to one (Mayes et al, 1988).

Description

This disorder is characterized by repeated voluntary regurgitation and rechewing of food, without apparent nausea or associated gastrointestinal illness, accompanied by weight loss or failure to make expected weight gain. Some forms of repetitive vomiting may be variants of this symptom. Rumination appears to be an enjoyable source of pleasurable stimulation or a means of tension release. When not ruminating, the child may appear apathetic and withdrawn, irritable and fussy, or quite normal.

Differential Diagnosis

Medical causes of vomiting include gastroesophageal reflux (due to esophageal sphincter dysfunction or hiatal hernia), gastrointestinal infections, congenital malformations (such as pyloric stenosis), or hyperactive gag reflex. Failure to gain weight may result from inadequate feeding, malabsorption syndromes, systemic infection, or inborn errors of metabolism.

Etiology

About one-third of infants with rumination disorder have a history of obstetrical complications; one-fourth have developmental delays attributed to mental retardation or pervasive developmental disorder. Abnormalities in parental caretaking have been implicated, either understimulation with neglect or excessive stimulation out of phase with the infant's needs, accompanied by harsh handling. Cases with no apparent abnormalities in the infant or in the mother–child relationship may represent habit disorders that were encouraged by characteristics of the child's gastrointestinal physiology or triggered by a transient medical illness.

Rumination appears to require several components: impaired regulation by affected individuals of their internal state of satisfaction; a physical propensity to regurgitate food; and learned association that regurgitation helps relieve internal states of dissatisfaction. Assessment of the child needs to address these factors, as well as medical and maternal (caretaker) characteristics.

Evaluation

Pediatric hospitalization is usually required for evaluation, with a search for possible causes and for sequelae such as dehydration, electrolyte imbalance, and malnutrition. Calorie counts and weight should be recorded. A detailed history is taken of physical and emotional development and of feeding. Upper gastrointestinal contrast and esophageal motility studies may be indicated. The mother–child interaction is observed during times of feeding and playing. It is important not to confuse the anxiety, frustration, and disgust the child's constant vomiting and unrewarding weight gain *induce* in the mother with dysfunctional mothering that may have *caused* the disorder. Some infants are so irregular and unpredictable in their rhythms and labile in their responses that the best parent has a difficult time. The child should be evaluated for developmental delay and the parents for possible primary psychiatric disorders and parenting skill deficits.

Treatment

Psychotherapy. Supportive psychotherapy for the parents, with attention to any psychopathology that may have become apparent in the evaluation, is indicated. Parents and child may be seen together to model feeding techniques and ways of interacting with the baby that will be rewarding to both.

Behavior Modification. Treatment programs using social social rewards such as cuddling and playing that are combined with mild appropriate punishments (brief ignoring, scolding) for rumination may be useful. The parents may benefit from developing alternate strategies to manage the child's eating behavior and needs. Caretakers often do best with clear, specific, and reasonable expectations regarding feeding and weight goals.

Environmental Interventions. Pediatric hospitalization may be necessary to restructure the feeding behavior of both parent and child and to reduce parental anxiety. A visiting nurse or homemaker may be arranged to support a mother who is overwhelmed. Developmentally delayed infants may benefit from an organized stimulation program. If parents refuse to cooperate with treatment, or parenting ability is so impaired that the infant is in danger, laws in all states mandate reporting to a child protective services agency.

Role of the Primary Care Physician

The pediatrician is the key player in cases of rumination disorder, conducts the medical evaluation, and works together with social services and the child psychiatrist on psychosocial evaluation and treatment. These families require close and prolonged pediatric care to monitor progress and mobilize additional resources.

Anorexia Nervosa and Bulimia Nervosa

These disorders are covered in detail in Chapter 12. Anorexia nervosa typically begins at puberty or in early adolescence and bulimia in late adolescence. The immediate and long-term medical sequelae are often more serious in young patients than in adults. Family treatment has a more central role in the care of adolescents compared with adults. The 12 step programs commonly used in adult treatment are generally not relevant for teenagers with eating disorders, whose dynamics more commonly relate to separation–individuation issues than addictive mechanisms.

Obesity

Obesity in childhood and adolescence has not been systematically studied; as a result, there are few scientific data to guide assessment and treatment. It appears to be a heterogeneous syndrome with multiple contributing factors, including emotional, socioeconomic, genetic, developmental, and neurological components. Obesity virtually always has its onset in childhood. It is not a psychiatric disorder, but it has significant psychosocial, as well as medical, sequelae. (Overeating that affects a patient's medical status can be designated under Psychological Factors Affecting Medical Conditions in DSM-IV.) An estimated 10 to 35% of American children and adolescents are overweight; many suffer from low self-esteem and impaired peer relationships as a result. Obese youngsters are typically physically inactive and spend many hours watching television and snacking. The majority of obese children over the age of 10 become persistently obese adults (see Chapter 24). Genetic and medical syndromes (i.e., Prader-Willi Syndrome, hypothyroidism) as a cause of obesity are rare.

Asssessment should include a basic medical evaluation with vital signs, physical examination, and laboratory tests as indicated. Information should be obtained on age of onset, duration, degree of obesity, family history of obesity, presence of medical illness- or syndrome-associated obesity, and family functioning. Caloric restriction below the recommended amounts for height, age, and sex is rarely indicated. Instead, the primary goal is to arrest continued weight gain until the child's or adolescent's height and weight are proportional.

The most effective treatment programs actively involve both parents and child and include education, a balanced diet, regular exercise, and peer activities (Epstein et al, 1990, 1996). Contingency management programs may be useful for children, while adolescents benefit from cognitive strategies such as those used for adults.

TOURETTE'S DISORDER

Tourette's disorder is the most severe and chronic of the tic disorders (Table 16–16). The others are chronic or transient vocal or motor tic disorders. Tourette's disorder is defined by chronic and frequent motor and vocal tics that typically change in location, pattern, frequency, and severity. A tic is an involuntary, sudden, rapid, recurrent, nonrhythmic, stereotyped motor movement or vocalization (words or sounds) (American Psychiatric Association, 1994).

Table 16–16 **Tourette's Disorder**

Characteristics
Onset in childhood
Commonly associated with ADHD and/or OCD*

Diagnosis
Chronic and frequent motor and vocal tics
Occur many times a day
More than a year's duration

Epidemiology
Estimated prevalence of 0.03–1.6%
Male predominance
Strong genetic etiology

Treatment
Identification and treatment of comorbid psychiatric disorders
Medication: neuroleptics, alpha-adrenergic agents
Behavior management
Education for family and school

* ADHD, attention deficit–hyperactivity disorder; OCD, obsessive–compulsive disorder.

Tics may be temporarily suppressed by conscious effort and typically diminish markedly during sleep. Estimated prevalence of Tourette's disorder is 0.03 to 1.6%, with a male predominance of three to one. Etiology is strongly genetic (autosomal dominant with incomplete, gender-specific penetrance and variable expression), but a variety of environmental influences can affect severity. Often far more disabling than the tics themselves are the commonly associated symptoms of hyperactivity, impulsiveness, distractibility, defiance, or obsessions and compulsions. It is controversial whether these problems are a part of Tourette's disorder per se or whether they are accounted for by genetic links with ADHD and OCD.

Initial treatment requires education of the child, family, teachers, and peers regarding the nature of the disorder. This often drastically reduces patient distress and school and family disruption. A variety of psychotherapeutic and behavior modification interventions may be helpful in reducing tics or other specific target symptoms, as well as secondary depression, anxiety, and low self-esteem. Special education may be useful. Low doses of haloperidol, pimozide, or clonidine may reduce tics and behavioral problems. Obsessions and compulsions may respond to clomipramine or fluoxetine. The use of stimulants to treat symptoms of ADHD in children with Tourette's disorder should be carefully considered. Recently, there has been interest in utilizing some of the newer neuroleptics; one open trial demonstrated the efficacy of risperidone in children and adolescents with TS who had been unresponsive to haloperidol or clonidine (Lambroso et al, 1995). Other drugs that have been tried include guanfacine, calcium channel blockers, opioid antagonists, clonazepam, nicotine, and nonsteroid androgen receptor blocking agents (e.g., flutamide) with some promising results. Because of the chronic waxing and waning course of Tourette's disorder and the high frequency of medication side effects, pharmacological treatment is best used sparingly.

SUBSTANCE-RELATED DISORDERS

Substance abuse in adolescents is a serious public health problem. Recent surveys of teenagers reveal increased experimentation and regular use of multiple drugs, including marijuana, hallucinogens, tobacco, alcohol, cocaine, and others. Compared with adults, adolescents abuse multiple drugs and have a higher incidence of unresolved comorbid disorders even after periods of abstinence. Approximately 40 to 90% of adolescents with a substance abuse or dependency diagnosis have at least one other comorbid psychiatric disorder. Substance use in adolescence has been associated with delinquency, early sexual activity, and school failure and nonattendance. Risk factors for adolescent substance abuse include genetic, constitutional, psychological, and sociocultural (family, peer, school, community) factors.

The issue of substance use should be routinely addressed with adolescents. In addition to obtaining historical information, laboratory testing for drugs may be indicated. Given the high incidence of comorbid conditions, all adolescents with substance problems should be evaluated psychiatrically. Interventions vary, depending on the scope and severity of the adolescent's drug problems, presence of other psychiatric disorders, and family functioning. Choices include both in- and outpatient treatment programs; many of these include elements of supportive psychotherapy (family, group, and individual), behavioral modification, educational/vocational remediation, and programming based on the Alcoholics Anonymous 12-step model (see Chapter 10).

MENTAL RETARDATION

Epidemiology
Individuals with mental retardation are considered to have deficits in their cognitive and functional abilities. Practically, classification has been based largely on IQ scores. IQ scores are distributed as a bell curve with the leftward tail (lower scores) being longer than the right. The prevalence of mental retardation is determined solely by the location of the cutoff point on the leftward tail of IQ. If the cutoff point is 2 SD from the mean (corresponding to a Weschler IQ of 70), 2.28% of the population is classified as mentally retarded. Males predominate 1.5 to 1. Individuals with IQs just above the cutoff point (70 to 84) are considered to have borderline intellectual functioning.

Description

Mental retardation is a syndrome characterized by global cognitive impairment. The DSM-IV diagnostic criteria are the following: 1) having significantly subaverage general intellectual functioning; 2) demonstrating significant deficits in adaptive living skills; and 3) having an onset prior to age 18. These criteria are modeled on those of the American Association of Mental Retardation (AAMR), but are not the same. Individuals are judged to meet the first criterion if they have an IQ of less than 70 on a standardized intelligent test (i.e., WAIS, WISC-IIIR) and the second criterion if they get a similar score on a measure of daily functioning. The four degrees of severity of mental retardation are seen in Table 16–17. Most retarded individuals are in the mild category. Educational and community agencies and institutions may use other labels or classifications (i.e., mentally handicapped, special needs, exceptional).

Differential Diagnosis

While attempts have been made to standardize and norm the IQ tests so that they are applicable for all children and adolescents regardless of their racial, cultural, and socioeconomic background, these tests are not unbiased, and individuals may test in the retarded range for reasons other than their cognitive abilities. Children who have been severely *neglected* may test in the retarded range. True intellectual capacity can only be assessed after a period of appropriate stimulation and remediation. Children with *specific developmental disorders* have delays in circumscribed areas with normal functioning in other areas. Children and adolescents who have *other major psychiatric disorders* (i.e., ADHD, major depression, psychosis) can appear cognitively impaired. The DSM V code *borderline intellectual functioning* is used for children with IQ scores between 71 and 84. These youngsters are impaired primarily in the school setting.

Children with *autistic disorder* have uneven developmental delays and qualitative abnormalities of behavior and emotions. Many have mental retardation *in addition* to autistic disorder. Some children identified by schools as having *ADHD* are, in fact, mentally retarded or have a borderline IQ. For children with *sensory impairments* such as deafness or blindness or *neuro-*

Table 16–17 **Classification of Mental Retardation***

DESCRIPTION	IQ RANGE	PROPORTION OF RETARDED POPULATION
Mild ("educable")	50–55 to 70	85%
Moderate ("trainable")	35–40 to 50–55	10%
Severe	20–25 to 35–40	3–4%
Profound	<20–25	1–2%

* Adapted from DSM-IV (American Psychiatric Association, 1994)

logical disorders such as cerebral palsy, expert psychological evaluation is needed to distinguish mental retardation from interference resulting from the disabilities. This assessment is particularly problematic in younger children because many of the important cognitive/developmental milestones have physical components.

Etiology

Intelligence appears to have a significant genetic component, with 45 to 80% of the variation in IQ scores being attributable to heritable factors (best explained by polygenic models). Mental retardation is a diverse category with a large number of etiologies. Identifiable organic causes are more common (estimated 60 to 75%) in those with moderate-to-profound retardation (IQ below 50) and include single gene or chromosomal abnormalities and metabolic, traumatic, and toxic etiologies. Organic and genetic etiologies can be classified as occurring in the prenatal, perinatal, or postnatal periods (see Table 16–18 for some of the more common types). Prenatal causes predominate, with the others accounting for approximately 10 to 25% of the more severe cases of mental retardation.

Table 16–18 **Some Causes of Mental Retardation**

Prenatal Factors

Chromosomal abnormalities
   Klinefelter's syndrome
   Turner's syndrome
   Neurofibromatosis
Genetic errors
   Down's syndrome
   Fragile X syndrome
   Phenylketonuria (PKU)
Toxins
   Alcohol
   Illicit drugs
Maternal infections
   Rubella
Physical alterations of brain structure or functioning
   Hydrocephalus

Perinatal

Fetal distress
Anoxia
Prematurity complications

Postnatal

Central nervous system infections
Hypothyroidism
Malnutrition
Trauma
Toxin exposure (lead)

One of the most important nongenetic etiologies of mental retardation is alcohol exposure in utero. Maternal consumption of alcohol during pregnancy can produce significant abnormalities in the child; the extent of symptomatology varies, with fetal alcohol syndrome being the most severe form and less severe types being described as fetal alcohol effects. The full syndrome consists of prenatal growth deficiency, characteristic dysmorphic facial features, and central nervous system effects. Cognitive abilities vary, but generally correlate with the amount of alcohol exposure and severity of the syndrome. Most affected individuals are in the mildly retarded range. They also have an increased incidence of ADHD, anxiety, depression, stereotypies, speech abnormalities, and eating disorders (see Chapter 10).

The two most common genetic causes of mental retardation are Down's syndrome and fragile X syndrome. Down's is an autosomal chromosomal defect that occurs in 1 of 700 births; three forms (trisomy 21, translocation 18, and mosaicism) have been identified. These individuals can have characteristic cardiac and musculoskeletal abnormalities, and there is a high incidence of Alzheimer's disease. Fragile X syndrome has an incidence of 1/1,000. The degree of mental retardation ranges from mild to severe with associated anomalies of a large, prominent jaw, large ears, and enlarged testes (in postpubescent males). Symptoms of autism and hyperactivity have been noted in this population.

In mild retardation, etiology is often attributed to a genetic endowment at the low end of the normal distribution and/or to psychosocial factors such as poverty and lack of stimulation. Many cases are idiopathic.

Evaluation

Intelligence testing is administered by a psychologist skilled in working with children in a setting that will encourage the child's cooperation. Commonly used tests of intellectual functioning are listed in Table 16–4. These tests measure skills that are related primary to successful performance in educational settings. Adaptive functioning (daily living skills) is evaluated by history, clinical observation, and standardized evaluation forms. One instrument commonly used is the well-standardized and normed Vineland Adaptive and Maladaptive Behavior Scales; it uses information from a caretaker on the child's or adolescent's abilities in social and functional areas of adaptive development and skills. Another measure is the AAMR Adaptive Behavior Scale for Children and Adults, which tends to be used for more severely retarded persons. A medical evaluation is indicated to seek causative disorders, sensory handicap, and associated physical problems such as congenital malformations, inborn errors of metabolism, or epilepsy. Genetic evaluation may be important in counseling the parents regarding risk to future children.

Psychiatric evaluation may be necessary to define associated psychiatric disorders, which are three to four times as common in the retarded as in the general population. Retarded children and adolescents can have the same psychiatric disorders as nonretarded youth. Determining diagnoses can be complicated since symptom profiles may not exactly fit DSM-IV criteria, due to developmental and cognitive factors. Generally, it is beneficial to start the clinical interview with an assessment of the child's or adolescent's cognition and perspectives. Retarded children and adolescents vary a great deal in their ability to understand and participate in an evaluation. Often, the pace of the interview needs to be slower, with more structure, less complex questions, and some toys or games to play (even if not appropriate for the individual's chronological age). Most mildly and some moderately retarded children and adolescents should be able to participate adequately in an evaluation. Generally, those with lower IQs do better with more structured, nonverbal techniques (i.e., play, drawing, games).

Treatment

Retarded children and adolescents can benefit from the same therapy modalities and approaches that are used with the nonretarded, although modifications for different cognitive levels may be necessary. Treatment choices should be based on the child's or adolescent's psychiatric symptoms or disorder.

Psychotherapy. Individual, family, and/or group psychotherapy or parent counseling may be useful to deal with developmental or situational crises or in the treatment of coexisting psychiatric disorders. Goals can include identifying and utilizing strengths; identifiying and working on reasonable, attainable goals; identifying and altering maladaptive behaviors; learning to express anger appropriately; and separating and in individuating from caretakers. Parents may need assistance to deal with their grief over having a "defective" child and to help the patient achieve an appropriate level of individuation and separation, even though most will require some level of structure, supervision, and support for all of their lives.

Behavioral Modification. These children, adolescents, and families often benefit from learning behavior modification techniques. Generally, affected individuals do better in structured and supervised situations with clear expectations and consequences. Particular behaviors may become more problematic as the child or adolescent grows older, since differences from nonretarded peers become more obvious. Specific behavioral programs are useful in teaching adaptive behaviors and reducing stereotypic behaviors, aggression, and self-injury.

Psychopharmacological Treatment. Generally, medications have efficacy against the same symptoms in the retarded and nonretarded populations; often, there is an increased incidence of side effects and poorer response rate in those with lower IQs. Medications should be used conservatively in situations in which the patient has a psychiatric diagnosis and targetable symptoms that are potentially responsive to medication. Responses and side effects should be carefully monitored. Polypharmacy should be avoided if possible.

Approximately 10 to 20% children with mental retardation have ADHD symptoms. *Stimulants* have been shown to be effective in treating ADHD target symptoms with a 60 to 75% response rate and side profiles similar to those of typical children, except somewhat more motor tics and emotional withdrawal (Gadow, 1985; Handen et al, 1992, 1994).

Neuroleptics have been used a great deal in the retarded population, especially for those who have been institutionalized. Often, the medication appears to be for behavioral control rather than for a specific psychiatric symptom or diagnosis. The studies on the effectiveness of neuroleptics for behavioral problems have been equivocal (Campbell and Cueva, 1995a). A recent open trial with the antipsychotic risperidone showed some benefits (Hardan et al, 1996). Their use must be weighed against their potential side effects, which include cognitive impairment, akathisia, and TD. Approximately 15 to 35% of mentally retarded patients on chronic neuroleptics have TD. Schizophrenia affects 1 to 2% of the mentally retarded population, and these individuals can be treated effectively with neuroleptics. Treatment-resistant schizophrenic mentally retarded individuals may respond to atypical antipsychotics. Alternative medications for aggression and self-injurious behavior should be considered.

Antidepressants have been used to treat depressive symptoms in retarded children and adolescents; case reports indicate that these medications are effective. Clomipramine was studied in an open trial for individuals with mental retardation and OCD and demonstrated positive effects (Barak et al, 1995).

Lithium has demonstrated effectiveness in reducing the frequency and severity of affective cycles in aggressive and self-injurious patients (Craft, 1987). In several studies, *naltrexone and naloxone* have had variable results in decreasing self-injurious and stereotypical behaviors. *Propranolol* has been effective in open trials in some cases of explosive, destructive behavior in this population (Campbell and Cueva, 1995a).

Environmental Interventions. Most of the services specifically for retarded children and adolescents are based in the educational system. Moderately to profoundly retarded youth benefit from comprehensive multidisciplinary habilitation programs. Specialized infant stimulation and preschool programs can reduce intellectual and adaptive deficits. Institutionalization is now indicated only for the most severely affected, usually those with accompanying medical disorders or severe behavior problems. Most communities have been making considerable efforts to keep retarded children and adolescents in community settings. Adolescents and young adults benefit from vocational training programs, sheltered workshops, and group homes in the community. An important aspect of care is intervening early to optimize the child's or adolescent's level of functioning and planning for young adulthood so that there is a smooth transition from educationally based services to more vocational and community-based interventions.

The Association for Retarded Citizens, a national organization, has state and local chapters that provide assistance to retarded persons and their families.

PERVASIVE DEVELOPMENTAL DISORDERS

These disorders are rare, especially the severe form. Affected children and adolescents have a global type of developmental delay with significant social, communicative, and behavioral manifestations. The most severe forms are diagnosed as Autistic Disorder (AD); those individuals with less severe features are considered to have Pervasive Developmental Disorder Not Otherwise Specified (PPDNOS). These patients are characterized by an uneven pattern of development that includes both severe delays and qualitative abnormalities (Table 16–19).

Epidemiology

AD occurs at a rate of 4/10,000 persons, and PDD at a rate of 10 to 20/10,000. There is a male predominance of three to four to one.

Table 16–19 **Pervasive Developmental Disorders**

Characteristics
Fundamental abnormality in social relationships
Often associated with significant language and cognitive abnormalities
Wide variability in functional impairment and symptom presentation

Diagnosis
Spectrum of disorders
Deficits in reciprocal social interaction, communication, and patterns of behavior
Developmental abnormalities

Epidemiology
Severe form (autistic disorder) occurs at a rate of 4/10,000
Significant genetic component
Male predominance

Treatment
Identify and treat comorbid psychiatric disorders
Early educational and environmental interventions
Psychotherapy to deal with specific psychological symptoms or issues (higher functioning patients and families)
Behavior modification
Structured and supervised environments
Medications useful for specific, targeted symptoms

Description

These disorders are characterized by severe and sustained impairment (relative to chronological and mental age) in reciprocal social interaction, communication, and patterns of behavior, activities, and interests. The onset is in infancy or early childhood with a variable age of diagnosis. These disorders are probably best considered to be in a spectrum, with AD being the most severe form and PPD NOS describing a heterogenous group of children and adolescents who have varying degrees of handicap in these areas. These children and adolescents demonstrate significant social dysfunction that seems to result from a lack of any emotional connection between themselves and others. They do not appear to consider other people as entities with thoughts, feelings, or emotions. Even those children and adolescents who have adequate speech and language skills still have difficulty communicating, often with language and speech that is distinctive and idiosyncratic. They tend to have restrictive, stereotyped patterns of behavior and activity. Children and adolescents who are severely affected do not relate to others, do not talk or communicate, and engage in repetitive, sometimes self-injurious behavior. Individuals with milder forms of PPD can interact with others in some ways and demonstrate less obvious communicative and behavior abnormalities, but still have clear deficits when assessed carefully.

Development may be markedly abnormal from early infancy, with indifference or aversion to cuddling. Eye contact may be absent or present, but impersonal. Some children may initially appear normal, with symptoms appearing at age 2 or 3 years as more complex communication and social interaction are expected. Children with the more severe forms tend to be diagnosed earlier; the milder forms may not be noticed until the child reaches elementary school and cannot make friends.

Differential Diagnosis

Children with pure *mental retardation* have a more even pattern of delays and do not have bizarre behaviors or deficits in social relatedness. Many children with PDD also have mental retardation, usually in the moderate range. In *aphasia, developmental language disorders,* or *deafness,* the deficits in language are partially compensated for by nonverbal gestures; social interest is normal. *Degenerative neurological diseases* may transiently resemble PDD.

History and clinical examination can distinguish PDD from *reactive attachment disorder of infancy* or severe reactions to trauma or separation from parents. With stimulation and a stable, appropriate environment, traumatized children and those with reactive attachment disorder should improve. In very young or nonverbal children, the symptoms of autism and *schizophrenia* may be difficult to distinguish (Watkins et al, 1988).

Etiology

Currently, the autism spectrum of disorders is considered to have a significant genetic component to its etiology. Pedigree studies have indicated a genetic contribution to the spectrum that includes PDD, language disorders, dyslexia, and mental retardation. In some families, autosomal recessive inheritance appears likely. Having one child with autism significantly increases the risk of having another. There is no evidence that child-rearing practices contribute to the development of this disorder. PDD is more common in children with certain chromosomal abnormalities (such as fragile X syndrome) and can follow a wide range of infections (especially maternal rubella during pregnancy) and traumatic insults to the central nervous system. Neuroanatomic imaging findings have been inconsistent.

Evaluation

Medical evaluation is needed to seek sensory deficits, possible treatable metabolic disorders, and degenerative diseases. A genetic evaluation may be useful for counseling family members about plans for future children. The physician should be alert to the possibility of epilepsy; major or minor motor or complex partial seizures develop in 20 to 35% of patients with autism by age 20. In evaluating family dynamics, the reciprocal effects on parents of the child's behavior must be taken into account. Baseline measurements are taken of cognitive level, social communication skills, language function, and additional psychiatric symptoms such as hyperactivity, aggression, severe anxiety, compulsions, depression, or mania.

Treatment

Psychotherapy. Group therapy with autistic or normal peers may significantly improve social functioning for higher functioning children and adolescents. Supportive psychotherapy may be of benefit to parents. Behavioral techniques are valuable in increasing learning and in reducing maladaptive or injurious behaviors. These management strategies should be taught to parents and incorporated into the school setting.

Psychopharmacological Treatment. No medications are known to affect autistic disorder per se, and medication should not be used as the sole treatment. Generally, medications have been effective against specific symptoms (i.e., overactivity, stereotypies), but medication use has been complicated by an increased occurrence of idiosyncratic reactions in these children and adolescents.

Neuroleptics. In some hyper-or normoactive autistic children, haloperidol (in doses of 0.5 to 3.0 mg/day) decreases behavioral target symptoms such as hyperactivity, aggression, temper tantrums, withdrawal, and stereotypies. In combination with a structured behavioral/educational program, it may enhance language acquisition. In general, hypoactive autistic children do not respond well to haloperidol (Campbell et al, 1985). Other neuroleptics, including risperidone (Demb, 1995), have improved aggression and other behavioral symptoms (see the section on schizophrenia for the use of neuroleptics in children and adolescents.)

Stimulants. Contrary to previous belief, recent reports indicate that methylphenidate in doses similar to those used to treat ADHD may reduce overactivity in autistic children and improve attention span without producing psychosis or increasing stereotyped behaviors (Birmaher et al, 1988; Strayhorn et al, 1988).

Other Medications. Clomipramine or fluoxetine may be useful in decreasing the compulsive rituals and perservative behaviors that often appear in persons with autism. Naltrexone has been found to be useful in the treatment of some children and adolescents with autistic disorder by decreasing withdrawal and self-injurious behavior and increasing communicative speech and social relatedness on global assessments, but improvement was not seen on more systematic measures (Campbell et al, 1990; Kolmen et al, 1995; Williamson-Swinkels et al, 1995).

Environmental Interventions. The best outcome is obtained with a specialized therapeutic educational program that integrates social, language, and behavioral components and that begins as early as possible (age 2 to 4 years). Sufficiently intensive early treatment can avert institutionalization for all but the most handicapped. Adolescents and young adults can benefit from sheltered workshops, vocational training programs, and group homes in the community. Support and advocacy groups for parents (such as a local chapter of the Autism Society of America) are useful.

Role of the Primary Care Physician

The pediatrician is usually the first to whom parents bring their concerns about a child with a PDD, often in the first 18 months of life. It is essential for the physician to take these concerns seriously. Whenever possible, referral should be made to a center with experience in this rare disorder where a multidisciplinary team assessment can be conducted. The primary physician will maintain an important role in coordinating medical care for these patients. The physician must be aware that parents of autistic children, driven to desperation by the severity of the disorder and the absence of curative treatments, are at risk for pursuing unconventional, unproven, and perhaps even harmful interventions that promise miraculous results.

SPECIFIC DEVELOPMENTAL DISORDERS

Description

This group of disorders is characterized by developmental delay in a specific domain (relative to that expected for mental age) that results in functional impairment. The delay must not be due to a diagnosable physical disorder, a visual or hearing impairment, a pervasive developmental disorder, mental retardation, or inadequate educational opportunities. It is common for a child to have more than one specific developmental disorder (Table 16–20). Frequent secondary symptoms include low self-esteem, demoralization, refusal to exert effort in school, and behavior problems.

Etiology

Genetic factors are suggested by the clustering of specific developmental disorders in families. Etiology is presumed to relate to delayed or abnormal maturation of or damage to local areas of the cerebral cortex. Substantial genetic contributions to dyslexia (developmental reading disorder) have been demonstrated.

Evaluation

Early diagnosis is crucial in facilitating remediation and reducing secondary emotional and behavioral symptoms. Assessment requires psychological testing (Table 16–4) to establish IQ, followed by academic achievement tests and tests of specific language, speech, and motor functions. Visual and hearing impairment must be ruled out. A careful history should be taken of school attendance and performance and of the quality of teaching. Schools overidentify boys and fail to identify girls with developmental reading disorder (Shaywitz et al, 1990).

Treatment

Children do not simply grow out of learning disabilities, but retain some degree of impairment into adulthood.

Table 16–20 Specific Developmental Disorders

DISORDER	ESTIMATED PREVALENCE* (AGE 5 TO 12)
Academic Skills Disorder	
Developmental Arithmetic Disorder	Unknown
Developmental Expressive Writing Disorder	2–8%
Developmental Reading Disorder (Dyslexia)	7–9%†
Language and Speech Disorders	
Developmental Articulation Disorder	5–10%
Developmental Expressive Language Disorder	3–10%
Developmental Receptive Language Disorder	3–10%
Motor Skills Disorder	
Developmental Coordination Disorder	6%
Developmental Disorder Not Otherwise Specified	Unknown

* American Psychiatric Association, 1987.
† Shaywitz et al, 1990.

Psychotherapy. Supportive psychotherapy may be required to deal with low self-esteem, passivity, lack of motivation, anxiety, or depression resulting from the learning difficulties. Family therapy can deal with sequelae of parental criticism and child academic failure. Behavioral techniques may be useful in motivating children to practice and learn skills that are difficult for them.

Educational and Adjunctive Interventions. Most important is specific remediation of the deficits, using teaching techniques tailored to the child's strengths and weaknesses. Special educational programs may be needed, ranging from tutoring to a resource room several periods a week, to full-time special classes. The most severe cases may require a special school or residential treatment program. Articulation or language therapy is indicated for language and speech disorders. Physical or occupational therapy may be needed.

MEDICAL ILLNESS IN CHILDREN AND ADOLESCENTS

Response of Child and Family to Physical Illness

Infancy

When infants less than 6 months old are hospitalized, they are usually most upset by changes in their usual routine. It is helpful to have the parents do as much of the care as possible and to arrange for consistency of nurses. For the older infant who has formed strong differential attachments, separation is traumatic, especially in the unfamiliar hospital environment and when accompanied by physical discomfort and medical procedures. Stranger anxiety adds to the baby's distress. The infant's immature language development exacerbates the problem since explanations are not useful in understanding the situation.

The constant presence of a parent is extremely important. In the absence of an attachment figure, the baby's thrashing, refusal to eat, and inability to sleep may have serious medical consequences. Fortunately, most pediatric hospital settings not only permit, but encourage parents to "live in" while their young child is hospitalized.

Early Childhood

Hospitalized children aged 1 to 3 years react primarily to separation from their parents. They may react by rejecting parents when they visit, being aggressive toward physicians and nurses, regressing in bowel and bladder control, and refusing to eat. If parents are absent, children may develop depression, sleep disturbance, diarrhea, or vomiting. Toddlers also have great concern for the intactness of their bodies and may be extremely fearful of minor procedures such as blood-drawing. Maximizing parental presence and providing the child with familiar items from home are helpful.

For children aged 3 to 5 years, separation from parents by hospitalization is still difficult, even for a child who is comfortably able to separate in other circumstances. Anesthesia and surgery are especially frightening because this is a time of normal fears of bodily injury. Children believe that illness and painful treatments are punishment for real or fantasized misbehavior. When possible, preparation by simple explanations and a visit to the hospital may help. Constant presence of a parent is important.

School Age

Children aged 6 to 12 years usually tolerate acute illness and hospitalization relatively well, especially if they are prepared, if parents visit daily for substantial periods, and if preceding development was normal. They may still have irrational explanations of illness (i.e., they are being punished or that their parents were unable to protect them). Behavioral regression or oppositional behavior often occurs.

Adolescence

Adolescents have more realistic fears regarding the outcome of illness, especially regarding changes in appearance or inability to continue favorite activities. An injury may make impossible a planned career (such as professional sports or the military). Loss of autonomy and privacy are especially painful, as are differences from peers.

Parents

At the time of diagnosis, the parents of a chronically ill or handicapped child must go through a period of mourning. The stages are similar to those following a death: anger, denial, grief, and resignation. Medical problems in a child may be viewed by the parent (and others) as a negative reflection on the parent. Parents feel guilty, especially for genetic diseases or complications that may be attributed (rightly or wrongly) to maternal behavior. The parent's anger, resentment, guilt, and/or denial may interfere with their ability to work together with the pediatric team. Realistic additional caretaking and financial burdens may stress parents beyond their ability to cope. (Regressive behavior in adults precipitated by physical illness is discussed in Chapter 20.)

Chronic Illness

Sequelae of chronic illness include interference with normal developmental tasks attained through school, peers, sports, and other activities. Autonomy and control of the child's own body are jeopardized. Children and adolescents with chronic illness, but without disability, are twice as likely as controls to have a psychiatric disorder. Those with disability as well as chronic illness are even more likely to have emotional problems, attention-deficit disorders, social isolation, or school performance problems. The majority of chronically ill youngsters do not, however, have psychiatric disorders or major difficulties with social or school adjustment (Cadman et al, 1987).

Compliance

Lack of compliance with medical regimens (e.g., medication, diet, exercise) is a major problem in the care of children and adolescents. Factors that contribute to noncompliance are seen in Table 16–21. Attention to and remediation of specific cause of noncompliance will improve medical management. (General issues in noncompliance are discussed in Chapter 20.)

Table 16–21 **Noncompliance**

Patient Factors

Denial or lack of acceptance of the disorder
Frustration with the outcome or nature of treatment
Wish to obtain parental attention or special privileges via symptoms
Wish to regain control
Rebellion against parents
Lack of knowledge or skills
Inability to resist peer pressure
Lack of relationship or miscommunication with health care team
Psychopathology
  Depression
  Suicidal intent
  Attention deficit–hyperactivity disorder
  Oppositional defiant disorder
  Conduct disorder
  Anorexia nervosa or bulimia

Family Factors

Unresolved guilt, denial, anger, and/or fear
Lack of knowledge and skills
Inability to encourage adolescent independence
Competition with medical personnel
Lack of support system
Other stressors on family
Family conflict acted out through the child's medical care
Rivalry between patient and healthy siblings

Treatment-Related Factors

Interference with usual activities
Side effects of drugs (pain, nausea, weight gain, hair loss)
Lack of clarity of connection between noncompliance and sequelae
Disinterested, inconsistent medical personnel

Specific Interventions for Medically Ill Children and Adolescents

A child and adolescent psychiatrist or pediatric psychologist can offer consultation and treatment for emotional and behavioral problems. Coexisting psychiatric disorders are treated as in medically healthy children, although modifications are often needed.

Psychotherapy

Supportive individual, family, and/or group psychotherapy is often valuable for both patient and parents. Instruction in social problem solving and coping skills may also be beneficial.

Behavior Modification

Techniques such as behavioral contracting with contingency management and self-monitoring with self-reinforcement are invaluable in improving medical and behavioral compliance. Children who refuse or are unable to swallow oral medication can be taught to take pills using instruction, modeling, contingent rewards, and shaping pill-swallowing using successively larger candies or placebos (Pelco et al, 1987).

Behavioral medicine techniques have been adapted for the level of the youngster's cognitive or emotional development. Relaxation training has been used in the treatment of pediatric migraine, juvenile rheumatoid arthritis, hemophilia, asthma, and hyperventilation in patients with cystic fibrosis. Hypnosis can be used in the treatment of physical symptoms with a psychological component or to help a child manage severe pain or nausea associated with a physical disorder or its treatment (Williams, 1979).

Behavioral therapy techniques in the management of chronic pain include operant techniques, self-monitoring, and stress management planning. Emphasis is placed on fostering a sense of control and mastery and on promoting normal functioning in spite of pain (Masek et al, 1984; Varni et al, 1986).

"Stress inoculation" uses education, modeling, systematic desensitization, hypnosis, contingency management, and training and practice in coping skills such as imagery and breathing exercises. It is useful in the prevention of stress and anxiety in children before medical and dental procedures and in chronically ill children for reduction of anxiety, pain, or other discomfort connected to repeated procedures such as spinal taps, bone marrow aspirations, and chemotherapy infusions (Melamed et al, 1984; Varni et al, 1986).

Psychopharmacological Treatment

The approach to treating psychiatric symptoms and disorders with medication is the same in the medically ill population, with some modifications. Psychopharmacological agents produce similar responses in medically ill children and adolescents. Careful attention must be paid to the interaction between the illness, medical treatment, and chosen psychotrophic; at times, some psychiatric drugs may be contraindicated for certain diseases or in combination with other medications. Often, medically ill children and adolescents will require lower doses or different dosing schedules.

Environmental Interventions

Peer activities and school should be normalized as much as possible. Chronically ill children may benefit greatly from special camps and recreation programs with medical supervision. Families may require concrete assistance to provide for an ill child.

Role of the Physician

Members of the medical team will be more successful if they are able to deal with their own feelings of guilt, helplessness, inadequacy, and anxiety. Staff support groups may be useful. Medically ill youth and their families generally do best when there is consistency in their medical providers. Generally, children, adolescents, and their families benefit from participating in frequent, ongoing discussions of the medical problems and treatments that include information both obtained from and given to them. Children and adolescents should always be included in the process at a developmentally appropriate level. In dealing with adolescents, efforts to respect and reinforce the patient's competence and autonomy, to give information in a way that permits the adolescent to understand and to save face, and to encourage questions will be rewarded with improved compliance and psychological adjustment. Children and adolescents with potentially fatal illnesses appreciate accurate information, titrated to their ability to understand and emotional readiness to hear.

CLINICAL PEARLS

Emotional and behvioral reactions should be anticipated.
- Medical providers should be as consistent as possible.
- Explain in advance as much as the child's age, coping style, and medical situation allow.
- Minimize separations from parents, especially for children under 8 years old.
- Try to understand the meaning of the illness to the child and correct her or his misconceptions.
- Understand that the child or adolescent needs to control *something* in the environment and arrange the milieu so that this will not interfere with treatment.
- Do not criticize or blame the child or parents for regressive behavior.

ANNOTATED BIBLIOGRAPHY

General

Adams PL, Fras I: Beginning Child Psychiatry. New York, Brunner/Mazel, 1988

> An introductory text.

Dulcan MK, Martini DR: Concise Guide to Child and Adolescent Psychiatry, 2nd ed Washington, DC, American Psychiatric Press, in press

> A brief paperback handbook. Manageable, comprehensive coverage of the diagnosis and treatment of psychiatric disorders of childhood and adolescence.

Lewis M, Volkmar F: Clinical Aspects of Child and Adolescent Development, 3rd ed. Philadelphia, Lea & Febiger, 1990

> Good coverage of both normal and pathological development.

Lewis M (ed): Child and Adolescent Psychiatry: A Comprehensive Textbook, 2nd ed. Baltimore, Williams & Wilkins, 1996

> A complete, clinically focused textbook. Chapters on assessment, treatment, all Axis I and II disorders, and special issues such as abuse and suicide.

Evaluation and Treatment

Adams PL: A Primer of Child Psychotherapy, 2nd ed. Boston, Little, Brown, 1982

Canino IA, Spurlock J: Culturally Diverse Children and Adolescents: Assessment, Diagnosis, and Treatment. New York, Guilford Press, 1994

Dulcan MK, Bregman J, Weller, EB, Weller, R: Treatment of childhood and adolescent disorders. In Schatzber AF and Nemeroff CB (eds): American Psychiatric Press Textbook of Psycho-pharmacology, 3rd ed. Washington DC, American Psychiatric Press, 1997

Rosenberg DR, Hottum J, Gershon S: Textbook of Pharmacotherapy for Child and Adolescent Psychiatric Disorders. New York, Brunner/Mazel, 1994

Simmons JE: Psychiatric Examination of Children, 4th ed. Philadelphia, Lea & Febiger, 1987

Wiener JM (ed): Diagnosis and Psychopharmacology of Childhood and Adolescent Disorders, 2nd ed. New York, John Wiley & Sons, 1996

Attention-deficit Hyperactivity Disorder

Barkley RA: Attention-deficit Hyperactivity Disorder: A Handbook for Diagnosis and Treatment. New York, Guilford Press, 1990

Cantwell DP: Attention deficit disorder: a review of the past 10 years. J Am Acad Child Adolesc Psychiatry 35:978-987, 1996

Oppositional Defiant Disorder

Forehand R, McMahon RJ: Helping the Non-Compliant Child: A Clinician's Guide to Parent Training. New York, Guilford Press, 1981

Anxiety Disorders

Bernstein GA, Borchardt CM, Perwien AR: Anxiety disorders in children and adolescents: a review of the past 10 years. J Am Acad Child Adolesc Psychiatry 35:1110–1119, 1996

Eth S, Pynoos RS (eds): Posttraumatic Stress Disorder in Children. Washington, DC, American Psychiatric Press, 1985

Ollendick TH, Francis G: Behavioral assessment and treatment of childhood phobias. Behav Modif 12:165–204, 1988

Reiter S, Kutcher S, Gardner D: Anxiety disorders in children and adolescents: clinical and related issues in pharmacological treatment. Can J Psychiatry 37:432–438, 1992

Wolff RP, Wolff LS: Assessment and treatment of obsessive–compulsive disorder in children. Behav Modif 15:372–393, 1991

Elimination Disorders

Howe AC, Walker CE: Behavioral management of toilet training, enuresis, and encopresis. Pediatric Clin North Am 39:413–432, 1992

Levine MD: Encopresis. In Levine MD, Carey WB, Crocker AC (eds): Developmental–Behavioral Pediatrics, 2nd ed, pp 389–397. Philadelphia, WB Saunders, 1992

Rappaport LA: Enuresis. In Levine MD, Carey WB, Crocker AC (eds): Developmental–Behavioral Pediatrics, pp 384–388. Philadelphia, WB Saunders, 1992

Mood Disorders

Birmaher B, Ryan ND, Williamson DE et al: Childhood and adolescent depression: a review of the past 10 years. Part I. J Am Acad Child Adolesc Psychiatry 35:1427–1439, 1996

Birmaher B, Ryan ND, Williamson DE, Brent DA, Kaufman J: Childhood and adolescent depression: a review of the past 10 years. Part II. J Am Acad Child Adolesc Psychiatry 35:1575–1583, 1996

Kutcher SP, Marton P: Parameters of adolescent depression: a review. Psychiatr Clin North Am 12:895–918, 1989

Schizophrenia

Cantor S: Childhood Schizophrenia. New York, Guilford Press, 1988

Volkmar FR: Childhood and adolescent psychosis: a review of the past 10 years. J Am Acad Child Adolesc Psychiatry 35:843–851, 1996

Eating Disorders

Casey PH: Failure to thrive. In Levine MD, Carey WB, Crocker AC (eds): Developmental–Behavioral Pediatrics, 2nd ed, pp 375–383. Philadelphia, WB Saunders, 1992

Chatoor I, Kickson L, Einhorn A: Rumination: etiology and treatment. Pediatr Ann 13:924–929, 1984

Kreipe RE: Eating disorders among children and adolescents. Pediatr Rev 16:370–9, 1995

Woolston JL (ed): Eating and growth disorders. Child Adolesc Psychiatr Clini North Am 2:1–95, 1993

Obesity

Neumann CG, Jenks BH: Obesity. In Levine MD, Carey WB, Crocker AC (eds): Developmental–Behavioral Pediatrics, pp 354–363. Philadelphia, WB Saunders, 1992

Tourette's Disorder

Cohen DJ, Brunn RD, Leckan JF (eds): Tourette's Syndrome and Tic Disorders: Clinical Understanding and Treatment. New York, John Wiley & Sons, 1988

Substance-Related Disorders

Jaffe SL (ed): Adolescent substance abuse and dual disorders. Child Adolesc Psychiatr Clin North Am 5:1–261, 1996

Mental Retardation

Bregman JD, Hodapp RM: Current developments in the understanding of mental retardation. Part I: Biological and phenomenological perspectives. J Am Acad Child Adolesc Psychiatry 30:707–719, 1991

Bregman JD: Current developments in the understanding of mental retardation. Part II: Psychopathology. J Am Acad Child Adolesc Psychiatry 30:861–872, 1991

Volkmar FR (ed): Mental retardation. Child Adolesc Psychiatr Clin North Am 5:769–977, 1996

Autistic Disorder/Pervasive Developmental Disorder

Denckla MB, James LS (eds): An update on autism: a developmental disorder. Pediatrics 87:5(suppl), 1991

Campbell M, Schopler E, Cueva JE, Hallin A: Treatment of autistic disorder. J Am Acad Child Adolesc Psychiatry 35:134–143, 1996

Specific Developmental Disorders

Silver L: The Misunderstood Child: A Guide for Parents of Learning Disabled Children. New York, McGraw-Hill, 1984

Medically Ill Children

Van Dongen-Melman JEWM, Sanders-Woudstra JAR: The chronically ill child and his family. In Cohen DJ, Schowalter JE (eds): Child Psychiatry. Vol. 2. Philadelphia, JB Lippincott, 73:1–9, 1985

Van Dongen-Melman JEWM, Sanders-Woudstra JAR: The fatally ill child and his family. In Cohen DJ, Schowalter JE (eds): Child Psychiatry. Vol. 2. Philadelphia, JB Lippincott, 74:1–11, 1985

REFERENCES

Abramowitz AJ, O'Leary SG: Behavioral interventions for the classroom: implications for students with ADHD. School Psychol Rev 20:220–234, 1991

Achenbach TM: Manual for the Child Behavior Checklist/4–18 and 1991 Profile. Burlington, University of Vermont Department of Psychiatry, 1991a

Achenbach TM: Manual for the Youth Self-Report and 1991 Profile. Burlington, University of Vermont Department of Psychiatry, 1991b

Achenbach TM: Manual for the Teacher's Report Form and 1991 Profile. Burlington, University of Vermont Department of Psychiatry, 1991c

Ackerman DL, Greenland S, Bystritsky A, et al: Predictors of treatment response in obsessive–compulsive disorder: multivariate analyses from a multicenter trial of clomipramine. J Clin Psychopharmacol 14:247–254, 1994

Allen AJ, Leonard HL, Swedo SE: Case study: a new infection-triggered, autoimmune subtype of pediatric OCD and Tourette's syndrome. J Am Acad Child Adolesc Psychiatry 34:307–311, 1995

Ambrosini PJ, Emslie GJ, Greenhill LL, et al: Selecting a sequence of antidepressants for treating depression in youth. J Child Adolesc Psychopharmacol 5:233–240, 1995

American Academy of Child and Adolescent Psychiatry: Practice parameters for the assessment and treatment of anxiety disorders. J Am Acad Child Adolesc Psychiatry 32:1089–1098, 1993

American Psychiatric Association: Diagnostic and Statistical Manual of Mental Disorders, 3rd ed. revised. Washington, DC, American Psychiatric Press, 1987

American Psychiatric Association: Diagnostic and Statistical Manual of Mental Disorders, 4th ed. Washington, DC, American Psychiatric Press, 1994

Anderson CM, Hogarty GE, Reiss DJ: Family treatment of adult schizophrenic patients: a psycho-educational approach. Schizophr Bull 6:490–505, 1980

Anderson JC, Williams S, McGee R, Silva PA: DSM-III disorders in preadolescent children: prevalence in a large sample from the general population. Arch Gen Psychiatry 44:69–76, 1987

Apter A, Fallon TJ, King RA, et al: Obsessive-compulsive characteristics: from symptoms to syndrome. J Am Acad Child Adolesc Psychiatry 35:907–912, 1996

Arredondo DE, Docherty JP, Streeter BA: Bupropion treatment of adolescent depression. Presentation, Annual Meeting of American Psychiatric Association, 1993

Barak Y, Ring A, Levy D, et al: Disabling compulsions in 11 mentally retarded adults: an open trial of clomipramine SR. J Clin Psychiatry 56:526–528, 1995

Barkley RA: Attention-Deficit Hyperactivity Disorder: A Handbook for Diagnosis and Treatment. New York, Guilford Press, 1990

Barrickman LL, Perry PJ, Allen AJ, et al: Bupropion versus methylphenidate in the treatment of attention-deficit-hyperactivity disorder. J Am Acad Child Adolesc Psychiatry 34:649–657, 1995

Bartels MG, Varley CK, Mitchell J, Stamm SJ: Pediatric cardiovascular effects of imipramine and desipramine. J Am Acad Child Adolesc Psychiatry 30:100–103, 1991

Beach PS, Beach RE, Smith LR: Hyponatremic seizures in a child treated with desmopressin to control enuresis. Clin Pediatrics 31:566–569, 1992

Bernstein GA, Garfinkel BD, Borchardt CM: Comparative studies of pharmacotherapy for school refusal. J Am Acad Child Adolesc Psychiatry 29:773–781, 1990

Biederman J: Sudden death in children treated with a tricyclic antidepressant. J Am Acad Child Adolesc Psychiatry 30:495–498, 1991

Biederman J, Baldessarini RJ, Goldblatt A: A naturalistic study of 24-hour electrocardiographic recordings and echocardiographic findings in children and adolescents treated with desipramine. J Am Acad Child Adolesc Psychiatry 32:805–813, 1993

Biederman J, Baldessarini RJ, Wright V, Knee D, Harmatz JS: A double-blind placebo controlled study of desipramine in the treatment of ADD: I. Efficacy. J Am Acad Child Adolesc Psychiatry 28:777–784, 1989

Biederman J, Munir K, Knee D, et al: A family study of patients with attention deficit disorder and normal controls. J Psychiatr Res 20:263–274, 1986

Biederman J, Thisted RA, Greenhill LL ,et al: Estimation of the association between desipramine and the risk for sudden death in 5- to 14-year old children. J Clin Psychiatry 56:87–93, 1995

Birmaher B, Quintana H, Greenhill LL: Methylphenidate treatment of hyperactive autistic children. J Am Acad Child Adolesc Psychiatry 27:248–251, 1988

Birmaher B, Waterman GS, Ryan N, et al: Fluoxetine for childhood anxiety disorders. J Am Acad Child Adolesc Psychiatry 33:993–999, 1994

Black B, Uhde TW: Treatment of elective mutism with fluoxetine: a double-blind, placebo-controlled study. J Am Acad Child Adolesc Psychiatry 33:1000–1006, 1994

Botteron KN, Vannier MW, Geller B, Todd RD, Lee BCP: Preliminary study of magnetic resonance imaging characteristics in 8- to 16-year-olds with mania. J Am Acad Child Adolesc Psychiatry 34:742–749, 1995

Cadman D, Boyle M, Szatmari P, Offord DR: Chronic illness, disability, and mental and social well-being: findings of the Ontario Child Health Study. Pediatrics 79:805–813, 1987

Campbell M, Adams PB, Small AM, et al: Lithium in hospitalized aggressive children with conduct disorder: a double bind and placebo-controlled study. J Am Acad Child Adolesc Psychiatry 34:445–453, 1995

Campbell M, Anderson LT, Small AM, et al: Naltrexone in autistic children: a double-blind and placebo-controlled study. Psychopharmacol Bull 26:130–135, 1990

Campbell M, Cueva JE: Psychopharmacology in child and adolescent psychiatry: a review of the past seven years. Part I. J Am Acad Child Adolesc Psychiatry 34:1124–1132, 1995a

Campbell M, Cueva JE: Psychopharmacology in child and adolescent psychiatry: a review of the past seven years. Part II. J Am Acad Child Adolesc Psychiatry 34:1262–1272, 1995b

Campbell M, Green WH, Deutsch, SI: Child and Adolescent Psychopharmacoloy. Beverly Hills, Sage Publications, 1985

Campbell M, Silva RR, Kafantaris V, et al: Predictors of side effects associated with lithium administration in children. Psychopharmacol Bull 27:373–380, 1991

Campbell SB: Hyperactivity in preschoolers: correlates and prognostic implications. Clin Psychol Rev 5:405–428, 1985

Cantor S, Kestenbaum C: Psychotherapy with schizophrenic children. J Am Acad Child Psychiatry 25:623–630, 1986

Carlson CL, Pelham WE, Milich R, Dixon J: Single and combined effects of methylphenidate and behavior therapy on the classroom performance of children with attention-deficit hyperactivity disorder. J Abnorm Child Psychol 20:213–232, 1992

Carlson GA, Kashani JH: Phenomenology of major depression from childhood through adulthood: analysis of three studies. Am J Psychiatry 145:1222–1225, 1988

Chappell PB, Riddle MA, Scahill L, et al: Guanfacine treatment of comorbid attention deficit hyperactivity disorder and Tourette's syndrome: preliminary clinical experience. J Am Acad Child Psychiatry 34:1140–1146, 1995

Coffey BJ: Anxiolytics for children and adolescents: traditional and new drugs. J Child Adolesc Psychopharmacol 1:57–83, 1990

Conners CK, Casat CD, Gualtieri CT, et al: Bupropion hydrochloride in attention deficit disorder with hyperactivity. J Am Acad Child Psychiatry 35:1314–1321, 1996

Costello EJ, Arnold A, Burns BJ, et al: The Great Smoky Mountains Study of Youth: goals, design, methods, and the prevalence of DSM-III-R disorders. Arch Gen Psychiatry 53:1129–1136, 1996a

Costello EJ, Arnold A, Burns BJ, et al: The Great Smoky Mountains Study of Youth: goals, functional impairment and serious emotional disturbance. Arch Gen Psychiatry 53:1137–1143, 1996b

Costello EJ, Pantino T: The new morbidity: who should treat it? Dev Behav Pediatr 8:288–291, 1987

Craft M, Ismail IA, Krishnamurti D, et al: Lithium in the treatment of aggression in mentally handicapped patients: a double blind trial. Br J Psychiatry 150:685–689, 1987

Cueva JE, Overall JE, Small AM, et al: Carbamazepine in aggressive children with conduct disorder: a double blind and placebo-controlled study. J Am Acad Child Adolesc Psychiatry 35:480–490, 1996

Dell ML, Dulcan MK: Childhood and adolescent development. In Stoudemire A (ed): Clinical Psychiatry for Medical Students, 3rd ed. Philadelphia, JB Lippincott, 1998

Demb HB: Risperidone in young children with pervasive developmental disorders and other developmental disabilities. J Child Adolesc Psychopharmacol 6:79–80, 1996

Derivan A, Agular L, Upton GV, et al: A study of venlafaxine in children and adolescents with conduct disorder. Presented at the 42nd Annual Meeting of the American Academy of Child and Adolescent Psychiatry, New Orleans, LA, October 1995

DeVane CL, Sallee FR: Serotonin selective reuptake inhibitors in child and adolescent psychopharmacology: a review of published experience. J Clin Psychiatry 57:55–66, 1996

Dorsett PG: Behavioral and social learning psychology. In Stoudemire A (ed): Human Behavior: An Introduction for Medical Students, 2nd ed. Philadelphia, JB Lippincott, 4:85–112, 1994

Douglas VI: Attentional and Cognitive Problems. In Rutter M (ed): Developmental Neuropsychiatry. New York, Guilford Press, 14:280–329, 1983

Dulcan MK (ed): Information for parents and youth on psychotropic medications. APPI, in press

Dulcan MK, Benson RS: AACAP Official Action. Summary of the practice parameters for the assessment and treatment of children, adolescents, and adults with ADHD. J Am Acad Child Adolesc Psychiatry. 32:1089–1098, 1997

Dulcan MK, Bregman J, Weller EB, Weller R: Treatment of childhood and adolescent disorders. In Schatzber AF and Nemeroft CB (eds): American Psychiatric Press Textbook of Psychopharmacology, 3rd ed. Washington, DC, American Psychiatric Press, 1997

Elia J, Borcherding BG, Rapoport JL, Keysor CS: Methylphenidate and dextroamphetamine treatments of hyperactivity: are there true nonresponders? Psychiatry Res 36:141–155, 1991

Emery G, Bedrosian R, Garber J: Cognitive therapy with depressed children and adolescents. In Cantwell DP, Carlson GA (eds): Affective Disorders in Childhood and Adolescence: An Update. New York, Spectrum Publications, 19:445–471, 1983

Emslie G, Weinberg W, Kowatch R, et al: A double-blind, placebo-controlled study of fluoxetine in depressed children and adolescents. Presentation at the Symposium on SSRIs in Children and Adolescents. Program Book, Annual Meeting of the New Clinical Drug Evaluation Unit (NCDEU), Orlando, Florida, May 31–June 3, 1995, p 26

Epstein LH, Coleman KJ, Myers MD: Exercise in treating obesity in children and adolescents. Med Sci Sports Exerc 28:428–435, 1996

Epstein LH, Valoski A, Wing RR, McCurley J: Ten-year follow-up of behavioral, family-based treatment for obese children. JAMA 264:2519–2523, 1990

Evans RW, Clay TH, Gualtieri CT: Carbamazepine in pediatric psychiatry. J Am Acad Child Adolesc Psychiatry 26:2–8, 1987

Evans RW, Gualtieri CT, Hicks RE: A neuropathic substrate for stimulant drug effects in hyperactive children. Clin Neuropharmacol 9:264–281, 1986

Famularo R, Kinscherff R, Fenton T: Propranolol treatment for childhood posttraumatic stress disorder, acute type. Am J Dis Child 142:1244–1247, 1988

Fenichel RR: Combining methylphenidate and clonidine: the role of post-marketing surveillance. J Am Acad Child Adolesc Psychiatry 5:155–156, 1995

Flament MF, Whitaker A, Rapoport JL, et al: Obsessive-compulsive disorder in adolescence: an epidemiological study. J Am Acad Child Adolesc Psychiatry 27:764–771, 1988

Forehand RL, McMahon RJ: Helping the Noncompliant Child: A Clinician's Guide to Parent Training. New York, Guilford Press, 1981

Fras I, Major LF: Clinical experience with risperidone. J Am Acad Child Adolesc Psychiatry 34:833, 1995

Gadow KD: Prevalence and efficacy of stimulant drug use with mentally retarded children and youth. Psychopharmacol Bull 21:291–303, 1985

Geller B, Cooper TB, Chestnut BS: Preliminary data on the relationship between nortriptyline plasma level and response in depressed children. Am J Psychiatry 143:1283–1286, 1986

Ghaziuddin N, Alessi NE: An open clinical trial of Trazodone in aggressive children. J Am Acad Child Adolesc Psychiatry 2:291–297, 1992

Graae F, Milner J, Rizzotto L, Klein RG: Clonazepam in childhood anxiety disorders. J Am Acad Child Adolesc Psychiatry 33:372–376, 1994

Green WH: Child and Adolescent Clinical Psychopharmacology. 2nd ed. Baltimore, Williams and Wilkins, 3–55, 1995

Greenhill LL, Solomon M, Pleak R, et al: Molindone hydrochloride treatment of hospitalized children with conduct disorder. J Clin Psychiatry 46:20–25, 1985

Grizenko N, Vida S: Propranolol treatment of episodic dyscontrol and aggressive behavior in children. Can J Psychiatry 33:776–778, 1988

Grob CS, Coyle JT: Suspected adverse methylphenidate-imipramine interactions in children. J Dev Behav Pediatr 7:265–267, 1986

Handen BL, Breaux AM, Janosky J: Effects and noneffects of methylphenidate in children with mental retardation and ADHD. J Am Acad Child Adolesc Psychiatry 31:455–461, 1992

Handen BL, Janosky J, McAuliffe S, et al: Prediction of response of methylphenidate among children with mental retardation and ADHD. J Am Acad Child Adolesc Psychiatry 33:1185–1193, 1994

Hardan A, Johnson K, Johnson C, Hrecznyj B: Case study: risperidone treatment of children and adolescents with developmental disorders. J Am Acad Child Adolesc Psychiatry 35:1551–1556, 1996

Henggeler SW, Borduin CM: Family Therapy and Beyond: A Multisystemic Approach to Treament of the Behavior Problems of Children and Adolescents. Pacific Grove, CA, Brooks/Cole, 1990

Herskowitz J: Development toxicology. In Popper C (ed): Psychiatric Pharmacosciences of Children and Adolescents. Washington, DC, American Psychiatric Press, 4:81–123, 1987

Horrigan JP, Barnhill LJ: Guanfacine for treatment of attention-deficit hyperactivity disorder in boys. J Child Adolesc Psychopharmacol 5:215–223, 1995

Hunt RD, Capper S, O'Connell P: Clonidine in child and adolescent psychiatry. J Child Adolesc Psychopharmacol 1:87–102, 1990

Hynes AFM, Vickar EL: Case study: neuroleptic malignant syndrome without pyrexia. J Am Acad Child Adolesc Psychiatry 35:959–962, 1996

Jacobsen LK, Giedd JN, Vaituzis AC, et al: Temporal lobe morphology in childhood-onset schizophrenia. Am J Psychiatry 153:355–361, 1996

Jensen PS, Hoagwood K, Petti T: Outcomes of mental health care for children and adolescents: II. Literature review and application of a comprehensive model. J Am Acad Child Adolesc Psychiatry 35:1064–1077, 1996

Johnston HF, Fruehling JJ: Using antidepressant medication in depressed children: an algorithm. Psychiatr Ann 24:348–356, 1994

Kafantaris V, Campbell M, Padron-Gayol MV, et al: Carbamazepine in hospitalized aggressive conduct disorder children: an open pilot study. Psychopharmacol Bull 28:193–199, 1992

Kagan J, Reznick JS, Snidman N: Biological bases of childhood shyness. Science 240:167–171, 1988

Kashani JH, Carlson GA, Beck NC, et al: Depression, depressive symptoms, and depressed mood among a community sample of adolescents. Am J Psychiatry 144:931–934, 1987

Kashani JH, Orvaschel H: A community study of anxiety in children and adolescents. Am J Psychiatry 147:313–318, 1990

Kazdin AE, Siegel TC, Bass D: Cognitive problem-solving skills training and parent management training in the treatment antisocial behavior in children. J Consult Clin Psychol 60:733–747, 1992

Kemph JP, DeVane Cl, Levin GM, et al: Treatment of aggressive children with clonidine: results of an open pilot study. J Am Acad Child Adolesc Psychiatry 32:577–581, 1993

Kendall PC, Braswell L: Cognitive-Behavioral Therapy for Impulsive Children. New York, Guilford Press, 1985

Kernberg PF, Chazan SE: Children with Conduct Disorders: A Psychotherapy Manual. New York, Basic Books, 1991

King RA, Riddle MA, Chappell PB, et al: Emergence of self-destructive phenomena in children and adolescents during fluoxetine treatment. J Am Acad Child Adolesc Psychiatry 30:179–186, 1991

Klauber GT: Clinical efficacy and safety of desmopressin in the treatment of nocturnal enuresis. J Pediatr 114:719–722, 1989

Kolman BK, Feldman HM, Handen BL, Janosky JE: Naltrexone in young autistic children: a double blind, placebo-controlled cross-over study. J Am Acad Child Adolesc Psychiatry 34:223–231, 1995

Kovacs M, Feinberg TL, Crouse-Novak MA, et al: Depressive disorders in childhood: I. A longitudinal prospective study of characteristics and recovery. Arch Gen Psychiatry 41:229–237, 1984a

Kovacs M, Feinberg TL, Crouse-Novak MA, et al: Depressive disorders in childhood: II. A longitudinal study of the risk for a subsequent major depression. Arch Gen Psychiatry 41:643–649, 1984b

Kumra S, Frazier JA, Jacobsen LK, et al: Childhood-onset schizophrenia: a double bind clozapine-haloperidol comparison. Arch Gen Psychiatry 53:1090–1097, 1996

Kuperman S, Johnson B, Arndt S, et al: Quantitative EEG differences in a nonclinical sample of children with ADHD and undifferentiated ADD. J Am Acad Child Adolesc Psychiatry 35:1009–1017, 1996

Kutcher SP, MacKenzie S, Galarraga W, Szalai J: Clonazepam treatment of adolescents with neuroleptic-induced akathisia. Am J Psychiatry 144:823–824, 1987

Kutcher SP, Marton P: Parameters of adolescent depression: a review. Psychiatr Clin North Am 12:895–918, 1989

Kutcher SP, Reiter S, Gardner DM, et al: The pharmacotherapy of anxiety disorders in children and adolescents. Psychiatr Clin North Am 15:41–67, 1992

Lambroso PJ, Scahill L, King RA, et al: Risperidone treatment of children and adolescents with chronic tic disorders: a preliminary report. J Am Acad Child Adolesc Psychiatry 34:1147–1152, 1995

Last CG, Perrin S, Hersen M, Kazdin AE: A prospective study of childhood anxiety disorders. J Am Acad Child Adolesc Psychiatry 35:1502–1510, 1996

Last CG, Strauss CC, Francis G: Comorbidity among childhood anxiety disorders. J Nerv Ment Dis 175:726–730, 1987

Latz SR, McCracken JT: Neuroleptic malignant syndrome in children and adolescents: two case reports and a warning. J Child Adolesc Psychopharmacol 2:123–129, 1992

Laughren TP: Regulatory issues in pediatric psychopharmacology. J Am Acad Child Adolesc Psychiatry 10:1276–1282, 1996

Leckman JF, Ort S, Caruso, et al: Rebound phenomena in Tourette's syndrome after abrupt withdrawal of clonidine. Arch Gen Psychiatry 43:1168–1176, 1986

Leonard HL, March L, Rickler KC, Allen AJ: Pharmacology of the selective serotonin reuptake inhibitors in children and adolescents. J Am Acad Child Adolesc Psychiatry 36:725–736, 1997

Leonard HL, Meyer MC, Swedo SE, et al: Electrocardiographic changes during desipramine and clomipramine treatment in children and adolescents. J Am Acad Child Adolesc Psychiatry 34:1460–1468, 1995

Liberthson RR: Sudden death from cardiac causes in children and young adults. N Engl J Med 334:1039–1044, 1996

Loeber R: Development and risk factors of juvenile antisocial behavior and delinquency. Clin Psychol Rev 10:1–41, 1990

Lombroso PJ, Pauls DL, Leckman JF: Genetic mechanisms in childhood psychiatric disorders. J Am Acad Child Adolesc Psychiatry 33:921–938, 1994

Loof D, Grimley P, Kuller F, et al: Carbamazepine for PTSD. J Am Acad Child Psychiatry 34:703–704, 1995

Lyons JA: Posttraumatic stress disorder in children and adolescents: a review of the literature. Dev Behav Pediatr 8:349–356, 1987

Mandoki MW: Risperidone treatment of children and adolescents: increased risk of extrapyramidal side effects? J Child Adolesc Psychopharmacol 5:49–67, 1995

March JS, Mulle K, Herbel B: Behavioral psychotherapy for children and adolescents with obsessive–compulsive disorder: an open trial of new protocol-driven treatment package. J Am Acad Child Psychiatry 33:333–341, 1994

Marriage K, Fine S, Moretti M, Haley G: Relationship between depression and conduct disorder in children and adolescents. J Am Acad Child Adolesc Psychiatry 25:687–691, 1986

Masek BJ, Spirito A, Fentress DW: Behavioral treatment of symptoms of childhood illness. Clin Psychol Rev 4:561–570, 1984

Mayes SC, Humphrey FJ, Handford HA, Mitchell JF: Rumination disorder: differential diagnosis. J Am Acad Child Adolesc Psychiatry 27:300–302, 1988

McConville BJ, Minnery KL, Sorter MT, et al: An open study of the effects of sertaline on adolescent major depression. J Child Adolesc Psychopharmacol 6:41–51, 1996

McDaniel KD: Pharmacologic treatment of psychiatric and neurodevelopmental disorders in children and adolescents (Part 1). Clin Pediatr 25:65–71, 1986

McKenna K, Gordon GT, Rapaport JL: Childhood-onset schizophrenia: timely neurobiological research. J Am Acad Child Adolesc Psychiatry 33:771–781, 1994

Melamed BG, Klingman A, Siegel LJ: Individualizing cognitive behavioral strategies in the reduction of medical and dental stress. In Meyers AW, Craighead WE (eds): Cognitive Behavior Therapy with Children. New York, Plenum Press, 1984

Milich R, Wolraich M, Lindgren S: Sugar and hyperactivity: a critical review of empirical findings. Clin Psychol Rev 6:493–513, 1986

Mufson L, Moreau D, Weisman MM, Klerman G: Interpersonal Therapy for Depressed Adolescents. New York, Guilford, 1993

Ollendick TH, Francis G: Behavioral assessment and treatment of childhood phobias. Behav Modif 12:165–204, 1988

O'Regan S, Yazbeck S, Hamberger B, Schick E: Constipation: a commonly unrecognized cause of enuresis. Am J Dis Child 140:260–261, 1986

Patterson GR: Families: Applications of Social Learning to Family Life. Champaign, IL, Research Press, 1975

Patterson GR, DeBaryshe BD, Ramsey E: A developmental perspective on antisocial behavior. Am Psychol 44:329–335, 1989

Pelco LE, Kissel RC, Parrish JM, Miltenberger RG: Behavioral management of oral medication administration difficulties among children: a review of literature with case illustrations. Dev Behav Pediatr 8:90–96, 1987

Pelham WE, Greenslade KE, Vodde-Hamilton M, et al: Relative efficacy of long-acting stimulants on children with attention-deficit hyperactivity disorder: a comparison of standard methylphenidate, sustained-release methylphenidate, sustained-release dextroamphetamine, and pemoline. Pediatrics 86:226–237, 1990

Pelham WE, Hoza J: Behavioral assessment of psychostimulant effects on ADD children in a summer day treatment program. Adv Behav Assess Child Fam 3:3–34, 1987

Pelham WE, Murphy HA: Attention deficit and conduct disorders. In Hersen M (ed): Pharmacological and Behavioral Treatment: An Integrative Approach. New York, John Wiley & Sons, 6:108–148, 1986

Pelham WE, Sturges J, Hoza J, et al: The effects of sustained release 20 and 10 mg Ritalin b.i.d. on cognitive and social behavior in children with attention deficit disorder. Pediatrics 80:491–501, 1987

Peterson BS: Neuroimaging in child and adolescent neuropsychiatric disorders. J Am Acad Child Adolesc Psychiatry 12:1560–1576, 1995

Peterson SE, Myers KM, McClellan J, Crow S: Neuroleptic malignant syndrome: three adolescents with complicated courses. J Child Adolesc Psychopharmacol 5:139–149, 1995

Pfefferbaum B, Overall JE, Boren HA, et al: Alprazolam in the treatment of anticipatory and acute situational anxiety in children with cancer. J Am Acad Child Adolesc Psychiatry 26:532–535, 1987

Piven J, Arndt S, Bailey J, Andreasen N: Regional brain enlargement in autism: a magnetic resonance study. J Am Acad Child Adolesc Psychiatry 35:530–536, 1996

Pleak RR, Birmaher B, Gavrilescu A, et al: Mania and neuropsychiatric excitation following carbamazepine. J Am Acad Child Adolesc Psychiatry 27:500–503, 1988

Popper CW, Zimmitzky B: Sudden death putatively related to desipramine treatment in youth: a fifth case and review of speculative mechanisms. J Child Adolesc Psychopharmacol 5:283–300, 1995

Preskorn SH, Weller EB, Hughes CW, Weller RA: Relationship of plasma imipramine levels to CNS toxicity in children. Am J Psychiatry 145:897, 1988

Preskorn SH, Weller EB, Hughes CW, et al: Depression in prepubertal children: dexamethasone nonsuppression predicts differential response to imipramine vs. placebo. Psychopharmacol Bull 23:128–133, 1987

Puig-Antich J: Major depression and conduct disorder in prepuberty. J Am Acad Child Adolesc Psychiatry 21:118–128, 1982

Puig-Antich J, Lukens E, Davies M, et al: Psychosocial functioning in prepubertal major depressive disorders: II. Interpersonal relationships after sustained recovery from affective episode. Arch Gen Psychiatry 42:511–517, 1985

Pynoos RS, Eth S: Witness to violence: the child interview. J Am Acad Child Adolesc Psychiatry 25:306–319, 1986

Pynoos RS, Frederick C, Nader K, et al: Life threat and posttraumatic stress in school-age children. Arch Gen Psychiatry 44:1057–1063, 1987

Quintana H, Keshavan M: Case study: risperidone in children and adolescents with schizophrenia. J Am Acad Child Adolesc Psychiatry 34:1292–1296, 1995

Realmuto GM, Erickson WD, Yellin AM, et al: Clinical comparison of thiothixene and thioridazine in schizophrenic adolescents. Am J Psychiatry 141:440–442, 1984

Reiter S, Kutcher S, Gardner D: Anxiety disorders in children and adolescents: clinical and related issues in pharmacological treatment. Can J Psychiatry 37:432–438, 1992

Riddle MA, Geller B, Ryan N: Another sudden death in a child treated with desipramine. J Am Acad Child Adolesc Psychiatry 32:792–797, 1993

Riddle MA, King RA, Hardin MT, et al: Behavioral side effects of fluoxetine in children and adolescents. J Child Adolesc Psychopharmacol 5:205–214, 1995

Rutter M: Syndromes attributed to "Minimal Brain Dysfunction" in childhood. Am J Psychiatry 139:21–33, 1982

Ryan ND: Heterocyclic antidepressants in children and adolescents. J Child Adolesc Psychopharmacol 1:21–31, 1990

Ryan ND: The pharmacologic treatment of child and adolescent depression. Psychiatr Clin North Am 15:29–40, 1992

Ryan N, Meyer VA, Dachille S, et al: Lithium antidepressant augmentation in TCA-refractory depression in adolescents. J Am Acad Child Adolesc Psychiatry 27:371–376, 1988a

Ryan ND, Puig-Antich J, Rabinovich H, et al: MAOIs in adolescent major depression unresponsive to tricyclic antidepressants. J Am Acad Child Adolesc Psychiatry 27:755–758, 1988b

Ryan ND, Williamson DE, Iyengar S, et al: A secular increase in child and adolescent onset affective disorder. J Am Acad Child Adolesc Psychiatry 31:600–605, 1992

Safer DJ, Krager JM: A survey of medication treatment for hyperactive/inattentive students. JAMA 260:2256–2258, 1988

Schuster CR, Lewis M, Seiden LS: Fenfluramine: neurotoxicity. Psychopharmacol Bull 22:148–151, 1986

Shaywitz SE, Shaywitz BA, Fletcher JM, Escobar MD: Prevalence of reading disability in boys and girls: results of the Connecticut Longitudinal Study. JAMA 264:998–1002, 1990

Simeon JG, Carrey NJ, Wiggins DM, et al: Risperidone effects in treatment resistant adolescents: preliminary case reports. J Child Adolesc Psychopharmacol 5:69–79, 1995

Simeon JG, Ferguson HB: Recent developments in the use of antidepressant and anxiolytic medications. Psychiatr Clin North Am 8:893–907, 1985

Simeon JG, Ferguson HB, Fleet JVW: Buproprion exacerbates tics in children with attention-deficit hyperactivity and Tourette's syndrome. J Am Acad Child Adolesc Psychiatry 26:285–290, 1990

Simeon JG, Ferguson HB, Knott V, et al: Clinical, cognitive, and neurophysiological effects of alprazolam in children and adolescents with overanxious and avoidant disorders. J Am Acad Child Adolesc Psychiatry 31:29–33, 1992

Simeon JG, Knott V, Dubois C, et al: Buspirone therapy of mixed anxiety disorders in childhood and adolescence: a pilot study. J Child Adolesc Psychopharmacol 4:159–170, 1994

Spencer TJ, Biederman J, Harding M, et al: Growth deficits in ADHD children revisited: evidence of disorder associated growth delays? J Am Acad Child Adolesc Psychiatry 35:1460–1469, 1996

Steingard RJ, Renshaw PF, Yurgelun-Todd D, et al: Structural abnormalities in brain magnetic resonance images of depressed children. J Am Acad Child Adolesc Psychiatry 35:307–311, 1996

Strayhorn JM, Rapp N, Donina W, Strain PS: Randomized trial of methylphenidate for an autistic child. J Am Acad Child Adolesc Psychiatry 27:244–247, 1988

Strober M, Carlson G: Bipolar illness in adolescents with major depression: clinical, genetic, and psychopharmacologic predictors in a three- to four-year prospective follow-up investigation. Arch Gen Psychiatry 39:549–555, 1982

Terr LC: Chowchilla revisited: the effects of psychic trauma four years after a school-bus kidnaping. Am J Psychiatry 140:1543–1550, 1983

Terr LC: Childhood psychic trauma. In Call JD, Cohen RL, Harrison SI, Berlin IN, Stone LA (eds): Basic Handbook of Child Psychiatry, Vol. V. New York, Basic Books, Vol. 5, Ch. 44, 414–420, 1979

Terr LC: Treatment of psychic trauma in children. In Call JD, Cohen RL, Harrison SI, Berlin IN, Stone LA (eds): Basic Handbook of Child Psychiatry, Vol. V. New York, Basic Books, 1987b

Valleni-Basile LA, Garrison CZ, Jackson KL, et al: Frequency of obsessive-compulsive disorder in a community sample of young adolescents. J Am Acad Child Adolesc Psychiatry 33:782–791, 1994

Valleni-Basile LA, Garrison CZ, Waller JL, et al: Incidence of obsessive-compulsive disorder in a community sample of young adolescents. J Am Acad Child Adolesc Psychiatry 35:898–906, 1996

Varley CK: Effects of methylphenidate in adolescents with attention deficit disorder. J Am Acad Child Psychiatry 4:351–354, 1983

Varni JW, Jay SM, Masek BJ, et al: Cognitive-behavioral assessment and management of pediatric pain. In Holvman AD, Turk ED (eds): Handbook of Psychological Treatment Approaches. New York, Pergamon Press, 1986

Venkataraman S, Naylor MW, King CA: Mania associated with fluoxetine treatment in adolescents. J Am Acad Child Adolesc Psychiatry 31:276–281, 1992

Watkins JM, Asarnow RF, Tanguay PE: Symptom development in childhood onset schizophrenia. J Child Psychol Psychiatry 29:865–878, 1988

Weller EB, Weller RA, Fristad MA: Lithium dosage guide for prepubertal children: a preliminary report. J Am Acad Child Psychiatry 25:92–95, 1986

Weller EB, Weller RA, Fristad MA: Bipolar disorder in children: misdiagnosis, underdiagnosis, and future directions. J Am Acad Child Psychiatry 34:709–714, 1995

Wender EH: The food additive-free diet in the treatment of behavior disorders: a review. J Dev Behav Pediatr 7:35–42, 1986

Werry JS, Aman MG (eds): Practitioner's Guide to Psychoactive Drugs for Children and Adolescents. New York, Plenum Medical Book Company, 3–21, 1993

West SA, Keck PE, McElroy SL, et al: Open trial of valproate in the treatment of adolescent mania. J Child Adolesc Psychopharmacol 4:263–267, 1994

Wilens TE, Biederman J, Baldessarini R, et al: Cardiovascular effects of therapeutic doses of tricyclic antidepressants in children and adolescents. J Am Acad Child Adolesc Psychiatry 35:1491–1501, 1996

Willemsen-Swinkels SH, Buitelar JK, Weijnen FG, Van Engeland H: Placebo-controlled acute dosage naltrexone study in young autistic children. Psychiatry Res 16:203–215, 1995

Williams DT: Hypnosis as a psychotherapeutic adjunct. In Harrison SI (ed): Basic Handbook of Child Psychiatry, Vol. 3. New York, Basic Books: Vol. 3, Ch. 6, 108–116, 1979

Williams DT, Mehl R, Yudofsky S, et al: The effect of propranolol on uncontrolled rage outbursts in children and adolescents with organic brain dysfunction. J Am Acad Child Psychiatry 21:129–135, 1982

Wolraich ML, Wilson DB, White JW: The effect of sugar on behavior or cognition in children: a meta-analysis. JAMA 274:1617–1621, 1995

Zohar AH, Ratzoni G, Paul DL, et al: An epidemiological study of obsessive compulsive disorder and related disorders in Israeli adolescents. J Am Acad Child Psychiatry 31:1057–1061, 1992

17 The Psychotherapies: Basic Theoretical Principles and Techniques

Robert J. Ursano,
Edward K. Silberman,
and Alberto Diaz, Jr.

Psychotherapy is the "talking cure." Through the use of words to create understanding, guidance, and support and lead the patient to new experiences, the psychotherapist aims to eliminate symptoms and increase the patient's productivity and enjoyment of life. The brain itself is the target of psychotherapy. Behavior, thoughts, and emotions derive from brain activity and have a neuroanatomical, neurochemical, and neurophysiological basis. The psychotherapies aim to alter brain "patterning" and function. Psychopathology frequently limits a patient's ability to see and experience options and choices. The patients' behaviors, thoughts, and feelings are constricted by their psychiatric illness. Through the various psychotherapies, the therapist attempts to increase the patients' insight into their own lives and their range of behavioral options and decrease painful constricting symptoms.

Psychotherapeutic approaches to psychopathology vary widely and reflect different concepts and theories of mental life, personality development, abnormal behavior, and the role of environmental and biological determinants. Psychotherapy is both cost effective and efficacious (Lazar, 1998). Recent studies show that patients receiving psychotherapy achieve significant benefits when compared to controls. The increasing understanding of the nature of the interaction of human beings with each other as individuals and as members of social groups has facilitated the application of some of the principles of mental life and behavior to the psychotherapeutic relationship as a treatment tool. Experience indicates that an *integrated* approach to treatment is the most successful strategy, combining medications with psychological therapy. Different patients benefit from different types of psychotherapy, just as they may benefit from different types of psychotropic medications. Because of this, the medically trained psychiatrist can provide the most comprehensive evaluation for combining medication with psychotherapeutic treatment. The psychiatrist can use combined medication and psychotherapeutic treatments and is trained to recognize and manage the potential interactions of these two treatments. The psychiatrist also is alert to changes in the patient's medical status that can be a cause of or a result of psychiatric illness. Patients with significant medical illness as part of their health history (e.g., migraine, ulcers, psychosomatic illnesses, and so forth) are best treated by the psychiatrist who, as a physician, is knowledgable of these disorders and their effects on feelings, behaviors, and life adjustment and is a skilled psychotherapist. Often, the seriously depressed or psychotic patient may also be more comfortable with a psychiatrist, who is trained in managing life-and-death issues, chronic illness, and the medical side effects of medication.

In the following pages, the major psychotherapies are reviewed. An understanding of these techniques and their theoretical concepts used in patient selection is important to the treatment armamentarium of inpatient, outpatient, and consultation–liaison psychiatric practices, as well as general medical practice.

PSYCHOANALYTIC PSYCHOTHERAPIES

Psychoanalysis

Psychoanalysis was developed by Sigmund Freud in the late 19th century. Freud found that his patients' life difficulties were related to unrecognized (unconscious) conflicts that arise in the course of child development and continue into adult life. Such conflicts are typically between libidinal (sexual and/or emotional) and aggressive wishes and the fear of loss, condemnation retaliation, the constraints of reality, or the opposition of other incompatible wishes. "Libidinal wishes" are longings for both sexual and emotional gratification. Sexual gratification in psychoanalysis refers to the broad concept of bodily pleasure, the state of excitement and pleasure experienced by various bodily sensations beginning in infancy. Aggressive wishes may be either primary destructive impulses or arise in reaction to perceived frustration, deprivation, or attack. Such (neurotic) conflicts may give rise to a variety of manifestations in adulthood, including anxiety, depression, and somatic symptoms, as well as work, social, or sexual inhibitions and maladaptive ways of relating to other people.

The goal of psychoanalysis is to understand the nature of the patient's childhood conflicts (the "infantile neurosis") and their consequences in adult life. This goal is accomplished through reexperiencing these conflicts in relation to the analyst (the "transference neurosis"). This is a major undertaking that requires a great deal of the patient to sustain the treatment. Psychoanalytic patients must be able to access their fantasy lives in an active and experiencing manner and be able to "leave it behind" at the end of a session. Psychoanalysis is frequently criticized for being used to treat reasonably healthy people; however, all medical treatments require certain innate capacities of the patient (e.g., an intact immune system for successful antibiotic therapy) for the patient to use the treatment successfully and not be injured by it. As with a generally healthy person with a relatively focal, yet painful physical disorder that impairs their functioning, a generally healthy person may have painful neurotic conflicts that interfere with both their work and personal life and, therefore, require treatment.

Psychoanalysis focuses on the recovery of childhood experiences as they are recreated in the relationship with the analyst (Sandler et al, 1973). This recreation in the doctor–patient relationship of the conflicted relationship with a childhood figure is called the "transference neurosis" (Table 17–1). In the therapeutic relationship with the analyst, the emotional conflicts and trauma from the past are relived. The feelings and conflicts that were part of the relationship with major figures in the child's development, most frequently the parents, are "transferred" to the analyst. When the transference neurosis is present, the patient emotionally experiences and reacts to the analyst in a very real manner "as if" the analyst was the significant figure from the past. Frequently, this experience is accompanied by other elements of the past being experienced in the patient's life. Countertransference, the analyst's transference response to the patient, is increased by life stress and unresolved conflicts in the analyst. It can appear as either an identification with or a reaction to the patient's conscious and unconscious fantasies, feelings, and behaviors (Racker, 1968). Understanding their own countertransference reactions can allow

Table 17–1 **Psychoanalysis**

Goal	Resolution of symptoms and major reworking of personality structures related to childhood conflicts
Patient selection criteria	No psychotic potential
	Able to use understanding
	High ego strength
	Able to experience and observe intense emotional states
	Psychiatric problem derived from childhood conflicts
Techniques	Focus on fantasies and the transference
	Free association
	Couch
	Interpretation of defenses and transference
	Frequent meetings
	Neutrality of the analyst
Duration	3–6 years

analysts to recognize subtle aspects of the transference relationship and to understand the patient's experience better.

Psychoanalytic treatment attempts to set up a therapeutic situation in which the patient's observing capacity can be used to analyze the transference neurosis. *Transference reactions occur throughout life in all areas and are a frequent accompaniment of the doctor–patient relationship in the medical setting;* however, psychoanalysis is unique in its efforts to establish a setting in which the transference, when it appears, can be analyzed and worked through in an intense manner to facilitate recovery from psychiatric illness by understanding patterns of feelings, fantasies, and interpersonal behaviors.

Modern psychoanalysis requires four to five sessions a week (45 to 50 minutes per session) continued, on the average, for 3 to 6 years. This frequency of sessions is necessary for patients to develop sufficient trust to explore their inner life and their subjective experience. Likewise, given the number of events that occur daily in one's lifetime, the frequent meetings are necessary for the patient to be able to explore fantasies, dreams, and reactions to the analytic situation instead of focusing only on daily reality-based crises and stresses. Individuals who are in severe crisis and are, therefore, focused on the crises in their life, are generally not candidates for psychoanalysis. If major crises do occur during analysis, formal analysis may be temporarily suspended for a more supportive psychotherapeutic approach. In general, psychoanalytic patients are encouraged to use a recumbent position on the couch to facilitate their ability to freely associate and verbalize their thoughts and feelings. In addition, the analyst usually sits out of the patient's view to assist the process of *free association.*

Free association, the reporting of all thoughts that come to mind, is a core technique in psychoanalytic treatment. Free association is difficult to attain, and much of the work of psychoanalysis is based on identifying those times when free association breaks down (the occurrence of a defense, clinically experienced by the analyst as "resistance"). When the patient is able to free associate easily, the neurotic conflicts have been largely removed and the termination of treatment is near.

Early in treatment, the analyst establishes a *therapeutic alliance* with the patient that allows for a reality-based consideration of the demands of the treatment and for a working collaboration between analyst and analysand (patient) directed toward understanding the patient. The analyst points out the defenses the patient uses to minimize awareness of conflicts and disturbing feelings. Dreams, slips of the tongue, and symptoms provide avenues to the understanding of unconscious motivations, feelings, and ideas.

The specific treatment effects of psychoanalysis result from the progressive understanding of defensive patterns and, most important, the feelings, cognitions, and behaviors that are "transferred" to the analyst from patterns of relationships with significant individuals in the patient's past. In the context of the arousal associated with the reexperiencing of these figures from the past and the simultaneous understanding of the experience, behavioral change occurs. Interpretation is an important technical procedure in this process. An interpretation links the patient's current experience with the analyst to an experience with a significant childhood figure during development.

The analyst operates under several rules that facilitate the analysis of the transference. These include the *rule of neutrality,* by which the analyst favors neither the patient's wishes (id) nor the condemnations of these wishes (superego), and the *rule of abstinence,* whereby the analyst does not provide to the patient emotional gratification similar to that of the wished-for childhood figure.

Medications are infrequently used in psychoanalysis, although some analysts are increasingly integrating psychoanalytic treatment with medication, particularly for mood disorders. In these cases, psychoanalysis is directed toward aiding the change in behaviors that may have been learned over a long time and may be interfering with the return of good psychosocial functioning. In general, however, the necessity for the use of medication may indicate the patient's need for greater support and structure than can be provided in the psychoanalytic treatment.

The assessment of a patient for psychoanalysis must include diagnostic considerations, as well as an assessment of the patient's ability to make use of the psychoanalytic situation for behavior change. A patient's ability to use psychoanalysis depends on the patient's psychological mindedness, the availability of supports in their real environment to sustain the psychoanalysis, which can be felt as quite depriving, and the patient's ability to experience and simultaneously observe highly charged emotional states. Because of the frequency of the sessions and the duration of the treatment, the cost of psychoanalysis can be prohibitive; however, low-fee training clinics frequently make a substantial amount of treatment available to some patients who could not otherwise afford it. Psychoanalysis has been useful in the treatment of obsessional disorders, conversion disorders, anxiety disorders, dysthymic disorders, and moderately severe personality disorders. Individuals with chaotic life settings and an inability to establish long-term, close relationships are usually not good candidates for psychoanalysis. In the present cost-effective climate, psychoanalysis is more frequently recommended after a course of brief psychotherapy has proved either ineffective or insufficient. Little empirical research is available on the efficacy of psychoanalysis compared with other psychotherapies. In general, those patients who can use understanding, introspection, and self-observation to modify their behavior find the treatment beneficial and productive.

Intensive (Long-Term) Psychoanalytically Oriented Psychotherapy

Psychoanalytically oriented psychotherapy, also known as psychoanalytic psychotherapy, psychodynamic psychotherapy, and explorative psychotherapy, is a psychotherapeutic procedure that recognizes the concepts of transference and resistance in the psychotherapy setting (Bruch, 1974; Reichmann, 1950). Both long-term and brief psychodynamic psychotherapy are possible. (See following section for brief psychodynamic psychotherapy.) Psychoanalytic psychotherapy is usually more focused than is the extensive reworking of personality undertaken in psychoanalysis. In addition, psychoanalytic psychotherapy is somewhat more "here and now" oriented, with less attempt to reconstruct the developmental origins of conflicts completely.

The psychoanalytic techniques of interpretation and clarification are central to psychoanalytic psychotherapy. Psychoanalytic psychotherapy makes more use of supportive techniques—such as suggestion, reality testing, education, and confrontation—than does psychoanalysis. This allows for its application to a broader range of patients, including those with the potential for severe regression.

Patients in long-term psychoanalytic psychotherapy are usually seen one, two, or three times a week. Patient and therapist meet in face-to-face encounters with free association encouraged. Psychoanalytic psychotherapy may extend for several months to several years, at times being as long as a psychoanalysis. The length is determined by the number of focal problem areas undertaken in the treatment. Medications can be used in psychoanalytic psychotherapy and may provide another means of titrating the level of regression (the experience of feelings, thoughts, and actions from childhood being readily accessed) a patient may experience.

The same patients who are treated in psychoanalysis can be treated in psychoanalytic psychotherapy (Table 17–2). The psychosocial problems and internal conflicts of patients who cannot be treated in psychoanalysis, such as those with major depression, schizophrenia, and borderline personality disor-

Table 17–2 **Psychoanalytically Oriented Psychotherapy**

Goal	Understanding conflict area and particular defense mechanisms used
	More "here and now" than psychoanalysis
Patient selection criteria	Similar to psychoanalysis
	Also includes personality disorders with psychotic potential (Borderline, Narcissistic)
	Some major depressions and schizophrenia may be helped when combined with medication during periods of remission for the treatment of psychosocial features
Techniques	Face to face–sitting up
	Free association
	Interpretation and clarification
	Some supportive techniques
	Medication as adjunct
Duration	Months to years

der, can be addressed in a long-term psychoanalytic psychotherapy. In long-term psychoanalytic psychotherapy, the regressive tendencies of such patients can be controlled with greater support, medication, and reality feedback through the face-to-face encounter with the therapist. Few empirical data are available on the efficacy of psychoanalytically oriented psychotherapy, although it is highly valued by many clinicians and patients. Recent studies tend to support the importance of working with the transference to create behavioral change (Luborsky and Crits-Cristoph, 1990). Interpersonal psychotherapy (IPT) (Klerman et al, 1984) has many psychodynamic principles and has been shown to be effective in studies using combined psychotherapy and medication interventions.

Brief Psychodynamic Psychotherapy

Following World War II, there was a rapid growth in the demand for psychotherapy that considerably increased the pressure upon psychiatrists to develop briefer forms of psychotherapy. In addition, the community mental health movement and, more recently, the increasing cost of mental health care and managed care have stimulated efforts to find briefer forms of psychotherapy. Brief psychotherapy is a necessary, efficacious, and central part of the psychiatrist's armamentarium (Crits-Christoph, 1992).

The goals of brief psychotherapy are described by most authors as facilitation of health-seeking behaviors and the mitigation of obstacles to normal growth. From this perspective, brief psychotherapy focuses on the patient's continuous development throughout adult life in the context of conflicts relating to environment, interpersonal relationships, biological health, and developmental stages. This picture of brief psychotherapy supports modest goals and the avoidance of "perfectionism" by the therapist.

While many of the selection criteria emphasized in the literature of brief psychotherapy are common to all kinds of psychodynamic psychotherapy, certain unique selection criteria are required because of the brief duration of treatment (Table 17–3). Patients in brief psychodynamic psychotherapy must be able to engage quickly with the therapist and terminate therapy in a short period. The necessity of greater independent action by the patient mandates high levels of emotional strength, motivation, and responsiveness to interpretation. The importance of rapidly establishing the therapeutic alliance underlies a substantial number of the selection and exclusion criteria.

Some exclusion criteria for brief psychotherapy were developed by Malan (1975). He excludes patients who have had serious suicidal attempts, drug addiction, long-term hospitalization, more than one course of electroconvulsive therapy (ECT), chronic alcoholism, severe chronic obsessional symptoms, severe chronic phobic symptoms, or gross destructive or self-destructive behavior. Patients who are unavailable for therapeutic contact or those who need prolonged work to generate motivation, penetrate rigid defenses, deal with complex

Table 17–3 **Brief Psychodynamic Psychotherapy**

Goal	Clarify and resolve focal area of conflict that interferes with current functioning
Patient selection criteria	High ego strength
	High motivation
	Can identify local issue
	Can form strong interpersonal relationships, including with therapist, in a brief time
	Good response to trial interpretations
Techniques	Face to face
	Interpretation of defenses and transference
	Setting of time limit at start of therapy
	Focus on patient reactions to limited duration of treatment
Duration	12–40 sessions; usually 20 sessions or less

or deep-seated issues, or resolve intense transference reactions are also not likely to benefit from brief psychotherapy and may have negative side effects.

The importance of focusing on a circumscribed area of current conflict in brief psychotherapy is mentioned by most authors (Davanloo, 1980; Malan, 1975; Mann, 1973; Sifneos, 1972). They also emphasize the importance of the evaluation sessions to determine the focus of treatment. The formulation of the focus to the patient may be, for example, in terms of the patient's conscious fears and pain, but it is important for the therapist to construct the psychodynamic focus at a deeper level to understand the work being done. Maintaining the focus is the primary task of the therapist. This enables the therapist to deal with complicated personality structures in a brief period of time. Resistance is limited through "benign neglect" of potentially troublesome but nonfocal areas of personality. The elaboration of techniques of establishing and maintaining the focus of treatment is critical to all brief individual psychodynamic psychotherapies.

Transference interpretations (that is, making comments that link the patient's reactions to the therapist to feelings for significant individuals from the patient's past) are generally accepted as important in brief psychotherapy; however, the manner and rapidity in which transference is dealt with varies considerably.

There is remarkable agreement on the duration of brief psychotherapy. Although the duration ranges from 5 to 40 sessions, authors generally favor 10 to 20 sessions. The duration of treatment is critically related to maintaining the focus within the brief psychotherapy. When treatment extends beyond 20 sessions, therapists frequently find themselves enmeshed in a broad character analysis without a focal conflict. Change after 20 sessions may be quite slow. Clinical experience generally supports the idea that brief individual psychodynamic psychotherapy should be between 10 and 20 sessions unless the therapist is willing to proceed to long-term treatment of greater than 40 or 50 sessions.

COGNITIVE PSYCHOTHERAPY

Cognitive psychotherapy is a method of brief psychotherapy developed over the last two decades by Aaron T. Beck and his colleagues at the University of Pennsylvania primarily for the treatment of mild and moderate depressions and for patients with low self-esteem (Beck, 1976; Rush and Beck, 1988). It is similar to behavior therapy in that it aims at the direct removal of symptoms rather than the resolution of underlying conflicts, as in the psychodynamic psychotherapies; however, unlike traditional behavioral approaches, the subjective experience of the patient is a major focus of the work. Cognitive therapists view the patient's conscious thoughts as central to producing and perpetuating symptoms such as depression, anxiety, phobias, and somatization. Both the content of thoughts and thought processes are seen as disordered in people with such symptoms. Therapy is directed toward identifying and altering these cognitive distortions.

The cognitive therapist sees the interpretations that depressed persons make about life as different from those of nondepressed individuals. Depressed people tend to make negative interpretations of the world, themselves, and the future (the negative cognitive triad). Depressed individuals interpret events as reflecting defeat, deprivation, or disparagement and see their lives as filled with obstacles and burdens. They view themselves as unworthy, deficient, undesirable, or worthless, and they see the future as bringing a continuation of the miseries of the present. These evaluations are the result of the negative biases inherent in depressive thinking and applied regardless of the objective nature of the individual's circumstances. Other psychiatric conditions have their own characteristic cognitive patterns that determine the nature of the symptoms. The "thinking" distortions in depression include arbitrary inferences about an event, selective use of details to reach a conclusion, overgeneralization, overestimating negative and underestimating positive aspects of a situation, and the tendency to label events according to one's emotional response rather than the facts.

Such cognitions (verbal thoughts) often feel involuntary and automatic. This kind of thinking is so automatic in response to many situations—and the resultant cognitions so fleeting—that people may often be virtually unaware of them. Such automatic thoughts differ from unconscious thoughts in that they can easily be made fully conscious if attention is directed to them. A large portion of the work of cognitive psychotherapy is to train patients to observe and record their automatic thoughts.

Cognitive theory postulates a chronic state of depression-proneness that may precede the actual illness and remain after the symptoms have abated. Depression-prone individuals have relatively permanent depressive cognitive structures ("cognitive schemas") that determine how new stimuli are perceived and conceptualized. Typical schemas of depression include "I am stupid," or "I cannot exist without the love of a strong person." Unlike automatic thoughts, patients are not typically aware and cannot easily become aware of such underlying general assumptions. These must be deduced from many specific examples of distorted thinking. Schemas such as "I am stupid" may lie dormant much of the time, only to be reactivated by a specific event, such as difficulty in accomplishing a task. These enduring self-concepts and attitudes are assumed to have been learned in childhood on the basis of the child's experiences and the reactions of important family members. Once formed, such attitudes can be self-perpetuating.

Just as depressive thoughts can be triggered by events, episodes of depressive illness may, from the cognitive perspective, be triggered by sufficient stress. Such stresses may be specific to the individual and her or his particular sensitivities developed in childhood. Alternatively, sufficient degrees of nonspecific stress may precipitate depression in vulnerable individuals. Experiences of loss, a setback in a major goal, a rejection, or an insolvable dilemma are especially common precipitants of depression. The onset of medical illness, with its attendant limitations and associated meanings, is also seen as likely to trigger depression in many people.

Researchers have accumulated considerable evidence that depressed individuals do indeed manifest negative biases in their views of themselves, their experiences, and the future. In addition, they have attitudes (schemas) that distinguish them from nondepressed subjects, as well as distortions in logic and information processing. It is less clear whether all depressed people show the thinking distortions that Beck has described. Much of the cognitive depression research has been criticized because the studies have been on nonpatient populations, such as student volunteers, with relatively mild degrees of depression. These individuals may be very different from actual psychiatric patients. Whether cognitive distortions are a predisposing factor to depression is also unclear. Most researchers have found that most distorted thinking disappears when depression is successfully treated, even with antidepressant medication. The findings suggest that these distortions are a symptom of depression rather than an enduring trait of depression-prone people. Clearly, further research is needed to test the causality of cognitive factors in depression.

Technique of Cognitive Psychotherapy

Cognitive psychotherapy is a directive, time-limited, multidimensional psychological treatment. The patient and therapist together discover the irrational beliefs and illogical thinking patterns associated with the patient's depressive affects (Table 17–4). They then devise methods by which patients themselves can test the validity of their thinking. The therapist helps patients to become aware of their irrational beliefs and distorted thinking ("automatic thoughts").

Cognitive psychotherapy was developed for unipolar, nonpsychotic, mild to moderately depressed outpatients. The presence of bipolar illness, delu-

Table 17–4 **Cognitive Psychotherapy**

Goal	Identify and alter cognitive distortions

Patient selection
  criteria
	Unipolar, nonpsychotic depressed outpatients
	Contraindications include delusions, hallucinations, severe
	  depression, severe cognitive impairment, ongoing substance
	  abuse, enmeshed family system

Techniques	Behavioral assignments Reading material Taught to recognize negatively biased automatic thoughts Identify patients' schemas, beliefs, attitudes
Duration	Time limited: 15–25 sessions

sions or hallucinations, or extremely severe depression is a contraindication for cognitive psychotherapy as the sole or primary treatment modality. Other contraindications include the presence of underlying medical illness or medications that may be causing the depression, the presence of a neurologically based mental disorder, or an ongoing problem of substance abuse. In addition, cognitive psychotherapy may not be indicated as the sole form of treatment for major or "endogenous" depression (which may be accompanied by endocrine, sleep, or other biological abnormalities in which antidepressant medication or ECT is needed) or for patients enmeshed in family systems that maintain a fixed view of themselves as helpless and dependent. Cognitive psychotherapy may be useful in patients who refuse to take, fail to respond to, or are unable to tolerate medication, as well as those who prefer a psychological approach in the hope of greater long-term benefits.

Cognitive psychotherapy is generally conducted over a period of 15 to 25 weeks in once-weekly meetings. With more severely depressed patients, two or three meetings per week are recommended for the first several weeks. While cognitive psychotherapy was developed and is usually administered as an individual treatment, its principles have also been successfully applied to group settings.

A course of cognitive psychotherapy proceeds in a succession of regular stages. The first stage is devoted to introducing the patient to the procedures and rationale of the therapy, setting goals for the treatment, and establishing a therapeutic alliance. The therapist may assign reading material on the cognitive theory of depression. In the next stage, the therapist begins to demonstrate to the patient that cognitions and emotions are connected. Patients are taught to become more aware of their negatively biased automatic thoughts and to recognize, both during and outside of the psychotherapy hours, that negative affects are generally preceded by such thoughts. Behavioral assignments may be used.

In the next phase, which normally comprises the majority of the work, the emphasis shifts to a detailed exploration of the patient's cognitions and their role in perpetuating depressive feelings. In the final stage of psychotherapy, patients will have had a great deal of experience in recognizing their habitual thought patterns, testing their validity, and modifying them when appropriate, with the result of substantial symptomatic relief. Psychotherapy then focuses on the attitudes and assumptions that underlie the patient's negatively biased thinking. For example, the patient might assume that, "If I'm nice, bad things won't happen to me." A logically equivalent assumption would then be, "If bad things happen to me, it is my fault because I am not nice." Target symptoms that might be the focus of a session include intense sadness, pervasive self-criticism, passivity and avoidance, sleep disturbance, or other affective, motivational, or cognitive manifestations of depression. The therapist repeatedly formulates the patient's beliefs and attitudes as testable hypotheses and helps the patient to devise and implement ways of verifying them. The therapist maintains an inquiring attitude toward the patient's reactions to the therapist and the therapeutic procedures. Such reactions are explored for evidence of misunderstanding and distortion, which are then dealt with in the same way as the patient's other cognitions.

A great variety of different techniques are used by cognitive therapists to break the cycle of negative evaluations and dysfunctional behaviors. Behavioral methods are often useful in the beginning of psychotherapy, particularly when the patient is severely depressed. Activity scheduling, mastery and pleasure exercises, graded task assignments, cognitive rehearsal, and role-playing may all be used.

More cognitively oriented methods are applied in the middle and late stages of psychotherapy as psychotherapy progresses. The therapist and patient explore the patient's inner life in a spirit of adventure. Patients become more observant of their peculiar construction of reality and usually focus more on actual events and their meanings. The fundamental cognitive technique is teaching patients to observe, record, and validate their cognitions.

Efficacy of Cognitive Psychotherapy

In contrast to most other psychotherapies, there is a growing literature on the efficacy of cognitive psychotherapy. Although the number is still relatively small, all studies examining the outcome of cognitive psychotherapy have found it to be an effective treatment, at least in ambulatory outpatients with mild-to-moderate degrees of depression. Cognitive psychotherapy has been shown to be more effective than no psychotherapy in treating both depressed volunteers and psychiatric patients with diagnoses of depression.

It should be emphasized that the choice of treatment for a depressed patient should often involve a combination of both psychotherapy and antidepressant medication. To withhold antidepressants from patients who have a clear biological component to their depression, based on their signs and symptoms and family history, because of a "bias" toward one sort of psychotherapy or another is unjustifiable on clinical grounds if not overtly unethical. Hence, integrated psychotherapeutic *and* pharmacological treatment is often indicated and should be considered in every patient, regardless of the orientation of the psychotherapist.

SUPPORTIVE PSYCHOTHERAPY

Supportive psychotherapy aims to help patients maintain or reestablish the best level of functioning, given the limitations of their illness, personality, native ability, and life circumstances (Table 17–5). In general, this goal distinguishes supportive psychotherapy from the change-oriented psychotherapies that aim to reverse primary disease processes and symptoms or restructure personality.

The line between supportive and "change-oriented" psychotherapy, however, is frequently not so clear. The situation is somewhat analogous to the medical treatment of viral versus bacterial infections. Treatment of the former is basically supportive in that it aims to maintain normal bodily functions (e.g., fever reduction, control of cerebral edema, dietary compensation for liver failure) in the face of infection, while in the latter, the aim is to eliminate the infection. In addition to the supportive aspects of treating bacterial infections, however, antibiotic treatment itself is supportive in the sense that it works as an adjunct to the body's natural immune system, without which it is relatively ineffective. There are supportive elements, however, in all effective forms of psychotherapy, and the terms "supportive" and "change-oriented" merely describe the balance of efforts in a particular case.

Patients who are generally very healthy and well adapted, but who have become impaired in response to stressful life circumstances, as well as those

Table 17–5 **Supportive Psychotherapy**

Goal	Maintain or reestablish best level of functioning
Patient selection criteria	Very healthy individuals exposed to stressful life circumstances (e.g., Adjustment Disorder)
	Individual with serious illness, ego deficits, e.g., Schizophrenia, Major Depression (psychotic)
	Individuals with medical illness
Techniques	Available, predictable therapist
	No/limited interpretation of transference
	Support intellectualization
	Therapist acts as a guide/mentor
	Medication frequently used
	Supportive techniques: suggestion, reinforcement, advice, teaching, reality testing, cognitive restructuring, reassurance
	Active stance
	Discuss alternative behaviors, social/interpersonal skills
Duration	Brief (days–weeks) to very long term (years)

who have serious illnesses that cannot be cured, can receive supportive psychotherapy. Supportive psychotherapy may be brief or long term. The "healthy" individual, when faced with overwhelming stress or crises (particularly in the face of traumas or disasters), may seek help and be a candidate for supportive psychotherapy. The relatively healthy candidate for supportive psychotherapy is a well-adapted individual (with good social supports and interpersonal relations, flexible defenses, and good reality testing) who is in acute crisis. This individual continues to show evidence of well-planned behaviors and a healthy perspective on the crisis. The person makes use of social supports, does not withdraw, and anticipates resolution of the crisis. Although the patient is functioning below his or her usual level, this patient remains hopeful about the future and makes use of resources available for problem-solving, respite, and growth. This patient uses supportive psychotherapy to reconstitute more rapidly, to avoid errors in judgment by "talking out loud," to relieve minor symptomatology, and to grow as an individual by learning about the world.

The more typical candidate for supportive psychotherapy has significant deficits in ego functioning, including poor reality testing, impaired impulse control, and difficulties in interpersonal relations. Patients who have less ability to sublimate and are less introspective are frequently treated in supportive psychotherapy, where more directive techniques and environmental manipulation can be used.

Ego strength and the ability to form relationships may be more important than diagnosis in the selection of patients for supportive psychotherapy (Werman, 1984; Rockland, 1989). The ability of the patient to relate to the therapist, a past history of reasonable personal relationships, work history and educational performance, and the use of leisure time for constructive activity and relaxation bear importantly on the treatment recommendation. Almost no information is known regarding which characteristics of the patient may predict a good result from supportive psychotherapy rather than merely a poor response to the change-oriented psychotherapies. Delineation of the minimum level of personal strengths needed to benefit from supportive individual psychotherapy is an important task for future research.

Technique of Supportive Psychotherapy

Psychoanalytic theory provides the major contributions to the theory of the supportive psychotherapy. In-depth psychological understanding of patients in supportive psychotherapy is as necessary as in the change-oriented, explorative psychotherapies (Rockland, 1989; Pine, 1986; Werman, 1984). Understanding unconscious motivation, psychic conflict, the patient–therapist relationship, and the patient's use of defense mechanisms is essential to understanding the patient's strengths and vulnerabilities. This knowledge is critical to providing support, as well as insight.

Therapists who are predictably available and safe (i.e., who accept the patient and put aside their own needs in the service of the treatment) assume some of the holding functions of the "good parent." In such a therapeutic situation, the patient is able to identify with and incorporate the well-functioning aspects of the therapist, such as the capacity for self-observation and the ability to tolerate ambivalence (Pine, 1986).

The containment of affect and anxiety is an important supportive function. Patients in need of supportive psychotherapy typically fear the destructive power of their internal rage and envy. They are helped to modulate their emotional reactions by the reliable presence of the therapist and the therapeutic relationship that remains unchanged in the face of emotional onslaughts.

The therapist fosters the supportive relationship by refraining from interpreting positive transference feelings and waiting until the intensity of feelings has abated before commenting about negative transference feelings. Interpretations of the negative transference are limited to those needed to ensure that the treatment is not disrupted. While maintaining a friendly stance toward the patient, the therapist respects the patient's need to establish a comfortable degree of distance. The therapist must not push for a more intimate or emotion-laden relationship than the patient can tolerate. The rapport with the patient, which the supportive psychotherapist tries to establish, differs from the "therapeutic alliance" of insight-oriented therapy. The doctor–patient relationship does not require the patient to observe and report on her/his own feelings and behavior to the same extent as in the change-oriented, explorative psychotherapies. The therapist acts more as a guide and a mentor.

There is virtually unanimous agreement among writers on supportive psychotherapy that fostering a good working relationship with the patient is the first priority. The therapist must be available in a regular and predictable manner. Rather than approach the patient as a "blank screen," the therapist actively demonstrates concern, involvement, sympathy, and a supportive attitude. The therapist serves as an "auxiliary ego" for the patient. The auxiliary ego functions of the therapist can be seen in the therapist's use of suggestion, reinforcement, advice, teaching, reality testing, cognitive restructuring, and reassurance. In taking such an active stance, it is especially important for the therapist to guard against grandiosity and personal biases so as not to "become an omnipotent decision maker." The therapist rather acts as "a strong, benign individual who is reasonably available when needed." To the extent that the patient develops the capacity to observe him- or herself, the psychotherapy may proceed beyond support and take on features of the explorative and change-oriented psychotherapies.

The defenses of denial and avoidance are handled by encouraging the patient to discuss alternative behaviors, goals, and interpretations of events. Reassurance has a variety of forms in supportive psychotherapy, including supporting an adaptive level of denial (such as a patient may employ in coping with a terminal illness); the patients' experience of the therapist's empathic attitude; or the therapist's reality testing of the patients' negatively biased evaluations of themselves or their situation. Reassuring a patient is not easy. Reassurance requires a clear understanding of what the patient fears. Overt expressions of interest and concern may be reassuring to a patient who fears rejection, but threatening to one who fears intrusion. Interpretations in supportive psychotherapy are limited to those that will decrease anxiety and strengthen (rather than loosen) defenses, particularly the defenses of intellectualization and rationalization.

The therapist's expressions of interest, advice giving, and facilitation of ventilation reinforce desired behaviors. Expressions of interest and solicitude are positively reinforcing. Advice can lead to behavioral change if it is specific and applies to frequent behaviors of the patient. Desired behaviors are rewarded by the therapist's approval and by social reinforcement. Ventilation of emotions is useful only if the therapist can help the patient safely contain and limit them, thus extinguishing the anxiety response to emotional expression. Cognitive and behavioral psychotherapeutic interventions that strengthen the adaptive and defensive functions of the ego (e.g., realistic and logical thinking, social skills, containment of affects such as anxiety) contribute to the supportive aspects of the psychotherapy.

Efficacy of Supportive Psychotherapy

Most data on the effectiveness of supportive psychotherapy come from studies in which supportive psychotherapy has been used as a control in testing the efficacy of other treatments. In such studies, the procedures used in supportive psychotherapy tend to be poorly specified, and no attempts are made to correlate individual supportive techniques with outcome. There are no studies in which supportive psychotherapy is compared with no treatment or minimal treatment. Despite its limitations, however, the research literature offers some evidence that supportive psychotherapy is an effective treatment, particularly when combined with medication. This conclusion appears to be true in the treatment of depression, anxiety disorders, and schizophrenia.

There is a body of research indicating that supportive psychotherapy is an effective component of the treatment of patients with a variety of medical illnesses, including those with ulcerative colitis or myocardial infarction and cancer patients undergoing radiation treatment. In general, patients in supportive psychotherapy improve emotionally and have fewer days in the hospital, fewer complications, and more rapid recovery.

The evidence to date, although preliminary, suggests that supportive psychotherapy can be effective in both psychiatric and medical illnesses and is frequently more cost effective than more intensive psychotherapies for some disorders. More research is needed on the indications, contraindications, and techniques of supportive psychotherapy.

BEHAVIORAL THERAPY

Behavioral therapy (behavior modification) is based on the concept that all symptoms of a psychological nature are learned maladaptive patterns of behavior in response to environmental or internal stimuli. It does not concern itself with the intrapsychic conflicts or with reconstructing the patient's life story and unconscious dynamics that are the focus of the psychodynamically oriented psychotherapies. Rather, it uses the concepts of learning theory to eliminate the involuntary, disruptive behavior patterns that constitute the essential features of psychopathology and substitutes these with highly adaptive and situation-appropriate patterns (Lazarus, 1971). Behavioral therapy has been useful in a wide range of disorders when specific behavioral symptoms can be targeted for change and this change is central to recovery. Eating disorders, chronic pain syndromes and illness behavior, phobias, sexual dysfunction, paraphilias, and conduct disorders of childhood are frequently treated with behavioral therapy techniques.

Techniques of Behavioral Therapy

A variety of techniques exist that permit the modification of undesirable and unwanted behaviors when applied by therapists skilled in their use (Table 17–6). These approaches require careful history taking and behavioral analysis to identify the behaviors to be targeted for extinction or modification. Often, adjunctive techniques, such as the use of hypnosis and drugs, are used to facilitate behavior modification, but are not requisite for therapeutic success. Present-day behavioral therapists are usually alert to interpersonal and emotional aspects of psychiatric symptoms and the doctor–patient relationship. Psychodynamic, cognitive, and interpersonal techniques are frequently integrated into the therapy, but are not seen as central to the therapeutic effect. Four of the more common behavioral techniques are described here.

Table 17–6 **Behavioral Therapy (Behavioral Modification)**

Goal	Eliminate involuntary disruptive behavior patterns and substitute appropriate behaviors
Patient selection criteria	Habit modification
	Targeted symptoms
	Phobias
	Some psychophysiological responses: headache, migraine, hypertension, Raynaud's phenomena
	Sexual dysfunction
Techniques	Systemic desensitization
	Implosion therapy and flooding
	Aversive therapy
	Biofeedback
Duration	Usually time limited

Systematic Desensitization

Systematic desensitization refers to a technique whereby individuals suffering primarily from phobic responses are gradually exposed to anxiety-provoking situations or objects in small increments. The therapist first identifies a hierarchy of behaviors directed to approaching the phobic object or situation. Relaxation techniques are used to decrease anxiety at each stage of the hierarchy. The patient moves up to the next level of intensity when the stimulus no longer provokes intense anxiety. This particularly effective technique is useful in an office setting as well, because experience has demonstrated that the patient can confront the anxiety-provoking stimulus in his imagination with very much the same effects. Again, a hierarchy of increasingly anxious imaginary scenes is constructed. The patient visualizes each scene, reexperiences the anxiety associated with it, and then uses relaxation techniques to become more comfortable with the fantasy gradually. Patients move up the hierarchy of images until they are able to visualize fully the phobic object/situation without undue anxiety. Usually, this in vitro technique will be accompanied by in vivo practice exposures. Hypnotic procedures and the use of anxiolytic drugs are useful adjuncts in certain types of patients. There is some controversy regarding the mechanisms underlying the effect of systematic desensitization. Various explanations have been suggested regarding the underlying mechanisms. It is possible, for example, that the graduated exposure to the anxiety-provoking situation represents nothing more than a sequential or progressive "flooding" technique (see next section). It is also possible that by exposing the individual to only small, and therefore more tolerable, amounts of anxiety, the individual is able to develop more appropriate and successful coping mechanisms. Other authors have suggested that the key to systematic desensitization lies in the suppression of anxiety, which is achieved by evoking a competitive physiological response such as deep muscle relaxation.

Implosion Therapy and Flooding

These two techniques vary only in the presentation of the anxiety-eliciting stimulus. Animal behaviorists discovered early on that avoidant behavior, which by its very nature can be expected to be highly resistant to extinction, could be extinguished rather rapidly by submitting the subject to a prolonged conditioned stimulus while restraining it and making the expression of the avoidant behavior impossible. In the therapeutic situation, the patient is directly exposed to the stressful stimulus until the anxiety subsides. This is in contrast to the graded exposure of systematic desensitization. In theory, each session should result in ever-decreasing intervals between exposure and cessation of anxiety. In implosion therapy the patient uses mental images as substitutes for the actual feared object or situation, whereas in the flooding approach, the therapist conducts the procedure in vivo. Results appear to indicate that both approaches are equally effective. Some have questioned the ethics of submitting patients to such painful experiences, especially when other alternatives are available. A risk associated with this technique is the danger that the patient may refuse to submit to such an uncomfortable experience and may terminate the exposure prior to the abatement of the anxiety. This will result in a successful "escape" and will therefore reinforce the phobic response.

Aversive Therapy

This treatment modality has its roots in classical and operant conditioning. Controversial by its very nature, it has nevertheless found acceptance as a potentially useful avenue of therapy for a narrow range of disorders and unwanted habits. Perhaps the most common form of aversive therapy is the use of disulfiram (Antabuse) in alcoholics. This treatment approach is based on the fear of an extremely unpleasant, and indeed sometimes fatal, physiological response (the unconditioned stimulus) when someone who has been taking Antabuse then imbibes alcohol (which becomes the conditioned stimulus). In theory, the alcoholic patient on Antabuse therapy will avoid alcohol to avoid the alcohol–Antabuse reaction. The use of mild aversive stimuli has also been found to be useful in smoking-cessation programs. Because of safety considerations, and to ensure continued patient participation, aversive stimuli used under these conditions are often mild and may not constitute much more than having to hold the smoke in the oral cavity for a prolonged period of time. Various aversive techniques have also been used in the treatment of sexual offenders and have included the use of such stimuli as mild electric shocks and unpleasant odors. Ethical considerations, understandable patient reluctance to participate in treatment, and pejorative associations by the general public with torture and other forms of maltreatment have resulted in rather limited applications for these techniques. In addition, its effectiveness has been more variable than that of other behavioral techniques.

Biofeedback

Biofeedback is not a type of behavioral therapy per se, but rather a tool or technique that can be integrated with other operant procedures for the management of a number of psychophysiological disorders. Some of the conditions in which there is documented short-term efficacy for biofeedback are hypertension, migraine headaches, tension headaches, some cardiac arrhythmias, and Raynaud's phenomenon. This approach presumes that many pathological psychophysiological responses could be subject to modification if the individual could become aware of their existence and of positive changes incurred as a result of learned responses (Gaarder and Montgomery, 1977). For the conditioned response to be reinforced and for learning to take place, the organism must be aware that a response has taken place. The biofeedback techniques consist of the use of sophisticated instrumentation to detect changes in skin temperature, muscle tension, or heart rate. Biofeedback first burst on the scene amid great publicity and exaggerated claims regarding its efficacy. This was followed by an expected period of disenchantment and skepticism. Nevertheless, for selected patients, especially those suffering from psychophysiological disorders characterized by measurable vascular and neuromuscular changes, such as chronic tension headaches, this approach may be of some use either by itself or in conjunction with other therapies, including medication and formal psychotherapy. Biofeedback is often administered in clinics by technicians. There is a paucity of evidence, however, that for tension-related syndromes such as chronic headache, it is any more effective than simple relaxation exercises.

Effectiveness of Behavioral Therapies

The behavioral approaches have proved to be of considerable value in the treatment of a wide spectrum of disorders, particularly phobias and muscle tension, as well as migraine headaches. They also may be considered as valuable adjunct techniques in the overall management of psychiatric and other medical conditions such as headaches and eating disorders. Often, much time and effort are devoted to discussing the relative merits of the behavioral techniques versus the psychodynamic therapies. Elements from each approach play a significant factor in the other. Even in the most dynamically oriented therapy situation, the achievement of new insights, improvements in the quality of life, and the lessening of anxiety facilitate the progress toward wellness. Similarly, there has been little research into the nature of the relationship between the patient and her or his behavioral therapist. The degree to which conflicts between the behavioral therapist and the patient may recreate past relationships, how this is handled, and how this influences treatment progress are not well known.

GROUP THERAPIES

In its most basic form, group therapy can be described as the attainment of therapeutic goals through the skilled manipulation of group processes or mechanisms. The changes effected can be limited and situation specific, or they can be far-reaching and foster personality development and growth. Family therapy and couples therapy are specific forms of group therapy directed to the family and the couple—usually the marital couple—in special group/interpersonal settings. In contrast to the individual therapies, the group therapies have direct access to the interpersonal processes of the patient with individuals of varying age and sex. Intrapsychic, interpersonal, communication, and system theories, as well as a knowledge of family and couple development and roles, are used to elucidate various aspects of behavior and increase the patient's awareness. In addition, new behaviors can be tried in the group with the therapist present (Yalom, 1986). The different types of group therapy emphasize different theoretical perspectives and may have different group compositions (Table 17–7). All groups provide members with support, a feeling of belonging, and a safe, secure environment where change can be effected and tried out first. The therapist uses the vast array of processes at work in a group to facilitate interaction among its members and to guide the work of the group toward the desired goal. Skill, training, and a keen understanding of group dynamics are required. Particular awareness of group fantasies, projections, scapegoating, and denial are a part of most group therapy work. Frequently, cotherapists run the group. This often increases the ability to attend to the many processes occurring in the group and aids in the avoidance of countertransference pitfalls.

Group Psychotherapy

Group psychotherapists use a variety of techniques derived from knowledge of the dynamics and behavior of social groups to foster desired change in the individual members (Yalom, 1986). The theoretical framework supporting the various therapeutic modalities, however, varies with the goals and purposes of the group, the type of group, and the composition of the group. A review of the literature reveals widely diverging definitions and classifications. Different approaches achieve a measure of fame and popularity, such as the so-called encounter groups, and then recede from the scene. In general, however, groups can be divided into three separate and distinct categories: (1) directive, (2) psychodynamic/interpersonal, and (3) analytic. This classification is based largely on the degree to which the group fosters the exploration and evocation of repressed, unconscious material. As a result, each group type will vary widely in approach, techniques, composition, conceptual model, and defined goals. Group psychotherapy occurs in both inpatient and outpatient settings.

Table 17–7 **Group Therapies**

Goal	Alleviation of symptoms
	Change interpersonal relations
	Alter specific family/couple dynamics
Patient selection criteria	Vary greatly based on type of group
	Homogeneous groups target specific disorders
	Adolescents and personality disorders may especially benefit
	Families and couples for whom the system needs change
	Contraindications: substantial suicide risk, sadomasochistic acting out in family/couple
Techniques	Directive/Supportive Group Psychotherapy
	Psychodynamic/Interpersonal Group Psychotherapy
	Psychoanalytic Group Psychotherapy
	Family Therapy
	Couples Therapy
Duration	Weeks to years; time limited and open-ended

Directive/Supportive Group Psychotherapy

These groups usually have very specific, well-defined, and relatively limited goals. Good examples are the Alcoholics Anonymous (AA) and Overeaters Anonymous groups. The groups function within a very narrow set of guidelines defined by a specific philosophy, set of values, or religious orientation. In the case of AA, for example, the members help each other achieve sobriety and cope with everyday problems of living by adhering to "The Twelve Steps" and entrusting their fate to a "Higher Power." The group leader serves as a role model, stressing common sense, reality-oriented solutions to problems while using the group to apply peer pressure, enhance self-esteem, foster a feeling of togetherness and belonging, and provide a supportive and nurturing environment. Members usually share at least one major attribute in common (for example, alcoholism), but in many other respects, the group is heterogeneous in composition. There may be a wide divergence in social background, education, personality types, and even the presence of major psychiatric disorders. Behavioral techniques often are applied in similar group situations to treat individuals with phobias while group support and encouragement is used to enhance efficacy.

Psychodynamic/Interpersonal Group Psychotherapy

These groups address the individual members' psychopathology, foster the development of insight, promote the development of better interpersonal and social skills, and, in general, promote improved coping skills for the here and now. Defenses are identified and challenged in an atmosphere of support and acceptance. Positive change is encouraged and reinforced. These groups may adhere to any of a wide variety of theoretical models (such as gestalt therapy, psychodrama, and so forth) or may be eclectic in their approach and incorporate aspects of these models into the system to fit the needs and characteristics of the group. They tend, however, to focus on the individual's subjective experience and interpersonal behaviors.

Psychoanalytic Group Psychotherapy

This type of group essentially uses the psychoanalytic approach, as applied in individual therapy. The therapist remains neutral and nondirective and thus promotes a transference neurosis that can be analyzed. Defenses are identified and resistances interpreted. The group focuses on past experiences and repressed unconscious material as the underlying factors in psychopathology. The therapist attempts to identify individual transferences of the members, as well as shared group fantasies or assumptions.

In general, most patients who benefit from individual psychotherapy benefit from group psychotherapy. Empirical data are lacking, except for directive/supportive group psychotherapy approaches (e.g., AA, Overeaters Anonymous, type A personality). The differences and similarities in behavior change following group and individual psychotherapy are largely unknown. Although there is no hard evidence for the greater or lesser efficacy of either technique applied to appropriate patients, not all patients will do well in all groups, and some patients should not be considered for inclusion in a treatment group under any circumstances. Specifically, severely depressed and suicidal individuals should not be assigned to outpatient groups. Their emotional state will prevent them from becoming integrated into the group, and the lack of an initial strong therapeutic relationship with a specific therapist may increase the risk of suicide. Such patients should be considered for individual and other more intensely supportive modalities and inpatient hospitalization when indicated. Manic patients tend to be disruptive to group process, and their impulsivity and lack of control prevent them from obtaining any real benefit from group work. Some types of personality disorders, such as explosive, narcissistic, borderline, and antisocial personalities, may also present insurmountable difficulties for treatment with this modality. Schizophrenics may do well in highly directive, structured groups with emphasis on reality testing and improving interpersonal coping skills. Group therapy can be used as an effective adjunct to either individual psychotherapy or psychotropic medications. Inpatient group psychotherapy is a very common treatment modality and differs from outpatient treatment because of the heterogeneity of the group and its frequent change in membership. Group psychotherapy may be particularly helpful with adolescents, who are highly sensitive to peer group support and influence. Groups also provide a powerful arena in which individuals with personality disorders can become increasingly aware of their interpersonal problems.

Family Therapy

In family therapy, psychological symptoms are considered to be the pathological expression of disturbances in the social system of the family. For the purposes of this discussion, the latter can include any members, ranging from the basic couple to children, grandparents, distant relatives, and, in some cases, even close friends of the family. The essential feature is the relationship among the various members and how their behavior can affect the group as a whole, as well as the individual family members. The theoretical models may run the whole gamut of therapeutic approaches, ranging from the psychoanalytic to the behavioral (Beels, 1988).

Most family therapists agree that family groups are extremely complex and dynamic systems with a definite hierarchical structure that is a result of cultural and societal proscribed roles, repetitive behavior patterns, and ingrained ways in which the family members have interrelated. Family structure can be seen as a self-regulating system with multiple control mechanisms designed to ensure some degree of a homeostatic equilibrium. The family system seeks stability and inherently resists change. When the system is subjected to internal or external stresses, the family may respond by "designating" one of its members as the "patient," and his or her "illness" may act as a safety valve to maintain system integrity. This same resistance to change will, of course, oppose any therapeutic efforts and may take the form of refusal to explore family issues by the other members of the family, missed appointments, no apparent therapeutic progress, and so forth. Some change does occur in any family as the passage of time thrusts on the system irresistible forces such as maturation of children, illness, death, old age, and, of course, personal growth and maturity. The family system may thus be conceived as three-dimensional: highly structured, homeostatic, but slowly evolving and changing its character over long periods of time.

The clinical indications for family therapy are very broad. Psychopathology in any member of a family will undoubtedly influence family dynamics, and vice versa. The treatment of children and adolescents frequently requires family therapy to deal with the environment that may be causing or sustaining the symptoms. Recent research indicates the particular value of family therapy in the treatment of schizophrenic patients in reducing rehospitalization rates. Practical considerations such as geographical distance, economic situation, or refusal to participate can rule out family participation. When family members are being extremely destructive to the family unit or important familial relationships, family therapy should not be instituted or should be suspended for a brief time. The treatment of childhood disorders, eating disorders, alcoholism, and substance abuse generally requires a family therapy intervention.

Each clinician brings to the field her/his own conceptual framework, clinical experience, philosophical orientation, and training background. The orthodox psychoanalyst may conceive of family therapy as the individual treatment of the symptomatic member, while at the other end of the spectrum, the social worker specializing in this form of treatment may include any or all members of the family in the sessions and may use a highly directive approach, including didactic presentations and environmental manipulation. The focus of most family therapy is on current issues (the here and now) and achievement of discrete changes toward an identifiable goal. Developmental conflicts, communication patterns, boundary management, flexibility, familial conflict resolution techniques, and roles accepted and proscribed by the system for each member are areas of therapeutic attention. Exploration of individual unconscious material is usually avoided. When an individual psychotherapy is stalled, the use of family (or couples) therapy can help resolve environmental and family system variables that are inhibiting further individual progress. In such cases, a course of family (or couples) therapy can frequently reestablish the momentum of an individual treatment. Family therapy can be an important adjunct to inpatient treatment to facilitate discharge and psychosocial readjustment.

No single technique or procedure dominates family therapy. Therapists may see one or two members of the family, or they may see the entire group. The family may be seen together by a single therapist, individually by different therapists, together by more than one therapist, or more than one family may be seen in special forms of multifamily group therapy. Similarly, the therapeutic techniques can range from inducing change by crisis to focusing on small aspects of how the family functions in order to create positive changes that the system can assimilate and incorporate over varying periods of time.

Couples Therapy

Couples therapy is the treatment of dysfunctional couples. In modern society, this includes both married and unmarried "dyads," as well as homosexual couples. It is very similar to, and, in fact, may be described as a form of, family therapy. The same theoretical concepts and treatment approaches described above apply. If the couple has an extreme sadomasochistic relationship, therapy may be blocked. During times when one partner is being overly destructive to the relationship or the other partner, the therapist may need to intervene directly. If destructive behavior cannot be limited in the treatment, a brief individual therapy with each partner may sufficiently resolve the tension to allow the couples therapy to continue. The goal of treatment may be to resolve conflict and to reconstruct the dyadic relationship or to facilitate disengagement in the least painful way possible.

SEXUAL DYSFUNCTION THERAPY

The term *sexual dysfunction therapy* encompasses the entire spectrum of accepted psychotherapies from the purely behavioral techniques to the psychodynamically oriented approaches. Treatment may be restricted to a single form of therapy or may consist of a combination of approaches. The focus, however, is the resolution of a specific sexual dysfunction, such as premature ejaculation, impotence, orgasmic dysfunction, or vaginismus (Masters and Johnson, 1970). Most sex therapists emphasize focusing on symptom relief with the use of behavior modification techniques, followed by attempts at resolution of underlying conflicts (which may represent the core of the disorder) by more traditional insight-oriented dynamic methods (Table 17–8). In general, the brief focused therapies, whether used singly or in combination with other forms, seem to have a greater success rate with specific symptom relief than do the longer term treatments.

The evaluation of sexual dysfunction should include a complete investigation of possible medical causes (see Chapter 14). A considerable number of physical illnesses, injuries, and congenital malformations can result in symptoms suggestive of a psychosexual disorder and, if not addressed, will render all other therapies useless (Kaplan, 1974). Intraabdominal adhesions and masses, for example, can result in pain during intercourse. Endocrine disturbances may affect sexual drive, and spinal injuries can inhibit penile erections and orgasm.

Table 17–8 **Sexual Dysfunction Therapies**

Goal	Resolution of specific sexual dysfunctions
Patient selection criteria	Couples
	Sexual dysfunction: impotence, premature ejaculation, vaginismus, orgasmic dysfunction
	Rule out medical causes
Techniques	Behavior modification techniques, including systematic desensitization, homework, education
	Psychodynamic approaches
	Hypnotherapy
	Group therapy
	Couples therapy as needed to deal with the system dynamics
Duration	Weeks to months

Similarly, a number of medications can result in dysfunctional symptoms, causing great distress to the patient. Thioridazine, a commonly used neuroleptic, is often associated with reversible retrograde ejaculation in the otherwise normal male. In this situation, simple counseling and reassurance may suffice to calm the patient. Thus, the role of careful history taking, a complete physical examination, and indicated laboratory testing cannot be overemphasized.

The human sexual response cycle may be divided into four distinct phases: (1) appetitive (baseline), (2) excitement, (3) orgasmic, and (4) resolution. For the purposes of our discussion, the last phase bears little relation to disturbances in sexual functioning. The psychosexual disorders may be grouped according to where the dysfunction occurs in the response cycle. Sexual desire disorders are part of the appetitive phase; sexual arousal disorders are part of the excitement phase; and orgasmic disorders are part of the orgasmic phase. Sexual pain disorders are difficult to assign, but may directly or indirectly affect the cycle at any level. This classification must be borne in mind when deciding on the most appropriate therapeutic regimen. Disorders affecting the orgasmic phase are readily treatable by simple behavioral techniques, and the results appear to be dramatic and long lasting. Disorders affecting the appetitive phase, however, reflect deep-seated conflicts and are much more resistant to therapeutic intervention. They often require the use of insight-oriented therapies and the uncovering of repressed material in conjunction with behavioral therapy. The disturbances of the excitement phase fall somewhere between these two in terms of prognosis and choice of treatment.

Choice of Therapeutic Approach for Sexual Dysfunction

Proponents of the various therapeutic approaches can make a case for the efficacy of their methods in the treatment of these disorders. A basic understanding of the more commonly used and successful treatments is essential for appropriate treatment planning or selection of optimal referral sources.

Individual Psychodynamic Therapy

Individual brief-term psychodynamically oriented psychotherapy remains one of the more useful and effective techniques available when dealing with psychosexual disorders that have complex intrapsychic conflicts at their roots with pervasive negative influences over many other aspects of the individuals' lives. In actual practice, individual psychotherapy by itself may not bring about the desired results, but its efficacy may be greatly enhanced by the application of one of the many behavioral therapies in conjunction with the more traditional approach.

Behavioral Therapy

The use of behavioral techniques such as systematic desensitization and, to a lesser degree, implosion or flooding therapy, is often extremely useful in treating sexual dysfunctions, particularly those associated with disturbances of the orgasmic phase (Masters and Johnson, 1970). The actual techniques differ very little from the tried and true methods used in other disorders amenable to treatment by these methods (see Chapter 14). The therapist performs a detailed behavioral analysis and develops a hierarchical list of anxiety-producing situations during the sexual act that culminate in the pathological response, be it premature ejaculation, retarded ejaculation, or inhibited orgasm. Through gradual exposure to the anxiety-provoking stimulus, the patient eventually learns to cope in a more appropriate fashion and to perform sexually in an enjoyable, rewarding fashion. As noted earlier, these techniques are particularly effective when dealing with disorders of the orgasmic phase, but their primary value when treating disturbances of the appetitive phase is as an adjunctive technique (Kaplan, 1974). Specific techniques of behaviorally oriented therapy for specific types of sexual dysfunction are discussed in Chapter 14.

Hypnotherapy

Hypnotic suggestion can be used effectively to convince a patient that he or she does not need to feel pain during intercourse and to relieve disabling anxiety that may impair performance or consummation and enjoyment of the sexual act.

Group Therapy

Group therapy may be of value for selected patients whose perceived inadequacies and concerns about their symptoms may make them feel "different," socially isolated, and unable to share their feelings, fears, and irrational fantasies. Support from other members of the group with whom they can relate and identify may result in decreased anxiety and improvement in symptoms and may make the patient more amenable to participation in other forms of treatment, such as behavioral therapy.

Dual Sex (Couples) Therapy

This variant of behavioral therapy was initially proposed by Masters and Johnson, and in its original form, approached sexual dysfunction disorders as a "dyad" issue, that is, a patient suffering from a psychosexual disorder did so in the context of his relationship with his sexual partner. The two would be treated together as members of the "dyad" unit by a team consisting of a male and a female therapist. The latter not only directed what was, for all intents and purposes, a behavioral treatment approach, complete with educational sessions and schedule of assignments (systematic desensitization), but also served as role models for the same-sex member of the "dyad." In recent years, adherence to the male–female team and male–female "dyad" concept has not been as strict, and the makeup of the participants has been tailored to fit individual circumstances. Nevertheless, it remains an extremely effective approach that uses education, behavioral modification, modeling, and couples therapy to effect change in sexual dysfunction.

SUMMARY

The psychotherapies are important components of the treatment plan for nearly all psychiatric illnesses. Both short- and long-term techniques are available. Which psychotherapy is most effective for which patient and with which therapist is less clear. Psychotherapy provides the patient with new problem-solving techniques. Some patients prefer one type of problem-solving or can learn one type and not another.

How the outcomes from the different psychotherapies may differ and what this may mean for long-range health/relapse warrant further research. Increasingly, data indicate the effectiveness of the psychotherapies in reducing hospitalization rates and in reducing the use of other medical resources. Studies on the use of psychotherapy as an adjunct in the treatment of various physical illnesses also tend to indicate cost benefits in overall medical care dollars. The ability to use a range of psychotherapies is important in the treatment of psychiatric illness and in obtaining maximum benefit from medical case management and from the therapeutic effectiveness of the doctor–patient relationship.

For the nonpsychiatric physician, a referral for psychiatric assessment is essential when psychotherapy may be indicated. The psychiatric consultant can evaluate the interplay of biological, psychological, and social context variables that may be causing or maintaining illness in the patient. A comprehensive treatment plan and goals can then be formulated. Prior to referring a patient, the physician should educate the patient. Many patients will have the belief that the general population views psychiatric illness as fake or imaginary. They should be reassured that their distress and pain are real and that there is a wide array of possible treatments. Patients are best prepared when they can understand the role of medication in providing possible relief of symptoms and the role of the psychotherapies in learning new ways to handle the problems that may be precipitating their distress. For instance, the physician refers a patient to physical therapy to learn a new way to walk when the patient has developed a limp to compensate for chronic pain. (The limp may persist even after the pain is relieved by medication.) Similarly, the psychotherapies teach, through various means, new problem-solving techniques to relieve patterns of behaviors, feelings, and thoughts that are causing or maintaining impairment.

Finally, as noted earlier, it should be emphasized that the best form of treatment is often integrated psychotherapy and pharmacotherapy. Psychiatrists or nonpsychiatric clinicians who are polarized one way or the other may offer a narrow range of treatment and overlook either a biological or psychological therapy that might potentially be dramatically effective for the patient. Hence, in making a referral for an initial evaluation, it is recommended that one consult a clinician who has a balanced, integrated approach. The success of a referral for psychiatric evaluation or psychotherapy is *critically* dependent on the attitude, confidence, and enthusiasm of the referring physician.

CLINICAL PEARLS

- It is important to exhibit confidence and enthusiasm when making a referral for psychiatric evaluation or psychotherapy. Patients will detect ambivalence and skepticism on the physician's part about the need for such treatment. It is usually helpful to recommend a psychiatrist or other health professional who is known *personally* by the physician.
- Always present the psychiatric referral as part of the patient's ongoing medical care. Some patients will view a psychiatric referral as meaning you are "dumping" them onto another doctor and as a "rejection." Patients should be reassured that any psychiatric treatment will occur in parallel with their ongoing medical care.
- Have the name and telephone number of your referral source readily available to give to the patient.
- Call the psychiatrist to explain personally the reason and need for the referral and what role you would like to continue to play in the patient's care.
- Make the appointment for the psychiatric evaluation while the patient is still in the office or clinic.
- Be sure to schedule a follow-up appointment after the date of the psychiatric evaluation to check on the patient's reaction to the referral and their response to initial treatment.

ANNOTATED BIBLIOGRAPHY

Balint M, Ornstein P, Balint E: Focal Psychotherapy. Philadelphia, JB Lippincott, 1972

This book is one of the first written in the area of brief psychodynamic psychotherapy. It is a superb demonstration of a case of brief psychotherapy in an individual with moderately severe psychopathology. The case illustrates the exceptional clinical skill and technical requirements needed to carry out a brief psychodynamic psychotherapy.

Bruch H: Learning Psychotherapy. Cambridge, Harvard University Press, 1974

This eloquent and well-written introduction to psychotherapy presents basic principles of psychotherapeutic relations of the management of psychotherapy that are applicable to nearly all psychotherapeutic endeavors. It is based on the author's extensive career as a psychotherapist. An excellent introduction to psychotherapy.

Coleman J: Aims and conduct of psychotherapy. Arch Gen Psychiatry 18:1–6, 1968

This is a clearly written, classic article that articulates without jargon the basic doctor–patient relationship, goals, and orientation maintained by the psychiatrist in conducting psychotherapy.

Gabbard G: Psychodynamic Psychiatry in Clinical Practice: The DSM IV Edition. Washington, DC, American Psychiatric Press Inc, 1994

Well-written, detailed application of psychodynamic principles to DSM-IV disorders.

Novalis PN, Rojcewicz SJ, Peele R: Clinical Manual of Supportive Psychotherapy. Washington, DC, American Psychiatric Press, 1993

An excellent practical guide to supportive psychotherapy

Sullivan HS: The Psychiatric Interview. New York, WW Norton, 1954

This excellent introduction to the psychiatric interview is written from the perspective of the interpersonal school of psychiatry. However, its basic presentation is applicable to all of the psychotherapies. It provides a basic science to the application of talk as a curative agent.

Ursano RJ, Hales RE: A review of brief individual therapies. Am J Psychiatry 143:1507–1517, 1986

This article is an overview of both individual and group brief psychotherapies. It has a detailed list of references and presents the psychotherapies as medical interventions with substantive technical and selection criteria. In addition, there is a brief overview of the cost-benefit issues in psychotherapy.

Ursano RJ, Silberman EK: Psychoanalysis, Psychodynamic Psychotherapy, and Supportive Psychotherapy. In Hales RE, Yudofsky SC, Talbot JA (eds): Textbook of Psychiatry. Washington, DC, American Psychiatric Press, 1035–1060, 1994

This chapter reviews psychodynamic and supportive psychotherapies. It contains an extensive review of supportive psychotherapy, perhaps the most widely used and understudied of all of the psychotherapies.

Ursano RJ, Sonnenberg SM, Lazar SG: Concise Guide to Psychodynamic Psychotherapy: Principles and Techniques in The Era of Managed Care. Washington, DC, American Psychiatric Press, 1997

This book is a concise, highly readable text on the techniques of psychodynamic psychotherapy. It includes a glossary and sections on supportive and brief psychotherapy.

Werman DS: The Practice of Supportive Psychotherapy. New York, Brunner/Mazel, 1984

This book is one of a very few that describe supportive psychotherapy in a technical manner. It is a substantive contribution to the literature and to the clinician's ability to learn supportive psychotherapy as a technique.

Yalom ID: The Theory and Practice of Group Psychotherapy. New York, Basic Books, 1985

This book is the basic text of group psychotherapy. It is a comprehensive review with technical directions for the application of the technique by clinicians.

REFERENCES

Beck AT: Cognitive Theory and the Emotional Disorders. New York, International Universities Press, 1976

Beels CC: Family Therapy. In Talbott JA, Hales RE, Yudofsky SC (eds): Textbook of Psychiatry. Washington, DC, American Psychiatric Press, 929–930, 1988

Bion WR: Experiences in Groups. New York, Basic Books, 1961

Bruch H: Learning Psychotherapy. Cambridge, Harvard University Press, 1974

Crits-Christoph P: The efficacy of brief-dynamic psychotherapy: a meta-analysis. Am J Psychiatry 149:151–158, 1992

Davanloo H (ed): Short-Term Dynamic Psychotherapy. New York, Jason Aronson Press, 1980

Fiore J, Stoudemire A, Kriseman N: The family in human development and medical practice. In Stoudemire A (ed): Human Behavior: An Introduction for Medical Students, 2nd ed. Philadelphia, JB Lippincott, 1994

Gaarder K, Montgomery P: Clinical Biofeedback. Baltimore, Williams & Wilkins, 1977

Kaplan HS: The New Sex Therapy. New York, Brunner/Mazel, 1974

Klerman GL, Weissman MM, Rounsaville BJ et al: Interpersonal Psychotherapy of Depression. New York, Basic Books, 1984

Lazar S: Epidemiology of mental illness in the United States: an overview of cost effectiveness of psychotherapy. Psychoanal Inquiry suppl 4–16, 1997

Lazarus A: Behavior Therapy and Beyond. New York, McGraw-Hill, 1971

Luborsky L, Crits-Cristoph P: Understanding Transference. New York, Basic Books, 1990

Malan DH: A Study of Brief Psychotherapy. New York, Plenum Press, 1975

Mann J: Time-Limited Psychotherapy. Cambridge, Harvard University Press, 1973

Masters WH, Johnson VE: Human Sexual Inadequacy. Boston, Little, Brown & Co, 1970

Pine F: Supportive psychotherapy: a psychoanalytic perspective. Psychiatr Annu 16:524–534, 1986

Racker H: Transference and Countertransference. New York, International Universities Press, 1968

Reichmann FF: Principles of Intensive Psychotherapy. Chicago, University of Ghicago Press, 1950

Rockland LH: Supportive Therapy: A Psychodynamic Approach. New York, Basic Books, 1989

Rush AJ, Beck AT (eds): Cognitive therapy. In Frances A, Hales RE (eds): American Psychiatric Press Review of Psychiatry. Washington, DC, American Psychiatric Press, 533–670, 1988

Sandler J, Dare C, Holder A: The Patient and the Analyst. New York, International Universities Press, 1973

Sifneos PE: Short-Term Psychotherapy and Emotional Crisis. Cambridge, Harvard University Press, 1972

Werman DS: The Practice of Supportive Psychotherapy. New York, Brunner/Mazel, 1984

Yalom I (ed): Group psychotherapy. In Frances A, Hales RE (eds): American Psychiatric Press Review of Psychiatry. Washington, DC, American Psychiatric Press, 655–764, 1986

18 Biological Therapies for Mental Disorders

Jonathan M. Silver,
Gerald I. Hurowitz,
and Stuart C. Yudofsky

GENERAL CONSIDERATIONS IN SELECTING A SOMATIC THERAPY

The use of a somatic treatment for a psychiatric illness is a decision that should be made only after careful consideration of many factors for that individual patient. Medication alone is never *the* treatment for a patient, rather medications may be important components of a larger overall treatment plan. All psychiatric patients require a skilled and thorough psychiatric, neurological, and physical evaluation. A key component of a well-considered decision to use a somatic treatment is the specification of *target symptoms.* One should list those specific symptoms that are designated for treatment and monitor response of these symptoms to treatment; however, a frequent and dangerous clinical error is the treatment of specific symptoms of a disorder with multiple drugs, rather than treating, more specifically, the underlying psychiatric disorder. For example, it is not uncommon for a psychiatrist to be referred a patient who is taking one type of benzodiazepine for anxiety, a different type of benzodiazepine for insomnia, an analgesic for nonspecific somatic complaints, and a subtherapeutic dose of an antidepressant (e.g., 50 mg/day of imipramine) for feelings of sadness. Often, the somatic complaints, insomnia, and anxiety are components of the underlying depression, which is aggravated by the polypharmaceutical approach inherent to symptomatic treatment. In such circumstances, full explanation to the patient of the syndrome of depression, with emphasis on the necessity of adequate doses and duration of treatment with an antidepressant, should precede discontinuation of the benzodiazepine and analgesic medications and the proper administration of an antidepressant agent. After the decision has been made to initiate psychopharmacological treatment, the clinician must select the specific drug. Usually, this choice is made on the basis of the patient's prior history of response to medication, the side effect profile of the drug chosen, and the patient's most likely response to those specific side effects.

Choice of Medication

Choice of a medication also involves an understanding of the *pharmaco-kinetics* of a particular drug, as well as a familiarity with the relative benefits of the available routes of administration of that medication. Most antidepressant and antipsychotic drugs have sufficiently long half-lives to permit a once-a-day dosing regimen, which may increase compliance. The choice of a particular medication may depend on whether that drug is available in injection and liquid forms in addition to tablet, pill, or capsule forms.

Once a decision has been made as to the need for and the choice of a specific drug, attention must be paid to issues related to patient information about indications for and risks and benefits of the medication. A general principle is that the more the patient understands about his or her illness and the reason that medications have been chosen to treat the illness, the more compliant the patient will be. The clinician must also consider the physical, intellectual, and psychological capacities of the patient and her or his caretakers when selecting a new medication. For example, impulsive patients with a history of suicide attempts and alcohol abuse may not safely or reliably be treated with a monoamine oxidase inhibitor because of the need to follow a strict dietary regimen. In general, the more complicated the instructions, the more medications that are prescribed, and the greater number of times per day the medication is to be taken, the more difficulty the patient will have in complying.

A major component of the treatment plan should comprise the evaluation of response and criteria for discontinuation of the medication. Far too frequently, medications are discontinued with the assumption of "failure of response to the medication" without an adequate (i.e., dose, serum level, and duration) drug trial. Different treatment approaches range from a second trial with a related class of medication to the use of complementary or different treatment modalities.

Finally, for those patients whose specific target symptoms do respond to somatic intervention, an end point for treatment must be determined. It is not uncommon for patients to be continued on medications beyond the point at which therapeutic benefit is derived. A common example is the use of benzodiazepines for the treatment of anxiety; patients may be maintained on this drug for years without periodic assessment of its therapeutic benefit by attempts at gradual discontinuation.

ANTIPSYCHOTIC DRUGS

Until quite recently, all neuroleptics were considered equally efficacious in the treatment of psychosis per se. Although many antipsychotic agents are available in parenteral, oral, and depot preparations, and this will at times have some bearing on the choice of agents, choosing the right drug has been determined largely by the drug's side effect profile and the ability of the individual patient to tolerate or benefit from those side effects. With the advent of clozapine, and the newer *atypical* neuroleptics, this situation has changed somewhat. The antipsychotic drugs that are commonly used are shown in Table 18–1.

Mechanisms of Action

For many years, the prevailing theory regarding the mechanism of action of antipsychotic drugs was based on the observation that all available neuroleptics had similar actions on the dopaminergic system: the blocking of dopamine binding to the postsynaptic dopamine receptor in the brain. More specifically, the dopamine-2 (D2) receptor, which, in distinction to the D1 receptor, is *not* linked to adenylate cyclase, was believed to be responsible for the action of this class of drugs. The theory that psychosis is a result of an excess of dopamine or of abnormal activity of certain dopamine receptors has been confirmed by the observation of increased dopamine concentrations and an increased number of D2 receptors in the brains of some patients with schizophrenia (see Chapter 4).

On the other hand, the theory that psychosis is a result of a simple excess of dopamine activity has always been suspect on the grounds that several dopaminergic pathways exist in the brain. The best studied of these, the nigrostriatal system, is involved in motor activity. When antipsychotics reduce dopamine activity in the nigrostriatum (via dopamine receptor blockade), extrapyramidal signs and symptoms result, such as those found in Parkinson's disease. This tendency of antipsychotics to mimic neurological illness led to the use of the term *neuroleptic.* A second locus of dopamine receptors exists in the pituitary and hypothalamus (the tuberoinfundibular system) and influences prolactin release, appetite, and temperature regulation. Because dopamine inhibits the release of prolactin, the antipsychotic drugs disinhibit, and thereby increase, prolactin levels.

Dopamine pathways also connect the limbic system, the midbrain tegmentum, septal nuclei, and mesocortical projections. These areas seem to play a pivotal role in the brain's capacity for thought and emotion. Revised "dopamine hypotheses" have focused on these various pathways and have amended the prevailing theory to accommodate many new findings from basic research. Dopamine receptors more recently discovered—the D3, D4, and D5 receptors—are limited to the frontal cortex and limbic, but not striatal, areas. Some researchers have found that the newer *atypical* neuroleptics (e.g., clozapine)

Table 18–1 **Selected Antipsychotic Drugs and Dosages (see also Table 5–4)**

CLASS/ GENERIC NAME	TRADE NAME	DOSE EQUIVALENT (mg)	USUAL MAINTENANCE DAILY ORAL DOSE (mg)*
Phenothiazine (Aliphatic)			
Chlorpromazine hydrochloride	Thorazine	100	200–600
Piperidine Phenothiazine			
Thioridazine hydrochloride	Mellaril	90–104	200–600
Mesoridazine besylate	Serentil	50–62	150–200
Piperazine Phenothiazine			
Trifluoperazine	Stelazine	2.4–3.2	5–10
Fluphenazine hydrochloride	Prolixin	1.1–1.3	2.5–10
decanoate enanthate		0.61	10 mg/day oral fluphen- azine = 12.5–25 mg/ 2 weeks fluphenazine decanoate
Perphenazine	Trilafon	8.9–9.6	16–24
Thioxanthenes			
Chlorprothixene	Taractan	36–52	75–200
Thiothixene	Navane	3.4–5.4	6–30
Butyrophenones			
Haloperidol	Haldol	1.1–2.1	2–12
Haloperidol decanoate			10 mg/day oral halo- peridol = 100–200 mg/4 weeks halo- peridol decanoate
Dibenzoxazepine			
Loxapine	Loxitane	10	20–60
Indole derivatives			
Molindone hydrochloride	Moban	5.1–6.9	15–60
Diphenylbutylpiperidine			
Pimozide	Orap	N/A	2–10
Dibenzodiazepine			
Clozapine (atypical)	Clozaril	50	200–900
Benzisoxazole			
Risperidone (atypical)	Risperdal	1–2	2–6
Thienobenzodiazepine (Zyprexa)			
Olanzapine (atypical)			5–20
Imidazolidinone			
Quetiapine Seroquel (atypical)			300–750

* Dose ranges required for patients vary. Adjustment in doses may be required depending on the patient's clinical status and responsiveness to medication.
[Silver JM, Yudofsky SC, Hurowitz G: Psychopharmacology and electroconvulsive therapy. In Hales RE, Yudofsky SC, Talbott JA (eds): The American Psychiatric Press Textbook of Psychiatry, 2nd ed. Washington, DC, American Psychiatric Press, 1994]

bind more effectively to these receptors than their older counterparts. Moreover, these newer medications are also less likely to cause extrapyramidal side effects (EPS) and do not elevate prolactin levels. (Clozapine also appears to carry no risk of tardive dyskinesia but can cause agranulocytosis in 1–2% of patients.) The specificity of the atypical antipsychotics for frontal and limbic dopamine receptor sites may account for their distinctive side effect profile and efficacy. Another important difference between the atypical and classical neuroleptics is that the newer drugs are potent 5-hydroxytryptamine (5-HT)2 (serotonin) receptor blocking agents. Meltzer (1995) has suggested that their combined (relatively weak) D2 and (potent) serotonin blockade is what accounts for the special properties of the atypical agents.

Indications and Efficacy

The most common use of antipsychotic drugs is in the treatment of acute psychotic exacerbations and in the maintenance of remission of these psychotic symptoms in patients with schizophrenia. Psychotic symptoms include abnormal thought content such as delusions, perceptual abnormalities such as hallucinations, and abnormal thought form such as disorganized speech.

The impressive data on the effectiveness of antipsychotic drugs as maintenance treatment for schizophrenia have been reviewed thoroughly by Davis and Andriukaitis (1986). Without continued treatment with antipsychotic medication after remission of acute psychotic symptoms, there is a relapse rate of approximately 8 to 15% a month for patients with schizophrenia (Davis and Andriukaitis, 1986). Patients maintained on drugs have a relapse rate ranging from 1.5 to 3% a month.

Antipsychotic drags are effective in ameliorating psychotic symptoms that result from diverse etiologies such as mood (affective) disorders with psychotic features, drug toxicities such as "steroid psychoses" (delirium), and brain disorders such as Huntington's disease or those that occur after head injury. The delusional disorders, including paranoia, delusional jealousy, erotomania, and monosymptomatic hypochondriacal psychosis, are treated with neuroleptic agents. Acute manic symptoms are effectively treated with antipsychotic drugs, with a more rapid response than with lithium. Patients with borderline and schizotypal personality disorders have been treated with antipsychotic drugs. Brief treatment with relatively low-dose antipsychotic drugs may be effective in alleviating the symptoms of somatization, anxiety, and psychotic ideation in these patients. Patients with psychotic or delusional depression may be successfully treated with a combination of antipsychotic and antidepressant drugs, but not with antipsychotic drugs alone.

The sedative side effect of antipsychotic drugs may often lead to their misuse in several clinical situations. These drugs frequently are improperly prescribed as hypnotic or anxiolytic agents. Because of the potential long-term risks of these drugs (see section on tardive dyskinesia), antipsychotics are *not* recommended for the treatment of anxiety or insomnia. In addition, the antipsychotic drugs are often administered to patients who are chronically agitated and violent. We emphasize that although they are valuable for acute episodes of agitation and aggression, these drugs should generally *not* be used for the treatment of chronic aggression and agitation in nonpsychotic patients.

Clinical Use

General Principles

Drug potency refers to the milligram equivalence of drugs, not to the relative efficacy. For example, although haloperidol is more potent than chlorpromazine (2 mg haloperidol = 100 mg chlorpromazine), therapeutically equivalent doses are equally effective (12 mg haloperidol = 600 mg chlorpromazine). These doses are listed in Table 18–1. By convention, the potency of antipsychotic drugs is compared with a standard 100-mg dose of chlorpromazine. As a rule, among the older, classic neuroleptics, *the high-potency antipsychotic drugs with an equivalent dose of less than 5 mg have a high degree of EPS and low levels of sedation and autonomic side effects* (e.g., haloperidol, thiothixene, fluphenazine). Low-potency antipsychotic drugs have an equivalent dose of greater 40 mg (e.g., chlorpromazine and thioridazine). These have a high level of sedation and autonomic side effects and a low degree of EPS. Those antipsychotic drugs with intermediate potency (equivalent dose between 5 and 40 mg) have a side effect profile that lies between these two groups (e.g., perphenazine). The new, atypical antipsychotics, such as quetiapine, diverge from this general principle. In their typical dosage ranges (Table 18–1), these agents have relatively high potency, but a low risk of promoting EPS.

Treatment with antipsychotic medication must be tailored to the individual patient. Flexible guidelines that are supported by scientific principles and research should be followed. These guidelines are outlined in Table 18–2.

Risks, Side Effects, and Their Management

Extrapyramidal Reactions

Serious side effects of antipsychotic use result from the blockade of the postsynaptic dopamine receptor. A variety of EPS may emerge, including acute dystonic reactions, parkinsonian syndrome, akathisia, akinesia, "rabbit syndrome," tardive dyskinesia, neuroleptic-induced catatonia, and the neuroleptic malignant syndrome.

Among the most disturbing and frightening adverse drug reactions that occur with the administration of antipsychotic drugs are *acute dystonic reactions.* This reaction most frequently occurs within hours or days of the initiation of antipsychotic therapy. *The most common feature of this syndrome includes uncontrollable tightening of the face and neck and spasm and*

Table 18–2 **Guidelines for Antipsychotic Drug Therapy**

1. Obtain thorough medical evaluation, including evaluation for tardive dyskinesia.
2. Select drug on the basis of side effect profile, risk/benefit ratio, and history of prior use and response.
3. Inform the patient and family of risk of tardive dyskinesia.
4. Initiate drug therapy at low dose [chlorpromazine (CPZ) equivalent 50 mg orally three times a day].
5. Use prophylactic anticholinergic medication with classic high-potency antipsychotic drugs or in patients younger than 40 years old.
6. Gradually increase dose (50–100 mg CPZ equivalent every other day) until improvement or usual maximum dose of 600 mg CPZ equivalent is reached.
7. Maintain maximum dose for 2–4 weeks.
8. Consider using sedative drugs or beta-blockers for agitation and akathisia.
9. If response is inadequate, obtain plasma level of drugs.
10. If level is low, increase dose to equivalent of 1,000 mg CPZ.
11. Maintain dose for 2–4 weeks. If improvement is inadequate, gradually decrease drug and substitute with an antipsychotic from a different class.
12. Monitor patient closely for therapeutic effects and side effects of treatment.
13. Decrease dosage of antipsychotic medications as soon as possible after initial control of psychotic symptoms.

[Silver JM, Yudofsky SC, Hurowitz G: Psychopharmacology and electroconvulsive therapy. In Hales RE, Yudofsky SC, Talbott JA (eds): The American Psychiatric Press Textbook of Psychiatry, 2nd ed. Washington, DC, American Psychiatric Press, 1994]

distortions of the head and/or back (opisthotonus). If the extraocular muscles are involved, an oculogyric crisis may occur, wherein the eyes are elevated and "locked" in this position. Laryngeal involvement may lead to respiratory and ventilatory difficulties.

Intravenous or intramuscular administration of anticholinergic drugs provides rapid treatment of acute dystonia. Table 18–3 lists the drugs and dosages used to treat dystonic reactions. Note that the anticholinergic drug given to reverse the dystonia will wear off after several hours. Since antipsychotic drugs may have long half-lives and duration of action, additional oral anticholinergic drugs should be prescribed for several days after the dystonic reaction has occurred.

The *parkinsonian syndrome* has many of the features of classic idiopathic Parkinson's disease: diminished range of facial expression (masked facies), cogwheel rigidity, slowed movements (bradykinesia), and "pill-rolling" tremor. The onset of this side effect is gradual and may not appear for weeks after neuroleptics have been administered. Drugs used in the treatment of the parkinsonian side effects of antipsychotic agents are listed in Table 18–3.

Akathisia is an extrapyramidal disorder consisting of an unpleasant feeling of restlessness and the inability to sit still. It is a common reaction and most often occurs shortly after the initiation of antipsychotic drugs. Unfortunately, *akathisia is frequently mistaken for an exacerbation of psychotic symptoms, anxiety, or depression.* The patient may pace or may become agitated

Table 18–3 **Drugs for Treatment of Extrapyramidal Disorders**

GENERIC NAME (TRADE NAME)	(STARTING DOSE)
Anticholinergic Drugs	
Benztropine (Cogentin)	P.O. 0.5 mg t.i.d.
	I.M./I.V. 1 mg
Biperiden (Akineton)	P.O. 2 mg t.i.d.
	I.M./I.V. 2 mg
Diphenhydramine (Benadryl)	P.O. 25 mg q.i.d.
	I.M./I.V. 25 mg
Ethopropazine (Parsidol)	P.O. 50 mg b.i.d.
Orphenadrine (Norflex, Disipal)	P.O. 100 mg b.i.d.
	I.V. 60 mg
Procyclidine (Kemadrine)	P.O. 2.5 mg t.i.d.
Trihexyphenidyl (Artane)	P.O. 1 mg t.i.d.
Dopamine Agonists	
Amantadine (Symmetrel)	P.O. 100 mg b.i.d.
Beta-Blockers (Akathisia)	
Propranolol (Inderal)	P.O. 20 mg t.i.d.

[Silver JM, Yudofsky SC, Hurowitz G: Psychopharmacology and electroconvulsive therapy. In Hales RE, Yudofsky SC, Talbott JA(eds): The American Psychiatric Press Textbook of Psychiatry, 2nd ed. Washington, DC, American Psychiatric Press, 1994]

or angry with the inability to control the symptoms associated with akathisia. If the dose of antipsychotic medications is increased, the restlessness continues or worsens. Consequently, *akathisia is a major cause of neuroleptic non-compliance.* Lowering the dose may improve the symptoms. Although in the past, anticholinergic drugs were suggested as the first line of therapy, they often are ineffective. Benzodiazepines, such as lorazepam, may be effective; however, the treatment of choice for akathisia is a beta-adrenergic blocking drug, particularly propranolol.

Akinesia (or the similar term, *bradykinesia*) is characterized by diminished spontaneity, few gestures, unspontaneous speech, and apathy. As with the parkinsonian syndrome, this may appear only after several weeks of therapy. This syndrome may be mistaken as depression in patients treated with antipsychotic agents. The anticholinergic drugs in the dose ranges suggested in Table 18–3 are effective in treating akinesia; however, akinesia also may be a manifestation of negative symptomatology in a patient with schizophrenia. In such cases, treatment strategies aimed at improving the negative symptoms will be necessary.

The "rabbit syndrome" consists of fine, rapid movements of the lips that mimic the chewing movements of a rabbit. This side effect occurs late in neuroleptic treatment and is treated effectively with anticholinergic drugs. It has been found to be present in approximately 4% of patients receiving neuroleptic therapy (without concomitant anticholinergic agents) (Yassa and Lal, 1986).

Tardive dyskinesia (TD) is a disorder characterized by involuntary movements of the face, trunk, or extremities. The syndrome is related to exposure to dopamine-receptor blocking agents, most frequently the classic antipsychotic agents (Table 18–4); however, the use of drugs such as the antidepressant amoxapine, the antiemetic agents metoclopramide and prochlorperazine, and other drugs with dopamine receptor blocking properties can result in TD. The American Psychiatric Association (APA) Task Force on Tardive Dyskinesia estimates that among patients receiving chronic neuroleptic treatment, 15 to 20% will have some evidence of this condition. The most commonly hypothesized mechanism for the development of TD is that postsynaptic dopamine receptor supersensitivity develops after use of dopamine receptor blocking drugs. Other hypotheses have also been proposed.

The most significant and consistently documented risk factor for the development of TD is *increasing age of the patient.* Women have been found to be at a greater risk for severe TD, although the evidence to date suggests that this finding is limited to geriatric populations. Other risk factors may include the dose of neuroleptic, total time on the drug, EPS early in the course of treatment, history of drug holidays (a greater number of drug-free periods is associated with an increased risk), time since the first exposure to antipsychotic drugs (including drug holidays), presence of brain damage, and presence of a mood disorder.

Table 18–4 **Clinical Features of Tardive Dyskinesia**

The following abnormal movements may be seen in tardive dyskinesia:

Facial and Oral Movements

Muscles of facial expression: involuntary movement of forehead, eyebrows, periorbital area, cheeks; involuntary frowning, blinking, smiling, grimacing
Lips and perioral area: involuntary puckering, pouting, smacking
Jaw: involuntary biting, clenching, chewing, mouth opening, lateral movements
Tongue: involuntary protrusion, tremor, choreoathetoid movements (rolling, wormlike movement without displacement from the mouth)

Extremity Movements

Involuntary movements of upper arms, wrists, hands, fingers: choreic movements (i.e., rapid, objectively purposeless, irregular, spontaneous), athetoid movements (i.e., slow, irregular, complex, serpentine). Tremor (i.e., repetitive, regular, rhythmic)
Involuntary movement of lower legs, knees, ankles, toes: lateral knee movement, foot tapping, foot squirming, inversion and eversion of foot

Trunk Movements

Involuntary movement of neck, shoulders, hips: rocking, twisting, squirming, pelvic gyrations

(Adapted from National Institute of Mental Health: Abnormal Involuntary Movement Scale. In Guy W: ECDEU Assessment Manual. Rockville, MD, U.S. Department of Health, Education, and Welfare, 1976)

The issue of informed consent with respect to antipsychotic medications and the risk of TD has been extensively reviewed (Munetz and Roth, 1985). It is usually difficult, if not impossible, to obtain informed consent from an acutely psychotic patient. A general guideline is to inform and educate the patient's family about the risks of TD before starting the antipsychotics and to educate the patient gradually about this disorder as soon as possible after agitation and psychosis remit. In many circumstances, true informed consent may be impossible to obtain from an acutely psychotic patient for several weeks. The psychiatrist also needs to be aware that some states legally mandate that informed consent be obtained from patients before the initiation of antipsychotic treatment (e.g., California and New Jersey). All such discussions with patients and their families should be documented in the patients' records. An informed consent that is exclusively in the written form has been shown to be less effective in communicating information to the patient than an oral consent obtained in conjunction with education of the patient (Munetz and Roth, 1985). The psychiatrist must allot adequate time to the question of informed consent, consistent with the confusional state and cognitive capabilities of the patient.

Prevention is the most important aspect of TD management. Periodic assessments must be made to determine the patient's requirement for continuing antipsychotic drug therapy. In addition, every 6 months a reevaluation is required to ascertain the lowest possible dose of antipsychotic drug that still proves to be effective in the treatment of psychotic symptoms.

There is no reliable treatment of TD other than discontinuing the antipsychotic medication; however, because neuroleptics remain the only effective treatment for most patients with schizophrenia, the case often arises in which a patient develops TD, but still requires the neuroleptic treatment to function. If discontinuation of the antipsychotic drug is possible, improvement in the TD may be gradual. Worsening of the involuntary movements often occurs initially with the withdrawal of neuroleptics. (Conversely, TD movements may be masked temporarily by increasing the dosage of neuroleptic medication, but will reemerge eventually, often in a more severe form.) However, while TD is often felt to be "permanent," a 50% reduction in dyskinetic movements is documented in most patients by 18 months after discontinuation of antipsychotic agents (Glazer et al, 1984).

For patients who develop TD and yet cannot be taken off neuroleptics, the most promising treatment is clozapine. Lieberman et al (1991) found at least 50% improvement in TD among 43% of patients switched from another neuroleptic to clozapine. Severe TD, and especially tardive dystonia, seem to respond best. In view of the risks of agranulocytosis with clozapine treatment (see below), this strategy must be investigated further.

Neuroleptic Malignant Syndrome. In rare instances, patients on antipsychotic medications may develop a potentially life-threatening disorder known as neuroleptic malignant syndrome (NMS). While most frequently occurring with the use of high-potency neuroleptics (haloperidol), this condition may emerge after the use of any antipsychotic agent. The patient with NMS becomes severely rigid and occasionally catatonic. There is fever, elevated white blood cell count, tachycardia, abnormal blood pressure fluctuations, tachypnea, and diaphoresis. Creatinine phosphokinase (CPK) levels are elevated due to muscle breakdown; CPK levels are an excellent parameter to check for the presence of the disorder and response to treatment.

NMS is most often associated with the initiation or increase of antipsychotic medication. Patients on stable doses of neuroleptics who develop NMS are usually suffering from dehydration. Concurrent lithium treatment may increase the risk appreciably, as may the presence of a mood disorder. Higher doses, rapid escalation of dosage, and intramuscular injections of neuroleptics all are associated with the development of NMS. A prodrome to neuroleptic malignant syndrome is *neuroleptic-induced catatonia,* wherein the prominent signs are EPS and a catatonic behavioral state that may be mistaken for a worsening of the psychosis. Neuroleptic-induced catatonia is best treated with amantadine 100 mg b.i.d. over several weeks.

The key treatment steps after recognition of NMS are discontinuation of all medications, thorough medical evaluation, and physical support, including intravenous fluids, antipyretic agents, and cooling blankets. Several treatments have been suggested to control NMS. These include amantadine, electroconvulsive therapy, benzodiazepines, and anticholinergic drugs. As noted above, amantadine appears to be more useful in the treatment of neuroleptic-induced catatonia than do the anticholinergic drugs. Dantrolene sodium (a direct-acting muscle relaxant) and bromocriptine (a centrally active dopamine agonist) appear to be the most successful agents in the treatment of NMS, but their efficacy over supportive care has not been definitively proved. Because these two agents may treat differing symptoms of NMS and may act through separate mechanisms, they also may be useful in combination. Unfortunately, no controlled clinical trials related to the somatic treatment of NMS have yet been conducted.

Anticholinergic Effects

In the treatment of a patient with antipsychotic drugs, anticholinergic side effects may be caused by either the neuroleptic or the anticholinergic drug that has been prescribed to alleviate EPS. Among the newer agents, clozapine has especially pronounced anticholinergic effects, whereas risperidone and olanzapine have only minor anticholinergic effects. Anticholinergic effects are categorized as peripheral or central. Among the peripheral side effects, the most common are dry mouth, decreased sweating, decreased bronchial secretions, blurred vision (due to inhibition of accommodation), difficulty in urination, and constipation. Central side effects of anticholinergic drugs include impairment in concentration, attention, and memory. In cases of toxicity, anticholinergic delirium—which includes hot, dry skin, dry mucous membranes, dilated pupils, absent bowel sounds, and tachycardia—may appear.

Other Side Effects

Blockade of alpha-adrenergic receptors can result in orthostatic hypotension and dizziness. Mesoridazine, chlorpromazine, thioridazine, and clozapine are the most potent alpha-1 blockers of the antipsychotic drugs. Changes in hormonal function have been reported to occur with neuroleptic treatment. Because of the dopamine blocking effect, prolactin levels increase, which may result in gynecomastia in both men and women. Galactorrhea, although unusual, also may occur. Additional neuroendocrine side effects of neuroleptics mediated by hyperprolactinemia include amenorrhea, weight gain, breast tenderness, and decreased libido.

Sexual dysfunction also may be caused by neuroleptic therapy. In men, difficulty in achieving or maintaining an erection, decreased ability to achieve orgasm, and changes in the quality of orgasm are reported. Thioridazine may cause painful retrograde ejaculation in which semen is ejected into the bladder. Women may experience changes in the quality of orgasm and decreased ability to achieve orgasm with antipsychotic use. Menstrual irregularities also may occur.

Pigmentary changes in the skin and eyes may occur, especially with long-term treatment. Pigment deposition in the lens of the eye does not affect vision. Pigmentary retinopathy, which can lead to irreversible blindness, has been associated specifically with the use of thioridazine. Pigmentary retinopathy has most often been reported with doses above the recommended dosage ceiling for thioridazine (i.e., 800 mg/day). Almost all patients on neuroleptics, especially the aliphatic phenothiazines (e.g., chlorpromazine), become more sensitive to the effects of sunlight, which can lead to severe sunburn. Especially in the summer months, patients should avoid excess sun exposure and use ultraviolet blocking agents, such as sunscreens that contain paraaminobenzoic acid.

Several of the antipsychotic medications have cardiac effects that can be detected on the electrocardiogram. For example, thioridazine is associated with prolonged QT intervals, and this change is related to plasma level concentration. There have been reports of other arrhythmias and sudden death with antipsychotic agents, probably due to their quinidine-like effects.

Increases in liver function enzymes have been associated with antipsychotic treatment. Many cases of this reaction were linked to impurities in the original formulation of chlorpromazine, and because the incidence has profoundly decreased over the years, it is now considered rare among the classical antipsychotic drugs. One notable exception to this finding of a low risk of liver dysfunction is the new atypical neuroleptic olanzapine. Olanzapine has been found to cause an elevation of serum transaminases in some patients, an effect that was transient and reversible on discontinuation of the medications. Transient leukopenia and, in rare cases, agranulocytosis have been associated with neuroleptic treatment. These are idiosyncratic reactions that usually occur within the first 3 to 4 weeks after the initiation of treatment with an antipsychotic drug. Clozapine has a much greater propensity for inducing agranulocytosis and, in order to be prescribed, requires special precautions to safeguard against it (see below).

The antipsychotic drugs have been shown to lower seizure threshold, a phenomenon that has been confirmed in animal models. Of all the antipsychotics, fluphenazine and molindone have been most consistently shown to have the lowest potential for lowering the seizure threshold. Clozapine is at the other end of the seizure-risk spectrum. The risk of seizures with clozapine is dose related: below 300 mg/day, the risk is just 1%, whereas between 300 and 600 mg/day, the risk is 2.7%, and above 600 mg/day, the risk jumps to 4.4% (Devinsky et al, 1991). Special precautions must be taken with the use of antipsychotic agents in those patients with a history of convulsions who are not on anticonvulsant therapy and in those patients with brain lesions associated with abnormal electroencephalographic (EEG) findings.

Antipsychotic drugs directly affect the hypothalamus and suppress control of temperature regulation. In combination with the alpha-adrenergic receptor and cholinergic receptor blocking effects of antipsychotics, this effect becomes particularly serious in hot, humid weather.

As a general guideline, antipsychotic drugs should be used in pregnant patients only if absolutely necessary, at the minimal dose required, and for the briefest possible time.

The treatment of refractory psychosis had been limited for many years by the fact that all the available antipsychotic medications were equally effective. The introduction of the atypical neuroleptic clozapine, for use in treatment-resistant schizophrenia, has changed this situation. Clozapine is atypical because it causes significantly fewer EPS, does not elevate serum prolactin, and has not been found to date to induce TD. Significant improvement has been found in up to 30% of patients with schizophrenia who have failed to respond to classic antipsychotic medications. Clozapine has been shown to be useful in refractory cases of schizoaffective disorder and psychotic mood disorders (McElroy et al, 1991). Moreover, because it appears to be devoid of parkinsonian side effects, clozapine is useful in low doses for Parkinson's patients with medication-induced psychoses.

Unfortunately, the use of clozapine is associated with potentially severe side effects. There is a 2 % risk of developing a potentially fatal agranulocytosis (apparently the risk is higher among Ashkenazic Jews). For this reason, weekly blood counts are required by the manufacturer for any patient prescribed clozapine. Patients being considered for clozapine treatment must be screened for illnesses associated with immunocompromise, including tuberculosis and human immunodeficiency virus infection.

To date, the newer atypical neuroleptics—risperidone, olanzapine, and quetiapine—have not been shown to be efficacious among patients refractory to treatment with the classic neuroleptic agents; however, several studies have suggested that, among schizophrenia patients who do respond to neuroleptic treatment, these atypical antipsychotics are superior overall to the older agents because of a clear edge they have in the treatment of the negative symptom syndrome.

ANTIDEPRESSANT DRUGS

The modern era of drug treatment of depression began in the 1950s when iproniazid, a monoamine oxidase inhibitor (MAOI) used for the treatment of tuberculosis, was noted to elevate the mood of these patients. Imipramine, the first of the tricyclic antidepressants (TCAs), was developed as a derivative of chlorpromazine with the hope that the drug would be more effective as an antipsychotic agent. Although imipramine did not exhibit antipsychotic efficacy, it was found to be effective in the treatment of depression.

Since that time, many other antidepressant drugs have been approved for use in the United States. Among this group are the secondary amine TCAs, drugs of the MAOI family, selective serotonin-reuptake inhibitors (SSRIs), and the so-called atypical antidepressants, trazodone (a triazolopyridine), bupropion (an aminoketone), venlafaxine (a bicyclic), nefazodone (a phenylpiperazine), and mirtazapine (Remeron). The currently available antidepressants in the United States are listed in Tables 18–5, and 18–6).

Mechanisms of Action

Antidepressant drugs acutely affect the serotonergic and catecholaminergic systems in the central nervous system. The TCAs and SSRIs block the presynaptic reuptake of 5-HT and/or norepinephrine, thereby increasing the availability of these neurotransmitters for activity at receptor sites. Like many of the TCAs, venlafaxine blocks the reuptake of *both* NE and 5-HT, but it is nearly devoid of the anticholinergic effects associated with the TCAs. Bupropion's main mode of action also involves reuptake inhibition, but in this case, the reuptake of dopamine is thought to be primarily affected. The MAOIs augment monoaminergic transmission by blocking the catabolism of several biogenic amines, including norepinephrine, 5-HT, tyramine, phenylephrine, and dopamine. Trazodone has mixed effects on the serotonin system, but apparently achieves an antidepressant effect through its antagonism of the postsynaptic 5-HT2 receptor. Nefazodone has a similar effect on the postsynaptic 5-HT2 receptor but, in addition, has mild serotonin and NE reuptake inhibition properties. Mirtazapine also has mixed effects on the serotonin system, including postsynaptic 5-HT1A agonist properties, but its antidepressant effects are believed to be a consequence of antagonism at the central noradrenergic alpha-2 receptor.

Table 18–5 **Selected Antidepressant Drugs and Dosages**

CLASS/GENERIC NAME	TRADE NAME	DOSE RANGE (mg)
Tertiary Amine Tricyclics		
Imipramine	Tofranil	75–300
	Tofranil PM	
	SK-Pramine	
Amitriptyline	Elavil	75–300
	Endep	
Doxepin	Adapin	75–300
	Sinequan	
Trimipramine	Surmontil	50–200
Secondary Amine Tricyclics		
Desipramine	Norpramin	75–300
	Pertofrane	
Nortriptyline	Aventyl	50–150
	Pamelor	
Protriptyline	Vivactil	10–60
Tetracyclic		
Maprotiline	Ludiomil	150–200
Dibenzoxazepine		
Amoxapine	Asendin	75–400
Triazolopyridine		
Trazodone	Desyrel	200–600
Unicyclic		
Bupropion	Wellbutrin	150–450
Selective Serotonin Reuptake Inhibitors		
Fluoxetine	Prozac	10–40
Sertraline	Zoloft	50–200
Paroxetine	Paxil	10–40
Fluroxamine	Lurox	50–300
Phenylpiperazine		
Nefazodone	Serzone	300–600
Bicyclic phenethylamine		
Venlafaxine	Effexor	75–375
Piperazinoazopine		
Mirtazapine	Remeron	15–45

The early observation of these acute effects of antidepressants on neurotransmitters led to the *catecholamine hypothesis* of depression, which postulated that depression was caused by a relative deficiency of catecholaminergic neurotransmitters that was "corrected" by antidepressant drugs. Because, at that time, the existing antidepressants affected serotonin and/or norepinephrine function to varying degrees, it was anticipated that depression subtypes would be discovered, depending on whether a patient was primarily deficient

Table 18–6 **Selected Monoamine Oxidase Inhibitors Drugs and Dosages**

CLASS GENERIC NAME	TRADE NAME	USUAL DAILY MAXIMUM ORAL DOSE (mg)
Hydrazines		
Phenelzine	Nardil	90
Isocarboxazid	Marplan	50
Nonhydrazines		
Tranylcypromine	Parnate	60
Pargyline	Eutonyl	150

[Silver JM, Yudofsky SC, Hurowitz G: Psychopharmacology and electroconvulsive therapy. In Hales RE, Yudofsky SC, Talbott JA (eds): The American Psychiatric Press Textbook of Psychiatry, 2nd ed. Washington, DC, American Psychiatric Press, 1994].

in serotonin or norepinephrine. However, no such diagnostic differentiation of depression has been discovered to date. More recently, these two neurotransmitter systems, serotonin ascending from the raphe nucleus and norepinephrine from the locus ceruleus, have been hypothesized to interconnect in a feedforward system, such that the induction of one serves to induce the other.

With further research, investigators discovered that, whereas the effects on reuptake inhibition are immediate, it is the effect of antidepressants on receptor sensitivity after chronic administration that most clearly parallels the well-known delayed clinical response to these agents. It appears that the presynaptic autoreceptors, the alpha-2 noradrenergic and the 5-HT1 and 5-HT2 serotonergic receptors, gradually develop a functional downregulation that enhances presynaptic neuronal firing and enhances neurotransmitter release.

Years of research have begun to elucidate the mechanism by which this downregulation occurs. It is fairly well established that, by increasing the amount of neurotransmitter in the synapse, antidepressants cause a *compensatory* downregulation of the receptors. However, there are reports that cultured cells exposed to antidepressants, but devoid of norepinephrine, still show evidence of downregulated beta-adrenergic receptors. Attention has now focused on the *second messenger* system of the cells in question, specifically on the effects of antidepressants on the coupling of G proteins (which include stimulatory and inhibitory subtypes), via adenylyl cyclase, with the various intracellular second messengers [e.g., cyclic adenosine monophosphate(cAMP)]. This research has demonstrated that antidepressants facilitate the coupling of the G_s protein with adenylyl cyclase, resulting in increased cAMP production. A cAMP-dependent protein kinase is thereby activated, which in turn may phosphorylate the receptor, serving to uncouple it from the G protein. This uncoupling of the receptor and G protein completes a cycle that results in receptor downregulation. In addition, the cAMP-dependent protein kinase enters into the cell nucleus where, through phosphorylation, it can affect protein transcription and gene expression.

The MAOIs have a mode of action that distinguishes them from the reuptake inhibitor antidepressants. The enzyme MAO inactivates biogenic amines such as norepinephrine, serotonin, dopamine, and tyramine through oxidative deamination. MAOIs block this inactivation and thereby increase the amount of these transmitters available for synaptic release. There are two types of MAO, types A and B. Type A (MAO-A) acts selectively on the substrates norepinephrine and serotonin, whereas type B (MAO-B) preferentially affects phenylethylamine. Both MAO types oxidize dopamine and tyramine. Because norepinephrine and serotonin have been hypothesized to play a major role in the pathophysiology of depression, MAO-A inhibition is, at least theoretically, the source of the therapeutic effects of the MAOIs.

Currently available MAOIs are either hydrazine or nonhydrazine derivatives. The hydrazine derivatives, isocarboxazid and phenelzine, are related to iproniazid. The nonhydrazine derivatives include tranylcypromine, the selective MAO-B inhibitor and anti-Parkinson's drug selegiline, and the antihypertensive drug pargyline (Table 18–6). MAO must be regenerated before the activity of the enzyme is reestablished. In practical terms, this means that the effects (including risks of drug and food interaction) of the "irreversible" MAO inhibitors will last until sufficient MAO has been regenerated. For this reason, the clinician must wait 10 to 14 days after discontinuation of these drugs before instituting other antidepressants or permitting certain drugs or foods that may interact adversely with the MAOIs. All the currently marketed MAOIs, with the exception of selegiline, are *nonselective* in that they inhibit both MAO-A and MAO-B. Selegiline, approved for use in the treatment of Parkinson's disease, is selective for MAO-B in doses up to 20 mg a day, but becomes nonselective at higher doses and shows some degree of MAO-A inhibition. At these higher doses, selegiline possesses antidepressant properties, although it is not used for the treatment of depression in the United States.

Indications and Efficacy

Although the antidepressant drugs have many potential therapeutic uses, the primary approved indication for these drugs is the treatment of depression that corresponds to the diagnosis of major depressive disorder. Approximately 70 to 80% of depressed patients respond to an adequate trial of an antidepressant. Among the other disorders that may respond to antidepressants are panic disorder, obsessive–compulsive disorder, enuresis, chronic pain, migraine headaches, bulimia, and attention-deficit hyperactivity disorder.

Patients with depression characterized by the symptoms of oversleeping, overeating, mood reactivity, and prominent anxiety ("atypical depression") may show a preferentially positive response to MAOIs, which have even been suggested as the treatment of choice in this group of patients.

For patients with recurrent unipolar depressions, maintenance TCAs with and without lithium are effective in decreasing the chance of relapse. The role of lithium in the prevention and treatment of episodes of bipolar illness is discussed in detail in a later section.

Several other disorders also respond to antidepressants, although in many of these cases, the Food and Drug Administration (FDA) has not approved the use of antidepressants for these conditions. Among these conditions are panic disorder (TCAs, SSRIs, and MAOIs), social phobia (MAOIs and SSRIs), obsessive–compulsive disorder (clomipramine and the SSRIs), post-traumatic stress disorder, bulimia (SSRIs), attention deficit hyperactivity disorder (bupropion, desipramine, tranylcypromine), peptic ulcer disease (TCAs), irritable bowel syndrome, enuresis (TCAs), migraine (TCAs and MAOIs), and chronic pain (TCAs and SSRIs).

Clinical Use of Antidepressants

The psychiatric history, current symptoms, physical examination, and mental status of patients with depressed mood are major factors in the choice of the appropriate therapeutic modality. Diagnostic factors that may influence the choice of antidepressant drug include a history of manic or hypomanic episodes, the presence of psychosis, the prior course of episodes of depression, and the presence of "atypical" symptoms.

A history of previous episodes of mania or hypomania should alert the clinician to the possible precipitation of these episodes with antidepressants. If hypomania occurs while the patient is on antidepressant therapy, a reduction in dosage should be attempted as a first effort to control these symptoms. Depending on the severity of the hypomania, a mood stabilizer also may be added. When there is evidence of a burgeoning mania, or when the hypomania persists, mood stabilizers should be used alone. Patients with bipolar disorder may experience more frequent mood cycling and general increases in resistance to treatment when treated chronically with antidepressants. Precipitation of hypomania or mania in a depressed patient treated with an antidepressant suggests that the patient has a bipolar mood disorder. Pretreatment with a mood stabilizer in usual therapeutic doses before the administration of antidepressant drugs should be considered in depressed patients who have experienced previous manic episodes; however, concurrent mood stabilization treatment will *not* guarantee by any means that the patient will not develop hypomania or mania, nor will it ensure that the patient will not have more frequent manic/depressive episodes (increased cycling).

As noted, chronic antidepressant has been shown to decrease the interval between affective episodes and to increase "cycling" in bipolar patients. For bipolar patients who develop mixed manic–depressive states or increased cycling on antidepressants, valproate (the drug of choice for *mixed states*), carbamazepine, or lithium should be started, and the antidepressant drug should be gradually tapered. Increasing cycle frequency should also be considered in unipolar depressed patients. Because of the demonstrated efficacy of lithium in the prevention of relapse in unipolar and bipolar patients (see section on lithium), lithium should be considered for patients with unipolar depression in whom the interval between episodes has been decreasing.

Patients with delusional (psychotic) depression respond poorly to treatment when antidepressant medications are used as the sole agent. Patients with delusional depression respond better to combined treatment of antidepressants *and* antipsychotics than to either alone, but they generally show the best response to electroconvulsive therapy.

Psychotherapy is vitally important in the treatment of patients with depression. Studies have demonstrated that the response to the combination of psychotherapy and medication is superior to that of either treatment as the sole modality (Conte et al, 1986).

Treatment of depressed patients with pharmacological agents must be guided by scientific principles that are tailored to the needs of individual patients. This requires guidelines for initiation of therapy (Table 18–7) in addition to an overall treatment strategy. As with the antipsychotic drugs, the choice of which antidepressant to use is often dependent on the side effect profile of the drug. Other factors involved in this decision include the patient's

Table 18–7 **Guidelines for Use of Antidepressant Drugs***

1. Complete a thorough medical evaluation, especially with regard to cardiovascular and thyroid status.
2. Select drug on the basis of side effect profile (stimulating effect, sedating effect, anticholinergic effect, and cardiovascular effect) and history of previous response.
3. Inform the patient and family of risks and benefits. Emphasize the expected 2–3-week "delay" in therapeutic response and anticipated side effects and their management.
4. Initiate and increase dose slowly. Initial dose is generally one-eighth to one-quarter of the eventual therapeutic dose.
5. Stabilize at low therapeutic dose for 2–5 weeks.
6. If there is no significant effect after 2–5 weeks, slowly increase dosage to maximum recommended dose (if the clinical condition allows).
7. If there is no significant improvement after 14–21 days, obtain plasma level (if appropriate) and electrocardiogram (if TCA) and adjust dose as needed. An electrocardiogram should be obtained before each dose increase (if TCA) in patients with severe heart disease. Serum levels stabilize on a given dose after 7–10 days. Therapeutic serum levels are best established for imipramine, desipramine, and nortriptyline.
8. A therapeutic trial is defined as a 6-week treatment with antidepressant, with at least 3 weeks with a therapeutic serum level. Then consider an antidepressant from another class, or go to ECT immediately. Reevaluate diagnosis.
9. Elderly and medically ill patient may require lower dose ranges than those noted above.
10. Most of the currently available antidepressants can be given once a day. SSRIs venlafaxine and protriptyline should be given early in the day. Bupropion and nefazodone require multiple daily doses. Most TCAs are best taken before bed.

* Note special exemptions *especially for fluoxetine.* MAOI, monoamine oxidase inhibitor; ECT, electroconvulsive therapy; SSRI, selective serotonin-reuptake inhibitor. [Silver JM, Yudofsky SC, Hurowitz G: Psychopharmacology and electroconvulsive therapy. In Hales RE, Yudofsky SC, Talbott JA (eds): The American Psychiatric Press Textbook of Psychiatry, 2nd ed. Washington, DC, American Psychiatric Press, 1994]

history of previous treatment response, the anticipation of the need for useful plasma levels, the medical status of the patient, and the risk of suicide by overdose. Finally, consideration of the overall treatment strategy (including the possibility of a future trial of an MAOI) and other drug interactions play a role in the initiation of treatment.

The side effects that impact on the choice of antidepressant most often are the anticholinergic effects, cardiovascular effects, sedation, and stimulation. (These are discussed in greater detail below.) In summary, among the TCAs, those with more potent effects on norepinephrine reuptake inhibition are more stimulating. Thus, desipramine may be poorly tolerated in agitated, depressed patients. TCAs with marked antihistaminic effects and predominantly serotonergic effects (clomipramine and doxepin) are sedating. The 5-HT-2 blocking agents nefazodone and trazodone are also quite sedating for many patients. This effect may be advantageous in patients with marked initial insomnia but undesirable in patients with psychomotor retardation. The SSRIs, bupropion, and venlafaxine are all more stimulating than the TCAs and have little or no anticholinergic effects. These drugs are also less likely to cause weight gain and occasionally will cause (usually mild) anorexia or weight loss. On the other hand, overstimulation and insomnia may become a problem, especially in anxious or agitated patients. The SSRIs, bupropion, and (especially) venlafaxine are associated with more gastrointestinal side effects such as nausea and/or diarrhea.

The initial therapeutic response of the depressed patient to medications may be detected as early as the first week with the patient showing improvement in sleep and energy. Mood, however, may not respond for 1 to 4 weeks after medication has been initiated. Of crucial importance is the fact that the patient may have a return of energy while still experiencing the hopelessness that characterizes the depression. Thus, the patient may be at an increased risk of suicide at this time, for she or he may regain the energy requisite to complete a suicidal act that was not present before treatment.

A complete trial of antidepressant medication consists of treatment with therapeutic doses of a drug for a total of 6 to 8 weeks. At the end of this period, the patient can be conceptualized as falling into one of three groups, depending on whether there has been a full response, a partial response, or no response at all. For those fortunate patients who achieve full remission, the dose of the antidepressant and the length of time necessary for continuance on the medication must be determined. Results from a National Institute of Mental Health collaborative study indicate that antidepressant therapy should not be withdrawn before 4 to 5 symptom-free months have passed (Prien and Kupfer, 1986). After the maintenance phase of treatment, antidepressants should be gradually tapered over several months and discontinued. In patients with chronic (unipolar) depression, longer periods of antidepressant treatment are warranted to protect against recurrence.

For patients who have not responded to an adequate trial of one particular antidepressant, it is recommended that the patient be switched to a drug from another *first-line* class of antidepressant (e.g., from an SSRI to a TCA, or vice versa). Sixty to 65% of patients who fail to respond to a TCA will respond to an SSRI, and vice versa (Preskorn and Burke, 1992).

For patients who achieve a partial response (or who have failed to respond to adequate trials of first- and second-line antidepressants), several augmentation strategies are advised. Augmentation involves the concurrent use of two antidepressants or the use of a single antidepressant in combination with lithium, thyroid hormone, or a psychostimulant. Of these strategies, lithium augmentation has received the most attention. Some patients manifest a rapid and dramatic response when lithium is added to their ongoing antidepressant therapy, but improvement may require 6 weeks. Patients often respond at doses of lithium that would be insufficient for the treatment of bipolar disorder. It has also been reported that thyroid hormone supplementation with T_3 preparations possibly potentiates antidepressant effects in TCA nonresponders. This technique is rarely used by clinicians and its efficacy is generally disappointing.

The use of more than one antidepressant is potentially beneficial in the treatment of refractory depression. Fluoxetine plus TCA combinations have been reported to be effective for patients who fail to respond to monotherapy and may bring a more rapid antidepressant effect. Fluoxetine causes an elevation of tricyclic plasma levels, but this effect does not account for the synergism between the two antidepressants; however, this elevation of TCA levels does raise the risk of accidental TCA toxicity when these drugs are combined with fluoxetine. We therefore recommend starting with low TCA doses (e.g., desipramine 25 mg) and proceeding only after plasma levels have been measured. The other SSRIs carry a lower risk of elevating plasma TCA levels, with sertraline apparently having the lowest risk; however, lower TCA doses and close monitoring are prudent. Combined use of antidepressants should be done only under the supervision of a psychiatrist.

Despite concerns over the severe reactions that may occur with concomitant treatment with TCAs and MAOIs, the combination may be safely prescribed, provided specific precautions are taken, such as starting the medications together and ensuring that frequent, daily blood pressure monitoring takes place during the "loading" phase of treatment. In low doses, an MAOI may be added to ongoing TCA treatment, but *please note that it is extremely hazardous to add the TCAs to *ongoing* MAOI treatment.* MAOIs can never be prescribed with SSRIs. Due to the long half-life of fluoxetine, MAOIs may not be initiated until 5 weeks after fluoxetine has been discontinued.

Risks, Side Effects, and Their Management

The side effect profile of a specific antidepressant drug in large part determines the selection of a particular drug for an individual patient. In addition, patients have varying reactions to side effects when they occur. For example, for some patients, the almost omnipresent anticholinergic effects (i.e., dry mouth, blurred vision) of most TCAs are intolerable, while other patients note the presence of these side effects without complaint.

The tricyclic antidepressant drugs vary greatly in their relative potential to produce anticholinergic side effects. Because of the anticholinergic effects, patients with prostatic hypertrophy and narrow angle glaucoma must be treated conservatively. The precautions and evaluations of these complications are outlined in the section on antipsychotic drugs. In practical terms, trazodone, nefazodone, venlafaxine, and the SSRIs (with the exception of paroxetine) have virtually no anticholinergic effects, yet dry mouth and blurred vision occur more frequently with these drugs than with placebo. Bupropion has no effect on the cholinergic system.

With the exception of trazodone, nefazodone, and mirtazapine, the relative sedating properties of the antidepressants parallel their respective histamine receptor binding affinities. Trazodone, trimipramine, amitriptyline, and doxepin are the most sedating antidepressants. If this property is adversely experienced by the patient, a less sedating antidepressant should be prescribed (e.g., desipramine, an SSRI, venlafaxine, bupropion).

The SSRIs, bupropion, venlafaxine, MAOIs, and certain TCAs, such as desipramine, are associated with excess stimulation in some patients. Such patients complain of "jitteriness," restlessness, tense feelings, and/or disturbed sleep. For patients prone to such reactions, starting the medication in low doses and increasing it slowly will often help. The short-term use of a benzodiazepine may also help the patient cope with overstimulation in the early stages of treatment until tolerance to this side effect develops. For antidepressant-induced insomnia, trazodone may often prove useful as a sedative–hypnotic before bed.

Orthostatic hypotension is the cardiovascular side effect that most commonly results in serious morbidity, especially in the elderly and in patients with congestive heart failure. The symptoms of orthostatic hypotension usually consist of dizziness or lightheadedness when the patient changes from a lying to sitting or sitting to standing position. Although orthostatic hypotension may occur from any TCA (especially the tertiary TCAs), nortriptyline has been found to cause less orthostatic hypotension than imipramine. Trazodone and the MAOIs also may cause significant hypotension. Although the incidence is much lower than that associated with the TCAs and MAOIs, fluoxetine has been rarely reported to cause bradycardia and syncope in patients with no history of cardiovascular disease. While bupropion and venlafaxine are not associated with orthostatic hypotension, buproprion, and venlafaxine carries a significant risk of inducing *hyper*tension.

Because TCAs at toxic levels can cause life-threatening arrhythmias, many clinicians believe that TCAs can cause dangerous arrhythmias at treatment doses. In actuality, TCAs are potent antiarrhythmic agents, possessing quinidine-like properties. The particular effects of the TCAs on the cardiac conduction system are of great clinical importance. Because prolongation of the PR and QRS intervals can occur with TCAs' use, these drugs should not be used in patients with preexisting heart block, such as second-degree heart block, or markedly prolonged QRS and QT intervals. In such patients, TCAs can lead to second- or third-degree heart block—a life-threatening condition. There is also evidence that using drugs with quinidine-like effects like the TCAs may increase mortality and morbidity following myocardial infarction. Patients with relatively focal, benign, and stable right bundle and left bundle branch blocks may at times be treated with TCAs after clearance by cardiology and dosing initiated in the inpatient setting with frequent cardiac monitoring. Information available to date suggests that bupropion and the SSRIs are free of clinically significant effects on the cardiac conductive system.

Sexual dysfunctions associated with antidepressants include impotence, ejaculatory dysfunction, anorgasmia, and decreased interest and enjoyment of sexual activities for both men and women. Trazodone and nefazodone are the only antidepressants that have been associated with priapism, which may be irreversible and require surgical intervention. While every class of antidepressants has been associated with sexual side effects, bupropion and nefazodone carry the lowest risk overall.

Patients treated with TCAs, MAOIs, and SSRIs may experience an undesirable weight gain. This does not appear to relate to improvement of mood, as changes in weight and appetite are not correlated to response to treatment. On the other hand, treatment of depressed patients with fluoxetine may actually be associated with weight loss.

As with most drugs, allergic and hypersensitivity reactions may occur with antidepressants, but are extremely rare and may be connected to those pill forms that contain yellow dye with tartrazine. For more serious skin eruptions, the drug should be discontinued, preferably over several days, to reduce the possibility of antidepressant withdrawal symptoms. Tremor is a common side effect of antidepressants, such as imipramine and desipramine, that affect predominantly the noradrenergic system. Dose reduction or changing the type of antidepressant may ultimately be required to alleviate the tremor.

In general, the potential of antidepressants to induce seizures is difficult to assess. Maprotiline has been associated with seizures in both therapeutic and toxic doses, but especially at doses above 200 mg/day. While there is an increased risk of seizures associated with the use of bupropion, this is low when single dosages do not exceed 150 mg and the total daily dosage is not greater than 450 mg. Similarly, a dose-related risk of seizures has been found with clomipramine, and this has led to a recommendation that its daily dose not exceed 250 mg. Patients with obvious risk factors for seizures (patients with epilepsy, head trauma, abnormal EEGs) should not be treated with these antidepressants unless special care is taken and the patient is prescribed anticonvulsant medication. Among the remaining antidepressants, amoxapine and desipramine may have a higher risk of seizures after overdosage. On the other hand, there are reports of fluoxetine improving seizure control in some epileptic patients when it was added to their existing anticonvulsant regimen.

Antidopaminergic effects, such as dystonia, parkinsonism, and akathisia are rare side effects of the antidepressants, with two notable exceptions.

Fluoxetine has been found to cause akathisia and may exacerbate parkinsonism. Amoxapine, which has a mild neuroleptic effect, is liable to cause extrapyramidal effects, akathisia, and even TD.

Because the incidence of suicide and suicide attempts is high in depressed patients, deliberate overdosage with antidepressant drugs is a common occurrence. As many as 10,000 cases of antidepressant overdoses each year are attributed to suicide attempts. It is unfortunate that a population that is at high risk for suicide is often trusted with drugs that have a low median lethal dose— a relatively low ceiling for toxic doses. This is especially true for the TCAs and MAOIs. For patients at high suicide risk, clinicians should consider giving only a week's supply of these antidepressants. The SSRIs, venlafaxine, and nefazodone are much less toxic in overdose situations compared with tricyclics. The greatest morbidity risk with bupropion overdose is seizures. While seizures per se are seldom life threatening, in association with driving, a fall, or other trauma-related event, a patient could harm or kill him- or herself or others.

The major complications from overdose with TCAs include those that arise from neuropsychiatric impairment, hypotension, cardiac arrhythmias, and seizures. Because most TCAs have significant anticholinergic activity, anticholinergic delirium often occurs when they are taken in high doses. Other complications of anticholinergic overdose include agitation, supraventricular arrhythmias, heart block, hallucinations, severe hypertension, and seizures. These drugs also lower the seizure threshold and can result in prolonged seizures.

Because the TCAs are metabolized by the liver, drugs that induce hepatic microsomal enzymes will result in a decrease in plasma levels of the antidepressant drugs. These agents include alcohol, anticonvulsants, barbiturates, chloral hydrate, glutethimide, oral contraceptives, and cigarette smoking. Antipsychotic drugs, methylphenidate, SSRIs, and increasing age are associated with increased plasma levels of the tricyclics. In general, the SSRIs are metabolized by the cytochrome P450 system, and through saturation of these enzymes, they may elevate the plasma levels of many other drugs (Harvey and Preskorn, 1996). SSRI interactions with the CYP2D6 and CYP3A4 enzymes may cause elevated levels of the TCAs and the antihistamine terfenadine (Seldane), respectively, both cardiotoxic at higher plasma levels. Although all the SSRIs will elevate plasma levels of these drugs to some degree, fluoxetine and paroxetine carry the greatest risk of causing clinically significant elevations, while sertraline can cause interactions as well. Furthermore, fluoxetine has been reported to increase bupropion levels and to double plasma phenytoin (Dilantin) levels. Through their effects on the CYP3A enzymes, sertraline, fluoxetine, and fluvoxamine can elevate plasma carbamazepine and alprazolam levels, and through CYP2C19, all three (but especially fluvoxamine) can boost diazepam levels. In addition, fluvoxamine has been found to elevate plasma warfarin (Coumadin) theophylline and clozapine levels. Effexor has little P450 effect and thus minimal drug interactions.

Most clinical concern regarding the use of the MAOIs stems from the reaction that occurs when ingested tyramine is not metabolized because of the

MAOI inactivation of intestinal monoamine oxidase. This reaction has been called the "cheese reaction" because tyramine is present in relatively high concentrations in aged cheese. Tyramine may act as a false transmitter and displace norepinephrine from presynaptic storage granules.

Patients receiving MAOI treatment should be instructed to avoid cheeses (except cottage cheese, ricotta, and cream cheese), beers and ales (*including nonalcoholic varieties*), yeast and protein extract (which are ingredients in many soups, gravies, and sauces), broad beans, fermented sausage, sauerkraut, shrimp paste, soy sauce, overripe or stewed figs, raisins, dates, and bananas (Shulman et al, 1989). Several foods formerly considered a danger are no longer included on the list of prohibited substances. For example, in moderation, most wines (with the possible exception of Chianti) and liquors are safe. Smoked fish, and beef and chicken liver, if fresh, are also safe; caffeine and chocolate are of concern only when consumed in large amounts.

Certain general anesthetics and drugs that have sympathomimetic activity—including certain decongestant sympathomimetics such as phenylpropanolamine—should not be taken while a patient is being treated with an MAOI. Two such agents, ephedrine and pseudoephedrine, are constituents of many over-the-counter cold and allergy remedies. Dextromethorphan, an ingredient in several over-the-counter cough syrups, also must be strictly avoided. Local anesthetics containing epinephrine, such as Novocaine (routine in dental procedures), must not be used. Appetite suppressants, and especially fenfluramine (Redux, Pondimin), must be avoided. Synthetic opioids should be used with caution because they may induce the serotonin syndrome. Meperidine (Demerol) must be avoided entirely for this reason.

The tyramine reaction can range from mild to severe. In the mildest form, the patient may complain of sweating, palpitations, and a mild headache. The most severe form manifests as a hypertensive crisis, with severe headache, increases in blood pressure, and possible intracerebral hemorrhage. The severity of this reaction cannot be predicted by MAOI dose, food type, amount ingested, or even prior history of a crisis. For example, a patient may ingest cheese without any reaction at one time, but may have a life-threatening hypertensive crisis on a subsequent occasion when he or she combines the same amount of cheese with the same dose of MAOI. For this reason, patients should be carefully instructed not only about prevention, but also about not gaining false confidence if dietary guidelines are broken without immediate consequences.

The calcium channel blocker nifedipine has received some attention as a possible treatment for mild-to-moderate cases of MAOI-induced hypertension; however, in a recent review of the use of this treatment, Grossman and colleagues (1996) uncovered reports of five myocardial infarctions, two of them fatal, related to the use of nifedipine for presumed MAOI-induced hypertension. Therefore, *nifedipine can no longer be recommended for patients on MAOIs.*

If a patient taking an MAOI experiences a severe or even moderately painful occipital headache, they should immediately seek medical attention, which will include having their blood pressure monitored. If the blood pressure is severely elevated, a drug with alpha-adrenergic blocking properties, such as intravenous phentolamine (Regitine) 5 mg or intramuscular chlorpromazine 25 to 50 mg, may be administered. Because treatment with phentolamine may be associated with cardiac arrhythmias or severe hypotension, however, this should be done only in an emergency room setting by qualified medical personnel with proper monitoring equipment. It is advisable to have patients on MAOIs carry an identification card or Medic Alert bracelet as notification to emergency medical personnel that the patient is currently taking MAOIs. Patients should always carry lists of prohibited foods and medications and should be told to notify physicians that they are taking an MAOI before accepting a medication or anesthetic.

ANXIOLYTICS, SEDATIVES, AND HYPNOTICS

Anxiety disorders are the most frequently diagnosed psychiatric illnesses in the general population, with a 6-month prevalence rate approaching 16% (Reich, 1986). Approximately one-third of the population suffers from insomnia during the course of a year, and 4% of adults use a medically prescribed drug to produce sleep (Mellinger et al, 1985).

Given these figures, it is to be expected that drugs that produce sedation and reduce anxiety historically have been the most widely used drugs. The commonly used anxiolytics and hypnotics and usual dosages are shown in Table 18–8.

Mechanisms of Action

The existence of benzodiazepine receptor binding sites has been confirmed by positron emission tomography using radiolabeled benzodiazepines. These receptors are intimately linked with the receptor for gamma-aminobutyric acid (GABA), the major inhibitory neurotransmitter in the brain. Administration of GABA results in an opening of chloride channels and a decrease in neuronal activity. Activation of the benzodiazepine receptor potentiates the action of GABA. Zolpidem is a *non*benzodiazepine hypnotic that also achieves its effects via the benzodiazepine receptor.

The azapirones, buspirone (Buspar) and gepirone (not currently marketed in the United States), are nonbenzodiazepine anxiolytics known to inhibit dopamine autoreceptors, but recent research indicates that their anxiolytic effect is mediated by a selective stimulation of the 5-HT1A (serotonin) receptor. Acute administration of the azapirones suppresses firing rates in the dorsal raphe through stimulation of this serotonin autoreceptor; however, with

Table 18–8 **Selected Anxiolytic Drugs: Dosages and Half-Lives**

CLASS/GENERIC NAME	TRADE NAME	USUAL DAILY DOSE (mg)	APPROXIMATE ELIMINATION $T\frac{1}{2}$ INCLUDING METABOLITES
Benzodiazepine Anxiolytics			
Alprazolam	Xanax	0.75–1.5, generalized anxiety disorder 2–6, panic disorder	12 hours
Chlordiazepoxide	Librium Libritabs	15–100	1–4 days
Clorazepate	Tranxene	15–60	2–4 days
Clonazepam	Klonopin	1–4	1–2 days
Diazepam	Valium Valrelease	4–40 15–45	2–4 days
Halazepam	Paxipam	40–160	2–4 days
Lorazepam	Ativan	2–6	12 hours
Benzodiazepine Hypnotics			
Estazolam	Prosom	1–2	10–24 hours
Quazepam	Doral	7.5–15	3 days
Oxazepam	Serax	30–120	12 hours
Prazepam	Centrax	20–60	2–4 days
Flurazepam	Dalmane	30	3 days
Temazepam	Restoril	30	12 hours
Triazolam	Halcion	0.125–0.25	4–6 hours
Barbiturates			
Phenobarbital		30–120	2–4 days
Amobarbital	Amytal	50–300	1–2 days
Secobarbital	Seconal	100–200	1–2 days
Nonbenzodiazepines/Nonbarbiturates			
Hydroxyzine hydrochloride	Atarax	75–400	Less than 4 hours
Hydroxyzine pamoate	Vistaril	200–400	
Diphenhydramine*	Benadryl	25–50	
Chloral hydrate		750 (sedation) 500–1,000 (hypnotic)	Less than 12 hours
Zolpidem	Ambien	5–10 mg	2.5 hours
Azapirone			
Buspirone	Buspar	15–60	2–7 hours

* Diphenhydramine, while an antihistamine, is also a hypnotic and has strong anticholinergic properties.
[Silver JM, Yudofsky SC, Hurowitz G: Psychopharmacology and electroconvulsive therapy. In Hales RE, Yudofsky SC, Talbott JA (eds): The American Psychiatric Press Textbook of Psychiatry, 2nd ed. Washington, DC, American Psychiatric Press, 1994]

chronic exposure to these drugs, these receptors become desensitized and raphe serotonin activity is thereby increased (Suranyi-Cadotte et al, 1990). This delayed effect is felt to account for the slow onset of therapeutic action when buspirone is administered clinically. As with the antidepressants, buspirone takes 2 to 4 weeks to work its anxiolytic effect, and so must be taken on a regular rather than p.r.n. basis.

Indications and Efficacy

Benzodiazepines

The efficacy of the benzodiazepines in the treatment of anxiety, including symptoms of worry, psychic anxiety, and somatic symptoms (gastrointestinal and cardiovascular), has been clearly and repeatedly demonstrated in many well-controlled studies.

Benzodiazepines have been shown to be effective in the treatment of panic attacks. Although the high-potency benzodiazepines alprazolam (Xanax) and clonazepam (Klonopin), have received more attention as antipanic agents, lorazepam (Ativan) and diazepam (Valium) have been shown to treat this condition effectively as well. Some clinicians have raised concerns about the development of dependency on these drugs when used in the long-term treatment of panic disorder.

Although only a few benzodiazepines have specific FDA-approved indications for the treatment of insomnia, almost all benzodiazepines may be used for this purpose. Over the past decade, temazepam (Restoril), triazolam (Halcion), and the nonbenzodiazepine zolpidem (Ambien) replaced flurazepam (Dalmane) as the most commonly prescribed hypnotic agent. Flurazepam was found to have a metabolite, desalkylflurazepam, with a very long elimination half-life. Accumulation of this metabolite is a liability, especially in elderly patients, because of the potential for adverse effects on mentation and motor performance; however, the pendulum then began to swing the other way: there have been numerous reports of adverse reactions to the short-acting benzodiazepine triazolam—severe rebound insomnia, amnestic effects, and aggressive outburst attributed to disinhibition. Although several reviews of this issue found these reports of danger somewhat exaggerated, public pressure has influenced prescribing practices, and triazolam prescriptions have dropped considerably since the late 1980s. Most experienced clinicians now avoid the use of triazolam, especially in the elderly. As will be reviewed later in this section, each benzodiazepine has a particular pharmacodynamic and pharmacokinetic profile that importantly influences its clinical indications and application.

Buspirone (Buspar)

Double-blind, controlled studies have shown that buspirone is efficacious in the treatment of generalized anxiety, and its efficacy is not statistically different from that of the benzodiazepines, provided the drug is given in therapeutic doses (20 to 60 mg/day) and for a sufficient period (at least 3 to 4 weeks). It is reported that buspirone, unlike the previously available anxiolytics, is not sedating, has no dangerous interactions with alcohol, has a low dependence liability, and does not impair psychomotor performance. At higher dosages, buspirone may have antidepressant effects. Common side effects include dizziness, nausea, headache, and increased anxiety; however, despite buspirone's usefulness in general anxiety, it appears to be ineffective in the treatment of panic disorder, except perhaps in an auxiliary role for the associated generalized anxiety. It is important to realize that buspirone will *not* treat benzodiazepine withdrawal, and so, in switching a patient, *the benzodiazepine must be tapered slowly to avoid a withdrawal syndrome (including the risk of seizures),* even when the patient's anxiety is well controlled once on the buspirone.

Clinical Use of Anxiolytic and Sedative Drugs

Pharmacotherapy of Generalized Anxiety Disorder

The first step in the treatment of a patient with anxiety is a thorough medical, neurological, and psychiatric evaluation. Many patients with the symptoms of generalized anxiety disorder either have or have had panic disorder. The presence of panic attacks changes the focus of treatment. Medications should be considered as only one component in the treatment of anxiety. Psychotherapy is required to help the patient understand and control the circumstances that surround the anxiety. For most patients, anxiolytic medications are indicated only for relatively short-term use (i.e., 1 to 2 months), although some patients may require more prolonged treatment. The benzodiazepines generally are contraindicated in patients with sleep apnea or other forms of respiratory suppression and in patients with a history of alcohol and drug abuse.

Because benzodiazepines frequently cause sedation, may impair performance on tasks that require a high degree of mental alertness, and may lead to dependence, this class of drugs should be used for as brief a period of time as possible in the lowest effective dose (Table 18–9).

Several clinically important facets of the anxiolytic response to buspirone differentiate it from the benzodiazepines. Buspirone does not interact with other sedating drugs (including alcohol), does not seem to impair mechanical performance such as driving, and is not associated with dependence, tolerance, or withdrawal. It also does not have muscle relaxant or anticonvulsant properties, as do the benzodiazepines. Studies suggest that response to buspirone occurs in approximately 2 to 4 weeks, compared with the more rapid onset associated with benzodiazepines.

Pharmacotherapy of Panic Disorder

Many patients who have the symptoms of generalized anxiety disorder either currently have or have had a history of panic disorder. Anxiety may

Table 18–9 **Guidelines for Anxiolytic Treatment with Benzodiazepines**

1. Complete a thorough medical evaluation, especially with regard to thyroid status, caffeine intake, and current medications. Include a thorough evaluation of drug and alcohol history. Patients with sleep apnea should not receive benzodiazepines.
2. Evaluate patient for psychodynamic and social factors that may contribute to or precipitate anxiety.
3. Initiate benzodiazepines at a low dose (e.g., diazepam 2 mg three times a day) and increase every few days until sedation or therapeutic effect is obtained (up to 15 mg three times a day).
4. Caution patient on sedative properties, performance impairment, dependence properties, and drug and alcohol interactions.
5. Set guidelines for duration of expected treatment clearly to the patient in advance.
6. Reevaluate need for medication every month. Avoid refills by telephone.
7. Taper medication as soon as possible, by approximately 10% per week for patients on long-term treatment (greater than 3 months).
8. In patients with chronic anxiety or prone to anxiety and requesting or needing chronic therapy, obtain a psychiatric consultation.

[Silver JM, Yudofsky SC, Hurowitz G: Psychopharmacology and electroconvulsive therapy. In Hales RE, Yudofsky SC, Talbott JA (eds): The American Psychiatric Press Textbook of Psychiatry, 2nd ed. Washington, DC, American Psychiatric Press, 1994]

---

develop in response to frequent spontaneous panic attacks, termed "anticipatory anxiety." Breier et al (1986) have reported that over 80% of patients with panic disorder or agoraphobia with panic attacks have anticipatory or generalized anxiety that is responsive to treatment with benzodiazepines.

Drugs from several families of psychotropic medications may be used in the treatment of panic disorder. The benzodiazepines, specifically alprazolam and clonazepam, have been shown to be effective. These medications should be initiated at relatively low doses (e.g., alprazolam 0.25 mg t.i.d. or clonazepam 0.5 mg b.i.d.) and increased gradually over 1 to 2 weeks. After successful treatment of panic disorder with alprazolam, withdrawal and discontinuation of medication are difficult because of increased panic attacks and occurrence of withdrawal symptoms, including malaise, weakness, insomnia, tachycardia, lightheadedness, and dizziness. Discontinuation of these medications should be extremely slow (10%/week). Because of its long half-life, taperings and dose reductions with clonazepam are typically much "smoother" than with alprazolam.

Because panic disorder usually requires a prolonged period for successful treatment, benzodiazepines may be associated with an increased risk of dependence. Therefore, we recommend that the use of antidepressants be considered as the initial treatment of panic disorder. Among the antidepressants, the SSRIs, the TCAs, and the MAOIs have all been shown to be effective treatments. There is evidence that the SSRIs as a class are superior to imipramine and alprazolam (Boyer, 1995); however, SSRIs must be started at low dosages (i.e., 2.5 to 5 mg of fluoxetine) since patients with panic attacks are highly sensitive to the anxiogenic effects of these drugs. For patients unable to tolerate SSRIs at any dose, imipramine, desipramine, or nortriptyline should prove effective. A decision as to which of these drugs to choose should be based on the same factors discussed in the section on antidepressant drugs. MAOIs are usually reserved for patients who have not responded to the first- and second-line antidepressants, although they may be used as a primary treatment, particularly if the patient also meets criteria for atypical depression. The doses, durations, and side effects of antidepressants used for the treatment of panic disorder parallel those described in the previous section for the treatment of depression.

Patients with panic disorder are exceedingly sensitive to a temporary exacerbation or worsening of symptoms in the first weeks of treatment with an SSRI or TCA. Therefore, doses should be started very low and increased in small increments. For highly anxious patients with panic disorder, alprazolam or clonazepam, begun concurrently with the antidepressant, often mitigate any excess stimulation due to the antidepressant and help to bridge the latency period until the onset of the therapeutic effect. Once a positive response to the antidepressant is established, the benzodiazepine may be tapered and discontinued. The treatment of panic and other anxiety disorders is discussed in detail in Chapter 8.

Pharmacotherapy of Insomnia

A complete medical, sleep, and psychiatric history is required before administration of drugs to produce sleep. There are multiple causes for insomnia, and the differential diagnosis of sleep disorders must be considered before the prescribing of any hypnotic. Among the common disorders associated with insomnia are depression, psychoses, anxiety, central nervous system disorders, and other medical illnesses associated with pain and discomfort. Stimulants (including caffeine), as well as alcohol, may lead to insomnia.

The individual hypnotic benzodiazepines have varying pharmacodynamic and pharmacokinetic profiles that importantly influence their use in clinical practice. While all of the currently available benzodiazepine hypnotics are absorbed relatively rapidly and achieve peak plasma levels in approximately 1.5 hours, affinity for the benzodiazepine receptor and elimination half-life both affect the clinical utility of these agents. For example, while flurazepam and quazepam are rapidly absorbed, they are metabolized into desalkylflurazepam, a compound with a half-life as long as 40 to 50 hours. This very long elimination half-life may result in daytime sedation and impaired motor performance. Accumulation of this compound in the body is especially worrisome for elderly patients. With a half-life of just 1.5 to 5 hours, triazolam is at the other end of the spectrum among the benzodiazepines. The rapid elimination of this drug reduces the risk of accumulation and of a morning-after "hangover" effect. On the other hand, there is the risk of rebound insomnia and early-morning awakening. Temazepam and estazolam have intermediate half-life values and, as a result, these agents have fewer day-after and rebound effects.

The nonbenzodiazepine hypnotic agent zolpidem acts selectively at the benzodiazepine *type 1* receptor, a receptor subtype that is touted as the site specific to the benzodiazepine sedation effect. In keeping with this, zolpidem is known to have only minor anticonvulsant and muscle relaxant effects; however, zolpidem is associated with many of the same adverse effects typical of short-acting benzodiazepines given at equivalent doses.

Pharmacotherapy of Obsessive–Compulsive Disorder

Anxiolytics and the older generation antidepressants are not generally effective in the treatment of obsessive–compulsive disorder (OCD). Clomipramine was the first agent studied extensively for the treatment of this disorder and was found to be clearly superior to the other TCAs and the MAOIs. A member of the TCA family with very potent serotonin-reuptake inhibitory effects, its major side effects are sedation and anticholinergic effects. Fluoxetine has been compared with clomipramine and found to have approximately equivalent antiobsessional effects. While some patients will respond to lower doses, many patients achieve optimal benefit at a dosage of 60 to 80 mg a day. All the SSRIs have demonstrated clinical efficacy in the treatment of OCD, but of the remaining agents, fluvoxamine has been the most extensively studied. In a daily dose of 100 to 300 mg, fluvoxamine is roughly equivalent in efficacy to fluoxetine and clomipramine.

Risks and Side Effects of Anxiolytic and Hypnotic Drugs

The production of sedation by benzodiazepines may be considered either a therapeutic action or a side effect. Hypnotics are expected and required to produce sedation to be efficacious; however, when the patient complains of sleepiness the following day, this therapeutic action becomes a side effect.

Physical dependence may occur when benzodiazepines are taken in dosages higher than usual or for prolonged periods of time. If precipitously discontinued, severe withdrawal symptoms (hyperpyrexia, seizures, psychosis, and death) may occur. Other symptoms of withdrawal may include tachycardia, increased blood pressure, muscle cramps, anxiety, insomnia, panic attacks, impairment of memory and concentration, and perceptual disturbances. These withdrawal symptoms may begin as soon as the day after discontinuing benzodiazepines and may continue for weeks to months.

As a general principle for all drugs, discontinuation should be accomplished gradually. For patients treated with benzodiazepines for longer than 2 to 3 months, we suggest that the dose be decreased by approximately 5 to 10% a week. Thus, for a patient receiving 4 mg/day of alprazolam, the dose should be tapered by 0.25 mg/day a week for 16 weeks. The last few dosage levels may be the most difficult to discontinue, and the patient will require increased attention and support from the physician at this time. Clonazepam may be substituted for alprazolam to assist with the discontinuation process.

Since clonazepam has a prolonged half-life, tapering can be accomplished with less rebound anxiety than occurs with alprazolam withdrawal.

Buspirone, when administered to subjects who had histories of recreational sedative abuse, showed no abuse potential. Buspirone has almost no abuse potential and is relatively nontoxic in overdose situations. The side effects that are more common with buspirone than the benzodiazepines are nausea, headache, nervousness, insomnia, dizziness, and lightheadedness. Restlessness has also been reported, which theoretically may be related to buspirone's activity at the dopamine receptor. The side effects are dose-related and can be managed by starting with a low dose and gradually increasing the dosage as tolerance develops over time.

Overdose

Benzodiazepines are remarkably safe when taken in overdose. Dangerous effects occur when the overdose includes several sedative drugs, especially alcohol. There now exists a safe and effective benzodiazepine antagonist, flumazenil, which may be used via intravenous injection in an emergency setting to reverse the effects of any potential overdose with a benzodiazepine; however, medical management of an overdose often will still require physical supportive measures, such as support of respiratory function. As with most medications, use of anxiolytics during pregnancy or when breastfeeding should be avoided whenever possible.

Drug Interactions

Most sedative drugs, including narcotics and alcohol, potentiate sedation from benzodiazepines. Cimetidine, oral contraceptives, acute alcohol intake, propranolol, and disulfiram inhibit the hepatic metabolism and increase the elimination half-life of benzodiazepines that are metabolized by oxidation, which include diazepam and chlordiazepoxide. Because of their specific effects on the cytochrome P450 enzymes, sertraline, fluvoxamine, and fluoxetine can significantly increase plasma alprazolam and diazepam levels; however, benzodiazepines such as lorazepam, oxazepam, and temazepam are metabolized by glucuronide conjugation, and therefore their half-life is not affected by liver disease, aging, and medication, all of which affect oxidative capacities in the liver associated with the drugs just cited. Buspirone does *not* appear to interact with alcohol to increase sedation or motor impairment.

Barbiturates

The use of barbiturates for the treatment of anxiety (and insomnia) has been largely supplanted by the much safer benzodizepines. With barbiturates, potentially fatal respiratory depression can occur at only several times the standard therapeutic dosages. Barbiturates are potent inducers of hepatic microsomal enzymes and, therefore, they interact with many other drugs that are metabolized in the liver.

The clinical use of barbiturates is determined by their respective onsets of action and half-lives. The ultra-short barbiturates thiopental (Pentothal) and methohexital (Brevital) are used primarily as intravenous agents for the induction of general anesthesia. Amobarbital (Amytal), pentobarbital (Nembutal), and secobarbital (Seconal) have been used as sedative agents. Amobarbital is also valuable for the acute management of agitated patients when administered parenterally in doses of approximately 250 mg. Phenobarbital, a long-acting barbiturate, may be used as an anxiolytic agent, although tolerance to this effect occurs after several weeks. The principal clinical application of phenobarbital is as an anticonvulsant drug.

Alcohol Detoxification

Because of the cross-tolerance of benzodiazepines and alcohol, the benzodiazepines are used frequently for the treatment of alcohol withdrawal and detoxification. A relatively simple procedure for treating alcohol withdrawal is the benzodiazepine loading dose technique. This technique takes advantage of the long half-life of benzodiazepines such as diazepam and chlordiazepoxide. Unit doses of 20 mg diazepam (or 100 mg chlordiazepoxide) are administered hourly to patients until there are no signs or symptoms of alcohol withdrawal. Thereafter, no further doses of benzodiazepines are administered. Because of the long half-lives of benzodiazepines, the therapeutic plasma level of the benzodiazepine is maintained during the period of risk for alcohol withdrawal symptoms (see also Chapters 10 by Dr. Swift and 19 by Dr. Dubin).

ANTIMANIC DRUGS

Over three decades of clinical investigation have conclusively demonstrated that lithium is effective in the prophylaxis of recurrent mood disorders. Research has also shown that antipsychotic drugs and electroconvulsive therapy are highly effective in the treatment of *acute* mania. Indeed, these treatments elicit responses more rapidly than does lithium carbonate, and they are often administered while awaiting the therapeutic response to lithium. Other classes of drugs with different chemical structures and with apparently different mechanisms of actions have been reported to be effective in the prophylaxis and treatment of mania. Among these are the anticonvulsant drugs valproic acid, carbamazepine, and lamotrigine; the calcium channel-blocking drug verapamil; the alpha-adrenergic agonist clonidine; the benzodiazepine anticonvulsant clonazepam; and the beta-adrenergic receptor-blocking drug propranolol. In this section, we will review the clinical use of lithium, valproic acid, and carbamazepine, for which the efficacy in bipolar disorder is well established (Table 18–10). The other drugs mentioned above are not routinely used to treat bipolar illness, and their efficacy is questionable.

Table 18–10 **Antimanic Drugs**

CLASS/GENERIC NAME	TRADE NAME	USUAL DOSE RANGE (mg/day)	PLASMA LEVELS
Lithium			
Lithium carbonate	Eskalith Lithane Lithonate Lithotabs	600–1,800	0.6–1.2 mEq/l
Time-release	Eskalith CR		
Lithium citrate (syrup)	Cibalith-S		
Carbamazepine	Tegretol	800–1,200	8–12 µg/ml
Valproic acid	Depakene Depakote	750–1,000	50–100 µg/ml
Lamotrigine*			

*Still under investigation.

Lithium

Mechanism of Action

Despite years of extensive study, our understanding of the mechanisms underlying the antimanic and antidepressant effects of lithium has developed very slowly. It is now believed that lithium acts at the level of the second messenger systems in a wide variety of cell types. Mania and depression may be viewed as overactive central nervous system processes, perhaps the excessive, mutually compensatory reactions of a homeostatic system gone awry. In keeping with this view, pathological excesses in the activity of several neurotransmitter systems have been implicated in mania and depression, and it now appears that lithium reduces the sensitivity of the various receptor types involved.

Among second messenger system constituents suspected of playing a role in mood disorders, the two most attractive candidates to date are adenylate cyclase and phosphoinositol. Lithium has been reported to inhibit the activation of adenylate cyclase by a number of neurotransmitters, while it does not suppress basal adenylate cyclase activity. Similarly, lithium interferes with phosphoinositol metabolism, a by-product of which is the production of the second messengers inositol trisphosphate and diacylglycerol. Through these second messengers, phosphoinositol may affect intracellular calcium utilization. It has been suggested that a dysequilibrium in calcium regulation is a critical element in the pathogenesis of bipolar illness. Both adenylate cyclase and phosphoinositol metabolism affect levels of protein kinase C (PKC), which is known to facilitate the release of a wide range of neurotransmitters, including those long thought to be involved in the development of mania and bipolar illness. Lithium's ultimate effect may be to attenuate PKC activity, as it has been found that the reduction of PKC levels parallels the time course for lithium's delayed onset of action (Manji et al, 1996).

Indications and Efficacy

Lithium, usually administered as the carbonate salt, has been shown to be efficacious in the treatment of many of the mood disorders. Acute manic episodes respond to treatment with lithium within 7 to 10 days. Because manic episodes have so great a potential for psychosocial disruption, behavioral control is usually desired before lithium becomes effective. Supplemental medication (most often benzodiazepines and antipsychotic drugs), therefore, is administered on an acute basis. Patients with less severe bipolar illness, such as cyclothymia or bipolar II disorder (episodes of major depression punctuated by periods of hypomania), may also exhibit improvement with lithium therapy.

Lithium may be effective in the prevention of future depressive episodes in patients with recurrent unipolar depressive disorder (Consensus Development Panel, 1985) and as an adjunct to antidepressants in patients only partially responsive to treatment with antidepressants alone (discussed in the section on antidepressants). Finally, lithium may be useful in the maintenance of remission of depression with antidepressants and after electroconvulsive therapy.

Clinical Use

Before the initiation of treatment, patients should be informed of side effects that occur commonly with lithium treatment, which include nausea, diarrhea, polyuria, polydipsia, thirst, fine hand tremor, and fatigue. While these side effects are often transient, in some patients, they may persist with therapeutic lithium levels. Women of childbearing age should have a pregnancy test and be advised that lithium has been reported to cause cardiac defects (Ebstein's anomaly) when taken in the first trimester.

Because of the narrow range between the therapeutic and toxic doses of lithium, the optimum dose for an individual patient cannot be based on the dosage administered, but rather should be based on the concentration of lithium in the plasma. Thus, appropriate use of lithium requires familiarity with its pharmacokinetics. Lithium is completely absorbed by the gastrointestinal tract and reaches peak plasma levels in 1 to 2 hours. The elimination half-life is approximately 20 to 24 hours. Steady-state lithium levels are obtained in approximately 5 days.

Therapeutic plasma levels for patients on lithium therapy range from 0.5 to 1.5 mEq/L. Although lower plasma levels are associated with less troubling side effects, there is strong evidence that levels in the range of 0.8 to 1.0 mEq/L provide better prophylaxis against relapse. Therefore, most clinicians now seek to establish levels of at least 0.8 mEq/L in treating acute mania. When intolerable side effects have not intervened, treatment with lithium should not be considered a failure in acute mania until plasma levels of 1.2 to 1.5 mEq/L have been reached and maintained for 2 weeks.

Most healthy patients may be conservatively started on a 300 mg b.i.d. dosage of lithium, and this dose may be increased by 300 mg every 3 to 4 days. Larger "loading" doses may be used in acute manic states (e.g., 1,200 mg/day in divided doses). Elderly patients are extremely sensitive to the neurotoxic side effects of lithium, such as ataxia, tremor, and delirium, and generally should be treated with doses of lithium that produce serum levels at the lower end of the therapeutic range. In the healthy patient with no renal function impairment, plasma level determinations are obtained biweekly. Since steady-state plasma levels are not obtained until the patient has been on a constant dose regimen for at least 5 days, this method may slightly underestimate the steady-state level. Lithium levels must consistently be obtained 12 hours after the last lithium dose. After therapeutic lithium levels have been established, levels should be monitored every month for the first 6 months and every 2 to 3 months thereafter. Gastrointestinal side effects can be minimized by having patients take their lithium after meals.

The frequency of lithium dosing needs to be considered individually for each patient. Since lithium has a serum half-life of approximately 24 hours, the administration of lithium as a single daily dose is possible. For example, for the patient receiving a maintenance dose of lithium of 1,200 mg/day, a dosing regimen of either 1,200 mg once a day or 300 mg four times a day is theoretically possible; however, the multiple dosing regimen will expose the kidneys to multiple peak levels of intermediate concentration, whereas a single daily dose results in a single peak of higher absolute concentration. Nephrotoxicity related to chronic lithium use (see discussion below) and acute lithium-induced polyuria seem to be related to the duration of exposure to peak lithium levels and not to the absolute level of any single peak. For this reason, many clinicians now favor once-a-day dosing. Although slow-release preparations of lithium are available, these are not necessary for adequate 24-hour plasma levels. The main advantage of sustained release lithium is that less lithium ion is released in the stomach, where it can act as an irritant, while more is released in the small intestines. For patients who experience nausea and gastric irritation, the slow-release formulations may protect them from this unpleasant side effect. On the other hand, diarrhea may be worse when relatively more lithium ion is released in the intestines. Of course, gastric irritation may be reduced by simply advising patients to take lithium on a full stomach (see Table 18–11).

Risks, Side Effects, and Their Management

Most of the effects of lithium on the kidney are reversible after discontinuation of the drug. Although permanent morphologic changes in renal structure have been reported, the exact clinical implications of these changes have yet to be established. Renal function tests are required before lithium therapy is initiated and at specified intervals throughout the course of treatment.

The most noticeable effect of lithium on renal function is the vasopressin-resistant impairment in the kidney's ability to concentrate urine. This is nephrogenic diabetes insipidus (NDI), and it may result in polyuria. Most patients on lithium therapy may complain of increased frequency of urination. Preventive and management strategies for NDI include once-daily dosing, decreasing the

Table 18–11 **Guidelines for Lithium Treatment**

1. Complete a thorough medical evaluation.
2. Complete appropriate medical laboratory evaluations.
3. Inform patient and family of proper use of lithium. Include common side effects, importance of monitoring lithium levels, exact procedures for accurate lithium monitoring, early signs and symptoms of toxicity, potential long-term side effects, and warnings regarding pregnancy during treatment (if patient is female).
4. Initiate therapy at 300 mg twice a day and increase by 300 mg every 3 to 4 days.
5. Obtain lithium levels (12 hours after last dose) twice a week, until lithium level is approximately 1.0 mEq/L.
6. Treatment of acute manic symptoms may require concomitant therapy with antipsychotic medications.
7. Repeat lithium levels every month for the first 6 months, then every 2 to 3 months.

[Silver JM, Yudofsky SC, Hurowitz G: Psychopharmacology and electroconvulsive therapy. In Hales RE, Yudofsky SC, Talbott JA (eds): The American Psychiatric Press Textbook of Psychiatry, 2nd ed. Washington, DC, American Psychiatric Press, 1994]

total daily dose, and increasing liquid intake. Amiloride 5 mg b.i.d. has been suggested as a treatment for polyuria. By blocking the absorption of lithium in the renal tubules, it prevents lithium from interfering with the action of vasopressin. Unlike many other diuretics, amiloride does not increase plasma lithium concentration (Battle et al, 1985). Nevertheless, it is prudent to continue to monitor serum lithium levels when amiloride is combined with lithium.

Lithium nephropathy, characterized by tubular interstitial nephritis, has been reported as a consequence of long-term lithium therapy. Although mild decreases in the glomerular filtration rate occur in some patients treated with lithium, there have been no published reports of irreversible renal failure as a result of chronic nontoxic lithium therapy.

In all patients treated with lithium, renal function tests should be monitored, but whether or not lithium has any nephrotoxic effects with long-term use is controversial. Preliminary laboratory evaluations include serum testing for blood urea nitrogen, creatinine, and electrolytes, and a urinalysis. Some conservative clinicians recommend a 24-hour collection of urine to measure the creatinine clearance. Impairment in concentrating urine may be assessed by the 12-hour fluid deprivation test, wherein the patient first refrains from drinking any fluid for 12 hours. After this time, a urine specimen is collected, and the urine osmolality is measured. A urine specific gravity of less than 1.010 may imply disordered kidney function and may indicate that further specific renal function studies are required.

Hypothyroidism may occur in as many as 20% of patients treated with lithium (Myers et al, 1985). Many patients have an elevation of thyroid antibody titer during lithium treatment. Lithium-induced hypothyroidism is more common in female patients, and among patients with thyroid antibodies or with exaggerated thyroid-stimulating hormone (TSH) response to thyroid-releasing hormone injection prior to lithium treatment.

Initial laboratory tests include T_3 resin uptake, T_4 radioimmunoassay, T_4 free thyroxine index, and TSH levels. TSH is the most sensitive of these tests for detecting hypothyroidism. Because of the association between the presence of antithyroid antibodies and the subsequent development of hypothyroidism, antithyroid antibodies should also be measured before lithium treatment. TSH should be reassessed after every 6 months of lithium therapy. If laboratory tests indicate the development of hypothyroidism (such as an elevated TSH level), the patient should be evaluated clinically for signs and symptoms of hypothyroidism. In collaboration with an endocrinologist, the psychiatrist should decide on the appropriate treatment, which may include low doses of supplementation of thyroid replacement.

The effects of lithium on calcium metabolism may be related to very rare reports of lithium-induced hyperparathyroidism and associated hypercalcemia. Hyperparathyroidism is associated with neuropsychiatric symptoms, which include mood changes, anxiety, psychosis, delirium, and dementia.

Lithium therapy may be associated with several types of neurological dysfunction. Fine resting tremor is a neurological side effect that may be detected in as many as one-half of patients in lithium treatment. Severe neurotoxic reactions occur with toxic lithium levels, and these symptoms include dysarthria, ataxia, and intention tremor, which also may occur with lithium levels in the therapeutic range. Complaints of impairment of memory and concentration are relatively infrequent. Elderly patients are much more sensitive to these reactions, and they occur at lower serum levels.

Mitchell and Mackenzie (1982) reported changes in T-wave morphology on the electrocardiogram (flattening or inversion) in 20 to 30% of patients on lithium. Although these changes are most likely benign, a medical evaluation should be completed to assess other possible etiologies. Lithium also may suppress the function of the sinus node and result in sinoatrial block. Patients with cardiac sinus disease or conduction defects, therefore, should not be treated with lithium. Before the initiation of treatment with lithium, all patients should have a complete cardiac evaluation, including history and physical examination pertinent to the cardiovascular system and an electrocardiogram in patients over 40 years old.

Weight gain is a frequent side effect of lithium treatment. Patients with polydipsia may drink fluids with a high caloric content, such as carbonated soft drinks, and thereby gain weight. Weight gain may also be a direct effect of lithium therapy. Possible mechanisms include influences on carbohydrate metabolism, changes in glucose tolerance, or changes in lipid metabolism.

The most frequent dermatological reaction is skin rash, which is reported in up to 7% of lithium-treated patients. Hair loss and hair thinning have also been reported.

Gastrointestinal difficulties are frequent, especially nausea and diarrhea. While these symptoms may be manifestations of toxicity, they also occur at lithium levels within the therapeutic range. Gastrointestinal symptoms may improve with reducing the dose, changing to a slow-release formulation, or ingesting lithium with meals.

The most frequent hematological abnormality detected in patients on lithium is leukocytosis (approximately 15,000 white blood cells/mm^3). This change is generally benign and may in fact be used to treat several conditions associated with depressed granulocytes. Lithium-induced leukocytosis is readily reversible with discontinuation of lithium therapy. Before initiation of therapy with lithium, a white blood cell count with differential should be obtained and should be repeated at yearly intervals thereafter.

Because of the narrow range between therapeutic and toxic plasma lithium levels, the psychiatrist must allow sufficient time to inform the patient and the family about the signs, symptoms, and treatment of lithium toxicity (Table 18–12). The patient must be made aware of circumstances that may increase the chances of toxicity, such as drinking insufficient amounts of fluids, becoming overheated with increased perspiration, or ingesting too much medication. The psychiatrist must emphasize the prevention of lithium toxicity through the maintenance of adequate salt and water intake, especially during hot weather and exercise. The signs and symptoms of lithium toxicity can be divided into those that usually occur with lithium levels at 1.5 to 2.0 mEq/L, 2.0 to 2.5 mEq/L, and more than 2.5 mEq/L; these are listed in Table 18–12. The drug should *not* be given to women who are pregnant or who are likely to become pregnant, due to possible toxic fetal effects.

Drug Interactions

Diuretics increase lithium levels and should be used with caution when treating lithium-induced diabetes insipidus. Some nonsteroidal antiinflammatory drugs such as indomethacin also can increase the plasma lithium level. Theophylline will increase renal clearance and result in a lower lithium level.

Lithium has been reported to increase the intracellular levels of some antipsychotic drugs and may aggravate the inherent neurotoxicity of these agents as well. Thiazide diuretics raise lithium levels and, if used, warrant close monitoring of lithium levels. Furosemide and spironolactone appear to affect lithium levels minimally.

Anticonvulsant Mood Stabilizers

Evidence from controlled studies indicates that the anticonvulsants valproic acid and carbamazepine, and possibly lamotrigine, are effective in both acute and prophylactic treatment of mania in some patients with bipolar disorder. These findings have largely been confirmed in bipolar patients unresponsive to lithium or in bipolar patients unable to tolerate lithium-induced side effects (Keck et al, 1992). Also, patients with frequent recurrences (including rapid cycling bipolar patients) and those who develop mixed mood states (e.g., dysphoric mania) may respond more favorably to these drugs.

Table 18–12 **Signs and Symptoms of Lithium Toxicity**

Mild-to-Moderate Intoxication (Lithium Level 1.5–2.0 mEq/L)
Gastrointestinal
  Vomiting
  Abdominal pain
  Dryness of mouth
Neurological
  Ataxia
  Dizziness
  Slurred speech
  Nystagmus
  Lethargy or excitement
  Muscle weakness

Moderate-to-Severe Intoxication (Lithium Level 2.0–2.5 mEq/L)
Gastrointestinal
  Anorexia
  Persistent nausea and vomiting
Neurological
  Blurred vision
  Muscle fasciculations
  Clonic limb movements
  Hyperactive deep tendon reflexes
  Choreoathetoid movements
  Convulsions
  Delirium
  Syncope
  Electroencephalographic changes
  Stupor
  Coma
  Circulatory failure (lowered blood pressure, cardiac arrhythmias, and conduction
    abnormalities)

Severe Lithium Intoxication (Lithium Level >2.5 mEq/L)
Generalized convulsions
Oliguria and renal failure
Death

Mechanism of Action

Carbamazepine and valproic acid have multiple effects on the central nervous system and act on numerous neurotransmitters and second messenger systems. The precise effects that account for the usefulness of these anticonvulsants as antimanic and mood-stabilizing drugs have yet to be adequately determined. Of particular interest, however, is the effect of carbamazepine and valproate on "limbic kindling" and the hypothesis that kindling underlies the pathophysiology of mood disorders. In the process of kindling, repetitive stimuli eventually may lead to either a behavioral or convulsive response. Carbamazepine and valproic acid have been shown to inhibit the development of this response.

As with lithium, valproate is known to reduce PKC activity. PKC is a second messenger system component that stimulates the release of several of the neurotransmitters implicated in mood dysregulation. Of interest is the finding that the attenuation of PKC activity occurs more rapidly with exposure to valproate than with lithium exposure (Manji et al, 1996). This finding may account for the observation that valproic acid has a more rapid onset of action against manic symptoms than does lithium. In another similarity with lithium, carbamazepine appears to inhibit adenylyl cyclase activity, which also results in reduced PKC production.

Clinical Use

Valproic acid is typically initiated at a dosage of 250 mg two or three times a day. The dose is increased by 250 mg approximately every 3 days until a plasma level between 50 and 100 µg/ml is obtained. Most patients will require a daily dose of 1,250 to 1,500 mg a day to achieve such a level. For the treatment of acute mania, some investigators have recommended rapid oral loading of this agent. An immediate dosage of 20 mg/kg/day may provide acute antimanic effects in as short a time as 3 days (McElroy et al, 1996), an effect not possible with lithium or carbamazepine. Carbamazepine should be initiated at a dosage of 200 mg twice a day. For acute mania, dose increments of 200 mg/day every 3 to 5 days should be made until a plasma level of 8 to 12 µg/ml is obtained. Too rapid increases in dose may lead to dizziness, ataxia, and other adverse reactions. Although the maximum dosage of carbamazepine recommended by the manufacturer is 1,200 mg/day, many patients will require higher daily doses to achieve a therapeutic plasma level. Treatment principles for the use of these anticonvulsants are listed in Table 18–13.

Risks, Side Effects, and Their Management

The side effect that is of most concern with the use of valproic acid is the development of hepatotoxicity. Fortunately, fatal cases of hepatotoxicity have been limited to children who have been treated with multiple anticonvulsants. On occasion, patients will have increases in liver function tests. These changes may normalize if the patient is maintained on valproic acid, although discontinuing the medication may be necessary. Valproate has been associated with changes in platelet count, but clinically relevant thrombocytopenia has rarely been documented. Coagulation defects have also been reported, but the risk of inducing a coagulation disturbance in an otherwise healthy adult is very low when the daily dose of valproate is maintained below 3,000 mg a day; however, in patients for whom anticoagulation is strictly contraindicated, or for patients receiving ongoing anticoagulation therapy, continuous monitoring of the coagulation profile and whole bleeding time is required. Other common side effects include drowsiness, weight gain, tremors, and alopecia. Elderly patients receiving chronic treatment may gradually develop parkinsonian side effects, including cognitive impairment.

Table 18–13 **Evaluation and Monitoring of Anticonvulsant Treatment of Bipolar Disorder**

1. Complete medical evaluation (see numbers 7 and 8).
2. Inform patient and family of potential side effects of treatment and of the importance of monitoring serum levels.
3. Initiate carbamazepine (CBZ) at 200 mg twice a day. Initiate valproic acid (VPA) at 250 mg twice a day.
4. Increase CBZ dose by 200 mg or VPA dose by 250 mg every 3–5 days.
5. Obtain serum levels every week until therapeutic levels are obtained (CBZ: 8–12 µg/ml; VPA: 50–100 µg/ml).
6. Monitor levels every month for the first 3 months and every 3 months thereafter.
7. Hematologic monitoring for CBZ: obtain complete blood count and platelet count every 2 weeks for the first 2 months of treatment and every 3 months thereafter.*
8. Liver function monitoring (CBZ and VPA): obtain SGOT, SGPT, LDH, and alkaline phosphatase every month for the first 2 months of treatment and every 3 months thereafter.†

* These are very conservative guidelines that in clinical practice have been relaxed due to the rarity of CBZ hematological problems.
† SGOT, serum glutamic-oxaloacetic transaminase; SGPT, serum glutamate pyruvate transaminase; LHD, lactate dehydrogenase.
[Silver JM, Yudofsky SC, Hurowitz G: Psychopharmacology and electroconvulsive therapy. In Hales RE, Yudofsky SC, Talbott JA (eds): The American Psychiatric Press Textbook of Psychiatry, 2nd ed. Washington, DC, American Psychiatric Press, 1994]

The most serious toxic hematological side effects of carbamazepine are agranulocytosis and aplastic anemia, which may be fatal. While carbamazepine-induced agranulocytosis or aplastic anemia is extremely rare—now estimated to occur in 1 in 125,000 patients (Pellock, 1987)—leukopenia (total white blood cell count of less than 3,000 cells/mm^3) is more common, with a prevalence of approximately 10%. Persistent leukopenia and thrombocytopenia occur in approximately 2% of patients, and "mild anemia" occurs in fewer than 5% of patients.

Hart and Easton (1982) originally recommended obtaining blood and platelet counts before carbamazepine therapy and complete blood counts every 2 weeks for the first 2 months, and quarterly thereafter (Table 18–13). Patients with abnormal results on baseline tests should be considered at high risk and require a risk–benefit assessment before treatment is initiated. During therapy, the development of leukopenia necessitates follow-up laboratory evaluations every 2 weeks. If the counts do not return to normal in 2 weeks, the drug dose should be reduced. If a patient on carbamazepine develops fever, infection, petechiae, weakness or pallor, and a white blood cell count of less than 3,000/mm^3 or an absolute neutrophil count of less than 2,000/mm^3, all drugs should be discontinued immediately. Consultation with a hematologist is also required at this point. The frequency of hematologic monitoring of patients on carbamazepine is slightly controversial, and clinicians should consult a neurologist for the most recently recommended guidelines.

The syndrome of inappropriate antidiuretic hormone secretion may be induced by carbamazepine treatment. When hyponatremia develops, it is often transient, yet persistent or more severe cases of this condition can often be managed by fluid restriction or the addition of lithium, demeclocycline, or doxycycline. Carbamazepine occasionally may result in hepatic toxicity. This is usually a hypersensitivity hepatitis that appears after a latency period of several weeks and is associated with elevations in serum glutamic-oxaloacetic transaminase, serum glutamate pyruvate transaminase, and lactic dehydrogenase (LDH). Cholestasis is also possible, with increases in bilirubin and alkaline phosphatase. Mild transient elevations of LDH and the transaminases can generally be monitored without discontinuation of the carbamazepine.

Carbamazepine has anticholinergic activity, which may lead to blurred vision, constipation, and dry mouth. In addition, patients may also complain of dizziness, drowsiness, and ataxia. These symptoms may often occur at therapeutic plasma levels, especially in the early phases of treatment. The development of rashes is also common. Weight gain does not appear to be a side effect of carbamazepine therapy. Concurrent use of the calcium channel blockers verapamil and diltiazem with carbamazepine can result in increases in carbamazepine that approach the toxic range. For this reason, these drugs should not be used concomitantly. Carbamazepine is essentially a tricyclic agent and, similar to the TCAs, has quinidinelike side effects on the heart.

PSYCHOSTIMULANTS

The use of psychostimulants, such as methylphenidate and dextroamphetamine, is primarily limited to treating attention-deficit hyperactivity disorder (see Chapter 16). In neurology, methylphenidate, dextroamphetamine, and pemoline are used to treat narcolepsy (see Chapter 22). Some psychiatric research has suggested that these drugs may be of benefit in depression or as an adjunct to antidepressants, or they may predict responsiveness to antidepressant treatment. Their use for these purposes, however, is not considered a part of standard care in psychiatric practice. Rather, psychostimulants are employed primarily in adjunctive polypharmacy regimens in refractory depressions.

Despite the very limited use for psychostimulants in most mood disorders, several clinical situations exist in which they may be of some definite benefit. Some general hospital psychiatrists advocate their use in anergic, apathetic, and withdrawn medical patients, such as those recovering from cerebrovascular stroke or other debilitating medical illnesses. The short-term use of methylphenidate 10 to 40 mg/day or dextroamphetamine 10 to 20 mg/day has been recommended to "activate" such anergic and apathetic patients. The clinical efficacy of such strategies has mostly been reported in short-term uncontrolled studies. More recently, the use of methylphenidate for depression associated with the acquired immunodeficiency syndrome has also received support (see Chapter 21).

Psychostimulant therapy entails the risk of causing restlessness, anxiety, agitation, and insomnia. Of particular concern, especially when amphetamines are used chronically, is the risk of paranoid reactions and dependency. In addition, a rebound depression is quite common after the drugs are discontinued in patients who have become dependent on them. For these reasons, the use of psychostimulants is still largely reserved for carefully selected patients.

ELECTROCONVULSIVE THERAPY

Electroconvulsive therapy (ECT) is the use of electrically induced convulsions (i.e., grand mal or motor seizures) to treat psychiatric illnesses such as depression and mania or psychiatric symptoms such as psychosis or catatonia. Although ECT was first used in the late 1930s, the treatment today remains clinically relevant because of its high degree of efficacy, safety, and utility.

Mechanisms of Action

The mechanisms of action of ECT are complex and not completely understood. Nevertheless, ECT has been found to affect many of those transmitters and receptors that have been implicated in depression and its treatment. In studies involving both humans and animals, ECT has been found to affect such brain transmitters as serotonin, GABA, endogenous opiates and their receptors, and catecholamines, including dopamine, norepinephrine, epinephrine, and their receptors. It also affects a wide variety of other neurotransmitters, neuropeptides, and neuroendocrine pathways.

Indications

ECT is primarily indicated in the treatment of severe depression—particularly depression in which symptoms are intense, prolonged, and accompanied by profound alterations in the patient's level of vegetative functioning, including sleep, appetite, libido, and activity level. As has been demonstrated in previous sections of this chapter, TCAs, SSRIs, and MAOIs are the primary somatic treatments for depression. In patients with major depression with psychotic features, severe obsessional features, or active suicidal ideation, ECT is considered by some clinicians as the first-line treatment. In general, among patients with schizophrenia, those with prominent affective and catatonic symptoms respond the best to ECT, while those patients with chronic (and especially negative) symptoms often fail to respond. There is no indication that ECT alters the fundamental psychopathology of schizophrenia.

Yudofsky (1981) outlined special clinical situations in which ECT may be advantageous over other treatment approaches and may be the first line of treatment. Among these situations are the following:

1. Patients whose severe mood disorders have not responded to adequate psychopharmacological treatment

2. Patients with delusional (psychotic) depression (see Chapter 7)

3. Patients who cannot tolerate the side effects of antidepressant or antipsychotic agents

4. Patients whose acute symptoms are so severe that a rapid and dramatic response is required

5. Patients with histories of depressive episodes that have responded successfully to previous ECT

ECT also may be used in the treatment of acute and chronic manic episodes resistant to medication.

Contraindications

The contraindications to ECT are relatively few. First, patients with clinically significant space-occupying cerebral lesions must not receive this treatment because of the risk of brain stem herniation. Second, patients with significant cardiovascular problems that may include recent (within 6 months) myocardial infarction, severe cardiac ischemia, and uncontrolled hypertension are at higher risk for complications. Such patients may or may not be safely given ECT and must be evaluated before treatment by a cardiologist and an anesthesiologist familiar with the potential side effects of ECT. Before the use of muscle relaxants in the ECT technique, degenerative diseases of the spine and other bones comprised a significant risk from ECT. Today, however, adequate anesthetic techniques render ECT generally safe in patients with these disorders. While it is generally suggested that patients should be discontinued from their MAOIs for at least 2 weeks before the initiation of ECT to prevent dangerous increases in blood pressure during treatment, ECT has been administered to patients currently treated with MAOIs without adverse effects (Wells and Bjorkstein, 1989). Pretreatment with betaandrenergic blockers to attenuate sympathetic autonomic cardic stimulates all but removes cardic toxicity from ECT.

Medical Evaluation Before Treatment

Before receiving ECT, a patient should have a complete medical and neurological examination, complete blood count, blood chemistry analysis, urinalysis, and electrocardiogram. A chest X-ray must be obtained because of the use of positive-pressure respiration during general anesthesia. Electroencephalogram and a computed tomographic scan may be required for patients with known or suspected brain disease such as stroke or brain tumors. X-ray of the lumbosacral region of the spine may be obtained if orthopedic problems are suspected.

Because of the high degree of fear and misinformation related to ECT, we encourage that ample time be devoted to discussion of the risks, benefits, and techniques of ECT with both patients and their families. Education of the patient and family are actually the most time-consuming aspects of administering ECT.

Technique

In the United States, ECT treatments are generally given on an every-other-day basis (three times a week) for 2 to 3 weeks for a total of 6 to 9 treatments on average. Seizure lengths of between 25 and 60 seconds per treatment are considered adequate for therapeutic purposes. Electrodes may be placed unilaterally on the nondominant cerebral hemisphere (i.e., the electrodes over the right hemisphere for a right-handed individual) or bilaterally over both temples. One technique of inducing seizures at the initial treatment session is to determine the seizure threshold, which is determined by administering relatively low dosages of current at first and increasing the current in a stepwise fashion until a seizure is elicited. For unilateral ECT, subsequent treatments are administered at a dosage of several times the threshold dosage. Bilateral treatments may be administered at minimally suprathreshold dosages. With these parameters, unilateral ECT is associated with much fewer cognitive side effects but may not be as rapidly efficacious as bilateral stimulation.

Side Effects

For each treatment there is an initial confusional period that lasts for approximately 30 minutes. Memory impairment that occurs with ECT is highly variable. While certain patients report no problems with their memory, others report that their memory "is not as good as it used to be" after receiving ECT. It has been found that for some patients who experience retrograde amnesia (i.e., diminished ability to recall information that was recently learned before ECT was administered) following bilateral ECT seem to have recovered complete memory function by 6 months after treatment, with little evidence that new learning ability is still deficient at this time. In some patients who do have memory impairment following bilateral ECT, information acquired during the days and weeks before, during, and for several weeks following ECT may be permanently lost. If the patient had cognitive dysfunction secondary to severe depression, memory may actually improve 4–6 weeks after ECT!

ECT remains an effective, if not preferred, treatment for those patients with severe depressions that include those with delusional and suicidal features. ECT is only one component of a larger treatment plan that includes psychosocial interventions. The optimum strategy for treatment of a patient after a course of ECT is not clear. While some patients will do well with maintenance antidepressant medications, other patients may require lithium, either alone or in addition to antidepressants. Finally, since patients who have been previously refractory to or intolerant of antidepressants receive ECT, it can be predicted that they will not respond to these drugs after ECT. Therefore, maintenance ECT, at a frequency of one treatment a month for a period of 6–12 months, may be given to maintain remission in patients who are at extremely high risk for relapse. Current clinical trials are being conducted to measure the efficacy and safety of maintenance ECT.

CLINICAL PEARLS

- A relatively easy way to remember the differential side effects of the classic antipsychotic or neuroleptic drugs is that the "low-potency" drugs such as chlorpromazine and thioridazine have relatively *high* anticholinergic and orthostatic hypotensive side effects and low EPS. The "high-potency" drugs such as haloperidol, thiothixene, and fluphenazine conversely have *low anticholinergic and orthostatic hypotensive side effects* and a high propensity for EPS. Hence, the side effects in the "high-potency" and "low-potency" drugs vary inversely in this respect. The newer atypical agents risperidone, olanzapine, and sertindole have more in common with the "high-potency" agents, except for their very low risk of inducing EPS. Clozapine should be classified as a "low-potency" agent; it is especially high in anticholinergic effects. The atypical agents in general carry the very lowest risks of EPS and TD.

- Monitoring serum CPK levels is an excellent way to identify the prodrome or the presence of neuroleptic malignant syndrome, as well as to monitor the course of the patient's recovery from it.

- It is imperative that patients being considered for long-term use with neuroleptic (antipsychotic) agents give informed consent, that they be monitored frequently for EPS using structured rating instruments such as the Abnormal Involuntary Movements Scale, and that the informed consent be updated every 6 months. Neuroleptic drugs should always be used in the lowest possible dose, and the need for continued treatment should be documented periodically.

- In respect to the antidepressant drugs, one should choose a drug based on its side effect profile, matching the side effects of the drug with the symptoms and physiological vulnerabilities of the patient. For example, patients with severe anxiety, agitation, and insomnia may better tolerate a relatively sedating antidepressant such as nortriptyline or nefazodone. Alternatively, patients who are more apathetic, anergic, and hypersomnolent may respond best to a more "stimulating" drug such as fluoxetine, bupropion, or desipramine.

- Most antidepressant drugs, with the exception of bupropion, should be given once a day, usually in the morning or before bedtime. Although nefazodone is currently recommended as twice-a-day agents, many psychiatrists find that one daily dose is effective and well tolerated. Because of their stimulant properties, the SSRIs, MAOIs, venlafaxine, and the tricyclic protriptyline are usually best given in the early parts of the day.

- The most common reasons for "refractory" depression are noncompliance with medication and treatment with inadequate doses of antidepressants for too brief a period of time.

- Patients who have Parkinson's disease with psychotic symptoms should be considered for treatment with clozapine or one of the newer atypical antipsychotics such as olanzapine. Clozapine not only has very few if any EPS that could possibly worsen the Parkinson's disease, but some investigators have reported that it actually improves the symptoms of Parkinson's disease due to its anticholinergic effects.

- The most problematic aspect of treating elderly patients with TCAs is the development of orthostatic hypotension. Of the traditional TCAs, nortriptyline has the fewest orthostatic side effects, and of the new antidepressants, bupropion, venlafaxine, and the SSRIs appear to have the definite advantage; however, venlafaxine has a clinically small but significant risk of hypertension.

- Of the traditional TCAS, desipramine appears to have the fewest anticholinergic side effects. Of the newer drugs, the SSRIs and bupropion have the advantage over both the older and newer drugs in this respect.
- The benzodiazepines can be best differentiated into two classes. Oxazepam, temazepam, and lorazepam all are primarily metabolized by conjugation, and therefore, their half-lives are not affected by aging or liver disease. Practically all the other drugs, with the exception of clonazepam, are metabolized by way of oxidative mechanisms and therefore may be affected by age, liver disease, or other medications that affect hepatic enzymatic activity. Clonazepam should also be avoided in patients with liver disease.
- Lorazepam and midazolam are the only two benzodiazepines that may be reliably absorbed by the intramuscular route and are the preferred benzodiazepines to be given intravenously.
- Shorter acting benzodiazepines such as midazolam, triazolam, and alprazolam may cause anterograde amnesia.
- In respect to the cardiovascular side effects, the TCAs all have quinidinelike side effects, and therefore may be arrhythmogenic in patients with heart block. Carbamazepine is also a tricyclic compound with quinidinelike side effects.
- ECT is often the safest and most predictable treatment for certain patients with profound (and especially psychotic) depressions. ECT is particularly useful for elderly or medically debilitated patients who may not be able to tolerate the side effects of antidepressant agents. ECT is *not* recommended for patients who have expanding intracranial mass lesions, nor for patients who have experienced a recent myocardial infarction. A careful assessment of risk versus benefit must be undertaken for patients with severe cardiovascular disease in which the hypertension and tachycardia associated with seizure activity may place an excessive demand on the myocardium. These latter side effects can usually be managed through appropriate autonomic blockade with agents such as labetalol, esmolol, or pretreatment with nifedipine.

ANNOTATED BIBLIOGRAPHY

American Psychiatric Association: Tardive Dyskinesia: A Task Force Report of the American Psychiatric Association. Washington, DC, American Psychiatric Association, 1992

    This report reviews current knowledge of assessment, risk factors, prevention, and treatment of tardive dyskinesia.

American Psychiatric Association: The Practice of Electroconvulsive Therapy: Recommendations for Treatment, Training, and Privileging A Task Force Report of the American Psychiatric Association. Washington, DC, American Psychiatric Association, 1990

    This is the state-of-the-art review of the current practice of ECT.

Dubovsky SC: Psychopharmacologic treatment in neuropsychiatry. In Yudofsky SC, Hales RE (eds): The American Psychiatric Press Textbook of Neuropsychiatry, 2nd ed., pp 411–438. Washington, DC, American Psychiatric Press, 1992

    This is a succinct review of the use of psychopharmacological agents in patients with neuropsychiatric disorders.

Kass FE, Oldham JM, Pardes H: The Columbia University College of Physicians and Surgeons Complete Home Guide to Mental Health. New York, Henry Holt, 1992

Bernstein JG: Handbook of Drug Therapy in Psychiatry. St. Louis, Mosby-Year Book, 1995
> A thorough review of psychopharmacology with an emphasis on practical applications.

Bloom FE, Kupfer DJ (eds): Psychopharmacology: The Fourth Generation of Progress. New York, Raven Press, 1995
> This is a superb and encyclopedic source on clinical psychopharmacology. It covers almost every aspect of clinical psychopharmacology from basic neuropharmacologic mechanisms to practical clinical applications. Excellent as a reference source for special study or complex clinical situations.

Schatzberg AF, Cole JO: Manual of Clinical Psychopharmacology, 3rd ed. Washington, DC, American Psychiatric Press, 1997
> This is an excellent short guide to practical clinical psychopharmacology that is well referenced and contains excellent tables.

Schatzberg AF, Nemeroff CB (eds): The American Psychiatric Press Textbook of Psychopharmacology. Washington, DC, American Psychiatric Press, 1995
> Another excellent, comprehensive source on clinical psychopharmacology. In addition to its thorough treatment of theoretical and basic science issues, it is a valuable, practical reference source for the clinician.

Silver JM, Yudofsky SC, Hurowitz G: Psychopharmacology and electroconvulsive therapy. In Hales RE, Yudofsky SC, Talbott JA (eds): The American Psychiatric Press Textbook of Psychiatry, 2nd ed. Washington, DC, American Psychiatric Press, 897–1008, 1994
> This is an expanded discussion of many of the basic principles discussed in this chapter.

Stoudemire A, Fogel BS, Gulley LR, Moran MG: Psychopharmacology in the medical patient. In Stoudemire A, Fogel BS (eds): Psychiatric Care of the Medical Patient. New York, Oxford University Press, 155–206, 1993
> This is an expanded and detailed discussion of the special modifications that must be made in the use of psychopharmacologic agents in medically ill patients. It deals on a specialty-by-specialty basis with each of the major organ systems and the possible vulnerabilities of medically ill patients to psychopharmacologic agents.

Yudofsky SC, Hales RE, Ferguson T: What You Need to Know about Psychiatric Drugs. New York, Grove Weidenfeld, 1991
> These books are excellent resources for patient education about psychiatric disorders and treatments.

REFERENCES

American Psychiatric Association: Diagnostic and Statistical Manual of Mental Disorders, 4th ed. Washington, DC, American Psychiatric Association, 1994

Battle DC, VonRiotte AB, Gaviria M, et al: Amelioration of polyuria by amiloride in patients receiving long-term lithium therapy. N Engl J Med 312:408–414, 1985

Boyer W: Serotonin uptake inhibitors are superior to imipramine and alprazolam in alleviating panic attacks: a meta-analysis. Int Clin Psychopharmacol 10:45–49, 1995

Breier A, Charney DS, Heninger GR: Agoraphobia with panic attacks: development, diagnostic stability, and course of illness. Arch Gen Psychiatry 43:1029–1036, 1986

Consensus Development Panel: Mood disorders: pharmacologic prevention of recurrences. Am J Psychiatry 142:469–476, 1985

Conte HR, Plutchik R, Wild KV, et al: Combined psychotherapy and pharmacotherapy for depression: a systemic analysis of the evidence. Arch Gen Psychiatry 43:471–479, 1986

Davis JM, Andriukaitis S: The natural course of schizophrenia and effective maintenance drug treatment. J Clin Psychopharmacol 6:2S–10S, 1986

Devinsky O, Honigfeld G, Patin J: Clozapine-related seizures. Neurology 41:369–371, 1991

Gelenberg AJ, Kane JM, Keller MB, et al: Comparison of standard and low serum levels of lithium for maintenance treatment of bipolar disorder N Engl J Med 321:1489–1493, 1989

Glazer WM, Moore DC, Schooler NR, et al: Tardive dyskinesia: a discontinuation study. Arch Gen Psychiatry 43:623–627, 1984

Grossman E, Messerli FH, Grodzicki T, et al: Should a moratorium be placed on sublingual nifedipine capsules given for hypertensive emergencies and pseudoemergencies? JAMA 276:1328–1331, 1996

Hart RG, Easton JD: Carbamazepine and hematological monitoring. Ann Neurol 11:309–312, 1982

Harvey AT, Preskorn SH: Cytochrome P450 enzymes: interpretation of their interactions with selective serotonin reuptake inhibitor. part II. J Clin Psychopharmacol 16:345–355, 1996

Keck Jr PE, McElroy SL, Nemeroff CB: Anticonvulsants in the treatment of bipolar disorder. J Neuropsychiatry Clin Neurosci 4:395–405, 1992

Lieberman JA, Saltz BC, Johns CA, et al: The effects of clozapine on tardive dyskinesia. Br J Psychiatry 158:503–510, 1991

Manji HK, Chen G, Hsiao JK, et al: Regulation of signal transduction pathways by mood-stabilizing agents: implications for the delayed onset of therapeutic efficacy. J Clin Psychiatry 57(suppl 13):34–46, 1996

McElroy SL, Dessain EC, Pope HG Jr, et al: Clozapine in the treatment of psychotic mood disorders, schizoaffective disorder, and schizophrenia. J Clin Psychiatry 52:411–414, 1991

McElroy SL, Keck PE, Stanton SP, et al: A randomized comparison of divalproex oral loading versus haloperidol in the initial treatment of acute psychotic mania. J Clin Psychiatry 57:142–146, 1996

Mellinger GD, Balter MB, Uhlenhuth EH: Insomnia and its treatment: prevalence and correlates. Arch Gen Psychiatry 42:225–232, 1985

Meltzer HY: Role of serotonin in the action of atypical antipsychotic drugs. Clin Neurosci 3:64–75, 1995

Mitchell JE, Mackenzie TB: Cardiac effects of lithium therapy in man: a review. J Clin Psychiatry 43:47–51, 1982

Munetz MR, Roth LH: Informing patients about tardive dyskinesia. Arch Gen Psychiatry 42:866–871, 1985

Myers DH, Carter RA, Burns BH, et al: A prospective study of the effects of lithium on thyroid function and on the prevalence of antithyroid antibodies. Psychol Med 15:55–61, 1985

National Institute of Mental Health: Abnormal Involuntary Movement Scale. In Guy W (ed): ECDEU Assessment Manual. Rockville, MD, U.S. Department of Health, Education, and Welfare, 1976

Pellock JM: Carbamazepine side effects in children and adults. Epilepsia 28(suppl):64–70, 1987

Preskorn SH, Burke M: Somatic therapy for major depressive disorder: selection of an antidepressant. J Clin Psychiatry 53(suppl):5–18, 1992

Prien RF, Kupfer DJ: Continuation drug therapy for major depressive episodes: how long should it be maintained? Am J Psychiatry 143:18–23, 1986

Reich J: The epidemiology of anxiety. J Nerv Ment Dis 174:129–136, 1986

Shulman KI, Walker SE, MacKenzie S, et al: Dietary restriction, tyramine, and the use of monoamine oxidase inhibitors. J Clin Psychopharmacol 9:397–402, 1989

Silver JM, Yudofsky SC, Hurowitz GI: Psychopharmacology and electroconvulsive therapy. In Hales RE, Yudofsky SC, Talbott JA (eds): The American Psychiatric Press Textbook of Psychiatry, 2nd ed. Washington, DC, American Psychiatric Press, 1994

Suranyi-Cadotte BE, Bodnoff SR, Welner SA: Antidepressant-anxiolytic interactions: involvement of the benzodiazepine-GABA and serotonin systems. Prog Neuropsychopharmacol Biol Psychiatry 14:633–654, 1990

Wells DG, Bjorkstein AR: Monoamine oxidase inhibitors revisited. Can J Anaesth 36:64–74, 1989

Yassa R, Lal S: Prevalence of the rabbit syndrome. Am J Psychiatry 143:656–657, 1986

Yudofsky SC: ECT in general hospital psychiatry: focus on new indications and technologies. Gen Hosp Psychiatry 3:292–296, 1981

19 *Psychiatric Emergencies: Recognition and Management*

William R. Dubin

Emergency management of psychiatric disorders is one of the unique areas of medicine in which physicians must have a broad knowledge of both medicine and psychiatry. The interplay between physical illness and psychological functioning is dramatic. This chapter's purpose is to provide an introduction to evaluating and treating psychiatric emergencies by highlighting the major syndromes most commonly seen in the emergency department (ED). Topics include the evaluation and treatment of psychosis; violence; suicide; rape; child, spouse, and elder abuse; and legal issues pertaining to emergency psychiatry. More general legal issues in psychiatry are discussed in Chapter 25.

ACUTE PSYCHOSIS: DIFFERENTIATING MENTAL DISEASE DUE TO MEDICAL, NEUROLOGICAL, AND TOXIC CAUSES FROM FUNCTIONAL PSYCHIATRIC ILLNESS

The most important decision in evaluating a psychotic patient is to differentiate mental disorders due to medical, neurological, or toxic causes from a "functional" psychiatric illness. Between 3.5 and 18.4% of patients considered to be primarily psychiatric in nature have undetected medical illness (Dubin and Weiss, 1984). Clinicians often make a premature psychiatric referral in the context of metabolically, neurologically, or toxin-induced brain dysfunction because of the following:

1. *Bias against psychiatric patients or patients with psychiatric symptoms.* Psychiatric patients often make physicians uncomfortable, anxious, fearful, and frustrated because of their bizarre or disruptive behavior. Physicians may not view such patients with the same urgency or seriousness as they do patients with cardiovascular disease or physical trauma. Too often, initial decisions are based on a single piece of datum, symptom, item of past history, or previous diagnosis (Leeman, 1975).

2. *Disordered perceptions.* A common misconception is that delusions, hallucinations, and disorganized thoughts are synonymous with psychiatric illness only. On the contrary, these symptoms, like pain or headache, are ubiquitous and occur in psychiatric *and* medical illness. Psychotic symptoms may occur transiently in certain personality disorders during times of emotional crisis.

3. *Violence.* Because violence makes clinicians anxious, they quickly tend to refer any violent or potentially violent patient for psychiatric evaluation; however, 17% of violence that occurs in psychiatric settings results from underlying medical or neurological illness (Tardiff and Sweillam, 1980). Violence, like disordered perceptions, is etiologically nonspecific.

4. *Self-induced illness.* The least-tolerated patients are those who are believed to create their own disease, such as alcoholics, drug abusers, or suicidal patients (Weissberg, 1979). Consequently, clinicians tend to minimize these patients' symptoms. An example is a patient who presents with a suicide attempt by overdose with antidepressants and who initially is fully alert and clinically stable. In patients like this, physicians tend to trivialize the seriousness of the overdose, yet half the patients who die from a tricyclic antidepressant overdose present fully alert and stable, but have a catastrophic deterioration within 1 hour after admission to the ED (Callahan and Kassel, 1985).

5. *Ageism.* Clinicians often fail to take seriously or follow up the complaints and illnesses of elderly patients and attribute these complaints to old age or hypochondriasis (Goodstein, 1985). This problem may be further exacerbated in the patient with dementia. The term *dementia* is used generically to describe chronic irreversible and progressive deterioration of higher intellectual functioning, but 30 to 40% of all patients who present with symptoms of dementia have potentially treatable and sometimes completely reversible underlying causes for their altered mental status (Dubin, 1984). Premature labeling can preclude the physical, neurological, and laboratory evaluation necessary to determine the etiology of a patient's cognitive dysfunction.

DELIRIUM, DEMENTIA, AND OTHER DISORDERS WITH COGNITIVE IMPAIRMENT

Delirium is commonly encountered in the ED. Delirium specifically refers to a (usually) reversible disturbance of cerebral functioning due to a toxic, neurological, or metabolic disturbance (see Chapter 4). The onset is acute, generally developing over a 6- to 96-hour period, and is characterized by impairment of alertness, thinking, memory, perception, concentration, and attention (Lipowski, 1967). The incidence varies from 5 to 15% (Wise, 1987). The level of consciousness is altered and fluctuates in a sine-wave fashion.

Several common clinical features are highly suggestive of delirium: clouding of consciousness, age over 40 with no previous psychiatric history, disorientation, abnormal vital signs, visual hallucinations, and illusions (Dubin et al, 1983; Hall et al, 1978).

The differential diagnosis of delirium is so extensive that physicians may tend to avoid searching for an etiology (Wise, 1987). For example, an elderly delirious patient may have multiorgan disease (e.g., pulmonary insufficiency, cardiac failure, preexisting brain damage) and may be taking multiple medicines (Wise, 1987). In such a patient, each problem is a potential contributor to the delirium and should be pursued and evaluated independently.

For the sake of differential diagnosis, clinicians should consider two categories of illness severity: *emergent* and *urgent.* Emergent conditions are life threatening; they require immediate attention and are of major concern to the psychiatrist (Table 19–1) (Anderson, 1987). Most other causes of delirium, while not life threatening, require urgent treatment (Table 19–2) (Dubin and Weiss, 1985).

Laboratory studies that will help rule out emergent illnesses include a complete blood count, glucose, serum electrolytes, blood urea nitrogen, chest radiograph, electrocardiogram, arterial blood gases, and urinary drug screen. Patients who present with an acute behavioral change and/or clouded consciousness unexplained by this laboratory evaluation may require computed tomography followed by a lumbar puncture.

Table 19–1 **Life-Threatening Causes of Delirium (Selected List)**

Meningitis and encephalitis
Hypoglycemia
Hypertensive encephalopathy
Diminished cerebral oxygenation
Anticholinergic intoxication
Intracranial hemorrhage
Wernicke's encephalopathy
Drug or alcohol withdrawal or intoxication

Table 19–2 **Selected Causes of Cognitive Dysfunction**

Cardiac	**Vitamin Deficiencies**
Arrhythmias	Thiamine
Congestive heart failure	Niacin
Myocardial infarction	Riboflavin
Pulmonary	Folate
Chronic obstructive pulmonary	Ascorbic acid
disease	Vitamin A
Pulmonary emboli	Vitamin B$_{12}$
Hepatic	**Drug Induced**
Cirrhosis	Alcohol
Hepatitis	Tranquilizers
Wilson's disease	Over-the-counter preparations
Renal	Any drug used to treat medical
Worsening of mild nephritis by urinary	illness, e.g., Dilantin, aminophylline,
tract infection	digitalis, steroids
Dehydration with elevation of blood	**Exogenous Toxins**
urinary nitrogen (BUN) over	Carbon monoxide
50 mg/dl.	Bromide
Vascular	Mercury
Subdural hematoma	Lead
Cerebrovascular accident	**Infections**
Endocrine Disease	**Tumors**
Thyroid disease	**Normal Pressure Hydrocephalus**
Cushing's disease	**Depression**
Diabetes	**Acquired Immunodeficiency Syndrome**
Addison's disease (hypoadrenalism)	
Hypoglycemia	
Electrolyte Imbalance	
Hyponatremia	
Hypernatremia	
Hypercalcemia	

At times, extreme agitation can significantly impede the evaluation. In these cases, pharmacological intervention (rapid tranquilization) will be helpful so that the appropriate medical–neurological examination can be completed. This procedure is discussed later under the section about violence.

In addition to medication, psychological support is important. Patients should have a staff member, if available, or a family member with them at all times during the evaluation. This can be reassuring to patients and can reduce mishaps such as pulling out intravenous lines or falling out of bed (Wise, 1987). Delirium is also discussed in Chapter 4.

Functional Psychiatric Illness

The ED physician's task is (1) to differentiate primary metabolically, neurologically, or toxin-induced brain dysfunction from psychiatric illness and to rule out any life-threatening causes of aberrant behavior; (2) to stabilize the patient medically and/or psychiatrically; and (3) to determine the most appropriate treatment setting (inpatient, outpatient, partial hospital). Ultimately, correctly diagnosing patients with psychiatric illness is essential because there are specific treatments for each illness (i.e., lithium for bipolar disorder, antidepressants for depression, antipsychotic medications for schizophrenia); however, for the few hours that the patient is in the ED, the treatment of aberrant behavior, agitation, excitement, and potential violence is the overriding priority. In this setting, the primary interventions include psychotherapy, pharmacotherapy, and, at times, physical restraints. While psychotropic medication has greatly enhanced our ability to attenuate the behavioral emergency effectively, verbal intervention remains an integral part of successful treatment.

THE EMERGENCY DEPARTMENT INTERVIEW

Treatment is inextricably interwoven with the evaluation process (Dubin and Weiss, 1991). The initial interview not only serves to elicit important diagnostic information, it may be therapeutic in itself. The goal of the interview is to gather information about the present illness, past psychiatric and medical history, family and occupational history, and drug and alcohol use. *The interviewer should not be distracted by the patient's bizarre behavior or verbalizations.* Such behavior often makes physicians feel uncomfortable; as a result, they are indifferent or overtly, defensively hostile. This approach may exacerbate the patient's symptoms. A controlled, patient professional composure on the physician's part is reassuring to psychotic patients, who may feel very much out of control. Even the most psychotic patient usually has enough self-awareness to form a rudimentary alliance when addressed with respect and dignity.

Emergency psychiatry work with hostile, uncooperative, or insulting patients can be especially difficult and frustrating. Hanke (1984) presents a thorough and comprehensive review of working with such difficult patients. She notes that the most common negative feelings are various forms of anger, anxiety, and despair. While clinicians may be aware of strong negative feelings, most commonly we express them in an indirect way that we may not recognize. Negative feelings may impede clinical judgment and decision making in the following ways:

1. *Arbitrary inferences,* or jumping to a conclusion based on inadequate or incorrect data ("Nothing will help this patient").
2. *All-or-nothing thinking,* or seeing situations as strictly black and white ("No one talks to me like that").
3. *Personalization,* or taking too much blame or too much credit without an objective reason ("With a little crisis intervention, I solved the patient's problem").

In general, if a clinician has an extremely negative reaction toward a patient, it suggests that the patient has struck an area of emotional vulnerability in the physician. Hanke (1984) suggests five guidelines to help manage negative responses to patients:

1. View the patient's maladaptive behavior as symptomatic of their condition, rather than as a personal attack.
2. View negative reactions as overreactions.
3. Find a rationale (reason) for overreactions by identifying the type of response (i.e., arbitrary inference, all-or-nothing thinking, or personalization).
4. Generate alternate reactions. For example, instead of viewing patients as "a manipulative sociopath," try to see them as pitiful or self-destructive, or as someone's son.
5. Maintain a larger perspective on negative reactions by attributing multiple causes to the negative reaction; for example, the negative feelings come from the patient's profanity (50%), the clinician's fatigue from being on call all night (25%), and the overcrowded waiting area (25%).

While it is difficult to eliminate negative feelings completely, clinicians should try to neutralize them to prevent distortion of their clinical judgment in a way that impedes optimum care.

To begin the interview, physicians should introduce themselves and address the patient as "Mr. Smith" or "Ms. Jones." If the patient does not pose an imminent risk, the physician should sit. Standing over the patient may impede rapport by implying domination or intimidation. To establish a friendly atmosphere, it often helps to offer the patient food or a drink (avoid hot liquids) or to offer to call a friend.

One of the major paradoxes in emergency medicine occurs in respect to emergency psychiatry. Most emergency departments focus on rapid intervention and disposition, but in emergency psychiatric interventions, *time is a major treatment variable.* The intensity of a patient's symptoms often diminishes in a structured, supportive environment with "tincture of time." Therefore, clinicians must restrain the impulse to "get right to the heart of the matter." The interview should begin with very nonspecific, less intrusive questions. After the patient begins to show some comfort with the interviewer, the physician can then start to ask about specific details. Questions should be open-ended to avoid simple "yes" or "no" answers. The physician should keep the interview format flexible, without trying to adhere to a predetermined rigid structure.

When interviewing an acutely disturbed agitated patient, the physician often must structure the interview by asking straightforward questions. If the patient begins to ramble, the interviewer should then restructure the interview to help patients to pick up the trend of their thinking. The interviewer should not take a passive role but should be an active, involved participant.

With patients having hallucinations or delusions, it is important not to use simple logic in an attempt to convince them that their perceptions are wrong. This maneuver tends to make patients feel more defensive and misunderstood and may destroy any rapport that may have developed.

Except with the extremely paranoid patient, "laying on of hands" often helps establish rapport. This can be done by asking patients if the interviewer can take their pulse or blood pressure or feel their forehead. Unless there is some reason not to do it, the physician should offer to shake the patient's hand during the introduction.

An important element of the interview is helping patients identify their feelings. The patients' need to protect their integrity and self-control may initially make them reluctant to engage in the interview. If patients are resistant to the idea of talking, it is useful to elicit their feelings about the situation and to try to understand their predicament of being in the hospital and not knowing what will happen.

When a psychotic patient does not respond to questioning, the interviewer should then use whatever data are available to make contact with the patient. Noting the patient's words, expressions, appearance, or behavior, as well as the physician's subjective reactions and feelings that are elicited by the patient can be helpful in this regard. Comments should be as specific as possible ("I don't know what Jesus says to you" or "I see you are in a bathrobe. I gather you were brought to the hospital unexpectedly.").

Despite the physician's most empathic and sensitive interventions, some patients will remain mute. Muteness is usually an angry response symbolizing an attempt to control the environment (Robbins and Stern, 1976). While medical and neurologic illnesses have been reported as etiologic for cases of mutism, it is rarely a sign of neurological disease (Wells, 1980). When patients are mute, the first step is to indicate that appropriate responses are expected. If the patient continues to remain silent, the interviewer then should pause and observe what the silence is communicating. At no time should the clinician indicate a sense of futility by angrily and repeatedly asking questions and getting no reply. If the clinician cannot engage the patient in conversation, she or he should try to gather diagnostic information from the patient's family, friends, or spouse. If time permits, a sodium amytal interview may sometimes lead to dramatic improvement. If muteness persists, admission to a psychiatric unit for evaluation and treatment is indicated.

The most difficult patients for even experienced psychiatrists to interview are the *paranoid* patients. Perry (1976) has outlined an excellent approach to interviewing paranoid patients. If the patient is frightening, physicians should *not* ignore their own fear. Patients can quickly sense this discomfort and may become frightened themselves, leading to an escalation of symptoms. Sometimes it is helpful for clinicians to acknowledge their fears by saying to the patient, "The way you're looking makes me feel that you're on the verge of striking out. What can we do to help you feel more in control of things?" If the physician remains professionally confident and in control, patients are usually reassured. The patient's anxiety can be further ameliorated if the interview is conducted with the door open or if additional staff are present.

It is important to be tactful with paranoid patients because they are defensive, irritable, and easily humiliated. Paranoid patients who are angry often begin with a tirade of accusations about being mistreated. The clinician may have to interrupt and say to the patient, "How do you feel I might help you?" With the angry, paranoid patient, the physician should always maintain a professional demeanor by not becoming too friendly, intrusive, or controlling and by avoiding jokes or patronizing reassurance.

Occasionally, paranoid patients can make the interviewer feel defensive and foolish by twisting the meaning of the interviewer's words, making it impossible for the interviewer to sustain any direction in the interview. Under these circumstances, the interviewer should alter the course of the interview by explaining to the patient that he or she is making the interviewer uncomfortable and suggesting that they discuss ways to help the patient feel more comfortable. If meaningful contact cannot be made, the interview should be terminated until the situation and the patient's condition permit a more productive interaction, usually after the patient has been medicated (see below).

THE VIOLENT PATIENT

The risk of violence in hospital settings appears to be increasing (Lavoie et al, 1988; Pane et al, 1991). In the EDs of teaching hospitals (With more than 40,000 patient visits a year) 32% had one verbal threat a day, 18% noted that weapons were displayed at least once each month, and 43% reported a physical attack on a medical staff member at least once a month (Lavoie et al, 1988). Forty-six percent of the hospitals in this study noted that weapons were confiscated at least once each month from patients or visitors. Against this backdrop, it becomes increasingly essential that clinicians learn the basic skills for management of aggressive patients. Patients can usually be successfully treated in the ED if the clinician approaches the patient in an objective, systematic manner and understands the dynamics of violence (Dubin, 1981). Simply stated, most patients tend to become violent when they feel helpless, passive, or trapped (Lion, 1972). Successful interventions often alleviate these feelings and diminish the chances of behavioral dyscontrol.

Usually, a prodromal pattern of behavior precedes overt violence. Fortunately, sudden, unexpected physical assault is rare, and most violence is a predictable culmination of a 30- to 60-minute period of escalation. This prodrome can often be observed in the patient's posture, speech, and motor activity. Most violence is preceded by a period of increasing restlessness and pacing. Hyperactivity itself may be a sign of a psychiatric emergency that requires immediate intervention. Patients who manifest rigid postures by literally "having their back up in the air," those who clench their fists and jaws, and those whose temporal arteries are visibly pulsating are in the early stages of escalation. As part of the prodromal syndrome, patients are often verbally abusive and profane. *The clinician's response to such verbal stridency is central to the outcome of the intervention.* When verbal abuse is personalized and the clinician reacts defensively or angrily, the risk of violence is increased. *It is important to remember that verbal abuse is an attempt by the patient to assert autonomy and diminish feelings of helplessness.*

Treatment of Violence

As with psychotic patients, verbal intervention can be strikingly effective with potentially assaultive patients. Even with patients who appear to be on the verge of total loss of control, appropriate and well-timed verbal interventions can have a positive impact on behavior. Patients are terrified of losing control and welcome therapeutic efforts to restore it and prevent their acting out (Lion and Pasternak, 1973). The agitated, fearful, panicky feeling that is especially common in psychotic patients prior to their assaultiveness can be attenuated by empathic verbal interventions. Talking gives the patient an outlet for the tension that is being generated and is important for ventilating angry, hostile feelings (Lion, 1972).

During the interview, the clinician should focus on the patient's underlying feeling state or affect. Efforts to calm a patient through rationalization and intellectualization are usually not therapeutic and may only increase the patient's frustration and feelings of being misunderstood. Physicians often are reluctant to have patients express their anger as they fear that this ventilation will only escalate their loss of emotional control. On the contrary, ventilating angry feelings reduces the agitation. Often the hostile feelings frighten the patient, and by acknowledging these feelings, some degree of emotional catharsis can be achieved and diminish the need for further aggression (Lion et al, 1972).

During the interview, the clinician should stay at least an arm's length from the patient. Never leave potentially violent patients alone, as this could be interpreted as rejection or could permit them to hurt themselves. An interviewer who feels anxious or unsure of how the patient will respond should ask the police, security personnel, or the family to remain nearby to help control the patient, if necessary. There is some disagreement as to whether the patient or the interviewer should be closer to the door during the interview; a compromise would be to have both equal distance from the door.

As noted earlier, as part of verbal intervention, it can be helpful to offer the patient food or a drink (again, avoiding hot liquids for obvious reasons). Offering food symbolizes friendship and caring and often helps alleviate a patient's angry affect. During the interview, it is also important to observe the patient's behavior; it may suggest that the patient is not as threatening as she or he may sound. When patients have their hands behind their backs or in their pockets or comply with all the interviewer's requests, they are less likely to become violent, despite their strident speech.

The ultimate threat comes from patients with weapons. If a patient admits to having a weapon, never immediately ask for it, but explore the fear that led the patient to arm himself or herself. A weapon symbolizes a defense against feelings of helplessness and passivity. An immediate request to give up a weapon may heighten these feelings and further exacerbate the threat. During the interview, if the patient agrees to give up the weapon, the interviewer should *never* accept the weapon directly from the patient. Instead, the patient should be asked to put the weapon on the table or the floor so that the interviewer can pick it up at the end of the interview. If the patient refuses to give up the weapon, the clinician should immediately notify hospital personnel. If the patient actually threatens the interviewer with the weapon, the clinician should avoid exacerbating the patient's feelings of helplessness and shame. Nonthreatening expressions of a desire to help, coupled with an expression of fear and submission, are the response most likely to avert physical harm ("I want to help you, but I'm too frightened to think with a gun pointed at me") (Dubin et al, 1988).

While staff often voice concern about the threat of armed patients, consideration must also be given to weapons, especially guns, carried by police officers and security personnel. Generally, it is preferable to have them disarmed while in the ED. There are several anecdotal reports of patients who have taken guns from police officers in such situations and injured themselves and/or others. In several instances, this scenario occurred with patients who were not under the supervision of the police. Table 19–3 summarizes basic techniques in managing the violent patient.

Table 19–3 **Dos and Don'ts of Treating Violent Patients**

DO	DON'T
Anticipate possible violence from hostile, threatening, agitated, restless, abusive patients or from those who lack control for any reason.	Don't ignore your "gut" feeling that a patient may be dangerous.
Heed your gut feeling. If you feel frightened or uneasy, discontinue the interview and get help.	Don't see angry, threatening, or restless persons right away.
Summon as many security guards or orderlies as possible at the first sign of violence. Patients who see that you take them seriously often will not act out further. If they do, you will be prepared.	Don't compromise your ability to escape a dangerous situation. Don't sit behind a desk or between a patient and the door.
Ask if the patient is carrying a weapon. These must be surrendered to security personnel. Never see an armed patient.	Don't antagonize the patient by responding angrily or being patronizing.
Offer help, food, medication. Bolster patients by commenting on their strength and self-control.	Don't touch or startle the patient or approach quickly without warning.
If restraint becomes necessary, assign one team member each to the patient's head and to each extremity. Be humane but firm, and do not bargain. Search the patient for drugs and weapons.	Don't try to restrain a patient without sufficient backup.
If the patient refuses oral medication, offer an injection after a few moments. Be prepared to administer it if the patient continues to refuse.	Don't neglect looking for medical causes of violence.
Keep a close eye on patients who are sedated and/or restrained. Restrained patients should never be left alone.	Don't bargain with a violent person about the need for restraints, medication, or psychiatric admission.
Hospitalize patients who state their intention to harm anyone, refuse to answer questions about their intent to harm, are abusing alcohol or drugs, are psychotic, have cognitive impairment, or refuse to cooperate with treatment.	Don't forget medical–legal concerns, such as full documentation of all interventions and the duty to warn and protect. If the patient is transferred, tell the admitting physician about any specific threats and victims.
Warn potential victims of threatened violence and notify the appropriate protection agencies.	Don't overlook family and friends as important sources of information
Follow up on any violent person and document this in the chart.	

(Used with permission from Dwyer B, Weissberg M: Treating violent patients. Psychiatric Times, p. 11, December 1988.)

Rapid Tranquilization

While verbal intervention is the mainstay of evaluation and treatment, medication is often necessary. In rapid tranquilization (RT), antipsychotic medication, usually in combination with a benzodiazepine, is given at 30- to 60-minute intervals; ideally, patients respond significantly within 30 to 90 minutes (Dubin et al, 1986). The target symptoms for RT include *tension, anxiety, restlessness, hyperactivity,* and *motor excitement.* Core psychotic symptoms such as hallucinations, delusions, and disorganized thought are usually not affected by RT and may require several days or weeks of appropriate antipsychotic drug treatment to attenuate. *The goal of RT is to calm patients so that they can cooperate in their evaluation, treatment, and disposition.* Occasionally, there is concern that RT will obscure the patient's mental status and that antipsychotic treatment should be withheld until a diagnosis is made. This specious argument can lead to withholding an effective treatment and may prolong the risk of violence. A psychiatric diagnosis is not made on a single mental status evaluation and, as stated earlier, definitive psychiatric treatment is not the primary task in the ED.

At times, clinicians also withhold medication for fear that it will obscure or worsen underlying medical conditions; instead, they physically restrain patients while they attempt a physical evaluation and laboratory workup. Besides the questionable accuracy of a physical examination done on a restrained, agitated patient, restraints carry significant medical risks (Gutheil and Tardiff, 1984; Johnson et al, 1987). With the exception of anticholinergic delirium (which can be worsened by RT due to the anticholinergic properties of some neuroleptics), the safety of RT in medically ill patients has been repeatedly demonstrated (Dubin et al, 1986).

RT is effective across all diagnostic categories, regardless of the etiology of the aggression. It is effective in psychosis secondary to functional psychiatric illness such as schizophrenia or mania, as well as in behavioral syndromes secondary to dementia, delirium, or alcohol and substance abuse or withdrawal (Dubin et al, 1986); however, in substance- and alcohol-abuse patients, RT should be used for behavioral dyscontrol only. Cross-tolerant agents such as benzodiazepines for alcohol withdrawal are preferred for treatment of the withdrawal syndrome itself.

Until recently, the mainstay of rapid tranquilization has been high-potency antipsychotics (i.e., thiothixene, haloperidol, fluphenazine, and loxapine); however, recent reports suggest that high-potency antipsychotic medication combined with a benzodiazepine (usually lorazepam) is more effective than either drug alone (Garza-Treviño et al, 1989; Barbee et al, 1992). Both medications are drawn up in the same syringe and given intramuscularly. The most common side effect of lorazepam includes sedation and ataxia (Dubin, 1988). The most common side effects of these high-potency neuroleptics are extrapyramidal symptoms, in contrast to the low-potency neuroleptics (e.g., chlorpromazine and thioridazine), whose primary side effects are hypotension and sedation (see Chapter 18).

The dosages used during RT are generally modest, and most patients respond in one to three doses given over 30 to 90 minutes (Table 19–4) (Dubin et al, 1986). While some patients may require higher doses, there are currently no predictive clinical variables for this subgroup. No ceiling doses have been established, and the ultimate number of doses is an empirical decision based on an assessment of the patient's clinical status. During RT, medication is given at 30- to 60-minute intervals; most studies have found 60-minute intervals sufficient. An important caveat is to try to use the minimum dosage over the maximum amount of time clinically feasible.

While RT was conceptualized as an ED procedure, its use has expanded to the intensive care unit (ICU) setting. In the ICU, the delirious agitation and combativeness of patients frequently impedes medical treatment and sometimes can be life threatening. Several studies have clearly demonstrated the efficacy and safety of RT in critically ill delirious patients in the ICU (Dudley et al, 1979; Adams, 1984; Sos and Cassem, 1980; Tesar et al, 1985).

Intravenous (IV) administration of medication is frequently the preferred route of choice in the ICU. Patients for whom IV administration may be useful include those with lowered cardiac output who will not absorb intramuscular medication, those incapable of taking oral medication, and those with extensive tissue damage, such as burn patients. While IV antipsychotic medication is safe and effective, the onset of action is variable. Some investigators used the IV route when a more rapid effect was desired (Clinton et al, 1987), while others found the onset of action variable (i.e., 10 to 40 minutes) (Tesar et al, 1985). The incidence of side effects from IV administration appears to be no greater than with other routes of administration. Patients who receive IV haloperidol may have a lower incidence of extrapyramidal symptoms compared with patients receiving oral medication (Menza et al, 1987). Goldstein (1987), in an excellent review of RT in the ICU, provides a useful guideline for the IV use of antipsychotics (Table 19–5). One caution: haloperidol is not

---

Table 19–4 Rapid Tranquilization of the Violent Patient*

Lorazepam (Ativan) 2–4 mg IM combined with haloperidol
  (Haldol) 5 mg IM or thiothixene (Navane) 5 mg IM
RT with an antipsychotic alone
Thiothixene (Navane) 10 mg IM or 20 mg concentrate orally
Haloperidol (Haldol) 5 mg IM or 10 mg concentrate orally
Loxapine (Loxitane) 10 mg IM or 25 mg concentrate orally

* All doses given at 30- to 60-minute intervals. Use half-dose for medically ill or older patients.

Table 19–5 **Treatment Guidelines for the Use of Intravenous Haloperidol in the Intensive Care Setting***

Starting Dose

Degree of Agitation	Dose
Mild	0.5 to 2.0 mg
Moderate to severe	2.0 to 10 mg

Titration and Maintenance:

Allow 20 to 30 minutes before the next dose.

If agitation is unchanged, administer double dose every 20 to 30 minutes until patient begins to calm.

If patient is calming down, repeat the last dose at the next dosing interval.

Adjust dose and interval to patient's clinical course. Gradually increase the interval between doses until the interval is 8 hours, then begin to decrease the dose.

Once stable for 24 hours, give doses on a regular schedule and supplement with p.r.n. doses.

Once stable for 36 to 48 hours, begin attempts to taper dose.

When agitation is very severe, very high boluses (up to 40 mg) may be required (Tesar et al, 1985).

* Haloperidol is not specifically approved by the Food and Drug Administration for the intravenous route; careful documentation for the necessity and rationale for its use should be made.
(Used with permission from Goldstein MG: Intensive care unit syndromes. In: Stoudemire A, Fogel BS, eds. Principles of Medical Psychiatry. Orlando: Grune & Stratton, 412, 1987)

specifically approved for IV use, and documentation of the rationale for this maneuver should be made.

Side Effects During RT. Side effects during RT are generally few, mild, and reversible. Most studies have found that fewer than 10% of patients develop extra-pyramidal symptoms (muscle rigidity, drooling, dystonias, akathisia, bradykinesia, etc.) within the first 24 hours of RT (Dubin et al, 1986). Extrapyramidal symptoms are not dose related and can occur even after one dose. By far the most common extrapyramidal symptoms are *dystonic reactions*, which are involuntary turning or twisting movements produced by massive and sustained muscle contractions (Mason and Granacher, 1980). Their suddenness in onset and bizarreness in presentation often leads to a misdiagnosis of (hysterical) conversion disorder. Dystonia usually involves muscles of the back, neck, and oral area. The back may be extended (opisthotonos), or the head may arch severely backward (retrocollis) or sideways (torticollis) (Hyman and Arana, 1987). The eyes may be pulled upward in a painful manner (occulogyric crisis). At times, patients may complain of thickness of the tongue or difficulty swallowing.

The most serious form of dystonia is laryngospasm. This contraction of the muscles of the larynx can compromise the airway and lead to severe respiratory distress. While it is extremely rare, clinicians should be alert for it.

A side effect that can be frequently misdiagnosed as a psychotic decompensation is *akathisia.* This Greek word literally means "inability to sit still." Patients feel uncomfortably restless, and pacing is their only relief. They will often say they feel "unable to relax," "tense," "all wound up like a spring," "irritable," or "like jumping out of my skin," or that they have "restless" legs (Van Putten and Marder, 1987). *Severe* akathisia can lead to a psychotic decompensation, and in its most severe manifestation, patients have committed suicide and homicide (Van Putten and Marder, 1987). In the ED, akathisia is likely to occur under one of the following scenarios:

1. A patient is being rapidly tranquilized, and after two or three doses, appears to be worsening behaviorally.
2. A patient responds to RT and then several hours later becomes agitated, with the psychosis appearing to break through.
3. A patient who is known to comply with drug treatment has been taking medication and is brought to the hospital because of an apparent relapse.

The treatment for dystonia and akathisia is the same: benztropine (Cogentin) 2 mg or diphenhydramine (Benadryl) 50 mg IM or IV. These doses can be repeated at 5-minute intervals, up to three doses. Generally, relief occurs within 1 to 3 minutes after injection. While the response is dramatic in most patients, a few may not respond. In these cases, diazepam (Valium) 5 mg IV or IM or lorazepam (Ativan) 2 to 4 mg IV or IM may be helpful. In severely thought-disordered, agitated patients, it may be impossible to differentiate akathisia from psychotic excitement (Van Putten and Marder, 1987). Occasionally, treating the patient first for akathisia will resolve the diagnosis if the patient has a positive response to benztropine or diphenhydramine.

The issue of prophylactic treatment during RT is unresolved (Dubin et al, 1986). In the first 24 hours after RT, the occurrence of extrapyramidal symptoms appears to be low, and most patients do not need antiparkinsonian agents, yet it is clinically appropriate to use prophylactic antiparkinsonian drugs with patients who have a previous history of extrapyramidal symptoms, who are reluctant to take medication for fear of extrapyramidal symptoms, or who are paranoid and in whom extrapyramidal symptoms may lead to noncompliance. If a patient is rapidly tranquilized in the ED and then admitted to the hospital, benztropine or diphenhydramine should be ordered on a p.r.n. ("as needed") basis since dystonia or akathisia can occur *several hours* after medication is given. If a patient is discharged from the ED, they should be given several 2-mg benztropine tablets, informed of the possible extrapyramidal side effects, and told when to take the benztropine.

Of major concern to many clinicians is *neuroleptic malignant syndrome* (NMS) (see also Chapter 18). This *extremely serious,* life-threatening idiosyncratic reaction to neuroleptics causes autonomic instability with hyperthermia, hypertension, and "lead-pipe" rigidity as hallmark symptoms (Mueller,

1985). It is an ill-defined sensitivity reaction that may occur in about 1% of patients on antipsychotic medication. Variables that place patients at risk for NMS are young, chronic, male patients who are dehydrated, malnourished, neurologically impaired, and placed in poorly ventilated seclusion rooms or in restraints (Mueller, 1985). To date, there have been no reports of this syndrome occurring with RT in the ED. There has been a single case report of a gynecology patient developing NMS after an injection of haloperidol 5 mg for sedation before surgery (Konikoff et al, 1984). Another case was recently reported of a psychiatric patient who developed NMS 18 hours after receiving a total of haloperidol 45 mg over 18 hours (O'Brien, 1987). Despite these reports, concern about NMS should not deter the clinician from using an effective treatment such as RT unless the patient has a history of NMS.

Hypotension is a major concern with the use of low-potency antipsychotics such as chlorpromazine. When it occurs, treatment consists of keeping the patient supine or in the reverse Trendelenberg position, administering IV fluids for hypovolemia, and giving only noradrenergic drugs such as levarterenol or metaraminol (Bassuk, et al, 1984). Mixed α and β- or β-adrenergic agonists such as isoproterenol and epinephrine should never be used because they could further reduce blood pressure (Bassuk et al, 1984).

The risk of *tardive dyskinesia* (TD) has not been well defined in RT patients; however, since most patients who develop TD have been on antipsychotic medication for long periods of time, it does not appear that a patient is at risk from RT. *Seizures* from antipsychotic medications are rare, with only two reported seizures occurring in patients on low-potency drugs during RT (Hamid and Wertz 1973; Man and Chen, 1973). Patients in alcohol withdrawal and drug intoxication do not appear to be at higher risk for seizures when treated for extreme agitation with antipsychotic medication (Dubin et al, 1986). There are no reports of sudden death related to RT. The cardiovascular safety of antipsychotic medication has been demonstrated repeatedly, often in patients with severe, unstable cardiovascular illness (Dubin et al, 1986) Other potential side effects generally develop from long-term use and are not of concern in RT.

Physical Restraint

At times, verbal intervention and rapid tranquilization will not be sufficient, and additional personnel may be necessary. A show of force often induces compliance. Security personnel should be called in a quiet, nonthreatening manner. Patients should never be threatened with, "Either you cooperate, or we are going to call security." The security force should never be presented as a challenge to a patient's masculinity or a threat to her or his passivity. When security guards are present, it is usually sufficient to have them visible, but not threatening; it is rarely necessary to have them in the interview room. The presence of security guards conveys to the patient that his or her impulses are going to be controlled and also allays the staff members' fears. When used in this manner, security guards should be unarmed, and they should should never approach patients while carrying weapons. The risk is too great that the patient may take the weapon if a physical struggle develops.

The ultimate method of behavior control is restraints, which should be used when patients may be harmful to themselves or others, or when they remain agitated and noncompliant, and violence seems imminent. Patients should not be threatened with restraints, but when they are inevitable, maximum force should be used immediately and without belligerence (Bell and Palmer, 1981). Restraints provide a sound means for calming patients who do not respond to medication. Contrary to most clinicians' concerns, restraining a patient does not interfere with the therapeutic alliance; in the end, patients are usually grateful that they were prevented from acting destructively. The procedure for using restraints is outlined in Table 19–6. In all restraint episodes, documentation should clearly outline the behavior requiring restraint, efforts that were made to attenuate the patient's behavior before the use of restraints, the use of all medication, continuous documentation of all efforts to remove the patient from restraints, and monitoring of the patient to prevent injury (5-minute checks of extremities to ensure adequate circulation and adequate hydration and exercise of limbs when appropriate). All clinicians should review and thoroughly understand restraint guidelines (Gutheil and Tardiff, 1984).

The final decision to be made in the ED is which setting (outpatient or inpatient) is most appropriate for continued treatment. Criteria for hospitalization are summarized in Table 19–7 (Dubin and Weiss, 1991). Psychiatric consultation is almost always indicated in this situation.

Table 19–6 **Guidelines for Using Restraints**

At least four, and preferably five, persons should be used to restrain the patient.
  Leather restraints are the safest and surest type of restraints.
Explain to patients why they are going into restraints.
A staff member should always be visible and reassuring the patient while they are
  being restrained. This helps alleviate the patient's fear of helplessness.
Patients should be restrained with legs spread-eagled and one arm restrained to
  one side and the other arm restrained over the patient's head.
Restraints should be placed so that intravenous fluids can be given if necessary.
Raise the patient's head slightly in order to decrease the patient's feelings of vul-
  nerability and reduce the possibility of aspiration if the patient vomits.
The restraints should be checked every 5 minutes for safety and comfort.
After the patient is in restraints, the clinician should begin treatment using verbal
  intervention or RT. Even in restraints, most patients still take antipsychotic medication in concentrated form.
After the patient is under control, one restraint at a time should be removed at
  5-minute intervals until the patient has only two restraints on. Both of these
  remaining restraints should be removed at the same time. It is inadvisable to
  have only one limb in restraints.
Document the rationale for using restraints and the exact details of the process.

(Adapted from Dubin WR, Weiss KJ: Psychiatric emergencies. In Michels R, Cavenar JO, Brodie HK, et al, eds: Psychiatry, Vol. 2. Philadelphia, JB Lippincott, 9, 1985.)

Table 19–7 **Criteria for Hospital Admission**

The patient shows no improvement with medication and interview.
The patient improves, but remains so psychotic that they cannot care for their daily needs (i.e., work, housing, grooming, etc).
The patient poses a physical threat.
The patient is having command hallucinations.
The physician is in doubt about the severity of the condition.
The patient is toxic from drugs and/or alcohol or prescribed medication.
The patient is psychotic and has exhausted caregivers or all sources of external support.

THE SUICIDAL PATIENT

Suicide is one of the most dire consequences of mental illness and occurs in all diagnostic psychiatric categories. The annual suicide rate in the United States averages 12.5 suicides/100,000 population. The suicide rate in users of psychiatric emergency services is ten times greater than that in the general population (Hillard, 1983). ED clinicians are frequently the first to encounter patients who have either completed suicide, attempted suicide, or have suicidal ideation. Important in the evaluation and treatment of these patients is knowing the risk factors for suicide and having the skill to elicit key clinical features that differentiate the truly suicidal patient from the attention-seeker. *Never dismiss any patient as a nonrisk before a thorough evaluation is completed, even if the patient is well known to the ED staff or has a previous history of multiple attempts.*

In assessing patients, a number of risk factors have been enumerated (Dubin and Weiss, 1991). These factors are only guidelines that can help the physician judge the ultimate risk of suicide for each individual patient. One of the most important risk factors is the *lethality of attempt.* For example, someone whose gun misfires during a suicide attempt has made a much more lethal attempt than someone who swallows five aspirin. *In general, the more lethal the attempt, the greater the risk of suicide.* The concept of lethality, however, must also be based on the patient's perspective (Dubin and Weiss, 1985). For example, many patients overdose on benzodiazepines, as they believe they are fatal; others overdose on aspirin as they think a household drug must be harmless. The benzodiazepine patient may be the more suicidal of the two, but the aspirin patient is more likely to die of medical complications.

Another important indicator of suicidal risk is the *imminence of possible rescue,* that is, the less imminent the chance of rescue, the greater the risk of suicide

Epidemiological studies have identified other risk factors (Cross and Hirschfeld, 1989). Males exceed females at levels for the risk of suicide.

Generally, the suicide rates increase directly with age in the general population and in the white male population. In nonwhites, the peak occurs in the late 20s to early 30s. In white females, the peak suicide rate occurs in the 45 to 54 age range. Whites are twice as likely as nonwhites to commit suicide, though in the 25 to 34 year age group, they are equal. Rates for the widowed, divorced, or separated are higher than for those who are married, and rates are highest in Protestants, intermediate in Jews, and lowest in Catholics.

Recent studies have identified new risk factors for suicide. Patients with comorbid psychiatric illness, especially mood disorder, substance-use disorder, and antisocial disorder are at greater risk for a serious suicide attempt (Beautrais et al, 1996). In children and adolescents, psychosocial factors increase the risk of suicide beyond that attributable to psychiatric illness (Gould et al, 1996). Psychosocial risks include school problems, a family history of suicidal behavior, poor parent–child communication, and stressful life events, i.e., suspension from school, appearance in juvenile court, or breakup with a girlfriend or boyfriend. Finally, a recent study compared two groups of elderly depressed patients (Szanto et al, 1996), one group with active suicidal ideation and the other with passive suicidal ideation. Patients with passive suicidal ideation experienced as high a degree of hopelessness as patients with active suicidal ideation and had a past history of suicide attempts. Therefore, the authors concluded that the distinction between active and passive suicidal ideation should not be overdrawn and that clinicians should maintain the same degree of clinical vigilance with both active and passive suicidal ideation.

Other factors that increase the risk of suicide are the following (Dubin and Weiss, 1991):

> Unemployment
> Poor physical health
> Past suicide attempts
> Depression resistant to treatment
> Family history of suicide, especially a parent
> Psychosis
> Alcoholism/drug abuse
> Chronic, painful disease
> Sudden life changes
> Patient living alone
> Anniversary of a significant interpersonal loss

Treatment

The ED treatment of the suicidal patient is a complex problem that should generally be managed by a psychiatrist. Suicide attempts, gestures, or thoughts are always tinged with ambivalence about death, and the patient's presence in the ED may be a manifestation of part of the desire to live (Dubin and Weiss, 1991).

It is important to instill hope in the patient. Confront the patient's sense of hopelessness by helping the patient to develop a realistic, concrete approach to his or her own problems. Emphasize the patient's past successes in dealing with similar situations. Point out that the patient's negative beliefs are a result of a viewpoint that is perhaps distorted and hopeless; things are not necessarily the way they appear to be. Stress the patient's positive traits and accomplishments. Mobilize the patient's support system by asking family, spouse, parents, and friends to come to the ED; this will enhance the patient's sense of self-esteem and will increase their feeling of being loved.

Approach the suicidal patient in an objective, nonjudgmental, and concerned manner. Do not reprimand the patient for the suicide attempt. When evaluating the suicidal patient, phrase questions concerning suicide in the general context of feelings of depression and hopelessness (i.e., How bad do you feel? What do you feel the future has in store for you? If you felt this bad before, can you describe what was happening?). Question the patient specifically about the suicide plan. *It is a myth that asking about specific suicide plans and thoughts will plant the idea of suicide.* Exploring the patient's feelings can be cathartic. Encouraging patients to discuss their feelings and fantasies often dispels the mystique of suicide, and they will begin to consider other alternatives to resolve their conflict.

The central issue in the treatment of suicidal patients is educating them about other solutions to their problems by listening to the patient and providing guidance, interpretation, and education. Involving significant others when appropriate can increase the patient's feelings of emotional support and control. Using ancillary systems such as social services, job programs, welfare assistance programs, and psychiatric outpatient and inpatient programs can further enhance support. The physician can also increase the patient's feelings of support by making such statements as, "I'm going to help you by giving you medication to relax you, by making an appointment for you, by calling your family, etc." The important phrase is "I'm going to help."

Nonverbal communication (i.e., a patient who comes to the emergency room with a bag packed and expects to be admitted) frequently gives clues to the nature of suicidal intent. Patients who recently made a will or straightened out their financial affairs may not be expecting to live too long. If the patient is in treatment, the treating psychiatrist or therapist should be notified of the suicidal gesture/attempt while the patient is in the ED. Patients can often provide information that will facilitate emergency treatment.

Disposition

Table 19–8 outlines the general indications for hospitalization of suicidal patients (Dubin and Weiss, 1991; Walker, 1983). If the patient is hospitalized, he or she should be continuously observed; a staff member should accompany the patient to the bathroom. The patient should wear a gown, and ties, belts, shoelaces, or stockings should be removed.

Table 19–8 **Indications for Hospitalization of Suicidal Patients**

Psychosis
Intoxication with drugs or alcohol that cannot be evaluated and
    treated over a period of time in the emergency department
No change in mood or symptoms despite the intervention of the
    physician, family, and friends
Command hallucinations
Low availability of outpatient resources
Family exhaustion
Escalating number of suicide attempts
Uncertainty about the risk of suicide

Under no circumstances should a suicidal patient be allowed to leave the ED until an evaluation by a psychiatrist is completed. If the patient insists on leaving before such an evaluation, they should be detained under the appropriate state legal guidelines until a reasonable assessment can be made. The patient's rights are secondary to this potentially life-threatening situation.

State laws permit involuntary commitment of a person who is demonstrably suicidal and refuses voluntary hospitalization. Physicians can be held liable for professional negligence if they fail to identify the suicide risk, do not try to detain a suicidal person, or prescribe medications that are later used by the patient to attempt suicide. *Thorough documentation of the patient's history, examination, and treatment plan are the best protection against charges of negligence.*

When a patient is discharged from the ED, all efforts should be made to have friends or relatives accompany the patient home and spend at least the next 24–48 hours with him or her. *Almost without exception, a patient who presents with suicidal ideation or gestures should not be sent home alone.* Patients should be given the name and phone number of the treating ED physician and reassured that they can call at any time. Ideally, the patient should have an outpatient appointment the next day, if outpatient treatment is deemed safe. All efforts should be made to avoid giving medication to patients who are being discharged; however, when it is clinically determined that medication would be of benefit, not more than three pills should be dispensed in total. Initially, definitive drug therapy is the responsibility of the physician who will be involved in the ongoing treatment of the patient.

ACUTE ALCOHOL AND DRUG INTOXICATION AND WITHDRAWAL

Substance-abuse emergencies are a common ED problem. The treatment of substance abuse is complicated because patients often ingest multiple substances. Intoxication and withdrawal states frequently present both a medical and behavioral emergency, requiring close collaboration between the psychiatrist and other ED physicians. Since substance abuse is extensively reviewed in Chapter 10 by Dr. Swift, only highlights pertaining to the ED will be addressed here.

Assessment

Many patients are brought to the ED because of acute alcohol intoxication. Treatment for such patients begins with the initial interview, which can strongly influence the course of treatment. Interviewers should be tolerant and nonthreatening and should accept the intoxicated patient just as they accept insults and rudeness as part of the illness. Food and support will often serve to calm the patient. The availability and presence of security personnel can deter the belligerent patient from violent outbursts and will help reassure the interviewer. The patient will respond in a calmer fashion if placed in a quiet room with minimal stimulation. Intoxicated patients should be prevented from harming themselves or others; physical restraints may be needed.

A physical examination is mandatory to rule out other medical conditions that may accompany alcohol intoxication, such as bleeding, cardiac arrhythmias, pneumonitis, and head injuries. Use caution with stuporous patients. Before letting them sleep it off, rule out head injury, or make sure the patient did not overdose with other drugs.

Usually, the preferred disposition is to send patients home with support of family and friends and refer them to an alcohol program the next day. Part of the follow-up includes a referral to Alcoholics Anonymous. No ataxic patient should ever be discharged. Criteria for hospitalizing a patient withdrawing from alcohol are summarized in Table 19–9 (Greenblatt and Shader, 1977).

A frequently misdiagnosed syndrome in the ED is the Wernicke-Korsakoff syndrome, which is characterized by ophthalmoplegia, nystagmus, impaired recent memory, peripheral neuritis, and ataxia (Reuler et al, 1985). Patients require immediate intervention, as many of the neurological signs are reversible if treated in a timely fashion. Treatment usually begins in the ED with thiamine 100 mg intramuscularly, which should be continued throughout treatment. The patient should be hospitalized and withdrawn from alcohol and should receive vigorous vitamin therapy (see also Chapter 10).

Patients in delirium tremens (DTs) or alcohol withdrawal delirium are often referred to psychiatrists because of their extreme agitation and hallucinations. DTs is a serious withdrawal syndrome that occurs 3 to 4, or as late as 10, days after cessation of drinking. Mortality has been reported between 1 and 10%, with hyperthermia and peripheral vascular collapse as the usual causes of death. Symptoms of DTs are similar to those found in delirium, with waxing and waning of symptoms, visual hallucinations, disorientation, gross tremors,

Table 19–9 **Criteria for Hospitalization of a Patient Withdrawing From Alcohol**

Alcohol withdrawal delirium (delirium tremens)
Hallucinosis
Seizure in patient with no known seizure disorder
Presence of acute Wernicke's and/or Korsakoff's syndrome (alcohol amnestic disorder)
Fever over 101°F
Head trauma with a period of unconsciousness or altered sensorium
Clouding of sensorium
Presence of major medical illness (e.g., respiratory failure or infection, hepatic decompensation, pancreatitis, gastrointestinal bleeding, severe malnutrition)
Known history of delirium, psychosis, or seizures in previous untreated withdrawal episodes

[Reprinted with permission from Greenblatt DJ, Snader RI. Treatment of the alcohol withdrawal syndrome. In Snader RI (ed.): A Manual of Psychiatric Therapeutics. Boston, Little, Brown, 214, 1977]

and elevated autonomic signs. DTs is a medical emergency requiring immediate, aggressive intervention.

In a comprehensive review of inpatient management of alcohol withdrawal and DTs, Frances and Franklin (1987) note that benzodiazepines are clearly the medication of choice because of their relatively high therapeutic safety index, the option of oral, IM, or IV administration, and their anticonvulsant properties. All benzodiazepines are equally efficacious; special circumstances may favor a particular drug (Frances and Franklin, 1987). The long half-lives of chlorodiazepoxide and diazepam (24 to 36 hours) give an advantage of a smooth induction and gradual decline in blood levels so that there are fewer symptoms on discontinuation of lower dosage. Chlorodiazepoxide gives greater sedation, while diazepam has greater anticonvulsant activity, which may make it more preferable for patients with a history of seizures. In elderly patients or those with liver diseases, lorazepam or oxazepam, which have short half-lives, are preferred. Lorazepam also has the advantage of being the only benzodiazepine other than midazolam that has rapid and complete absorption following IM administration. Relative potencies are as follows: diazepam 10 mg = chlorodiazepoxide 25 mg = lorazepam 1 mg. A standard management regimen for alcohol withdrawal, as suggested by Frances and Franklin (1987), is outlined in Table 19–10.

Drug Intoxication and Withdrawal

The evaluation of patients intoxicated or withdrawing from controlled substances can pose one of the more complex problems in the ED. Frequently,

Table 19–10 **Treatment of Alcohol and Substance Intoxication and Withdrawal States**

SYMPTOM	TREATMENT
Alcohol Withdrawal States*	
	Chlorodiazepoxide 25–100 mg p.o. q.i.d. on first day; 20% decrease in dose over 5 to 7 days plus 25–50 mg p.o. q.i.d. p.r.n. for agitation, tremors, or change in vital signs; or substitute
	Lorazepam 2 mg orally q2hr for elderly patients or patients with liver disease
	Thiamine 100 mg p.o. q.i.d.
	Folic acid 1 mg p.o. q.i.d.
	Multivitamin one per day
	Magnesium sulfate 1 mg IM q6h x 2 days (if status postwithdrawal seizures)
Extreme agitation†	Lorazepam 2–4 mg IM q1h or rapid tranquilization (see Table 19–14)
Barbiturate Withdrawal	
	Pentobarbital challenge test:
	Give pentobarbital 200 mg p.o. and observe patient for 1 h. if:
	patient asleep—not barbiturate-dependent
	no effect —repeat 200 mg hourly until nystagmus or drowsiness develops
	nystagmus and/or
	drowsiness—total dosage is starting point for detoxification with 10% reduction each day, tapered over 10 days
Cocaine and Amphetamine Intoxication	
Mild-to-moderate agitation	Diazepam 10 mg orally q8h
Severe agitation	Thiothixene 20 mg concentrate or 10 mg IM
	Haloperidol 10 mg concentrate or 5 mg IM
Phencyclidine (PCP) Intoxication	
	Ammonium chloride 2.75 mEq/kg/dose in 60 ml of saline given by nasogastric tube in conjunction with ascorbic acid (2 g/500 ml IV) q6h until urine pH is below 5
Hyperactive, mild agitation, tension, anxiety, excitement	Diazepam 10–30 mg orally
	Lorazepam 3–4 mg (0.05 mg/kg) IM may be considered as an alternative in uncooperative patients

(continued)

Table 19–10 *(continued)*

SYMPTOM	TREATMENT
Phencyclidine (PCP) Intoxication (cont.)	
Severe agitation and excitement with hallucinations, delusions, bizarre behavior	Haloperidol 5–10 mg IM q 30–60 min.
Opioid Withdrawal	
	Methadone 10–20 mg orally, titrated by 10%/day
	Clonidine 0.1 mg b.i.d. or t.i.d. may be used as an adjunct to methadone or alone to decrease the hyperadrenergic symptoms
Anticholinergic Delirium	
	Use of phystostigmine has been questioned; should be used with the supervision of a medical consultant in doses of 1–4 mg IM or IV

* Frances and Franklin, 1987; Hyman and Arana, 1987.
† Rapid tranquilization in alcohol withdrawal states is for severe agitation and behavioral dyscontrol. The actual treatment of withdrawal is with a cross-tolerant medication.

patients ingest multiple medications; at other times, they may self-medicate their withdrawal, thereby presenting a confusing picture.

Drug screening can be helpful with a confusing clinical presentation, atypical signs and symptoms, or when there is a vague clinical history. Urine screening is noninvasive and the most frequently used method of drug screening. In assessing the results of drug screening, the clinician must be knowledgable as to the procedure used by the laboratory. Most clinicians assume that a "routine drug screen" detects all abused drugs; however, many laboratories use the inexpensive and relatively insensitive thin-layer chromatography (TLC) method (Vereby, 1992). Routine TLC only detects high levels of certain drugs and is not sensitive enough to detect marijuana, PCP, mescaline, LSD, MDA, MDMA, and fentanyl (Verebey, 1992). Therefore, a negative screen does not mean that the patient has not used drugs. Screens performed by enzyme immunoassay (EIA) such as the enzyme multiplied immunoassay test (EMIT), radioimmunoassay (RIA), or fluorescent polarization immunoassay (FPIA) have greater sensitivity and detect a greater range of drugs than the TLC method (Verebey, 1992).

Often, because of the patient's agitated behavior, treatment is necessary before the results of toxicology screens are available. The most common problem is extreme agitation secondary to intoxication from cocaine, amphetamines, or phencyclidine. Treatment interventions are outlined in Table 19–10 (Dubin et al, 1986). The signs and symptoms of intoxication and withdrawal with various drugs are outlined in Table 19–11 and are discussed in Chapter 10.

Table 19–11 **A Triage Approach to Drug Abuse***

	CANNABIS	COCAINE AND OTHER CNS STIMULANTS	PHENCY-CLIDINE	OPIOID WITHDRAWAL	OPIOID INTOXICATION	SEDATIVE INTOXICATION AND ALCOHOL INTOXICATION	SEDATIVE WITHDRAWAL	HALLUCI-NOGENS
Autonomic Signs								
Hypertension		O	O				O	
Hypotension						O	O	
Tachycardia		O	O				O	
Hyperthermia		O	O				O	O
Hypothermia	O				O	O		
Nausea and vomiting	O	O	O		O		O	O
Neurological Signs								
Dilated pupils		O		O				O
Pinpoint pupils					O			
Nystagmus			O			O	O	O
Hyperreflexia			O					
Hyporeflexia					O	O		
Ataxia			O			O		
Psychological Symptoms								
Hallucinations	O	O	O					O†
Delusions	O	O	O					O

* While awaiting laboratory analysis of a urine sample, a clinician can make a reasonable clinical assessment as to the drug ingested using autonomic and neurological signs and psychological symptoms. Adulterated drug samples or multiple drug ingestion will complicate the clinical picture.
† Visual.

VICTIMS OF VIOLENCE

Rape

Rape is an act of aggression and hostility in which victims are often brutalized; if ED diagnostic and treatment procedures are handled in an insensitive, disrespectful manner, a clinical "second rape" may occur (Goodstein, 1984). Evaluations are often undertaken without offering an explanation to the patient or without getting the patient's consent. Multiple questions from clinical personnel, family, and legal staff are often asked in a negative tone and may involve off-color comments by the interviewer. The legal aspects of the case are often delayed and protracted, and newspapers may publish the victim's name and address (25% of the cases). Clinical follow-up for pregnancy, venereal disease, and vaginal infections may be lengthy. This entire process psychologically prolongs the trauma.

In approaching the rape victim, it is important to realize that patients have several important psychological, medical, and legal needs. The phenomenon of the acquired immunodeficiency syndrome has cast another specter over the trauma of rape.

Evaluation and Treatment

Psychological Interventions. The victim's response may vary widely from confusion, guilt, agitation, and terror to some evidence of fear and anxiety. Some patients may display complete calm and even occasionally smile, indicating they are essentially still in a state of emotional shock. Since patients may resent the offer of psychiatric help, immediate psychiatric intervention should be reserved for complicated cases or for dealing with families; however, psychological care begins the moment the patient arrives. The patient should have immediate attention and privacy and should be asked to sign consent forms for examination and future release of medical records. *Police officers should not be present during the history and physical examination, nor should family members and friends.* However, rape patients should never be left alone, and a female should be with female victims.

Many patients tend to blame themselves for their handling of the rape encounter. Patients will need support and reassurance that whatever they did was appropriate because it helped them come out of the encounter alive. At times, patients will need to repeat the story continuously. An important task is to listen and to allow patients to share their feelings of pain, anger, and embarrassment. Patients who are unwilling to talk about the experience and their feelings even after being encouraged to do so should be respected.

Burgess and Holmstrom (1980) describe two phases of psychological reaction to a rape: disorganization and gradual reorganization. In the disorganization phase, emotions may be expressed openly (crying, shaking, inappropriate smiling) or victims may feel numb and empty and unable to express emotion. Fear and physical symptoms are prominent. The reorganization phase usually begins 2 to 3 weeks after the rape. Victims may change the locks on their doors, move to a new residence, or change their phone number. Nightmares, phobias, and hyperactivity may occur. The victim may resort to maladaptive solutions such as drugs, alcohol, or suicidal or homicidal plans. During the reorganization phase, symptoms gradually diminish and, within months to years, the victim returns to normal functioning.

Before being discharged from the ED, patients should be counseled as to the potential psychological sequelae of the rape and told where they can receive psychological help, if necessary (perhaps the name of a psychiatrist and information about Women Organized Against Rape, a local counseling center, or support groups). Patients should not be sent home alone. To provide continued emotional support, all efforts should be made to arrange for family or friends to be with the victim for at least 24 hours after they are discharged.

Medical Interventions. Hanke (1984) outlines the following steps for the treatment of the physical trauma of the rape:

1. Obtain the patient's permission to have needed physical exams done, specimens collected, photographs taken, and releases of information completed.
2. Before doing the physical exam, be sure the patient will agree to it. If patients are reluctant to allow an exam, reassure them of the need for the exam for their physical safety and legal defense.
3. Obtain specimens from the vaginal pool for the police laboratory to test. Obtain cervical and rectal cultures for gonorrhea, and obtain a serology for syphilis. (Obtain HIV testing with informed consent.)
4. *Establishing that a rape occurred is a legal decision, not a medical diagnosis.* Record the history in the patient's own words, document laboratory work, and save all clothing. Defer the diagnosis of rape.
5. To prevent pregnancy, offer a 5-day course of medroxyprogesterone or diethylstilbestrol. If the patient is taking oral contraceptives or has an intrauterine device, medication is not needed.
6. To protect the patient against venereal disease, penicillin should be given. If the patient is allergic to it, use oral tetracycline or intramuscular streptomycin.
7. Obtain medical consultation for HIV prophylaxis.

Spouse Abuse

Spouse abuse is generally wife abuse. It is rarely the presenting complaint, and many women will not volunteer information unless asked. Spouse abuse occurs in all social classes and ethnic groups, but the highest incidence is among the poor. Specific recommendations for clinical recognition of wife abuse include the following (Goodstein, 1984):

1. Consider abuse in women who present with injuries to the head, face, back, and arms. Familiar excuses for bruises and lacerations are "I walked into a door" or "I fell off a chair."
2. Suspect abuse if there are chronic injuries or a substantial delay between the time of injury and presentation for treatment.
3. Ask patients wearing sunglasses to remove them, as they may be used to hide black eyes.
4. Ask about abuse in women who come for treatment with strong themes of separation anxiety from the spouse or who have the triad of trauma, depression, and problems with children.
5. Inquire about other violence at home, especially child abuse and incest.

Emergency treatment centers around caring for any acute trauma and ensuring the immediate safety of the woman and her children. If it is not safe for them to go home, they can be referred to emergency shelters for abused women. Hospitalization is not indicated unless trauma requires it or the woman is seriously suicidal or homicidal. ED treatment is difficult because the patient will be distressed by the intensity and range of her feelings, which include loss of control, helplessness, fear, anger, shame, doubts about sanity, and ambivalence about the abuser. It is very unlikely that an abusive cycle can be broken during a single emergency visit, but the first step toward intervention in a dangerous relationship can be taken. Referral to private therapy, a mental health agency, or community service should be made from the ED. If therapy is not possible for the couple, the victim should be encouraged to seek help alone. In an excellent review of the battered-wife syndrome, Goodstein (1984) outlines in depth a variety of psychosocial interventions.

Child Abuse

There are four types of child abuse: *physical abuse, sexual abuse, neglect,* and *emotional abuse.* ED clinicians should be familiar with their state laws; most states require that reports of suspected abuse or neglect be filed immediately. Interviews with family about child abuse should be handled in a nonthreatening, supportive, empathic manner and should involve both the child and the broader family unit. Hanke (1984) suggests leading up to the question of physical abuse by obtaining more general information, such as difficulties during pregnancy, labor, or delivery, feeding or sleeping problems, and presence of colic. Other initial questions include whether the child is provocative, is always getting into trouble, has temper tantrums, or gets into fights with siblings and peers. Questions about actual abuse should aim at getting a clear picture of the parent's and child's behavior before, during, and after an episode of abuse.

Parents may become angry or defensive and deny that they have harmed the child or have done anything wrong. The task is not to blame the parents or to get them to admit to wrongdoing, but to make sense of the history and physical findings. The interview should focus on how the child's behavior leads the parents to overreact. The clinician should avoid trying to rescue the child from parents. The main focus of the interview is to convince the parents that physical abuse of the child is a family problem with which you would like to help them. When all data point to child abuse as the most likely diagnosis, or there is other evidence to reasonably suspect the diagnosis, it is wise to review the case with a social work consultant and to file a report as specified by state law.

Sexual abuse in children should be suspected in the following situations (Hanke, 1984):

1. Gynecological symptoms in prepubertal children
2. Pregnancy in a girl under 12 years old
3. Abrupt changes in behavior or school performance
4. Suicidal behavior in a preadolescent girl
5. Vague somatic complaints from the child or the mother
6. Overstimulation between father and daughter (bathing together, wrestling, excessive physical contact).

Sexual abuse is a sensitive topic. The interview should be conducted in a nonjudgmental and empathic, but fact-finding manner. The procedure for data collection is the same used in suspected child abuse. ED interventions are directed toward protecting the child and family from further abuse and engaging the family in treatment.

Elder Abuse

Research on domestic violence has focused primarily on child and spouse abuse. Until recently, neglect and abuse of elderly persons has received little attention in the medical literature. Conservatively, there are 1.1 million elderly people who are victims of moderate to severe abuse annually (Bourland, 1990). To intervene and effectively prevent cases of elder abuse, physicians must be aware that the problem exists and that detection of elder abuse requires a high index of suspicion (Jones et al, 1988).

The majority of victims of elder abuse are white, widowed women, usually older than 75 years of age, and without the sufficient income to live independently (Bourland, 1990; Jones et al, 1988). In addition, victims tend to be more dependent on the caregiver for carrying out the activities of daily living. Abused victims have significantly greater cognitive impairment and are more likely to display such problematic behaviors as incontinence, nocturnal shouting, wandering, or manifestations of paranoia (Bourland, 1990). The abuser more often is a relative and frequently lives in the same household. About 40% of abusers are spouses, and about 50% are children or grandchildren (Bourland, 1990). The caregiver is likely to be under great stress. Alcoholism, marital problems, unemployment, financial difficulties, social isolation, drug abuse, a family history of violence, or the presence of mental illness or mental retardation or dementia in the family caregiver are all risk factors for elder abuse and neglect (Bourland, 1990).

Abuse can take various forms and usually falls into one of several categories (Bourland, 1990; Jones et al, 1988). Physical abuse is an act of violence that results in bodily harm or mental distress. Such abuse can be detected by signs of physical injury, including injuries that are in various stages of healing. Common are lesions consistent with the shape of a weapon or located in areas normally covered by clothing. Injuries may occur around the mouth, face, or eyes and should raise suspicion of abuse. Alopecia and hemorrhaging at the nape of scalp are findings that strongly suggest hair pulling. Bruises, burns, and human bite marks should also arouse suspicion. Ambulation that appears to be painful or an unusual gait may be symptoms of sexual assault or other hidden injuries.

Physical neglect is the deliberate or unintentional withholding of assistance vital to the performance of activities of daily living. Physical neglect is far more common than physical injury and should be suspected in elderly patients who exhibit signs such as pallor, wasting, dehydration, and decubitus ulcers. Improper care of medical problems, untreated injuries, or poor hygiene may also indicate that no one is attending to the patient's basic needs.

Psychological abuse is repeated verbal abuse and threats of deprivation of property or services resulting in emotional suffering. The caregiver may threaten nursing home placement or withdrawal of financial support or may resort to simple name-calling. When psychological abuse occurs, there may be no physical signs of abuse; however, behavioral findings may include depression, withdrawal, anger, infantile behavior or agitation, or the expression of ambivalent feelings toward family.

In addition to a physical examination, certain studies can be helpful in detecting patients who are suspected victims of elder abuse (Jones et al, 1988). These studies include a radiological screen for fractures or evidence of physical abuse; a metabolic screening for nutritional, electrolyte, and endocrine abnormalities; and a toxicological and drug level screen to determine over- or undermedication. Hematological screening for coagulation defect is important when abnormal bleeding or bruising is documented; computed tomography may be necessary if there has been a major change in neurological status or head trauma.

The intervention when one suspects elder abuse will depend on the type of abuse present, its severity, and the caregiver's interest in improving the home environment. Clinicians must take responsibility for educating themselves about various local community, social, and health services. Unlike abused children, abused elderly persons can refuse protective services. Intervention without the caregiver's consent is protected when there is probable cause of suspected abuse and the elderly victim either consents to intervention or is incapable of giving informed consent. In such instances, the physician should contact the adult protective services division of the local service agency, if the community has one, or the local law enforcement agency. If the patient is discharged from the ED, follow-up arrangements should be made immediately with the guarantee of a home visit by a visiting nurse or social worker.

FORENSIC ISSUES: COMPETENCY AND COMMITMENT

Commitment laws vary throughout the United States, and clinicians must be familiar with the commitment laws of their state. There are two types of commitment (Hanke, 1984). In *voluntary commitment,* a patient agrees to be admitted to a psychiatric unit for hospitalization. Generally, patients are admitted to unlocked units. Criteria for release from the unit vary from state to state; some states require the patient to request discharge in writing, after which he or she may be allowed to leave or may be detained for variable periods of time. *Involuntary commitment* is undertaken when a patient is mentally ill and refuses to be admitted voluntarily for treatment. In the broadest sense of the term, most involuntary commitments are allowed when patients either pose a danger to themselves or others or demonstrate a lack of ability to care for themselves to such an extent that without intervention they would be at medical risk for death. The evidence needed to determine or predict dangerous behavior is controversial: some state laws require evidence of an imminent act, while others require that a threatened act or steps toward commission of an act be documented. Some states actually require that suicidal or homicidal acts be committed before involuntary commitment can take place. Since most states require that psychiatric treatment occur in the least restrictive setting, involuntary commitment is viewed as a treatment of last resort when other treatments or approaches have failed.

COMPETENCE

Under the law, all adults are presumed to be competent unless judged by a court to be incompetent (Dubin and Weiss, 1991); however, in a psychiatric emergency, waiting for a court to act is rarely feasible. Therefore, the patient's ability to make decisions regarding treatment and/or hospitalization is based on clinical competence. The main criteria used by clinicians to assess the patient's clinical competence are orientation to time, place, person; awareness of the psychological condition under consideration; understanding the potential benefits and risk of proposed treatment; and understanding the consequences of refusing treatment (Dubin and Weiss, 1991). A patient who is delirious, grossly psychotic, demented, or intoxicated, is probably not competent to make decisions. In such cases, consent for treatment should be obtained from family members. If the patient is dangerous, consent issues are less important because most state laws permit treatment of dangerous patients against their will. If alternative consent is not available, the clinician can, in good faith, treat a severely psychotic patient. Failure to do so could be considered negligence.

INFORMED CONSENT

There are three basic elements to informed consent: information, competence, and voluntariness (Dubin and Weiss, 1991). A patient cannot be expected to consent to or refuse treatment without having enough information to weigh the risk and benefits. The clinician is responsible for providing this information, including whatever the patient might want to know about the treatment side effects, legally known as material risk. To satisfy the legal requirement for informed consent, the clinician cannot merely recite a list of side effects. Rather, the clinician must discuss all treatment side effects that could reasonably make a difference with the patient about whether to accept or reject treatment. Furthermore, one cannot withhold treatment information for fear that the patient will refuse treatment based on the information. A useful decision tree (Groves and Vaccarino, 1987) outlines an approach for obtaining informed consent (Figure 19–1.)

Competence, as discussed above, is the ability of the patient to understand treatment information and make a decision.

Voluntariness means that the consent to treatment must be given voluntarily, that is, with free will. The concept of free will—the absence of being forced to choose—is practical rather than philosophical. To say "sign this admission paper or I will call the police" is a type of coercion that negates voluntariness. Any treatment given under conditions of a threat could be seen by a court as assault or battery.

Initial consent procedures should become an automatic part of every clinical interaction. At a minimum, there should be documentation that the proposed benefits and the potential risks of treatment were discussed with the patient. Consent should not be set aside except under conditions of manifest danger to the patient or others. Even then, when the emergency subsides, the patient usually retains the right to refuse treatment and be supplied with information about potential risks. To ensure that all patients are assessed for competence and that they are provided with sufficient information to give an informed consent, the following procedure should be followed during the initial examination (Dubin and Weiss, 1991):

1. The patient's orientation to time, place, and person should be assessed, as well as the patient's understanding of the emergency visit. Informed consent can only be given by a competent patient.
2. The patient should be informed of the clinician's role, the clinician's understanding of the clinical situation, and how the assessment for the need for treatment will be conducted.

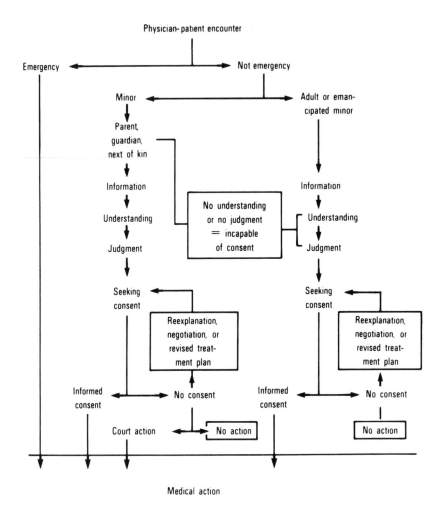

Figure 19–1. *Seeking and obtaining informed consent. (Reproduced with permission from Groves JE, Vacarino JM. Legal aspects of consultation. In: Hackett TP, Cassem NH, eds. Massachusetts General Hospital Handbook of General Hospital Psychiatry, 2nd ed, p 601. Littleton, MA: PSG, Publishing Co., 1987)*

3. The clinician should explain the clinical findings, what they mean, and what can be done to remedy the situation.
4. The patient should reiterate in her/his own words the explanation for the situation and then solicit questions or comments.
5. If possible, the treating physician should obtain written consent from the patient.
6. The consent must be witnessed.

CLINICAL PEARLS

Suspect a medical, neurological, or substance-induced mental syndrome if the patient has one of any of the following: clouded consciousness, age over 40 with no previous psychiatric history, disorientation, abnormal vital signs, visual hallucinations, or illusions.

- The most common emergent life-threatening illnesses that present as psychiatric emergencies can usually be detected by a complete blood count, glucose, serum electrolytes, blood urea nitrogen, chest radiograph, electrocardiogram, arterial blood gases, and urinary drug screen.
- The most common drug combination for rapid tranquilization is haloperidol 5 mg with 2 to 4 mg of lorazepam given intramuscularly in the same syringe.
- The target symptoms of rapid tranquilization are tension, anxiety, restlessness, and hyperactivity.
- No patient who presents suicidal should be discharged home alone.
- Head injuries, bruises, lacerations, dehydration, or broken bones should trigger suspicion of spouse abuse, elder abuse, or child abuse.
- When patients are a danger to themselves or others, informed consent can be set aside; however, it should be obtained once the emergency subsides.

ANNOTATED BIBLIOGRAPHY

Dubin WR, Weiss KJ: Handbook of Psychiatric Emergencies. Springhouse, PA, Springhouse Corporation, 1991

This handbook is comprehensive without overwhelming the reader with detail. It is designed in a very practical manner so that information is readily obtainable and usable. The format is designed to lead the reader through the process of evaluation, treatment, and disposition. Each clinical problem is discussed in the following manner: how to identify the problem, interpersonal interventions, pharmacological interventions, educational intervention, disposition, and medical/legal considerations. The key clinical points in each chapter are summarized in attractive charts and graphs.

Dubin WR, Weiss KJ, Dorn JM: Pharmacotherapy of psychiatric emergencies. J Clin Psychopharmacol 6:210–222, 1986

This article is a comprehensive review of most of the studies in the literature that have addressed drug management of psychiatric emergencies. In addition to this comprehensive review, the authors propose basic guidelines for the drug management of psychiatric emergencies. The extensive, comprehensive bibliography is useful for those who wish to read the literature on rapid tranquilization.

Tardiff KJ: Management and Treatment of the Violent Patient. Washington, DC, American Psychiatric Press, 1996

This book is a well-written, concise presentation of the principles and clinical issues involved in the management of aggressive patients. This book is easily readable, and the information is immediately applicable to most emergency department clinical situations. This book includes an excellent chapter on recognition of potentially aggressive patients, and gives a good overview of interpersonal and pharmacological interventions for managing aggressive patients.

Van Putten T, Marder SR: Behavioral toxicity of antipsychotic drugs. J Clin Psychiatry 48 (9 suppl):13–19, 1987

> This article presents an excellent discussion of the antipsychotic drug side effects of akathisia and akinesia. Of importance is the excellent discussion of akathisia, which is often misdiagnosed in the treatment of psychiatric emergencies. The discussion is clinically pertinent with excellent clinical examples. The discussion on akinesia is also comprehensive in its clinical description and clinical vignettes. This is an important article for clinicians who will be using antipsychotic drugs in their daily practice.

REFERENCES

Adams F: Neuropsychiatric evaluation and treatment of delirium in the critically ill cancer patient. Cancer Bull 36:156–160, 1984

Anderson WH: The emergency room. In Hackett TP, Cassem NH (eds): Massachusetts General Hospital Handbook of General Hospital Psychiatry, 2nd ed. Littleton, MA, PSG Publishing Co., 419–437, 1987

Barbee JG, Mancuso DM, Freed CR, et al: Alprazolam as a neuroleptic adjunct in the emergency treatment of schizophrenia. Am J Psychiatry 149:506–510, 1992

Bassuk EL, Panzarino PJ, Schoonover SC: General principles of pharmacologic management in the emergency setting. In Bassuk EL, Birk AW (eds): Emergency Psychiatry: Concepts, Methods, and Practices. New York, Plenum, 61–75, 1984

Beautrais AL, Joyce PR, Mulder RT, et al: Prevalence and comorbidity of mental disorders in persons making serious suicide attempts: a case-control study. Am J Psychiatry 153:1009–1014, 1996

Bell CC, Palmer JM: Security procedures in a psychiatric emergency service. J Natl Med Assoc 73:835–842, 1981

Bourland MD: Elder abuse: from definition to prevention. Postgrad Med 87:139–144, 1990

Burgess AW, Holmstrom LL: Rape trauma syndrome. Am J Psychiatry 137:1336–1347, 1980

Callaham M, Kassel D: Epidemiology of fatal tricyclic depressant ingestion: implications for management. Ann Emerg Med 14:1–9, 1985

Clinton JE, Sterner S, Stelmachers Z, et al: Haloperidol for sedation of disruptive emergency patients. Ann Emerg Med 16:319–322, 1987

Cross CK, Hirschfeld RMA: Epidemiology of disorders in adulthood: suicide. In Michels R et al (eds): Psychiatry, 2nd ed. Vol. 3. Philadelphia, JB Lippincott, 1–15, 1989

Dubin WR: The evaluation and management of the violent patient. Ann Emerg Med 10:481–484, 1981

Dubin WR: Assessment and management of psychiatric manifestations of organic brain disease. In Dubin WR, Hanke H, Nickens HW (eds): Clinics in Emergency Medicine: Psychiatric Emergencies. New York, Churchill Livingstone, 21–33, 1984

Dubin WR: Rapid tranquilization: antipsychotics or benzodiazepines. J Clin Psychiatry 49 (suppl):S-11, 1988

Dubin WR, Weiss KJ: Diagnosis of organic brain syndrome: an emergency department dilemma. J Emerg Med 1:393–397, 1984

Dubin WR, Weiss KJ: Psychiatric emergencies. In Michels R, Cavenar JO, Brodie HK, et al (eds): Psychiatry, Vol. 2. Philadelphia, JB Lippincott, 1–15, 1985

Dubin WR, Weiss KJ: Handbook of Psychiatric Emergencies. Springhouse, PA, Springhouse Corporation, 1991

Dubin WR, Weiss KJ, Dorn JM: Pharmacotherapy of psychiatric emergencies. J Clin Psychopharmacol 6:210–222, 1986

Dubin WR, Weiss KJ, Zeccardi J: OBS: The psychiatric imposter. JAMA 249:60–62, 1983

Dubin WR, Wilson S, Mercer C: Assaults against psychiatrists in outpatient settings. J Clin Psychiatry 49:338–345, 1988

Dudley DL, Rowlett DB, Loebel PJ: Emergency use of intravenous haloperidol. Gen Hosp Psychiatry 1:240–246, 1979

Dwyer B, Weissberg M: Treating Violent Patients. Psychiatric Times, p 11, December 1988

Frances RJ, Franklin JE: Alcohol-induced organic mental disorders. In Hales RE, Yudofsky SC (eds): Textbook of Neuropsychiatry. Washington, DC, American Psychiatric Press, 141–156, 1987

Garza-Treviño ES, Hollister LE, Overall JE, et al: Efficacy of combinations of intramuscular antipsychotics and sedative-hypnotics for control of psychotic agitation. Am J Psychiatry 146:1598–1601, 1989

Goldstein MG: Intensive care unit syndromes. In Stoudemire A, Fogel BS (eds): Principles of Medical Psychiatry. Orlando, Grune & Stratton,403–421, 1987

Goodstein RK: Situational emergencies. In Dubin WR, Hanke N, Nickens HW: Clinics in Emergency Medicine: Psychiatric Emergencies. New York, Churchill Livingston, 169–207, 1984

Goodstein RK: Common clinical problems of the elderly camouflaged by ageism and atypical presentation. Psych Ann 15:299–312, 1985

Gould MS, Fisher P, Parides M, et al: Psychosocial risk factors of child and adolescent completed suicide. Arch Gen Psychiatry 53:1155–1162, 1996

Greenblatt DJ, Shader RI: Treatment of the alcohol withdrawal syndrome. In Shader RI (ed): A Manual of Psychiatric Therapeutics. Boston, Little Brown, 211–235, 1977

Groves JE, Vaccarino JM: Legal aspects of consultation. In Hackett TP, Cassem NH (eds): Massachusetts General Hospital Handbook of General Hospital Psychiatry, 2nd ed. Littleton, MA, PSG Publishing Co., 1987

Gutheil T, Tardiff K: Indications and contraindications for seclusion and restraint. In Tardiff K (ed): The Psychiatric Uses of Seclusion and Restraints. Washington, DC, American Psychiatric Press, 17–20, 1984

Hall RCW, Popkin MK, DeVaul RA, et al: Physical illness presenting as psychiatric disease. Arch Gen Psychiatry 35:1315–1320, 1978

Hamid TA, Wertz WJ: Mesoridazine versus chlorpromazine in acute schizophrenia: a double-blind investigation. Am J Psychiatry 130:689–692, 1973

Hanke N: Handbook of Emergency Psychiatry. Lexington, MA, The Collamore Press, 1984

Hillard JR: Emergency management of the suicidal patient. In Walker JI (ed): Psychiatric Emergencies: Intervention and Resolution. Philadelphia, JB Lippincott, 101–123, 1983

Hyman SE, Arana GW: Handbook of Psychiatric Drug Therapy. Boston, Little Brown, 1987

Johnson SB, Alvarez WA, Freinhar JP: Rhabdomyolysis in retrospect: are psychiatric patients predisposed to this little-known syndrome? Int J Psychiatry Med 17:163–171, 1987

Jones J, Dougherty J, Schelble D, et al: Emergency department protocol for the diagnosis and evaluation of geriatric abuse. Ann Emerg Med 17:1006–1015, 1988

Konikoff F, Kuritzky A, Jerushalmi Y, et al: Neuroleptic malignant syndrome induced by a single injection of heloperidol (letter). Br Med J 289:1228–1229, 1984

Lavoie FW, Carter GL, Danzi DF, et al: Emergency department violence in United States teaching hospitals. Ann Emerg Med 17:1127–1233, 1988

Leeman CP: Diagnostic errors in emergency room medicine: physical illness in patients labeled "psychiatric" and vice-versa. Int J Psychiatry Med 6:533–540, 1975

Lion JR: Evaluation and Management of the Violent Patient. Springfield, IL, Charles C Thomas, 1972

Lion JR, Levenberg LB, Strange RE: Restraining the violent patient. J Psychiatr Nurs Ment Health Serv 10:9–11, 1972

Lion JR, Pasternak SA: Countertransference reactions to violent patients. Am J Psychiatry 130:207–210, 1973

Lipowski ZJ: Delirium, clouding of consciousness and confusion. J Nerv Ment Dis 145:227–255, 1967

Man PL, Chen CH: Rapid tranquilization of acutely psychotic patients with intramuscular haloperidol and chlorpromazine. Psychosomatics 14:59–63, 1973

Mason AS, Granacher RP: Clinical Handbook of Antipsychotic Drug Therapy. New York, Brunner/Mazel, 1980

Menza MA, Murray GB, Holmes VF, et al: Decreased extrapyramidal symptoms with intravenous haloperidol. J Clin Psychiatry 48:278–280, 1987

Mueller PS: Neuroleptic malignant syndrome. Psychosomatics 26:654–661, 1985

O'Brien PJ: Prevalence of neuroleptic malignant syndrome (letter). Am J Psychiatry 144:1371, 1987

Pane GA, Winiarski AM, Salness KA: Aggression directed toward emergency department staff at a University teaching hospital. Ann Emerg Med. 20:283–286, 1991

Perry S: Acute psychotic states. In Glick RT, Meyerson AT, Robbins E, et al (eds): Psychiatric Emergencies. New York, Grune & Stratton, 51–88, 1976

Reuler JB, Girard DE, Cooney TG: Wernicke's encephalopathy. N Engl J Med 16:1035–1039, 1985

Robbins E, Stern M: Assessment of psychiatric emergencies. In Glick RA, Myerson AT, Robbins E, et al (eds): Psychiatric Emergencies. New York, Grune & Stratton, 9–48, 1976

Salamon I: Violent and aggressive behavior. In Glick RA, Myerson AT, Robbins E, et al (eds): Psychiatric Emergencies. New York, Grune & Stratton, 1976

Sos J, Cassem NH: Managing postoperative agitation. Drug Ther 10:103–106, 1980

Swift RM: Alcohol and drug abuse in the medical setting. In Stoudemire A, Fogel BS (eds): Principles of Medical Psychiatry. Orlando, Grune & Stratton, 237–251, 1987

Szanto K, Reynolds CF, Frank E, et al: Suicide in elderly depressed patients. Am J Geriatr Psychiatry 4:197–207, 1996

Tardiff K, Sweillam A: Assault, suicide, and mental illness. Arch Gen Psychiatry 37:164–169, 1980

Tesar GE, Murray GB, Cassem NH: Use of high-dose intravenous haloperidol in the treatment of agitated cardiac patients. J Clin Psychopharmacol 5:344–347, 1985

Van Putten T, Marder SR: Behavorial toxicity of antipsychotic drugs. J Clin Psychiatry 48 (9 suppl):13–19, 1987

Vereby K: Diagnostic laboratory: screening for drug use. In Lowinson JH, Ruiz P, Millman RB (eds): Substance Abuse: A Comprehensive Textbook. Baltimore, Williams & Wilkins, 1992

Walker JI: Psychiatric Emergencies: Intervention and Resolution. Philadelphia, JB Lippincott, 1983

Weissberg MP: Emergency room medical clearance: an educational problem. Am J Psychiatry 136:787–790, 1979

Wells CE, Duncan GW: Neurology for Psychiatrists. Philadelphia, FA Davis, 1980

Wise M: Delirium. In Hales RE, Yudofsky SC (eds): Textbook of Neuropsychiatry. Washington, DC, American Psychiatric Press, 89–105, 1987

20 *Psychiatric Aspects of Medical Practice*

James L. Levenson

The goals of this chapter are to examine the sources and consequences of psychiatric symptoms and disorders specific to medical patients and to understand the physician's corresponding responsibilities and opportunities for treatment. This chapter is grounded in the biopsychological model of illness (see *Human Behavior: An Introduction for Medical Students,* edited by Dr. Stoudemire, and Chapters 1 and 2 of this text). Major psychiatric disorders that are often encountered in the medical setting are also discussed individually elsewhere in this book, including delirium, dementia, and other disorders with cognitive impairment (Chapter 4), personality disorders (Chapter 6), mood disorders (Chapter 7), somatoform disorders (Chapter 9), and substance abuse (Chapter 10).

This chapter focuses on special aspects of psychiatry in medical practice not discussed in depth in the earlier chapters. First, an overview is provided of *psychiatric disorders in medical patients.* Second, *psychological and emotional reactions to physical illness* are discussed, including the management of these reactions in the general medical setting. Third, the nature of *grief and mourning* and the *dying patient* are considered. Fourth, *drugs and medical disorders that can produce psychiatric symptoms* are reviewed. Finally, guidelines are provided for the evaluation of patients' *competency* and for *obtaining psychiatric consultation.*

Many aspects of this chapter reflect and expound upon topics discussed elsewhere in this volume, but are also an extension of areas discussed in the companion text to this volume, *Human Behavior: An Introduction for Medical Students* (Stoudemire, 1998). Specifically, students may wish to consult chapters in that text on psychological reactions to medical illness by Dr. Stephen Green, on the doctor–patient relationship by Dr. Susan Shelton, and on the biopsychological model in medical care by Drs. Cole and Levinson.

PSYCHIATRIC DISORDERS IN MEDICAL PATIENTS

Psychiatric disorders are common in medical patients, although the measured frequency varies depending on the criteria used. A reasonable estimate would be that 25 to 30% of medical outpatients and 40 to 50% of general medical inpatients have diagnosable psychiatric disorders (Table 20–1). The most common psychiatric syndromes are depression, anxiety, somatoform disorders, and substance abuse in medical outpatients (Von Korff et al, 1987, Spitzer et al, 1994) and disorders associated with cognitive impairment (delirium, dementia, etc.), depression, and substance abuse in medical inpatients (Wallen et al, 1987; Fulop et al, 1987). Psychiatric diagnoses are likely to be found in patients with unexplained physical symptoms (especially when multiple), and in those who are high utilizers of medical services. Most physicians underdiagnose and undertreat psychiatric disorders in the medically ill (Higgins, 1994; Saravay, 1996). This is unfortunate because (1) many patients

Table 20–1 **Prevalence (%) of Selected Psychiatric Disorders***

	COMMUNITY	PRIMARY CARE PATIENTS	MEDICAL INPATIENTS
All psychiatric disorders	15–20	25–30	40–50
Mood disorders	11	10–30	20–35
Major depression	10	5–16	5–10
Dysthymia	2.5	5–10	—
Bipolar disorder	1	1	1
Anxiety disorders	17	10–20	20–30
Panic disorder	2	3–6	—
Generalized anxiety disorder	5	5–10	—
Obsessive–compulsive disorder	1	1–3	—
Somatoform disorders	—	10–20	2–5
Alcohol abuse or dependence	10	5–20	5–20
Cognitive disorders			
Under age 65	1	—	15–20
Over age 65	5–10	15–20	30–50

* Sources include Kessler et al, 1994 and Spitzer et al, 1994.

with serious psychiatric illnesses depend on primary care physicians, not mental health professionals, for their mental health care (Regier et al, 1993); (2) without recognition and intervention, coincident psychopathology increases medical care utilization and costs (Levenson et al, 1990; Saravay and Lavin, 1994); and (3) there are effective interventions for psychiatric disorders in the medically ill (Levenson, 1992; Katon and Gonzales, 1994; Saravay, 1996).

There are a number of reasons why many patients with psychiatric disorders are seen by primary care (and nonpsychiatric specialist) physicians, rather than mental health professionals. Some are fearful of being stigmatized as mentally ill, and some prefer to confide in an already familiar trusted figure. The primary reason may be problems of access, i.e., inadequate available mental health services (especially in rural areas) or lack of knowledge regarding how to find them. Insurance barriers include less generous reimbursement for mental health care (higher cost for patient) and more restrictive "gatekeeping" by managed care.

The presence of psychiatric disorders alongside medical disorders adversely affects clinical outcomes and raises health care costs. Psychopathology in general is associated with longer length of hospital stay and more utilization of outpatient services (Levenson et al, 1990; Saravey, 1996; Spitzer et al, 1994). Depression results in higher morbidity and mortality in several medical disorders (e.g., myocardial infarction, chronic renal failure). Medically ill patients with delirium have a higher mortality rate and stay in the intensive care unit longer than those without delirium, and they are more likely to remove their own tubes and assault their caregivers. Patients with somatization are especially high users of medical care, while remaining among those least satisfied with their care. Psychopathology erodes medical outcomes and raises healthcare costs through a variety of mechanisms. Psychiatric comorbidity decreases functional capacity, amplifies somatic symptoms, decreases motivation and compliance, promotes maladaptive risk behaviors, delays seeking healthcare, and strains doctor–patient relationships.

Fortunately, there are a range of effective interventions for psychiatric disorders in the medically ill. First, improved identification has been necessary to enable effective interventions, and this been accomplished through various forms of feedback to nonpsychiatric physicians and other healthcare professionals. The presence of a consultation–liaison psychiatrist enhances identification of psychopathology in the medically ill (Katon and Gonzales, 1994). There are also many useful screening instruments for psychopathology in medical settings. Some are designed to identify general psychopathology (e.g., the General Health Questionnaire), some to make any of several diagnoses (e.g., the PRIME-MD), some to screen for specific dysfunctions (e.g., the CAGE for alcohol abuse/dependence, the Beck Depression Inventory for mood disorders, and the Mini-Mental Status for Examination for cognitive dysfunction).

Psychiatric interventions with demonstrated effectiveness in the medically ill include psychiatric medication, individual or group psychotherapy, and consultation–liaison interventions. For example, antidepressant therapy for major depression in diabetic patients improves their glycemic control. Group therapy has improved quality of life in cancer patients and may even have beneficial effects on longevity. A consultation–liaison psychiatrist's feedback to primary care physicians regarding how to manage their patients with somatization disorder better dramatically reduced their (inappropriate) utilization of healthcare resources (Smith, 1986).

COMMON PSYCHOLOGICAL REACTIONS TO MEDICAL ILLNESS AND TREATMENT

Regression and Dependency

Regression, a return to more childlike patterns of behavior and feeling, is a universal human reaction to illness. Sick patients wish to be comforted, cared for, and freed from the responsibilities of adult life. In moderation this is adaptive, as the ill patient must give up some control over their bodies and lives and accept some dependency on others. Regression is problematic when it becomes more extreme. It is difficult to care for a patient who has minimal pain tolerance, cannot tolerate being alone, is infantile, overly needy, whining, and easily upset or frustrated.

Not all patients regress in the same fashion. The varieties of regression are similar to the developmental phases of early childhood. Like young infants, some regressed patients are overdependent and seem to want "feeding" on demand, constantly pushing the nurses' call button in the hospital or, as outpatients, telephoning the physician too much. They let others make decisions, complain petulantly about their care, and avoid sharing responsibility.

Other regressed patients resemble children in the "terrible twos." They have an excessive need to control their medical care in the hospital environment and get into struggles over less critical elements of their care. They may have tantrums over getting their way and tend to be perfectionistic and intolerant of any irregularities, disarray, or tardiness.

Like many 3- to 4-year-olds, some patients who regress need to feel powerful and admired. They tend to be aggressive and narcissistic, oblivious to the needs of other patients around them. They may be sexually provocative, particularly if the illness has assaulted their sense of self-esteem and power (e.g., acute paraplegia or myocardial infarction).

These developmental descriptions of regression are illustrations that do appear as described, but also appear at milder, more easily tolerated levels. When ill, we all regress more or less along each of these lines: the need to be cared for, the need for control and order, the need for increased self-esteem. Some patients find such regression comfortable (ego-syntonic), particularly if it elicits comforting responses from those around them. Others are very uncomfortable with their regression (ego-dystonic), feeling embarrassed at the unexpected emergence of childlike feelings or actions.

Sources

As noted, moderate regression is adaptive. In the face of illness, adults hope to receive the nurturance, reassurance, and care provided by parents during childhood. Patients who regress behaviorally to an extreme often have preexisting psychopathology, particularly personality disorders. Those who use a narrow range of inflexible defenses become more helpless and regressed when serious illness overwhelms them. Patients who find regression too comfortable have usually received significant secondary gain from previous illnesses. Those who suffered serious deprivation in childhood, with emotionally or physically absent or dysfunctional parents, may experience the care of physicians and nurses as the only nurturing experiences they have ever had. As adults, they unconsciously yearn to recreate this experience and so may regress excessively when ill.

Intervention

When regression is marked, physicians and nurses become impatient and angry, especially with those patients whom they feel should not act "childishly" (e.g., patients who are health care professionals). As with other reactions to illness, physicians should avoid scolding or shaming patients (a parallel regression in the physician). Instead, the physician can explain to the patient that feeling more dependent or needy is part of an expected reaction to illness. Patients who make repeated, unreasonable, or unrealistic demands may require behavioral limit-setting. While tolerating some necessary regression, the physician takes steps to mobilize the patient physically and emotionally to participate in treatment and rehabilitation. Psychiatric consultation should be sought if regression is too great or persists too long, creating significant interference in treatment, distress for the patient, or unnecessary invalidism.

Anxiety

Anxiety occurs with the same symptoms in the medically ill as in healthy individuals, but a correct diagnosis is more difficult with coexistence of physical disease because the signs of anxiety may be misinterpreted as those of physical disease, and vice versa. Many somatic pathophysiological events share symptoms with anxiety states, such as tachycardia, diaphoresis, tremor, shortness of breath, or abdominal or chest pain. Panic attacks present with so many prominent somatic symptoms that they are routinely misdiagnosed as a wide variety of physical illnesses. On the other hand, autonomic arousal and anxious agitation in a medically ill patient may be prematurely attributed by the physician to "reactive anxiety," when they also can be signs of a pulmonary embolus or cardiac arrhythmia.

Physicians tend to become desensitized in working with seriously ill patients and may lose sight of the spectrum of normal anxiety reactions. For example, having diagnosed diabetes mellitus in an asymptomatic young adult patient, the physician may assume that a diagnosis of "just chemical diabetes" ought not to cause too much anxiety. The physician may not notice that the patient is frightened, or if the physician does notice, she or he may conclude that the patient is responding with pathological anxiety. The patient may be thinking about serious complications (amputations, blindness, and kidney failure) witnessed in relatives with the disease, leading to more anxiety than the physician expected.

Sources

There are many reasons for anxiety in the medically ill patient. Different individuals will react to the same diagnosis, prognosis, treatment, and complications with widely varying concerns. Patients may be very aware of some fears, but simultaneously affected by less conscious ones. Ideally, the physician explores concerns with the patient by inquiring about those aspects of the illness that are causing anxiety and by observing the patient's behavior.

Fear of death frequently occurs during the course of an illness, but not necessarily in proportion to the severity of disease. Many other factors may magnify or diminish this fear (e.g., previous losses, religious beliefs, personality, intractable pain, and previous experiences in the medical care system, including witnessing other patients' deaths). While for some patients with minor illness the fear of death can be overwhelming, for others, with major or even terminal illness, it may be less important than other fears.

Fear of abandonment ("separation anxiety") occurs in the medically ill as the fear of being alone. It may occur under the same circumstances that give rise to the fear of death, but here an individual is less concerned about the end of life and more concerned with the thought of being separated from loved ones. For some individuals who are immature, overly dependent, or overwhelmed, being hospitalized may itself precipitate acute separation anxiety. The patient must leave the security of home, family, and friends for the impersonal and anonymous institution of the modern hospital.

Closely related to separation anxiety is the *fear of strangers* ("stranger anxiety"). Visiting a physician when ill requires a patient to answer personal questions and to be physically examined by and put one's trust in (usually) previously unknown physicians and other members of the health care team. As patients become more acutely ill or face a terminal illness, the fear of abandonment tends to be much greater than the fear of strangers. The sick and dying very rarely wish to be left alone. Not recognizing how important they have become to their patients, residents and interns are often surprised at how anxious and depressed some patients become when it comes time for physicians to rotate to a new service each month. What has become routine for the house staff is a repetitive source of anxiety and depression for patients.

The morbidity and disability caused by physical disease produce a number of other fears. *The fear of loss of, or injury to, body parts or bodily functions* includes fear of amputations, blindness, and mutilating scars and is particularly highly charged when directed at the genitalia ("castration anxiety"). *The fear of pain* is universal, but the threshold varies greatly among individuals. Some patients experience intense *fear of loss of control.* They may also fear that they will no longer be able to manage a career, family, or other aspects of their life. Directed inwardly, individuals may be frightened by loss of control over their own bodies, including fear of incontinence or metastasis. Closely related is the *fear of dependency.* Here, it is not so much the loss of control of one's body or life that frightens the patient but having to depend on others. For some, this fear of dependency is part of a more general *fear of intimacy.* Certain individuals (particularly schizoid, avoidant, paranoid, and some compulsive personalities) are frightened of getting close to people in any setting. Physical illness is very threatening to them because they must allow physicians and nurses to penetrate the interpersonal barriers they have constructed.

Finally, some patients experience *guilty fears* ("superego anxiety") related to their anticipation that others will feel angry or disappointed at them. This is particularly common with illnesses attributable to patients' habits (smoking, diet, alcohol, etc.) and in situations in which patients have not complied with physicians' advice. Some patients may feel their illness is a punishment from God or has some special punitive significance for past "sins."

Consequences

Some degree of anxiety is adaptive during physical illness because it alerts the individual to the presence of danger and the need for action. An appropriate and tolerable amount of anxiety helps patients get medical help and adhere to physicians' recommendations. The total absence of anxiety may be maladaptive, promoting a cavalier attitude of minimizing disease and the need for treatment. In most such cases, however, the absence of anxiety is only an apparent one—the patient is often extremely anxious unconsciously and is resorting to defenses like denial (see below) in order not to be overwhelmed by the illness. Too much anxiety is also maladaptive, leading to unnecessary invalidism. Becoming paralyzed with fear of disease progression or relapse, such patients give up functioning occupationally, socially, and/or sexually. In most diseases, a modicum of anxiety is expectable and adaptive, but occasionally even a normal amount of anxiety can pose some risk. For example, immediately after an acute myocardial infarction, any anxiety-associated increases in heart rate and blood pressure may be considered dangerous and warrant treatment.

Intervention

First, the physician should explore the particular patient's fears. If the physician wrongly presumes to know why the patient is anxious without asking, then the patient is likely to feel misunderstood. Facile, nonspecific reassurance can undermine the physician–patient relationship, as the patient is likely to feel the physician is out of touch with and not really interested in what they are actually feeling.

Knowing the patient's specific fears leads the physician to appropriate therapeutic interventions. Unrealistic fears can be reduced by cognitive interventions. For example, the patient who is frightened of having intercourse after a heart attack can be reassured that it is unnecessary to give up sex. Fears of closeness can be reduced by taking extra care to respect the patient's privacy. When fears of pain, loss, or injury to body parts are not unrealistic, it is helpful for the physician to emphasize the ways in which medical care can reduce suffering and enhance functioning through rehabilitation. Physicians should tell patients about disease-specific support organizations for patients and families, which provide a continuing antidote for anxiety.

When clarifying the patient's anxieties and intervening in one of these ways is insufficient, the judicious, short-term use of benzodiazepines may be helpful (see Chapters 8 and 18); however, drug therapy for anxiety is no substitute for the reassurance and support that can be provided through the doctor–patient relationship. Antianxiety medication is best directed at new symptoms of anxiety that have been precipitated by an identifiable recent stressor (e.g., hospitalization). Drug therapy for anxiety in the medically ill should be time limited (usually 1 to 3 weeks), because tolerance and dependence may develop with long-term use. If benzodiazepines are abruptly discontinued, significant withdrawal symptoms may occur, including rebound anxiety and insomnia, agitation, psychosis, confusion, and seizures. While benzodiazepines are relatively safe in the medically ill, their most common side effect, sedation, may intensify confusion in delirium and dementia, suppress respiratory drive in severe pulmonary disease, and interfere with optimal participation by patients in their medical care. Sustained use of benzodiazepines or other sedatives will aggravate depression. Antianxiety medication prescribed during a medical hospitalization should not be automatically continued after discharge.

In deciding whether psychiatric consultation and intervention are required, it is important to distinguish normal, expectable anxiety from more serious "pathological" anxiety. Anxiety is usually a symptom of a psychiatric disorder when it remains unrealistic or out of proportion, despite the physician's clarification and reassurance, as described above. Other signs that anxiety requires psychiatric intervention are sustained disruption of sleep or gastrointestinal functions, marked autonomic hyperarousal (tachycardia, tachypnea, sweating), and panic attacks. Psychiatric consultation should also always be requested when anxiety fails to respond to low doses of benzodiazepines, is accompanied by psychosis, or renders patients unable to participate in their medical care (including those who threaten to leave against medical advice).

Depression

In addition to clinical psychiatric depressions, depressed states in the medically ill may include grief, sadness, demoralization, fatigue, exhaustion and psychomotor slowing. The same pitfalls of under- or overdiagnosis described for anxiety also occur with depression. The vegetative signs and symptoms of depression (e.g., anorexia, weight loss, weakness, constipation, insomnia) may be incorrectly attributed to a physical etiology and lead the physician to undertake unnecessary diagnostic evaluations. On the other hand, the physician must also guard against prematurely concluding that somatic symptoms are due to depression, as an occult medical disease (e.g., malignancy) may be missed. Desensitization to illness and suffering may make physicians unaware of, or impatient with and intolerant of, normal reactive depression. Physicians sometimes err in the other direction and regard a serious (and treatable) coexisting psychiatric depression as merely a "normal" response to physical illness.

Sources

Medically ill patients feel sad or depressed about many of the same issues discussed above under anxiety. When a feared event has not yet taken place, patients are anxious; when the loss or injury has already occurred, the patient becomes depressed. Thus, depression may arise secondary to loss of relationships, loss of body parts or functions, loss of control or independence, chronic pain, or guilt. Hospitalization, which results in separation of the patient from loved ones, is a potential source for depression, especially for young children and mothers of infants. Medical illness also may reawaken dormant grief and sadness when a patient recalls the parent or sibling who died from the same disease the patient has. Patients who cannot express anger, either because they have always had difficulty doing so or because they are afraid of offending those with whom they are angry (e.g., physicians), are at higher risk for depression.

Another explanation for depression in the medically ill is *learned helplessness,* a behavioral model derived from animal experiments. When repeatedly exposed to painful or other aversive stimuli while being prevented from controlling or escaping from such stimulation, many species become passive, withdrawn, and unmotivated. In patients, the course of physical illness, particularly when there are multiple relapses, relentless progression, and/or treatment failure, may produce a very similar state of helplessness, giving up, and the perception that one has no control over one's fate. Both experimentally and clinically, learned helplessness can be reduced by increasing the subject's sense of control. Physicians may unwittingly add to some patients' helplessness by not actively eliciting patients' participation and preferences in decision making about their health care.

Consequences

In the face of disease and disability, patients frequently feel discouraged, dejected, and helpless and need physicians who are able and willing to listen to such feelings. When feelings of sadness become too great and demoralization or clinical depression occurs, a number of maladaptive consequences may ensue, including poor compliance, poor nutrition and hygiene, and giving up prematurely. If severe, patients may become actively or passively suicidal (e.g., a transplant patient who deliberately misses doses of maintenance immuno-suppressive drugs). Recognizing these serious consequences helps the physician to distinguish pathological depression from normal depressive reactions, including grief (see below).

Intervention

As with the anxious patient, the first step for the physician is to listen and understand. Physicians can help patients by encouraging them to openly express sadness and grief related to illness and loss. Physicians should avoid premature or unrealistic reassurance or an overly cheerful attitude as this tends to alienate depressed patients, who feel that their physician is insensitive and either does not understand or does not want to hear about their sadness. Physicians *should* provide specific and realistic reassurance, emphasize a constructive treatment plan, and mobilize the patient's support system. For patients who seem to be experiencing learned helplessness, enabling them to have a sense of more control over their illness will be helpful. Physicians can accomplish this by encouraging patients to express preferences about their health care, by giving them more control over the hospital and nursing routines, and by emphasizing active steps patients can undertake, rather than to just passively accept what is prescribed by others for them. Patients who are demoralized before beginning treatment or who are at the start of major treatment (e.g., transplantation, amputation, dialysis, chemotherapy, colostomy) can benefit from speaking with successfully treated patients who have had the same disorder.

Normal depressive reactions to illness must be differentiated from pathological depression, which requires psychiatric consultation and intervention (antidepressants and psychotherapy). Patients experiencing normal degrees of depression retain their abilities to communicate, make decisions, and participate in their own care when encouraged to do so. Depression usually constitutes a psychiatric disorder when depressed mood, hopelessness, worthlessness, withdrawal, and vegetative symptoms (e.g., insomnia, anorexia, fatigue) are persistent *and* out of proportion to coexisting medical illness. Urgent psychiatric referral should always be obtained when the patient is thinking about suicide (see below) or has depression with psychotic symptoms. Psychiatric consultation should also be obtained if less serious depression fails to improve with the physician's support and reassurance and becomes prolonged, if antidepressant medication is needed, or if patients remain too depressed to participate in their own health care and rehabilitation. The treatment of depression is discussed from the biological standpoint in Chapters 7 and 18, and psychotherapy for depression is discussed in Chapter 17.

Assessing Suicide Risk in Medical Patients

All physicians should be able to screen patients for suicide risk in the medical setting. Chapter 19 addresses assessment of suicide in the emergency setting. Suicide is a common preventable cause of death in the medically ill, and patients frequently drop hints to their physicians about suicidal impulses or plans. Chronic illness and chronic pain are risk factors for suicide. The physician's concern should increase when other risk factors are present. These include major mood disorder, alcoholism, schizophrenia, disorders associated with impaired cognition, recent loss of a loved one, divorce, loss of a job, or a family history of suicide.

Whenever patients appear depressed or despondent, physicians should explicitly ask about suicidal feelings and plans. Physicians are sometimes reluctant because they fear that they will "put ideas into the patient's head" or offend the patient. Others simply are not sure how to ask. The great majority of patients who are experiencing suicidal thoughts are relieved to discuss them with a caring physician. The physician should ask gradually and directly, with a series of questions like: "How bad have you been feeling? Have you ever felt bad enough to not go on with life? Have you ever thought of doing something about it? What did you think of doing?" Ominous signs indicative of serious suicide risk include:

1. The motive behind the suicidal wish is entirely self-directed, with no apparent intent to influence someone else.
2. Detailed suicide plans are contemplated over an extended period of time.
3. Lethal means have been considered by and are available to the patient.
4. A suicide attempt was made in an isolated setting where the individual was unlikely to be discovered.
5. The individual is putting affairs in order, i.e., making out a will, reviewing life-insurance coverage, or giving away prized possessions.
6. Hints or direct statements are made about feeling suicidal. Spontaneous statements like "I'm going to kill myself" should never be dismissed as "just talk," but always carefully and thoroughly explored by the primary physician.

The presence of any suicidal ideation, with or without any attempt, is an indication for psychiatric consultation, and it is the physician's responsibility to ensure that it is obtained. Physicians must also guard against unwittingly providing the means for suicide: for significantly depressed patients, physicians should prescribe all medications in carefully monitored, small supplies (usually 1 week at a time).

Denial

Denial is a defense mechanism that reduces anxiety and conflict by blocking conscious awareness of thoughts, feelings, or facts that an individual cannot face. Denial is common in the medically ill, but varies in its timing, strength, and adaptive value. Some patients are aware of what is wrong with them but consciously suppress this knowledge by avoiding thinking about or discussing it. Others cope with the threat of being overwhelmed by their illness by unconsciously repressing it and thereby remain unaware of their illness. Physicians may sometimes misperceive as deniers patients whose lack of awareness stems from not having been sufficiently informed about and/or not understanding the nature of their disease. While denial of physical disease may accompany and be a symptom of a major psychiatric disorder (e.g., schizophrenia), outright denial also occurs in the absence of other significant psychopathology. Marked denial, in which the patient emphatically refuses to accept the existence or significance of obvious symptoms and signs of a disease, may be seen by the physician as an indication that the patient is "crazy," because the patient seems impervious to rational persuasion. In the absence of other evidence of major psychopathology (e.g., paranoid delusions), such denial is not often a sign of psychosis, but rather is a defense against overwhelming fear.

Denial also occurs as a direct consequence of disease of the central nervous system, commonly in dementia along with other cognitive deficits and, rarely, as an isolated finding with parietal lobe lesions (anosognosia).

Sources

Denial is a defense mechanism used in the face of intolerable anxiety or unresolved conflict. The medically ill patient, threatened with any of the fears outlined above, may resort to denial. Individuals who deny other life stresses, such as marital or occupational problems, are particularly likely to use denial in the face of clinical illness. Denial is also common in individuals who are threatened by dependency associated with illness, for whom the sick role is inconsistent with their self-image of potency and invulnerability.

To avoid fear and conflict, the patient may deny all or only part of the disease and its consequences. Some will deny that they are ill at all; others will accept the symptoms but deny the particular diagnosis (usually displacing it to a more benign organ system, e.g., interpreting angina as indigestion), the need for treatment, or the need to alter lifestyle.

Consequences

Denial is not always a pathologic defense and may serve several adaptive purposes. When denial occurs as part of the initial shock upon learning of a serious diagnosis or complication, it allows the individual sufficient time to adjust to the bad news and to avoid overwhelming, full, immediate awareness.

A lesser, continuing degree of denial helps patients function without being overly preoccupied with full consciousness of the morbidity or mortality associated with their diseases.

The adaptive value of denial may vary, depending on the nature or stage of illness. For example, myocardial infarction and sudden death may occur when denial prevents an individual with symptoms of coronary artery disease from acknowledging the symptoms and promptly seeking medical care. Those who delay going to the hospital after the acute onset of coronary symptoms have greater morbidity and mortality. Physicians seldom have an opportunity to affect denial at that stage of illness (that is, prior to seeking medical care), except by educating the general public. Moderate denial during hospitalization may be very adaptive, perhaps even reducing morbidity and mortality in some diseases (Levenson et al, 1989). If not excessive, such denial reduces anxiety, but does not prevent the patient from accepting and cooperating with medical treatment.

Denial after hospital discharge may also be helpful or harmful. Too little denial may leave the patient flooded with fears of disability and death and result in unnecessary invalidism; however, excessive denial may result in the patient's rushing back to full-time work, disregarding the rehabilitation plan, ignoring modifiable risk factors, and adopting a cavalier attitude toward medication or other treatment.

Intervention

When a patient's denial does not preclude cooperation with treatment, the physician should leave it alone. The physician does have an ethical and professional obligation to ensure that the patient has been informed about his/her own illness and treatment. Following that, if the patient accepts treatment but persists in what seems an irrationally optimistic outlook, the physician should respect the patient's need to use denial to cope. For some, the denial is fragile, and the physician must judge whether the defense should be supported and strengthened, or whether the patient would do better by giving up the denial to discuss fears and receive reassurance from the physician. The physician should not support denial by giving the patient false information, but rather by encouraging hope and optimism.

When denial is extreme, patients may refuse vital treatment or threaten to leave against medical advice. Here, the physician must try to help reduce denial, but not by directly assaulting the patient's defenses. Since such desperate denial of reality usually reflects intense underlying anxiety, trying to scare the patient into cooperating will intensify denial and the impulse to flight. A better strategy for the physician is to avoid directly challenging the patient's claims, while simultaneously reinforcing concern for the patient and maximizing the patient's sense of control. Involving family members should be considered, as they may be more successful in convincing the patient that accepting medical care is in his/her own best interests. Psychiatric consultation is very helpful in cases of extreme or persistent maladaptive denial and should always be obtained if the denial is accompanied by symptoms of a major psychiatric disorder (see also Chapters 5 and 14 in Stoudemire, 1998).

Noncompliance

Noncompliance with medical treatment is a frequent behavioral response to medical illness. It may occur in up to 90% of those receiving short-term medication regimens and probably averages about 50% in the drug treatment of patients with chronic disease (Eraker et al, 1984). Misled both by wishful thinking and by stereotypes of the noncompliant patient, physicians generally underestimate its occurrence. Noncompliance is common in patients who poorly understand their treatment, in those who are hostile to medical care, in those with major psychiatric disorders, and in those who flatly deny their illness; however, noncompliance also occurs in "ideal" patients and is not confined to any socioeconomic or ethnic group. Physicians are also misled because patients overestimate their compliance when asked. They may be embarrassed by their failure to stick to the regimen, frightened of the consequences (including fear of angering their physician), or unconscious of the problem. The physician will be more likely to get accurate information by asking in a friendly, nonjudgmental way without any threats, accusations, or anger. The physician must avoid shaming or infantilizing the patient through scolding or patronizing.

Labeling a patient as "noncompliant" implies that the physician's recommendations are entirely correct, but sometimes our instructions are unnecessary, debatable, or even wrong. Physicians must also avoid concluding noncompliance whenever there is unexplained failure of the patient to respond to the usual treatment. This may be an appropriate time to suspect noncompliance, but the physician should not reach a conclusion without evidence.

A patient is noncompliant when the patient and physician both share the belief that treatment is warranted, but the patient fails to follow through; however, physicians must remember that patients have their own value and belief systems that guide their actions. Scientific principles and the medical literature are not as compelling for most patients as they are for physicians. Religious beliefs, cultural values, and the patient's own theories of causation and treatment, which may be culture bound or idiosyncratic, all influence patient responses to physicians' recommendations.

Noncompliance is not a monolithic behavior. While some patients are globally noncompliant, others are only noncompliant with a particular aspect of treatment. Some have difficulty keeping appointments, others with taking medication. Many have difficulty complying with recommended changes in habits or lifestyle, including patterns of work and sleep, smoking, diet, and exercise. Others may follow recommendations coming from one trusted doctor (often a primary care physician), while ignoring the advice of unfamiliar consultants. Some individuals are only intermittently noncompliant (for example, only during periods of depression).

Sources

As suggested above, preexisting beliefs the patient has about diagnosis and treatment are a major source of deviation from the treatment plan. Many ethnic subcultures have their own traditional theories of disease and therapy that may influence how members take medications. Such patients tend to hide their beliefs from physicians who are not members of the same ethnic/cultural group because the patients think their beliefs will not be accepted or because they are embarrassed to acknowledge "old-fashioned," "superstitious" ideas. A similar phenomenon is seen with those who believe various "counterculture" theories of disease, like homeopathy or naturopathy, and with followers of religions that practice faith-healing. Some patients have deep and powerful beliefs about the right and wrong way to treat their illness, based on past personal or family experience. If a severe side effect has previously occurred with dire consequences or, alternatively, the patient knows someone who did well despite refusing treatment, the physician may find the patient very reluctant to accept treatment.

Noncompliance is more likely to occur when the treatment regimen is too complex (i.e., multiple drugs on different dosage schedules), expensive, inconvenient, or long term, or if it requires alteration of lifestyle. Misunderstanding or lack of knowledge may be the most common source of apparent noncompliance. Physicians widely overestimate patients' understanding of the reasons for treatment, the method and schedule prescribed, and the consequences of not following through. Physicians tend to assume that they are understood by patients, when they often are not. One study showed that "q6 hours" was correctly understood by only 36% of the patient sample (Mazzullo, 1976).

The previously described emotional and defensive reactions to illness (anxiety, depression, denial, and regression) are also major causes of noncompliance. Patients may be frightened by the treatment itself or simply avoid carrying out the treatment or habit-change because it reminds them of the feared disease. Patients who are depressed may do a poor job of following treatment recommendations because of poor concentration, low motivation, pessimism, or acting out of suicidal feelings. Individuals who need to feel strongly in control of their lives may get into struggles with physicians over compliance as a way of maintaining a sense of power over their lives and disease.

Consequences

Noncompliance results in inadequate treatment, poor follow-up, and failure to reduce risk factors, with consequent increased morbidity and mortality. Noncompliance also causes much frustration and consternation for the physician and strains the doctor–patient relationship. A vicious circle may be established in which the patient, finding that the physician becomes angry over incomplete compliance, volunteers less and less information about it. The physician in turn feels increasingly upset that the patient seems to be ignoring instructions and is not being forthright.

Intervention

Trying to scare the patient into compliance is rarely successful. Patients who are noncompliant because they are already frightened will become even more anxious and more resistant. The physician should inform patients of the consequences of not following recommendations, but preferably by emphasizing the benefits of treatment. Positive reinforcement to motivate behavior is almost always more effective than negative reinforcement or punishment, a truism well established in behavioral psychology. Scolding, shaming, or threatening seldom has a beneficial effect. It is also important to maintain a nonjudgmental, nonpunitive attitude when a patient confesses noncompliance, so that the patient will be open about deviations later in the course of treatment.

Physicians can also enhance compliance by careful attention to treatment recommendations. The regimen should be simplified by minimizing the number of drugs and the number of times per day they need to be taken. Even the most highly motivated patients will have difficulty if they must take one drug q.i.d., one t.i.d., one b.i.d., and one every other day. When a regimen remains necessarily complex, the physician should help the patient determine which aspects of treatment are most important. It is also helpful to implement the complex regimen gradually, adding one drug at a time, and to tailor dosage schedules to the patient's lifestyle. Compliance is also enhanced by incorporating the patient's preferences, which may be based on realistic factors (e.g., differing side effect profiles) or on less objective beliefs (e.g., the drug that the patient's sister did well on).

Physicians should also exercise some restraint pursuing therapeutic goals. While physicians have an ethical responsibility to maximize patients' health, therapeutic perfectionism fails to recognize that, for a particular patient, other values may counterbalance some aspects of treatment. Physicians have an ethical responsibility to respect the individual patient's autonomous wishes and not to ignore them in the pursuit of an ideal therapeutic outcome. Compromise with the patient is not only ethically justified, but is also a practical way of enhancing compliance with the most essential aspects of treatment.

Psychiatric consultation is appropriate whenever noncompliance appears linked to a major psychiatric disorder. Consultation may also be very helpful whenever physician and patient are at a standoff, although the physician should not expect the psychiatrist to compel the patient to become compliant. Instead, the psychiatrist helps arbitrate the dispute by eliciting the patient's values and motivation, recognizing psychological factors like anxiety or a personality disorder that may be interfering, and repairing misunderstandings in the patient's relationship with the primary physician (see also Cole and Levinson, in Stoudemire, 1998).

Discharges Against Medical Advice

Leaving the hospital against medical advice (AMA) might be viewed as a drastic extension of noncompliance. Approximately 1% of all general hospital discharges are AMA. Patients who leave AMA have many different motives. Some are patients whose psychological reactions to illness are so intense that they try to flee (e.g., a patient phobic about undergoing general anesthesia who leaves AMA the night before surgery). Some patients are angry, feeling mistreated, misinformed, ignored, or insulted by medical or nursing staff members. Such perceptions may conform to actual experience, may be distortions arising from a patient's disordered personality or more often may be both. Any patient who suddenly, and for no apparent reason, wishes to leave during the first few days of hospitalization may be dependent on alcohol or other substances. Agitation and irritability may reflect early withdrawal symptoms and the patient may wish to leave the hospital to gain access to the abused substance and avoid further withdrawal. Another segment of potential AMA discharges are patients who are delirious or demented. If the physician has not recognized that the patient has a neurological syndrome, the patient's attempt to leave the hospital may be misperceived as rationally motivated, when instead, it results from the patient's confusion and misperception of reality.

The direct consequence of AMA discharges is the disruption or cessation of medical care. Such discharges are rarely if ever amicable, leaving patients, physicians, and other hospital staff resentful, hurt, and indignant. Rather than approaching the widening breach in the relationship as something to be repaired, physicians and staff may respond in a legalistic and bureaucratic manner. Patients may in turn become more upset, feeling further misunderstood and not cared for.

When a patient first expresses the intention of leaving the hospital AMA, the physician should not coerce, threaten, or try to scare the patient into remaining. The first step is to try to restore the alliance by listening to the patient's grievances, giving them legitimate consideration, and trying to work out compromises. Suspected withdrawal syndromes should be appropriately treated. If the patient still wishes to leave, the physician should calmly explain the potential consequences and emphasize the benefits further hospitalization can offer.

If these initial steps do not lead to constructive negotiations, psychiatric consultation is indicated. The actual AMA form used by many hospitals should not be overvalued: while it serves an administrative purpose, it is unnecessary and is insufficient to protect against future lawsuits. The physician's ethical and legal obligation in such a situation is to ensure that the patient is making an informed choice. The patient's reasons for leaving and the physician's concerns that have been communicated to the patient should be documented in the patient's chart. If it appears that the patient is incapable of understanding the need for continued treatment due to mental illness or severe medical illness or both, this too should be documented and the possibility of involuntary medical treatment should be considered.

Doctor-Shopping

Physicians commonly encounter patients who appear to be shopping around for medical care, either visiting a succession of doctors or several simultaneously for the same complaints. Some are patients with strong psychological motivations for staying in the sick role (e.g., hypochondriacs). Others may be seeking a particular diagnosis, treatment approach, or personality style in their physician and will continue searching until they find it. A few are unconsciously gratified by frustrating and defeating the efforts of physicians (e.g., factitious disorder, a variant of which is called Munchausen's syndrome). Of course, there are also those who shop around because they have received bad medical care elsewhere and/or have an illness that has defied correct diagnosis. Certain medical and psychiatric diagnoses are notorious for eluding diagnosis, and it is not unusual for the patient to have visited many physicians before being correctly diagnosed. Panic disorder is typically misdiagnosed as various medical illnesses because of the prominent somatic symptoms; myasthenia gravis, in its early stages, is often mistaken for "stress" or depression because routine physical and laboratory examinations are normal.

On first seeing a patient who appears to have been doctor-shopping, the physician should carefully and objectively consider the chief complaint and previous evaluation and treatment. The physician should not pursue extensive diagnostic evaluation or aggressive treatment solely because of strong pressure from the patient to "do something!" There is neither an ethical nor a legal obligation to duplicate workups when they are not clinically indicated. Were the patient's evaluation and treatment elsewhere adequate? Were they optimal? What led the patient to change physicians? Some patients are shopping around not because they want more procedures, but because they are looking for a physician who will spend adequate time listening to them.

In all cases, one should temper enthusiasm with moderation. The physician should not tell the patient that "there is nothing wrong," nor should the physician be overconfident. Do not promise that you will "certainly find out what is wrong and take care of it." This is particularly important for patients who have visited several good physicians and are still frustrated. Acknowledging the limitations of medicine is often better than promising too much. Psychiatric consultation is indicated if the physician suspects underlying primary psychopathology, such as depression or panic disorder. The physician must recognize that many doctor-shoppers may refuse psychiatric consultation, particularly those who are receiving substantial secondary gain by staying in the sick role. Doctor-shopping is also discussed in the context of the somatoform disorders in Chapter 9.

NORMAL AND PATHOLOGICAL GRIEF

Normal Grief

Grief is the psychological response to loss. We are most familiar with grief following the death of a loved one, but analogous reactions follow other losses (e.g., body parts or functions, independence, affection). Grief, and the mourning process through which it is resolved, follow a typical course with recognizable manifestations (Fig. 20–1) (Brown and Stoudemire, 1983). Psychological symptoms of grief begin with an initial state of shock and disbelief, followed by painful dejection, despair, helplessness, protest, and anger. Social dysfunction occurs, with loss of interest in life's activities, social withdrawal, apathy, and inertia. While some individuals retreat into silent sadness, others are affectively very demonstrative and cry. Somatic symptoms accompanying grief

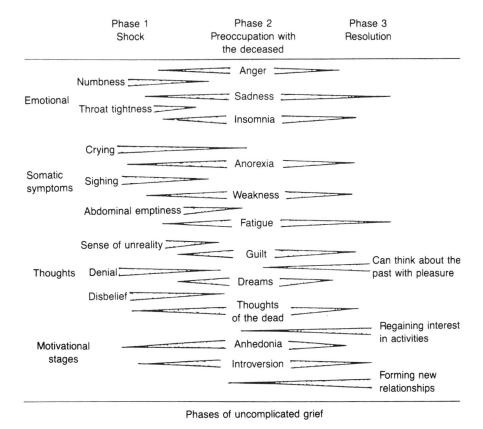

Phases of uncomplicated grief

Figure 20–1. *Phases of grief. (Reproduced with permission from Brown JT, Stoudemire A. Normal and pathological grief. JAMA 250:378, 1983)*

include insomnia; anorexia and weight loss; tightness in the throat, chest or abdomen; and fatigue.

The initial phase of shock and numbness lasts for days and is followed by a period of preoccupation with the deceased. During the day, thoughts focus on recalling the life of the deceased and on one's own relationship with the deceased. Anger, jealousy, and resentment about the lost loved one may resurface, along with guilt over unresolved conflicts and regret over missed opportunities. The living experience self-blame, wishing they had acted or felt differently in the past, ruminating over why they have been the ones to survive, and wondering if they should have done something more during the terminal illness. Sleep is delayed by these obsessive thoughts and is often interrupted by dreams about the deceased. Fleeting hallucinations may occur in which the dead seem to appear at one's bedside or in a crowd, or in which the deceased's voice calls out, usually the name of the living.

The length and intensity of the phases of shock and preoccupation are affected by the suddenness of the death. When there has been no warning, the period of shock and disbelief is prolonged and intense; when death has been long expected, much of the mourning process may occur while the loved one is still alive, leaving an anticlimactic feeling after the death. In normal grief, the intensity of symptoms gradually abates, so that by 1 month after the death, the mourner should be able to sleep, eat, and function adequately at work and at home. Crying and feelings of longing and emptiness do not disappear, but are less intrusive. By 6 to 12 months most normal life activities will have been gradually resumed. For major losses, the grieving process continues throughout life, with the reappearance of the symptoms of grief on anniversaries of the death or other significant dates (family holidays, wedding anniversaries, birthdays). "Normal" reactions demonstrate a wide range of variability, and there is not a "right way" to mourn applicable to everyone (e.g., not all must "get out" their feelings of grief in verbal form).

The type or cause of death can greatly influence the character of grief and mourning. Grief is least likely to be complicated following anticipated deaths of elderly patients with diseases without social stigma. Those mourning a victim of suicide or homicide usually have more anger, angst, religious conflicts, and guilt. Anger toward a family member or close friend who has committed suicide is particularly difficult to "metabolize" in the mourning process. Grief following a death from the human immunodeficiency virus/acquired immunodeficiency syndrome (HIV/AIDS) may be complicated by fear, shame, hopelessness, sexual conflicts, recrimination, isolation, and stigma. Disasters may result in multiple deaths and community upheaval and disorder, with the grieving process simultaneously both disrupted by social chaos and facilitated by communally shared feelings. Loss of an infant to sudden infant death syndrome (SIDS) results in especially intense shock and grief. The parents must also face questions regarding the possibility of abuse or neglect. Even though there is no abuse in most apparent cases of SIDS, the grieving parents often blame themselves for not somehow preventing the death. A neonatal death is a loss of hopes, dreams, plans, and a relationship that has already started unilaterally in the parent's mind. While usually not quite as intense, similar grief follows miscarriage, stillbirth, termination of pregnancy for severe congenital abnormality, and even at the point of prenatal diagnosis of such an abnormality.

Grief and mourning also occur following losses other than deaths. Grief follows loss of body parts (e.g., amputation, mastectomy) and loss of bodily functions (e.g., blindness, paraplegia). Caregivers for a patient with Alzheimer's disease experience grief long before the patient's death because "his personality died long before he did." Even the loss of time may produce grief, e.g., an individual who overcomes long-standing substance abuse and who then in abstinence feels the full weight of his/her wasted years.

The experience of grief changes developmentally over the life span. While young children usually do not fully comprehend death's permanence, they certainly experience grief. Sleep disturbance, developmental regression (e.g., enuresis), behavior problems, and magical thinking are common. Older children and adolescents have a fuller understanding of death; decline in school performance, strained peer relations, sleep disturbance (especially hypersomnia), and acting out are common. Young adults have full intellectual comprehension of death, but denial of death's personal relevance is typical. At this stage of life, grief over the death of an elderly relative is very different from grief over the unexpected death of a peer, the latter breaking through the defensive denial of death. For the elderly, accumulating experiences of loss and death are desensitizing; grief and mourning become more ritualized and less intense. This easing of intensity of grief is offset against increasing loneliness, as well as closer identification with the deceased—an older person thinks "that could have been me," while the younger reassure themselves "that was not me."

Distinguishing Grief from Depression

Many of the psychological, social, and vegetative symptoms of depression also occur in grief (Table 20–2). Distinguishing them is important for physicians, for the indicated interventions are quite different. As noted, in normal grief, severe symptoms should abate after several months, while in depression, symptoms persist longer. While wishes to join the deceased are normal in acute grief, frank suicidal ideation (especially with a plan) is not and suggests a major depression. Transient hallucinatory experiences occur with grief, but not more sustained psychotic symptoms (e.g., delusions of decay, nihilism, or guilt) indicative of a psychotic depression. Crying and intense feelings of sadness and loneliness occur in both grief and depression, but in grief, they occur as "pangs" interspersed with periods of more normal feeling; in depression, they are more continuous. Self-reproach is experienced in both, but not equivalently. In grief, self-blame is focused on the deceased, e.g., what one could have done differently. The depressed are primarily negative about themselves, feel-

Table 20–2 **Distinguishing Grief from Major Depression***

	GRIEF	MAJOR DEPRESSION
Time course	Severe symptoms ≥1–2 months	Longer
Suicidal ideation	Usually not present	Often present
Psychotic symptoms	Only transient visions or voice of the deceased	May have sustained depressive delusions
Emotional symptoms	Pangs interspersed with normal feelings	Continuous pervasive depressed mood
Self-blame	Related to deceased	Focused on self
Response to support and ventilation	Improvement over time	No change or worsening

* It should be noted that depressive *symptoms* are a pervasive part of the grief response and that a clear delineation of grief versus depression is not always possible.

ing worthless, guilty, and helpless, not just in regard to the deceased. Finally, grief and depression respond differently to intervention. The grieving welcome emotional support from others, congregate with them, and feel better after ventilating their feelings. Those who have major depression tend to withdraw from reassurance and feel worse when encouraged to ventilate.

Pathological Grief

In some individuals, grief and mourning do not follow the normal course. Grieving may become too intense or last too long; be absent, delayed, or distorted; or result in chronic complications. Risk factors for pathological grief in the mourner include sudden or terrible deaths, an ambivalent relationship with or excessive dependency on the deceased, traumatic losses earlier in life, social isolation, and actual or imagined responsibility for "causing" the death. Grief that is too intense or prolonged exceeds the descriptions given of normal grief and can lead to an inability to function occupationally or socially for months. *Absent or delayed grief* occurs when the feelings of loss would be too overwhelming and so are repressed and denied. Such avoidance or repression of affect tends to result in the later onset of much more prolonged and distorted grief and in a higher risk for developing a major depression, especially at later significant anniversaries. Physicians should be careful not to assume that grief is absent just because the individual is quiet and not affectively demonstrative. This may be a matter of personal or cultural style; what counts is the individual's internal experience of grief.

Grief that is still symptomatic 1 year after the death is called *chronic grief* and occurs in approximately 10% of grief reactions. Some chronic persistence of active mourning is expectable after the closest losses (child, spouse, or life partner) but is considered abnormal if the mourner is unable to resume full social and occupational functioning eventually. Risk factors for chronic grief include major unresolved conflicts with the deceased, overdependence, and dysfunctional individual personalities or families characterized by chronic hostility. Chronic grief may evolve into a chronic depression; the boundary between them is not sharp.

Anticipatory grief is grief experienced in anticipation of a death, sometimes long before the terminal phase of an illness. For example, an asymptomatic person who learns they are HIV positive may experience a full-blown grief reaction, with an acute sense of a foreshortened future, even though it may be years before any illness develops. Anticipatory grief is not necessarily pathological, but would be considered so when it promotes "giving up/given up" feelings or when the grief inappropriately interferes with adaptation to life, medical treatment, or planning for death.

Distorted grief occurs when any one facet of grieving becomes disproportionate in magnitude or duration. "Survival guilt" refers to the feeling that one does not deserve to have outlived the deceased and is especially common in those who have shared a traumatic experience with the deceased (e.g., same organ transplant program, airplane crash, or concentration camp). It is normal in moderation, but can become so pronounced that the survivors remain too guilty to ever return to full lives.

Some degree of identification with the deceased is also normal. Grief is partly resolved through intensification of traits shared with or admired in the deceased and the treasuring of special inherited possessions. When conscious or unconscious identification is too strong, it leads to a variety of maladaptive outcomes. The living may abdicate personal life or identity to pursue the interests of the deceased. Through a process of conversion, mourners may develop symptoms identical to those of the loved one's illness. When denial of the loss is very pronounced, there may be an attempt to maintain the deceased's room and belongings entirely unchanged.

Prolonged pathological grief results in chronic complications, including major depression, substance dependency, hypochondriasis, and increased morbidity and mortality from physical disease.

The Physician's Role

Physicians are in a critically important position to identify and help manage grief, especially if they have long-established relationships with patients and their families. During the acute phase of shock following a death, the physician can help the family accept the reality of the loss and provide a calm and reassuring presence that facilitates both the release of emotion and the planning necessary by those grieving. The physician must sit down, not stand, when talking with anyone experiencing acute grief; otherwise, the physician will be perceived as too busy or uncomfortable or eager to leave. Patients frequently seek out their personal physicians when they are acutely suffering from grief and often focus on the somatic manifestations. The physician can explain the normal symptoms and process of grief and mourning and reassure patients that they are not "losing their minds" (a common fear, especially if vivid nightmares or fleeting hallucinatory phenomena have been experienced). Family members who wish should be allowed (but never pressured) to see the body of the deceased in the hospital after the physician prepares them for any distortion of appearance due to the fatal disease, accident, or treatment.

The physician's role in the management of grief has expanded in importance in recent years. The physician should address resuscitation status, advance directives, and related treatment issues with patients who are competent and with their families when the patients no longer are. Besides the medical, ethical, and legal reasons for doing so, there are psychological benefits in making patients and families feel heard, respected, and able to contribute to terminal care. Discussion regarding the patient's wishes, e.g., organ donation, is another vital responsibility of physicians that may provide a source of hope and meaning in the face of senselessness and despair.

Physicians should resist the temptation to sedate the individual suffering from acute grief, since this tends to delay and prolong the mourning process. Antidepressants should not be prescribed for acute grief, but rather reserved for a possible subsequent major depression. If insomnia is severe and not spontaneously improving after several days, a brief course of a benzodiazepine hypnotic may be prescribed, but extended use will be more harmful than beneficial.

THE DYING PATIENT

Helping dying patients is a major responsibility of the physician. Elizabeth Kubler-Ross drew professional attention to this long-neglected subject 20 years ago and described a model of five sequential stages that characterize the typical response to impending death: denial, anger, bargaining, depression, and acceptance (Kubler-Ross, 1969). As we have learned more, there does not appear to be a unique, correct, or necessarily sequential order to this process. Individual patients will experience each of these reactions (and others) in varying degrees, combinations, and sequences. How a patient copes with the knowledge that she or he has a fatal illness generally reflects the style used to cope with other life stresses. A compulsive patient may become obsessed with statistical prognostic information, while a histrionic one exhibits dramatic emotional outbursts. Usual coping styles may become exaggerated or markedly change. Some variability in patients' psychological responses to dying derives from the nature of the illness (e.g., acute versus chronic, occult versus easily visible) and beliefs about the illness (e.g., viewing the illness as a punishment).

Cultural and religious background profoundly influence how patients respond when they learn they are dying. Knowing this background is important for the physician, but it can also be misleading, as the prospect of death may produce abrupt changes in the patient: an agnostic may become deeply religious; a lifelong skeptic of medicine may become obsessed with medical progress; patients who have been very distant from their families may seek to reunite; and those who have been close may begin to withdraw from their relationships in anticipation of ultimate separation. Most patients take comfort through some form of sustaining hope, including hopes for miraculous cures, new medical discoveries, the resolution of personal conflicts or alienated relationships before death, leaving a legacy, or something as simple as enough improvement to leave the hospital briefly and walk in the garden.

Physicians' Reactions to the Dying Patient

Physicians' reactions are also important in the management and support of the dying patient. Many physicians, as do most people, have an aversion to death. The dying patient may make the physician feel like a failure, since treatment has been ineffective and it appears that there is nothing more to offer the patient. The physician's feeling of failure is especially likely to occur with younger patients because it is harder for the physician to resort to fatalistic rationalizations (e.g., "she lived a full life" or "he died due to the inevitable progression of old age"). Even experienced physicians feel sad if the dying patient has become well known to them. Sadness in the physician is also likely if the physician is reminded of a personal loss in his or her own life. Sadness, helplessness, and a feeling of failure in the physician may interfere with optimal care in a number of ways. The physician may avoid the patient spend little or no time with them while on rounds, and rationalize this behavior as not wanting to disturb the patient. Avoidance is particularly unfortunate because most patients have a fear of dying alone and because the physician is less available to provide specific comfort-care measures. The secure belief that the physician's attention will continue unceasingly until death is a benefit to patients often underestimated by physicians. Support through human contact often is most meaningful and invaluable to the patient precisely when technological treatment options have been exhausted.

Some physicians take an overly cheerful approach in an effort to instill hope. When cheerfulness is excessive, it alienates patients, who contrast their fate with that of the seemingly happy physician, and creates a gulf between them. Believing that they ought to be truthful, some physicians are overly blunt and announce to the patient, "Nothing more can be done; we have done everything we can think of." This message robs patients of hope. It is possible to be truthful without being so disheartening. Needlessly prolonging death, some physicians have difficulty accepting that further treatment is useless and resort to excessive heroics. Finally, many well-meaning physicians, sensing a patient's need to talk about dying, may prematurely refer the patient to a psychiatrist, social worker, or chaplain. At best, the patient will take the referral as a sign that the physician is uncomfortable discussing these issues; at worst, the patient may worry that the physician thinks there is something wrong with how the patient is reacting or that the feelings are too unimportant for the physician's attention. Most patients prefer talking about death and dying directly with their primary physician.

Intervention

How to inform a patient of a grave diagnosis and prognosis is part of the art of medicine. Taking into account the patient's intellectual abilities and emotional and physical state, the physician must gauge how much to tell and at what rate. The questions the patient asks are an indicator of whether the physician is going too fast or too slow. Important information may require repetition within the same session and over several visits. Shock induced by the initial pronouncement may interfere with the patient's registering other needed information. Physicians must balance their truthtelling obligation with some respect for different patients who want to know more or less about the details of a grave prognosis.

Another important responsibility for the physician is to discuss the patient's preferences and values regarding future treatment decisions, particularly those involving the termination of aggressive treatment. This should not be raised too quickly after the patient has been first told of a serious diagnosis, both because the patient may be too overwhelmed to participate meaningfully in such a discussion and because the patient may misinterpret the discussion as a sign that the physician is ready to give up; however, physicians tend to err in delaying such discussion until the patient's illness has progressed to the point when it can no longer be avoided. Unfortunately, by then, the patient may no longer be competent and the physician will feel less certain that the patient's preferences have not been unduly influenced by physical discomfort, family pressure, or financial worries. This problem is avoidable by initiating discussion before the final stages of illness. Physicians should also allow the patient the opportunity to include family members in the discussion.

In the face of serious illness, physicians feel better "doing something." Anticipating a patient's inevitable and impending death, physicians should focus on what can be done. Quality of life during the process of dying can be significantly improved through adequate pain control (which is often underprescribed), attention to bowel and bladder function, hygiene, sleep, and other comfort measures. For some patients, comfort is the primary goal, while other patients may be willing to sacrifice some comfort for greater mobility and the chance to even briefly leave the hospital. Physicians should encourage patients to make wills and put their affairs in order with legal assistance, help mobilize the patient's support system, and discuss options like hospice care.

Patients with grave illnesses often have questions about what to tell their children. Most children do not develop a firm concept of the finality of death until between ages 8 and 11, but children, like adults, vary in the intellectual and emotional maturity necessary to comprehend death. Patients and families should be urged to gauge their answers by the nature of their children's questions. Questions spontaneously asked by a child of any age should be answered truthfully in language the child can understand. The adult should indicate his or her continued availability for further questions and comfort. Should children attend funerals? If the child wishes to go, this wish should be respected and supported. If the child appears very reluctant or refuses, this, too, should be respected. When in doubt, it is probably helpful for the child to attend, as funerals are rituals that have evolved in our cultures to help us collectively deal with death.

As noted, psychiatric consultation should not be sought prematurely as a substitute for direct conversation between patient and physician. Psychiatric consultation is indicated for the terminally ill patient when suicidal ideation appears, for assistance with management of intractable pain, and for the emergence of major unresolved emotional conflict.

The fundamental fear of dying patients is usually not the fear of death itself, but the fear of being abandoned or deserted by others, including their physician, and dying alone. Perhaps the most reassuring comment that a physician can make to a patient with a terminal illness is, "No matter what happens or how bad things get, we're in this thing together, and I'll stick by you no matter what happens. You don't have to worry about suffering alone. As long as you are ill, I'll be here to help you with whatever comes, including making sure you'll be comfortable and kept out of pain." Issues related to death and dying are discussed in the companion text to this volume on human behavior, particularly in the chapter on adult development by Drs. Wolman and Thompson (in Stoudemire, 1998).

DRUGS THAT CAUSE PSYCHIATRIC SYMPTOMS

Drugs used to treat medical illnesses frequently cause psychiatric symptoms or side effects through a variety of mechanisms. Most drugs at toxic levels produce signs of central nervous system disturbance, including drugs that are normally benign with few side effects, such as aspirin. Certain medications frequently cause psychiatric symptoms even at therapeutic drug levels (e.g., L-dopa). Symptoms may occur via a direct effect of the drug on the central nervous system (e.g., lidocaine), a metabolic effect of the drug (e.g., hypokalemia caused by thiazide diuretics), or drug interactions. Some drugs may precipitate an underlying psychiatric disorder in vulnerable patients, such as reserpine-induced depression or sympathomimetic-induced panic attacks. Physicians must be vigilant for the possibility of psychiatric side effects induced by medications the patient may be taking without the doctor's knowledge, particularly if the patient is doing this surreptitiously and is embarrassed to tell the physician (e.g., the excessive use of over-the-counter nasal decongestants or inhalers).

Table 20–3 shows many of the drugs that can cause psychiatric symptoms. Most of these can cause a wide variety of symptoms, influenced by the patient's premorbid psychopathology and personality style, metabolic status, and pre-existing central nervous system pathology. When the effect on the brain is mild to moderate, most of the listed drugs can cause anxiety, depression, sleep disorders (insomnia, hypersomnia, nightmares), and sexual dysfunction. When severe, psychosis (schizophreniform, manic, or depressive), delirium, or dementia may occur, sometimes resulting in seizures and coma (see also Chapter 4). A recent text covers all the known psychiatric side effects of prescription and over-the-counter medications (Brown and Stoudemire, 1998).

MEDICAL DISORDERS THAT CAUSE PSYCHIATRIC SYMPTOMS

Many medical disorders produce psychiatric symptoms as part of their pathophysiology, sometimes as the initial presentation of the disease. Here we focus on psychiatric symptoms that are a consequence of the disease process itself through either direct effects on the central nervous system or derangement in metabolism or homeostatic regulatory mechanisms. Some diseases cause a wide range of different neuropsychiatric symptoms in different individuals, largely determined by which areas of the brain have been affected by the disease. These disorders are listed in Table 20–4. Table 20–5 shows diseases that commonly cause specific psychiatric symptoms. While most of these also can cause a range of symptoms, they typically present with the indicated psychiatric syndromes. Symptoms and signs in other organ systems serve as clinical clues to help the clinician suspect a particular cause, but psychiatric symptoms may precede the onset of other clinical signs in most disorders.

When a patient presents with unexplained psychiatric symptoms, certain clues should heighten the physician's suspicions that an underlying medical disorder may be responsible. An underlying medical disorder as etiology should be considered whenever: (1) psychiatric symptoms increase and decrease in concert with prominent physical symptoms; (2) when the "vegetative symptoms" of an apparent psychiatric disorder are disproportionately greater than the psychological symptoms (e.g., a patient with a 50-lb. weight loss and only mild depressive ideation is unlikely to have major affective disorder as the explanation for the weight loss); (3) when significant cognitive abnormalities are present in the mental status examination, particularly changes in level of consciousness, attention, and memory; (4) when the age of onset or course of psychiatric illness is very atypical (e.g., new onset of "schizophrenia" in an 85-year-old patient); and (5) whenever there are objective findings of central nervous system disease (e.g., pathological reflexes, abnormal electroencephalogram, computed tomography scan, or magnetic resonance image, or changes in spinal fluid). As with drug-induced psychiatric symptoms, medical illnesses may cause mild-to-moderate changes in affect, personality, sleep, or sexual function, which can be easily missed or misattributed. When severe, medical illnesses produce psy-

Table 20–3 **Drugs That May Cause Psychiatric Symptoms***

Depression

Antihypertensives (especially reserpine, methyldopa, beta-blockers, clonidine)*
Amphotericin B
Corticosteroids*
Anticonvulsants
Sedative–hypnotics*
Oral contraceptives
Antipsychotics
Metoclopramide
Interferon-alpha*

Indomethacin (and other non-steroidal anti-inflammatory drugs)
Antineoplastic drugs
  Procarbazine
  Tamoxifen
  Vinblastine
  Asparaginase
Ethionamide
Acetazolamide

Mania

Corticosteroids*
Sympathomimetics (esp. non-prescription decongestants and bronchodilators)
Isoniazid
Tramadol

Dopamine agonists
Antidepressants
Zidovudine (AZT)

Stimulants

Anxiety

Sympathomimetics*
Theophylline*
Caffeine*

Stimulants
Antidepressants (SSRIs)
Sedative–hypnotics (withdrawal)*

Psychosis (Hallucinations or Delusions)

Anticholinergics*
Antihistamines (cimetidine, ranitidine, diphenhydramine, etc)
Antiarrhythmics (esp. lidocaine, tocainide, mexiletine, quinidine)
Dopamine agonists*
  L-dopa
  Bromocriptine
  Amantadine
Corticosteroids*
Digitalis
Antidepressants
Opiates
  Meperidine
  Pentazocine
Antimalarials
Anticonvulsants
Beta-blockers

Antiviral drugs
  Acyclovir
  Vidarabine
  Interferon
  Zidovudine (AZT)
  Podophyllin
Antineoplastic drugs
  Asparaginase
  Methotrexate
  Vincristine
  Cytarabine
  Fluorouracil
Disulfiram
Sympathomimetics
Metrizamide
Methysergide
Baclofen
Cycloserine
Cyclosporine
Interleukin (IL-Z)

* Denotes especially "high-risk" drugs for causing symptoms in question.

Table 20–4 **Medical Disorders Causing a Wide Range of Psychiatric Symptoms**

Traumatic brain injury
Stroke
Systemic lupus erythematosus and other forms of cerebral vasculitis
Brain tumor (primary or metastatic)
Encephalitis (acute or chronic)
AIDS/HIV encephalopathy
Infectious endocarditis

chosis, delirium, or dementia, which are less likely to be missed but whose nature or causation may still be misinterpreted (see Chapters 1 and 4).

The physician should also keep in mind those diseases that do not produce psychopathology per se but may be mistaken for it. Recurrent pulmonary emboli may be misdiagnosed as anxiety or panic attacks because of episodic autonomic arousal. Early myasthenia gravis is often mistaken for depression or a conversion disorder because the clinician finds a normal examination in a patient who complains of weakness and fatigue whenever they work too hard. Multiple sclerosis may be misdiagnosed as conversion disorder because the pattern of the patient's symptoms seems changing and inconsistent and does not conform to simple neuroanatomical localization.

COMPETENCY

When a patient refuses diagnostic procedures or treatment or seems unable to make medical care decisions, physicians often question whether the patient is competent. Strictly speaking, "competency" is a legal concept and is determined by the court; physicians, including psychiatrists, render opinions about competency, based on their clinical assessment of the patient's mental status. What physicians must decide is whether the patient appears to have the capacity to participate in rational and reasoned decision making (President's Commission, 1982). Are limited intelligence, a psychiatric disorder, or a medical disease preventing the patient from thinking rationally about medical care? Most determinations of this kind are made by clinicians at bedside; frequency and the need for timely resolution make it impractical to seek judicial action on every case.

While psychiatric consultation is often requested to help determine if the patient is competent, primary physicians can determine competency themselves in most cases. Does the physician actually suspect impaired mental capacity, or do the patient and the physician simply disagree? The test of whether a patient possesses the capacity to participate in health care decision making is a simple, functional one: does the patient understand the particular decision at hand? First, the physician must ensure that the patient has been fully informed. Then, the following questions should be asked, taking into account that patients will answer in their own language, not in "medically correct" terms: (1) Can the patient describe what the physician believes is wrong with the patient? (2) Does the patient understand the diagnostic procedure or treatment proposed and the reasons for it? (3) Does the patient understand any alternative procedures or treatments that may exist? and (4) Does the patient understand the risks and benefits of each course of action, including the consequences of refusing treatment? If the answer is "yes" to all of these questions, the patient possesses the capacity for decision making. To be viewed as competent, the patient does not necessarily have to have a good reason for disagreeing with the physician, but the patient must be able to demonstrate an understanding of the physician's advised plan.

Since this clinical competency test focuses on particular proposed treatments, it is possible that some patients may be judged able to make some but not all decisions, or that their ability varies over time. Others may be so mentally impaired that it is obvious that they entirely lack decision-making capacity.

Some patients will give answers that demonstrate their ability to understand what the physician has said, but they will persist on an irrational course, based on psychotic delusional thinking. This, too, may be grounds for a determination of incompetence and indicates the need for psychiatric consultation. Psychiatric consultation is also helpful if the primary physician remains unsure of the patient's level of understanding, if there is disagreement among the physicians caring for the patient, or if legal action is considered likely.

If the physician determines that the patient does not possess sufficient capacity, a surrogate decision-maker will be required. If the surrogate is a family member as it is in most circumstances, this does not necessitate going to court. A court-appointed guardian should be sought when the family members remain intractably divided over health care decisions, when they appear unable to act in the best interests of the impaired patient, or when the treatment is controversial (see also Fig. 19–1 in Chapter 19).

PSYCHIATRIC CONSULTATION

From the other parts of this chapter, it is evident that there are many reasons for a physician to seek psychiatric consultation. Unfortunately, some physicians are reluctant to do so or do not ask for psychiatric assistance very effectively. Some physicians fear that seeing a psychiatrist will upset the patient, who may feel that the physician thinks he or she is crazy. Other physicians approach patients with the belief that all medical pathology should be absolutely ruled out before considering psychological explanations for symptoms. It is certainly reasonable to avoid prematurely concluding that a patient's symptoms are psychogenic, but the relentless pursuit of a physical etiology is

Table 20-5 **Psychiatric Presentation of Selected Medical Disorders**

	PSYCHIATRIC PRESENTATION	CLINICAL CLUES	SCREENING DIAGNOSTIC EVALUATION*
Endocrine Disorders			
Hypothyroidism	Retarded depression (± psychosis)	Weight gain, fatigue, cold intolerance, hoarseness, bradycardia, constipation, hair loss	Free T_4, TSH
Hyperthyroidism	Anxiety, panic attacks, agitated depression (often retarded in the elderly)	Tremor, tachycardia, heat intolerance	Free T_4, T_3-RIA, TSH
Hyperadrenalism (Cushing's)	Depression or mania	Hypertension, diabetes, hirsutism, moon facies, weight gain	Dexamethasone suppression test
Hypoadrenalism (Addison's)	Depression	Postural hypotension, nausea, vomiting, skin pigmentation, weight loss	Cosyntropin stimulation test
Pheochromocytoma	Panic attacks, anxiety	Labile hypertension, headache, sweating, nausea, palpitations	24-Hour urinary catecholamines and metanephrines
Metabolic Disorders			
Hypoglycemia	Anxiety, panic attacks	Sweating, tachycardia, headache	Blood glucose during symptoms
Hypokalemia	Depression	Weakness, ECG changes	Serum K^+
Hyponatremia	Depression, psychosis	Weakness, nausea, vomiting, seizures	Serum Na^+
Hypercalcemia	Retarded depression	Weakness, nausea, confusion	Serum Ca^{2+}
Hypocalcemia	Anxiety	Tremor, tetany, paresthesias	Serum CA^{2+}
Hypermagnesemia	Retarded depression	Hypotension, nausea, vomiting	Serum Mg^{2+}
Hypomagnesemia	Anxiety, psychosis	Tremor, tetany	Serum MG^{2+}, Ca^{2+}
Hypophosphatemia	Depression	Weakness, paresthesias	Serum PO_4^{2-}
Vitamin B_{12} deficiency	Psychosis, dementia	Megaloblastic anemia, peripheral neuropathy, myelopathy (but may occur in absence of these)	Serum B_{12}
Hepatic encephalopathy	Confusion, psychosis	Asterixis, jaundice	Liver function tests, serum NH_3

Uremia	Depression, dementia	Anemia, nausea, edema	BUN, creatinine
Porphyria (acute intermittent)	Psychosis	Episodic abdominal pain with nausea and vomiting, constipation, neuropathy	Blood and urine porphyrin screen
Lead poisoning	Personality change, depression	Colic, anemia, peripheral neuropathy	Serum FEP
Neurological Disorders			
Normal pressure hydrocephalus	Depression, dementia	Gait apraxia, urinary incontinence	CT or MRI scan
Multiple sclerosis	Depression	Multiple intermittent neurological symptoms over time	Neurological evaluation, MRI, CSF (oligoclonal bands)
Huntington's disease	Personality disorder, psychosis	Movement disorder, family history	Neurological exam
Parkinsonism	Depression, dementia	Bradykinesia, tremor, rigidity	Neurological exam
Wilson's disease	Psychosis	Movement disorder, liver disease, Kayser-Fleischer rings	Slit-lamp exam, serum ceruloplasmin
Neoplastic Disorders			
Pancreatic cancer	Depression	Weight loss, abdominal pain	Abdominal CT or MRI scan
Paraneoplastic limbic encephalitis (usually associated with small-cell carcinoma of the lung)	Psychosis, dementia	Seizures, fluctuating course	EEG, lumbar puncture
Infectious Diseases			
Infectious mononucleosis	Depression	Lymphadenopathy, hepatosplenomegaly, sore throat, malaise	CBC, Monospot
Viral hepatitis	Depression	Anorexia, fatigue, jaundice, malaise, hepatomegaly	Liver function tests, serologies
Encephalitis	Psychosis	Fever, seizures	EEG, lumbar puncture
Whipple's disease	Depression, dementia	Diarrhea, weight loss, arthritis, lymphadenopathy	Malabsorption studies, small bowel biopsy

* TSH, thyroid-stimulating hormone; RIA, radioimmunoassay; BUN, blood urea nitrogen; FEP, free erythrocyte protoporphyrin; CT, computed tomography; MRI, magnetic resonance imaging; CSF, cerebrospinal fluid; EEG, electroencephalogram; CBC, complete blood count.

costly, exposes patients to unnecessary risks, reinforces a disregard for psychological factors by the patient, and neglects treatable psychiatric disorders.

Some physicians hesitate to obtain psychiatric consultation simply because they are unsure how to tell the patient. It is a mistake to ask for consultation without telling the patient, since this action makes it more likely that the patient will misunderstand the physician's intentions. If not told, patients may well wonder if their physician thinks them mentally ill or may believe that their physician is frustrated and wants to transfer their care to someone else. Several studies have demonstrated that when patients are informed by physicians of the purpose of a psychiatric consultation, the great majority have little difficulty accepting it.

The physician should explain that the psychiatrist is a consultant who will advise the patient and the physician and that the physician is still the primary doctor committed to helping the patient recover. The specific purpose for the consultation should be explained in terms the patient can understand (e.g., "Besides having heart failure, your spirits seem very low. I'd like to have our psychiatrist see if there is anything we can do to help you feel better emotionally, as well as physically").

The physician should always formulate a specific question or problem for which the consultant's help is desired (Table 20–6). If the physician is unsure whether psychiatric consultation would be helpful, the physician should discuss the concern with the consultant. Occasionally, the physician may anticipate problems in persuading the patient to see a psychiatrist. Here, too, discussion with the consultant ahead of time will be helpful. With careful explanation and a respectful approach, a skilled psychiatric consultant can persuade the great majority of patients who initially refuse consultation to agree to be interviewed.

Table 20–6 **Common Indications for Psychiatric Consultation**

Suicidal ideation or behavior
Verbal threats or dangerous behavior
Psychosis (hallucinations, delusions, thought disorder)
Need for psychiatric medication or change of dose
Psychiatric disorder in need of treatment
Psychiatric disorder complicating medical illness
Psychiatric symptoms thought to be caused by medical illness
Psychiatric symptoms thought to be due to medication
Competency evaluations
Noncompliance, AMA* discharges
Significant problems in doctor–patient relationship
  (or nurse-patient relationship)
Evaluation of cognitive dysfunction (delirium, dementia)

* AMA, against medical advice.

When the patient has unexplained symptoms, physicians should avoid "either/ or" thinking (that is, considering the symptoms as either physical or psychological). Otherwise, the physician may be misled into thinking too narrowly about causation. Physicians should never diagnose by exclusion (i.e., conclude that symptoms must be psychogenic because physical and laboratory examinations have revealed only "normal" results). A medical disease may still be present. Psychiatric diagnoses should be made on the basis of positive criteria, not solely on the absence of identifiable physical pathology. In evaluating symptoms of unclear causation, when the physician suspects the possibility of psychogenic origin, psychiatric consultation should not be delayed until the end of hospitalization. Such delays are unfortunate because they leave little time for psychiatrists to do their job, they reinforce the patient's (possibly false) belief that the symptoms are physical, they promote unnecessary diagnostic testing, and they leave the patient with the implied message that the physician is at the end of their rope and is giving up the patient to the care of a psychiatrist.

Even when symptoms clearly appear to be due to conversion, hypochondriasis, or malingering, the physician should never tell the patient, "There's nothing wrong" or "It's all in your head." Patients experience such remarks as humiliating and insulting, and consequently, the doctor–patient relationship is seriously strained. Instead, patients can be reassured that extensive diagnostic testing has not turned up any grave or malignant etiology for their illness and that it appears they have a physical symptom exacerbated by stress for which help is available.

Indications for Psychiatric Referral

While patients often bring psychiatric and psychosocial problems to their primary care physicians, some patients should be referred for primary management and treatment by psychiatrists (and/or other mental health professionals). Nonpsychiatric physicians will individually vary in expertise and desire to manage psychiatric disorders themselves, but some general rules guide who should be referred. Patients with depression who are suicidal, psychotic, or so depressed that they cannot maintain normal daily functioning should be referred to a psychiatrist, as should those who have failed to improve with standard antidepressant therapy. Depressed individuals with a personal or family history of bipolar illness should be referred to a psychiatrist for evaluation for mood-stabilizing medications. Patients with severe incapacitating anxiety disorders and anxiety disorders with a history of substance abuse should be referred to a psychiatrist. Patients with chronic phobias, obsessive–compulsive disorders, or agoraphobia should be referred to a mental health clinician with expertise in behavioral therapy. Schizophrenia, mania, and other psychoses should be managed by psychiatrists. Anorexia nervosa and bulimia require involvement of a primary care physician, psychiatrist, and psychotherapist. Dementia requires psychiatric management primarily when behavioral complications like psychosis, depression, or severe agitation develop. Abuse of tobacco and caffeine usually can be managed by primary care physicians, although referral to a substance-abuse specialist is indicated for intractable abuse despite serious medical complications. Addiction to alcohol, sedatives, or illicit drugs are best treated through referral to specialized (usually outpatient) substance-abuse treatment programs.

Severity of illness is not the only factor that may indicate the need for referral. Time constraints prevent most primary care physicians from providing more than very limited counseling. Psychological problems requiring further attention should be referred to a mental health professional. In addition, some patients are not comfortable discussing adjustment and relationship problems with their primary care physician (especially if this physician also cares for other members of the same family), so that even "minor" problems sometimes require referral to a mental health professional.

ANNOTATED BIBLIOGRAPHY

Cassem NH (ed): Massachusetts General Hospital Handbook of General Hospital Psychiatry, 3rd ed. St. Louis, Mosby Year Book, 1991

> This compact handbook provides a ready and portable reference for managing the most common psychiatric disorders encountered in general hospital patients.

Stoudemire A, Fogel BS (eds): Psychiatric Care of the Medical Patient. Second edition. New York, Oxford University Press, 1998

> This is a definitive reference source for dealing with the psychiatric problems of the medically ill. Each major subspecialty is covered in terms of biological, psychological, and sociologic factors relevant to medical illness that may affect psychiatric functioning. It contains detailed discussions of diagnostic and psychopharmacologic treatment issues in treating the medically ill patient with psychiatric disturbances.

REFERENCES

Brown JT, Stoudemire GA: Normal and pathological grief. JAMA, 250:378–382, 1983
Brown TM, Stoudemire A: Psychiatric Side Effects of Prescription and Over-the-Counter Medications. Washington, DC, American Psychiatric Press, 1998
Eraker SA, Kirscht JP, Becker MH: Understanding and improving patient compliance. Ann Intern Med 100:258–268, 1984
Fulop G, Strain JJ, Vita J, et al: Impact of psychiatric comorbidity on length of hospital stay for medical/surgical patients: a preliminary report. Am J Psychiatry 144:878–882, 1987
Higgins ES: A review of unrecognized mental illness in primary care: prevalence, natural history, and efforts to change the course. Arch Fam Med 3:908–917, 1994
Katon W, Gonzales J: A review of randomized trials of psychiatric consultation-liaison studies in primary care. Psychosomatics 35:268–278, 1994.
Kessler RC, McGonagle KA, Zhao S, et al: Lifetime and 12-month prevalence of DSM-III-R psychiatric disorders in the United States. Results from the National Comorbidity Survey. Arch Gen Psychiatry 51:8–19, 1994
Kubler-Ross E: On Death and Dying. London, Macmillan, 1969

Levenson JL: Psychosocial interventions in chronic medical illness: an overview of outcome research. Gen Hosp Psychiatry, 14S:43–49, 1992

Levenson JL, Hamer RM, Rossiter LF: Relation of psychopathology in general medical inpatients to use and cost of services. Am J Psychiatry 147:1498–1503, 1990

Levenson JL, Mishra A, Hamer R, Hastillo A: Denial and medical outcome in unstable angina. Psychosom Med 51:27–35, 1989

Mazzullo J: Methods of improving patient compliance. In Lasagna L (ed): Patient Compliance. Mount Kisco, NY, Futura Publishing, 21–30, 1976

President's Commission for the Study of Ethical Problems in Medicine and Biomedical and Behavioral Research: Making Health Care Decisions: A Report on the Ethical and Legal Implications of Informed Consent in the Patient-Practitioner Relationship. Washington, DC, U.S. Government Printing Office, 1982

Regier DA, Narrow WE, Rae DS, et al: The de facto U.S. mental and addictive disorders service system. Epidemiologic catchment area prospective 1 year prevalence rates of disorders and services. Arch Gen Psychiatry 50:85–94, 1993

Saravay SM: Psychiatric interventions in the medically ill. Outcome and effectiveness research. Psychiatr Clin North Am 19:467–480, 1996

Saravay SM, Lavin M: Psychiatric comorbidity and length of stay in the general hospital. A critical review of outcome studies. Psychosomatics 35:233–252, 1994

Smith GR Jr, Monson RA, Ray DC: Psychiatric consultation in somatization disorder: A randomized controlled study. N Engl J Med 314(22):1407–1413, 1986

Spitzer RL, Williams JBW, Kroenke K, et al: Utility of a new procedure for diagnosing mental disorders in primary care: The PRIME-MD 1,000 study. JAMA 272:1749–1756, 1994

Stoudemire A (ed.): Human Behavior. An introduction for Medical Students, 2nd ed. Philadelphia, J.B. Lippincott, 1998

Von Korff M, Shapiro S, Burke JD, et al: Anxiety and depression in a primary care clinic. Arch Gen Psychiatry 44:152–156, 1987

Wallen J, Pincus HA, Goldman HH, Marcus SE: Psychiatric consultations in short-term general hospitals. Arch Gen Psychiatry 44:163–168, 1987

21 Psychiatric Aspects of Acquired Immune Deficiency Syndrome

Michael G. Moran

At the turn of the century, the saying "By knowing syphilis, one knows medicine" was common in medical circles. As we approach the new century, the disease that includes more of medicine than any other, demands more of the physician than any other and taxes our society more than any other is surely acquired immune deficiency syndrome (AIDS). By knowing AIDS, one will know much of medicine, including psychiatry. This syndrome is a psychological malignancy: the patient's defenses and coping mechanisms are attacked and eroded by repeated assaults on livelihood, relationships, sense of integrated identity, and, in the end, on sanity and the very ability to think. AIDS presents myriad psychiatric pictures and complications. A patient may be angry, inhibited, depressed, manic, psychotic, or demented as a result of AIDS and its sequelae.

The broad scope of this syndrome confronts physicians with their personal and therapeutic limitations, sometimes in a brutal way. Diagnostic efforts can seem endless and futile. Avenues of treatment may appear few in number and without substance. There are certain principles, however, that can help the physician conduct a thorough search for treatable causes of the psychological dilemmas and psychiatric complications of AIDS. This chapter seeks to introduce the medical student to current approaches and techniques in the psychiatric management of these patients. An outline of the most common complications of the illness and the complications of treatment is given. A section is included on how and when a psychiatric consultation may be helpful. Following the chapter is a brief list of the current review literature on the psychiatric aspects of AIDS for students with a special interest in this area.

EPIDEMIOLOGY AND DEMOGRAPHICS OF INFECTION WITH HUMAN IMMUNODEFICIENCY VIRUS

Human immunodeficiency virus (HIV), the causative agent of AIDS, is transmitted chiefly through the exchange of body fluids (Table 21–1). It is the leading cause of death in U.S. adults aged 25–44 years. The most common routes of exchange are male homosexual intercourse, especially anal intercourse; use of contaminated needles during the intravenous administration of drugs; and administration of contaminated blood and blood products. An infected pregnant woman can also transmit the virus to her unborn fetus.

The virus is lymphotropic and neurotropic. It attacks the CD4+ T lymphocyte and causes a time-dependent and progressive destruction of that cell. The clinical results are the development of severe, often life-threatening infections with organisms against which the CD4+ T lymphocyte usually defends or helps defend. The clinical results of the neurotropism are seen in almost all levels of the neuraxis, but cerebral involvement is the most common.

Subacute encephalitis or subcortical dementia are the most common neuropsychiatric presentations. Heightened susceptibility to deliria from a variety of causes may then ensue. It should be noted that primary central nervous system (CNS) infection with HIV may occur before overt systemic signs of immunosuppression appear. This is a critical factor that will be discussed in more detail later in this chapter.

Nationwide, homosexual and bisexual men account for about 51% of all AIDS cases; intravenous drug users, about 24%; and women, about 18%. Most of the women are intravenous drug users, and the rest are prostitutes or sex-

---

Table 21–1 **High-Risk and Low-Risk Behavior Concerning HIV Contagion**

High-Risk Behavior

Sharing drug needles and syringes
Anal sex, with or without a condom
Vaginal or oral sex with someone who shoots drugs or engages in anal sex
Sex with strangers (a pickup or a prostitute) or with individuals with a history of multiple indiscriminately chosen sexual partners
Unprotected sex (without a condom) with an infected person

Safe Behavior

Not having sex (abstinence)
Sex with one mutually faithful, uninfected partner
Not injecting drugs

(Adapted from: U.S. Department of Health and Human Services. Understanding AIDS. Public Health Service, 1988)

ual partners of men at risk. Hemophiliacs and other recipients of blood and blood products constitute less than 1% of AIDS patients (Centers for Disease Control, 1996). Children comprise 2% of AIDS patients.

The prevalence of "triply diagnosed" patients (with AIDS, chronic mental illness, and drug use) is increasing (Kelly, 1997). Parenteral drug abuse appears to be a more common risk factor for acquiring HIV than does homosexual behavior, at least among psychiatrically hospitalized patients (Volavka et al, 1991).

Half of the people infected with HIV are unaware of the fact. A new oral test that samples mucosal transudate may make testing more available and accessible (Graham, 1997)

PSYCHIATRIC ASPECTS OF AIDS: THE CLINICAL PICTURE

The Changing Picture for Survival

The advent of new HIV protease inhibitors (nelfinavir, ritonavir, saquinavir, mesylate, and indinavir sulfate) and a diagnostic assay for serum levels of HIV viral copies have provided physicians with powerful new tools and patients with a chance for a "second life" (Rabkin and Ferrando, 1997). The restructuring of lives and expectations resulting from altered prognoses will present new psychological dilemmas to the patient and the treatment team. In addition there are unanswered questions regarding the new drugs, including their possible psychiatric side effects and their interactions with psychotropic medications.

AIDS-Related Impairment of Cognition

After infection with HIV, the clinical presentations are shaped by the target systems of the virus's attack (the immune system and the nervous system, especially the brain) and by the psychiatric reactions to the diagnosis of the illness and to its immunological and neurological complications. The psychiatric problems resulting primarily from immune dysfunction are chiefly deliria that stem from severe infections, their metabolic complications, and the measures used to treat them. The psychiatric problems that arise from the *neurotropism* of the virus can be seen as a species of dementia. The dementia then renders the patient more susceptible to the insults that cause the aforementioned deliria, and some of the causes of the deliria, if they are prolonged, can add to or produce a picture of dementia. Less common manifestations of neurological complications of AIDS include a vacuolar myelopathy, similar to that of cobalamin deficiency; cranial nerve syndromes, often caused by localizations of systemic infections; and Landry-Guillain-Barré syndrome. All told, central nervous system disease occurs in *at least* 40% of AIDS patients and is the initial symptom of the syndrome in at least 10% (Table 21–2).

To complicate this picture further, sequelae of the immune deficiency, namely certain neoplasms, can occur in the CNS and cause neurological dis-

Table 21–2 **Neuropsychiatric Complications of HIV Infection**

Delirium

Infectious causes: viral (incl. HIV), mycobacterial, parasitic, bacterial
Metabolic: volume depletion, electrolyte disturbances
Medications: CNS depressants and anticholinergics
Intracranial mass lesions: hematoma, neoplasm

Dementia

Sequelae of chronic deliria; see above
HIV infection of the brain
    Subcortical dementia is most common
    No specific treatment
    May present initially as aseptic meningitis

Vacuolar Myelopathy

Resembles cobalamin deficiency
Mechanism is unknown

Peripheral Nervous System Involvement

Local infections or neoplasms
HIV polyneuropathy

ease; examples are Kaposi's sarcoma and lymphomas of various types, including lymphomas involving the CNS. Other psychiatric symptoms are best characterized as psychological and are associated with the meanings of the events already catalogued here. These are discussed in a later section.

Delirium in AIDS

Delirium, or acute confusional state, is caused in AIDS by many potential factors; accurate diagnosis requires meticulous and careful clinical investigative work. It occurs in about one-third of hospitalized patients with AIDS. Sometimes no specific etiology is found and empiric treatment must be instituted in any case. More often, more than one candidate can be found as a cause for the delirium. Intracranial and systemic infections (often presenting as a diffuse encephalopathy), electrolyte and volume abnormalities, hypoxemia, and medication side effects are the chief offenders (Glatt et al, 1988). The delirious patient may be only mildly disoriented and agitated, in which case a careful mental status exam may be the key to detecting the disorder. The spectrum of delirium can range, however, to combativeness and psychosis, with hallucinations and visual illusions. Misdiagnosis of the patient as "schizophrenic" or "manic" in this setting can result in improper treatment. Undiagnosed delirium is a cause of significant morbidity and mortality. Once delirium is suspected, a search for the infectious agent or metabolic derangement should begin. Some of the most common infectious causes of delirium are discussed below.

Pneumocystis carinii pneumonia (PCP) affects more than 80% of patients. It is the most frequent AIDS-defining diagnosis. Progressive dyspnea with chest pain, fatigue, and fever constitute the clinical picture. Hypoxemia from the pneumonia can be severe, and when cerebral functioning is already marginal because of an intracranial infection or dementia, delirium can result.

Systemic infections can be caused by viruses (probably including HIV), fungi, parasites, and bacteria (including *Mycobacterium* species). Sites of entry into the systemic circulation include focal infections, such as pneumonia, as well as less localized sites such as erosions of the gastrointestinal tract and skin. In such settings, delirium can accompany fever, seeding of the bloodstream with the infectious agent(s), metabolic and fluid derangements caused by diarrhea, nausea and vomiting, and decreased ability or desire to eat and drink. These infections are diagnosed by blood culture, as well as by examination and culture of the appropriate body fluid.

Toxoplasma gondii causes a focal encephalitis, characterized by a picture ranging from mild headache and fever to seizures, neurological deficits, delirium, and coma (Glatt et al, 1988). Extracerebral involvement is unusual. Computed tomography (CT) and magnetic resonance imaging (MRI) scans may show the characteristic but nonspecific constellation of multiple lesions in the cortical and subcortical regions, enhancing with contrast.

Cryptococcal meningitis is most often unimpressive in AIDS patients in its first stages. It may resemble depression, with lethargy, fatigue, and irritability. A devastating and rapidly progressive illness with meningitic signs, severe delirium, and eventual extraneural involvement is uncommon. CT scan is not helpful in making the diagnosis.

Infections with mycobacteria, especially *Mycobacterium avium-intracellulare*, are common in AIDS patients. *M. tuberculosis* infections are usually reactivations of earlier acquired disease and are most common in patients with a high background prevalence of the illness. Atypical presentations of *M. tuberculosis* infection are common, and bronchoscopy with biopsy of lung tissue, or biopsy of other tissue suspected of involvement, may be necessary for diagnosis. Intermediate-strength purified protein derivative tuberculin skin tests are too insensitive to be reliably helpful, and late in the course of the illness, the patient may not be able to mount the inflammatory immune response that gives the positive reaction.

M. avium-intracellulare (MAC) is an infective complex that is usually found in immunocompromised hosts. The presentation is generally that of a chronic pulmonary infection that responds poorly to antibiotics, even when in vitro sensitivity has been demonstrated. In AIDS patients, the infection can be disseminated widely, affecting the lungs, liver, bone marrow, and lymph nodes. Biopsy of these tissues yields the diagnosis, as can culture of the blood. A "wasting syndrome" is associated with *M. avium-intracellulare* infections in AIDS patients and consists of malaise, weakness, diarrhea, fatigue, weight loss, and fever (Hawkins et al, 1986). When the fever or diarrhea is severe, delirium can result, even without primary central nervous system infection. The prognosis for patients with *M. avium-intracellulare* infections is poor; there is no effective therapy at this time.

Cytomegalovirus (CMV) is commonly a disseminated illness in the AIDS patient. The organism probably causes a subacute encephalopathy with associated delirium, but can also cause colitis with diarrhea, adrenalitis, and retinitis.

HIV itself produces an acute encephalopathy very similar to that supposedly seen with CMV. Altered mentation, varying alertness, apathy, depressive affect, and decreased mental and verbal acuity and spontaneity are seen. The syndrome can progress and result in paranoid ideation, impulsive behavior, and psychotic symptoms of hallucinations and illusions. Delirium with prominant psychotic symptoms can be the initial presentation of AIDS. Only autopsy reveals the diagnosis with certainty. Other viruses that can cause acute meningitis and possibly encephalopathic presentations include several in the herpes group: Epstein-Barr virus, varicella zoster, and herpes simplex. The latter commonly presents as an intracerebral mass lesion in patients without AIDS; in AIDS patients, such a picture is unusual. A more diffuse encephalopathic syndrome, or widespread mucocutaneous lesions without CNS involvement, can be seen.

Fluid, electrolyte, and oxygenation abnormalities, and *intravenous drug use* can have profoundly adverse effects on AIDS patients who are already suffering cerebral compromise. Sedating and anticholinergic medications (among others), at doses normally tolerated well by other patients, may induce confusion, disorientation, and psychotic symptoms in severely ill AIDS patients. The door toward diagnosing these problems is opened by a high index of suspicion. Careful attention to variations in mental status, laboratory values, and the list of medications the patient is taking is essential for uncovering the cause(s) of delirium.

Dementia in AIDS

Dementia can result from the chronic sequelae of most of the causes of delirium: severe electrolyte imbalance, hypoxemia, or meningitis, to name a few; however, cerebral infection with HIV probably causes a large proportion of cases of dementia seen in AIDS patients. The exact percentage of patients who become demented is hard to estimate, but studies suggest that over one-third of patients with debilitating dementia had evidence of active HIV infection at autopsy. The virus has been recovered even from patients who have neurological symptoms and signs, but do not have AIDS or any evidence of immune deficiency. Early detection of subtle HIV-induced neuropsychological impairment requires sophisticated testing. Subjective complaints and neurological signs do not correlate reliably with subtle deficits. Even mild atrophy on brain CT, diffuse electroencephalographic (EEG) slowing, and nonspecific hyperdensities on brain MRI are usually unreliable indices (Perry, 1990).

The neuropathological picture is rather distinct, as is the early clinical presentation: *subcortical dementia.* Subcortical and white matter changes dominate in these cases; gray matter is relatively spared. Macrophages, lymphocytes, and perivascular collections of multinucleated giant cells further characterize the microscopic appearance. Inclusion bodies are present in those infected with CMV, which can cause dementia in AIDS patients, too, but is probably less common as a true etiology for the dementia and occurs after CNS infection with HIV.

Clinical features of subcortical dementia (of any origin) include mental slowness, apathy, impaired cognition, and depressive affect (see Chapter 4 for a general description of subcortical dementias). The bedside mental status examination is not sensitive enough to detect impairment early in the course. Asymptomatic HIV-positive men who are not intravenous drug users may show early deficits in memory (Stern et al, 1992). In rapidly progressive or in advanced cases, disorganization and delirium may be evident. The cortical dementias, of which Alzheimer's disease may be said to be the prototype, cause more debilitating intellectual deficits, and the affected patients are more likely to show amnesia, agnosia, and aphasia. Motor abnormalities (dysarthria, ataxic gait, abnormal involuntary movements, and leg weakness) are more common with subcortical dementia.

Rapid deterioration is the rule. Progressive slowing of mentation brings on muteness and severe confusion, interfering with the accurate communication of needs. There may be periods of severe agitation if the patient becomes delirious; hallucinations and sensory illusions can occur. With advancement of the motor deficits, truncal ataxia can appear, as can spastic weakness, paraplegia, and quadriparesis.

The diagnosis of subcortical dementia is a clinical exercise; HIV dementia itself can be diagnosed definitively only at autopsy. The virus can be grown from the cerebrospinal fluid (CSF) of a fraction of the patients. The CSF is often normal, but may reveal a slight mononuclear pleocytosis and a mild elevation of protein. As mentioned earlier, the MRI and CT scans can be abnormal even before there are clinical manifestations of the dementia. Atrophy and ventricular enlargement can occur early in the course of the illness. Small white matter lesions are better revealed by MRI than by CT scan. There are as yet no known scan features that are pathognomonic for HIV brain infection.

The previously discussed neuropsychiatric factors can undermine patients' capacity to modulate and manage their own mood states and adaptive responses to the news of the diagnosis and the evidence of illness progression. For example, delirious or demented patients may be relatively disinhibited and may be more likely to self-treat impulsively with alcohol or other drugs, further impairing their efforts at adapting appropriately to psychological insults. In vitro and in vivo evidence of immune suppression as a result of substance use, coupled with coexistent psychiatric illness, makes substance use especially destructive in patients with a lethal communicable disease (Flavin and Frances, 1987).

Psychological Aspects of AIDS

Early Phases

Even when free of HIV infection, members of groups at high risk for contracting AIDS face considerable anxiety and interpersonal tension because of the threat of the disease. Pressure, which at times can seem to these persons unreasonable and coercive, may be exerted by others in an attempt to change the lifestyles and sexual behavior of the members of the risk group. Persons at little risk for the disease also have psychological reactions to AIDS that powerfully determine their behavior, sometimes with phobias or unnecessary discrimination toward persons with AIDS. Psychosocial characteristics that raise the risk for a severe psychological reaction to infection include past psychiatric history, positive family psychiatric history, high school education or less, and low support from one's spouse, family, or friends (Dew et al, 1990). Other events with powerful meaning and serious impact include the inherent personal and vocational losses, debilitation, probability of isolation, sense of loss of control, and potential for loss of self-esteem seen in persons with AIDS (indeed, in most chronic, debilitating illnesses). Medical personnel need to be acutely aware of their attitudes about AIDS and the persons in the groups at highest risk in order to give the best medical care to affected patients.

The *psychological* reactions to the *meanings* of the illness form an important part of the clinical presentation. The psychological "malignancy" of the syndrome exerts powerful effects on the patient, care-givers, family and other intimates in the patient's life (Walcott et al, 1986). Members of high-risk groups may respond to the risk of infection by changing their behavior (either toward reducing or increasing their risk), changing their mood and self-image, and altering their view of their lifestyle. Fear of the illness and its effects may be so intense that these feelings either are acted on destructively or are projected onto others, with resultant near-paranoia. Some persons who are not in high-risk groups can foster such projections by baiting and criticizing risk-group members, especially homosexual men. The fear of contracting an incurable illness that is associated with wasting, misery, and ostracism is a nightmare in itself. In a setting fueled by prejudicial fantasies and minimal factual information, irrational thought predominates. The crucial role of the physician as a provider of information, an educator, and a role model can help stem the destructive effects of phobic behavior and discrimination.

Increasing knowledge of the effects of physical and emotional stress on the immune system and on the progress of (or susceptibility to) physical illness may provide new insights about AIDS management (Rabkin and Ferrando, 1997; Cole and Kemeny, 1997). Stressors appear to exert their effects via a variety of mechanisms, including immune-derived cytokines, hypothalamic-pituitary-adrenal axis disturbances, and the possibly resulting neural dysregulation of inflammation (Anisman et al, 1996; Luster, 1998; McEwen, 1998). Certain psychological characteristics may determine differential disease progression (Cohen and Herbert, 1996).

The Decision to Be Tested: A Painful Dilemma

Counseling for AIDS testing, for those persons who wish to know their serological status, is described at length in a superb review (Perry and Markowitz, 1988). Pretest counseling involves giving information about the test, its usefulness, and its limitations and assessing the patient's strengths and psychological vulnerabilities. Making such an assessment allows the physician to figure the risk–benefit ratio for the test (as should be done for any medical procedure). The complexity of the decision to test and its potential for adverse consequences are well examined in the case illustrations of the paper mentioned.

Patients' abilities to use their own coping capacities and outside support can best be assessed before the test results are given. The physician must systematically seek to understand why patients want the test now, what they expect the result to be, how they plan to react to positive or negative results, whom they plan to tell, and how they expect them to react. After this assessment, patients usually can better tolerate the interviewer's questions about their current state of health, including specific questions about symptoms of HIV infection.

Lastly, recommendations can be made to patients about how to use the strengths and resources already available to them, regardless of the test results. It is important to emphasize the need for personal tailoring of the approach to counseling and testing: no single approach will work for all patients (Sikkema and Bissett, 1997).

Posttest counseling includes reducing the stress of those who are seropositive and explaining methods to prevent transmission. This is also the time to arrange proper follow-up care. The first 6 months after learning of positive test results is a high-risk period for deliberate self-harming behavior (Gala et al, 1992). A past psychiatric history or past self-harming behavior in any context raises the likelihood of other such incidents.

The test results for HIV seropositivity are powerful information: the patient discovers whether he or she has a lethal illness. It comes as no surprise that such information could powerfully affect his or her risk-taking behavior. The prospect of a positive result can make some members of risk groups avoid obtaining test results: in one study of homosexual men who were offered the chance to be tested, only 67% elected to do so. Those found to be seronegative decreased risk-taking behavior by a significantly smaller margin than the seropositive patients did (Fox et al, 1987). In another study, over 2,000 homosexual men were tested for HIV, and then asked by mail if they wanted their results. Among the responders, there was no difference between those who chose to learn the result and those who refused; however, there was a significant difference between those who responded and those who did not: the latter group tended to be younger, nonwhite, and less educated. The group that refused to learn the results said they declined because they felt the test was not predictive of the development of AIDS or they were concerned about the worry that a positive result would cause them (Lyter et al, 1987).

Most discussions on AIDS prevention emphasize that giving information, especially about modes of infection, is the way to modify the high-risk activities of certain groups. The nationwide mailing of the Department of Health and Human Services pamphlet "Understanding AIDS" in 1988 is an example of this kind of logic and intervention. Health-related behaviors have been shown to be related to possession of clear, consistent information, but other important factors impinge on such behavior. Peer-group opinions and support also play a major role in maintaining or altering health-related behavior. When the risk behaviors of a group of homosexual male physicians and college students were studied, the authors concluded that such multifactorial determinants of behavior were at work and that precise intervention was necessary if behaviors were to be changed. The authors suggested that programs for older, well-educated homosexual men should be designed so as to increase the sense of control over outcome (that is, to promote the notion that changing habits is *effective*). For young, well-educated men, programs aimed at appealing to peer-group norms were thought most likely to succeed.

This summary of the study is not meant to serve as a comprehensive list of interventions for groups at risk. For example, no mention is made here (nor was any made in the study) of intervention with drug users or prostitutes. The point is that in order to make a substantive change in the intended audience, the intervention will probably need to be tailored specifically to each group. Information, no matter how clearly presented, is usually not enough to change behavior.

Being in a high-risk group can itself be associated with severe psychological distress in the current setting of the AIDS epidemic. Symptoms are usually dominated by anxiety and can include panic attacks. Vigilant self-observation, when fostered by fear about a physical illness, can result in inordinate preoccupation with physical signs and symptoms. When these symptoms become severe enough, they can interfere with social and work functioning (Faulstich, 1987).

"Malignant" Progression of Psychological Symptoms

Once diagnosed, the psychological developments in AIDS patients closely resemble the sequence seen in terminal cancer patients. Many patients are filled with denial and disavowal at the news of their seropositivity or clinical immune deficiency. Anger, despair, and expressed or enacted hopelessness and helplessness are common. As mentioned before, an antecedent personality disorder, especially coupled with substance use, can render the patient prone to living out fantasized solutions to his or her situation or wishes for revenge and restitution. Some of the sense of being endangered and invaded (by the virus) is projected; care-givers are seen as the problem, or at least as inadequate. News reports that suggest slow progress with experimental treatments and minimal attention by the medical establishment to the concerns of affected persons and their associated high-risk groups promote these externalizations. The patient may feel and act overtly hostile to family members, physicians, and other intimates (Faulstich, 1987). If the patient acquired or suspects acquisition of the disease from a lover, that relationship can obviously come under the intense burdens of guilt, fault-finding, and desire for revenge. Other individuals find in the crisis an opportunity for increased emotional intimacy and work together against a common enemy. Such a response is usually founded on the earlier presence of a solid and loving relationship. Ironically, AIDS patients appear to be less suicidal than HIV-positive patients. The brain dysfunction in AIDS-related CNS disorders may reduce suicidality among AIDS patients (McKegney and O'Dowd, 1992). Risk factors include alcohol and drug abuse, and severe neuropsychiatric impairment (Starace, 1995).

Reports suggest that both homicidal and suicidal impulses can lead to sexually risky behavior among distressed infected persons. Alcohol, serving as an anxiolytic, may facilitate the living out of "love suicide" fantasies, in which the uninfected person tries to acquire HIV infection and the infected person tries to infect others. Intravenous drug users with the same conscious and unconscious wishes (to spread the infection or to commit suicide) may display the same kind of behavior by knowingly using and trading contaminated needles. Anecdotal reports suggest that similar behavior occurred in epidemics of polio, tuberculosis, and syphilis (Flavin et al, 1986).

Existential Issues

The existential issues of *worth, control,* and *lovability* are paramount in the psychological picture of this illness. Every attentive physician will be able to see the patient striving to regulate her or his feelings of being worthless, out of control, and unlovable. As the patient's ability to function at work or in other settings is eroded, they may become desperate to find a way to prove their worth or demand a show of being valued from others. This may take the form of seeming entitled and demanding with medical caregivers and others.

Chronic, debilitating physical illness is the prototype of an attack on control of one's life. AIDS patients lose their ability to control their bodies (even bowel and bladder function), their place of residence (through repeated hospitalizations), and their sensorium and level of awareness (because of delirium); usually, these relentlessly worsen. The patient's reactions to such loss of control can include what may appear to be a childish attempt to control others or to fight medical care.

The illness severely strains the patient's sense of being lovable. As mentioned, the strain usually invades intimate relationships. The partners must struggle with questions of sexual intimacy and how to handle the new risk imposed by the disease. If one partner is uninfected and gives any evidence of withdrawal or unavailability in the relationship amid the many medical and psychological crises that ensue, the patient will probably feel unloved. Family and friends who are frightened by the fear of easy contagion or who reject the patient's lifestyle (most often seen with male homosexual patients) may also withdraw. Usually, the patient is at some level aware of the feelings of these others, and major disruptions in the family can ensue. Feeling unloved, the angry and hurt patient may retaliate in an attempt to make others feel the same way. Such actions may serve only to further the avoidant and angry feelings and behavior of family and other loved ones. In other families, such intense evidence of feeling on both sides may provide the opportunity for reviewing the situation of the illness and for allowing appropriate planning and support for the future. Such a scenario is uncommon in the early phases of the illness, during which denial, disavowal, and projection of feelings dominate.

As with any patient faced with a virtually inevitable and fatal outcome, death and the meaning of ending one's life become issues with which to reckon.

Most patients affected with AIDS are young men, usually healthy, before the occurrence of the illness. For them especially, contemplating death is a horror, so out of alignment with "expectable" concerns at their stage in the life cycle. After working through these issues to some extent, other fears often become apparent: many patients are less afraid of death per se than they are of suffocating, being alone as they die, or being left in agonizing pain. The latter is actually less common in the final stages of AIDS. As we have seen, however, PCP and interpersonal strife are real and may lend extra credence to the chances of an isolated or suffocating death.

TREATMENT OF NEUROPSYCHIATRIC AND PSYCHOLOGICAL ASPECTS OF AIDS

This section presents treatment issues regarding the problems arising from neuropsychiatric sequelae (chiefly, delirium and dementia) and from psychological sequelae of AIDS. See Chapter 4 for a systematic overview of the treatment of delirium and dementia.

Treatment and Prevention of Delirium and Dementia

Specific medical treatment of the different infectious and metabolic complications of AIDS, the most common antecedents to delirium, is beyond the scope of this chapter, but details of a working approach are presented. Preventive quarantine, in an effort to isolate the patient from potential carriers of superinfecting pathogens, is bound to fail; as mentioned before, most infections are reactivations of a previously acquired organism. Similarly, most AIDS patients with opportunistic infections do not represent an infectious threat to others. The only exceptions are infections due to *M. tuberculosis,* herpes, and perhaps salmonella (Glatt et al, 1988). Thus, the delirium caused by infections and the accompanying fever, bacteremia, and viremia generally cannot be treated by prophylaxis, but rather requires specific treatment of the infection once clinically evident, and by supportive measures.

Persistence of the delirium in spite of what seems to be appropriate treatment should alert the physician to another cause of infection or a separate cause for the delirium, such as a medication, volume depletion, or an intracranial mass. An acute change in sensorium or the appearance of new neurological signs should prompt the consideration of a complete system review and new physical examination. Rarely, CT and MRI scans might be useful when routine laboratory procedures or bedside examinations show no cause for the new delirium, but the scans are rarely diagnostic.

PCP responds to appropriate antimicrobial treatment in 60 to 80% of the cases. The infection, and the potential for the associated delirium, recurs in

65% of patients after 18 months. Toxoplasmosis and cryptococcosis also are rarely cured; relapse is the rule. Thus, previous history of pulmonary or disseminated infection with either of these agents should prompt investigation for their presence in the setting of a new delirium.

M. avium-intracellulare infections are not cured in HIV patients by current methods. *M. tuberculosis* may be somewhat more likely to invade the CNS and can do so despite appropriate therapy.

The other common causes of delirium are sometimes forestalled with meticulous maintenance and supportive care. Avoiding *medications* with psychotropic activity—especially sedative–hypnotics, anxiolytics, and drugs with high anticholinergic side effects—is an important cautionary step. If necessary, low starting doses (for example, half the dose for a young, otherwise healthy person) should be the rule. The nursing staff should be alerted to early signs of toxicity, such as sedation, confusion, or, in the case of anticholinergic drugs, dry mouth and urinary retention; however, CNS side effects can occur without these peripheral signs.

Vital signs can help track *volume status* and *oxygenation.* Patients with diarrhea who have impeded access to fluid replenishment, or who are too demented to ask for fluids, are at greatest risk for hypotension and accompanying cerebral dysfunction. Falls also are more likely then. Patients with pneumonia or antecedent lung disease might require arterial blood gases or saturation monitors to follow oxygenation status. Bedridden patients need close nursing attention to help avoid bedsores, another site for entry of infectious pathogens.

Those cases characterized by severe agitation or psychotic symptoms may require the addition of a high-potency neuroleptic, such as haloperidol, in low doses. The physician must remember that the AIDS patient has an increased susceptibility to extrapyramidal side effects and probably neuroleptic malignant syndrome because of the preexistent brain disease (see also Chapter 18).

Many principles that apply to HIV-associated infections (Glatt et al, 1988) are useful in the clinical management of delirium:

1. Most of the infections are incurable and require long-term suppressive therapy. Likewise, delirium may be chronic in many patients and require symptomatic, long-term treatment. A thorough search for reversible infectious, metabolic, and drug-induced causes can allow specific treatment of the delirium. The essential points here are the need for a high index of suspicion for the causes listed, careful elimination and treatment of the specific causes when possible, and judicious use of a neuroleptic in selected cases. The use of neuroleptics will be discussed in the section on treatment. (See Chapter 4 for further details on the diagnosis and treatment of delirium.)
2. These patients rarely have just one infection. Similarly, the causes of delirium are often multiple. The physician's search

for etiology should be thorough, and vigilance for changes in mental status should be maintained throughout the care of the patient. Clinical "failure" in the treatment of delirium may result not from clinical error, but from a second cause.

3. Certain infections occur at their observed frequency in AIDS patients because of the prevalence of asymptomatic infection in the local population (e.g., histoplasmosis and cryptococcosis). Likewise, behavior that antedates the HIV infection, seen in the groups at highest risk for AIDS, may play a role in the susceptibility of AIDS patients for delirium. Examples of such behaviors include habitual alcohol or drug use preceding the onset of AIDS. If these behaviors are repeated after the cerebral compromise (from whatever specific etiology) is present in a case of AIDS, the patient is much less likely to tolerate the CNS effects of such behavior than before the HIV infection began. In the setting of depression and hopelessness, self-destructive or suicidal behavior can then occur because of decreased impulse control (Flavin et al, 1986).

To the extent that dementia is caused, in any one patient, by factors that show up early as delirium and are reversible, dementia might be forestalled or prevented. If caused by HIV, there is no current treatment. Whatever the cause, dementia in AIDS is generally managed through supportive measures. Here again, nursing care and meticulous attention to metabolic parameters and medications is preeminent. Cognitive deficits can be symptomatically improved by use of stimulants, such as methylphenidate or dextroamphetamine. Doses generally have to be individualized. Improvement usually takes the form of more organized thinking, improved memory, and more spontaneity and animation (Angrist et al, 1992).

Treatment of the psychological problems associated with AIDS can rarely be divorced from the nonpsychological or purely physiologically oriented treatments, for several reasons. First, symptoms of brain dysfunction from medical and neurological causes can masquerade as functional psychiatric disorders. An approach that arbitrarily separates the patient into two camps, mind and body, will fail in managing the illness. Second, the psychological reactions, if not addressed, will affect the patient's ability to care for herself or himself and to participate in medical treatment and may adversely affect immunocompetence. The death of an intimate partner is particularly stressful, and has immunological consequences (Kemeny et al, 1995). Third, the psychological effects of the illness extend to the caregivers. If physicians are unaware of or deny the ways they can be affected by working with these patients, appropriate care of the patient will be impossible.

The treatment of *depression* in the AIDS patient is complex and filled with pitfalls. First, the presentation is rarely that of a classic vegetative depression: anger, self-criticism, projection of self-hatred, and preoccupation with somatic symptoms are rather common. In addition, as with any chronic or wasting disease, the absolute diagnosis *or* exclusion of depression is often impossible. The clinician, however, must maintain a high index of suspicion for depression and must be ready to deal with this treatable illness: indeed, mood disorder is a common reason for psychiatric referral of AIDS patients (Seth et al, 1991). Treatment includes psychotherapy, mobilization of the family and other supports, and antidepressants with low (desipramine) or no (fluoxetine or sertraline) anticholinergic effects. Antidepressants must be used carefully because of their anticholinergic, sedating, and hypotensive effects. Studies are in progress to evaluate these drugs systematically in AIDS patients. A number of reports have advocated the use of psychostimulants such as methylphenidate 10 to 40 mg/day given in divided doses early in the day as a treatment of depression in AIDS patients.

Treatment of pain in AIDS patients must be a priority of care. Prevalent among AIDS patients, pain is often undertreated and contributes heavily to the psychological and functional morbidity of the illness. A multidisciplinary approach (including accurate characterization and work up of the pain, ruling out of infection and malignancy, thorough history and physical examination, and use of adequate dosages of pain medication) provides the largest array of resources (Lefkowitz, 1996).

TREATMENT DECISIONS IN IRREVERSIBLE ILLNESS

Early in the course of the illness, soon after diagnosis, involvement of the support system of the patient (family, lover, friends) can be helpful. If this seems impossible, *support groups,* most readily available for homosexual men, are valuable resources. The physician's willingness to discuss the need for referral and support is in itself a supportive act and can help pave the way for a useful experience working with the referral agency or specialist. Since substance use has such an augmenting effect on destructive behavior in this population, the physician should try to help the patient pay special attention to such behavior and obtain appropriate *counseling* and perhaps *disulfiram treatment.*

Emphasis on legal needs is also an important aspect of the counseling at this point. Attention to putting the patient's affairs in order, such as drawing up a will, may be too much for the patient in the acute setting, but dealing with such issues should not be inordinately delayed. Other considerations include designating a close *friend* or *relative* who could serve as legal guardian. Establishing individualized, clear-cut criteria for the timing of need for *hospice care* or decisions about remaining at home for treatment should be considered. Consultation with *social services* can help in making the appropriate referrals.

In making decisions about major treatment and resuscitative efforts, the physician can be a help and guide for the distressed patient and family. Most patients want the physician to spare them the risk of unnecessary and potentially harmful procedures and drugs; however, such wishes may be obscured by a more overtly expressed and persistent fantasy about cure. If the physician has her or his own fantasies about "rescuing" the patient, the combination can yield a fruitless and futile zeal for treatment. At some point in the course of the illness, a frank discussion with the patient, and perhaps with family or lovers, should focus on these issues. A treatment approach aimed at aggressive palliation of discomfort and symptoms, rather than at unattainable symbols of "cure," is usually experienced as reassuring and supportive (Cassem, 1987; Wachter et al, 1988).

In addition, AIDS patients may be frightening: they have a severe infectious disease, and even education about the level of risk of contagion may not stem associated fears in medical personnel. Additionally, the patient may be hostile because of low self-esteem and fears of dying and be out of control because of delirium.

Most AIDS patients are male homosexuals, intravenous drug users, or prostitutes. If the physician is shocked, offended, or disgusted by such persons and is not in control of those feelings, many reactions could occur. In an attempt to disavow such feelings, the physician may adopt an intense therapeutic zeal, aimed at giving "the best" to a hated patient. Such feelings could result in "working everything up," a futile and destructive approach in the context of end-stage irreversible illness (see the earlier discussion). In a less-subtle form, hostility toward the patient may take the form of unnecessary intramuscular injections, invasive procedures, or restraints. Among nursing staff, these reactions may appear in a nurse's slowness to respond to the patient's calls, restrictions on visitation, and "forgetting" to take vital signs. Being aware of one's attitudes toward these patients, informal discussions with colleagues, and in-service training sessions can be helpful.

Physicians' Reactions to AIDS Patients

To render the best care, physicians must be aware of their own reactions to this devastating illness. Many of these patients are young men, healthy and active before contracting the disease. Overidentifying with the patient is a common and hazardous response that can contribute to rescue fantasies, doomed to fail in this context. The intense investment of time and emotional energy by physicians and staff can leave them vulnerable to repeated assaults on their self-esteem when the patient dies (O'Dowd and McKegney, 1990). In addition, the wish to avoid the illness can impede taking a history, such as for needed family planning and sexual practices (Coverdale and Aruffo, 1992). Anger at patients who fail to reduce their high-risk behaviors can interfere with proper follow-up and counseling (Carlson et al, 1989).

ROLE OF THE PSYCHIATRIST

The *psychiatrist* can assist in the treatment in several ways: in those situations in which the primary physician needs help constructing and implementing a differential diagnostic approach to delirium and dementia; when the patient manifests a major psychiatric illness, such as depression, mania, or delirium; as a referral source for psychotherapy for patients or family members; when psychiatric hospitalization is required for psychotic or suicidal patients; and to help manage the reactions of support staff in their dealings with AIDS patients.

Many patients experience referral to a psychiatrist as a rejection or as a criticism by the primary physician. They may feel the primary doctor is saying, "It's all in your head." An open discussion with the patient about the importance of the care for his or her psychological state can reduce these concerns. The primary care physician's unbiased attitude toward psychiatric care is essential. One approach that may be used is to speak of the referral as being helpful *to the primary care physician* in further helping the patient. It is important to arrange a follow-up visit with the primary care physician soon after the psychiatric appointment. Sometimes the patient will refuse to see the psychiatrist. The primary care physician may then elect to proceed with the consultation through personal discussions of the case with the psychiatrist.

CLINICAL PEARLS

- Neuropsychiatric complications of AIDS can be the *first* presentation of the illness. They can also masquerade as functional psychological problems. Persons in high-risk groups and those who appear to be depressed, confused, disoriented, psychotic or merely easily fatigued should be elevaluated for active HIV infection, dementia, and delirium, as well as functional psychological illness.
- Heterosexuals (outside the high-risk groups of drug users, prostitutes, and hemophiliacs) are at high risk for HIV infection, albeit at an undetermined level. HIV testing, when otherwise clinically indicated, should not be deferred merely because the person is heterosexual. Careful counseling and informed consent are required for HIV testing.
- Vigilance in diagnostic and therapeutic zeal must be tempered at some point in the illness with a consideration for what fate awaits the patient after treatment of the acute problem. Physicians treating AIDS patients need to acquaint themselves thoroughly with various strategies for dealing with irreversible illness.
- Some reports suggest that depression in patients with HIV infection responds to psychostimulants such as methylphenidate.
- About 4% of AIDS patients seen for psychiatric consultation demonstrate violent behavior. Most are demented or delirious (Travin et al, 1990).
- Physicians should educate themselves about local laws that address HIV testing, confidentiality of testing results, and duty to protect unsuspecting third parties about exposure to HIV (Haimowitz, 1989).
- A large number of AIDS patients use "complementary" therapies (e.g., yoga, meditation, herbal treatments, and acupuncture).

ANNOTATED BIBLIOGRAPHY

Cohen S, Herbert TB: Health psychology: psychological factors and physical disease from the perspective of human psychoneuroimmunology. Ann Rev Psychol 47:113, 1996

> This article examines the effects of stress and depression on the immune system, and the consequences for human illness.

Emanuel EJ: Do physicians have an obligation to treat patients with AIDS? N Engl J Med 318:1686–1690, 1988

> This is a thought-provoking examination of a question for every physician.

Ernst E: Complementary AIDS therapies: the good, the bad and the ugly [editorial]. Int J STD & AIDS 8:281, 1997

> More money is spent on unconventional care in the US than on conventional. This article examines the implications for AIDS patients and their physicians.

Graham NM: Epidemiology of acquired immunodeficiency syndrome: advancing to an endemic era. Amer J Med 102:2, 1997

> Graham reviews HIV distribution in the US population, and examines clues as to its prevention and spread.

McDonald CK, Kuritzkes DR: Human immunodeficiency virus type 1 protease inhibitors. Arch Intern Med 157:951, 1997

> This is a review of the most recently approved drugs used to treat HIV infection.

Rabkin JG, Ferrando S: A "second life" agenda. Psychiatric research issues raised by protease inhibitor treatments for people with the human immunodeficiency virus or the acquired immunodeficiency syndrome. Arch Gen Psychiatry 54:1049, 1997

> This is an excellent review of the most recent diagnostic and therapeutic innovations, with a discussion of their impact on patient care.

Ruark JE, Raffin TA, the Stanford University Medical Center Committee on Ethics: Initiating and withdrawing life support. N Engl J Med 318:25–30, 1988

> This thoughtful, scholarly review presents Stanford's approach to the difficult problem of initiating and withdrawing life support.

REFERENCES

Angrist B, d'Hollosy M, Sanfilipo M, et al: Central nervous system stimulants as symptomatic treatments for AIDS-related neuropsychiatric impairment. J Clin Psychopharmacol 12:268–272, 1992

Anisman H, Baines MG, Berczi I, et al: Neuroimmune mechanisms in health and disease: 2. Disease. Can Med Assoc J 155:1075, 1996

Carlson GA, Greeman M, McClellan TA: Management of HIV-positive psychiatric patients who fail to reduce high-risk behaviors. Hosp Community Psychiatry 40:511–514, 1989

Cassem NH: Treatment decisions in irreversible illness. In Hackett TP, Cassem NH (eds.): Massachusetts General Hospital Handbook of General Hospital Psychiatry, 2nd ed. Littleton, MA, PSG Publishing Co., 1987

Centers for Disease Control: HIV/AIDS Surveillance Report. 8:8, 1996

Centers for Disease Control: Revision of the case definition of acquired immune deficiency syndrome. MMWR 36:1S–15S, 1987

Cohen S, Herbert TB: Health psychology: psychological factors and physical disease from the perspective of human psychoneuroimmunology. Ann Rev Psychol 47:113, 1996

Cole SW, Kemeny ME: Psychobiology of HIV infection. Crit Rev Neurobiol 11:289, 1997

Coverdale JH, Aruffo JF: AIDS and family planning counseling of psychiatrically ill women in community mental health clinics. Community Ment Health J 28:13–20, 1992

Dew MA, Ragni MV, Nimorwicz P: Infection with human immunodeficiency virus and vulnerability to psychiatric distress: a study of men with hemophilia. Arch Gen Psychiatry 47:737–744, 1990

Faulstich ME: Psychiatric aspects of AIDS. Am J Psychiatry 144:551–556, 1987

Flavin DK, Frances RJ: Risk-taking behavior, substance abuse disorders, and the acquired immune deficiency syndrome. Adv Alcohol Subst Abuse 6:23–32, 1987

Flavin DK, Franklin JE, Frances RJ: The acquired immune deficiency syndrome (AIDS) and suicidal behavior in alcohol-dependent homosexual men. Am J Psychiatry 143:1440–1442, 1986

Fox R, Odaka NJ, Brookmeyer R, et al: Effect of HIV antibody disclosure on subsequent sexual activity in homosexual men. AIDS 1:241–246, 1987

Gala C, Pergami A, Catalan J, et al: Risk of deliberate self-harm and factors associated with suicidal behavior among asymptomatic individuals with human immunodeficiency virus infection. Acta Psychiatr Scand 86:70–75, 1992

Glatt AE, Chirgwin K, Landesman SH: Treatment of infections associated with human immunodeficiency virus. N Engl J Med 318:1439–1448, 1988

Goedert JJ, Biggar RJ, Weiss SH, et al: Three-year incidence of AIDS in five cohorts of HTLV-III risk group members. Science 231:992–995, 1986

Graham NM: Epidemiology of acquired immunodeficiency syndrome: advancing to an endemic era. Amer J Med 102:2, 1997

Haimowitz S: HIV and the mentally ill: an approach to the legal issues. Hosp Community Psychiatry 40:732–736, 1989

Hawkins CC, Gold JWM, Whimbey E, et al: *Mycobacterium avium* complex infections in patients with the acquired immunodeficiency syndrome. Ann Intern Med 105:184–188, 1986

Kelly JA: HIV risk reduction interventions for persons with severe mental illness. Clin Psychol Rev 17:293, 1997

Kemeny ME, Weiner H, Duran R, Taylor SE, Visscher B, Fahey JL: Immune system changes after the death of a partner in HIV-positive gay men. Psychosom Med 57:547–554, 1995

Lefkowitz M: Pain management for the AIDS patient. J Florida Med Assoc 83:701, 1996

Luster AD: Chemokines—Chemotactic cytokines that mediate inflammation. New Engl J Med 338:436, 1998

Lyter DW, Valdiserri RO, Kingsley LA, Amoroso WP, Rinaldo CR Jr: The HIV antibody test: why gay and bisexual men want or do not want to know their results. Public Health Rep 102:468–474, 1987

McEwen BS: Protective and damaging effects of stress mediators. New Engl J Med 338:171, 1998

McKegney FP, O'Dowd MA: Suicidality and HIV status. Am J Psychiatry 149:396–398, 1992

Moran MG, Dubester SN: Connective tissue diseases. In Stoudemire A, Fogel BS (eds): Psychiatric Care of the Medical Patient, pp 739–756. New York, Oxford University Press, 1994

O'Dowd MA, McKegney FP: AIDS, patients compared with others seen in psychiatric consultation. Gen Hosp Psychiatry 12:50–55, 1990

Perry SW: Organic mental disorders caused by HIV: update on early diagnosis and treatment. Am J Psychiatry 147:696–710, 1990.

Perry SW, Markowitz JC: Counseling for HIV testing. Hosp Commun Psychiatry 39:731–739, 1988

Rabkin JG, Ferrando S: A "second life" agenda. Psychiatric research issues raised by protease inhibitor treatments for people with the human immunodeficiency virus or the acquired immunodeficiency syndrome. Arch Gen Psychiatry 54:1049, 1997

Seth R, Granville-Grossman K, Goldmeier D, et al: Psychiatric illness in patients with HIV infection and AIDS. Br J Psychiatry 159:347–350, 1991

Sikkema KJ, Bissett RT: Concepts, goals, and techniques of counseling: review and implications for HIV counseling and testing. AIDS Education & Prevention 9:14, 1997

Starace F: Epidemiology of suicide among persons with AIDS. AIDS Care 7 (suppl 2):123–128, 1995

Stern RA, Singer NG, Silva SG, et al: Neurobehavioral functioning in a nonconfounded group of asymptomatic HIV-Seropositive homosexual men. Am J Psychiatry 149:1099–1102, 1992

Travin S, Lee HK, Bluestone H: Prevalence and characteristics of violent patients in a general hospital. NY State J Med 90:591–595, 1990

Volavka J, Convit A, Czobor P, et al: HIV seroprevalence and risk behaviors in psychiatric inpatients. Psychiatry Res 2:109–114, 1991

Wachter RM, Cooke M, Hopewell PC, et al: Attitude of medical residents regarding intensive care for patients with the acquired immunodeficiency syndrome. Arch Intern Med 148:149–152, 1988

Wheelan MA, Kricheff II, Handler M, et al: Acquired immunodeficiency syndrome: cerebral computed tomographic manifestations. Radiology 149:477–484, 1983

Wolcott DL, Fawzy F, Pasnau RO: Acquired immune deficiency syndrome (AIDS) and consultation–liaison psychiatry. Gen Hosp Psychiatry 7:280–292, 1986

22 The Evaluation and Management of Sleep Disorders

Karl Doghramji

THE SCOPE AND CONSEQUENCES OF SLEEP DISORDERS

Sleep-related complaints rank among the highest reported ailments in the population. In a recent large-scale demographic survery, sleep difficulties were voiced by 47% of the population; 35% experienced them on an occasional basis and 12% on a frequent basis (National Sleep Foundation Report, 1995). Sleep difficulties are also among the most frequently encountered problems in clinical medicine; in one study, 80% of the medical patients of a general hospital who received psychiatric consultation complained of disturbed sleep (Berlin et al, 1984). In another study, 58% of psychiatric outpatients reported sleep difficulties, compared with 21% of nonpatients.

Despite the ubiquity of sleep disturbances, scientists and physicians are only now beginning to understand the debilitation, misery, and suffering that sleep disorders cause. We now know, for example, that insomniacs have an increased risk for the development of emotional disturbances, most notably depressive and anxiety disorders (Ford and Kamerow, 1989; Tan et al, 1984). Sleep disorders also seem to be associated with impairments in proper mental functioning; 53% of chronic insomniacs complain of memory difficulties, and patients with obstructive sleep apnea syndrome have significant impairments in performance on complex motor tasks (Findley et al, 1986). It is not surprising, therefore, that inadequate sleep is associated with decreased work efficiency and impaired industrial productivity (Johnson and Spinweber, 1983) as well as an increased risk of traffic accidents (Mitler et al, 1988). Finally, sleep disorders seem to enhance the propensity for cardiovascular disease (Partinen et al, 1982) and increase the risk of death (Wingard and Berkman, 1983). Physicians should, therefore, be familiar with the techniques for the diagnosis and management of sleep disorders.

NORMAL HUMAN SLEEP

Sleep Stages and Architecture

Owing to the milestone discovery of rapid eye movement (REM) sleep by Aesrinsky and Kleitman in 1953, we now know that sleep is not simply the absence of wakefulness, but a complex behavioral, physiological, and psychological state that is the product of active and coordinated brain processes. One manifestation of these changes is the stages of sleep, which repeat in cyclical fashion throughout the night, forming a pattern widely known as sleep architecture.

Proper characterization of sleep stages necessitates the simultaneous monitoring of the numerous physiological parameters, a process known as polysomnography. Minimally required are the electroencephalogram (EEG), electrooculogram (EOG), and electromyogram (EMG) of skeletal muscle, usually the submentalis. EEG patterns for the sleep of a young adult are depicted in Figure 22–1. The EEG of individuals who are awake and attentive exhibits a pattern of low voltage and mixed ("random") frequencies. However, during relaxed wakefulness or drowsiness, the EEG reveals a preponderance of rhythmic alpha activity (8 to 12 cps). The transition from wakefulness to stage 1 sleep is marked by the disappearance of rhythmic alpha and the establishment of relatively low voltage and mixed frequency pattern with the prevalence of theta (3 to 7 cps) activity.

During stage 2, two characteristic waveforms are noted: *sleep spindles* (12 to 14 cps activity lasting 0.5 to 1.5 seconds) and *K complexes* (negative sharp waves followed by a slower positive component lasting 0.5 seconds or greater). Low-voltage *mixed-frequency* activity persists in the background. Sleep spindles are synchronized waveforms, i.e., have a uniform oscillatory pattern resulting from the simultaneous activation of a large number of neurons by one or more synchronizing pacemakers located in the thalamus. Spindles are found in all mammals and are identical in all species. They develop before the age of 3 months in humans and may be slower to develop in mental retardation. The significance of K complexes is unknown; they may occur spontaneously or in response to environmental noise.

During stages 3 and 4, high-amplitude *slow delta activity* (less than 2 cps) dominates the record. During stage 3 sleep, 20 to 50% of the tracing is comprised of delta waves, whereas during stage 4 sleep, more than 50% of the record is comprised of delta waves. Stages 3 and 4 sleep are collectively

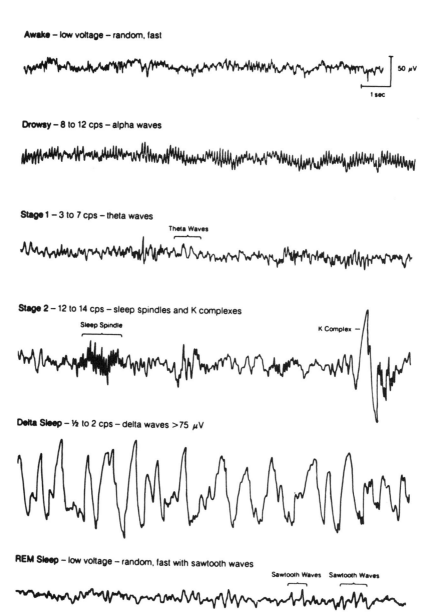

Awake – low voltage – random, fast

50 μV

1 sec

Drowsy – 8 to 12 cps – alpha waves

Stage 1 – 3 to 7 cps – theta waves

Theta Waves

Stage 2 – 12 to 14 cps – sleep spindles and K complexes

Sleep Spindle

K Complex –

Delta Sleep – ½ to 2 cps – delta waves >75 μV

REM Sleep – low voltage – random, fast with sawtooth waves

Sawtooth Waves   Sawtooth Waves

Figure 22–1.

referred to as *delta sleep, deep sleep,* and *slow wave sleep.* Well-formed delta waves are not seen until 2 to 6 months after birth. The emergence of delta sleep is a reflection of maturation in brain structure and function.

Although the eyes are still (other than occasional eye blinks) during relaxed wakefulness, involuntary ocular activity occurs just prior to the onset of stage 1 sleep (Fig. 22–2). On the EOG, this is noted as slow ("rolling") eye movements. These usually persist during the initial portions of stage 1. Eye movements are absent during stages 2, 3, and 4 (Fig. 22–3). During wakefulness, the EMG reveals phasic (episodic) bursts of activity. However, as individuals wind down prior to sleep, EMG tone (amplitude) gradually diminishes and continues to do so as sleep progresses through the various stages. Stages 1 through 4 are collectively referred to as non-REM (NREM) sleep and constitute approximately 75% of total sleep time in adults.

During REM sleep, the EEG again displays low-voltage mixed frequencies. However, characteristic rapid eye movements are noted on the EOG, and the EMG displays the lowest amplitude of the night, a reflection of skeletal muscle atonia mediated through active CNS inhibition (Fig. 22–4).

Sleep is typically entered through stage 1, and an orderly progression from stages 1 through 4 occurs within 45 minutes of falling asleep. Within 90 minutes, the first REM period occurs. This NREM–REM pattern, referred to as a sleep cycle, lasts approximately 90 minutes and recurs continuously throughout the night (Fig. 22–5). Although this cycle is present at birth, each cycle lasts 50 to 60 minutes in neonates.

Delta sleep is most prominent in the first third of the night and virtually disappears during the last third of the night. Greater periods of prior sleep deprivation result in longer periods of delta sleep in the beginning of the night on

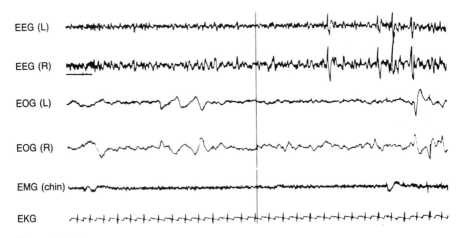

Figure 22–2.

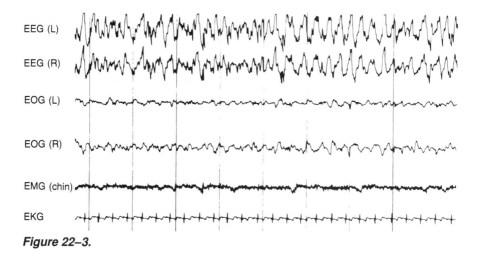

Figure 22–3.

subsequent nights. In contrast, REM sleep periods, although initially brief in duration, lengthen with each subsequent sleep cycle such that REM sleep is most prominent in the last third of the night. This pattern is relatively independent of prior sleep deprivation and is thought to be controlled by a circadian oscillator in the brain, one that also controls body temperature, the concentration of plasma cortisol, and other biological cycles.

The percentage distribution of sleep stages in a young adult is outlined in Table 22–1. Many factors alter these percentages. For example, conditions that

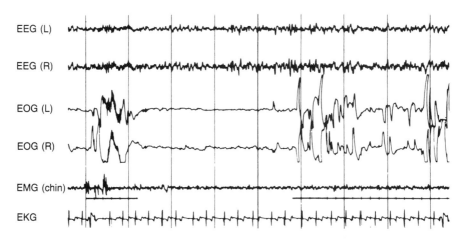

Figure 22–4.

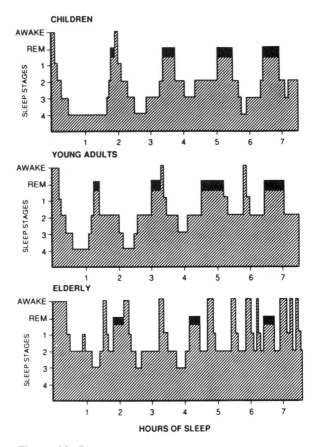

Figure 22–5.

produce sleep disruption, such as disease states and environmental noise, cause an increase in the proportion of stage 1 sleep and a decrease in delta sleep. Age also has profound effects on sleep. Delta sleep is maximal in children and diminishes markedly with age, especially during adolescence. Seniors may have little or no delta sleep. The loss of delta sleep with age may be a consequence of the diminution in cortical synaptic activity. In contrast, stage 1

Table 22–1 **Percentage of Sleep Stages in a Young Adult**

REM	25
NREM	75
Stage 1	(5)
Stage 2	(45)
Stages 3 and 4	(25)

sleep increases with age. With aging, there is a general tendency toward sleep fragmentation, characterized by an increase in the frequency of awakenings and brief arousals.

Sleep Depth

The arousal threshold is lowest for stage 1 sleep, i.e., the volume of environmental sound needed to awaken a sleeper from this stage is the lowest. The arousal threshold is highest for delta sleep (hence the synonym "deep" sleep) and variable for REM. Delta sleep also appears to be the most refreshing, and deprivation of this sleep stage often results in daytime sleepiness despite adequate length of sleep. The sense of unrefreshing sleep reported by the elderly is often related to low percentages of delta sleep.

Sleep Needs

Although the precise function of sleep is unknown, Rechtschaffen and his colleagues (1989) recently demonstrated that the lack of sleep leads to serious physical harm and even death in laboratory animals. One day of sleeplessness in humans has minimal effects on cognitive function the following day. However, with greater deprivation of sleep, performance on tasks is impaired. Therefore, adequate time spent asleep is desirable. Nevertheless, the need for sleep is highly variable from person to person. Although the average nightly sleep duration is approximately 8 hours, children obtain about 10 hours and the elderly less than 7 hours. Sleep lengths vary even within similar age groups, with some individuals requiring as little as 3 hours of nightly sleep. The most prudent answer to the question "How much sleep do I need?" is the amount of sleep that results in optimal daytime alertness and a sense of mental efficiency and well-being.

When discussing sleep needs, consideration should also be given to the need for optimal sleep quality, as this also contributes to daytime alertness. Sleep quality refers to the integrity of the sleep architectural pattern. Impairments in sleep quality appear polysomnographically as an increase in the number of arousals (brief awakenings and stage changes), awakenings, and body movements; an increase in the shallow stages of sleep (1 and 2); a decrease in deep (delta) sleep; and a decrease in the number of well-formed sleep cycles.

Sleep Deprivation and Rebound

On the first night following total sleep deprivation, a rebound of delta sleep is noted first, i.e., delta sleep is recovered at the expense of other sleep stages. REM rebound occurs later during the night or on subsequent nights.

These and other findings are the bases for the belief of many sleep researchers that delta sleep is related to the maintenance of important biological functions. Additionally, selective deprivation of either delta or REM sleep for long periods of time also results in a subsequent rebound in the proportion of that particular sleep stage. For example, REM rebound is often seen following the abrupt discontinuation of drugs that suppress REM activity, such as certain antidepressant agents, and is often experienced as vivid dreaming and nightmares.

Cognitive and Behavioral Aspects of Sleep

Cognitive mental processes seem to be at a low level during stage 1 sleep as sleepers who are awakened from it usually report experiencing thought fragments or vague images. Most individuals awakened from delta sleep report no mental activity at all. In contrast, most sleepers report dreams when awakened from REM sleep. Dreaming also occurs during REM sleep in laboratory animals. Dreaming is only one facet of a host of complex biological processes that are activated during REM sleep and that affect almost every bodily function. These produce, among other things, rapid eye movements, bursts of tachycardia, penile tumescence, and peripheral skeletal muscle atonia. The observation of a highly active mind superimposed on a picture of a motionless paralyzed body led earlier researchers to refer to REM sleep as "paradoxical" sleep.

The onset of sleep is characterized by a reduced responsiveness to environmental stimuli. Individuals asked to respond to sound or light have an increased reaction time as they approach sleep and no longer react following established sleep. Consequently, sleep-deprived automobile drivers tend to react sluggishly to traffic hazards and are more vulnerable to traffic accidents. Nevertheless, responsiveness to important stimuli is typically maintained during normal sleep, as in the case of a sleeping mother's selective sensitivity to her baby's crying. Sleep also produces retrograde amnesia; memory for events just prior to the onset of sleep is lost if ensuing sleep lasts for more than a few minutes. This phenomenon is the basis for not recollecting the moment of sleep onset or the events that occur during brief awakenings during the course of the night.

POLYSOMNOGRAPHY

Polysomnography is typically performed in specialized facilities called sleep disorder centers or sleep laboratories. Many are staffed by physicians specializing in sleep disorders medicine. In preparation for polysomnography, patients are introduced to their sleeping quarters during their initial office-based evaluation, and provisions are made for special needs. On the night of the test, they arrive at the laboratory well in advance of the study time in order to acclimate to the new environment. Studies are conducted in noise-free and private rooms, and comfort is maximized by making rooms esthetically pleasing. Contrary to their commonly expressed concerns, most patients experience their sleep in the laboratory to be the same as, and at times even better than, their sleep at home.

As noted above, characterization of sleep stages requires, at the minimum, the EEG, EOG, and EMG of the submentalis. However, a typical clinical polysomnogram also includes monitors for airflow at the nose and mouth, respiratory effort strain gauges placed around the chest and abdomen, and noninvasive oxygen saturation monitors that function by introducing a beam of light through the skin. Other parameters include the electrocardiogram and EMG of the anterior tibialis muscles, which are intended to detect periodic leg movements. Finally, patients' gross body movements are continuously monitored by audiovisual means.

The most commonly employed form of polysomnography, referred to as the nocturnal polysomnogram (NPSG), is conducted during the typical sleeping hours of the patient and identifies pathological processes during sleep. Another form is the multiple sleep latency test (MSLT). This test provides an objective measure of daytime somnolence. Objectively derived assessments of the severity of daytime somnolence are of great clinical importance since sleepy patients often cannot accurately estimate the severity of their own sleepiness. For example, patients who are so sleepy that they regularly succumb to involuntary sleep attacks—sleep episodes that strike without warning—may deny feeling sleepy. The procedure is appropriately performed in any disease state associated with daytime somnolence. The MSLT is also necessary to establish the diagnosis of narcolepsy definitively. During the MSLT, patients are monitored polysomnographically in a darkened room while lying down in their sleep laboratory beds and are instructed not to resist the urge to fall asleep. They are allowed these opportunities to nap at 2-hour intervals throughout the day. The speed of falling asleep during naps, referred to as the sleep latency, is an indicator of the severity of daytime sleepiness. An average sleep latency of less than 10 minutes indicates, by convention, a clinically significant degree of daytime sleepiness, and one less than 5 minutes implies the presence of a severe degree of daytime sleepiness and an increased risk of sleep attacks. The maintenance of wakefulness test (MWT) is another test that measures daytime somnolence. In contrast to the MSLT, during the MWT, patients are instructed to remain awake while sitting in a dimly lit room. The MWT strives to assess the ability of individuals to resist the urge to fall asleep as they are engaged in soporific activities of daily life, such as driving or reading. Normative values for the MWT have been established (Doghramji et al, 1997); the inability to remain awake for longer than 11 minutes is abnormal. Additional specialized forms of polysomnography include nocturnal penile tumescence monitoring for the assessment of impotence and gastroesophageal pH monitoring for the assessment of sleep-related gastroesophageal reflux.

Ambulatory (home) monitoring was recently introduced, whereby patients are monitored in their natural settings, such as the home or hospital bed. Ambulatory monitoring has the advantage of minimizing the artifactual contributions of the laboratory environment and makes polysomnography possible for those who cannot travel to a laboratory. Cost-containment efforts have also seen a greater reliance on ambulatory screen studies, i.e., studies performed with a minimal number of channels (such as oximetry) and not attended by a technician. Concerns remain regarding the potential for errors of omission. Therefore, the role of screen studies remains, at present, unclear.

SPECIFIC SLEEP DISORDERS

The disorders listed below adhere to the nomenclature of the International Classification of Sleep Disorders (Diagnostic Classification Steering Committee, 1990). (DSM-IV also has a nomenclature for sleep disorders.)

Inadequate Sleep Hygiene

Many individuals unknowingly engage in habitual behaviors that harm sleep. Insomniacs, for example, often compensate for lost sleep by delaying their morning awakening time or by napping, which actually have the effect of further fragmenting nocturnal sleep. Instead, insomniacs should be advised to adhere to a regular awakening time, regardless of the amount of sleep, and to avoid naps. Other sleep hygiene measures are outlined in Table 22–2. These measures, in written form, are often helpful when given to patients by physicians for home use.

Table 22–2 **Sleep Hygiene Measures**

---

1. Sleep as much as needed to feel alert during the day, but not more. Curtailing the time in bed seems to solidify sleep; excessive time spent in bed seems to fragment sleep.
2. Establish in the morning a regular awakening time that you can adhere to every day, including weekends and vacations. Such regularity strengthens circadian cycling.
3. Exercise performed regularly, but not too close to bedtime, probably deepens sleep.
4. Excessive noise may disturb sleep; insulate your room against loud noises.
5. Excessive warmth disturbs sleep. Keep the room temperature at a comfortable level.
6. A light snack prior to bedtime may improve sleep, although a large meal and excessive fluids close to bedtime may have the opposite effect.
7. Caffeinated beverages disturb sleep, even though you may not be aware of their effect.
8. Alcoholic beverages, which may assist in falling asleep, can significantly fragment sleep.
9. If you feel angry and frustrated because you cannot fall asleep, don't try harder to fall asleep. Instead, leave the bedroom and do something not very stimulating, like reading a boring book.
10. The chronic use of tobacco and alcohol disturbs sleep.

Insufficient Sleep Syndrome

Persons affected with this disorder voluntarily curtail their time in bed, usually in response to social and occupational demands. Although sleep reduction may be as little as 1 hour per night, over long periods of time, such a pattern may lead to daytime hypersomnolence and result in impairment. Sleep logs usually reveal extended bedtime hours on weekends and holidays, during which individuals often awaken spontaneously in the morning. Treatment with stimulant agents is rarely warranted, as no degree of accruing chronic sleep debt can be overcome by stimulant agents. Instead, sufferers, usually younger adults, should be urged to extend bedtimes on a daily basis.

Adjustment Sleep Disorder

This common disorder is caused by acute emotional stressors such as a job loss or a hospitalization. The result is an insomnia, typically a difficulty in falling asleep, mediated through tension and anxiety. Symptoms usually remit shortly following the abatement of the stressors. Treatment is warranted if daytime sleepiness and fatigue interfere with functioning or if the disorder lasts for more than a few weeks. Treatment modalities are similar to those outlined for psychophysiological insomnia (see below).

Psychophysiological Insomnia

Although insomnia may be *initiated* by a wide variety of stressors and conditions, it may persist well beyond the resolution of these factors, due to the emergence of *perpetuating* factors such as conditioned arousal at bedtime. Patients develop *anticipatory anxiety* over the prospect of another night of sleeplessness followed by another day of fatigue. Anxiety typically *increases* as bedtime approaches and reaches maximum intensity following retiring to bed. Sufferers often spend hours in bed awake focused on and brooding over their sleeplessness, which, in turn, aggravates their insomnia even further. Persistent psychophysiological insomnia often complicates other sleep disorders.

The diagnosis of psychophysiological insomnia is supported by a history of difficulty in falling asleep selectively related to the patient's own bedroom. Patients also report approaching bedtimes at home with intense anxiety and dread. Although they may have "hard-driving" personalities, psychiatric evaluations usually do not uncover diagnosable psychopathology.

During the clinical examination, patients may appear tense. Personality inventories such as the Minnesota Multiphasic Personality Inventory reveal patterns consistent with somatization of tension. Although polysomnography is not usually necessary to confirm the diagnosis, it can be useful in ruling out other concurrent sleep disorders.

Behavioral and pharmacological treatments are available for the disorder. The former usually take a longer time to implement, yet have the advantage of longer lasting benefit. Pharmacological treatments, in contrast, provide rapid relief from symptoms, yet may not provide definitive resolution unless combined with behavioral and psychotherapeutic measures. The most commonly utilized behavioral measure is relaxation training. There are many types, and the choice of therapy depends on the patient's preference. EMG biofeedback training strives to reduce muscle tension. During this treatment, the EMG tension of skeletal muscle, typically the temporalis, is monitored electronically and translated into an auditory tone to the patient. The heightened awareness of muscle tension gives the patient direct feedback while engaging in progressive relaxation exercises. These methods are then practiced at home prior to bedtime. This is usually supplemented by cognitive psychotherapy, which strives to identify and dispel thoughts that are tension producing and that have a negative effect upon sleep, such as the preoccupation with unpleasant work experiences or examinations at school (see Chapter 17). During sessions, patients' fears regarding sleeplessness can be overcome by reassurance and by suggestions that they deal with anxiety-producing thoughts during sessions and at times other than bedtime.

Stimulus control therapy, introduced by Bootzin et al (1991), is also effective and strives to interrupt the learned association between the bedroom setting and tension. The most salient features of stimulus control therapy are to ask patients to use the bed only for sleep (not for reading or watching television) and to not stay in bed trying to sleep for more than 10 minutes at a time, but to go into another room and to return to bed only after feeling sleepy. Patients repeat this maneuver as many times as necessary without extending their time in bed beyond their usual arising time. They are also urged to avoid napping. Compliance with these measures is monitored by sleep logs. Other forms of therapy include insight-oriented psychotherapy, which strives to enhance patients' awareness of ongoing psychological conflicts that stem from prior years and that contribute to sleeplessness through the production of anxiety. Also highly effective for this type of insomnia are hypnotic agents that afford patients a few nights' sleep and, by so doing, diminish concerns regarding the potential for relentless insomnia that are at the heart of the disorder. Hypnotic agents can be gradually discontinued after a brief period of nightly treatment. Finally, sleep hygiene measures should be closely adhered to during and after the termination of treatment, regardless of type.

Sleep Apnea Syndromes

The two types of sleep apnea syndrome are *obstructive sleep apnea syndrome* (OSA) and *central sleep apnea syndrome* (CSA). Their prevalence has been estimated at 1 to 3% of the population (Lavie, 1983). In OSA, the pharyngeal walls collapse repetitively during sleep, causing intermittent sleep-related upper airway obstruction and cessation in ventilation (apneas). In CSA, cessation of ventilation is related to a concomitant loss of inspiratory effort. Isolated cases of pure CSA are rare; instead, CSA usually coexists with OSA, in which case the latter is considered to be the primary pathological entity.

Upper airway closure in OSA is thought to occur because of a failure of the genioglossus and other upper airway dilator muscles. Apneas are accompanied by cyclic asphyxia (hypoxemia, hypercarbia, and acidosis), which, in turn, often results in cardiac arrhythmias. Pulmonary and systemic hypertension are evident during apneas. Cardiac output falls during apneas and rises to normal levels following their termination.

Apneas are terminated by arousals, which are sudden generalized activations of the brain that result in transient disruptions of sleep. Arousals also lead to profound sleep fragmentation and poor sleep quality, which are thought to be responsible for the daytime hypersomnolence and emotional consequences of the disorder, discussed further below.

The major presenting symptoms of OSA are summarized in Table 22–3. Snoring is a source of embarrassment and may place significant strain on interpersonal relationships as spouses resort to sleeping in separate beds or bedrooms. Since patients are unaware of their own snoring, bedpartners and family members must be questioned in this regard during the evaluation of OSA. Naps, although frequent, are usually not refreshing. Less commonly, patients complain of repeated awakenings during the course of the night. Many adopt unusual positions during sleep, such as sitting up in bed or kneeling at the bedside, usually in association with severe hypoxemia. Sleepwalking and nocturnal vocalizations are common, as are profuse sweating, sleep-related enuresis, and gastroesophageal reflux. Many patients awaken in the morning with frontal headaches, possibly as a result of episodic asphyxia and consequent cerebral vasodilatation, and with mouth dryness, resulting possibly from the continuous flapping of the upper airways during snoring. Most patients are obese at the time of presentation and report gaining weight gradually over the years, often despite heroic attempts to curb this process through diet and exercise. However, normal weight does not preclude the diagnosis. OSA has been diagnosed in normal weight individuals, particularly those with oral phyrangeal airway anomalies.

Cardiovascular diseases are common in individuals suffering from OSA. Inhibited sexual desire, impotence, and ejaculatory impairment are reported

Table 22–3 **Major Symptoms of Obstructive Sleep Apnea Syndrome**

Loud snoring
Reports of prolonged pauses in respiration during sleep
Daytime hypersomnolence
Disturbed, nonrefreshing sleep
Weight gain

by nearly a third of patients. If left untreated, the illness may be associated with increased mortality (He et al, 1988). Depression is also common and is often accompanied by marked irritability, agitation, heightened anxiety, and occasionally aggressiveness leading to violent outbursts (Doghramji, 1993). Spouses often are alarmed by sudden changes in personality as the condition escalates in severity. Many patients misuse alcohol to control anxiety and stimulants to stay awake.

OSA sufferers demonstrate deficits in attention, motor efficiency, and graphomotor ability (Greenberg et al, 1987) as well as in concentration, complex problem-solving, and short-term recall (Findley et al, 1986) in proportion to the severity of the hypoxemia. OSA patients have been found to hit a greater number of road obstacles than controls when operating driving simulators (Findley et al, 1989) and are known to have a high rate of auto accidents (Findley et al, 1988).

In a recent study by Kales and colleagues (1985), 66% of patients reported a deterioration in interpersonal relationships, and 64% reported marital discord that they attributed to the disorder; 84% reported occupational impairment, 62% had fallen asleep on the job, and 13% had left their jobs because of the condition. Many also reported academic difficulties secondary to sleepiness.

The male to female ratio is 10 to 1, yet the prevalence increases among females following menopause, presumably related to weight gain. The onset of symptoms is usually in the third decade of life to middle age and the prevalence increases dramatically with age and ranges from 31 to 67% in elderly men (Smallwood et al, 1983). Nevertheless, OSA has been identified in children.

Factors that predipose individuals to OSA are summarized in Table 22–4. Sedating pharmacological agents, including alcohol and benzodiazepine anxiolytic agents such as diazepam and alprazolam, tend to increase the duration and frequency of apneas. Therefore, benzodiazepines are contraindicated for untreated patients.

Table 22–4 **Predisposing Factors for Obstructive Sleep Apnea Syndrome**

Nasal obstruction
Large uvula
Low-lying soft palate
Retrognathia, micrognathia, and other craniofacial abnormalities
Excessive and redundant pharyngeal tissue
Pharyngeal masses such as tumors or cysts
Macroglossia
Tonsilar hypertrophy
Vocal cord paralysis
Obesity
Hypothyroidism
Acromegaly

If the disorder is suspected following the office-based evaluation, nocturnal polysomnography should be performed so that the diagnosis can be conclusively established. This test reveals obstructive apneas, defined as cessations in air flow through the nares or mouth lasting 10 seconds or greater with the concomitant resumption of inspiratory efforts. It also reveals obstructive hypopneas in which air flow diminishes, yet does not completely cease. The syndrome is often polysomnographically defined by a frequency of breathing abnormalities [respiratory disturbance index (RDI)] of more than 5 per hour of sleep. However, this threshold is based on convention; therefore, a lower RDI in the presence of severe oxyhemoglobin desaturation and frequent cardiac dysrhythmias may be sufficient to warrant a clinical diagnosis of OSA.

Many options exist for the management of the syndrome. Continuous positive airway pressure (CPAP) applied via a nasal mask is the most commonly utilized because of its greatest efficacy and least potential for adverse effects. Recently, laser-assisted uvuloplasty (LAUP), an office-based procedure performed with local anesthesia, has largely replaced the uvulopalatopharyngoplasty surgery, an intraoperative procedure performed under general anesthesia. In both, portions of the uvula and soft palate are removed. Although both are highly effective for the elimination of snoring, both also suffer from lower efficacy than CPAP for pathogenic apneas. Furthermore, studies attempting to identify preoperatively characteristics of patients that would predict postoperative success have been disappointing (see, for example, Doghramji et al, 1995).

Although tracheostomy can provide definitive resolution of pathogenic apneas, it is reserved for cases of severe apnea that cannot be managed by CPAP or LAUP. Nasal surgery can be helpful in patients with mild-to-moderate OSA who also have some degree of nasal airway compromise. Dental devices that prevent mandibular collapse or tongue retrusion during sleep have also seen a recent increase in popularity. Pharmacological agents may be effective in mild cases; many antidepressants are also REM suppressants and, if apneas occur mostly during REM sleep, their use can diminish the frequency of these REM-related apneas. Serotonergic mechanisms have been implicated in the control of respiration during sleep, and the use of serotonin-reuptake inhibtor antidepressants such as fluoxetine may, therefore, also diminish apnea frequency independently of their effects on REM. Oxygen has also been reported to be efficacious in certain cases. Weight loss is also recommended as it may lead to diminution of severity in some patients, although it cannot be relied on as the sole treatment measure, as results are unpredictable. Patients must also be urged to refrain from using alcohol, hypnotic agents, and other central nervous system (CNS) depressant agents, as these can exacerbate the condition. Regardless of treatment type, polysomnography should always be performed following treatment to ensure that pathogenic events have resolved or diminished.

CPAP is an ambulatory device that introduces room air at a high flow rate into the upper airway via a nasal mask. The optimum pressure required to eliminate apneas is determined through polysomnography with a variable pressure device, following which patients utilize CPAP at a constant pressure at home while asleep. The primary complication in the use of CPAP is noncompliance; half of patients prescribed it actually use it regularly (Kribbs et al, 1993). Patterns of noncompliance range from using the treatment for portions of each night to not using it at all. Reasons for noncompliance are numerous and include complaints of upper airway irritation that can often be adequately managed with humidification, discomfort at the mask site, and feelings of suffocation, among others. A number of CPAP variants have been recently introduced to enhance comfort, including bilevel positive airway pressure devices that deliver lower pressures during expiration than inspiration, and demand-pressure devices that tailor the pressure delivered to the severity of apneas on an ongoing basis.

Concurrent depression and psychosocial and marital difficulties can be addressed by psychotherapy. If psychiatric symptoms are severe, they should be treated aggressively since they can also impact on the effectiveness of the management of the OSA by causing noncompliance. Antidepressants that are alerting, such as protriptyline, fluoxetine, or bupropion, are presumably best suited to manage depression, which is often accompanied by daytime hypersomnolence. Chronic anxiety, which may complicate the picture, should not be managed with benzodiazepines; instead, the nonbenzodiazepine anxiolytic buspirone, which does not appear to aggravate OSA, is often effective, as are behavioral techniques.

If CSA is diagnosed, an attempt should be made to uncover underlying conditions. Although many cases of CSA are idiopathic, it can also be seen in congestive heart failure, nasal obstruction, certain neurological disorders, and following trips to high altitudes. Treatment is directed at the specific abnormality if one is uncovered. However, treatment of the idiopathic variety is often inadequate. Acetazolamide, protriptyline, clomipramine, medroxyprogesterone, and oxygen have met with variable results. Diaphragmatic pacing or mechanical ventilation must be considered in refractory cases. Regardless of the approach chosen, monitoring the course of treatment with polysomnography is essential, as some treatments such as oxygen may actually exacerbate the condition. CNS depressants such as hypnotic agents and alcohol may have a similar effect and must therefore be avoided.

Narcolepsy

Narcolepsy is a lifelong condition that affects more than 250,000 Americans. It is idiopathic, yet thought to be related to neurochemical abnormalities in the brain. Its peak age of onset is the second decade. A genetic basis for the disorder has long been suspected since a familial pattern has been noted in certain breeds of narcoleptic dogs. More recently, clarification of human narcolepsy genetics has been provided by the near 100% association between narcolepsy and the DQB1-0602 and DQA1-0102 (DQ1) human leukocyte antigen (HLA) genes (Mignot et al, 1994). In contrast, the incidence of these genes in the general population is lower.

The five major symptoms of narcolepsy, summarized in Table 22–5, include the following:

1. Persistent daytime sleepiness, the most common presenting complaint. It is usually accompanied by daytime naps that, unlike the case of OSA, are brief (typically 15 minutes) and result in increased alertness. Naps are often accompanied by vivid dreams.

2. Cataplexy, an abrupt paralysis or paresis of skeletal muscles that usually follows waking hour emotional experiences such as anger, surprise, laughter, or physical exercise. It may be generalized, in which case the patient typically collapses, or isolated to an individual muscle group, resulting in transient loss of function. The episode typically lasts a few minutes, during which the patient is awake. Following its termination, the patient typically regains function without any residual impairment. Although cataplexy is the pathognomonic symptom of narcolepsy, it can only be elicited in up to 50% of interviews. Cataplexy should not be confused with its near-homonym *catalepsy*, or *waxy flexibility*, an unrelated phenomenon noted in schizophrenia of the catatonic type. Catalepsy is also not an epileptic phenomenon.

3. Hypnagogic (or hypnopompic) hallucinations, which are vivid and often frightening dreams that occur shortly after falling asleep (or upon awakening).

4. Sleep paralysis, a transient global paralysis of voluntary muscles that usually occurs shortly after falling asleep and lasts a few seconds or minutes. Cataplexy, hypnagogic hallucinations, and sleep paralysis are thought to be manifestations of an underlying aberration in the control of the timing of REM sleep, which, in turn, results in "attacks" of REM sleep during wakefulness. These, in turn, result in the occurrence of the physical

Table 22–5 **Major Symptoms of Narcolepsy**

Persistent daytime sleepiness
Cataplexy
Hypnagogic or hypnopompic hallucinations
Sleep paralysis
Restless and disturbed sleep

and cognitive manifestations of REM sleep while individuals are awake.

5. Disturbed and restless sleep, characterized by numerous awakenings and arousals.

Narcoleptics develop significant psychosocial impairments, such as job loss and interpersonal difficulties, as a result of daytime hypersomnolence. They are also susceptible to auto accidents and to sustaining injuries as a result of falling asleep in inappropriate situations. Many develop depression, anxiety, and substance-use difficulties.

Other than the obvious behavioral manifestations of excessive daytime sleepiness (yawning, drooping eyelids, psychomotor retardation), physical examination is typically unrevealing in narcolepsy. If the diagnosis is suspected, it must be confirmed by an NPSG, followed by an MSLT. The former is performed to ensure adequate nocturnal sleep and the lack of intrinsic sleep disorders. The NPSG often reveals a very short REM latency and sleep fragmentation caused by numerous awakenings and arousals. The average MSLT sleep latency in narcoleptics is usually less than 10 minutes and often less than 5 minutes. Additionally, the MSLT reveals REM episodes during at least two naps, an abnormal phenomenon that is highly diagnostic for the disorder.

Treatment of narcolepsy is directed at daytime somnolence, REM-related aberrations, and psychosocial consequences. In milder cases, excessive sleepiness can be managed with conservative measures, such as spending an adequate time in bed, taking two or three daily naps, and avoiding alcohol and other sedating substances. Even in more severe cases, judiciously timed naps may minimize the dosage of medication required to control symptoms. Commonly utilized medications for excessive sleepiness include pemoline 18.75 to 112.5 mg/day, methylphenidate 5 to 60 mg/day, and dextroamphetamine 5 to 60 mg/day. In refractory cases, mazindol 3 to 6 mg/day, a tricyclic compound with anorexic properties, may be utilized. Tolerance may be minimized by prescribing the lowest effective dose and asking patients to take regular drug holidays on days when their need for alertness is lowest. Modafinil is a stimulant that may be introduced for clinical use in the United States, and the first compound specifically indicated for narcolepsy. With single doses of 200 and 400 mg, it appears to be an effective alerting agent and may prove to be less likely to produce tolerance after extended use than the amphetamines and methylphenidate (Buguet et al, 1995). Despite improvement in the subjective sense of daytime alertness, many clinicians remain concerned regarding the potential for impairments in alertness while patients are engaged in critical tasks such as driving and operating heavy machinery; sleep attacks in such settings can jeopardize the health of the patient, as well as that of others. In such cases, follow-up MWTs may be helpful.

The REM-related symptoms of cateplexy—hypnagogic hallucinations and sleep paralysis—can be controlled with REM-suppressant medications, such as tricyclic antidepressants. The ones more commonly utilized are those with the least likelihood of producing sedation, such as protriptyline. The serotonin-specific reuptake inhibitor antidepressants, fluoxetine, sertraline, and paroxetine, may also be effective in this regard and may also provide partial relief for daytime somnolence since they are, for the most part, alerting agents. Many narcoleptics also require emotional support. Education also plays a key role in management, as peers, parents, teachers, and patients themselves may confuse the effects of drowsiness with laziness or lack of motivation.

Idiopathic Hypersomnolence

This is a lifelong and incurable disorder that has a variable age of onset. Its mode of acquisition, whether acquired or inherited, is unclear. The most prominent symptom is unrelenting daytime somnolence. Patients spend lengthy periods of time sleeping at night only to awaken feeling more sleepy. They take frequent and lengthy daytime naps. However, unlike narcoleptics, they awaken from these feeling unrefreshed. Additionally, naps are rarely accompanied by dreams. As a result of their chronic debilitation, patients experience lifelong impairment in relationships and employment. In fact, many cannot support themselves financially. Many suffer from depression.

Polysomnography reveals long nocturnal sleep without evidence of other sleep pathology. The MSLT reveals pathologically short sleep latencies without REM periods. Treatment principles are similar to those outlined for narcolepsy. However, treatment is often unsatisfactory.

Periodic Limb Movement Disorder (Nocturnal Myoclonus)

Also referred to as nocturnal myoclonus, this disorder is characterized by the repetitive (usually every 20 to 40 seconds) twitching or kicking of the lower extremities during sleep. Patients usually present with the complaint of unrelenting insomnia, most often characterized by repeated awakenings following sleep onset. A minority complain of chronic daytime hypersomnolence. In either case, they are unaware of the movements and the brief arousals that follow and have no lasting sensation in the extremities. The disorder is more common in middle and older age. Although often idiopathic, the disorder can be seen in association with drug withdrawal states, sleep apnea syndrome, narcolepsy, chronic renal and hepatic failure, and during treatment with certain medications such as tricyclic antidepressants. Movements are often exacerbated by stress.

Bedpartners should be questioned for kicking or jerking movements on the part of the patient. Other factors and conditions related to the disorder should be searched for via a thorough history, physical examination, and blood tests. Polysomnography will confirm the diagnosis.

Treatment of the idiopathic syndrome is indicated if symptoms interfere with daytime functioning or psychological well-being. Agents that have been shown to have clinical efficacy in methodologically sound clinical trials include baclofen 20 to 40 mg, triazolam 0.125 to 0.25 mg, clonazepam 0.5 to 1.0 mg, and carbidopa 25 mg with levodopa 100 mg. Clonazepam is the most widely utilized. Since the disorder is usually chronic in course, long-term treatment may be necessary; weekly drug holidays may be effective in minimizing tolerance.

Restless Legs Syndrome

The hallmark of this disorder, also referred to as Ekbom's disease, is a "creeping" sensation in the lower extremities and irresistible leg kicks that affect patients upon reclining, prior to falling asleep. Unlike the previous disorder, patients are all too aware of these phenomena and resort to moving the affected extremity by stretching, kicking, or walking to relieve symptoms. As a result, they complain of intense difficulty in falling asleep. Many patients are depressed, irritable, and angry. Psychosocial impairment such as job loss and relationship difficulties is quite common.

The disorder is more common in later age and is exacerbated by pregnancy, fatigue, environmental temperature extremes, the intake of caffeinated beverages and tricyclic antidepressants, and drug withdrawal states. Akathisia from neuroleptics or fluoxetine should also be considered (see Chapter 18). It is usually idiopathic, yet has been noted in association with a variety of medical disorders, including pernicious anemia (vitamin B_{12} deficiency), iron deficiency, uremia, leukemia, rheumatoid arthritis, and fibromyositis (or fibromyalgia—a syndrome of nonspecific "aches and pains" without evidence of immunological dysfunction).

Polysomnography almost always reveals periodic leg muscle bursts during quiet wakefulness and sleep, the latter associated with arousals and awakenings. The syndrome should be distinguished from nocturnal leg cramps that involve pain in the deep muscles of the lower extremities and that are independent of sleep. The treatment of the disorder is essentially the same as periodic limb movement disorder.

Drug-Related Sleep Disorders

Recreational, over-the-counter, and prescription drugs can cause disturbed sleep and excessive daytime somnolence, as summarized in Tables 22–6 and 22–7. It should be noted that, although the agents listed in Table 22–6 are associated with insomnia following short-term use, their cessation following long-term administration at high dosages often results in withdrawal symptoms, including sleepiness, lassitude, and irritability. Similarly, the cessation of agents associated with daytime sleepiness (Table 22–7) can, after prolonged use, result in insomnia. It should also be noted that although caffeine has a

Table 22–6 **Pharmacological Agents That Can Cause Insomnia**

Monoamine oxidase inhibitors
Selective serotonin-antidepressants (SSRIs)
Bupropion
Anticancer agents
Steroids
Decongestants
Bronchodilators
Weight loss agents
Thyroid preparations
Xanthine derivatives (caffeine, theophylline, etc.)
Nicotine
Stimulants (cocaine, ephedrine, methylphenidate,
   amphetamines, etc.)

half-life in plasma of 3 to 7 hours, its absorption from the gastrointestinal tract can be erratic, and there are wide variations in individual sensitivity to it. Therefore, caffeinated beverages consumed even early in the day can still negatively affect sleep quality at night.

Circadian Rhythm Sleep Disorders

This group of disorders features a disturbance in the coordination between internal and environmental circadian rhythms involving the sleep–wake cycle. Thus, patients typically present with complaints of insomnia, excessive daytime somnolence, or both. These conditions are commonly associated with peptic ulcer disease, gastritis, irritability, and depression. Patients often misuse alcohol and hypnotic agents to promote sleep and stimulants to stay awake (Segawa et al, 1987).

One of the most common disorders in this group is *time zone change (jet lag) syndrome,* caused by rapid travel across time zones and resulting in a mismatch between the sleep schedules of the body and that of the new envi-

Table 22–7 **Pharmacological Agents That Can Cause Excessive Daytime Sleepiness**

Alcohol
Antihypertensive agents
Sedative–hypnotic agents
Anxiolytic agents
Antipsychotic agents
Trazodone, some tricyclic antidepressants
Opioids and other analgesic agents
Cannabis

ronment. Eastward flight results in more severe symptoms than westward travel. The severity of symptoms is also related to the number of time zones crossed; travel across more than two to three time zones surpasses the adaptive capabilities of the body. Such travel often leads to a desynchronization between internal body rhythms as well, such as those of temperature, sleep, and hormone secretion. When coupled with the curtailment of sleep length and the disturbance of sleep quality caused by any new environment, this leads to the symptoms of the disorder.

Jet lag countermeasures include the utilization of short-acting hypnotic agents for brief periods following arrival in the new locale. A safer and more effective method, however, is simply to maximize exposure to daylight in the new locale, which has the effect of resetting circadian rhythms with the environment. Individuals should also be urged to shift their sleep/wake schedules gradually prior to travel to coincide approximately with those of their destination.

Another circadian rhythm sleep disorder is *shift work sleep disorder*. Most problematic is variable shift work in which shifts are rotated or changed frequently; sleep times typically must be changed accordingly. This often leads to poor sleep quality immediately following the new shift, which is followed by a period of adaptation. The severity of symptoms is proportional to the frequency with which shifts are changed, the magnitude of each change, and the frequency of counterclockwise (phase-advancing) changes. However, even fixed-shift workers who must sleep during the day experience difficulties since daytime noise and light often interfere with the quality of their sleep and since they often change their sleep times for social or family events.

One-quarter of the work force is involved in variable shift work, and this proportion is climbing at a rate of 3% a year (Gordon et al, 1986). The elderly are more profoundly affected by rapidly changing shifts. Shift work is also associated with impaired job productivity and performance (Mitler et al, 1988). Job productivity seems to be at its lowest during time periods when individuals are naturally more sleepy, i.e., early morning (about 2 to 7 am.) and midafternoon (about 2 to 5 p.m.).

Shift workers should be advised to maximize their exposure to sunlight at times when they should be awake and to ensure that the bedroom is as dark and quiet as possible when they are asleep, which is often during the day. Bright artificial light emanating from especially constructed boxes, when administered at critical times, can enhance adaptation of internal rhythms to the new shift (Czeisler et al, 1990). If symptoms are not responsive to conventional countermeasures, it may be necessary to devise more rational shift schedules.

In *delayed sleep phase syndrome*, individuals fall asleep later than normal evening bedtime hours and awaken later than desired, often extending their bedtimes well into the afternoon. Thus, they typically complain of both insomnia and daytime sleepiness. Sufferers are usually young adults who present for treatment because of diminished school performance resulting from daytime sleepiness or missed morning classes. Prior history reveals a tendency for individuals to be night owls who prefer to work and play well into the night. They can be distinguished from people who stay up late by choice because of social or occupational needs in that they cannot fall asleep earlier even if they were to try.

Attempts to advance the sleep/wake cycle by retiring earlier are uniformly unsuccessful. Instead, delaying bedtimes even further by increments of 3 hours a day are often successful, a process referred to as chronotherapy (Weitzman et al, 1981). More recently, Rosenthal and his colleagues (1990) demonstrated that bright light therapy, when administered for a duration of 2 hours early in the morning, resulted in an advance of biological rhythms on subsequent nights and progressively earlier sleep times.

In *advanced sleep phase syndrome,* sleep/wake times are advanced in relationship to socially desired schedules. The disorder is more common in the elderly and is responsive to treatment with bright lights when administered in the evening.

Parasomnias

Patients present with complaints regarding disturbing events that occur during sleep or that are aggravated by sleep. Clinical aspects of the most common parasomnias are summarized in Table 22–8.

Medical/Psychiatric Sleep Disorders

There is a close association between disturbed sleep and psychiatric disorders, most notably depression (see Chapter 7). For example, 90% of patients affected with major depression demonstrate clinical evidence of sleep disturbance (Reynolds and Kupfer, 1987). Conversely, a majority of chronic insomniacs (between 60 and 69%) are affected by at least one major psychiatric disorder, most commonly mood disorders, which includes depression (Jacobs et al, 1988; Tan et al, 1984). Therefore, it is imperative that physicians keep a high index of suspicion for underlying psychopathology with an emphasis on mood disturbances whenever confronted with the complaint of insomnia. This is also true for patients assessed as having a "routine" or "primary" insomnia, who often suffer from undetected depression. Symptomatic management of the insomnia in such patients with, for example, hypnotic agents alone, can lead to treatment failure since the underlying disorder, in this case depression, remains unaddressed.

Although it was once thought that early morning awakening was the hallmark sleep-related symptom of depression, more recent data with large groups of depressives have shown that difficulties in falling asleep in the beginning of the night, repeated nocturnal awakenings, and early morning awakening are equally prevalent in depressives (Perlis et al, 1997). The absence of early morning awakening should not, therefore, rule out a diagnosis of depression, and the presence of initial insomnia as the only sleep-related symptom is con-

Table 22–8 **Parasomnias**

PARASOMNIA	CLINICAL FEATURES	POLYSOMNOGRAPHIC FINDINGS	TREATMENT
Sleepwalking	Ambulation in sleep Age affected: prepubertal children Difficulty in arousal during episode Amnesia for the episode Episodes occur in first third of night	Sleepwalking out of delta sleep	Prevention: removal of sharp objects, floor mattresses, etc.; reassurance of parents, psychiatric evaluation for adults
Sleep terror	Sudden, intense scream during sleep with evidence of intense fear Other features similar to sleepwalking	Sleep terror beginning during delta sleep	Stress reduction Psychiatric evaluation for adults
Nightmares	Sudden awakening with intense fear Recall of frightening dream content Full alertness on awakening Usually occur in latter half of night Frequent nightmares can be indicative of psychiatric conditions	Abrupt awakening from REM Tachycardia and tachypnea during episode	Psychotherapy Hypnosis
REM sleep behavior disorder	Violent or injurious behavior during sleep Body movement associated with dreams Dreams are enacted while they occur Neurologic evaluations with MRI of the brain and evoked potentials may reveal structural lesions; most cases idiopathic	Excessive EMG tone or phasic twitching in REM Body movements or complex behaviors during REM	Clonazepam Protective measures Psychotherapy
Sleep bruxism	Tooth grinding or clenching during sleep Tooth wear and jaw discomfort	Bursts of jaw EMG activity	Dental examination Mouth guards Relaxation training Psychotherapy

Table 22–9 **Polysomnographic Findings in Major Depression**

Increased sleep latency and frequency of awakenings during sleep
Diminished proportion, and absolute amount, of delta sleep
Shift of delta sleep activity from the first to the second sleep cycle
Shortened REM latency
Increased frequency of rapid eye movements in the first half of the night
Increased REM sleep time in the first half of the night

sistent with a diagnosis of depression. In contrast, in certain depressive conditions such as bipolar mood disorder and seasonal affective disorder, sleep is uninterrupted, yet patients complain of unrelenting daytime sleepiness. Hypersomnia is also characteristic of the sleep of younger depressives.

Depression has profound and predictable effects upon objectively monitored sleep, as well. Polysomnographic patterns of patients with major depression in the acute phase of the illness are summarized in Table 22–9. Many of these patterns are so characteristic that they can be utilized diagnostically with a high degree of accuracy. In addition to being indicative of current depression, some are thought to be trait markers, i.e., indicative of the potential for future depression in otherwise healthy individuals. The persistence of polysomnographic abnormalities following the resolution of depressive episodes has also been noted to correlate with a greater probability of relapse.

Although sleeplessness is often thought of as a consequence of depression, emerging evidence suggests that it can also be a cause of depression, or, at least, foment underlying depressive tendencies. Results of the hallmark study into the prevalence of emotional disorders (Ford and Kamerow, 1989) indicated that insomniacs who had no evidence of baseline depressive disorders were much more likely to develop depression during the course of a year-long insomnia than those who did not have insomnia. Such evidence suggests that insomnias caused by disorders other than depression may, if left unaddressed, eventually lead to the development of new depression. Although studies have not conclusively demonstrated that treatment of the insomnia itself can avert the onset of depressive episodes, such studies suggest that clinicians should be attentive to the symptom of insomnia in depressed patients and treat it aggressively.

If depression is accompanied by sleeplessness, serious consideration should be given to choosing an antidepressant agent that promises to ameliorate sleep-related symptoms. The effects of antidepressants on polysomnographic sleep vary (for a review, see Winokur and Reynolds, 1994). In general, the sedating tricyclic antidepressants such as nortriptyline and doxepin enhance sleep continuity and depth, yet, because of long half-lives, tend to cause daytime drowsiness. The monoamine oxidase inhibitors, in contrast, can enhance nocturnal awakenings and diminish sleep continuity, yet their activating properties make them better suited for the depressive with hypersomnia. The selective serotonin-reuptake inhibitors (fluoxetine, paroxetine, sertraline) tend to worsen sleep discontinuity and, in the case of fluoxetine, produce an excessive amount of slow-rolling eye movements and arousals (Armitage et al, 1995a). Bupropion also tends to have sleep-disruptive effects. In contrast, trazodone, nefazodone, and mirtazepine enhance sleep continuity and diminish the proportion of shallow sleep stages such as stage 1.

These effects of antidepressants apply, in general, to the acute (8 weeks) stages of treatment, and little is known about their effects on sleep when used over longer periods of time. If sleeplessness persists during treatment with an antidepressant, however, consideration should be given to the addition of low doses of another sleep-promoting antidepressant such as trazodone (Armitage et al, 1995b). However, this practice enhances the possibility of adverse effects such as daytime somnolence and a paradoxical activation with autonomic changes referred to as "the serotonin syndrome." Therefore, small doses should be utilized (25 to 150 mg), and the patient should be monitored frequently for such adverse effects. The combination of antidepressants with hypnotic agents is also a valid clinical practice; hypnotics are discussed further below. When patients require this degree of complex medication management, a psychiatrist should be involved.

Mania, in the acute phase, is associated with a decrease in total sleep time. Therefore, decreased sleep in a depressed bipolar patient can herald an impending switch into mania and signals the need for close observation. Some researchers have presented evidence indicating that decreased sleep may itself be a precipitant and not just a consequence of mania; thus, situational stressors such as a relationship failure that result in an adjustment sleep disorder can precipitate a manic episode in a depressed bipolar patient (Wehr et al, 1987).

Sleep in other psychiatric disorders has been extensively studied, but is of greater interest to researchers than clinicians. Almost any disorder, however, that is associated with psychic activation or anxiety can produce sleep loss and fragmentation. In addition, many medical and neurological conditions also cause sleep disturbances. For a review of these disorders, as well as strategies for management, readers are referred to Moran and Stoudemire (1992).

THE CLINICAL APPROACH TO SLEEP-RELATED COMPLAINTS

Most sleep-disordered patients present for clinical attention with the complaints of insomnia and excessive daytime sleepiness. An important dictum is that insomnia and sleepiness are not disorders in and of themselves, but are *symptomatic manifestations* of a host of underlying sleep disorders. Therefore, the physician confronted with these complaints should strive to identify the underlying disorder(s) prior to treatment. Following their identification, specific treatment can be instituted with confidence. Table 22–10 lists the most common sleep disorders and their most probable presenting complaints.

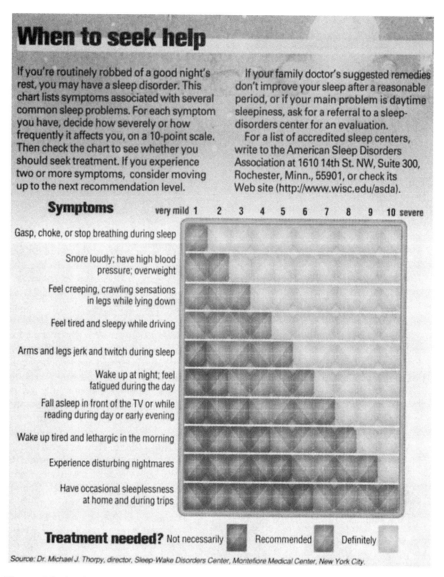

When to seek help

If you're routinely robbed of a good night's rest, you may have a sleep disorder. This chart lists symptoms associated with several common sleep problems. For each symptom you have, decide how severely or how frequently it affects you, on a 10-point scale. Then check the chart to see whether you should seek treatment. If you experience two or more symptoms, consider moving up to the next recommendation level.

If your family doctor's suggested remedies don't improve your sleep after a reasonable period, or if your main problem is daytime sleepiness, ask for a referral to a sleep-disorders center for an evaluation.

For a list of accredited sleep centers, write to the American Sleep Disorders Association at 1610 14th St. NW, Suite 300, Rochester, Minn., 55901, or check its Web site (http://www.wisc.edu/asda).

Symptoms   very mild 1   2   3   4   5   6   7   8   9   10 severe

Gasp, choke, or stop breathing during sleep

Snore loudly; have high blood pressure; overweight

Feel creeping, crawling sensations in legs while lying down

Feel tired and sleepy while driving

Arms and legs jerk and twitch during sleep

Wake up at night; feel fatigued during the day

Fall asleep in front of the TV or while reading during day or early evening

Wake up tired and lethargic in the morning

Experience disturbing nightmares

Have occasional sleeplessness at home and during trips

Treatment needed? Not necessarily ▨   Recommended ▨   Definitely ▢

Source: Dr. Michael J. Thorpy, director, Sleep-Wake Disorders Center, Montefiore Medical Center, New York City.

Figure 22–6. *A patient self-assessment rating scale of sleep quality.*

The diagnostic process, summarized in Table 22–11, begins with a thorough history, with particular attention directed toward the hallmark symptoms of the major sleep disorders outlined above. In most cases, it is beneficial also to interview the bedpartner, who is more likely than the patient to be aware of unusual events during sleep. If the presenting symptom is daytime sleepiness, its severity should be carefully evaluated. Patients almost invariably misjudge

Table 22–10 **The Most Commonly Encountered Sleep Disorders**

DISORDER	PRIMARY PRESENTING COMPLAINT	
	Insomnia	EDS[a]
Inadequate Sleep Hygiene	*	*
Insufficient Sleep Syndrome		*
Adjustment Sleep Disorder	*	
Psychophysiological Insomnia	*	
Obstructive Sleep Apnea Syndrome		*
Central Sleep Apnea Syndrome	*	
Narcolepsy		*
Idiopathic Hypersomnolence		*
Periodic Limb Movement Disorder	*	*
Restless Legs Syndrome	*	
Drug-Dependent Sleep Disorders	*	*
Circadian Rhythm Sleep Disorders	*	*
Parasomnias		
Medical/Psychiatric Sleep Disorders	*	*

[a] EDS, excessive daytime sleepiness

the extent of sleepiness; therefore, direct questioning regarding how sleepy an individual feels often is not helpful. The propensity for falling asleep is more accurate a measure; in severe cases, individuals fall asleep while actively engaged in complex tasks, such as speaking, writing, or even eating. They may also experience sleep attacks, whose occurrence mandates rapid clinical inter-

Table 22–11 **The Clinical Evaluation of Sleep Disorders**

Patient interview
    Chief complaint: insomnia, EDS, or parasomnia?
    History of present illness
    Sleep/wake habit history
    Sleep hygiene history: meal and exercise times, ambient noise,
      light and temperature, etc.
    Pattern of consumption of recreational substances (especially
      caffeine and alcohol) and medications
    General medical, psychiatric, and surgical history
Sleep diary
Inventories for daytime sleepiness/alertness
Psychological inventories
Bedpartner interview
Physical and mental status examination
Serum laboratory tests
Polysomnography

vention. Milder levels of daytime sleepiness result in falling asleep in passive situations, such as while reading or watching television. The Epworth Sleepiness Scale (Johns, 1991; Table 22–12) assesses the tendency to fall asleep in various situations of daily living; a cumulative score of 10 or greater is considered to represent an abnormally high level of daytime somnolence. Although a useful screening tool, this is a subjective scale and not as reliable a test for daytime sleepiness as the MSLT and MWT.

If the history is positive for naps, the possibility that they are related to narcolepsy should be examined by determining whether they are refreshing, brief in duration, or accompanied by dreams. The timing of naps also should be determined as this may alert the physician to the possibility of circadian rhythm disorders.

If the presenting symptom is that of insomnia, its duration should be determined. Disorders causing acute insomnia are usually transient in nature and are more likely to resolve with conservative intervention and treatment with hypnotic agents. On the other hand, chronic and unrelenting insomnia, i.e., that which lasts more than a few months, usually requires a more careful investigation and more complex treatments. A determination also should be made as to whether the patient's difficulty is in falling asleep or maintaining sleep. The former may be related to circadian rhythm disorders or chronic psychophysiological insomnia, and the latter is more consistent with major depression, central sleep apnea syndrome, and periodic limb movement disorder, among others.

Sleeping habits should be carefully reviewed, including the patient's usual bedtime, times spent awake in bed prior to and following the onset of sleep, and final morning awakening and arising times. Sleep logs completed daily over 2 weeks prior to the evaluation often are more revealing and accurate in this regard. The history also should include the pattern of drug, med-

Table 22–12 **The Epworth Sleepiness Scale**

How likely are you to doze off or fall asleep in the following situations? Use the following scale to choose the most appropriate number for each situation:

0 = would never doze   1 = slight chance of dozing
2 = moderate chance of dozing   3 = high chance of dozing

Situation				
Sitting and reading	0	1	2	3
Watching TV	0	1	2	3
Sitting, inactive, in a public place	0	1	2	3
Passenger in a car for an hour without a break	0	1	2	3
Lying down to rest in the afternoon	0	1	2	3
Sitting and talking to someone	0	1	2	3
Sitting quietly after a lunch with no alcohol	0	1	2	3
In a car, while stopped for a few minutes in the traffic	0	1	2	3

ication, and recreational substance use, as well as potential sleep hygiene difficulties.

Most intrinsic disorders of sleep do not exhibit diagnostic signs on physical examination. However, when symptoms are unremitting and severe, a physical examination should be performed to assess the potential for contributory medical and neurological illnesses. A thorough psychiatric history and mental status examination also are important. Finally, serum laboratory tests, including thyroid function studies, should be considered if they have not been performed within 6 months prior to the evaluation.

The above office-based diagnostic process is occasionally inconclusive. In fact, studies with insomnia patients have shown that it is insufficient for the proper diagnosis in 50% of cases (Jacobs et al, 1988). When the diagnosis is in doubt, polysomnography is recommended. Polysomnography is also warranted when seemingly adequate treatment of the *presumed* disorder does not result in the alleviation of symptoms. Polysomnography should always be performed when the office-based evaluation raises the possibility of intrinsic sleep disorders, such as obstructive sleep apnea syndrome or narcolepsy; their presence and severity must be established prior to management.

HYPNOTIC AGENTS

A wide array of compounds have been utilized for their sleep-promoting qualities over the years. Alcohol may be one of the most widely utilized agents by insomniacs because it enhances sleepiness and decreases sleep latency. However, it is a poor choice inasmuch as it alters sleep architecture and often results in further daytime somnolence. Patients also report unrefreshing and disturbed sleep during use and frequent nocturnal awakenings following discontinuation (Kay and Samiuddin, 1988). As noted above, alcohol can also result in further impairment in sleep-related respiration in patients with obstructive sleep apnea syndrome, a disorder commonly seen in insomniacs. Antihistamines and over-the-counter products cannot be wholeheartedly recommended either, since they have unpredictable effects on sleep and since they can cause adverse systemic effects, due to their anticholinergic, sympathomimetic, and other properties. Although barbiturates and barbituratelike drugs (chloral hydrate and glutethimide, among others) were utilized as hypnotics in the past, they, too, can no longer be recommended since they have a far greater potential for significant sedation and even death in overdoses, when compared with the benzodiazepines. Melatonin is a hormone released by the pineal gland whose secretion peaks during sleep. It has long been suspected as being helpful for sleep and has witnessed extraordinary popularity in recent years among insomniacs as an over-the-counter sleep aid. Unfortunately, the evidence for the efficacy of melatonin as a general sleep aid is scant. Melatonin may, however, be useful in affecting positive changes in circadian rhythm disorders such as jet lag or shift work sleep disorder, although more definitive studies are necessary in these areas, as well. In addition, concerns exist regarding its safety, and questions have been raised regarding the purity of certain melatonin preparations. Because of the lack of methodologically rigorous dose–response studies, the proper dosage is unknown, as well. Despite its enormous public popularity and the anecdotal reports of miraculous cures following its ingestion, it appears that its use cannot be fully supported by clinical evidence at the present time (Brzezinski, 1997).

Recently introduced hypnotic agents have proved to be far safer and more efficacious than previously available agents. Hypnotic agents can be distinguished on the basis of elimination half-life, a measure of the rate of drug disappearance from the plasma after distribution equilibrium has been attained. Those with a longer half-life include flurazepam (Dalmane) and quazepam (Doral). Those with an intermediate half-life include estazolam (ProSom) and temazepam (Restoril). Presently, the only short half-life hypnotics available for clinical use in the United States are triazolam (Halcion) and zolpidem (Ambien). All these agents fall within the benzodiazepine class of compounds, with the exception of zolpidem, an imidazopyridine. At the cellular level, zolpidem and quazepam (parent compound only) have a selective affinity for a subtype of gamma amino butyric acid receptors, whereas the other hypnotics do not. It is not clear whether this pharmacodynamic property is associated with clinical features that might distinguish these two agents from the others. The soon-to-be introduced compound zaleplon also is a nonbenzodiazepine hypnotic. It seems to have the shortest elimination half-life of all the hypnotic agents available in the United States. (Benzodiazepines are also discussed in Chapters 8 and 18.)

There are many factors influencing the decision as to which hypnotic to use in an individual clinical situation. The propensity for residual daytime somnolence is one such factor. Agents with greater elimination half-lives tend to be associated with a greater potential for daytime carryover effect and sleepiness on the day following administration, clearly a negative feature. Of the agents available for clinical use, triazolam and zolpidem have the least potential for residual daytime carryover effects if administered at bedtime. Triazolam has fallen out of favor because of problems with unterograde amnesia and rebound insomnia. Zaleplon promises to have even fewer negative effects on daytime alertness, even when taken in the middle of the night within a few hours of morning awakening time. Agents that are more lipophilic have a higher brain clearance rate and a more rapid redistribution from brain and blood into adipose tissue and other inactive storage sites and have, therefore, a shorter duration of action (Greenblatt, 1991). The most lipophilic hypnotic agent of the benzodiazepine class is quazepam. This may, in part, be responsible for its minimal tendency for daytime somnolence after single-dose nocturnal administration (Dement, 1991). Higher dosages also contribute to daytime somnolence, as do longer periods of continued use.

A second factor influencing the choice of hypnotics is the propensity for tolerance and rebound insomnia, the latter referring to a transient sleep disturbance (relative to baseline sleep) that occurs with abrupt discontinuation of the medication. Rebound can be controlled by gradually tapering when discontinuing the drug. It may occur, however, if patients discontinue the medication on their own accord. Tolerance and rebound were once thought to be sole functions of elimination half-life, since they tend to be more likely with the use of short elimination half-life benzodiazepine agents (Roth and Roehrs, 1992) and have been most widely reported with triazolam. However, there is little evidence for either difficulty with extended use of the short half-life agents zolpidem (Scharf and colleagues, 1994) and zaleplon. They can, nevertheless, be minimized by utilizing the medication at the lowest effective dose and for brief periods of time (days to weeks). If prolonged use is warranted, intermittent dosing, i.e., administration on 4 or 5 nights per week only, may be beneficial. With a few exceptions, hypnotic medications should be taken on predetermined nights; making the decision on a night-by-night basis enhances the possibility of further escalating anxiety caused by the focus on internal tension as patients lie in bed prior to ingestion of the hypnotic. Zaleplon may be an exception because of its very short half-life.

Hypnotic agents can be utilized in a wide array of disorders, including adjustment sleep disorder, psychophysiological insomnia, periodic limb movement disorder, time zone change (jet lag) syndrome, shift work sleep disorder, and even as adjunctive treatments in the insomnia of depression. However, as discussed above, hypnotic agents alone are inappropriate for the treatment of the insomnia of depression. *Regardless of the disorder, however, hypnotic agents should be utilized for brief periods of time and at the lowest effective doses.* During the course of treatment, physicians should carefully monitor patients for adverse effects, such as daytime somnolence, memory difficulties and performance decrements, and habituation and tolerance. Hypnotics are contraindicated in patients suspected of having obstructive sleep apnea syndrome and other sleep-related breathing disorders, in pregnant women, and in heavy alcohol users, and should be utilized with caution in any chronic disorder.

CONCLUSIONS

Sleep-related complaints such as insomnia and excessive daytime sleepiness can no longer be regarded as disorders in and of themselves, as they are now known to represent symptoms of a variety of underlying conditions. Thus, their evaluation should include the physician's systematic assessment of the specific sleep-related complaint, guided by a knowledge of the many possible pathological entities. Once the diagnosis is established, treatment can be conducted with confidence. This approach is the most gratifying not only for physicians, but for patients, as well.

CLINICAL PEARLS

- The first task in the management of sleep-related complaints such as insomnia, disturbed sleep, and daytime somnolence is to establish the diagnosis. Symptomatic management is often complicated by treatment failure and can even harm the patient.
- Depression is often overlooked in sleep-disordered patients, especially in insomniacs who are not consciously aware of their depressed feelings. Therefore, the clinician should carefully search for the diagnosis of depression during the routine evaluation of insomnia.
- The patient's bedpartner or another household member should be interviewed whenever possible. This can be especially helpful when the patient's clinical interview and examination are inconclusive. The bedpartner can provide invaluable ancillary information about the patient's sleep, such as the presence of snoring, breathing pauses, and unusual body positions or movements.
- Paper-and-pencil inventories often are helpful in the evaluation of sleep-related complaints. These inventories include 2-week logs for sleep/wake habits, the Epworth Sleepiness Scale, the Minnesota Multiphasic Personality Inventory, and the Beck Depression Inventory.
- The vast majority of sleep-disordered patients benefit from advice regarding sleep hygiene measures. In some cases, nothing more needs to be done. Tips on improving sleep can be given to patients in written form, and compliance can be assessed during follow-up visits.
- Prior to treatment with hypnotic agents, it is important to rule out the possibility of sleep-related breathing disorders, such as obstructive sleep apnea syndrome. Hypnotic agents can increase the frequency and length of breathing abnormalities during sleep.
- Excessive daytime sleepiness often is the product of three potential factors: (1) alterations in sleep quality by various sleep disorders, poor sleep hygiene, medications, and medical illnesses; (2) acute and chronic prior restriction in sleep length; and (3) improper timing of sleep.
- Important guidelines for treatment with hypnotic agents include the utilization of the lowest effective dose; regular monitoring for adverse effects, such as daytime somnolence and decrements in daytime performance; limiting the duration of treatment to prevent the development of tolerance; and gradually tapering the dosage during the discontinuation phase.

ANNOTATED BIBLIOGRAPHY

Bootzin RR, Epstein D, Wood JM: Stimulus control instructions. In Hauri PJ (ed): Case Studies in Insomnia, pp 19–28. New York, Plenum, 1991

> This chapter reviews instructions to patients regarding stimulus control therapy. The textbook also provides a thorough summary of behavioral and psychiatric treatment strategies for the insomniac patient.

Consensus Development Conference Statement: Drugs and insomnia: the use of medications to promote sleep. JAMA 251:2410–2414, 1984

> Outlines the consensus of experts in the field regarding critical questions confronting physicians who wish to utilize hypnotic agents.

Diagnostic Classification Steering Committee, Thorpy MJ (ed): International Classification of Sleep Disorders: Diagnostic and Coding Manual. Rochester, American Sleep Disorders Association, 1990

> This is the most comprehensive and up-to-date listing of disease entities in sleep disorders as well as their diagnostic criteria.

Greenblatt DJ: Benzodiazepine hypnotics: sorting the pharmacokinetic facts. J Clin Psychiatry 52(suppl 9):4–10, 1991

> Provides some pharmacokinetic considerations that may be of assistance in the selection of a hypnotic agent.

He J, Kryger MH, Zorick FJ, et al: Mortality and apnea index in obstructive sleep apnea. Chest 94:9–14, 1988

> Reviews data regarding the mortality of obstructive sleep apnea patients and how this is affected by various treatment options.

Kryger MH, Roth T, Dement WC (eds): Principles and Practice of Sleep Medicine, 2nd ed. Philadelphia, WB Saunders, 1994

> The most comprehensive reference textbook for the physician and scientist interested in sleep and its disorders.

Mitler MM, Carskadon MA, Czeisler CA, et al: Catastrophes, sleep, and public policy: consensus report. Sleep 11:100–109, 1988

> Reviews data regarding the impact of sleep disorders and daytime sleepiness on health, safety, and industrial productivity.

Moran MG, Stoudemire A: Sleep disorders in the medically ill patient. J Clin Psychiatry 53(suppl 6):29–36, 1992

> Summarizes the effects of miscellaneous medical conditions on sleep and outlines strategies in the management of altered sleep in these populations.

Reynolds CF, Kupfer DJ: Sleep research in affective illness: state of the art circa 1987. Sleep 10:199–215, 1987

> Reviews major findings in the sleep of depressed patients.

Tan TL, Kales JD, Kales A, et al: Biopsychobehavioral correlates of insomnia, IV: Diagnosis based on DSM-III. Am J Psychiatry 141:357–362, 1984

> Presents data regarding psychiatric conditions that are associated with chronic insomnia.

REFERENCES

Armitage R, Trivedi M, Rush AJ: Fluoxetine and oculomotor activity during sleep in depressed patients. Neuropsychopharmacology 12:159–65, 1995a

Armitage R, Yonkers K, Rush AJ, et al: Nefazodone improves sleep efficiency and has little effect on REM sleep in depressed patients. Sleep Res 24A:382, 1995b

Berlin RM, Litovitz GL, Diaz MA, et al: Sleep disorders in a psychiatric consultation service. Am J Psychiatry 141:582–584, 1984

Bootzin RR, Epstein D, Wood JM: Stimulus control instructions. In Hauri PJ (ed): Case Studies in Insomnia, pp 19–28. New York, Plenum, 1991

Brzezinski A: Melatonin in humans. N Engl J Med 336:186–195, 1997

Buguet A, Montmayeur A, Pigeau R, et al: Modafinil, d-amphetamine and placebo during 64 hours of sustained mental work. II. Effects on two nights of recovery sleep. J Sleep Res 4:229–241, 1995

Consensus Development Conference Statement: Drugs and insomnia: the use of medications to promote sleep. JAMA 251:2410–2414, 1984

Czeisler CA, Johnson MP, Duffy JR, et al: Exposure to bright light and darkness to treat physiologic maladaptation to night work. N Engl J Med 322:1253–1259, 1990

Dement WC: Objective measurements of daytime sleepiness and performance comparing quazepam with flurazepam in two adult populations using the multiple sleep latency test. J Clin Psychiatry 52(suppl 9):31–37, 1991

Diagnostic Classification Steering Committee, Thorpy MJ (ed): International Classification of Sleep Disorders: Diagnostic and Coding Manual. Rochester, American Sleep Disorders Association, 1990

Doghramji K: Emotional aspects of sleep disorders: the case of sleep apnea syndrome. New Dir Ment Health Serv 57:39–50, 1993

Doghramji K, Jabourian ZH, Pilla M, et al: Predictors of outcome for uvulopalatopharyngoplasty. Laryngoscope 105:311–314, 1995

Doghramji K, Mitler MM, Sangal RB, et al: A normative study of the maintenance of wakefulness test (MWT). Electroencephalogr Clin Neurophysiol 1997, in press

Findley L, Unverzagt M, Suratt P: Automobile accidents involving patients with obstructive sleep apnea. Am Rev Respir Disease 138:337–340, 1988

Findley LJ, Barth JT, Powers ME, et al: Cognitive impairment in patients with obstructive sleep apnea and associated hypoxemia. Chest 90:686–690, 1986

Findley LJ, Fabrizio MJ, Knight H, et al: Driving simulator performance in patients with sleep apnea. Am Rev Respir Disease 140:529–530, 1989

Ford DE, Kamerow DB: Epidemiologic study of sleep disturbances and psychiatric disorders. JAMA 262:1479–1484, 1989

Gordon NP, Cleary PD, Parker CE, et al: The prevalence and health impact of shiftwork. Am J Public Health 76:1225–1228, 1986

Greenberg GD, Watson RK, Deptula D: Neuropsychological dysfunction in sleep apnea. Sleep 10:254–262, 1987

Greenblatt DJ: Benzodiazepine hypnotics: sorting the pharmacokinetic facts. J Clin Psychiatry 52(suppl 9):4–10, 1991

He J, Kryger MH, Zorick FJ, et al: Mortality and apnea index in obstructive sleep apnea. Chest 94:9–14, 1988

Jacobs EA, Reynolds CF, Kupfer DJ, et al: The role of polysomnography in the differential diagnosis of chronic insomnia. Am J Psychiatry 145:346–349, 1988

Johns MW: A new method for measuring daytime sleepiness: The Epworth Sleepiness Scale. Sleep 14:540–545, 1991

Johnson LC, Spinweber CL: Good and poor sleepers differ in navy performance. Mil Med 148:727–731, 1983

Kales A, Caldwell AB, Cadieux RJ, et al: Severe obstructive sleep apnea—II: Associated psychopathology and psychosocial consequences. J Chron Dis 38:427–434, 1985

Kay DC, Samiuddin Z: Sleep disorders associated with drug abuse and drugs of abuse. In Williams RL, Karacan I, Moore CA (eds): Sleep Disorders: Diagnosis and Treatment, pp 315–372. New York, John Wiley & Sons, 1988

Kribbs NB, Pack AI, Kline LR: Objective measurement of patterns of nasal CPAP use by patients with obstructive sleep apnea. Am Rev Respir Dis 147:887–958, 1993

Kryger MH, Roth T, Dement WC (eds): Principles and Practice of Sleep Medicine, 2nd ed. Philadelphia, WB Saunders, 1994

Lavie P: Sleep apnea in industrial workers. Sleep 6:127–135, 1983

Mignot E, Lin X, Arrigoni J: DQB1*0602 and DQA1*0102 (DQ1) are better markers than DR2 for narcolepsy in Caucasian and black Americans. Sleep 17 (8 suppl):S60–76, 1994

Mitler MM, Carskadon MA, Czeisler CA, et al: Catastrophes, sleep, and public policy: consensus report. Sleep 11:100–109, 1988

Moran MG, Stoudemire A: Sleep disorders in the medically ill patient. J Clin Psychiatry 53(suppl 6): 29–36, 1992

National Sleep Foundation Report: Sleep in America, 1995.

Partinen M, Putkonen PTS, Kaprio J, et al: Sleep disorders in relation to coronary heart disease. Acta Med Scand Suppl 660:69–83, 1982

Perlis ML, Giles DE, Buysse DJ, et al: Which depressive symptoms are related to which sleep electroencephalographic variables? Biol Psychiatry (in press), 1997

Rechtshaffen A, Bergmann BM, Everson CA, et al: Sleep deprivation in the rat: X. Integration and discussion of the findings. Sleep 12:68–87, 1989

Reynolds CF, Kupfer DJ: Sleep research in affective illness: state of the art circa 1987. Sleep 10:199–215, 1987

Rosenthal NE, Joseph-Vanderpool JR, Levendosky AA, et al: Phase-shifting effects of bright morning light as treatment for delayed sleep phase syndrome. Sleep 13:354–361, 1990

Roth T, Roehrs TA: Issues in the use of benzodiazepine therapy. J Clin Psychiatry 53(suppl 6): 14–18, 1992

Scharf MB, Roth T, Vogel GW, et al: A multicenter, placebo-controlled study evaluating zolpidem in the treatment of chronic insomnia. J Clin Psychiatry 55:192–199, 1994

Segawa K, Nakazawa S, Tsukamoto Y, et al: Peptic ulcer is prevalent among shift workers. Dig Dis Sci 32:449–453, 1987

Smallwood RG, Vitiello MV, Giblin EC, et al: Sleep apnea: relationship to age, sex, and Alzheimer's dementia. Sleep 6:16–22, 1983

Sweetwood H, Grant I, Kripke D, et al: Sleep disorder over time: psychiatric correlates among males. Br J Psychiatry 136:456–462, 1980

Tan TL, Kales JD, Kales A, et al: Biopsychobehavioral correlates of insomnia, IV: Diagnosis based on DSM-III. Am J Psychiatry 141:357–362, 1984

Wehr TA, Rosenthal NE: Sleep reduction as a final common pathway in the genesis of mania. Am J Psychiatry 144:201–204, 1987

Weitzman ED, Czeisler CA, Coleman RM, et al: Delayed sleep phase syndrome. A chronobiological disorder with sleep-onset insomnia. Arch Gen Psychiatry 38:737–746, 1981

Wingard DL, Berkman LF: Mortality risk associated with sleeping patterns among adults. Sleep 6:102–107, 1983

Winokur A, Reynolds CF: The effects of antidepressants on sleep physiology. Prim Psychiatry November/December:22–27, 1994

23 *Basic Principles of Pain Management*

Robert J. Boland
and Richard J. Goldberg

Pain is a subjective, private experience. There is no questionnaire, blood test, or technology that can objectively quantify the amount of pain that someone feels. Pain is a complex product with contributions from personality, learning, memory, fantasy, and cultural traditions in the context of neurophysiological processes. Pain serves an important signaling function in the organism and often leads to recognition of some underlying disorder that can be medically or surgically treated. However, despite the available technology, pain often remains inadequately treated at times because of underlying patient or physician attitudes and sometimes because of medical or psychosocial misunderstandings.

In this chapter, we will review current research about pain. We will briefly examine the physiology of the pain experience. Most of this chapter is then devoted to techniques of assessment and pain management.

THE PHYSIOLOGY OF PAIN

One has only to examine the physiology of pain to realize how complex the pain experience is. Any desire we might have to trivialize a person's pain (with statements such as "the pain cannot be explained by the physical findings") is nullified by even a cursory examination of current research on pain mechanisms. Such research is briefly reviewed here and is available in more detail through a number of sources (e.g., Brose and Spiegel, 1987).

Origin of the Stimulus

Nociceptors

The pain experience usually begins with the nociceptors. These are afferent nerves that respond to noxious stimulation. Different nociceptors may preferentially react to a specific kind of noxious stimuli, such as mechanical or temperature sensation. Different types of nociceptors may be found in different sites: for example, the most common cutaneous receptor is the polymodal C fiber, which responds to pressure, temperature, and chemical stimuli, whereas skeletal muscle contains mostly chemoreceptors. All nociceptors have an initial high threshold to noxious stimuli, which decreases (at least initially) with repeated stimuli.

Stimulus Transmission

It is tempting to stop at this point and treat pain as a simple reflex, in which the nociceptor receives a noxious response and transmits it to the brain. Much pain treatment is based on this naive assumption. It is, in reality, a long and complicated journey between the nociceptor and the brain.

Signals from the nociceptor are transmitted to the spinal cord. This is done mainly by two fibers: A^d and C fibers. A^d fibers are myelinated and provide the initial pain response. C fibers are unmyelinated and probably cause the slower response felt several seconds after an injury.

Most of these fibers enter the spinal cord through the dorsal root ganglion and terminate in the dorsal horn of the spinal cord. Generally, they terminate ipsilaterally, but a small number will cross to the contralateral side. The clinical significance of this is not clear, but it may explain the incomplete pain relief seen after unilateral surgical ablation of this area.

The dorsal horn is organized into areas, called *laminae,* and certain pain fibers will predictably go to specific laminae. In the laminae, the fibers synapse with second-order neurons, which take various pathways to the brain. The best understood pathways are the *spinothalamic* and *spinoreticular* pathways. These pathways are named after their points of origin and termination.

Termination of the Stimulus

After processing (in the thalamus and other areas), the pain stimulus arrives in the limbic system and cortex. Different areas determine various aspects of the pain. For example, projections from the thalamus to the parietal lobe are involved with localization of pain, whereas projections to the limbic system are involved in qualitative aspects of pain. The somatosensory cortex receives input from most spinal pain tracts and is the primary cortical region for the perception of noxious information.

Modulation of the Stimulus

Local Chemicals

No "pain transmitter" has been identified. However, many substances can modulate a nociceptor's response to noxious stimuli. The best understood is substance P, which may work indirectly through vasodilatory effects. Other chemicals that have a role in pain modulation include prostaglandin, serotonin, histamine, acetylcholine, bradykinin, slow-reacting substance of anaphylaxis, calcitonin-gene-related peptide, and potassium.

Higher Downmodulation

Virtually every part of the pain system can reciprocally affect other parts, and the system should be envisioned as bidirectional. The cortex, in particular, can influence all previous stages of pain transmission through a variety of means. The most obvious is through attentional processes. Most of us are familiar with stories of combat victims who performed heroic acts after injury, apparently unaware of their pain until hours later. More common are reports from chronic pain patients that their pain seems to get worse at night, presumably when there is less distraction. The meaning of pain can also influence its perception—for example, pain perceived as jeopardizing health (e.g., cancer pain) can seem worse than pain that is not life threatening. Finally, a variety of learned phenomena, such as cultural factors, can affect one's perception and expression of pain.

ASSESSMENT OF PAIN

Pain is always subjective. It is the result of a variety of factors. The assessment of pain, therefore, must rely on methods that are necessarily subjective and multidimensional. Currently, there is no universal gold standard for pain assessment, and it is not our purpose here to outline a blueprint for such an assessment. However, any approach must acknowledge the many different dimensions of the pain experience. These dimensions are discussed in this section. A broader discussion is available in a number of sources (e.g., Turk and Melzack, 1992)

The Immediate Pain Experience

When a patient complains of "pain," we must first attempt to better understand what they mean. We would like to quantify and qualify the nature of their experience. Any clinician is familiar with basic questions to ask regarding any symptom: location and duration, for example. Often we ask the patient to apply adjectives to the pain: "burning," or "stabbing." Such an approach, although helpful, may only add to the subjectivity of the exam. We may not all agree what these adjectives actually feel like, particularly without firsthand experience of being severely burned or stabbed. (The use of adjectives remains important, however, as different descriptions of pain may characterize distinct conditions.) Thus, we must try to better understand the pain experience in ways that are both reliable for the individual and generalizable to others.

Intensity

Most commonly, we wish to quantify the intensity of the pain. A variety of approaches are used. We might give the patient a list of adjectives to describe the pain, usually listed in order of increasing intensity. Alternately, we might ask the patient to give a numerical value to the pain intensity. In the latter case, we often ask patients to rate the pain from zero to ten, zero being no pain and ten the most pain they can imagine. The latter approach is particularly practical in that it is rapid and easy to do, and most patients can readily understand the task. This can help us track changes in intensity over time, for example, in response to treatment. However, such scales are ordinal, and the distance between intervals is not clear. We cannot assume, for example, that the difference between a one and two in pain intensity is the same as the interval between an eight and nine. Patients may remember previous responses and try to be consistent in their reports. Also, patients may supply their own meaning to the numbers—they may assume, for example, that we will only raise their analgesic medication for pain reports over a five. Still, such methods are very practical at the bedside.

Another approach is to employ visual analog scales, in which a patient is asked to indicate the intensity of their pain with a mark on a line. The line is usually 10 to 15 cm long, and has no numbers on it except at the ends ("no pain" on one end, and "the most intense pain imaginable" on the other). This approach has the benefit of being very reliable and generalizable. When tested, it seems to be better than the other methods at reflecting reliable ratios along the line. It also is very sensitive to changes in pain intensity. The major drawback of this approach is the extra time involved in scoring the result: the clinician has to measure the mark (usually in millimeters).

The Affective Response to Pain

Individuals usually can distinguish between the intensity of pain and their feelings associated with the pain. An *affective response* involves many dimensions, but, generally, it represents the *degree of unpleasantness*. This response differs from pain intensity in that it is more influenced by the context of the pain. One can imagine that a woman in labor may experience pain that is just as intense as that of a cancer patient, but the pain may seem much less unpleasant. Not surprisingly, research studies have validated such contrasts.

Using the same methods as for pain intensity, including either verbal, numerical, or visual analog scales, we can assess the affective component of pain.

Location

Pain location is usually assessed graphically. Patients are shown figures of a human body, and they draw on them the locations of their pain. Different symbols can represent different qualities of pain (for example oo for "pins and needles" or xx for "burning"), or different depth locations (for example, E for external, and I for internal pain).

Composite Scales

Several scales combine several different dimensions of the pain experience. Examples include the McGill Pain Questionnaire (Fig. 23–1)and the Short-Form McGill Pain Questionnaire (Fig. 23–2) (Melzack and Katz, 1992).

Physical Functioning

We wish to assess how patients' pain affects their ability to do different activities. This task is necessarily subjective, and it often relies on self-report. It is important, however, as it is often the basis of any determination of financial compensation.

In evaluating physical function, we must distinguish among concepts of *impairment, functional limitation,* and *disability.*

Impairment refers to any objective abnormality or loss. These losses and abnormalities can be anatomic (e.g., loss of limb, physical deformity), physiological (e.g., decreased cardiac output, muscle weakness), or psychological (e.g., changes in cognition). They can usually be objectively measured.

Functional limitations are any restrictions in an individual's normal functioning. They are the practical result of impairment. In evaluating for functional limitations, we attempt to measure bodily functioning quantitatively in several activities judged necessary for daily living. There is no agreement on exactly what activities these are. Most evaluations include measurements of the range of motion at major joints, strength testing in major muscle groups, and endurance for specific tasks.

Disability refers to the inability to do one's usual activities or duties in response to impairment. It is task specific, and we should not speak of *global disability,* but rather of whether a person is disabled from doing a particular task. Again, there is no gold standard of assessment. The different organizations that evaluate and compensate disability (such as Social Security or Worker's Compensation) will require that specific factors are assessed. Each system emphasizes different concepts of disability. For example, Social Security relies primarily on objective measures of impairment over subjective symptoms such as pain.

McGill Pain Questionnaire

Patient's Name _____ Date _____ Time_____am/pm

PRI: S_____ A_____ E_____ M_____ PRI(T)_____ PPI_____
     (1–10)   (11–15)   (16)   (17–20)   (1–20)

1 FLICKERING QUIVERING PULSING THROBBING BEATING POUNDING	11 TIRING EXHAUSTING
2 JUMPING FLASHING SHOOTING	12 SICKENING SUFFOCATING
3 PRICKING BORING DRILLING STABBING LANCINATING	13 FEARFUL FRIGHTFUL TERRIFYING
4 SHARP CUTTING LACERATING	14 PUNISHING GRUELLING CRUEL VICIOUS KILLING
5 PINCHING PRESSING GNAWING CRAMPING CRUSHING	15 WRETCHED BLINDING
6 TUGGING PULLING WRENCHING	16 ANNOYING TROUBLESOME MISERABLE INTENSE UNBEARABLE
7 HOT BURNING SCALDING SEARING	17 SPREADING RADIATING PENETRATING PIERCING
8 TINGLING ITCHY SMARTING STINGING	18 TIGHT NUMB DRAWING SQUEEZING TEARING
9 DULL SORE HURTING ACHING HEAVY	19 COOL COLD FREEZING
10 TENDER TAUT RASPING SPLITTING	20 NAGGING NAUSEATING AGONIZING DREADFUL TORTURING

BRIEF ___ MOMENTARY ___ TRANSIENT ___	RHYTHMIC ___ PERIODIC ___ INTERMITTENT ___	CONTINUOUS ___ STEADY ___ CONSTANT ___

E = EXTERNAL
I = INTERNAL

PPI
0 NO PAIN
1 MILD
2 DISCOMFORTING
3 DISTRESSING
4 HORRIBLE
5 EXCRUCIATING

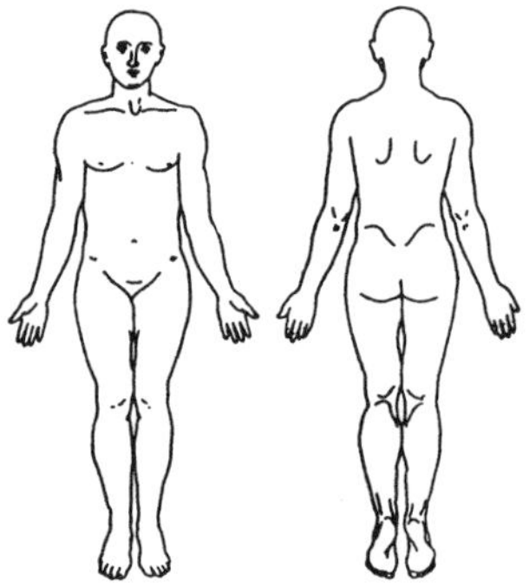

COMMENTS:

Figure 23–1. *The McGill Pain Questionnaire. Copyright 1975 by Ronald Melzack. Used with permission.*

SHORT-FORM McGILL PAIN QUESTIONNAIRE
RONALD MELZACK

PATIENT'S NAME: _____   DATE: _____

	NONE	MILD	MODERATE	SEVERE
THROBBING	0) _____	1) _____	2) _____	3) _____
SHOOTING	0) _____	1) _____	2) _____	3) _____
STABBING	0) _____	1) _____	2) _____	3) _____
SHARP	0) _____	1) _____	2) _____	3) _____
CRAMPING	0) _____	1) _____	2) _____	3) _____
GNAWING	0) _____	1) _____	2) _____	3) _____
HOT-BURNING	0) _____	1) _____	2) _____	3) _____
ACHING	0) _____	1) _____	2) _____	3) _____
HEAVY	0) _____	1) _____	2) _____	3) _____
TENDER	0) _____	1) _____	2) _____	3) _____
SPLITTING	0) _____	1) _____	2) _____	3) _____
TIRING-EXHAUSTING	0) _____	1) _____	2) _____	3) _____
SICKENING	0) _____	1) _____	2) _____	3) _____
FEARFUL	0) _____	1) _____	2) _____	3) _____
PUNISHING-CRUEL	0) _____	1) _____	2) _____	3) _____

NO
PAIN ├──┤ WORST
POSSIBLE
PAIN

P P I

0	NO PAIN	_____
1	MILD	_____
2	DISCOMFORTING	_____
3	DISTRESSING	_____
4	HORRIBLE	_____
5	EXCRUCIATING	_____

Figure 23–2. *Short-Form McGill Pain Questionnaire. Copyright 1984 by Ronald Melzack. Used with permission.*

Psychological Factors

No pain should ever be viewed as either "physical" or "psychological." Unfortunately, we often look only for the psychological factors contributing to pain after all biological contributors are ruled out. Psychological evaluation is important for any pain patient. It is important in predicting a patient's outcome, and it may be more accurate as an outcome predictor than other more "objective" measures of a patient's injury.

In performing a psychological assessment with a pain patient, we must look for any factors that may affect a person's perception of pain and subsequent response to the pain. Our goal is to find factors that *influence* pain, rather than *cause* it. It may be helpful to make these goals clear to the patient, who may be skeptical of psychological questions. Most patients will be defensive at the implication that the pain is "just in their head." They are usually quite willing, however, to consider how life stresses may influence pain.

In the past, much attention was devoted to notions of particular psychological profiles that were more vulnerable to pain syndromes (the "pain-prone personality"); however, this correlation has never been well validated.

A proper assessment often includes both the patient and other significant persons. A typical interview will examine a number of psychosocial areas. We should try to identify events that mediate pain. Also, we should review a patient's usual daily activities and appraise how these activities have changed because of the pain. We wish to learn how a patient copes with pain. Possible sources of reinforcement of the pain, whether financial, interpersonal or avoidance related, should be tactfully explored. We should ask about past significant events, which may resonate with the current situation. For example, Drossman and colleagues (1990), interviewing women who presented to a gastrointestinal clinic for abdominal pain, found that almost half of those with a functional disorder (irritable bowel syndrome, chronic abdominal pain, or nonulcer dyspepsia) had a history of physical or sexual abuse. Likewise, we should look for family histories of similar pain problems. Any psychiatric illnesses, such as depression and anxiety, may affect pain, and we should ask about these. Finally, we should try to understand the patient's beliefs about the pain. Such beliefs can include those about etiology, such as issues of purpose (i.e., retribution or blame). They also may include beliefs about etiology: one can imagine that patients will interpret a pain differently if they think it represents the progression of a serious disease.

Standard instruments generally fall into categories of general psychological measurements and ones that are specifically designed to measure psychological factors in pain patients. The former are more widely used and accepted, but they may not have been well validated for pain patients.

Pain Behavior

Besides the subjective pain experience, patients can exhibit predictable behaviors associated with their pain. These behaviors have the advantage of being readily observable. They also are reinforced over time, that is, they are *learned behaviors.* Most important, they represent potential targets for behavioral intervention.

Assessment of pain behavior is best done through observation, as patients may not even be aware of their behavior.

One can observe for verbal and nonverbal behavior associated with the pain experience. Examples of verbal behavior include complaining of pain or using other vocalizations (e.g., moaning). Nonverbal behavior can be general, involving movement (e.g., pacing) or position, or it may be more specific (e.g., guarding or rubbing a painful joint). Although different researchers emphasize particular behaviors as "more valid" indicators of pain, the behavioral expression of pain is probably very personal.

Physical Components of Pain

It would be very useful to have objective physical measurements that would correlate well with a patient's subjective pain experience. The existence of such measures is implied each time we hear a clinician say that "the patient is having pain beyond what can be explained by the physical findings." Unfortunately, no such statement is justifiable, as the relationship between organic pathology, physiological functioning, and pain report is poorly understood. Any correlations between these objective and subjective factors are weak and difficult to predict.

Several physiological measures are used in pain evaluations. Most remain only research tools, but some have clinical value. Examples include the use of electromyography in evaluations of tension headaches and temporomandibular joint syndrome. In each case, they serve as adjuncts, not substitutes, for the subjective evaluation.

DIAGNOSTIC ISSUES

Advocacy for Proper Diagnosis

Proper evaluation of the patient with pain includes a review of medical, diagnostic, and management issues pertinent to the pain complaint. For example, a careful review of history and physical examination in an elderly patient with multiple somatic complaints may lead to recognition of the need for evaluation of possible hip fracture. The history and physical examination of patients with low back pain syndromes must always be reviewed carefully with attention to the results of electromyography, nerve conduction studies, myelogram, and computed tomography or magnetic resonance imaging findings. Pain in patients with a history of malignancy should be carefully evaluated with a high index of suspicion that the pain complaint, presumed to require psychological management, is actually associated with cancer progression or cancer treatment (Foley, 1985a).

Patients with a known or presumed history of drug abuse are at special risk for having a medical basis for their pain overlooked because the medical team often assumes that these patients' pain complaints are simply drug-seeking behaviors. Similarly, patients with chronic schizophrenia or mental retardation may not be able to communicate pain complaints in a way that leads to proper medical diagnostic evaluation. The psychiatrist should be especially careful before taking a symptomatic treatment approach in these populations. The drug abuser who gets into a motor vehicle accident and is admitted to an orthopedic unit may have complaints of foot pain that are dismissed as drug-seeking behavior, but that actually represent early symptoms of a compartment syndrome from an excessively tight cast.

Certain other groups may be prone to receiving inadequate pain management, for example, minorities, the elderly, and women (Cleeland et al, 1994).

Categorization of Pain

Pain is usually categorized by its course. Usually, we differentiate whether pain is *acute* or *chronic*. Acute pain is not only brief, but it is usually associated with clear injury or disease. An example of acute pain is postsurgical pain, in which the source of injury is clear, and we can expect the pain to lessen as the surgical wound heals. Chronic pain is more complicated: although it often is associated initially with an injury, the association is less clear over time. Chronic pain may persist beyond the usual length of injury and be more self-perpetuating than acute pain.

One can further subdivide types of pain. Beyond acute pain, there is *acute recurrent pain*. Acute recurrent pain occurs when a person experiences brief periods of pain interspersed with periods of no pain. This is seen, for example, with migraine headaches or in sickle cell anemia.

Chronic pain also can be subdivided. Many patients will experience extended periods of pain associated with a chronic disease process (e.g., rheumatoid arthritis) or chronic injury (e.g., back injury). Chronic pain also may be caused by a progressive disease and is then called *chronic progressive pain*. In the latter case, as the disease worsens, so does the pain. In such illnesses as cancer or the acquired immune deficiency syndrome, the type of pain experienced may differ by the nature and site of the disease.

Differentiating between these types of pain is important, as it will have important treatment implications. Acute pain is addressed primarily by treating the injury or disease that is causing the pain. Secondarily, acute pain is treated symptomatically with analgesic medications to reduce the pain stimuli arising at the site of damage. Treating chronic pain is much more difficult. We cannot be sure that treating the injury associated with the pain will alleviate the pain. Furthermore, traditional analgesics may not be as effective in treating chronic pain, since they work best at alleviating pain that arises from noxious stimuli transmitted by nociceptors.

DSM and Pain Disorders

In DSM-III (American Psychiatric Association, 1980), a Psychogenic Pain Disorder had to be either incompatible with organic disease, or "grossly in excess" of what one would expect from the physical findings. It also stipulated that psychological factors were judged to be "etiologically related" to pain development. Obviously, these criteria were difficult to use. Most patients with chronic pain have some organic pathology, and it is impossible to say what pain is "in excess" of the pathology. Furthermore, psychological factors are *always* related to pain expression. DSM-III-R (American Psychiatric Association, 1987), therefore, dropped this last criterion, and renamed the disorder Somatoform Pain Disorder.

DSM-IV (American Psychiatric Association, 1994) simplified the name to Pain Disorder and suggested three main criteria: (1) pain is the predominant focus of clinical attention, (2) it causes substantial distress or impairment, and (3) psychological factors are judged to have a role in the pain's onset or expression (Table 23–1). The disorder is further subtyped based on whether it is associated with just psychological, or psychological and medical factors. It is also subtyped according to whether it is acute or chronic.

This further revision continues to present problems for the clinician treating patients with chronic pain. It invites value judgments, as one must decide the relative importance of psychological factors. It can be argued that psychological factors are *always* important in the expression of pain, and it is likely that *any* patient with chronic pain would meet the criteria of this disorder.

TREATMENT OF PAIN

Alleviating pain is one of our most fundamental roles. At times, this can be complex and frustrating. Often, however, through understanding some fundamental principles of pain management, even the inexperienced clinician can give some relief to the suffering patient. What follows is a brief overview of the common options for pain treatment.

PHARMACOLOGICAL TREATMENT FOR PAIN

Most patients who seek medical attention for pain will receive medication at some point. As with all treatments, it is important to follow a clear rationale in using pain medication. The physician and patient must have mutually understood goals and a plan of what to do when relief is not adequate.

All regimens must be individualized to the patient. It is best to begin with the least potent medication, the simplest dosing regimen, and the least invasive route of administration, and to work up from there.

Table 23–1 **Diagnostic Criteria for Pain Disorder***

A. Pain in one or more anatomical sites is the predominant focus of the clinical presentation and is of sufficient severity to warrant clinical attention.
B. The pain causes clinically significant distress or impairment in social, occupational, or other important areas of functioning.
C. Psychological factors are judged to have an important role in the onset, severity, exacerbation, or maintenance of the pain.
D. The symptom or deficit is not intentionally produced or feigned (as in Factitious Disorder or Malingering).
E. The pain is not better accounted for by a Mood, Anxiety, or Psychotic Disorder and does not meet criteria for Dyspareunia.

Code as follows:
307.80 Pain Disorder Associated With Psychological Factors: psychological factors are judged to have the major role in the onset, severity, exacerbation, or maintenance of the pain. (If a general medical condition is present, it does not have a major role in the onset, severity, exacerbation, or maintenance of the pain.) This type of Pain Disorder is not diagnosed if criteria are also met for Somatization Disorder.
Specify if:
  Acute: duration of less than 6 months
  Chronic: duration of 6 months or longer

307.89 Pain Disorder Associated With Both Psychological Factors and a General Medical Condition: both psychological factors and a general medical condition are judged to have important roles in the onset, severity, exacerbation, or maintenance of the pain. The associated general medical condition or anatomical site of the pain (see below) is coded on Axis III.
Specify if:
  Acute: duration of less than 6 months
  Chronic: duration of 6 months or longer

Note: The following is not considered to be a mental disorder and is included here to facilitate differential diagnosis.
Pain Disorder Associated With a General Medical Condition: a general medical condition has a major role in the onset, severity, exacerbation, or maintenance of the pain. (If psychological factors are present, they are not judged to have a major role in the onset, severity, exacerbation, or maintenance of the pain.) The diagnostic code for the pain is selected based on the associated general medical condition if one has been established (see Appendix G) or on the anatomical location of the pain if the underlying general medical condition is not yet clearly established, for example, low back (724.2), sciatic (724.3), pelvic (625.9), headache (784.0), facial (784.0), chest (786.50), joint (719.4), bone (733.90), abdominal (789.0), breast (611.71), renal (788.0), ear (388.70), eye (379.91), throat (784.1), tooth (525.9), and urinary (788.0).

* DSM-IV criteria (American Psychiatric Association, 1994).

The World Health Organization (WHO) has suggested a rational titration of pain medication, called the WHO ladder (Fig. 23–3). This stepwise approach was devised for the treatment of cancer pain, but is applicable for many other pain situations.

The first step in the approach is the use of nonsteroidal antiinflammatory drugs (NSAIDs) for mild-to-moderate pain. Adjuvant drugs also may be used at any step. When pain persists, a low-potency opioid (e.g., codeine or hydrocodone) should be added to this regimen. The NSAID should be maintained as it may provide additive analgesia. Pain that persists despite this regimen should be treated with more potent opioids (for example, morphine, hydromorphone, methadone, fentanyl, or levorphanol). For pain that is moderate to severe at the outset, opioids should be the first choice.

This approach emphasizes the importance of simplicity, both in drug choice and in dose scheduling. Single agents are more easily titrated, and their side effects are more predictable. Adjuvants should be added only when indicated. Several combination preparations have been used, the most famous

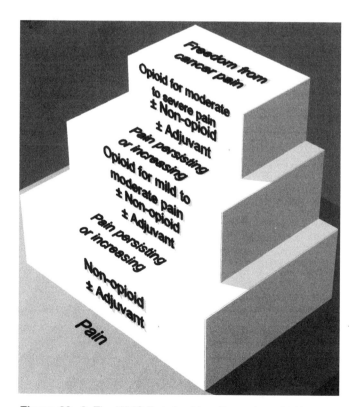

Figure 23–3. The WHO Pain Ladder. Reproduced with permission from Cancer pain relief, 2nd ed. Geneva, World Health Organization, 1996.

being *Brompton's cocktail,* which is a mixture of morphine, cocaine, and a phenothiazine. Despite anecdotal reports, no study has demonstrated any benefit of such mixtures over using single opioids. As they can also cause additive side effects, they should not be used.

Simple dosing, using a knowledge of a drug's pharmacokinetics, is equally important. To order a short-acting agent such as morphine or meperidine to be given every 4 to 6 hours is an overestimation of the drug's likely length of effect. Similarly, medications for persistent pain should be treated using scheduled around the clock doses to ensure a constant effective blood level. As-needed (i.e., p.r.n.) medications can be added to the regimen, but should not be used alone, as they can result in erratic levels of medication. There are a number of other important reasons for preferring scheduled doses over p.r.n. medication: scheduled doses based on the half-life of the narcotic prevent the reemergence of pain; the dose required to treat reemergent pain is often larger than what is needed to prevent its recurrence on a fixed schedule; patients on a p.r.n. schedule are in a dependent position, requiring them to ask for medication, which can create preoccupation with and delays in administration, and elderly and cognitively impaired patients may have difficulty in initiating appropriate requests for medication (Goldberg and Tull, 1983).

Another issue in the timing of narcotic doses pertains to special procedures. It is important to note whether the patient's pain problem is the result of an intermittent procedure such as debridement, dressing changes, or physical therapy. In such instances, the most important intervention may be to ensure that the patient receives an adequate narcotic dose prior to such an intervention.

Opioid Analgesia

Opioids remain the gold standard of pharmacological treatment for the patient with pain.

Mechanism of Action

In their action, narcotics mimic the effect of endogenous opioids, the most potent being beta-endorphin (Ferranta, 1996). All opioids, endogenous and exogenous, bind to specific opioid receptors in the brain and peripheral nervous system. Most of the opioids bind to the mu receptors. The potency of opioids is related to their affinity for the receptor.

There are two classes of mu receptor, mu-1 and mu-2. The first is involved in analgesia, and the second is responsible for respiratory depression. There is no opioid that can bind only with mu-1. Of the other receptors, the most important are delta and kappa, which are important in spinal analgesia.

It is important to understand the different relationships a compound may have at the opioid receptor. *Agonists* (Table 23–2) produce their response through receptor binding. Morphine is a prototypic mu agonist. *Partial agonists* incompletely bind to the receptor, exerting less than maximal effect, even at high concentrations. Buprenorphine is an example of a partial mu agonist.

Table 23–2 **Opioid Agonists***

NAME	BRAND NAME	PO	IV	PR
Alfentanil	Alfenta		X	
Morphine	Astramorph, Duramorph, Infumorph, Kadian, MSIR, RMS, Roxanol	X	X	X
Propoxyphene	Darvon	X		
Meperidine	Demerol	X	X	
Hydromorphone	Dilaudid	X	X	X
Fentanyl	Sublimaze		X	
Levophanol	Levo-Dromoran	X	X	
Methadone	Methadone	X		
Oxymorphone	Numorphan		X	X
Levo-alpha-acetymethadol (LAAM)	Orlaam	X		
Oxycodone	Roxicodone	X		
Sufentanil	Sufenta	X		

* Drug data for all tables derived from Physician's Desk Reference, 1996; Jacox et al, 1994; and Acute Pain Management Guideline Panel, 1992.

Opioids may also have different actions at different receptors. For example, pentazocine is a weak mu receptor agonist, but a strong kappa agonist; therefore, it is labeled an *agonist–antagonist* (Table 23–3). Partial agonists and agonist–antagonists are less preferable than pure agonists for pain management, given their weaker binding affinities for the mu receptor. Agonist–antagonists are especially problematic, as they can precipitate withdrawal when given to patients dependent on opioids. A number of opioids are also commonly prescribed in combination preparations (Table 23–4).

Indications

Opioids are the most effective agents available for treating acute pain, that is, pain associated with acute injury to the body.

Table 23–3 **Opioid Agonist–Antagonists**

NAME	BRAND NAME	PO	IV	IN
Buprenorphine	Buprenex		X	
Dezocine	Dalgan		X	
Nalbuphine	Nubain		X	
Butorphanol	Stadol		X	X
Pentazocine	Talwin	X		

Table 23–4 **Opioid Combinations Drugs**

NARCOTIC	+ ACETOMINOPHEN	+ ASPIRIN
Dihydrocodeine	DHC plus*	
Propoxyphene	Darvocet, Wyegesic	
Codeine	Tylenol with Codeine #s 2–4, Fiorect*,†	Fiorinal*,†
Hydrocodone	Hydrocet, Lorcet, Lortab, Vicodin, Zydone	
Oxycodone	Percocet, Tylox	Percodan
Pentazocine‡	Talacen	

* Also contains caffeine.
† Also contains butalbital.
‡ Agonist–antagonist.

Treatment Approach

Although pharmaceutical companies expend great energy in opioid development, it is unlikely we will see a "better" opioid in the foreseeable future. Apparent differences in potency are more often due to pharmacokinetic rather than pharmacodynamic differences, that is, all opioids can be made equipotent by adjusting their dose or route of administration. Thus, the student attempting to understand the proper use of opioids better should concentrate on understanding the pharmacology of opioids as a class, rather than the intricacies of individual drugs.

Perhaps most central to the use of opioids is the idea of *minimum effective concentration* (MEC). The MEC is a hypothetical plasma concentration below which a drug is ineffective. The MEC for an opioid (that is, the plasma level at which analgesia is effective) can vary greatly among different individuals. Thus, when choosing an opioid dose for a patient, we cannot know what the effective dose will be before we use the drug. The only way to find the proper dose is by titrating until the patient responds to the drug. Therefore, any table of "recommended doses" can be only a rough guideline for beginning therapy (Tables 23–5 and 23–6). Similarly, tables of relative potencies among opioids are rough estimates (Table 23–7).

Side Effects

Beyond deciding an appropriate dose for an individual, the titration of opioids usually involves the management of side effects. The most common opioid side effects are nausea and sedation. The most problematic side effect is respiratory depression, which is due to a reduction in brain stem responsiveness to PCO_2, and to the depression of pontine and medullary centers,

Table 23–5 **Opioid Agonists: Usual Adult Starting Doses (for Opioid-Naive Individuals)**

DRUG	ORAL	PARENTERAL	TRANSDERMAL
Alfenta		8–20 µg/kg*	
Morphine	30 mg q3–4 h	10 mg q3–4h	
Morphine controlled-release	90–120 mg q12h		
Propoxyphene	65 mg q4h		
Hydromorphone	6 mg q3–4h	1.5 mg q3–4h	
Levo-alpha-acetymethadol (LAAM)[†]	20–40 mg q48–72h		
Levorphanol	4 mg q6–8h	2 mg q6–8h	
Meperidine	Not recommended	100 mg q3h	
Methadone	20 mg q6–8h	10 mg q6–8h	
Oxymorphone		1 mg q3–4h	
Fentanyl		2–50 µg/kg*	Not recommended[‡]
Oxycodone	Immediate release: 10–30 mg q4h Controlled release: not recommended[‡]		
Sufentanil		1–8 µg/kg*	

* Usually used only for general anesthesia. Please see the package insert for dosing guidelines.
† Generally indicated only for the treatment of opioid dependence.
‡ Neither transdermal fentanyl nor oxycodone controlled-release are recommended for initial use.
In each case, it is preferable to start an immediate-release opioid and then convert to a continuous release preparation.

which are involved in the regulation of breathing. Fortunately, respiratory depression can be reversed by naloxone. When it is necessary to use naloxone, it is best administered in a dilute solution (0.4 mg in 10 ml of saline) slowly given intravenously, titrated against the patient's respiratory rate (Foley, 1985b). Patients receiving this treatment must be closely followed with frequent respiratory rate checks because naloxone has a short half-life, and patients may have to be redosed if taking longer acting narcotics such as methadone.

Opioids can also cause alterations in mood, tolerance, and alertness. They decrease gastrointestinal peristalsis and increase sphincter tone, causing constipation. This effect on sphincter tone also can increase biliary pressure and urinary retention. Opioids also can rarely depress cardiac function and cause bradycardia (although meperidine can cause tachycardia via its antimuscarinic effect).

The incidence and severity of side effects seen with different opioids are probably similar at equianalgesic doses (meperidine may be an exception

Table 23–6 **Opioid Combinations: Usual Adult Starting Doses (Opioid Naive)**

DRUG	DOSE (OF NARCOTIC)
Dihydrocodeine + acetaminophen	32 mg q4h
Propoxyphene + acetaminophen	100 mg q4h
Codeine + aspirin or	
acetaminophen	60 mg q3–4h
Hydrocodone + acetaminophen	10 mg q3–4h
Oxycodone + aspirin or	
acetaminophen	10 mg q3–4h
Pentazocine + acetaminophen	25 mg q4h

and is discussed separately). Thus, changing to a different opioid is less likely to improve side effects, and the clinician should be familiar with the symptomatic treatment of these side effects. In some cases, such as treating constipation associated with opioids, the prophylactic use of laxatives is often preferred.

Table 23–7 **Opioid Agonists: Approximate Equipotent Dose**

DRUG	ORAL	PARENTERAL	TRANSDERMAL
Morphine	Single/intermittent dose: 60 mg q3–4h Repeated (around the clock) dose: 30 mg q3–4h	10 mg q3–4h	
Morphine controlled-release	90–120 mg q12h		
Codeine	180–200 mg q3–4h	130 mg q3–4h	
Fentanyl			~100 µg/hr
Hydrocodone	30 mg q3–4h		
Hydromorphone	7.5 mg q3–4h	1.5 mg q3–4h	
Levorphanol	4 mg q6–8h	2 mg q6–8h	
Meperidine	300 mg q2–3h	100 mg q3h	
Methadone	20 mg q6–8h	10 mg q6–8h	
Oxycodone	Immediate release: 30 mg q4h Controlled release: 80 mg q12h		
Oxymorphone		1 mg q3–4h	
Propoxyphene	120–200 mg q3–4h		

Meperidine

Certain treatment strategies, including some in common use, are not recommended. Perhaps the most common problem is the continued overreliance on meperidine for pain management. Meperidine has a very short duration of action, making it inappropriate for all but brief courses of treatment. It is low in potency and often underdosed in patients (the common choice of 75 mg of meperidine is probably inadequate for most patients). Its metabolite normeperidine can be toxic, causing central nervous system irritation and can accumulate over time and lead to dysphoria, delirium, and even seizures. Structurally, meperidine is similar to atropine and may share many of atropine's anticholinergic effects. For these reasons, meperidine is best avoided unless a patient cannot tolerate other high-potency opioids.

The continued use of meperidine comes not only from force of habit, but from a belief that it has certain benefits over other opioids. Most common is the belief that it causes less sphincter spasm. Meperidine, therefore, remains the preferred opioid for patients undergoing endoscopic procedures at the pancreatic or bile duct. The evidence for such a belief, however, is weak. Thune and colleagues (1990) found that meperidine did not increase phasic contractions at the sphincter of Oddi, whereas morphine did cause a dose-dependent increase. It is significant, however, that neither opioid affected the basal sphincter pressure, and the study used subanalgesic doses of both medications. Using analgesic doses, Elta and Barnett (1994) did find that meperidine increased phasic contractions at the sphincter of Oddi. Again, there was no significant change in sphincter pressure. In the latter study, only meperidine was used, and we do not know how other opioids would have compared. In a recent editorial review of the literature on opioids and the sphincter of Oddi, Sherman and Lehman (1994) continue to advise against routine use of meperidine for these procedures.

Tolerance, Physical Dependence, and Addiction

The greatest barrier to opiate use is physicians' fear of causing addiction. In understanding this fear, it is important to distinguish among tolerance, dependence, and withdrawal. *Tolerance* is the decline in potency of an opioid experienced with continued use, so that higher doses are needed to achieve the same effect. This is a receptor-mediated effect and is common to all opioids. *Physical dependence* refers to the development of *withdrawal* symptoms once a drug is stopped. Typical symptoms of opioid withdrawal include yawning, diaphoresis, lacrimation, coryza, and tachycardia, followed by abdominal cramps, nausea, and vomiting.

Tolerance and dependence are physiological phenomena and are not the same as addiction. *Addiction* is a compulsion to use a drug, usually for its psychic, rather than therapeutic, effects. Thus, it implies a behavioral problem, with psychological, as well as physical, dependence. One can have tolerance or dependence without addiction, and the reverse is true, as well.

Clearly, individuals with histories of opiate addiction are at risk of continued addictive use if they are prescribed opioids. The question remains, however, whether we can cause opioid addiction by administering it to a patient without such history. In clinical investigations of the question, it appears that iatrogenic (hospital or clinic related) addiction is a very rare event. In a large review of over 11,000 Medicare inpatients who received narcotics, only four cases of iatrogenic narcotic addiction were documented (Porter and Jick, 1980). Patients who legitimately need pain medication almost never become addicted to them.

Route of Administration

An understanding of the different ways to deliver an opioid to a patient is as important as fluency with the different available opioids.

Oral Administration. Drugs administered into the gastrointestinal tract go through the portal circulation to the liver. In the liver, opioids are extensively metabolized (*first-pass* metabolism) to inactive products. Therefore, most of the oral dose never reaches the target receptor.

The amount of active medication that is available after first-pass metabolism varies greatly for different agents and varies among individuals. Heroin, for example, is completely metabolized orally, whereas 80% of ingested methadone remains available after first-pass metabolism. Morphine's oral bioavailabity can range from 10 to 65%, making for great variability in an individual's oral dose requirement. Generally, the oral to parenteral potency ratio for morphine is 1:6 for acute use, and 1:2 to 3 for chronic use.

Several compounds are available in sustained-release form (Table 23–8), and pharmaceutical companies have given much attention to the development of these compounds. In the United States, sustained-release preparations are available for morphine and for oxycodone. It remains a great challenge to develop agents that will maintain a stable blood level over time. Factors such as eating and physical activity also may alter a sustained-release drug's kinetics.

Sublingual Administration. Opioids given sublingually are directly absorbed into the systemic circulation, thereby avoiding first-pass metabolism. This route may be particularly useful for individuals who cannot tolerate oral medication because of nausea and vomiting. Buprenorphine, a partial agonist, is available in a sublingual preparation.

Rectal Administration. Like oral administration, substances absorbed rectally undergo first-pass metabolism. Suppositories can be useful for patients who cannot swallow or are likely to vomit after oral administration of the opioid.

Table 23–8 Opioid Agonists: Slow Release Preparations

NAME	BRAND NAME	PO	TD	PR
Morphine	MS Contin, Oramorph	X		
Fentanyl	Duragesic		X	
Oxycodone	Oxycontin	X		

Intramuscular Administration. Although very commonly used, intramuscular administration of opioids is often erratic, and patients may alternate between periods of toxicity and undertreatment. Such injections can be painful, particularly if they must be used continuously. This method of administration generally should be reserved for the unusual case in which no other method of administration is feasible.

Subcutaneous Administration. Although they have been used for years, we know surprisingly little about the pharmacokinetics of subcutaneous opioids. For morphine, the blood levels achieved with subcutaneous administration are probably comparable to those of intravenous administration. This is not as well understood for other opioids. This route of administration is becoming more compelling with the development of portable pumps that can deliver continuous infusions.

Intravenous Administration. IV administration remains the most rapid and effective means of delivering opioids to the systemic circulation. Most commonly, an IV dose is given at regular intervals. Proper use of this method requires understanding the pharmacokinetics of a drug, to ensure that the blood level does not go below the MEC for that drug. Several newer methods for IV administration are also available, as outlined below.

Continuous Infusion. This method of IV administration is becoming more popular. It can be a very efficient way to provide long-term pain relief. It should be remembered, however, that the blood level of the drug must always be kept above the MEC to provide effective pain relief continuously. This can be particularly difficult at the beginning of continuous therapy, as a drug requires four to five half-lives to achieve steady-state concentration. Therefore, a loading dose is required before starting continuous infusion.

Patient-Controlled Analgesia. In patient-controlled analgesia (PCA), the patient can decide when to give a dose and the timing between doses. The physician still decides the particular drug and dosing and timing limits. The advantage of such a system is that it acknowledges the subjectivity of a patient's perception and allows the patient freedom in making some treatment choices. It also avoids the potential struggles that can occur when a patient must ask someone for each dose. It has potential disadvantages, however, as patients can be just as likely as physicians to underdose themselves. Proper patient education in the use of the PCA (for example, that it is better to treat the pain at onset, rather than waiting until it gets very intense) is essential (Acute Pain Management Guideline Panel, 1992).

Transdermal Administration. The transdermal patch offers another method of delivering continuous analgesia. Currently, fentanyl is available in this formulation. Fentanyl is a potent, short-acting opioid that can be released slowly from the patch. From skin absorption, the fentanyl enters systemic circulation. Peak serum concentration begins to level off between 1 to 2 days after initial administration and remains relatively constant for 3 days. The various patches are labeled with the approximate dose delivered per hour. Because it offers a less cumbersome alternative to continuous IV administration, it is becoming popular among physicians for use in ambulatory chronic pain patients.

Transnasal Administration. Theoretically, this may be another practical method of delivering medication into the systemic circulation. However, only butorphanol (an agonist–antagonist) is available in a nasal spray. This agent is primarily used for acute headache and is not recommended for chronic pain (Jacox et al, 1994).

Spinal Administration. Direct administration of opioids to receptor sites is possible through intrathecal, epidural, and intracerebroventricular administration. Spinally administered opioids migrate to all areas of the spinal cord; therefore, they can be appropriate for many types of pain. Enthusiasm for this technique is tempered, however, by the occurrence of severe delayed-onset respiratory depression, which occurs in perhaps 1 in 1,000 patients receiving epidural morphine.

Tramadol

Tramadol hydrochloride (Ultram) is a centrally acting analgesic. Though marketed as a "nonopioid analgesic," it appears to act primarily as a μ-receptor agonist. It is also a weak norepinephrine and serotonin reuptake inhibitor. It may have a lower abuse potential than standard opioid analgesics. However, it has been shown to cause both physical dependence, withdrawal, and delirium. It is indicated for moderate to moderately severe pain, in a manner analogous to low-potency opioids, and is usually initiated at a dose of 50–100 mg every 4–6 hours, not to exceed 400 mg per day.

Nonsteroidal Antiinflammatory Drugs

Mechanism of Action

All NSAIDs inhibit cylooxygenase, which is an enzyme responsible for the synthesis of prostaglandins. Prostaglandins are metabolized from arachidonic acid. This process occurs at sites of tissue damage and seems to help sensitize nociceptors to painful stimuli. Acetaminophen usually is included in this group. Although not as potent an antiinflammatory agent, it has similar analgesic potency to the NSAIDs.

Indications

NSAIDs are helpful for treating many types of pain, ranging from minor aches and sprains to bony metastases.

Treatment Approaches

Unlike opioid analgesics, there is no clear relationship between serum levels of NSAIDs and analgesia. Although they are often used alone, their mechanism of action is different from that of opioids, and they can act syner-

Table 23–9 **Acetaminophen and NSAIDs: Usual Adult Starting Doses**

DRUG	DOSE
Acetaminophen	650–975 mg q4h
Aspirin	650–975 mg q4h
Choline magnesium (Trilisate)	1,000–1,500 mg b.i.d.
Diflunisal (Dolobid)	1,000-mg initial dose followed by 500 mg q12h
Etodolac (Lodine)	200–400 mg q6–8h
Fenoprofen calcium (Nalfon)	200 mg q4–6h
Ibuprofen (Motrin, Advil, others)	400 mg q4–6h
Ketoprofen (Orudis)	25–75 mg q6–8h
Magnesium salicylate	650 mg q4h
Meclofenamate sodium (Meclomen)	50 mg q4–6h
Mefenamic acid (Ponstel)	250 mg q6h
Naproxen (Naprosyn)	500-mg initial dose followed by 250 mg q6–8h
Naproxen sodium (Anaprox)	550-mg initial dose followed by 275 mg q6–8h
Salsalate (Disalcid, others)	500 mg q4h
Sodium salicylate	325–650 mg q3–4h
Ketorolac tromethamine (Toradol)	IM: 30 or 60 mg IM initial dose followed by 15 or 30 mg q6h Oral: 10 mg q6–8h

gistically with opioids. Typical doses are recommended in Table 23–9; these data are derived from long-term use in rheumatological disease.

Side Effects

The most common side effect is gastric irritation. The decrease in prostaglandin caused by NSAIDs results in a decrease in gastric mucus and an increase in gastric acidity. Acetaminophen is an exception.

Other side effects include salt and fluid retention, platelet inhibition, and tinnitus. An advantage of acetaminophen is its mimimal effect on platelet function. The drugs are excreted renally, and patients with renal insufficiency may be at risk for toxicity. NSAIDs may decrease renal blood flow and may cause renal failure. The latter effect is of most concern in patients who are elderly, or volume depleted, or taking other nephrotoxic drugs, or who have preexisting renal impairment, heart failure, or hepatic dysfunction (Jacox et al, 1994). Acetaminophen carries the additional hazard of possible liver damage from an overdose.

Route of Administration

Most NSAIDs are available only orally. An exception is ketorolac, which can be given parenterally and is useful in the management of postoperative pain. Ketorolac has been associated with nephrotoxicity with chronic use and therefore is used for acute pain.

Adjunctive Medications

Opioids and NSAIDs remain the most important pharmacological options in pain management. All other options must be considered secondary. The data and rationale for any of these agents are much weaker than that for opioids or NSAIDs, and much of it is anecdotal. Many are only useful in combination with standard analgesia. However, there remains a sizable group of patients for whom opioids or NSAIDs are either inadequate, intolerable, or inappropriate. Thus, the search for alternative analgesics continues.

Antidepressants

Antidepressants are the most commonly used adjunctive agents. They have become common in the treatment of certain types of pain.

Mechanism of Action. A variety of mechanisms have been suggested. Monoamine neurotransmitters, such as norepinephrine and serotonin, may influence the transmission of pain. This influence is thought to be a central phenomenon. However, sympathetic neurons are located near nociceptors and may play a role in peripheral pain modulation.

It remains uncertain whether antidepressants have a primary analgesic effect, or whether they simply relieve pain-associated depression. Some studies find a strong association between simultaneous improvement of both pain and depression. Other studies show independent effects. Similarly, some studies suggest that effective analgesic doses for antidepressants are much less than those used for depression; other studies suggest that both disorders require similar doses.

Indications. Antidepressants are most frequently used for neuropathies, such as that caused by diabetes mellitus. Other studies have shown their usefulness in treating migraine headaches. Beyond that, there are isolated accounts— usually anecdotal— of their use in almost every pain imaginable. It appears that the best antidepressants for pain treatment are those that increase both norepinephrine and serotonin (e.g., nortriptyline). In one comparison of several antidepressants in patients with diabetic neuropathies (Max et al, 1992), the tricyclic antidepressants amitriptyline and desipramine were superior to placebo. The use of tricyclics like nortriptyline and doxepin are mainstays in the management of chronic pain syndromes. The serotonin-reuptake inhibitor fluoxetine was less effective in pain relief than the other two, and no different from placebo. In this study, pain relief was independent of antidepressant effect.

Serotonin-reuptake inhibitors, however, may have some adjunctive role in pain management. Using animal models, one study demonstrated that morphine analgesia was potentiated by fluoxetine, without a concomitant increase in respiratory depression (Haynes and Fuller, 1982). Similarly, nefazodone was shown to potentiate morphine analgesia in certain animal models of pain (Pick et al, 1991).

Anticonvulsants

Anticonvulsants also are used for neuropathic pain (Swerdlow, 1984). For example, carbamazepine is considered by some to be the first-line treatment for trigeminal neuralgia (Tomson and Bertilsson, 1984). Anticonvulsants may act by suppressing neuronal firing in the area of damaged neurons. Usually, they are started slowly and gradually increased in dose to minimize side effects. Common side effects include dizziness, ataxia, drowsiness, blurred vision, and gastrointestinal irritation. Specific organ toxicities also can present a problem: carbamazepine can cause bone marrow suppression, and sodium valproate can very rarely cause liver toxicity. Both drugs require blood monitoring. Gabapentin and lamotrigine, although potentially useful, have not yet been extensively studied for pain treatment.

Local Analgesics

Lidocaine and 2-chlorprocaine are used for peripheral neuropathies. There is some suggestion that patients who describe their neuropathic pain as "constant" are more likely to benefit from these agents, whereas those with episodic pain benefit more from anticonvulsants. These agents are generally given intravenously; however, oral use of lidocaine derivatives (e.g., mexiletine and tocainide) has been reported to be useful in some patients (Dejard and Peterson, 1988).

Another locally acting agent is capsaicin, an alkaloid irritant derived from chili peppers. It is available as a cream (Zostrix) that is applied topically to painful areas. It appears to work by depleting substance P. It has been shown to be effective for a number of syndromes, including diabetic neuropathy, osteoarthritis, postherpetic neuralgia, and psoriasis (Zhang and Po, 1994).

Antihistamines

Hydroxyzine is most often used among the antihistamines for pain control. The use of hydroxyzine in combination with meperidine is so common that it is surprising how few data exist to justify this practice. Antihistamines are probably weakly analgesic, but they are quite inconsistent in their ability to potentiate the analgesic effects of opioids (Jacox et al, 1994). Moreover, they are probably much more effective at potentiating opioid side effects, such as sedation and confusion. They may have some use in modulating the anxiety caused by pain, but are unlikely to be preferable to other available agents.

Antipsychotics

Although rarely used as single agents, antipyschotics are thought to potentiate the action of opioids. Most of the support for this theory is anecdotal. The phenothiazines are most often used. Haloperidol also has been used as an antiemetic and to decrease opioid-associated confusion. Protracted use of these agents must be balanced against the risk of tardive dyskinesia and other long and short term side effects.

Benzodiazepines

Benzodiazepines do not appear to have any analgesic properties. They may, however, modify the affective experience of pain. They also act as muscle relaxants, which can be useful in musculoskeletal pain.

Stimulants

Stimulants include the amphetamines, caffeine, and cocaine. All act as sympathomimetics, and they can potentiate the action of opiates. It is not clear whether this effect is long or short term. Amphetamines have been combined with opiates, and caffeine has been used to potentiate NSAIDs. An advantage of stimulants is that they often act quickly, and their efficacy can often be judged after only a few days.

Cannabinoids

With the passage of Proposition 215 in California and Proposition 200 in Arizona, we can anticipate a new vigor in the debate over the medical uses of marijuana. Cannabinoids do appear to have some analgesic effect. This effect is probably mediated by nonopioid receptors, which may argue for an adjunctive role in pain management. The side effects associated with marijuana (dysphoria, drowsiness, hypotension, bradycardia, loss of coordination, impairment of judgment, and sensory disturbances) probably outweigh possible benefits (Jacox et al, 1994). Whether other cannabinoids, such as the orally available synthetic cannabinoid dronabinol, offer similar benefits while reducing the ill effects is a matter worthy of investigation.

Placebos

Occasionally, a clinician will administer placebo pills or injections when they are skeptical of the patient's pain. We believe that any attempt to deceive a patient is always inappropriate. Furthermore, the fact that a patient responds to a placebo analgesic does not prove that the pain was "in their head." The placebo response is a very real phenomenon, and 30 to 40% of the population are placebo responders (achieve pain relief), even in the presence of severe disease (Beecher, 1955).

PROCEDURAL TREATMENTS

Nonsurgical Procedures

Cutaneous Stimulation

Cutaneous stimulation involves the application of heat, cold, or mechanical pressure to a superficial area. Heat may decrease pain through vasodilation and by decreasing joint stiffness. Cold causes vasoconstriction and local hyperesthesia, which reduces inflammation in an affected area. Mechanical pressure is typified by massage, which can relax muscular aches.

Electrical Stimulation

The rationale for electrical stimulation to modulate pain is based on the gate theory of pain. Electrical charge excites large peripheral fibers, and other nociceptive information is blocked in the process. Transcutaneous electrical nerve stimulation uses low-intensity stimulation of muscle and skin in a particular segmental distribution. Dorsal column stimulation uses a high-frequency current over the dorsal spinal cord and has been useful in deafferentation pain syndromes. Electrical stimulation is used both solely and in combination with other treatments.

Acupuncture

Theoretically, acupuncture analgesia is very similar to that of electrical stimulation, except that manual stimulation is used. The stimulation is produced through rotation of small needles at certain body sites. The resulting sensation (*teh chi*) confers not only local analgesia, but also a more generalized phenomenon. This generalized effect may result from stimulation of chemical modulators. Although there are anecdotal reports of great benefit from acupuncture, systematic evidence demonstrating general efficacy for this technique is lacking.

Exercise

In cases of acute pain, immobilization often is needed. Prolonged immobilization, however, can cause joint contractures, muscle atrophy, and cardiovascular deconditioning, and it should be avoided whenever possible. Appropriate exercises depend on the specific injury or pathology and can range from passive motion and positional change to weight-bearing exercises and aerobic conditioning. Referral for physical therapy is an excellent strategy to mobilize patients and help with musculoskeletal pain syndromes.

Surgical Procedures

Neural Blockade

Typically, nerve transmission to an area is blocked through injection of an agent. The injection sites can be around the peripheral nerves or somatic plexuses and at the dorsal roots. Short-acting agents (e.g., lidocaine) can be used for acute pain, whereas more permanent blockade (e.g., alcohol) is used for chronic pain. In the latter case, diagnostic blocks are done first, in which short-acting agents can help localize the pain pathway.

Surgical lesions can also be used to block a pain pathway permanently. Side effects of this treatment mainly result from the fact that it is not possible to isolate the pain fibers. Therefore, other motor and sensory information may be lost, as well.

The efficacy of treatment is unpredictable, and neuronal block is often unreliable in chronic pain situations. When weighing the above side effects against a questionable benefit, permanent neuronal block is not usually appropriate in chronic pain situations. It also is not appropriate for nonnociceptive pain, such as neuropathic pain. Neurodestructive techniques sometimes worsen neuropathic pain. Such techniques may be appropriate when the life expectancy is short. Even then, it should be considered only when other approaches to pain management have been exhausted.

PSYCHOLOGICAL TREATMENTS

Psychoeducation

Properly educating patients about pain treatment can help make them active participants in their own pain management. Education can lessen potential misunderstandings about pain treatment. For example, patients may fear that if they ask for too much pain medication, they may become addicted. Similarly, patients often believe that they should avoid asking for pain medication until they can no longer bear their pain. Proper education can allay their fears about addiction and help them understand that their pain is probably better prevented early than when it reaches peak intensity.

Hypnosis

We have known for over a century that hypnosis can help treat pain. It remains, however, an underused option for pain management. Hypnosis works through a combination of effects, including relaxation, distraction, and perceptual alteration. Clearly, muscle relaxation and distraction (i.e., from other competing sensations) can be helpful in modulating the pain response. We are most intrigued, however, by the ability of hypnosis to alter perceptions. This seems to give hypnosis an almost mystical quality. The phenomenon is hardly mystical. Most individuals can learn to alter their sensations somewhat, and this ability improves with practice. Typically, an individual will receive the suggestion that the pain sensation is another sensation, such as a sense of warmth. An advantage of hypnosis is that, with training, patients can learn to hypnotize themselves.

Behavioral Treatment of Pain

This treatment is derived from learning theory, in which most behavior is assumed to be learned. For pain treatment, the focus is on the behavior associated with the pain experience, or *pain behavior.* The goal of treatment is to decrease the factors that are encouraging or "reinforcing" such behavior. A simple example is on hospital wards, where the staff pay more attention to patients with pain problems and thus may reinforce the pain behavior.

Furthermore, it is assumed that potential responses to situations, such as reacting with anxiety, may result in pain. In this sense, pain may be a *conditioned response* to a variety of circumstances. Several behavioral techniques are used to approach these problems.

Relaxation Training

Relaxation training is a simple behavioral technique that involves teaching patients to relax each of their muscle groups systematically. This can be useful in a variety of pain conditions, particularly when muscle tension may play a role (e.g., tension headaches). Usually patients also are taught to imagine a pleasant scene. With practice, the patient can perform this technique without assistance.

Biofeedback

In biofeedback, imperceptible physiological responses are amplified and made accessible. Once made aware of these responses, an individual can attempt to modify them. For example, a patient with tension headaches might hear an audible electromyogram representing the frequency of muscle contractions in selected muscle groups and then learn to reduce such contractions.

Cognitive–Behavior Therapy

In cognitive–behavior therapy, the focus is on both pain behavior and the conscious thoughts that influence such behavior. Typically, the therapist thoroughly explores all aspects of the pain experience, including thoughts and feelings preceding, accompanying, and following the experience. The goal is less one of eliminating pain and more of lessening the disability associated with the pain. Given the complexity of the pain experience and biopsychosocial interactions, it is not unusual for patients to perceive some lessening in pain intensity, as well.

Unlike pharmacological treatments, psychological treatments clearly require a great deal of time and motivation. There is a significant rate of nonresponse in many studies. A good predictor of response, however, may be one's motivation to persevere with treatment.

MULTIDISCIPLINARY PAIN REHABILITATION

Perhaps the best treatment for chronic pain can be given only by a multidisciplinary group. The multidisciplinary approach is in contrast to the traditional medical system, in which different consultants act in relative isolation from each other and the primary medical doctor. A multidisciplinary rehabilitation program employs professionals from various disciplines, including physical therapy, working in tandem. Usually, the goals of treatment are multiple, as well, simultaneously including decreasing pain intensity, increasing activity level, decreasing medication use, and decreasing use of medical services. Such a program is expensive, although it may be cost effective when compared with traditional medical/surgical interventions and diagnostic procedures. Unfortunately, studies proving such cost effectiveness are preliminary and use small numbers of participants.

SOME SPECIFIC PAIN SITUATIONS

Headaches

Headaches are probably the most common pain complaint. They account for tens of millions of patient visits and hundreds of millions of lost productivity days.

When a patient presents with headache complaints, it is important to rule out important signs that might suggest a serious cause of a headache (Table 23–10). Most headaches, however, fall into one of several categories of primary disorders. The International Headache Society has created a classification system for headaches (Table 23–11) with accompanying diagnostic criteria. This

Table 23–10 **"Danger Signs" in Headache Pain Patients**

1. Headache is a new symptom for the individual in the past 3 months, or the nature of the headache has changed markedly in the past 3 months.
2. Presence of any sensory or motor deficits preceding or accompanying headache other than the typical visual prodromata of migraine with aura. Examples include weakness or numbness in an extremity, twitching of the hands or feet, aphasia, or slurred speech.
3. Headache is one sided and has always been on the same side of the head.
4. Headache is due to trauma, especially if it follows a period of unconsciousness (even if only momentary).
5. Headache is constant and unremitting.
6. For patient-reported tension-type headache-like symptoms:
   a. Pain intensity has been steadily increasing over a period of weeks to months with little or no relief.
   b. Headache is worse in the morning and becomes less severe during the day. Headache is accompanied by vomiting.
7. Patient has been treated for any kind of cancer and now has a complaint of headache.
8. Patient or significant other reports a noticeable change in personality or behavior or a notable decrease in memory or other intellectual functioning.
9. The patient is over 60 years of age, and the headache is a relatively new complaint.
10. Pain onset is sudden and occurs during condition of exertion (such as lifting heavy objects), sexual intercourse, or "heated" interpersonal situation.
11. Patient's family has a history of cerebral aneurysm, other vascular anomalies, or polycystic kidneys.

(From Andrasic F, Baskin S: Headache. In Morrison RL, Bellack AS (eds): Medical Factors and Psychological Disorders: A Handbook for Psychologists. New York, Plenum, 325–349, 1987)

Table 23–11 **Classification of Headaches**

1. Migraine
    1.1. Migraine without aura
    1.2. Migraine with aura
    1.5. Childhood periodic syndromes that may be precursors to or associated with migraine
2. Tension-type headache
    2.1. Episodic tension-type headache
        2.1.1. Episodic tension-type headache associated with disorder of pericranial muscles
        2.1.2. Episodic tension-type headache unassociated with disorder of pericranial muscles.
    2.2. Chronic tension-type headache
        2.2.1. Chronic tension-type headache associated with disorder of pericranial muscles
        2.2.2. Chronic tension-type headache unassociated with disorder of pericranial muscles
3. Cluster headache and chronic paroxysmal hemicrania
    3.1. Cluster headache
        3.1.1. Cluster headache periodicity undetermined
        3.1.2. Episodic cluster headache
        3.1.3. Chronic cluster headache
4. Miscellaneous headaches unassociated with structural lesion
5. Headaches associated with head trauma
    5.1. Acute posttraumatic headache
        5.1.1. With significant head trauma and/or confirmatory signs
        5.1.2. With minor head trauma and no confirmatory signs
    5.2. Chronic posttraumatic headache
        5 2.1. With significant head trauma and/or confirmatory signs
        5.2.2. With minor head trauma and/or confirmatory signs
6. Headache associated with vascular disorder
7. Headache associated with nonvascular intracranial disorder
8. Headache associated with substances or their withdrawal
    8.1. Headache induced by acute substance use or exposure
        8.1.1. Nitrate/nitrite-induced headache
        8.1.2. Monosodium glutamate-induced headache
        8.1.3. Carbon monoxide-induced headache
        8.1.4. Alcohol-induced headache
        8.1.5. Other substances
    8.2. Headache induced by chronic substance use or exposure
        8.2.1. Ergotamine-induced headache
        8.2.2. Analgesic abuse headache
        8.2.3. Other substances
    8.3. Headache from substance withdrawal (acute use)
        8.3.1. Alcohol withdrawal headache (hangover)
        8.3.2. Other substances
    8.4. Headache from substance withdrawal (chronic use)
        8.4.1. Ergotamine withdrawal headache
        8.4.2. Caffeine withdrawal headache
        8.4.3. Narcotics abstinence headache
        8.4.4. Other substances
    8.5. Headache associated with substances but with uncertain mechanism
        8.5.1. Birth control pills or estrogens
        8.5.2. Other substances
9. Headache associated with noncephalic infection
10. Headache associated with metabolic disorder
11. Headache or facial pain associated with disorder of cranium, neck, eyes, ears, nose, sinuses, teeth, mouth, or other facial or cranial structures
12. Cranial neuralgias, nerve trunk pain, and deafferentation pain
13. Headache nonclassifiable

[From Headache Classification Committee of the International Headache Society: Classification and diagnostic criteria for headache disorders, cranial neuralgias, and facial pain. Cephalalgia 8(suppl 7):13–17, 1988]

Table 23–12 **Headache Diagnostic Criteria: Migraine**

Migraine Without Aura

A. At least five attacks fulfilling criteria B–D
B. Headache attacks lasting 4–72 hours (2–48 hours for children below age 15), untreated or unsuccessfully treated
C. Headache has at least two of the following characteristics:
1. Unilateral location
2. Pulsating quality
3. Moderate or severe intensity (inhibits or prohibits daily activities)
4. Aggravation by walking stairs or similar routine physical activity
D. During headache at least one of the following:
1. Nausea and/or vomiting
2. Photophobia and phonophobia
E. At least one of the following:
1. History, physical, and neurological examinations do not suggest one of the disorders listed in groups 5–11 in Table 23–11
2. History and/or physical, and/or neurological examination do suggest such disorders, but they are ruled out by appropriate investigations
3. Such disorder is present, but migraine attacks do not occur for the first time in close temporal relation to the disorder

Migraine With Aura

A. At least two attacks fulfilling criterion B
B. At least three of the following four characteristics:
1. One or more fully reversible aura symptoms indicating focal cerebral cortical and/or brain stem dysfunction
2. At least one aura symptom develops gradually over more than 4 minutes or two or more symptoms occur in succession
3. No aura symptom lasts more than 60 minutes. If more than one aura symptom is present, accepted duration is proportionally increased
4. Headache follows aura with a free interval of less than 60 minutes. It may also begin before or simultaneously with the aura
C. Same as Migraine Without Aura, criterion E

[From Headache Classification Committee of the International Headache Society: Classification and diagnostic criteria for headache disorders, cranial neuralgias, and facial pain. Cephalalgia 8(suppl 7):13–17, 1988]

classification system includes traditional causes of headaches, such as migraine (Table 23–12), tension (Table 23–13), and cluster (Table 23–14) headaches, but adds some previously underappreciated causes of headaches, such as headaches associated with substance use or withdrawal (Table 23–15). The most common substances producing headaches are the analgesics and the ergotamines. Both of these substances can lead to rebound headaches when overused. *Overuse* is difficult to define, however; as an example, a person who is using ergotamines for more than 2 days a week to treat headaches is probably overusing the substance. *Rebound* refers both to the phenomena of the worsening of a headache as the medication wears off and to typical withdrawal phenomena. In either case, a self-perpetuating situation is created as patients attempt to use more of the medication to alleviate the headaches that the medication itself is causing.

Table 23–13 **Headache Diagnostic Criteria: Tension-Type Headaches**

Episodic Tension-Type Headache

A. At least ten previous headache episodes fulfilling criteria B–D. Number of days with such headache <180/year (<15/month)
B. Headache lasting from 30 minutes to 7 days
C. At least two of the following pain characteristics:
    1. Pressing//tightening (nonpulsating) quality
    2. Mild or moderate intensity (may inhibit, but does not prohibit activities)
    3. Bilateral location
    4. No aggravation by walking stairs or similar routine physical activity
D. Bother of the following:
    1. No nausea or vomiting (anorexia may occur)
    2. Photophobia and phonophobia are absent, or one but not the other is present.
E. Same as Migraine Without Aura, criterion E

Chronic Tension-Type Headaches

As above, but:
    Average headache frequency ≥15/month (180 days/year) for ≥6 months
    Criterion C from above not needed
    No more than one of the following: nausea, photophobia, or phonophobia (and no vomiting)

Subtypes for Both Episodic and Chronic Tension-Type Headaches

Associated with disorder of pericranial muscles:
A. Fulfills criteria for tension-type headache (episodic or chronic)
B. At least one of the following:
    1. Increased tenderness of pericranial muscles demonstrated by manual palpation or pressure algometer
    2. Increased electromyographic (EMG) level of pericranial muscles at rest or during physiological tests
Unassociated with disorder of pericranial muscles:
A. Fulfills criteria for tension-type headache (episodic or chronic)
B. No increased tenderness of pericranial muscles; if studied, EMG of pericranial muscles shows normal levels of activity

[From Headache Classification Committee of the International Headache Society: Classification and diagnostic criteria for headache disorders, cranial neuralgias, and facial pain. Cephalgia 8(suppl 7):13–17, 1988]

Stress traditionally is assumed to be a major cause of headaches. In reality, it probably does not precipitate many severe headaches, but instead, may make an individual more vulnerable to the onset of an episode. Surprisingly, it seems that it is not severe stressors, but rather normal life stressors, that can predispose to such conditions as migraine headaches.

Assessment

As with all pain syndromes, the evaluation of headaches is subjective. One technique often used is the *headache diary*. Here, a patient keeps a daily journal, recording the time of headache occurrences, the intensity of the headache, other sensations, and the psychosocial context of the event.

Table 23-14 **Headache Diagnostic Criteria: Cluster Headache**

A. At least five attacks, fulfilling migraine criteria B–D
B. Severe unilateral orbital, supraorbital, and/or temporal pain lasting 15–180 minutes untreated
C. Headache is associated with at least one of the following signs, which have to be present on the pain side:
   1. Conjunctival injection
   2. Lacrimation
   3. Nasal congestion
   4. Rhinorrhea
   5. Forehead and facial sweating
   6. Miosis
   7. Ptosis
   8. Eyelid edema
D. Frequency of attacks from one every other day to eight a day
E. Same as migraine criterion E

[From Headache Classification Committee of the International Headache Society: Classification and diagnostic criteria for headache disorders, cranial neuralgias, and facial pain. Cephalalgia 8(suppl 7):13–17, 1988]

Treatment

Pharmacological and nonpharmacological approaches seem to be equally effective in the treatment of migraine and tension-type headaches. For cluster headaches and menstrual migraines, pharmacological approaches are probably more effective. Clearly, for substance-related headaches, the offending substance must be withdrawn. Often, such patients can be very reluctant to believe that the one thing they feel helps, even if insufficiently, is

Table 23-15 **Headache Diagnostic Criteria: Substance-Related Syndromes**

Headache Induced by Chronic Substance Use or Exposure

A. Occurs after daily doses of a substance for ≥3 months
B. A certain required minimum dose should be indicated
C. Headache is chronic (15 days or more a month)
D. Headache disappears within 1 month after withdrawal of the substance

Ergotamine-Induced Headache

A. Is preceded by daily ergotamine intake (oral ≥2 mg, rectal ≥1 mg)
B. Is diffuse, pulsating, or distinguished from migraine by absent attack pattern and/or absent associated symptoms

Analgesic Abuse Headache

A. One or more of the following:
   1. ≥50 g aspirin a month or equivalent of other mild analgesics
   2. ≥100 tablets a month of analgesics combined with barbiturates or other nonnarcotic compounds
   3. One or more narcotic analgesics

[From Headache Classification Committee of the International Headache Society: Classification and diagnostic criteria for headache disorders, cranial neuralgias, and facial pain. Cephalalgia 8(suppl 7):13–17, 1988]

what must be taken away. Often, withdrawal is only successful in an inpatient setting.

Sumatriptan. Sumatriptan is a selective serotonin agonist (5-HT1) that causes vasoconstriction in cerebral arteries. It is effective at relieving acute migraine headaches (with or without aura). It is not indicated for hemiplegic or basilar migraines. It is administered in a subcutaneous injection or in oral form.

Although sumatriptan is an important advance in the treatment of migraines, the question arises of whether it can be misused or cause dependence. Premarketing studies showed no evidence of dependency or misuse. A number of case studies reported after the drug became available suggest that some patients may indeed become dependent on or misuse sumatriptan and may even resell the drug illegally (Gaist et al, 1994; Kaube et al, 1994; Osborne et al, 1994). The best predictor of misuse was previous misuse of other migraine treatments.

Pain, Mood, and Anxiety

The relationship between pain and depression is complicated, and both can reciprocally affect the other. In experimental conditions, subjects who are depressed have a lower threshold for pain. In clinical situations, patients with depression may have a poorer response to analgesics. Also, chronic pain can cause depression.

Pain and anxiety are also closely linked. In both clinical and experimental settings, the two correlate highly. The question ultimately arises of whether this correlation represents a *mislabeling phenomenon* in which an individual cannot distinguish pain from anxiety. Some studies suggest a classical conditioning model in which pain becomes paired with anxiety. Anxiety can worsen pain, through both psychological (worsening the context of the pain) and physical mechanisms (through, for example, increased muscle tension).

The clinician often confronts a "chicken or egg" dilemma: it can be difficult to sort out whether the pain is the cause of the anxiety/depression or vice versa. It usually is not productive to try to sort out this dilemma definitively. Instead, the consultant should identify signs and symptoms of significant anxiety/depression and explain to the patient (and staff) that anxiety/depression and pain often coexist in a feedback loop in which they reinforce each other. The clinical strategy is to intervene in both areas. Treat the physical basis for the pain as aggressively as possible and simultaneously address the anxiety/depression.

Pain in Children

Pain syndromes have long been recognized in children; however, there has been little attempt to study pain in children. Nonspecific limb and muscle aches, "growing pains," are common and usually do not reach medical attention. The most common pain complaint in children is probably that of headaches. Also common is *recurrent abdominal pain,* defined as three or more episodes of pain severe enough to affect activities and occurring for longer than 3 months. The vast majority of these cases have no identifiable pathology and are caused by problems with normal physiological functioning (e.g., stool retention). They often relate to stressful life events, such as family pathology. With or without clear family pathology, treatment of childhood pain syndromes involves a psychosocial approach that must include family involvement.

Pain Treatment in the Opioid-Addicted Patient

In situations involving pain treatment in the narcotic addict, it is often helpful to keep the management of the addiction separate from the management of the pain. For example, the patient's underlying narcotic addiction can be managed with methadone. Most street addicts can be adequately managed on an oral dose of methadone between 20 and 40 mg/day (or an IM dose between 10 and 20 mg/day). With methadone used for maintenance of the underlying addiction, the pain then can be treated as a separate issue, using a different narcotic at doses 50% greater than normal.

Chronic Pain

In addressing a pain problem, the consultant always should try to decide, "Does this presumed acute pain management problem actually represent a chronic pain syndrome?" It is not unusual for a psychiatric consultation to be requested for a patient whose pain problem has exhausted other providers. Such situations are common with low back pain patients admitted for a myelogram that is read as questionable or negative or with chronic abdominal pain patients who have multiple surgeries and "million-dollar" workups. Medical patients and providers are used to thinking of pain in terms of an acute paradigm (i.e., "What can be done now?"). They often overlook the broader picture and can miss the fact that what they are dealing with is better conceptualized as a chronic pain syndrome. Instead of more diagnostic testing or battles over dose or drug, a shift in management philosophy is required.

Chronic pain may affect more than 50 million people in this country and cost many billions in lost productivity. In considering pain assessment and treatment, chronic pain remains one of the most controversial areas.

Part of this controversy relates to how we understand pain (Turk, 1996). Traditionally, we have viewed pain dichotomously: either it is somatogenic or psychogenic. If there is explainable pathology, we would consider the pain to be somatogenic. We would expect direct associations between physical pathology and reports of pain and would treat the pain by treating its cause. If the cause could not be treated, we would treat the symptoms, and it follows that the most humane treatment would be with opioids because they are most efficacious at treating somatogenic pain. If a physical reason for the pain cannot be found, the pain must then be psychogenic, and the treatment would then be psychological (with opioids contraindicated).

Unfortunately, pain is not that simple. We cannot always show clear pathology causing pain, even if we are convinced that the pain is a physical phenomenon. Some of the difficulty may represent limitations in our technology, as is presumed for migraine headaches. Even when pathology is proved, it often correlates poorly with pain reports. For example, lower back pain seems to correlate poorly with the degree of degenerative disc disease.

In a report commissioned by the Social Security Administration to examine the problems of pain, the Institute of Medicine concluded that

> the experience of pain is more than a simple sensory process. It is a complex perception involving higher levels of the central nervous system, emotional status, and higher order mental processes . . . . it is not always possible to identify the causes of pain, how it is expressed, and its behavioral and psychological reactions and consequences (Osterweis et al, 1987).

Thus, as already discussed, pain is subjective and biopsychosocial in nature.

Opioids and Chronic Pain

No issue is more hotly contested than whether opioids should be used in the treatment of chronic pain (Turk, 1996). Opinions in the literature range from complaints that opioids are underused to statements that they are totally inappropriate for the treatment of chronic pain.

Some of this controversy may be due to patient populations: clinicians in specialty pain clinics are often more critical of opioid use than those in cancer pain centers. There is little doubt now that in the treatment of cancer pain, opioids have a role. Thus, much of the controversy now revolves around chronic noncancerous pain.

Beyond moral or ethical issues, we should consider whether opioids are efficacious for chronic noncancerous pain. Unfortunately, to date, no convincing study conclusively supports or rejects the use of opioids. Most studies have methodological weaknesses. Furthermore, many studies come to different conclusions, with some showing reasonable response and others suggesting that opioids actually can worsen pain symptoms (e.g., with headache patients). We are, therefore, left without clear answers.

Several surveys have tried to learn what clinicians are doing. For example, the American Pain Society surveyed their membership to try to get a sense of how clinicians were treating chronic pain (Turk, 1996). They found that, while their members devoted a large part of their practice to treating chronic noncancerous pain (65%), only a small number (13%) did not use long-term opioids. The respondents tended to agree that the goal of treatment was to improve function rather than symptoms. This survey was limited by the small number of respondents (12% of their membership).

A larger survey of almost 2,000 physicians throughout the United States found that most did not often use long-term opioids (Turk, 1996). This practice differed by specialty (rheumatologists used the most long-term opioids, surgeons the least, and general practitioners somewhere in the middle) and by region (Midwestern physicians were the most conservative).

Unfortunately, there are no widely accepted rules to guide us in deciding what patient would be eligible for long-term opioids. Several guidelines have been proposed, but they differ widely on many issues. Opinions vary about what other interventions should first be tried, who should evaluate the patient, and whether a history of substance abuse is a contraindication. There is growing evidence that interdisciplinary pain clinics can be very useful in improving function and limiting opioid use. They must, however, still prove their cost effectiveness in this cost-conscious climate.

Ultimately, as Turk suggests, our decision to use long-term opioids is a judgment call, in which we ask ourselves, "How much suffering are we willing to accept to prevent what amount of abuse and negative side effects?" (Turk, 1996).

REFERENCES

Acute Pain Management Guideline Panel: Acute Pain Management Operative or Medical Procedures and Trauma. Clinical Practice Guideline. AHCPR Pub. No. 92-0032. Rockville, MD, Agency for Health Care Policy and Research, Public Health Service, US Department for Health and Human Services, Feb, 1992

American Psychiatric Association: Diagnostic and Statistical Manual of Mental Disorders, 3rd ed. Washington, DC, American Psychiatric Association, 1980

American Psychiatric Association: Diagnostic and Statistical Manual of Mental Disorders, 3rd ed., revised. Washington, DC, American Psychiatric Association, 1987

American Psychiatric Association: Diagnostic and Statistical Manual of Mental Disorders, 4th ed. Washington, DC, American Psychiatric Association, 1994

Andrasik F, Baskin S: Headache. In Morrison RL, Bellack AS (eds): Medical Factors and Psychological Disorders: A Handbook for Psychologists, pp 325–349. New York, Plenum, 1987

Beecher HK: The powerful placebo. JAMA 159:1602–1606, 1955

Brose WG, Spiegel D: Neuropsychiatric aspects of pain management. In Hales RE, Yudofsky SC (eds): Textbook of Neuropsychiatry. Washington DC, American Psychiatric Press, 1987

Cleeland CS, Gonin R, Hatfield AK, Edmonson JH, et al: Pain and its treatment in outpatients with metastatic cancer. N Engl J Med 330:592–596, 1994

Dejard A, Peterson P, Kestrup J: Mexiletine for the treatment of chronic painful diabetic neuropathy. Lancet 1:9–11, 1988

Drossman DA, Laserman J, Nachman G, et al: Sexual and physical abuse in women with functional or organic gastroenterological disorders. Ann Intern Med 113:828–833, 1990

Elta GH, Barnett JL: Meperidine need not be proscribed during sphincter of Oddi mamometry. Gastrointest Endosc 40:7–9, 1994

Ferranta FM: Principles of opioid pharmacotherapy: practical implications of basic mechanisms. J Pain Symptom Manage 11:265–273, 1996

Foley KM: The treatment of cancer pain. N Engl J Med 313:84–95, 1985a

Foley, KM: Non-narcotic and narcotic analgesics: applications. In Foley KM (ed): Management of Cancer Pain, pp 135–148. Syllabus of postgraduate course. New York, Memorial Sloan Kettering Cancer Center, 1985b

Gaist P, Sindrup S, Hallas J, Gram LF: Misuse of sumatriptan (letter). Lancet 344:1090, 1994

Goldberg RJ, Tull RK: The Psychosocial Dimensions of Cancer. New York, Free Press, 1983

Haynes MD, Fuller RW: The effect of fluoxetine on morphine analgesia, respiratory depression, and lethality. Drug Dev Res 2:033–042, 1982.

Headache Classification Committee of the International Headache Society: Classification and diagnostic criteria for headache disorders, cranial neuralgias, and facial pain. Cephalalgia 8(suppl 7):1–96, 1988

Jacox A, Carr DB, Payne R, et al: Management of Cancer Pain. Clinical Practice Guideline No. 9. AHCPR Pub. No. 94-0592. Rockville, MD, Agency for Health Care Policy and Research, Public Health Service, US Department for Health and Human Services, Feb, 1994.

Kaube H, May A, Diener HC, Pfaffenrather V: Sumatriptan (letter). BMJ 308:1573–1574, 1994

Max MB, Lynch SA, Muir J, et al: Effects of desipramine, amitriptyline, and fluoxetine on pain in diabetic neuropathy. N Engl J Med 326:1250–1256, 1992

Melzack R, Katz J: The McGill pain questionnaire: appraisal and current status. In Turk DC, Melzack R (eds): Handbook of Pain Assessment. New York, Guilford Press, 1992

Osborne MJ, Austin RCT, Dawson KJ, Lange L: Is there a problem with long term use of sumatriptan in acute migraine? (letter). BMJ 308:113, 1994

Osterweis M, Kleinman A, Mechanic D: Pain and Disability: Clinical, Behavioral, and Public Policy Perspectives. Washington, DC, National Academy Press, 1987

Physician's Desk Reference, 50th ed. Montvale, NJ, Medical Economics Data, 1996

Pick CG, Paul D, Eison MS, Pasternak GW: Potentiation of opioid analgesia by the antidepressant nefazodone. Eur J Pharmacol 211:375–381, 1992

Porter J, Jick H: Addiction rare in patients treated with narcotics. N Engl J Med 302:123, 1980

Sherman S, Lehman GA: Opioids and the sphincter of Oddi. Gastrointest Endosc 40:105–106, 1996

Swerdlow M: Anticonvulsant drugs and chronic pain. Clin Neuropharmacol 7:51–82, 1984

Thune A, Baker RA, Saccone GTP: Differing effects of pethidine and morphine on human sphincter of Oddi motility. Br J Surg 77:992–995, 1990

Tomson T, Bertilsson L: Potent therapeutic effect of carbamazepine-10, 11-epoxide in trigeminal neuralgia. Arch Neurol 41:598–601, 1984

Turk DC, Melzack R (eds): Handbook of Pain Assessment. New York, Guilford Press, 1992

Turk DC: Clinicians' attitudes about prolonged use of opioids and the issue of patient heterogeneity. J Pain Symptom Manage 11:218–230, 1996

Zhang WY, Li Wan Po A: The effectiveness of topically applied capsaicin. Eur J Clin Pharmacol 46:517–522, 1994

24 Behavioral Medicine Strategies for Medical Patients

Michael G. Goldstein,
Matthew M. Clark,
Laurie Ruggiero, Barrie J. Guise,
and David B. Abrams

It is now well established that lifestyle factors significantly contribute to more than half of the annual deaths in the United States (USDHEW, 1979; McGinnis and Foege, 1993). Behavioral medicine is the interdisciplinary field concerned with the application of behavioral principles and strategies to the modification of lifestyle patterns for the prevention of disease and enhancement of health.

It has become increasingly apparent that physicians have the opportunity to play a very important role in the area of prevention and health promotion (Grueninger et al, 1995; Marcus et al, 1995b). In this chapter, we define the physician's role in risk factor reduction, describe the barriers to physician involvement in this area, and provide a basic approach to risk factor reduction in the medical setting using two primary examples, smoking and obesity. Finally, we will use case histories of the assessment and treatment of these health risk factors.

THE PHYSICIAN'S ROLE IN RISK FACTOR REDUCTION

Physicians have the potential to play a very important role in the reduction of risk factors for disease. Over 75% of the population contact a doctor at least once each year, and more than 95% contact a physician at least once every 5 years. Thus, physicians have the opportunity to intervene with the vast majority of individuals who are at risk for disease.

Moreover, patients view their physicians as having considerable influence with respect to their preventive behavior. Something as simple as physician attention to a problem can be highly motivating to patients. In a study examining obese adults who either gained or lost weight over a 5-year period, researchers (Levy and Williamson, 1988) found that 81% of those who lost weight had been told by their physician they were overweight compared with only 46% of those who did not lose weight. Similar results have been found with smoking cessation. For example, smokers report that if they were asked by their physician to quit, 75% would give it a try (Fiore et al, 1996). Finally, physicians can be quite effective when they act to modify their patients' risk factors. Several smoking cessation strategies have been shown to be effective when used by physicians in the primary care setting (Fiore et al, 1996; Kottke et al, 1988). *Studies have also demonstrated that physician-delivered patient education and counseling can lead to improvement in patients' adherence to treatment regimens* (Inui et al, 1976; Mullen et al, 1985). Although a majority of physicians feel that they have an important role to play in health promotion, physicians are reluctant to engage in interventions to reduce risk factors for disease (Marcus et al, 1995b; Schwartz et al, 1991). Indeed, patient surveys indicate that only a relatively small percentage (27 to 50%) of smokers are advised to quit smoking by their physician (Anda et al, 1987; Gilpin et al, 1992), and only 10% of a sample of family physicians give advice about nutrition to more than 80% of their patients (Kottke et al, 1984). The barriers to physician involvement are discussed in the next section.

Barriers to Physician Involvement in Risk Factor Reduction

The barriers to physician involvement in counseling about risk factor reduction, listed in Table 24–1, fall within two domains: physician barriers and practice/organizational barriers. Although physicians are fairly well informed about the importance of health promotion and risk factor reduction, their *knowledge* of patient education and behavioral change interventions, materials, and resources is quite limited (Kottke et al, 1987; Orleans et al, 1985).

Lack of skills is a second important barrier to physician involvement in health promotion interventions (Clark et al, 1996; Kottke et al, 1987; Orleans et al, 1985). Skills required for effective health promotion and risk factor reduction include interviewing and assessment skills to enable the physician to make an accurate "diagnosis" of risk or educational need; patient education and counseling skills to enable the physician to intervene to help the patient reduce risk; and skills to help the patient maintain healthy behavior or prevent relapse (Green et al, 1988; Grueninger et al, 1995).

Medical education has neglected training in patient education and counseling skills, although it has been recognized that training in such

Table 24–1 **Barriers to Physician Involvement In Risk Factor Reduction**

Physician Barriers

Knowledge Deficit
Importance of risk factor reduction to health care
Effectiveness of physician intervention
Intervention methods
Resources for patients—materials and referrals
Skill Deficit
Interviewing/assessment/diagnostic skills
Patient education skills
Behavioral counseling skills
Maintenance/relapse prevention skills
Beliefs and Attitudes
Patients don't want to change or can't change
Perceived ineffectiveness in helping patients change
Lack of confidence in helping patients change
Emphasis on final outcomes
Disease-oriented biomedical approach
Paternalistic, directive style
Moralistic view of behavioral problems
Poor personal health habits
Dearth of role models practicing preventive care
Lack of commitment to risk factor reduction

Organization Barriers

Limited use of reminder systems, tracking logs
Little or no reimbursement for preventive services
Poor coordination with self-help and behavioral treatment programs
Limited involvement of office staff in health promotion activities

---

skills is needed (Preventive Health Care Committee, 1985). Attitudes and beliefs also play an important role in physicians' reluctance to provide health promotion interventions. Because of the deficits in knowledge and skills, physicians lack the confidence to intervene successfully with their patients to reduce or change risk factors (Kottke et al, 1987; Orleans et al, 1985). Physicians' self-perception of the ineffectiveness of such efforts is fueled by the low rates of successful behavior change among patients they try to help. An emphasis on final outcomes, such as smoking abstinence, leads to further frustration, because even the most effective physicians achieve 1-year abstinence rates of only 10 to 20% among their smoking patients.

The medical education process contributes to the development of attitudes that are not conducive to a preventive approach to patient care. Traditionally, physician training has emphasized a biomedical model, which is oriented toward diagnosis and treatment of diseases, rather than a systems model, which embraces prevention and health promotion (Engel, 1977; see also Chapters 1 and 2). As a result, many physicians continue to view health promotion activities as outside their role or as unchallenging and uninteresting (Nutting, 1986). Moreover, traditional medical training promotes a paternalistic and directive style that is less likely to lead to change in patient behavior than a collaborative and patient-centered style that involves the patient in the process of change. The dearth of role models in academia and the community who espouse and practice health promotion reinforces the attitude that prevention and health are not as important as more traditional forms of medical intervention. These and other negative attitudes and beliefs listed in Table 24–1 contribute to a lack of commitment to become more involved in risk factor reduction and health promotion activities. The *organizational barriers* that interfere with physician involvement in risk factor reduction are also listed in Table 24–1. Deficits in primary care physicians' knowledge, skills, and attitudes about health promotion interventions and systems/organizational barriers interact to limit the effective use of counseling for risk factor reduction in primary care.

A MODEL FOR RISK FACTOR REDUCTION IN THE MEDICAL SETTING

In this section, we describe a model for risk factor reduction in the medical setting that is adapted from models of patient education developed and described by Grueninger et al (1989) and Ockene and colleagues (1988). After describing the model, a practical step-by-step approach to risk factor assessment and intervention is outlined.

Grueninger and colleagues (1989) identify five levels of the patient education process (Fig. 24–1): (1) cognitive (knowledge, concepts, and awareness about risk factors); (2) attitudinal (beliefs, intentions, and readiness for change); (3) instrumental (instrumental skills); (4) behavioral (coping behavior and skills); and (5) social (social support). At each level, there is an opportunity for both assessment and intervention. *Assessment* involves gathering data to identify barriers and resources that may impede or facilitate patient education and behavior change. For example, assessment at the cognitive level might include asking the patient about his or her specific knowledge of risk factors and about his or her understanding of the relationship between risk factors and illness. *Intervention* involves providing the patient with the necessary information, skills, and support to help him or her overcome barriers and utilize resources. Thus, intervention at the cognitive level might include creating the individual's risk factors profile and informing the patient about his or her risk factors and what can be done to alter risk. This model also features a "patient-centered" approach to patient education and counseling, which emphasizes the importance of *tailoring the treatment plan* to each patient's specific needs (Grueninger et al, 1989, 1995; Ockene et al, 1988). Presently, most physicians do not have the knowledge and skills to assess and intervene effectively at each of

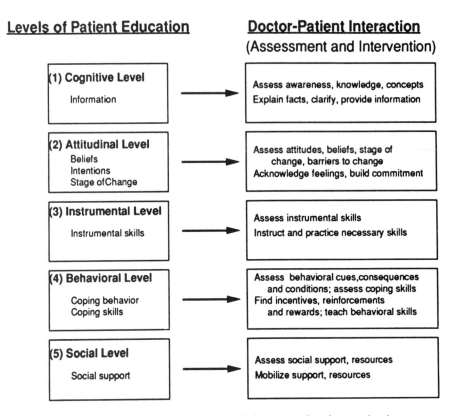

Figure 24–1. Levels of patient education and doctor–patient interaction in behavioral medicine.

the levels, especially the instrumental and behavioral levels. Although it may not be appropriate for the physician to intervene at each of these levels, knowledge of the assessment and intervention strategies used by others will help the physician to make appropriate referrals to those professionals who have these skills.

Identification of each patient's *stage of change,* a concept developed by Prochaska and DiClemente (1986), is an important element of patient assessment when counseling patients about lifestyle change. These investigators found that individuals making lifestyle changes, such as giving up smoking, move through predictable stages of change (Fig. 24–2). The five stages are precontemplation, contemplation, preparation, action, and maintenance.

Precontemplation is a stage of unawareness or denial of the problem or condition. This individual has no intention to change this problem behavior in the foreseeable future. This stage classifies the smoker who is not even considering quitting or the obese patient who has no intention to lose weight. These individuals may either deny the health risks associated with their

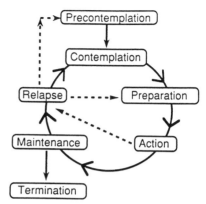

Figure 24-2. *Stages of patient change in risk factor reduction.*

behaviors or have low self-confidence because of past treatment failures. *Contemplation* is a stage of ambivalence, when pros and cons for change are weighed without definite commitment to taking action. *Preparation* is a stage in which the individual is aware that a behavior is problematic and intends to take action to change this behavior in the next month. In addition, individuals who are prepared for action report having made some changes in the problem behavior in the past year. Individuals who have reached the *action* phase have made a commitment to change and are actively attempting to change their behavior. *Maintenance* is the stage that is reached when the individual has successfully made a change but still needs to monitor behavior to prevent slips or relapses. For some problem behaviors, this stage may be lifelong. For example, many obesity researchers have advocated the adoption of a continuous care approach to obesity in which, similar to diabetes mellitus, patients are expected to require lifelong care (Perri et al, 1993).

Prochaska and DiClemente (1986) found that individuals may take several years to move through the stages of change; moreover, they may cycle repeatedly through the stages (Fig. 24–2). Ten specific processes of change have been identified. These include cognitive and behavioral strategies that facilitate change (Table 24–2). They also learned that individuals in a given stage respond best to specific change strategies (Table 24–3). For example, consciousness-raising is most useful for individuals in the contemplation stage, while behavioral strategies are most effective when provided to individuals in the action stage. Knowledge of these findings might help physicians to feel less frustrated when their patients return without having made a recommended change in their behavior. It is unrealistic to expect precontemplators, who are not fully aware of the nature of their problem, to take definitive action. It is especially frustrating, and not very useful, to provide precontemplators and contemplators with instructions to take action when they have not yet made a commitment to change. Moreover, because most individuals taking action are likely to relapse at least once, a relapse should be viewed as an opportunity for learning, rather than as a failure.

Table 24–2 **Titles, Definitions, and Representative Interventions of the Processes of Change**

PROCESS	DEFINITIONS: INTERVENTION
Consciousness raising	Increasing information about self and problem: observations, confrontations, interpretations, bibliotherapy
Self-reevaluation	Assessing how one feels and thinks about oneself with respect to a problem: value clarification, imagery, corrective emotional experience
Self-liberation	Choosing and commiting to act or believe in ability to change: decision-making therapy, New Year's resolutions, logotherapy techniques, commitment-enhancing techniques
Counterconditioning	Substituting alternatives for problem behaviors: relaxation, desensitization, assertion, positive self-statements
Stimulus control	Avoiding or countering stimuli that elicit problem behaviors: restructuring one's environment (e.g., removing alcohol or fattening foods), avoiding high-risk cues, fading techniques
Reinforcement management	Rewarding one's self or being rewarded by others for making changes: contingency contracts, overt and covert reinforcement, self-reward
Helping relationships	Being open and trusting about problems with someone who cares: therapeutic alliance, social support, self-help groups
Dramatic relief	Experiencing and expressing feelings about one's problems and solutions: psychodrama, grieving losses, role playing
Environmental reevaluation	Assessing how one's problem affects physical environment: empathy training, documentaries
Social liberation	Increasing alternatives for nonproblem behaviors available in society: advocating for rights of repressed, empowering, policy interventions

(Copyright 1991 by the American Psychological Association. Reprinted by permission from: Prochaska JO. DiClemente CC, Norcross, JC: In search of how people change: Applications to addictive behaviors. Am Psychologist 47:1102–1104, 1991)

An alternative to focusing exclusively on final outcomes is to focus on how to help individuals move more rapidly through the change process. Clinicians adopting this strategy can pick those interventions that are most likely to move the patient to the next stage. For example, for contemplators, helping the individual to recognize the benefits of change and offering personal support may facilitate movement to the action stage. Intermediate outcomes (i.e., movement to the next stage) become the goal of intervention. Further examples of the application of this patient-centered approach can be found in the sections on the management of smoking and obesity later in this chapter.

Table 24–3 **Stepwise Stages of Change In Which Particular Processes of Change Are Emphasized**

PRECON-TEMPLATION	CONTEM-PLATION	PREPA-RATION	ACTION	MAINTENANCE
Consciousness raising Dramatic relief Environmental reevaluation				
	Self-reevaluation			
		Self-liberation		
				Reinforcement management Helping relationships Counterconditioning Stimulus control

(Copyright 1991 by the American Psychological Association. Reprinted by permission from: Prochaska JO, DiClemente CC. Norcross JC: In search of how people change: Applications to addictive behaviors. Am Psychologist 47:1102–1104, 1991)

A PATIENT-CENTERED APPROACH
TO RISK FACTOR INTERVENTION

The step-by-step strategy for risk factor intervention that follows integrates aspects of the model of patient education described by Grueninger et al, (1995), the Prochaska and DiClemente model of stages of change, and a strategy for brief physician counseling, developed by the National Cancer Institute known as the "Four As" (Glynn and Manley, 1989). The patient education and counseling process is transformed into a rather simple sequence of specific tasks. The five tasks are: Address the Agenda, Assess, Advise, Assist, and Arrange Follow-up (listed in Table 24–4).

At the start of the counseling session, the physician begins by setting the agenda—bringing up the issue of risk factor assessment or reduction. Of course, it is important that the physician make sure that the patient's agenda has been addressed and his or her concerns answered. Then the physician involves the patient in the process by assessing his or her level of awareness of risk and stage of change. If the physician determines that the patient is not in the preparation or action stage, an attempt is made to increase the patient's awareness and build commitment for change. Personalized information, such as providing the patient with specific feedback about the relationship between a risk factor and the patient's health, is most likely to be effective in moving the patient toward action. If the patient is ready for action, the next task is

Table 24–4 **A Patient-Centered Approach to Risk Factor Intervention: The Five "A"s**

Address the Agenda
Attend to patient's agenda
Express desire to talk about risk factors

Assess
Assess knowledge, beliefs, concerns, feelings
Assess previous experience with change
Assess stage of change

Advise
Provide personalized information and advice

Assist
Provide support
Negotiate an intervention plan
Identify potential barriers and resources

Arrange Follow-up

(Adapted from Glynn and Manley, 1989: Grueninger et al, 1989: Levenkron et al, 1987; and Ockene, 1987)

the negotiation of an intervention plan with the patient. During this phase, the patient's resources are used as much as possible, and potential implementation problems are solved.

Table 24–5 describes the approach in more detail, delineating specific "skills" for each of the five tasks. Sample physician statements are provided for initiating dialogue with the patient. Clearly, there is more to each of these skills than just asking these questions and making these statements. Information should be provided using language that is at the patient's level of comprehension, checking frequently to ensure that the information is understood. Clarification of the patient's knowledge, beliefs, and feelings requires skill in interviewing. The physician also needs to know how to manage feelings when they are expressed by the patient. Development of rapport and establishment of a trusting therapeutic relationship will facilitate the process of change, especially when the physician is attempting to increase the patient's commitment.

When negotiating intervention plans to help patients change their risk-related behavior, the physician can choose from a variety of options. These options range from simple advice and provision of educational materials to face-to-face counseling by the physician and referral to a formal behavioral medicine treatment program. How does one choose among the various options? Careful assessment of the patient can help to provide the answer to this question.

Table 24–5 **A Patient-Centered Approach to Risk Factor Intervention: The Five "A"s (Expanded)**

Address the Agenda

Attend to patient's agenda
Express desire to talk about risk factors
  "I'd like to talk to you about _____"
Define problem
  "You have _____"
  "This means _____"

Assess

Assess and clarify patient's knowledge, beliefs and concerns
  "What do you know about _____?"
Assess and clarify patient's feelings about risk and change in behavior
  "How do you feel about _____?"
Assess patient's previous experience with change
  "What have you tried in the past?"
Assess stage of change and clarify patient's goals
  "Are you willing to _____ (e.g., stop smoking, change your diet) now?"
  "Are you considering changing _____ in the next few weeks?"
Assess pros and cons for change
  "What reasons do you have for wanting (and not wanting) to change?"

Advise

Provide personalized information regarding risk and benefits of change
Provide physiological feedback when available
  "Your test results (physical findings, etc.) indicate that _____
    is affecting your health"
Tell patient that you strongly advise change

Assist

Provide support, understanding, praise, and reinforcement
  "I can help you by _____"
  "It's often difficult to change _____"
  "It's great that you're considering _____"
Describe intervention options
Negotiate an intervention plan—match intervention to stage of change
  For Precontemplators and Contemplators:
Review patient's pros and cons for change: reinforce pros; express willingness to
  help patient and address cons
Provide more information, feedback
Address feelings
Encourage to consider change
  For Patients in Preparation and Action Stages:
Negotiate selection among options
Solve problems with implementation
"What problems might arise with _____?"
Provide resources (e.g., written materials)
Identity additional resources:
  "What (or who) might help you with _____?"
Teach skills/recommend specific strategies

(continued)

Table 24–5 **(continued)**

For Patients in Preparation and Action Stages:
Consider a written contract/prescription
Refer, when appropriate
Arrange Follow-up
Reaffirm plan
   "Now, what are you going to do?"
Arrange follow-up appointment or call
   "I'd like to see you again on _____"

(Adapted from Glynn and Manley, 1989; Grueninger et al, 1989; Levenkron et al,1987; and Ockene, 1987)

Patient characteristics that predict decreased likelihood of response to minimal interventions include being in an early stage of change (e.g., precontemplation), poor motivation, repeated failures during previous attempts to change, high levels of psychological dependence on the targeted risk behavior, poor social support, and high levels of physical dependence on the targeted risk behavior, when appropriate (e.g., nicotine dependence when smoking is the targeted risk factor). When one or several of these patient characteristics is present, it is likely that these patients will require a more intensive intervention or one that combines several modalities (e.g., behavioral, pharmacological, and social interventions). For other patients, a stepwise approach to treatment is reasonable, starting with a minimal intervention (e.g., provision of self-help materials) and moving to more intensive treatments if the minimal interventions are not effective.

As noted in the section of this chapter on the barriers to physician involvement in patient behavior change, most physicians don't feel they have the skills to engage in effective counseling in the area of risk factor reduction. Thus, most physicians are unlikely to provide face-to-face counseling to patients themselves. However, skills can be taught in this area if sufficient time and faculty effort are allocated to training (Levenkron et al, 1987; Ockene et al, 1988). It must also be recognized that even minimal physician-delivered counseling interventions can be quite effective, especially in the area of smoking cessation (Fiore et al, 1996; Kottke et al, 1988; Schwartz, 1987).

We have described a generic patient-centered approach to risk factor intervention, which stresses the importance of developing an understanding of the patient's readiness to engage in behavior change and also the need to build commitment in patients who are not yet ready to take action. In the next section, we describe some specific behavioral strategies that can be used to provide assistance to those patients who are ready to change their risk-associated behaviors. Case examples illustrate the approach to obese patients and patients who smoke.

ASSESSMENT AND TREATMENT OF OBESITY

Patient Assessment

In deciding when to intervene and at what level, several dimensions of patient characteristics are important: (1) level of obesity (e.g., body mass index); (2) biological factors and medical risk status; (3) behavioral factors, including eating and exercise habits; (4) psychological status (e.g., depression); (5) sociocultural–environmental factors, including support from friends, family, and the work environment; and (6) stage of readiness for changing eating and exercise habits to lose weight (see also Fig. 24–1) (Clark et al, 1993).

Biological and medical factors must be evaluated to help determine which program might be best for a particular patient. A review of the patient's health status and familial medical history can help determine how much weight a patient needs to lose to achieve health improvements (Goldstein, 1992). Attention to current eating habits is helpful. Patients may report eating in response to psychological factors (such as stress, depression, or social anxiety), or they may reveal fatigue, dizziness, or cravings for protein, carbohydrates, or sugar that could reflect biochemical imbalances (e.g., hypoglycemia). After completion of a history and physical, providing medical clearance for exercise or a referral for exercise stress testing can assist a patient in safely increasing their physical activity level.

Questions about current mood and functioning will be beneficial since some obese patients will have psychiatric comorbidity or psychological factors that require treatment prior to weight loss (King et al, 1996). Examples include current purging (vomiting, laxative abuse, etc.) or an active substance-abuse problem. Some psychological problems will warrant adjunctive treatment to enhance weight loss success but may be treated in conjunction with active weight loss. Binge Eating Disorder is an example since binge eating is a significant problem (Venditti et al, 1996), but many obese binge eaters benefit from obesity treatment (Marcus et al, 1995a).

Interpersonal and sociocultural–environmental factors should also be evaluated. Financial barriers or a stressful living environment may make it more difficult to change lifestyle. Social support (or lack of it) can also play a crucial role. Sometimes spouses, parents, or family are unaware of their power to support and sustain change; alternatively, they can unwittingly sabotage treatment efforts because of their own lifestyle habits or values. An assessment of the patient's environment often reveals a need to involve other members of the family in lifestyle change efforts.

Patients should be prepared for treatment by ensuring appropriate goals and expectations (Foster et al, 1997). One major barrier to successful weight loss is unrealistic expectations about the speed and ease of weight loss (Brownell and Wadden, 1992). Discussing reasonable goal weights and expected weekly weight loss with patients may help to prevent future frustration or discouragement (Clark et al, 1996). Patients should be discouraged from seeking rapid weight loss or "fad diets." Drawbacks of fad diets include high dropout rates (Clark et al, 1995): patients eventually feel deprived and must stop the diet. At this point, they typically return to their prior eating habits and regain weight.

A Step-Care Model of Treatment

Brownell and Wadden (1991) have proposed a step-care approach to weight loss that is perhaps the most rational and cost-effective way to proceed. Indeed, most experts recommend matching individuals to treatment (Schwartz and Brownell, 1995). The challenge to the physician is to determine which type of treatment is most appropriate for a particular patient (Fig. 24–3). Since cost, risk, and invasiveness increase with each step, it should be recommended that the patient begin at the lowest step not yet given a fair test. More costly and risky procedures should be reserved for those patients who have not responded to basic strategies.

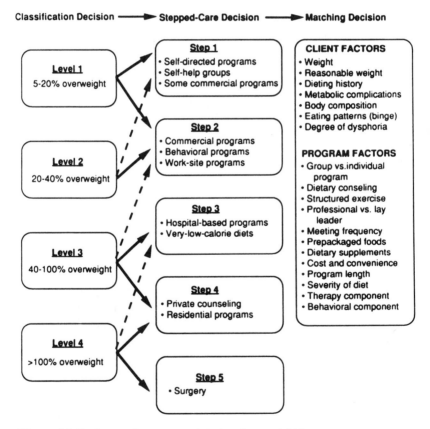

Figure 24–3. *A stepwise approach to treating weight loss.*

In general, mildly obese individuals should be encouraged to seek treatment in low-cost self-help programs, and moderately obese patients should be referred to behavioral programs. However, repeated unsuccessful efforts to lose weight can lead to adverse psychological effects, making each future attempt more difficult (Brownell and Wadden, 1991). Therefore, those who have tried and failed to lose weight on several occasions by these methods and those who are moderately to morbidly obese should be strongly encouraged to seek an intermediate level of care, such as a hospital-based behavior modification program (Clark et al, 1995).

The basic philosophy of behavior modification is that in order to lose weight and keep it off, a person must gradually replace old maladaptive eating behaviors and exercise habits with new health-promoting ones that can be maintained for a lifetime. Patients typically are taught to slow down their rate of eating, to use alternative skills in managing moods (e.g., relaxation training), to use social support (assertiveness), to apply problem-solving skills, to set task-oriented goals, to increase activity level, and to change their ways of thinking about food (cognitive restructuring). (For more details about clinical techniques, see Brownell, 1994.)

Severely overweight patients and those who have failed with a variety of conventional treatments might be appropriate candidates for a very-low-calorie diet (VLCD) (Clark et al, 1996) or gastroplasty surgery. These options are most appropriate when obesity poses a definite and sometimes imminent hazard to health because maximal interventions also carry a significant degree of risk in the form of side effects and/or complications. Behavior modification programs are now being combined with VLCDs and with gastroplasty to increase adherence/compliance and to improve the maintenance of weight loss (Wadden et al, 1992).

Maintenance of weight loss is the key problem, because long-term results (more than 1 year) have demonstrated that as many as 75% regain the weight lost in programs (Jeffrey, 1987). Research on maintenance (Perri et al, 1988) suggests that involvement in an ongoing intensive maintenance program—which includes continued contact with a professional, training in behavioral problem-solving skills, social support, and exercise—helps patients to maintain weight losses for at least 18 months after completion of an initial treatment program. As a result of findings like these, researchers have suggested that many obese individuals may need to remain in continuous care for their obesity. Furthermore, it has been suggested that obesity should be viewed as a chronic health problem, like hypertension or diabetes, and should be followed medically in a similar manner (Perri et al, 1993; Wing, 1992). By applying the approach outlined in this chapter, physicians can play a very important and unique role in the ongoing management of obese patients.

A CASE STUDY

A 46-year-old woman weighing 80% over ideal body weight presents to her physician because she is "feeling lousy." She reports experiencing fatigue and frequent headaches. The physician's examina-

tion reveals that she has a total cholesterol of 310 and a fasting blood sugar of 210. A dialogue that reflects a patient-centered approach to management follows.

Doctor: Ms. Jones, you've told me that you're fatigued and have frequent headaches. I think your symptoms are related to several factors. First, your blood sugar is elevated. In addition, your total cholesterol is 310. Both your blood sugar level and your cholesterol level need to be lowered, or else you stand an increased risk of heart attack, stroke, and the many complications of diabetes. Your weight has an important influence on your blood sugar and cholesterol. Therefore, the best way to reduce your cardiovascular risk is to lose weight and to eat a low fat diet. I can help you to select the best means of weight loss. Would you consider trying to lose weight in the next month?

Ms. Jones: If you think it would be a good idea.

Doctor: It would be a great idea if you're ready to give it a try. What do yon know about different weight loss methods?

Ms. Jones: Weight loss? I'm constantly on a diet. I know so much about weight loss I could write a book. I've been on everything. I've done Weight Watchers, the Scarsdale Diet, all-protein diets. . . . You name it, I've done it.

Doctor: I'm glad you're interested in losing weight. You have tried some methods of weight loss, but have you been on a medically supervised diet that incorporated principles of behavior modification and included calorie counting?

Ms. Jones: Well, my previous doctor told me that I should try to lose weight by sticking to 1,200 calories a day, but then I just went off. It didn't last much more than a week or two.

Doctor: So you've never really been closely supervised over an extended period of time. I have some ideas that may help you, but they involve a strong commitment on your part. Do you want to hear more today?

Ms. Jones: If you recommend a program, then I'll do my best.

Doctor: Very well, then. Here is my advice. Number one, with respect to your weight, losing 1 to 2 pounds a week over the next 3 months is a reasonable goal. Keep in mind that losing weight is often quite challenging, so don't be discouraged if you don't lose as fast as you might like. Research has shown that a 10% weight loss can have positive health benefits for someone like you. Number two, because your cholesterol is high, you need to reduce your intake of fatty foods. Number three, I recommend that you increase your activity level by getting into a formal exercise program. Given your current weight, your low activity level, and the amount of experience you have had at commercially available programs, I recommend that you go to a professionally led multidisciplinary behavior modification program. They will do a thorough assessment of your eating and exercise habits and come up with a treatment program that is tailored for you. They will also be able to help you make dietary changes to reduce your intake of fats. In addition, I can give you this table, which lists foods high and low in fat content. Finally, I will let them know you are able to start an exercise program. You need to begin exercising very modestly and gradually build up. If you like to walk or swim, either one would be fine for you. How do you feel about these options?

Ms. Jones: Fine. I'm happy to give it a try.

Doctor: What problems do you see that might arise with your attempt to follow through on this plan?

Ms. Jones: The main thing, Doctor, is my work. This is a very busy time of year, and it's hard for me to get away from the office. If I can't get an appointment time at the clinic that's suitable, that might get in the way of my following through. Also, trying to exercise when you're real busy at work is just not realistic.

Doctor: I'm glad you are aware of the possible problems you might run into. What might help you to overcome these obstacles and stick to a lifestyle change program that is really essential for your health at this time?

Ms. Jones: Well, I can ask my boss to let me come in a little earlier so that I can leave and make an afternoon appointment.

Doctor: That sounds like a good idea. Also, be sure to get in touch with me if you have any other questions or need clarification about this plan. So, once again, what exactly are you going to do?

Ms. Jones: I'll give the behavioral medicine clinic a call to set up an appointment as soon as possible. Changing the amount of fat I eat shouldn't be that hard, at least not when I'm home. Exercising will be tougher, but I guess I could walk in the evening after I get home from the office, maybe a mile at first and build up from there.

Doctor: That sounds like an excellent plan. I'd like to see you again in 3 months and check how much you have improved your cholesterol and blood sugar level. Let's aim for a 1- to 2-pound weight loss a week by then.

In this case, the physician was quickly able to determine that the patient was at the preparation stage. The appropriate intervention for this type of patient, given the severity of her medical problems and her previous experience, was at the intermediate level.

ASSESSMENT AND TREATMENT OF SMOKING

Patient Assessment for Smoking Cessation

It is helpful to assess patient characteristics before deciding on the appropriate level of intervention. Five major characteristics need to be evaluated. These are (1) stage of change or motivation, (2) degree of physiological addiction, (3) degree of psychological dependence, (4) history of attempts to quit, and (5) degree of positive social support end negative support (e.g., another smoker in the household).

If the patient is in the precontemplation or contemplation stage and not strongly motivated to change, then motivating her or him becomes the first priority before deciding on treatment options (Miller and Rolnick, 1991). Motivational strategies include: (1) providing personalized feedback on consequences of smoking; (2) developing a discrepancy between the patient's goals and the effects of smoking; (3) expressing empathy about the difficulties in being a smoker and giving up smoking; (4) providing a menu of options for treatment (including cutting down or limiting smoking in certain situations); and (5) accepting thinking about quitting as a positive step towards change (Miller and Rollnick, 1991).

Once an individual is ready for action, the rule of thumb is that smokers should receive a more intensive (maximal) treatment program if they (1) are more physiologically addicted (smoke more than 25 cigarettes a day, usually smoke within 30 minutes of awakening during the morning, and report having withdrawal symptoms during previous quit attempts); (2) are psychologically dependent (smoke for stress management, or to help cope with social interactions); (3) have associated psychiatric illness; or (4) have tried to quit on their own and failed.

In 1996, the Agency for Health Care Policy and Research (AHCPR) published a clinical practice guideline for smoking cessation (Fiore et al, 1996). Recent evidence reviewed by this panel found that all smokers, even those with low levels of nicotine dependence, may benefit from the use of nicotine replacement strategies (e.g., nicotine transdermal patches, nicotine chewing gum, nicotine nasal spray) even when no adjunctive behavioral treatment is provided (Fiore et al, 1996). This conclusion led the United States Food and Drug Administration (FDA) to release nicotine replacement products as over-the-counter drugs. However, the AHCPR panel also found that there was a dose–response relationship between the intensity of face-to-face smoking cessation counseling and smoking cessation outcomes. Although brief advice (less than 3 minutes) significantly increased cessation over no intervention (by about 20%), provision of more intensive counseling (i.e., greater than 10 minutes in any one session) more than doubled smoking cessation rates. In 1997, bupropion, an antidepressant with dopaminergic and noradrenergic activity, was approved by the Food and Drug Administration as a first-line agent for smoking cessation treatment (Goldstein, in press).

A review of the patient's previous attempts to quit can be revealing (Best, 1976). They may show, for example, that the patient was unable to quit even though he or she cut down (suggesting an important biological component to addiction), or that she or he quit for a period, but slipped back into smoking when stressed, angry, or depressed (suggesting a significant amount of psychological dependence). If the patient relapsed in a social situation, then social anxiety or lack of assertiveness may be a problem that needs correcting before the next quit attempt. Moreover, recent evidence suggests that a sizable proportion of smokers also suffer from a past or present psychiatric disorder (e.g., major depressive episode, alcohol or other psychoactive substance-use disorder, anxiety disorders) and that a majority of individuals with severe psychiatric disorders, such as schizophrenia, major depressive disorder, and bipolar disorder, smoke (Brown et al, 1993). Relapse to smoking may be precipitated by an exacerbation or reemergence of psychiatric symptoms in these patients.

A Step-Care Model of Treatment

By exploring the patient's status and history on biopsychosocial dimensions, one can decide how to move him or her in a stepwise fashion through three possible levels of treatment: (1) minimal interventions (self-help, brief physician counseling, over-the-counter nicotine replacement, commercial programs, hypnosis); (2) intermediate interventions (professionally led programs that feature behavior modification); and (3) maximal interventions (behavior modification plus pharmacological treatments and specialized programs that address psychiatric comorbidity, including other substance abuse).

Minimal Interventions

As noted above, several studies suggest the potential power of brief intervention in physicians' offices (Fiore et al, 1996). Strategies that increase the likelihood of success include face-to-face interventions, the combination of physician and nonphysician counselors, multiple sessions, and multiple intervention modalities (Kottke et al, 1988). Studies have demonstrated that physician interventions are particularly effective in patients with smoking-related illnesses or in those "at risk" for smoking-related disease (Schwartz, 1987). Physician advice is improved when follow-up is provided (Wilson et al, 1982). Other simple strategies that physicians can use in the office are listed in Table 24–6. As noted above, recent studies performed in the primary care setting have demonstrated the effectiveness of nicotine replacement and bupropion when brief counseling and several follow-up visits were also provided (Fiore et al, 1992, 1996; Goldstein, in press).

Other minimal interventions are listed in Table 24–6. Generally, it is the lighter, less-dependent smokers who are highly motivated to quit and who have excellent social support for quitting that are the preferred candidates for brief or minimal interventions.

Intermediate Interventions

If minimal interventions have been attempted without success, or if the individual is more physiologically or psychologically dependent on cigarettes, then formal behavioral treatment programs of several weeks' duration should be considered. These programs teach skills for quitting, as well as for managing, acute withdrawal and maintenance/preventing relapse (Abrams et al, 1991; Brown et al, 1993; Lichtenstein, 1982).

Behavioral approaches to quitting include stimulus control, aversive techniques, cognitive approaches to deal with urges and craving, and relax-

Table 24–6 **A Step-Care Model for the Treatment of Smoking**

I. **Minimal interventions**
Self-help programs
Physician counseling
  Advice
  Provide quitting materials (e.g., self-help manuals)
  Contracts
  Set quit date
  Follow-up visits or calls
  Nicotine nasal spray
  Bupropion
Over-the-counter nicotine replacement
  Nicotine transdermal patches (with brief behavioral counseling and follow-up)
  Nicotine gum
Commercial programs
Hypnosis/acupuncture
II. **Intermediate interventions**
Professionally led programs
  Nicotine fading
  Aversive techniques
  Behavior modification
    Self-monitoring of smoking behavior
    Goal setting and self-reinforcement
    Stimulus control
    Coping skills
      Cognitive restructuring
      Assertiveness training
      Problem solving
      Relaxation training
      Relapse-prevention training
III. **Maximal interventions**
Combined behavior modification/pharmacotherapy
  Nicotine resin complex
  Nicotine transdermal patches
  Clonidine
  Antidepressants
Outpatient treatment programs that address psychiatric comorbidity
Inpatient treatment programs

ation training. Gradual reduction of nicotine is designed to minimize withdrawal symptoms. Stimulus control involves rearranging the environment and self to make smoking more and more difficult (remove all ashtrays, smoke only in one room of the house, buy packs instead of cartons). Although aversive strategies are unlikely to be widely accepted by consumers, they have yielded some of the most successful outcomes. Most current programs include a variety of techniques rather than one strategy. Reviews of the behavioral literature indicate that at a 1-year follow-up, the average participant in the typical behavioral program has a 20 to 40% chance of being abstinent (Brown et al, 1993; Schwartz, 1987). Combined formal behavioral treatment and pharmacotherapy with approved agents should also be considered intermediate interventions.

Maximal Interventions

Programs that add other nonapproved pharmacological precedures (e.g., clonidine, other antidepressants) to behavior modification should be considered for the chronic and more "difficult to treat" heavy smoker who has tried to quit repeatedly without success (Abrams et al, 1991; Brown et al, 1993; Fagerstrom, 1978). Individuals with a past or present psychiatric disorder may require more intensive treatment to help them quit smoking, especially if they continue to have signs or symptoms of the disorder. Patients abusing alcohol or other psychoactive drugs are unlikely to quit smoking successfully until they stop abusing other drugs (Brown et al, 1993). A past history of depression may dispose an individual to experience depressive symptoms or a full-blown depression when their quit smoking (Brown et al, 1993). Therefore, outpatient or inpatient programs that address both smoking cessation and psychiatric comorbidity may be needed by smokers with these disorders.

Maintenance Strategies

Behavioral techniques for maintenance and prevention of relapse are of recent origin and hold much promise because 60% of those who quit smoking will relapse within the first 3 months of quitting (Marlatt and Gordon, 1985). Techniques for relapse prevention include a detailed analysis of "high-risk situations." These are people, places, or emotional states that the smoker feels are most likely to precipitate a return to smoking. Individuals are taught how to cope with these situations using rehearsal and other techniques to resist temptation. If they should have a slip back into smoking (one or two cigarettes), then they are provided with techniques to prevent the slip from becoming a full-blown relapse. Additional support and follow-up (e.g., telephone hot lines) are usually provided during the critical 3 to 6 months after quitting, when people are most vulnerable to relapse.

In summary, even a small amount of physician time can have a large impact on helping patients become motivated for quitting smoking and resisting relapse. A step-care plan can be adopted with every smoker in the office practice and in the hospital. Those who are not yet ready to quit are targeted for systematic counseling, education, and follow-up. More time and effort are spent on high-risk individuals and those who are willing to take action. Beyond physician advice (which can be very effective), self-help and comprehensive formal programs can be used. Helping patients to quit smoking can have a large impact on chronic disease and disability in the United States over the next decades. (Nicotine addiction is also discussed in Chapter 10).

A CASE STUDY

Ms. Williams is a 37-year-old, hard-working lawyer with two small children. She visits her physician complaining of productive coug *and fever for 3 days. After obtaining a history, performing a phy*

cal exam, and obtaining a chest X-ray, the physician returns to the
examining room to tell the patient that the chest X-ray is negative
and that she has bronchitis. He also notices from her chart that she
has been a chronic smoker. The dialogue that follows reflects a
patient-centered approach to smoking cessation.

Doctor: Your chest X-ray looks normal. I think you have bronchitis. I will discuss the treatment of your bronchitis with you, but first, I'd like to talk with you about smoking. Are you still smoking?

Ms. Williams: Yes, I'm ashamed to say.

Doctor: Have you thought about giving it up?

Ms. Williams: Yes, I'd like to quit, but smoking really helps me to relax and concentrate at work, and I have this big case coming up. I couldn't possibly try to quit till it's over.

Doctor: Hmm, it seems like you depend on cigarettes to help you deal with stress at work. Your work sounds pretty stressful right now. What reasons do you have for wanting to quit?

Ms. Williams: Well, I know it's not good for my health, especially since I keep getting bronchitis. Also, my father smoked, and he died of a heart attack. My husband is not a smoker, and he and the kids have been after me to quit, too.

Doctor: You've mentioned some good reasons for quitting. I think your infections would decrease if you quit, and your risk of developing heart disease will decrease dramatically when you quit. I know I've told you about the effects of passive smoke on your children's health, as well as the important influence you have on your kids as a role model. I'm glad you're willing to consider quitting, but it sounds like quitting now would be hard on you. I'd like to help you to quit when your case is over, though.

Ms. Williams: That would be fine. My case will be over in 2 months.

Doctor: Why don't you schedule an appointment with me in 2 months, then.

Ms. Williams: OK.

In this case, the physician (1) raised the issue of smoking and allowed the patient to express her ideas and feelings about quitting, (2) explored her reasons for quitting, as well as her reasons for continuing to smoke, and (3) recognized that the patient was contemplating quitting, but also that she was not ready for action. Therefore, the physician elected to reinforce the patient's reasons for quitting, personalize her risk, offer to help her quit, and ask her to schedule a follow-up appointment after her court case was over. It is likely that the physician helped to accelerate the patient's movement from the contemplation stage to the preparation or action stage with these interventions. If she returns in 2 months, or when she returns for any future visit, the physician can continue to build commitment, complete further assessment, and begin to suggest specific smoking cessation strategies.

ANNOTATED BIBLIOGRAPHY

Abrams DB, Emmons KM, Niaura RS, et al: Tobacco dependence: an integration of individual and public health perspectives. In Nathan PE, Langenbucher JW, McCrady BS, Frankenstein W (eds): Annual Review of Addictions Research and Treatment, Vol. 1. New York, Pergamon Press, 1991

> A comprehensive review of factors contributing to the development of tobacco dependence, with a description of the full range of potential interventions to prevent and treat tobacco dependence.

Brown RA, Goldstein MG, Niaura R, Emmons KM, Abrams DB: Nicotine dependence: assessment and management. In Stoudemire A, Fogel BS (eds): Psychiatric Care of the Medical Patient. New York, Oxford University Press, 877–902, 1993

> A detailed review of the assessment and management of nicotine dependence, with an emphasis on the role of the physician.

Brownell KD: The LEARN Program for Weight Control, 6th ed. Dallas, TX, American Health Publishing, 1994

> A comprehensive patient manual for weight management.

Clark MM, Ruggiero L, Pera V, Goldstein MG, Abrams DB: Assessment, classification, and treatment of obesity: a behavioral medicine perspective. In Stoudemire A, Fogel BS (eds): Psychiatric Care of the Medical Patient. New York, Oxford University Press, 1993

> A detailed review aimed at the medical practitioner.

Grueninger UJ, Duffy FD, Goldstein MG: Patient education in the medical encounter: how to facilitate learning, behavior change and coping. In Lipkin M Jr, Putnam S, Lazare A (eds): The Medical Interview: Clinical Care, Education, Research, pp 122–123. New York, Springer-Verlag, 1995

> Describes a comprehensive model for patient education and counseling in the medical setting as well as a practical patient-centered strategy for physician-delivered counseling.

Prochaskca JO, DiClemente CC: Towards a comprehensive model of change. In Miller WR, Heather N (eds): Treating Addictive Disorders: Processes of Change. New York, Plenum Press, 1986

> Description of a comprehensive model of behavioral change that includes an explanation of the stages and processes of change.

Russell ML: Behavioral Counseling in Medicine: Strategies for Modifying At-Risk Behavior. New York, Oxford University Press, 1986

> A practical primer for physicians in behavioral counseling techniques.

Sheridan DP, Winogrond IR (eds): The Preventive Approach to Patient Care. New York, Elsevier, 1987

> A text on the theory and practice of preventive medicine, using a life-cycle approach.

REFERENCES

Abrams DB, Emmons KM, Niaura RS, et al: Tobacco dependence: an integration of individual and public health perspectives. In Nathan PE, Langenbucher JW, McGrady BS, Frankenstein W (eds): Annual Review of Addictions Research and Treatment, Vol. 1. New York, Pergamon Press, 1991

Anda RF, Remington PL, Sienko DG, et al: Are physicians advising smokers to quit? The patient's perspective. JAMA 257:1916–1919, 1987

Best JA: Tailoring smoking withdrawal procedures to personality and motivational differences. J Consult Clin Psychol 4:1–8, 1976

Brown RA, Goldstein MG, Niaura R, Emmons KM, Abrams DB: Nicotine dependence: assessment and management. In Stoudemire A, Fogel BS (eds): Psychiatric Care of the Medical Patient. New York, Oxford University Press, 877–902, 1993

Brownell KD: The LEARN Program for Weight Control, 6th ed. Dallas, TX, American Health Publishing, 1994

Brownell KD, Wadden TA: The heterogeneity of obesity: fitting treatment to individuals. Behav Ther 22:153–177, 1991

Brownell KD, Wadden TA: Etiology and treatment of obesity: understanding a serious, prevalent, and refractory disorder. J Consult Clin Psychol 60:505–517, 1992

Clark MM, Guise BJ, Niaura RS: Obesity level and attrition: support for patient-treatment matching in obesity treatment. Obes Res 3:63–64, 1995

Clark MM, Pera V, Goldstein MG: Counseling strategies for obese patients. Am J Prev Med 12:266–270, 1996

Clark MM, Ruggiero L, Pera V, Goldstein MG, Abrams DB: Assessment, classification, and treatment of obesity: a behavioral medicine perspective. In Stoudemire A, Fogel BS (eds): Psychiatric Care of the Medical Patient. New York, Oxford University Press, 903–928, 1993

Engel GL: The need for a new medical model: a challenge for biomedicine. Science 196:129–136, 1977

Fagerstrom KO: Measuring degree of physical dependence to tobacco smoking with reference to individualization of treatment. Addict Behav 3:235–241, 1978

Fiore MC, Bailey WC, Cohen SJ, et al: Smoking Cessation. Clinical Practice Guideline No. 18. AHCPR Publication No. 96-0692. Rockville, MD, U.S. Dept. of Health and Human Services, Public Health Service, Agency for Health Care Policy and Research, April, 1996.

Fiore MC, Jorenby DE, Baker TB, Kenford SL: Tobacco dependence and the nicotine patch: clinical guidelines for effective use. JAMA 268:2687–2694, 1992

Foster GD, Wadden TA, Vogt RA, Brewer G: What is a reasonable weight loss? Patients' expectations and evaluations of obesity treatment outcomes. J Consult Clin Psychol 65:79–85, 1997

Gilpin E, Pierce J, Goodman J, Giovino G, Berry C, Bums D: Trends in physicians' giving advice to stop smoking, United States, 1974–87. Tobacco Control 1:31–36, 1992

Glynn T, Manley M: How to Help Your Patients Stop Smoking: The National Cancer Institute Manual for Physicians. Bethesda, MD, National Institutes of Health, 1989

Goldstein DJ: Beneficial health effects of modest weight loss. Int J Obes 16:397–415, 1992

Goldstein MG: Bupropion SR and smoking cessation. J Clin Psychiatry, in press

Green L, Eriksen M, Schor E: Preventive practices by physicians: behavioral determinants and potential interventions. Am J Prev Med 4(suppl):101–107, 1988.

Grueninger U, Duffy F, Goldstein M: Patient education in the medical encounter: how to facilitate learning, behavior change and coping. In Lipkin MJ, Putnam S, Lazare A (eds): The Medical Interview: Clinical Care, Education, Research, pp 122–133. New York, Springer-Verlag, 1995.

Grueninger UJ, Goldstein MG, Duffy FD: Patient education in hypertension: five essential steps. J Hypertens 7(suppl 3):593–598, 1989

Inui TS, Yourtee EL, Williamson JW: Improved outcome in hypertension after physician tutorials: a controlled trial. Ann Intern Med 84:646–651, 1976

Jeffrey RW: Behavioral treatment of obesity. Ann Behav Med 9:20–24, 1987

King TK, Clark MM, Pera V: History of sexual abuse and obesity treatment outcome. Addict Behav 21:283–290, 1996

Kottke TE, Battista RN, DeFriesse GH, Brekke ML: Attributes of successful smoking cessation interventions in medical practice: a meta-analysis of 39 controlled trials. JAMA 259:2882–2889, 1988

Kottke TE, Blackburn H, Brekke ML, Solberg LI: The systematic practice of preventive cardiology. Am J Cardiol 59:690–694, 1987

Kottke TE, Foels JK, Hill C, et al: Nutrition counseling in private practice: attitudes and activities of family physicians. Prev Med 13:219–225, 1984

Levenkron JC, Greenland P, Bowley N: Using patient instructors to teach behavioral counseling skills. J Med Educ 65:665–672, 1987

Levy BT, Williamson PS: Patient perceptions and weight loss of obese adults. J Fam Pract 27:285–290, 1988

Lichtenstein E: The smoking problem: a behavioral perspective. J Consult Clin Psychol 50:804–819, 1982

Marcus BH, Pinto BM, Clark MM, DePue JD, Goldstein MG, Simkin Silverman L: Physician-delivered physical activity and nutrition interventions. Med Exerc Nutr Health 4:325–334, 1995b

Marcus MD, Moulton MM, Greeno CG: Binge eating onset in obese patients with binge eating disorder. Addict Behav 20:747–755, 1995a

Marlatt GA, Gordon JR: Relapse Prevention. New York, Guilford Press, 1985

McGinnis J, Foege W: Actual causes of death in the United States. JAMA 270:2207–2212, 1993

Miller WR, Rolnick S: Motivational Interviewing: Preparing People to Change Addictive Behavior. New York, Guilford, 1991

Mullen PD, Green LW, Persinger GS: Clinical trials of patient education for chronic conditions: a comparative meta-analysis of intervention types. Prev Med 14:751–783, 1985

Nutting PA: Health promotion in primary medical care: problems and potential. Prev Med 15:537–548, 1986

Ockene JK: Physician-delivered intervention for smoking cessation: strategies for increasing effectiveness. Prev Med 16:723–737, 1987

Ockene JK, Quirk ME, Goldberg RJ, et al: A residents training program for the development of smoking intervention skills. Arch Intern Med 148:1039–1045, 1988

Orleans CT, George LK, Houpt JL, Brodie KH: Health promotion in primary care: a survey of US family practitioners. Prev Med 14:636–647, 1985

Perri MG, McAllister PA, Gange JJ, Nero AM: Effects of four maintenance programs on the long-term management of obesity. J Consult Clin Psychol 56:529–534, 1988

Perri MG, Sears SF, Clark JE: Strategies for improving the maintenance of weight loss: toward a continuous care model of obesity management. Diabetes Care 16:200–209, 1993

Preventive Health Care Committee, Society for Research and Education in Primary Care Internal Medicine: Preventive medicine in general internal medicine residency training. Ann Intern Med 102:859–861, 1985

Prochaska JO, DiClemente CC: Towards a comprehensive model of change. In Miller WR, Heather N (eds): Treating Addictive Disorders: Processes of Change. New York, Plenum Press, 1986

Schwartz JL: Review end Evaluation of Smoking Cessation Methods. The United States and Canada, 1978–1985. US Department of Health and Human Services, Public Health Service, National Institutes of Health, Natioual Cancer Institute, Division of Cancer Prevention and Control. Bethesda, MD, NIH Publication No. 87-2940, 1987

Schwartz JS, Lewis CE, Clancy C, Kinosian MS, Radany MH, Koplan JP: Internists' practices in health promotion and disease prevention: a survey. Ann Intern Med 114:46–53, 1991

Schwartz MB, Brownell KD: Matching individuals to weight loss treatments: a survey of obesity experts. J Consult Clin Psychol 63:149–153, 1995

US Department of Health, Education, and Welfare, Public Health Service: Healthy People: The Surgeon General's Report on Health Promotion and Disease Prevention. Washington, DC, Government Printing Office, 1979

Venditti EM, Wing RR, Jakicic JM, Butler BA, Marcus MD: Weight cycling, psychological health and binge eating in obese women. J Consult Clin Psychol 64:400–405, 1996

Wadden TA, Foster GD, Letizia KA, Stunkard AJ: A multicenter evaluation of a proprietary weight reduction program for the treatment of marked obesity. Arch Intern Med 152:961–966, 1992

Wadden TA, Stunkard AJ: Controlled trial of very low calorie diet, behavior therapy, and their combination in the treatment of obesity. J Consult Clin Psychol 54:482–488, 1986

Wilson D, Wood G, Johnston N, et al: Randomized clinical trial of supportive follow-up for smokers in family practice. Can Med Assoc J 126:127–129, 1982

Wing RR: Behavior treatment of severe obesity. Am J Clin Nutr 55:5455–5515, 1992

The authors wish to thank Barbara Doll for her secretarial assistance. The authors who contributed to the development of the model of patient education described by Grueninger, Duffy, and Goldstein are too numerous to list here. Readers are referred to the work by Grueninger, Duffy, and Goldstein for a complete list of references and acknowledgments.

25 *Legal Issues in Psychiatry*

Julie A. Rand
and Constance J. McKee

Forensic psychiatry is a subspecialty of psychiatry in which there is an intersection of two disciplines: law and psychiatry. The term *forensic* means belonging to the courts. In a psychiatric practice, there is a therapeutic alliance that develops between the patient and the psychiatrist. The psychiatrist primarily sees himself or herself in the role as a treating physician. If issues arise involving court and the psychiatrist is called to testify, he or she is considered a witness of fact. In contrast, a forensic psychiatrist often serves as an expert witness and renders opinions on a particular case or issue based on available data. The role of the expert witness usually involves an evaluation, not treatment. Forensic psychiatrists perform detailed assessments with all relevant data to render an opinion concerning the legal question. For success as a forensic expert, the psychiatrist must have good clinical skills and applications, along with the ability to draw conclusions from the data obtained.

Forensic psychiatry is divided into two areas, criminal and civil. Criminal forensics will be briefly discussed in this chapter; however, the focus of our discussion will be in the area of civil forensic psychiatry, which is most directly relevant to the practice of physicians in medical settings.

COMPETENCY: THE LEGAL CONCEPT AND ITS CLINICAL APPLICATIONS

Competence is the capacity of mental functioning necessary for decision-making to carry out a specific task (see also Chapters 19 and 20). There is a wide spectrum of competency ranging from competence to consent for medical treatment to competence to marry. Competence is a legal concept, which is determined by the courts, and all individuals, except for minors, are presumed to be competent unless legally adjudicated otherwise; however, patients often lack the capacity to make decisions concerning treatment, and psychiatrists are frequently called on to evaluate a patient's competency to refuse treatment. The psychiatrist often renders an opinion concerning a patient's "psychological capacity" rather than "legal competence" (Appelbaum and Roth, 1981). The opinion of the psychiatrist is important and can often prevent any unnecessary judicial hearing on the question of competency. When a hearing occurs, the judge often relies on the evaluation by the psychiatrist in making a decision concerning the patient's competence.

Criteria to Assess Capacity

In 1982, the President's Commission for the Study of Ethical Problems in Medicine and Biomedical and Behavioral Research emphasized the importance of assessing a patient's capacity to consent to medical treatment. Some have suggested that the legal standards for competence include communicating and maintaining a stable choice, understanding relevant information concerning a treatment decision, appreciating the current situation and its consequences, and manipulating information rationally, specifically when comparing the benefits and risks of various treatment options (Appelbaum and Grisso, 1988). There are some clinical factors that can affect the assessment of competency. These factors include a patient's psychodynamic issues, limited information provided by the patient, incomplete or confusing information provided by staff to the patient, a patient's fluctuating mental status, and the setting in which consent is to be obtained (Appelbaum and Roth, 1981).

Guidelines for Assessing
Decision-Making Capacity

When assessing competency, the clinician must perform a thorough evaluation of the patient, including a complete mental status examination with a detailed description of any cognitive deficits that may interfere with the functioning of the patient. It is most helpful to discuss the specific issues at hand with the treatment team and to review the patient's current medical record, along with previous medical records. With the patient's consent, the psychiatrist should speak with family members to obtain more history and to understand the patient's current situation. A psychiatric diagnosis should be made if one exists; however, even a diagnosis of schizophrenia or dementia does not necessarily mean that one lacks the capacity to consent to medical treatment. In fact, individuals with these diagnoses often understand the nature and consequences of certain procedures and should not be assumed to be incompetent.

During the evaluation, instead of direct questioning, the clinician should attempt to engage in conversation with the patient, which encourages the patient to express feelings and discuss issues concerning his or her situation. This enables the psychiatrist to obtain valuable information concerning the patient's thought process and cognition, including ability to reason and make a choice (Deaton et al, 1993). The dialogue approach often helps ally the patient with the psychiatrist; therefore, the psychiatrist is able to obtain more information to assess the patient's understanding of his or her medical problem and proposed treatment adequately, along with the risks and benefits of the proposed treatment and alternative treatments. The psychiatrist should then assess the patient's choice concerning treatment and the reasoning behind the choice.

After completing the evaluation, the psychiatrist should clearly document any cognitive or emotional deficits assessed during the evaluation and render an opinion concerning the patient's decision-making capacity for the task in question.

THE DOCTRINE OF INFORMED CONSENT

Since the establishment of common law, patients have been required to consent for treatment. In the 1914 case *Schloendorff v. Society of New York Hospital,* Justice Benjamin Cordozo stated that "Every human being of adult years and sound mind has a right to determine what shall be done with his own body." The informed consent doctrine was based on the issue of one's autonomy, and the doctrine developed as a part of the tort of battery, an unauthorized touching of the patient. The term *informed consent* was first introduced 40 years ago in a 1957 case, *Salgo v. Leland Stanford Junior, University Board of Trustees,* in which a court found that the patient's right to consent required adequate disclosure of necessary facts to make an informed decision.

The Fundamentals of Informed Consent

Informed consent requires three elements: competency, disclosure, and voluntariness. The issues concerning competency have been discussed in other sections of this text. Concerning disclosure, one must be informed of the nature of his or her illness and of the proposed treatment. In *Natanson v. Kline,* a landmark case in 1960, a Kansas court described the necessary disclosure for decision making by the patient. The required elements included information concerning the nature of the patient's illness and the proposed treatment, including the risks, benefits, likelihood of success, and alternative treatments. The court established the "reasonable medical practitioner" standard, which required the physician to disclose only that which the "reasonable medical practitioner" would disclose under similar medical circumstances. In 1972, the reasonable medical practitioner standard was challenged in *Canterbury v. Spence,* in which the court proposed that standards of disclosure be based on that which a "reasonable person" would find essential in decision making.

The third element of informed consent is voluntariness. Was the patient coerced into treatment? In the 1972 case of *Kaimowitz v. Michigan Department of Mental Health,* the court found that involuntary patients (whose discharge often is contingent on compliance with recommended treatment) are hospitalized in a "coercive institutional environment."

Exceptions to Informed Consent

The exceptions to informed consent include emergency situations, patient waivers, and therapeutic privilege (Schwartz, 1994). If a medical emergency exists, such as evidence of imminent danger of harm to the patient or others, the physician may treat immediately with implied consent, even against the will of the patient. Other exceptions to informed consent include the patient's desire to waive consent for a medical procedure and therapeutic privilege, which allows the physician to withhold information from a patient that could harm the patient.

Next-of-Kin Laws

If a medical emergency does not exist and the patient is incompetent, the clinician should consider a second opinion consultation and also consult with the hospital attorney. Depending on state laws, spouses, parents, children, and siblings may be able to consent to treatment for the incompetent patient; however, not all states have next-of-kin laws, and the patient's refusal often overrides the consent given by the next of kin. The laws concerning consent vary from state to state. Often, formal legal proceedings are necessary to designate a guardian or to determine who gives consent for the patient.

Guardianship

Many states provide for "emergency" guardianship, which can usually be obtained within 1 week or even for "emergency emergency" guardianship, which can be obtained within 1 to 2 days. Nonemergency guardianship often takes approximately 4 to 6 weeks. If there is not a family member available for the patient, the court can appoint a guardian. In many states, the duration of emergency guardianship is between 30 and 45 days, and termination occurs after this period. Concerning permanent guardianship, the guardian or ward can file a petition to terminate the guardianship. The guardianship terminates automatically when the ward dies (Overton, 1993).

CONFIDENTIALITY

Confidentiality is the clinician's obligation to avoid disclosing to a third party, without valid authorization, any information that was revealed in a professional relationship. This right continues even after the patient's death. Confidentiality is required by law and is based on the legal principle of the right to privacy. It is also required by medical licensing boards and by medical ethics; it is part of the Hippocratic Oath. A breach of confidentiality renders one liable for a malpractice suit and disciplinary action by licensing boards and professional organizations.

Confidentiality does not apply if there is no actual clinician–patient relationship, such as during an evaluation; however, there are ethical requirements to inform the patient of this exception before the evaluation. There are other significant exceptions to the confidentiality requirement (Table 25–1). The most common is a valid consent to release information. As in any other area of medicine in which a legal requirement could later be questioned, it is preferable to have this consent in writing. The consent should specify which information is authorized for release, and it should be recently signed, dated, and possibly witnessed. Before obtaining consent for the release of medical information, it is important to make sure that the patient has the capacity to give consent, as described in the informed consent section. If the patient does not have the capacity to consent to records release, as in the case of a minor or an incompetent patient, the legal guardian can be given information and becomes the authorizing person for the release of records on the patient's behalf. If the patient is deceased, the executor of the estate may give consent for records release.

Confidentiality is also waived within the clinical treatment circle. This means that one need not seek specific permission from the patient to discuss information with other staff members treating the patient, or with supervisors or consultants; however, disclosure of information to staff members does *not* include the casual sharing of patient information with friends or colleagues who are not currently involved in the patient's treatment. Also, note that the patient's family is not necessarily considered part of this circle; the patient's consent is required in order to share information with them, except in case of emergency, or if the patient is incompetent or a minor, as noted above.

Table 25–1 **Exceptions to Duty of Confidentiality**

No clinician–patient relationship (such as in an evaluation)
Valid consent
Clinical treatment circle
Mandatory reporting (such as Child Abuse)
Duty to protect others (Tarasoff duty)
Court order
Emergencies (dangerousness, to obtain consent, etc.)

Confidentiality is waived when it is necessary to reveal information in order to protect the patient or others. Examples include mandatory reporting, civil commitment, obtaining emergency consent for an incompetent patient, or in the Tarasoff duty to protect (see below). All states have mandatory reporting laws for the safety of society, such as the required reporting of contagious diseases, of firearm and knife wounds, of epilepsy patients who operate motor vehicles, and of child abuse. All states require that suspected child abuse be reported to the child protective agency of that state. Failure to report suspected child abuse can render a physician liable to criminal prosecution or to malpractice action, especially if further harm comes to the child. As with the Tarasoff duty, it is preferable, if possible, to inform the patient of the reporting requirement and to attempt to make the reporting part of the therapeutic process.

There is no obligation to report a past crime and no obligation to speak to law enforcement officials without a court order. To do so would constitute violation of confidentiality.

Privilege

A subpoena, although intimidating, is *not* an automatic exception from confidentiality. The patient has a right to bar the clinician from testifying about professionally obtained material in legal matters; this right of the patient is called *privilege.* Privilege laws vary in different state jurisdictions. If one receives a subpoena for records, a valid release should still be obtained; however, one *cannot* simply ignore a subpoena, *under penalty of law.* If the patient or his or her representative cannot or does not consent to the records release, the attorney issuing the subpoena should be contacted and informed that you do not have authorization to release the records. Additionally, the patient's or your own attorney could be consulted. These attorneys may seek to get the subpoena quashed, or see that a court order is issued. A court order for medical information is *always* an exception to confidentiality and must be obeyed.

CIVIL COMMITMENT

Civil commitment, also known as involuntary hospitalization, is the process of holding a person against his or her will in a psychiatric hospital because of mental illness.

Background of Civil Commitment

The United States Constitution entitles all citizens to life, liberty, and the pursuit of happiness. Depriving a person of liberty, however well intentioned, is a serious event and is therefore governed by law. Civil commitment is a deprivation of liberty. One legal basis on which physicians are legally able to violate an individual's liberty is called the doctrine of *parens patriae*. This concept originated with early monarchies, who believed that it is the role of the monarch, or government, to care for impaired citizens. An additional legal basis of civil commitment is the concept that government is authorized to use police powers to protect its citizens, even if this involves deprivation of liberty. Thus, civil commitment to a mental hospital is usually based on two criteria: whether a person needs hospital treatment, and whether he or she appears to be dangerous to him/herself or others.

Within these parameters, our society has vacillated with regard to how easy or how difficult it should be for an individual to be involuntarily hospitalized. Since the late 1960s, the pendulum has swung in the direction of stricter commitment criteria. This swing was a reaction to a period of relaxed civil commitment laws in the period following World War II. At that time, individuals could be hospitalized as long as doctors thought they needed treatment, making it difficult for the chronically mentally ill to be discharged. The average length of stay for a person with schizophrenia in 1958 was 13 years (Gutheil, 1994). These lengthy stays led to thousands of people being institutionalized in state hospitals. Ultimately, the courts became involved, ordering greater protection for individual liberties and establishing stricter criteria for civil commitment.

Clinical Guidelines for Patient Assessment

When the physician must make a decision about hospitalization for mental illness (Table 25–2), he or she must obtain an accurate history from sources in addition to the patient and do a mental status evaluation. It is not acceptable practice to admit or commit a patient without personally examining the patient. Even if the patient declines to speak, important information can be gathered by observing the patient and attempting an examination. It is also not advisable to accept the patient's word solely or information from the family or referral source solely about the patient's condition since significant disagreement may exist between the sources. If the physician determines that the

---

Table 25–2 Assessment Guidelines for Civil Commitment

History from the patient
Mental status exam of the patient
History from referring source, family
If patient needs hospitalization:
   Assess capacity to consent to voluntary hospitalization
If unable to consent to voluntary hospitalization or able to consent
   but refuses:
     Assess whether patient meets civil commitment criteria
If so, commit by signing applicable papers
If not, patient must be released

patient requires inpatient treatment, he or she should assess the patient for voluntary hospitalization. To be hospitalized voluntarily, the patient must have sufficient mental capacity to give informed consent to voluntary admission, as ruled on by the Supreme Court in the *Zinermon v. Burch* case in 1990. If the patient either refuses voluntary admission or lacks the capacity to consent to voluntary admission, the physician must determine whether the patient meets the civil commitment criteria that apply in the state. The specifics of the state laws vary, and the physician must be aware of the laws in his or her jurisdiction. Most civil commitment laws require that a person be mentally ill (or addicted to drugs or alcohol) and present a danger to him/herself or others. The physician must access the patient for suicidality, grave disability, and dangerousness toward others.

Assessment of the Suicidal Patient

There are approximately 30,000 suicides a year in the United States. Suicide is believed to be the eighth cause of death in this country and accounts for over 1% of all deaths in this country. Approximately 75% of the people who successfully commit suicide have told others that they intend to die, and approximately 50% have seen a physician during the month before their death (Simon and Sadoff, 1992). Patients are at higher risk during the first 3 months after a crisis, when he or she is reportedly improving. As the clinical depressive symptoms start to improve, the patient is often able to carry out the plans for suicide. From a forensic perspective, suicide and suicidal attempts are the most frequent causes for lawsuits against psychiatrists. Even though psychiatrists cannot predict future behavior with any high degree of certainty, they should be able to assess suicide risk factors and evaluate the patient's potential for suicide.

Concerning potential risk factors, suicide rates seem to vary with age. There is a higher risk for geriatric patients and for adolescents. For women, there is a steady increase in suicide rates until ages 45 to 54 and then a gradual decline. For men, there is a peak during ages 25 to 34, a decrease during ages 35 to 44, and then a gradual increase (Kaplan et al, 1994). Women attempt suicide three times as often as men do, and men commit suicide three times more often than women do. Men use lethal means more often than women. Caucasians commit suicide more often than non-Caucasians. Marital status is an important variable to consider. Married people with children have the lowest rate of suicide; separated or divorced individuals or those who live alone have a higher rate. Unemployment is a risk for suicide; however, employed professionals have a higher rate of suicide. Approximately 30% of individuals who commit suicide have made at least one previous attempt. It is important to know about all previous attempts, when the attempts occurred, and about the lethality of the attempt. A history of a previous inpatient psychiatric admission is an additional risk factor (see also Chapter 20).

Of most importance is assessment of current suicidal ideation and current plans. The patient should be asked about access to firearms and other means for carrying out the plan. Concerning risks related to psychiatric disorders, alcohol and substance-abuse history greatly increases suicide risk. Other psychiatric disorders that increase suicide risk include schizophrenia, bipolar disorder, major depression, and personality disorders. Patients with panic attacks or a high degree of anxiety, patients with a history of violent, impulsive behavior, and the medically ill all are at higher risk for suicide.

The physician must also assess the potential risk of harm to the patient from other sources, including a patient so mentally impaired that the individual could starve, freeze to death, walk into traffic, etc. The latter condition is referred to in many state commitment laws as "gravely disabled" and in those states is also a basis for civil commitment.

Assessment of the Dangerous Patient

The physician must also assess the patient's risk of violence toward others (Table 25–3). The mentally ill have an increased rate of violence compared with the general population. An epidemiological study of self-reported violence in the community (Swanson et al, 1990) showed the range to be 2% for those without a psychiatric diagnosis, 13% for those with a diagnosis of schizophrenia, and a 19 to 35% rate for those with diagnoses of alcohol or drug abuse. The occurrence of substance abuse with a mental illness greatly increases the risk.

Psychiatrists have shown poor accuracy at predicting violence in general. Although certain factors have been shown to assist in the short-term assessment of the risk of violence, the accuracy of long-term predictions remains problematic. The single *best predictor of future violence is past violence,* so a good history of past violent behavior must be taken, particularly from outside sources and records. Histories of substance abuse, paranoid thinking, antiso-

Table 25–3 **Factors Increasing Risk of Violence**

Any psychiatric diagnosis, especially paranoid disorders, substance abuse, antisocial personality disorder
Substance abuse combined with psychiatric diagnosis
Nature of threat: especially if specific, planned
Availability of potential victim
Availability of weapon
Motive (long-lasting grudge, perception of scorned love)
History of violence
History of victimization
Delinquency, gang membership
History of impulsivity
Other: male, low IQ, younger age

cial personality disorder, or head injury increase the risk of violence. Other risk factors for violence are whether the patient has made a specific threat and how serious that threat appears to be, the availability of the potential victim to the patient, the availability of a weapon, and having a motive, particularly one based on a long-lasting grudge or a perception of scorned love.

Duty to Protect: Tarasoff Duty

The Tarasoff case (*Tarasoff v. Board of Regents of the University of California*) set a now widely accepted duty for mental health professionals. A college student killed a young woman whom he felt had scorned his love. He had told a student health professional that he had such thoughts prior to the murder. In the final appeal of the legal case against the university, the court ruled in 1982 that if a threat is made by a patient to harm an identifiable person, the mental health professional must take "whatever steps are reasonably necessary to *protect* the potential victim." (Note that this is more than a duty to warn.) Some courts in other states have extended the duty to protect to the public in general, not just an identifiable victim.

Not all states have officially recognized a duty to protect, so the physician should determine the status of such a duty in his/her state. If the physician has determined after a thorough dangerousness assessment that a significant risk of harm toward others exists, the patient should be hospitalized until no longer dangerous. If the patient cannot be detained, attempts should initially be made, if possible, to work therapeutically with the patient, in the hope of helping him or her gain better control and avoiding the need for further actions. The physician should try to form an alliance with the part of the patient that feels ambivalent about the potential victim and that does not wish to harm the victim (Wulsin et al, 1983). If this is not possible or not successful, further steps should be taken. In conjunction with the medical team and legal counsel, the physician should consider notifying the police and giving written warning to the potential victim. Such steps may be considered exceptions to confidentiality; however, the psychiatrist should discuss proposed breaches of confidentiality with the patient and obtain informed consent whenever possible. The ultimate goal is to breach confidentiality as little as possible while protecting the endangered.

General Procedure for Civil Commitment

Once the decision is made to hospitalize a patient involuntarily, there are specific procedures and time frames to be followed, which vary in different states. Usually the physician must fill out an initial certificate that authorizes emergency detention for a brief period of assessment. Most states require that the commitment decision then be confirmed by a second physician in order to authorize commitment for an additional limited period for treatment. At the expiration of this period, if the treating physician believes that the patient still meets the civil commitment criteria, there must be a hearing, which is usually done under the jurisdiction of the probate court. The patient has a right to an attorney, and there is an established procedure for providing the patient and next of kin written notice about the hearing. If the judge does not think that hospitalization is indicated, the patient's release may be ordered.

Outpatient Commitment

Many states have provisions for legally requiring a patient to comply with treatment outside of the hospital; this is called *outpatient commitment*. It is usually imposed on those patients who have a history of repeated failure to take their medications as outpatients. These patients will usually have a history of repeated civil commitments related to their becoming psychotic and dangerous. Outpatient commitment usually allows the authorities to seek out and detain such patients when they have missed their medication appointments. This allows them to be rehospitalized before they become dangerous. It is also believed that when the patient realizes that consequences will definitely be imposed, he or she is more likely to be compliant with treatment.

PATIENTS' RIGHTS WITHIN A MENTAL HOSPITAL

Before the involvement of the courts and patients' advocates, patients who were civilly committed lost important rights as citizens. They were automatically considered incompetent and lost their rights to vote, to marry, or to handle their money. At times they lost the right to communicate with the outside world, and their living conditions were often inadequate. Numerous legal cases, most notably *Wyatt v. Aderholt* in Alabama in 1974, led to the establishment of patients' rights within a mental hospital. These rights include the rights to have visitors, to receive letters and phone calls, to be provided privacy, to handle funds, to be paid for work, etc. Patients' rights can be restricted for clearly documented clinical reasons, but cannot automatically be denied. Patients must have access to a patients' rights officer, who can assist a patient who feels his or her rights have been violated. Patients are also entitled to freedom from harm and freedom of movement; therefore, there are specific criteria governing the use of seclusion and restraint. Very important among these rights is the right to treatment in the "least restrictive alternative" available. This means that while being treated, patients must be given as much freedom as they can safely manage, including treatment outside the hospital.

Right to Refuse Treatment

All mental patients have a right to be free of unnecessary and excessive medication, and courts in numerous jurisdictions have ruled that patients have a right to refuse treatment. The legal basis for this ruling is the right to privacy. In these jurisdictions, medications may be forced under certain circumstances, which vary depending on the state and setting (hospital, jail, etc.). In many mental health settings, forced medication is allowed only if the patient is assessed to be dangerous to him/herself or others within the hospital itself. Thus, even when a patient is committed to a hospital because of dangerousness to self or others, medication cannot automatically be given if the patient refuses. Most jurisdictions have a review procedure for forced medications, which is usually conducted by nontreating professionals or by the courts. These reviews may also take into account the patient's competency and level of disability in addition to his dangerousness.

Patients' Right to Records

Medical records belong to the physician or hospital, but the information belongs to the patient. The patient has a right to have access to his or her medical records. However, this may be precluded if the physician thinks it would be harmful to the patient and documents this concern.

PSYCHIATRIC MALPRACTICE

Even though the number of lawsuits filed against psychiatrists continues to be low compared with other areas of medicine, the incidence has steadily increased during the past two decades. Malpractice is legally known as professional negligence that was unintentional. For a patient to file a malpractice claim, he or she must prove by preponderance of the evidence *the four "D"s* of malpractice:

1. There must be a *duty*.
2. There is a *dereliction* or breach of the duty.
3. The breach of duty is a *direct* cause of the damage.
4. There must be *damages* that were directly caused by the breach of the duty.

The plaintiff typically must find an expert physician who can give an opinion that the defendant deviated from the standard of care in his field.

The most frequent and expensive malpractice claims involve suicide and suicide attempts. Approximately 50% of suicides result in malpractice claims. Liability occurs during hospitalizations and after discharge; however, there is greater liability as an inpatient because staff are presumed to have control of the patient and the ability to protect the patient from harm. The physician should perform a comprehensive suicide assessment and provide means to observe and protect the patient, along with proper treatment to reduce the risk liability.

Electroconvulsive therapy and psychopharmacology are other sources for malpractice claims. It is important to obtain proper informed consent for electroconvulsive therapy and for all psychotropic medications. The psychiatrist should educate the patient about the potential risks of psychotropics, particularly the risk of tardive dyskinesia from antipsychotic medication. Other issues of negligence that often lead to litigation include failure to monitor and treat side effects, polypharmacy, and lack of indication for a particular prescription.

Negligence liability can also occur when using seclusion or restraints, which are tightly regulated in our society. If there is a violent episode, one has to weigh the risk of harm to self or others versus temporarily restraining a patient's movements to prevent any violence that could occur.

Malpractice claims based on sexual misconduct are uncommon, but they continue to occur. Sexual activity with a patient is a gross deviation from the standard of care under any circumstances. The relationship between a patient and a psychiatrist is one based on trust, and sexual exploitation of the patient is a breach of that trust and mismanagement of the transference. Other examples of exploiting a patient involve inability to set boundaries such as participating in social activities outside of appointments and making exceptions for the patient that are not typically done for other patients, such as charging lower fees or no fee and scheduling appointments after regular office hours. A psychiatrist found negligent for sexual misconduct can have his or her license revoked, and malpractice carriers can refuse to pay for damages. In some cases, the misconduct can result in criminal charges.

Other sources for malpractice claims are breaching confidentiality and failure to protect the endangered person from harm by not breaching confidentiality, as discussed in other sections of this chapter.

CRIMINAL ISSUES

The forensic psychiatry issues discussed so far in this chapter are in the civil area of law; however, forensic psychiatrists are also involved with assessments and treatment of individuals who are charged with crimes. Most notably, psychiatrists perform evaluations to determine whether defendants are competent to stand trial and whether they were criminally responsible for their actions (i.e., sane) at the time of the alleged crime.

An individual's competency to stand trial is based in general on whether he or she currently understands how the court works, the charges and the possible penalties, and whether he or she can assist the attorney in his or her own defense. In contrast, a criminal responsibility evaluation looks at the defendant's mental state at the time of the crime. States differ with regard to the standard used to determine criminal responsibility. The most famous standard for insanity, which is still in use in many jurisdictions, is called the M'Naghten Test. It was developed in England in 1843 following a trial in which Mr. M'Naghten was found not guilty by reason of insanity of killing the Prime Minister's secretary. For a defendant to be considered insane, the M'Naghten Test requires that at the time of the act, the defendant had "such a defect of reason, from disease of the mind, as not to know the nature and quality of the act he was doing; or . . . he did not know the difference between right and wrong . . . in respect to the act." Successful insanity defenses are rare, and individuals found insane often spend more time locked up in hospitals than they would have if they had been found guilty.

CLINICAL PEARLS

- Competence is a legal concept that is specific to a task. There is a wide spectrum of competency ranging from competence to consent for medical treatment to competence to marry.
- Informed consent requires three elements: competency, disclosure, and voluntariness. Exceptions to informed consent include emergencies, patient waivers, and therapeutic privilege.
- Maintaining confidentiality of information revealed in a professional relationship is the *clinician's obligation*. Privilege is the *patient's right* to bar the clinician from testifying about professionally obtained material in legal matters.
- Civil commitment usually is based on two criteria: the need for hospital treatment and whether he or she appears to be dangerous to self or others.
- The single best predictor of future violence is past violence.
- The Tarasoff Duty requires the mental health professional to take "whatever steps are reasonably necessary to protect the potential victim." This is more than a duty to warn the potential victim. Each state has its own law and the clinician should be aware of such a duty in his/her state.
- Even though a patient may be committed to a hospital because of dangerous behavior, medication cannot automatically be forced. In many hospitals, forced medication is only allowed if the patient is assessed to be dangerous to him/herself or others within the hospital itself.
- For a malpractice claim, there must be a *dereliction* of the *duty* which *directly* caused *damages*.

ANNOTATED BIBLIOGRAPHY

Appelbaum P, Grisso T: Assessing Patients' capacities to consent to treatment. N Eng J Med 319:1635–1638, 1988

   This article discusses in depth issues regarding the assessment of competency as it relates to consent for medical treatment.

Kaplan H, Sadock B, Grebb J: Synopsis of Psychiatry. Baltimore, MD, Williams & Wilkins, 1994

   The chapter on forensic psychiatry is an excellent, succinct review of the fundamental issues in criminal and civil forensic psychiatry.

Schwartz H: Informed consent and competency. In Rosner R (ed): Principles and Practice of Forensic Psychiatry, pp 103–110. New York, Chapman & Hall, 1994

> This is an expanded discussion with reference to landmark cases regarding the topics of competency and informed consent. This textbook is an excellent source for review of criminal and civil issues of forensic psychiatry.

Swanson JW, Holzer CE, Ganju VK, Jono RT: Violence and psychiatric disorder in the community: evidence from the Epidemiologic Catchment Area Surveys. Hosp Community Psychiatry 41:761–770, 1990

> This article provides a detailed discussion and a review of factors increasing the risk of violence, specifically psychiatric diagnoses.

Simon R, Sadoff R: Psychiatric Malpractice, Washington, DC, American Psychiatric Press, 1992

> This is an excellent guide and reference source for gaining an understanding of psychiatric malpractice. It covers the legal principles and clinical issues as it relates to the malpractice claims.

REFERENCES

Appelbaum P, Grisso T: Assessing patients' capacities to consent to treatment. N Eng J Med 319:1635–1638, 1988

Appelbaum P, Roth L: Clinical issues in the assessment of competency. Am J Psychiatry 138:1462–1467, 1981

Canterbury v. Spence, 464 F 2d 772, D.C. Circuit Court, cert denied, 409 US 1064, 1972

Deaton R, Colenda C, Bursztajn H: Medical-legal issues. In Stoudemire A, Fogel BS (eds): Psychiatric Care of the Medical Patient, pp 929–938. New York, Oxford University Press, 1993

Gutheil T: Confidentiality. In Forensic Psychiatry Review Course, American Academy of Psychiatry and the Law Annual Meeting, San Juan, Puerto Rico, 1996

Kaimowitz v. Michigan Department of Public Health, Div no 73-19434-AW, Circuit Court of Wayne County, Michigan, 1973

Kaplan H, Sadock B, Grebb J: Synopsis of Psychiatry. Baltimore, MD, Williams & Wilkins, 1994

Natanson v. Kline, 186 Kan 393, 350 P 2d 1093, clarified at 187 Kan 186, 354 P 2d 670, 1960

Overton W: Medical legal issues of dementia. In Stoudemire A, Fogel BS (eds): Psychiatric Care of the Medical Patient, pp 939–952. New York, Oxford University Press, 1993

Salgo v. Leland Stanford Junior University Board of Trustees, 154 Cal App 2d 560, 317 P 2d 170, 1st Dist, 1957

Schloendorff v. Society of New York Hospital, 211 NY 125, 105 NE 92, 1914

Schwartz H: Informed consent and competency. In Rosner R (ed): Principles and Practice of Forensic Psychiatry, 103–110, New York, Chapman and Hall, 1994

Simon R, Sadoff R: Psychiatric Malpractice, Washington, DC, American Psychiatric Press, 1992

Swanson JW, Holzer CE, Ganju VK, Jono RT: Violence and psychiatric disorder in the community: evidence from the Epidemiologic Catchment Area Surveys. Hosp Community Psychiatry 41:761–770, 1990

Tarasoff v. Board of Regents of the University of California, 17 Cal.3d 425; 551 P.2d 334; 131 Cal. Rptr. 14, 1976

Wulsin LR, Bursztajn HJ, Gutheil TG: Unexpected clinical features of the Tarasoff decision: the therapeutic alliance and the "duty to warn." Am J Psychiatry 140:601–603, 1983

Ricky Wyatt v. Charles Aderholt, (Commr. of Mental Health in Alabama, et al) 503 Fed. 2d 1305, U.S. Circuit Court of Appeals, 5th Circ, 1974

Zinermon v. Burch, 494 U.S. 113, 1990

Subject Index

NOTE: A *t* following a page number indicates tabular material, and an *i* following a page number indicates an illustration. Drugs are listed under their generic names. When a drug trade name is listed, the reader is referred to the generic name.